Frans P.G.M. van der Linden

Practical Dentofacial Orthopedics

Practical Dentofacial Orthopedics

Frans P.G.M. van der Linden, D.D.S., Ph.D.
Diplomate of the American Board of Orthodontics
Professor and Chairman
Department of Orthodontics 1962–1995
University of Nymegen, The Netherlands
Visiting Scientist
Center for Human Growth and Development
The University of Michigan, Ann Arbor, Michigan

John F. Jefferys, M.D., B.D.S.
Translator

quintessence books

Quintessence Publishing Co., Ltd.
London, Berlin, Chicago, São Paulo, Tokyo, Moscow,
Prague and Warsaw

Library of Congress Cataloguing-in-Publication Data

Linden, Frans P. G. M. van der
Practical dentofacial orthopedics
1. Orthodontics 2. Orthodontics, Corrective
I. Title
67.6'43

ISBN 1-85097-041-6

Typeset by Tek-Art, Croydon, Surrey, U.K.
Printed and bound by Bosch, Landshut
Lithographie by Bohn Stafleu Van Loghum, Houten/Zaventem
Printed in Germany

Preface

The demand for orthodontic treatment has increased considerably over the past few decades. Much of this treatment can be provided in general practice by dentists with sufficient interest and background in orthodontics. This requires accomplishments in several spheres: knowledge of diagnosis, understanding of the possibilities and limitations of the methods available, ability to handle not only the appliances but the patients, and an ability to appraise long-term results.

Practical Dentofacial Orthopedics is based on full documentation of 40 patients who have been chosen to illustrate the mentioned proposition. A point of considerable value is that most have been followed up for 10 to 20 years subsequent to the completion of treatment. In addition, this book can serve a useful purpose in providing illustrative material for patients and their families.

Most of the cases presented can be claimed to be successes; some have clear shortcomings, and a few cases are, in the long term, failures. The book can also be viewed as a collection of clinical lessons, and it contains experiences that have emerged not only from good, but also from faulty judgment and approaches. Misadventures are deliberately presented, since the didactic value of an unsuccessful case often can be greater than that of a successful one.

In the compilation of this book, it has been assumed that the reader is acquainted with previous works of the author, namely *Development of the Dentition, Facial Growth and Facial Orthopedics, Diagnosis and Treatment Planning in Dentofacial Orthopedics* (with H. Boersma), and *Problems and Procedures in Dentofacial Orthopedics*.

This volume could only have come into being thanks to the photographs that were taken by J.L.M. van de Kamp and H.A.W. Bongaarts, and the drawings that were provided by P.J. Wissink, M. Slooves, and H.C.M. Reckers. That applies also to the dental casts and orthodontic appliances provided by J.J.W. Siepermann and B.F. Bouwman. Much support and help over all those years were offered by the chairside assistants, radiographers and secretarial staff. J.C.M. Spijkers handled the collected records; M.J.Th. Cillessen-van Hoek prepared the manuscript. The author is very indebted to these people for their dedication, zeal, expertise and constructive and pleasant cooperation. That applies particularly to Prof.Dr. H. Boersma, Prof.Dr. A.M. Kuijpers-Jagtman, Dr. H.M.H.M. Ruiken, and Dr. J.F. Jefferys, who have gone through the manuscript critically and have suggested many improvements.

It is appropriate to mention again the contribution made by J.L.M. van de Kamp, who not only photographed all the dental casts and most of the clinical cases, but also printed and mounted all the photographs reproduced in this book. His professionalism and enthusiasm were a significant contribution to bringing this work to fruition.
Finally, it is fitting to offer a special word of thanks to those patients whose cases are presented in this book and who gave permission for their photographs to be published so that others could benefit from what they had undergone.

Introduction

The objective of this book is to provide clinical information on patients with orthodontic anomalies, to dentists who wish to treat them in their general practices. For that purpose, 40 cases have been selected, most of which have been followed up for 10, 15, and 20 years after treatment. In each case, the reasons for the use of particular appliances are given. The pros and cons of different treatment procedures are discussed. On the basis of the progress of treatment and its results both in the short and long term, a discussion follows of why therapy has been successful or why expected improvements were not achieved; at the same time, other treatment methods that might have secured better success are brought into focus.

The cases that are presented here have been selected according to the type of anomaly, the degree of difficulty, and the kind of appliances used. The first two cases were only kept under observation. Following them are simple cases that gradually lead to those anomalies that are more difficult to treat. The treatment methods are limited to removable plates, cervical and parietal headgears, lip bumpers, lingual arches, and partial fixed appliances in the maxillary arch. The treatment of anomalies for which extractions are indicated seldom is undertaken in this book. These often can only be satisfactorily treated with full fixed appliances, certainly in the mandible. That applies also to serious anomalies such as class II/2 anomalies.

Limiting the descriptions of cases to only those that have been followed up over a long period has its pros and cons. The greatest advantage is that it becomes clear whether or not a treatment result was stable, to what degree there has been any relapse, or what changes, desired or adventitious, might have taken place. Another advantage is that the influence of later growth on the treatment result can be analyzed. In the past, for example, many normal parameters derived from adults were applied to teenagers. It was not appreciated that in the course of normal growth of the face the dentition came to lie further back as a person became older. In this way, with teenagers — particularly boys — the dentition can dominate the face, yet with adulthood, it can assume a harmonious position. In such cases, premolar extractions can lead to a sunken mouth and a reduced facial animation at a later age. These examples indicate that a practitioner needs to realize what effects treatment might have in the long term. With that in mind, documentation of the situation existing at different times long after the conclusion of treatment has been included.

A disadvantage of presenting only cases that have been followed up over a long period is that the treatment has been carried out under conditions and following procedures and concepts that subsequently have been modified to some extent. For instance, in the past, the level of oral hygiene and dental care was lower than it now is. In the past, brackets were welded to metal bands and cemented to teeth, whereas brackets are now usually fixed directly to the enamel with composite resins.

The disadvantage of presenting patients who were treated a long time ago has been countered as far as possible by giving up-to-date information on techniques and concepts when pertinent. This applies especially to combined extraoral and functional therapy, with which at the present pronounced class II/1 anomalies can be improved remarkably in a relatively short time. Another example is the use of composite resins in treatment with removable plates, although it is not dealt with more than superficially.

The case presentation is based on facial photographs, both frontal and in profile. The occlusal conditions are portrayed with intraoral photographs as well as photographs of plaster casts of the dental arches and surrounding structures. To give an indication of the changes in facial expression and attractiveness, oblique photographs of the smiling patient have been taken. In addition, superimposed tracings of lateral skull radiographs are provided frequently to illustrate changes that have followed growth and treatment. Radiographs are only presented to a limited extent since this book is primarily devoted to treatment rather than diagnosis. Above all, a systematic reproduction of radiographs would have required a significant enlargement of this volume.

In assessing the occlusion of posterior teeth in intraoral photos as well as photos of dental casts, one needs to realize that the former were take somewhat obliquely from the front, and the latter perpendicular to the median plane. Therefore, neither photograph strictly corresponds with the picture of occlusion that is obtained by examining the relationship of teeth when looking at right angles to buccal surfaces of posterior teeth either by means of a mirror in the mouth or with dental casts held in the hand.

Each chapter contains a section in which relevant clinical matters are examined more deeply. A multiplicity of subjects and suggestions is examined, clarifying the use of particular appliances in detail.

Relatively little consideration is given in this book to the cooperation of the patient. Nonetheless, this aspect is enormously important in securing an easy passage along the course of treatment and in reaching a good result. It is an essential part of the task of the practitioner to generate such a degree of empathy with the patient and his/her family that the best possible cooperation will be maintained throughout what can be quite demanding treatment.

In the exact sciences, it is to a great extent possible to base activities on scientifically proven principles; in clinical disciplines, this is more or less impossible. A French physician once said that clinical thinking and procedures are based one-third on scientifically proven facts, one-third on tradition, and one-third on experience. Clinical fields are largely based on empiricism. If it is considered that a particular treatment led to an improvement, then it is applied subsequently to similar conditions. In education, methods that have been found to produce beneficial results have been passed down for centuries.

Each practitioner must also learn from his or her own experience. A clinical worker with a critical outlook can, through systematic observation and evaluation of treatment for which he or she is responsible, improve the standard of treatment in that area. In conjunction with that, communication with colleagues at scientific meetings and through professional (clinical) literature forms an important means by which practitioners may pass on the knowledge gained from their experiences.

People have a tendency to remember the positive aspects of the past, and so remember more easily the successes in their treatment and work in general. They also tend to speak more readily about their successes than their failures. At congresses and symposia, it is the success of particular therapies that is brought forward. Failures seldom are discussed, yet as a source of knowledge and experience, they can often be more important than successes. Together with the lack of longitudinal data, this has led to an excessively optimistic view of treatment methods and results when examined long term. Evaluation of therapies demands among other things a comparison of the initial condition with the end result. Orthodontics is privileged in that respect. With the best possible standardized facial and intraoral photographs, dental casts, and radiographs, the situation at a specific moment can be accurately recorded and compared with that at another moment in the course of treatment or years later.

The author has been involved in clinical orthodontics for 38 years, the last 33 years being at the University of Nymegen in the Netherlands. Among his duties have been the provision of undergraduate teaching for dental students and the postgraduate education of specialist orthodontists. Along with the experience gained in his practice, he increased his understanding of the possibilities of orthodontic therapy in teaching situations — particularly the treatment planning sessions associated with specialist training, and guiding the practical execution of what was deemed the most effective therapy during those sessions. In addition, useful information is obtained from the study of records systematically collected of patients whose treatment was completed 2, 5, 10, 15 and 20 years or more ago. Along with previous experiences, he has had ample opportunity to profit from the knowledge and expertise of colleagues both at home and abroad, personally and by attending scientific gatherings and participating in the sharing of knowledge through professional literature. It is also pertinent to mention the insight into the development of the dentition and facial growth that he was able to gain from research projects with which he was associated.

The author hopes that this book will contribute to the knowledge and understanding of those who undertake orthodontic treatment. Even more, he hopes that it will help those who need to undergo such treatment.

Contents

Chapter 1

Class II/1, double protrusion
No orthodontic treatment
Male: 12 years, 6 months to 40 years 6 months

A boy who was 12 years and 6 months old exhibited a mild class II/1 anomaly with a disto-occlusion of a quarter of a premolar crown-width (1/4 PW disto), double protrusion (DP), an anterior open bite, and crowding in the mandibular arch. All permanent teeth with the exception of the third molars had emerged. He was not able to keep his lips closed without effort. His teeth were a dominant feature of his face (Figs 1.1 and 1.2).

It was suggested that four first premolars be extracted, the disto-occlusion be corrected with a cervical headgear, and the extraction spaces be closed as much as possible to the distal with full fixed appliances. After extensive discussion with the boy and his parents, it was decided rather to refrain from orthodontic treatment because the anomaly was not considered to be disfiguring and the disadvantages of treatment would outweigh the benefits. Moreover, the parents were familiar with the phenomenon of "over-servicing" in the sphere of medicine.

It is clear from the records taken 28 years later, that he had developed a strong face. The originally small turned-up nose is now straight and large. The chin has grown ventrally. There is now normal relaxed lip closure. Because of the development of the surrounding structures the dentition is no longer a dominant feature and fits harmoniously into the face as a whole. There is still a mild disto-occlusion with an anterior open bite, indeed without associated functional or esthetic drawbacks (Figs 1.3, 1.4, and 1.5).

In hindsight, one may say with certainty that the decision not to treat was a correct one. Looking back, the question arises as to why complex treatment with four premolar extractions was proposed in the first place. Two reasons can be suggested. In the first place, it was considered in the 1960s by orthodontists who worked with full fixed appliances that in such a case of double protrusion the elimination of four premolars was the normal course. A second reason could be that up to that time, understanding and knowledge of the growth of the face were limited. As has already been stated in the introduction, it has since become clear that during puberty, and subsequently, the face develops markedly, especially in boys. Before, during, and directly after puberty, the dentition dominates the face. Only after some years has the growth of the surrounding tissues "built in" the dental structures. This goes together with the fact that the teeth when they are laid down already have their mature dimensions; because of that they predominate in the bony structures that

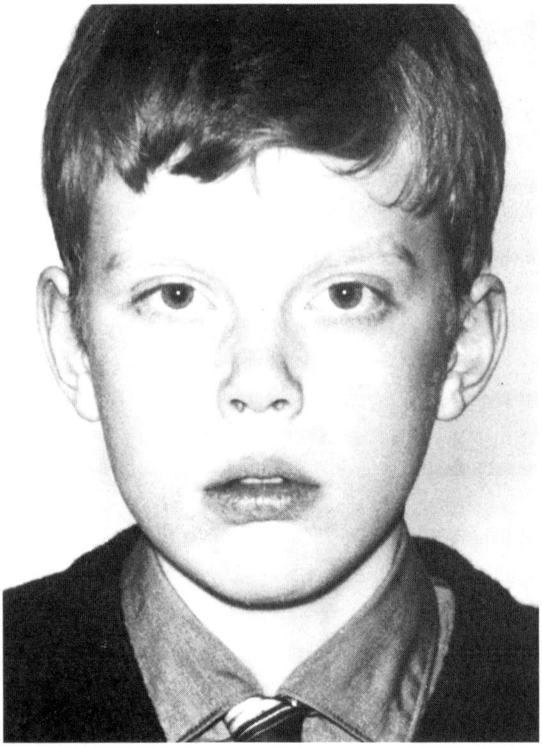

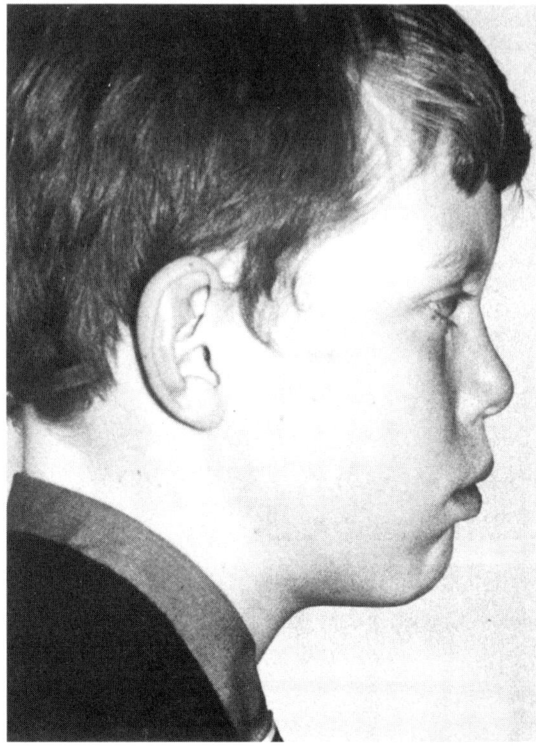

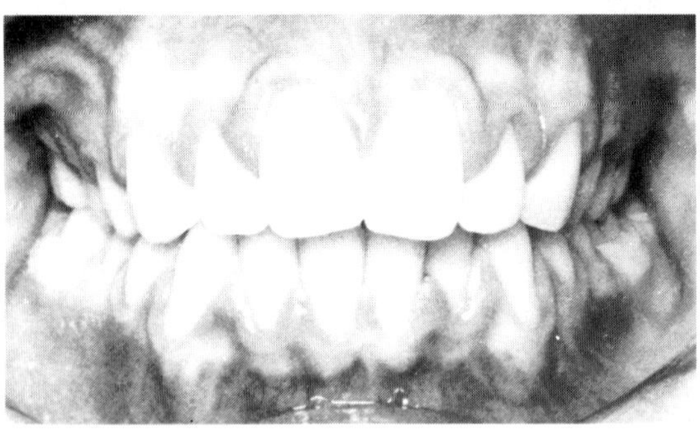

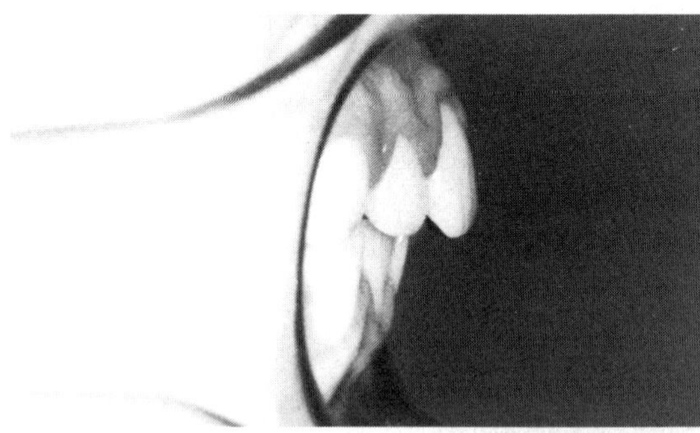

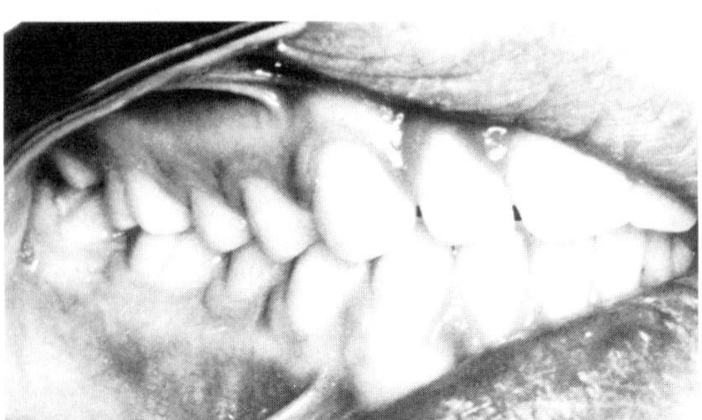

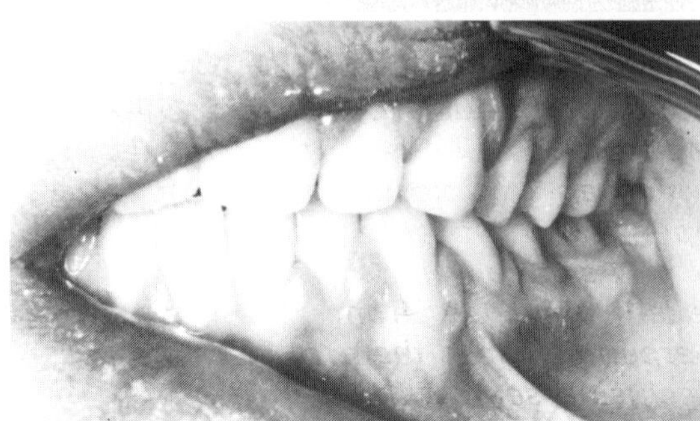

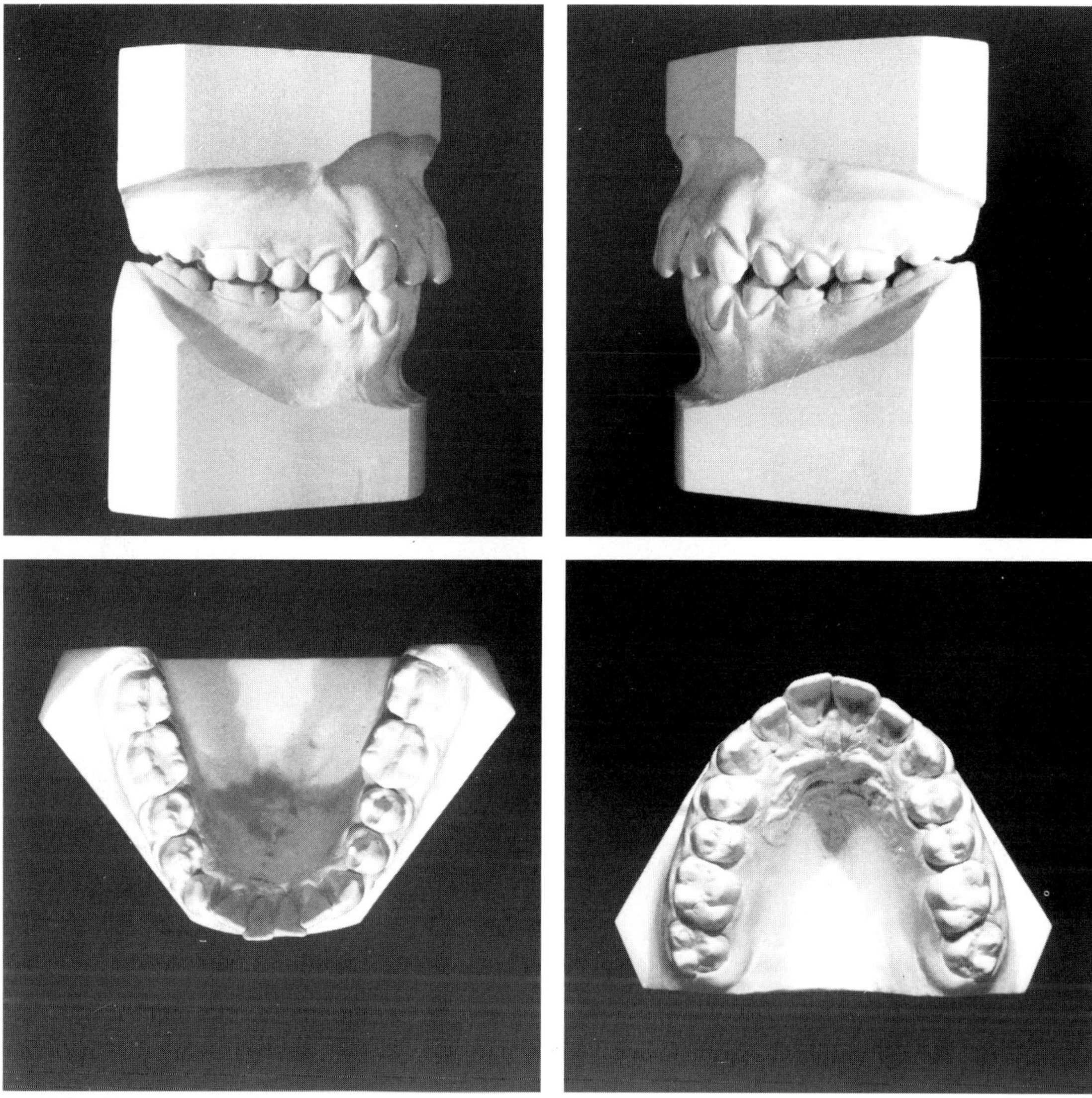

Figs 1-1 and 1-2 *Boy aged 12 y, 6 mo, with a mild class II/1 anomaly (¼ PW disto-occlusion), double protrusion, anterior open bite, mild crowding of the mandibular arch, and small nose with no obstruction. The dentition dominates the face. The lips, which are not closed, are prominent in relation to the nose and chin. The anterior open bite is associated with interposition of the tongue.*

N.B.: As stated in the introduction, the photographs of the posterior teeth have been taken obliquely from the front and those of the dental casts are obtained perpendicular to the median plane. Neither corresponds exactly with the view of the occlusion seen with a mirror in the mouth or models in the hand, when the cheek teeth can be seen at 90 degrees to their buccal surfaces.

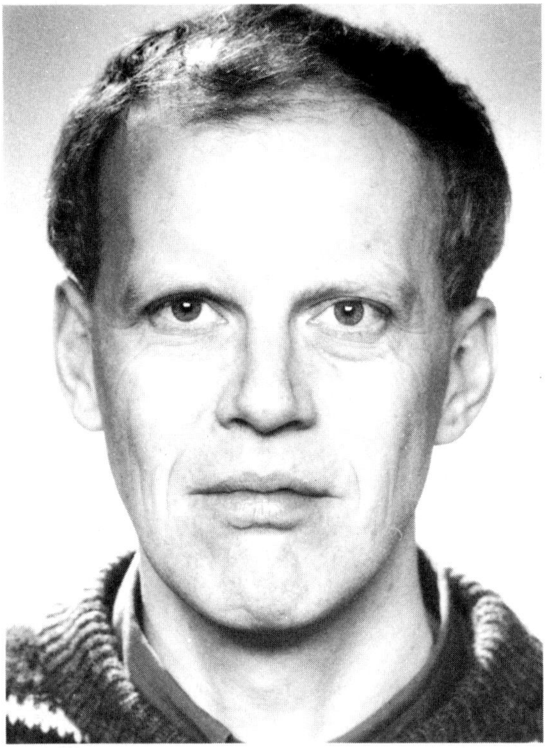
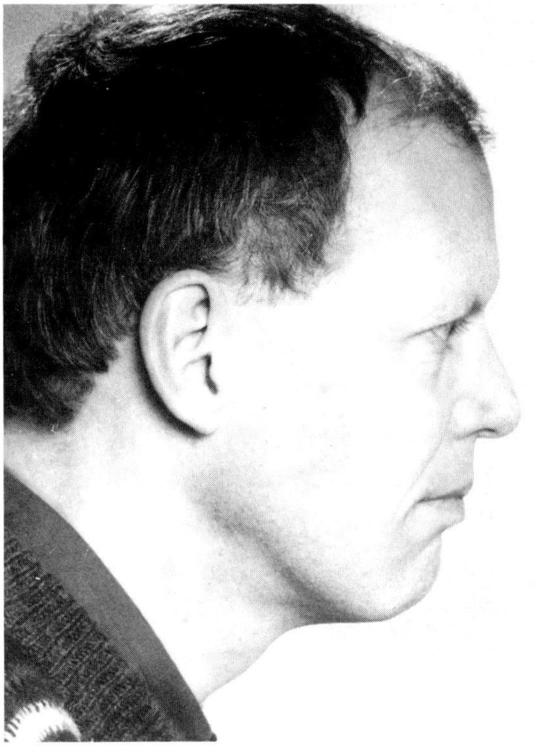
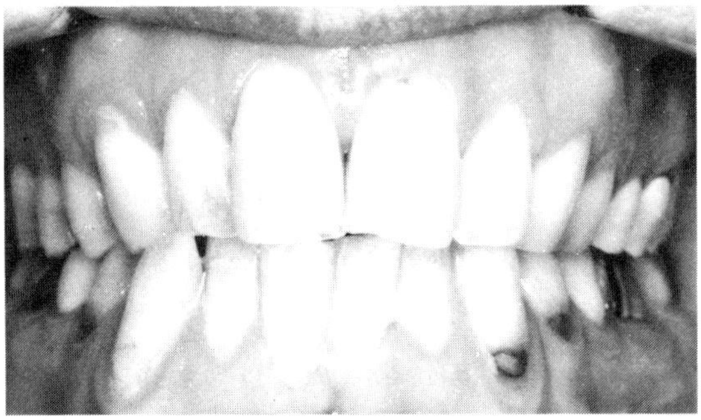
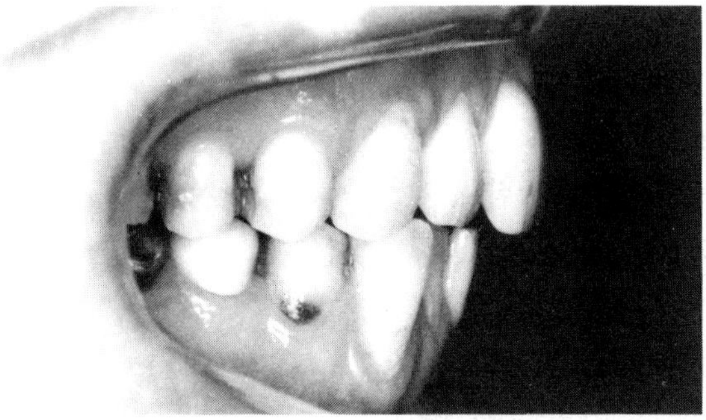
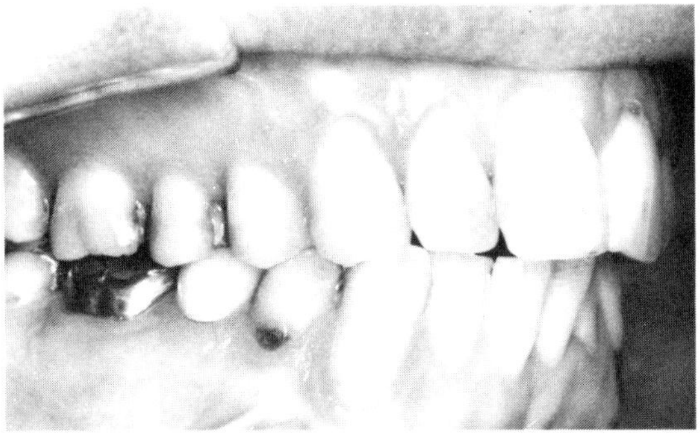
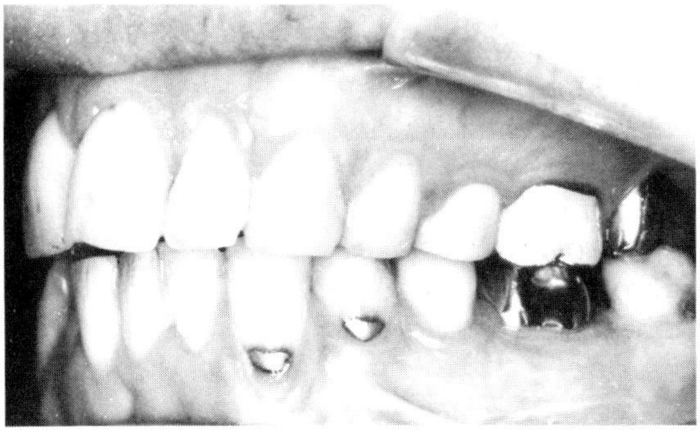

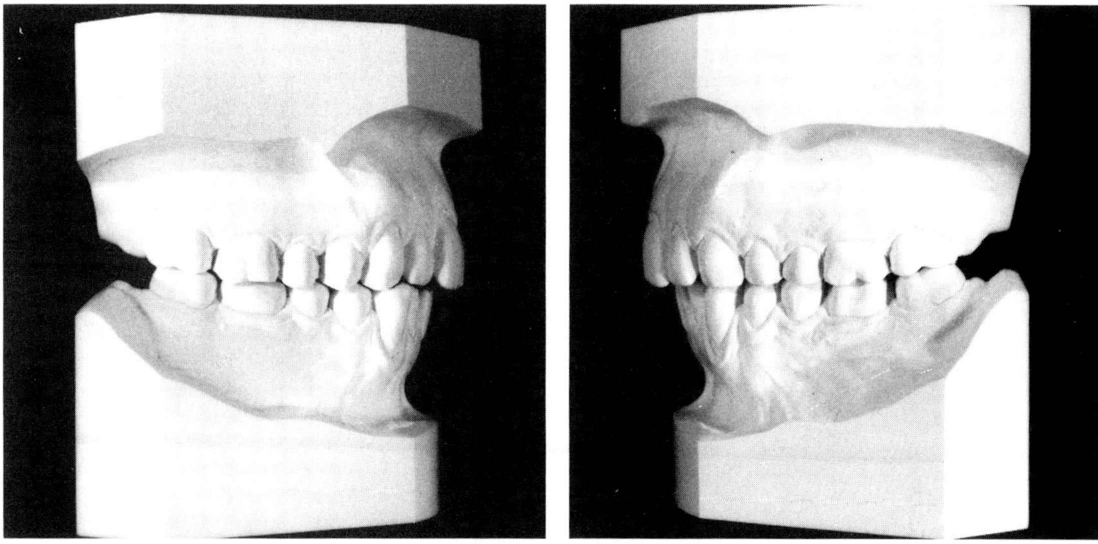

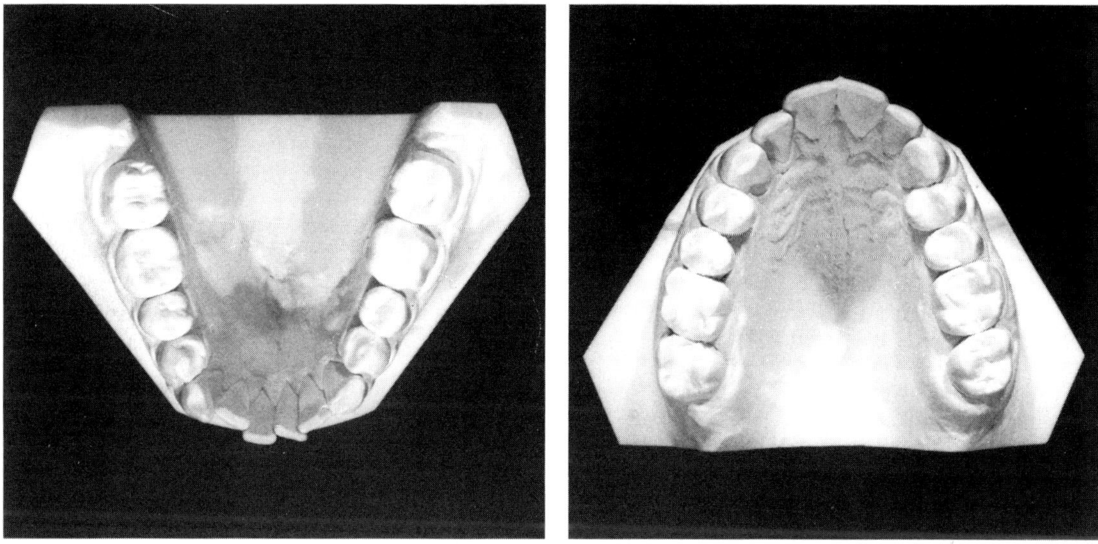

Figs 1-3 and 1-4 At the age of 40 y, 6 mo, the patients face is much larger, the nose and chin have developed, the lips are longer and function well. The mild disto-occlusion is still present, just as is the anterior open bite. The increased crowding of the mandibular incisors and the palatal position of the maxillary right lateral incisor are not considered objectionable.
The crowns and fillings in the teeth are representative of the type and number of restorations placed in the Netherlands during the 1960s and 1970s. In those years, little consideration was given to oral hygiene and toothpaste usually did not contain fluoride.

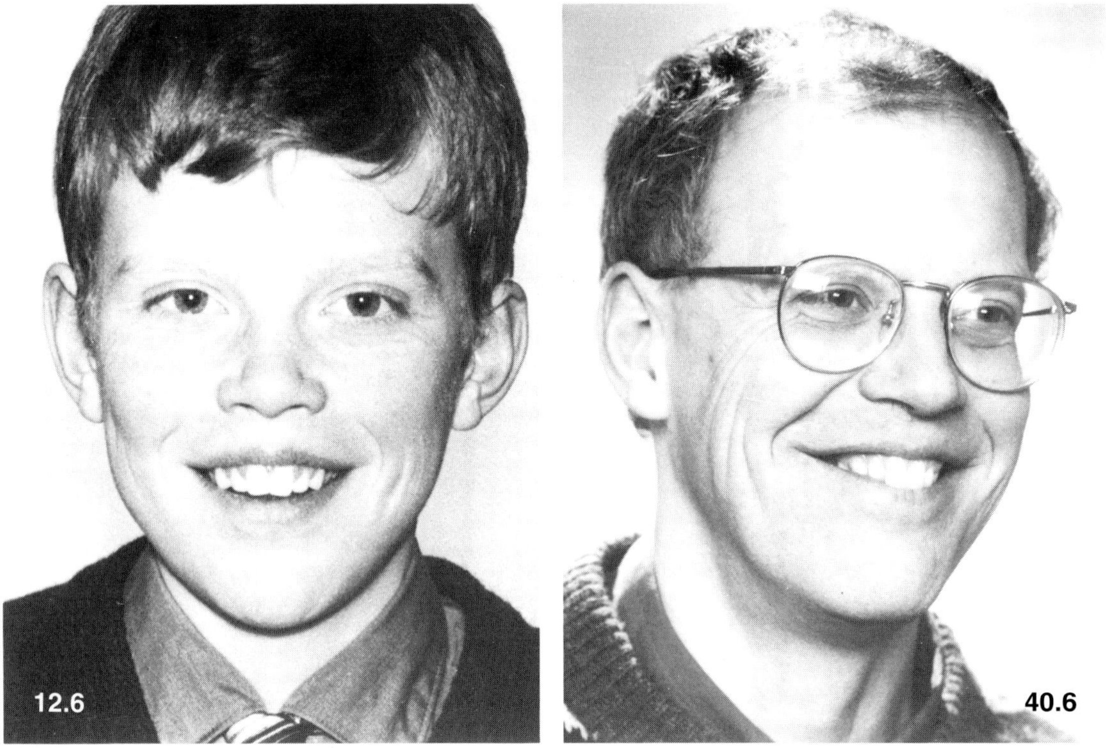

Fig 1-5 The face has gained character with maturity. Extraction of four first premolars would have been followed by the dentition falling back in relation to the face, narrowing of the maxillary arch in the region of the canines and premolars, a deeper nasolabial fold, and a reduction in facial expression.

have still a considerable amount of growth to undergo. Furthermore, together with the outward growth of the bony bases of the jaws, an uprighting of the axes of the incisor teeth is seen. The soft tissues do not reach their adult dimensions until after these processes. In many young teenagers, the lips are relatively short and incapable of relaxed closure. The mouth is often open, even when nose breathing is quite unimpeded. The typical order in which the three involved components achieve their growth to adult size — first the dentition, then the facial skeleton, and finally the soft tissues — makes it evident why the permanent teeth can be such a striking feature of the young face. That applies far more to boys than girls. Girls reach their adult size and proportions earlier than boys do, they grow distinctly less during adolescence and the changes continue for a shorter time.

Changes in the morphologic characteristics of the facial skeleton, in the position of the teeth, and in the soft tissues continue well after reaching adulthood (Fig 1.6). The profile becomes straighter, the upper lip becomes thinner and longer, and the lower lip becomes thicker and more prominent. The lip line falls in relation to the maxillary incisors. In addition, with age the tone and activity of the upper lip decrease so that

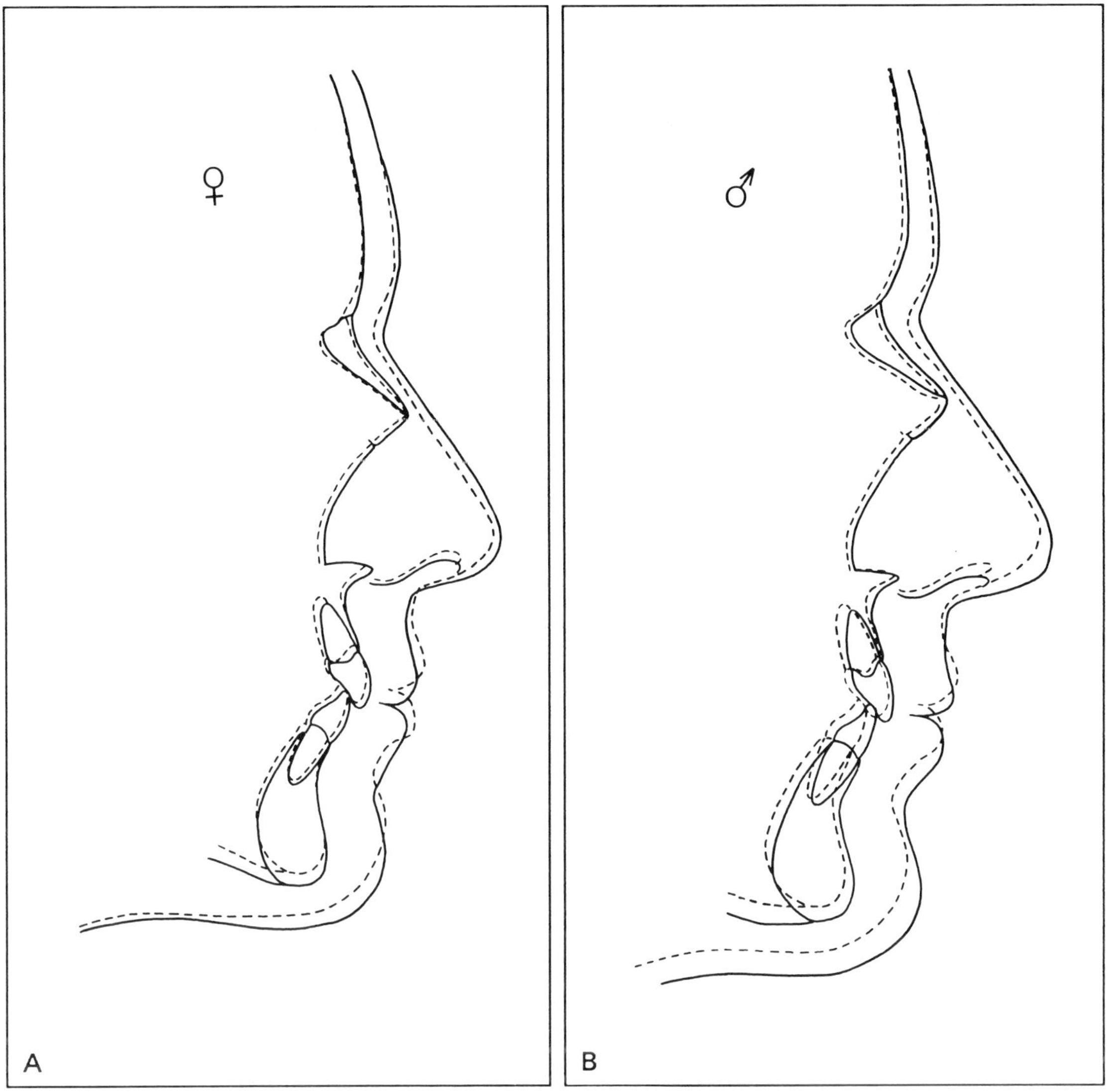

Fig 1-6 Superimposition of changes in contours of skeletal and dental structures, and of the profile, that occur during adulthood. The drawings are based on the average of the individual changes registered in 113 persons for whom a lateral cephalogram was available at approximate ages of 20 and 50 years.
In women (A), the mandible rotates backward and leads to an increase in the height of the lower face. The face also increases in height in men (B), and the mandible rotates forward, usually causing the chin to move ventrally.
In both sexes the nose becomes larger; the tip of the nose drops and becomes sharper. The lip line falls in relation to the maxillary incisors. The upper lip becomes longer and thinner, while the lower lip becomes thicker and more prominent. The latter applies also to the soft tissues that cover the chin.[2,11]

in speaking and smiling the maxillary front teeth are exposed less and the mandibular ones show more.
Orthodontists who continue to follow up their patients into adulthood sometimes notice unfavorable developments. That often applies to circumstances where at an earlier age four premolars were removed with the objective of reducing the dentition's dominance of the features. Certainly in the case of boys this can lead to the teeth lying too far back in the face by the time adult growth has been achieved, giving the appearance of a sunken mouth and less vital facial animation.
It is very seldom that ten years after orthodontic treatment is completed one regrets not having extracted teeth. In that respect, it has to be realized that removal of premolars or other teeth seldom reduces the chance of tertiary crowding occurring in the mandibular incisors, and also that if necessary, extraction can still be done.
A dentition that is well aligned and functions well is not always associated with an esthetically harmonious face. It might well be the reverse. For many people, an attractive and vital appearance is more important than dental arches with teeth in ideal alignment, particularly since as the person grows older they show their teeth much less. Moreover, esthetically disturbing malalignment can often be improved by selective grinding or by building up with composite resins.[25]
A high percentage of the population of the Netherlands (approximately 40%) have no vertical contact between their maxillary and mandibular front teeth. The question is whether or not a condition that is so prevalent can be described as abnormal, particulary as it seldom causes discomfort. It is clear that a situation that does not correspond with a standard ideal occlusion (that does not just include anterior open bites) by no means needs always to be corrected.

Chapter 2

Class III, agenesis 25, late development 15
No orthodontic treatment
Male: 9 years 4 months to 23 years, 7 months

A boy who was 9 years, 4 months old and who exhibited a class III anomaly with an anterior open bite, was examined. His mid-face was not underdeveloped and his mandible was large; his profile was straight. The incisal edges of maxillary and mandibular incisors were in an end-to-end position but were not in contact. On the right, the second deciduous molars were in crossbite. Radiographs showed that the maxillary left second premolar was agenetic and that the development of the one on the right side was quite retarded. Their predecessors were carious. The asymmetric anterior open bite could be attributed to thumb-sucking and tongue interposition (Fig 2.1).

The boy's father also had a class III anomaly with reversed incisor overjet, without ever having found it to present any difficulties. An older sister with a class II/1 malocclusion in which two maxillary permanent teeth were missing, exhibited such strong mandibular growth during treatment that it proved necessary to remove two mandibular premolars to be able to retract the mandibular incisors sufficiently to avoid a reversed incisor overjet developing.

It was decided in this young man's case to await further facial growth and at the appropriate time to make the decision not to treat, or to engage in dentofacial-orthopedic or indeed combined surgical-orthodontic treatment.

In the years that followed, there was no abnormal mandibular growth, nor did maxillary growth fall behind. The maxillary deciduous second molars were lost, after which the maxillary first permanent molars drifted mesially and rotated. The open bite became smaller once thumb-sucking stopped. The incisal edges of the maxillary and mandibular incisors came into contact in habitual occlusion. By the age of 17 years, a normal facial configuration existed without external symptoms of the class III anomaly (Fig 2.2).

In subsequent years, progressive mandibular growth did not show up. Nor did his adult face betray any indications of a class III anomaly, doubtless since the upper lip was clearly positioned in front of the lower lip and the nose had grown significantly forward. At the age of 23 years, a small positive overjet had developed. Meanwhile the maxillary right second premolar had emerged in endo-occlusion, probably as the result of lack of space (Fig 2.3).

It was thought that no treatment was needed during the entire period of observation. At no time was the anomaly considered to be disturbing esthetically, nor were the teeth thought to function inadequately.

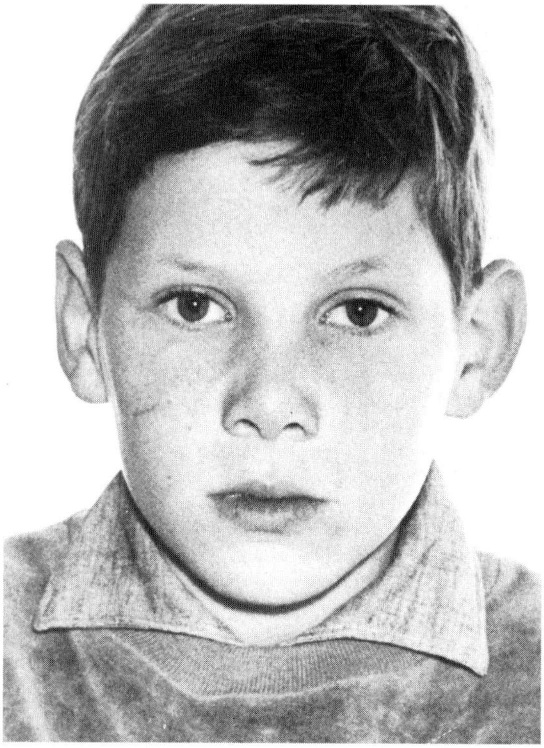

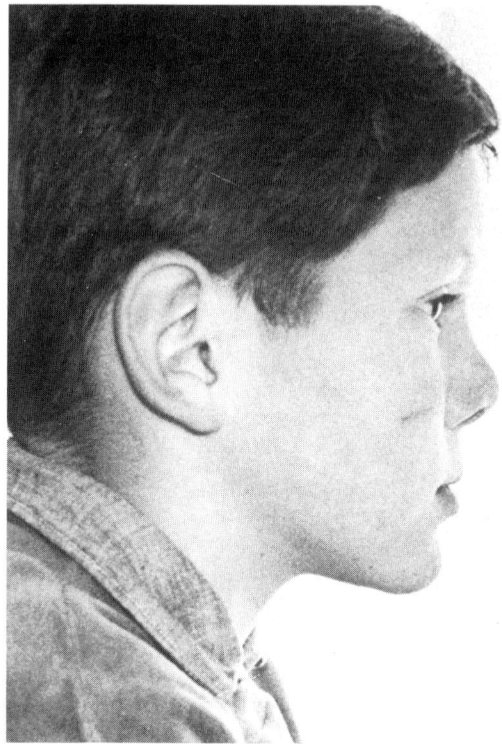

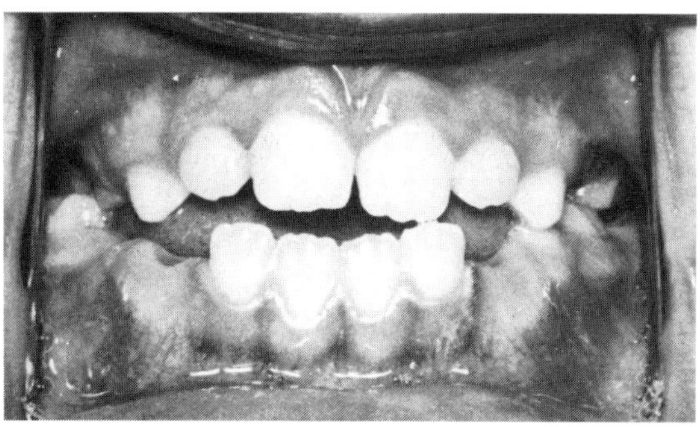

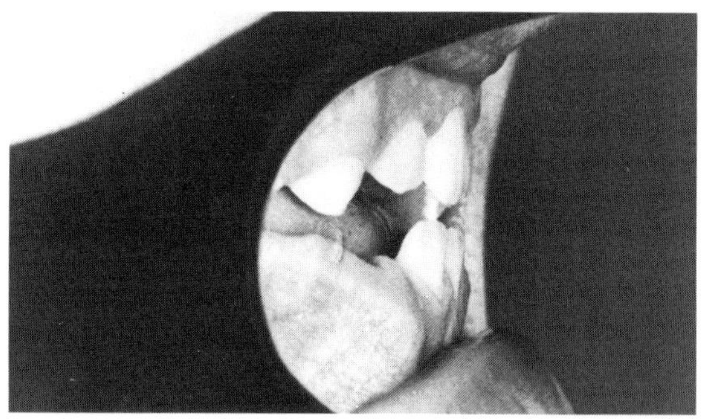

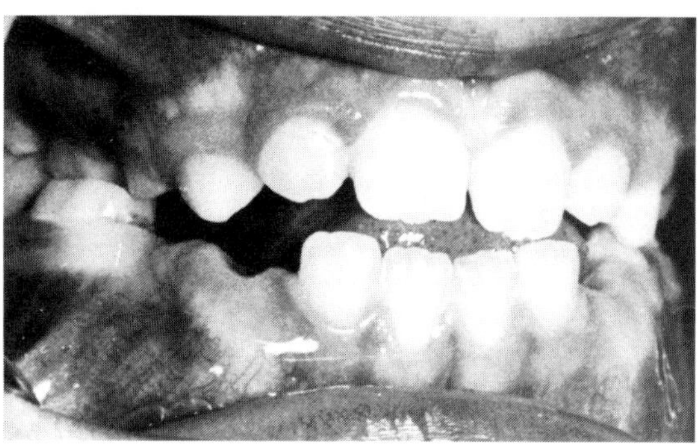

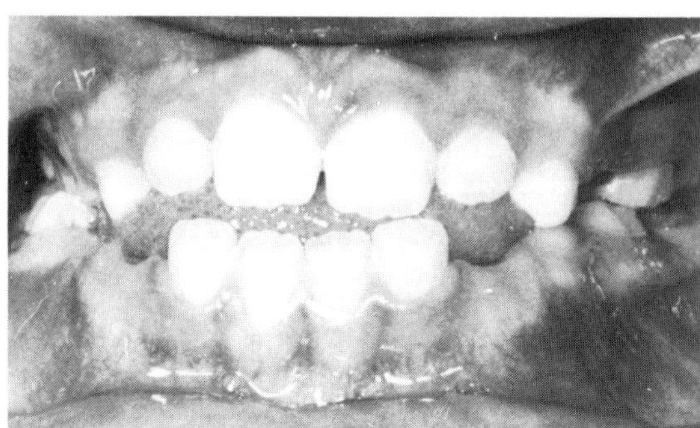

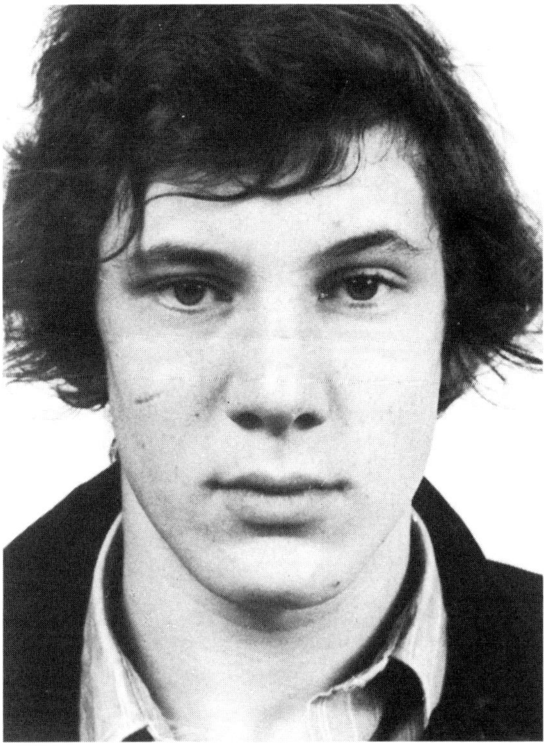
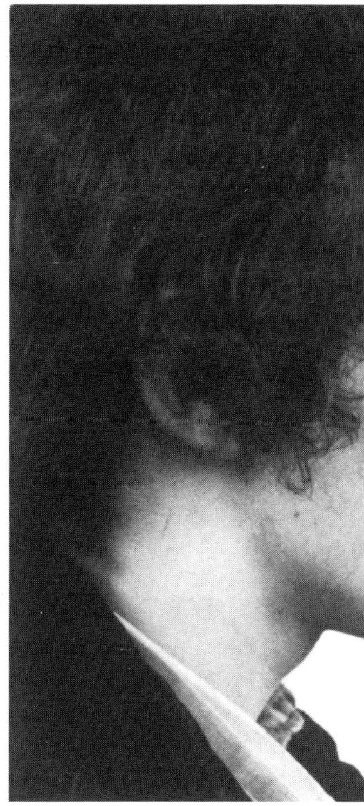
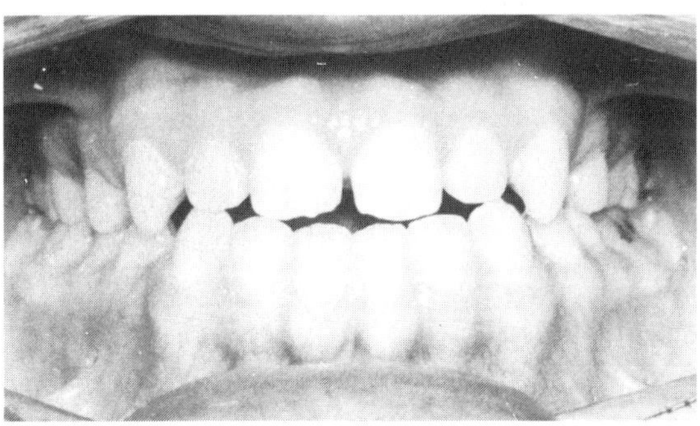
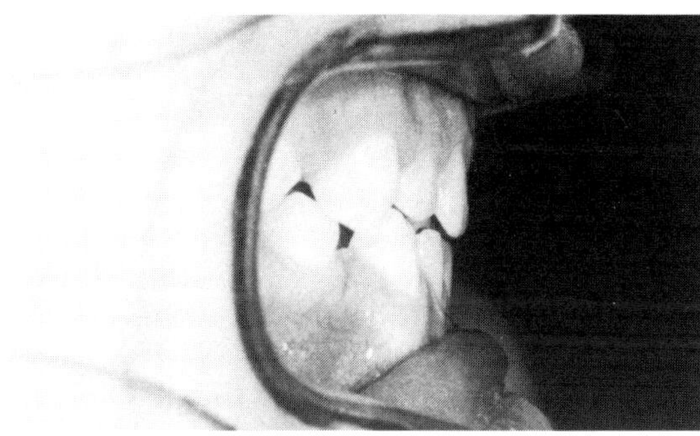
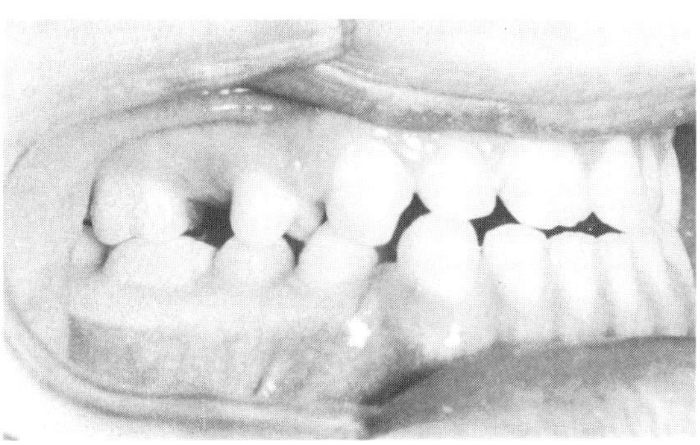
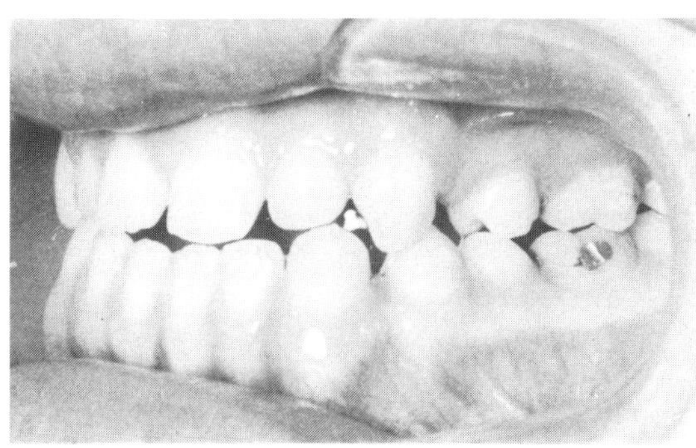

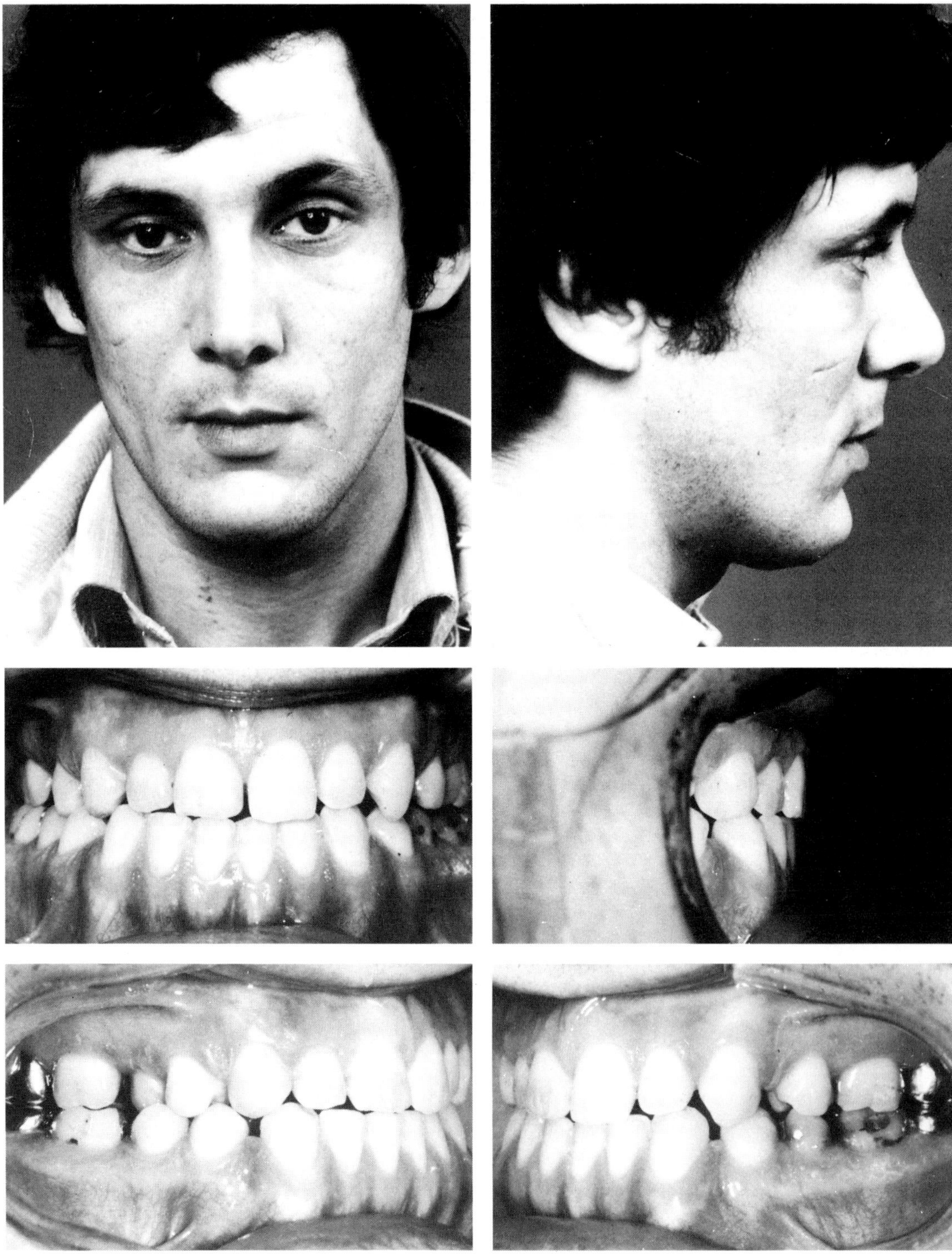

Fig 2-1 Boy aged 9 y, 4 mo, class III anomaly with anterior open bite, crossbite on the right, and tongue interposition. The maxillary left second premolar is agenetic, the one on the right is delayed in development. Despite a low attachment of the labial frenulum, no central diastema in the maxilla is present.

Fig 2-2 At the age of 17 y, a normal facial configuration exists; nothing in his outward appearance indicates a class III anomaly. The open bite has reduced. The occlusion has improved. Indeed a central diastema shows up now.

Fig 2-3 At the age of 23 y, 7 mo, a harmonious adult face is combined with normal lip relation and closure and a minimal overjet and overbite. The maxillary right second premolar has emerged in endo-occlusion.

Retrospectively, it can be said that dentofacial-orthopedic intervention would not have been likely to have contributed much to the beneficial development that occurred here. If ventral traction had been applied to the maxilla, then a satisfactory result might possibly have been attributed to the therapy.

It is difficult to guess whether or not a mild class III anomaly in a 10-year-old child will become worse, better, or change little. Progressive growth of the mandible can lead to serious deformity. It also can happen, as in this case, that the situation can improve even with an extra unfavorable factor such as agenesis of a maxillary premolar. In general, with doubtful class III cases it is better to maintain a watchful stance and carefully monitor development rather than begin treatment at once. For that purpose provision of dental casts and facial photographs at set intervals can be of great help.

Chapter 3

Class I, labioversion maxillary incisors
Maxillary removable plate
Female: 10 years, 9 months to 21 years, 5 months

A girl, 10 years and 9 months old, exhibited neutro-occlusion with, probably as the result of thumb-sucking, infraposition and eversion of the maxillary incisors. Diastemata were present between the maxillary incisors, and mild crowding could be seen in the mandibular anterior region. She had a harmonious facial appearance, normal lip position, adequate lip seal, and an unrestricted nasal airway (Figs. 3.1 and 3.2).

First of all, an attempt was made to discourage the thumb-sucking.[36] It would be expected that once the abnormal habit had ceased, spontaneous correction might obviate active orthodontic treatment. It can be seen that only the maxillary central incisors were in infraposition and too far to labial, while still sufficient room was available in the dental arch for achieving good alignment. The lateral incisors were in their correct places.

It was not only the maxillary central incisors that had been misplaced by the sucking habit; the slight linguoposition of the mandibular left central incisor could probably be attributed to it too.

Alas, it appeared that it was not possible to cease thumb-sucking. Consequently, two months later, it was decided that the sucking habit would be discouraged with use of a maxillary removable plate, which would procure the desired improvement in the positions of the maxillary incisors.

The plate was provided with retentive clasps and two divided labial arches to retract the central incisors.[4] Four months later, the goal had been reached (Figs 3.3 and 3.4). Retention was not provided. Tongue interposition and thumb-sucking had ceased and did not return.

Ten years later, the buccal occlusion appears improved. With facial growth , the mandibular arch moved further ventrally in relation to the maxillary arch. Indeed some rotation of the mandibular right central incisor occurred and tertiary crowding increased the amount of overlapping (Figs 3.5 and 3.6). However, the alignment of the mandibular incisors was not a matter for concern. Seen from the front it was hardly noticeable, even when smiling (Fig 3.7). The relatively small labiolingual dimensions of the proximal surfaces of the mandibular incisors permit overlapping to occur without leading to marked irregularities of the adjacent surfaces. On the other hand, these small dimensions also can lead more easily to overlapping since the approximal contacts in ideal alignment are narrow and fragile.

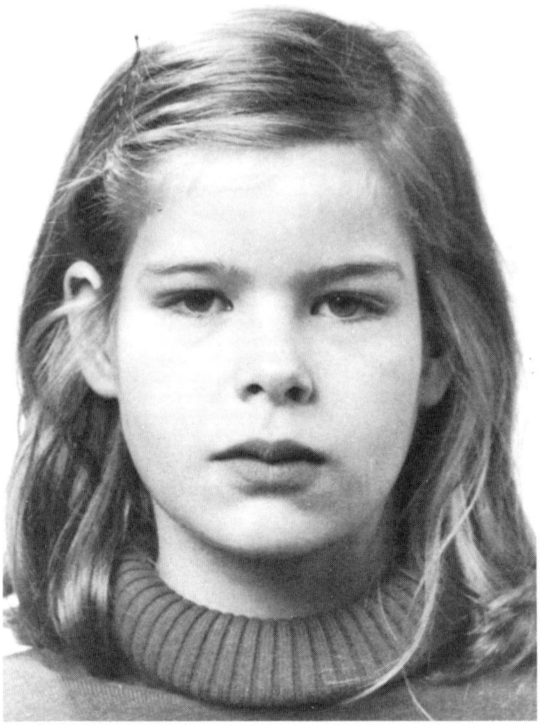

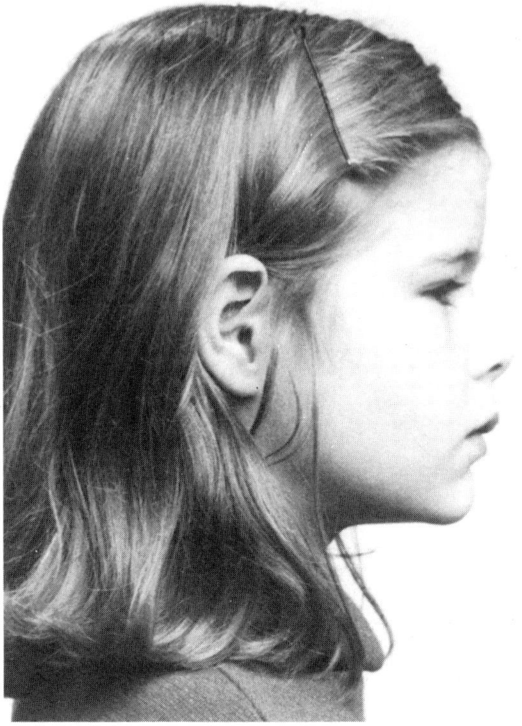

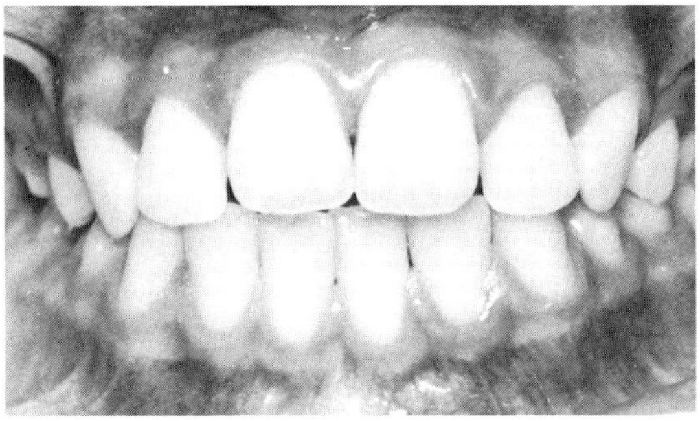

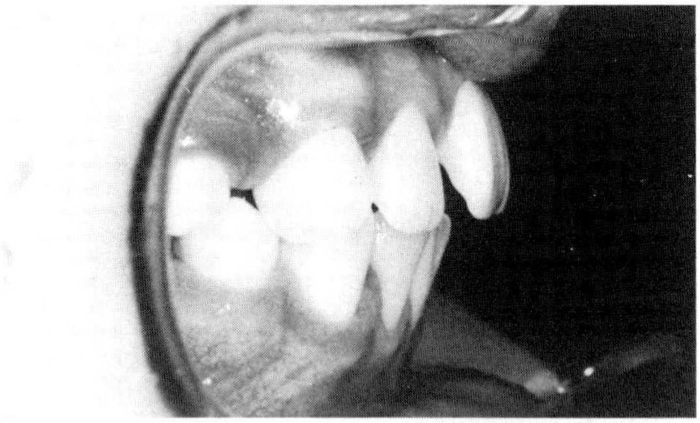

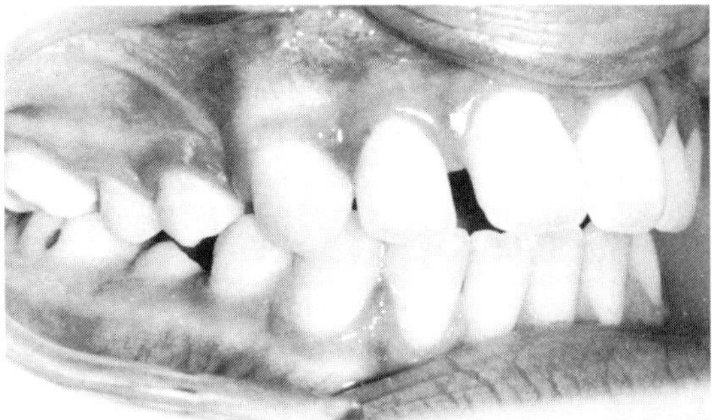

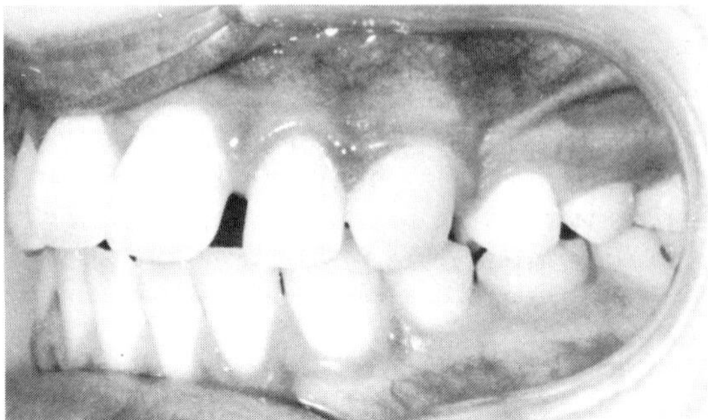

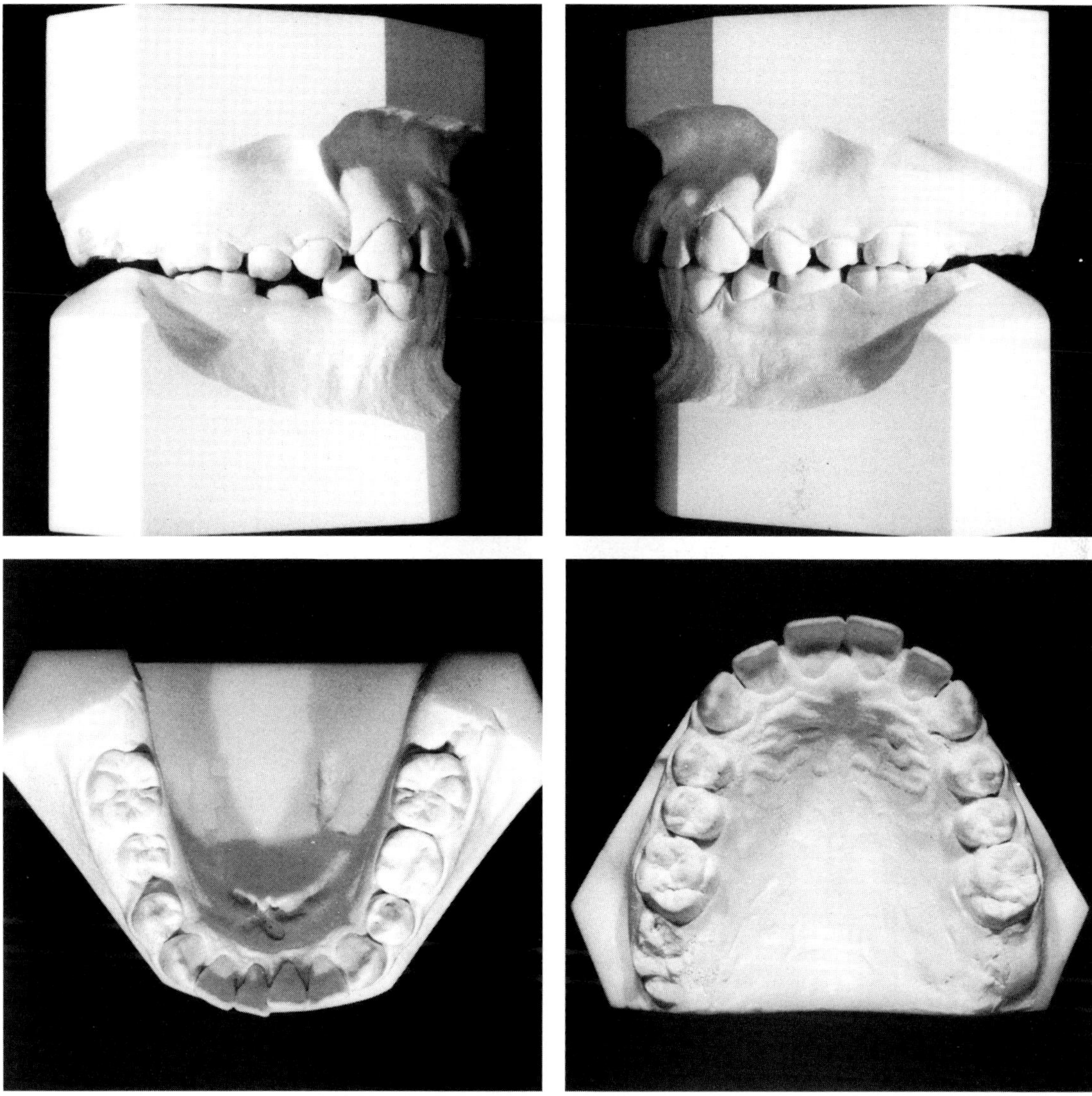

Figs 3-1 and 3-2 Girl aged 10 y, 9 mo, with harmonious face and good lip seal. She has a class I anomaly with eversion and infraposition of the maxillary central incisors as the consequence of thumb-sucking. The middle of the mandibular arch is located to the left of the maxillary arch center. Minor crowding of the mandibular incisors exists with the left central incisor slightly in linguoposition. Space is available around the recently emerged mandibular right second premolar; the mandibular left second deciduous molar is still present.

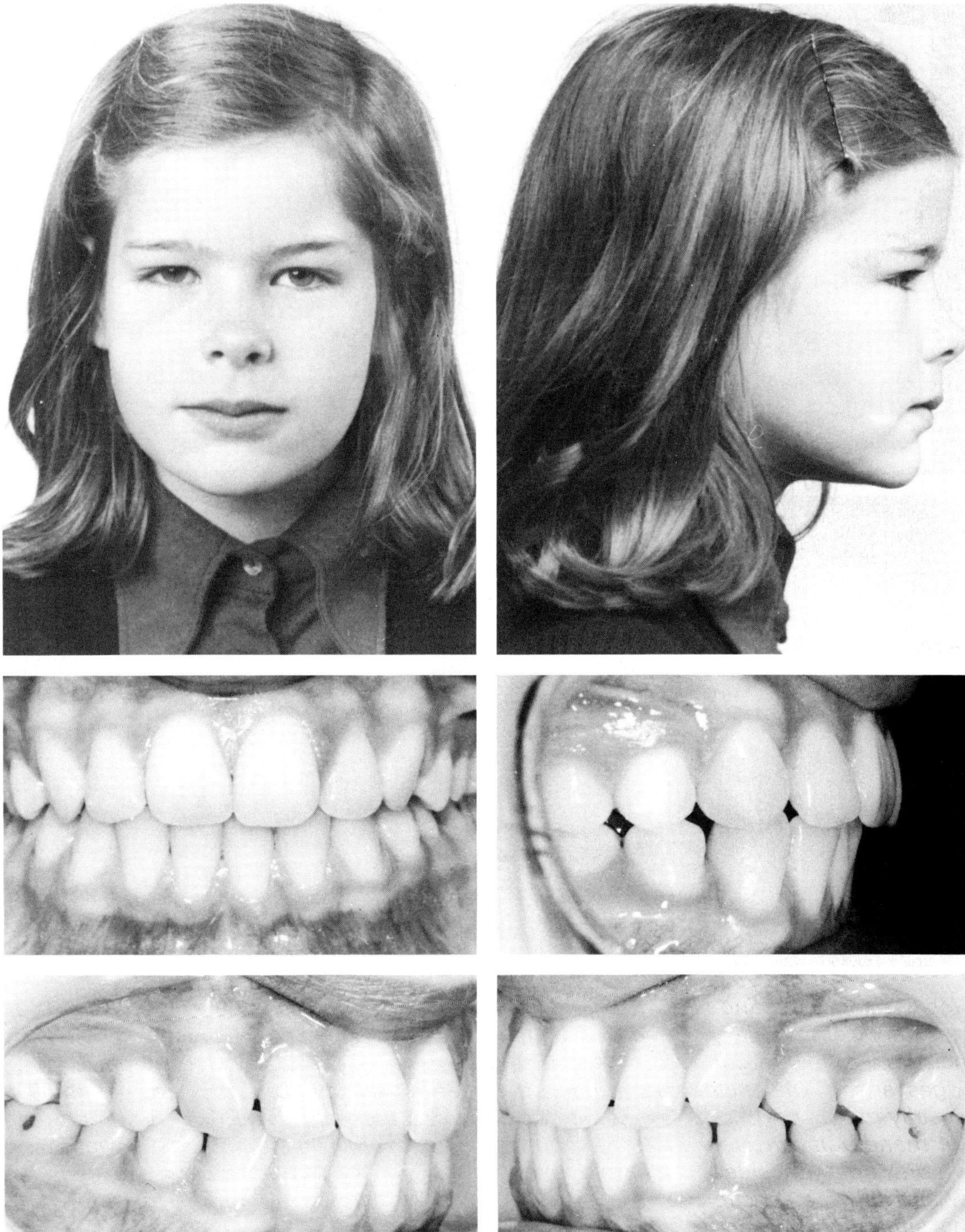

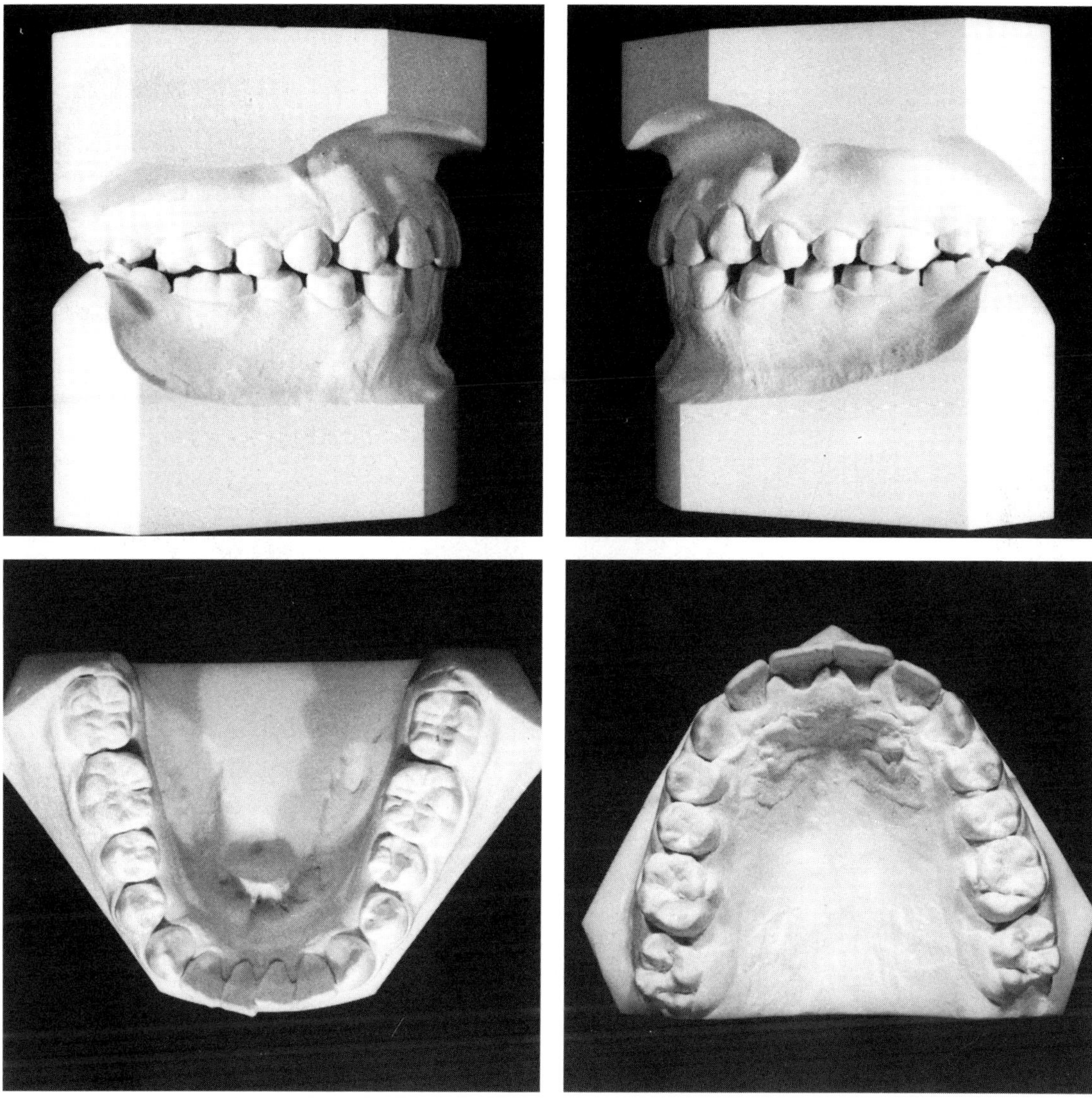

Figs 3-3 and 3-4 *The situation at 11 y, 3 mo, after four months of treatment with a maxillary removable plate with two divided labial arches. Both maxillary central incisors are now in good alignment and contact the mandibular incisors. Their incisal edges are a little lower than those of the lateral incisors, an arrangement that is visually more acceptable than when all four are at the same level. The overlapping in the mandibular incisors has not improved, despite the diastemata in the premolar regions on both sides. The gingiva palatal to the maxillary incisors had become hypertrophic, a reaction to wearing the plate; shortly after discarding the appliance this situation returned to normal.*

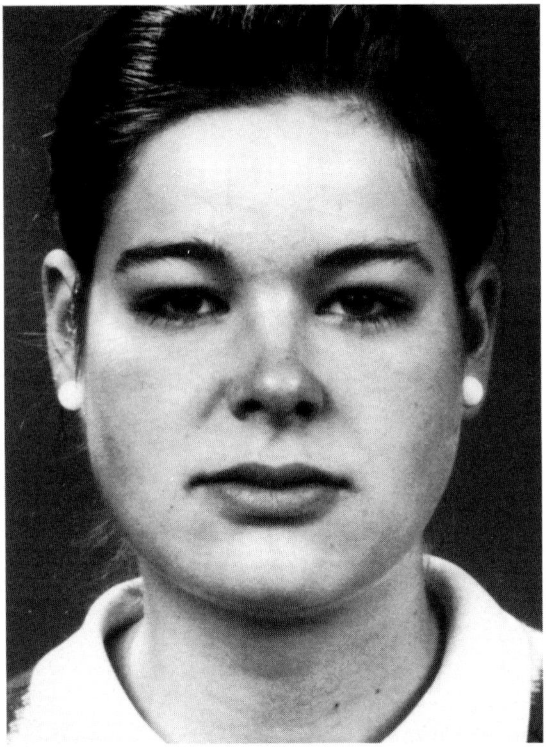
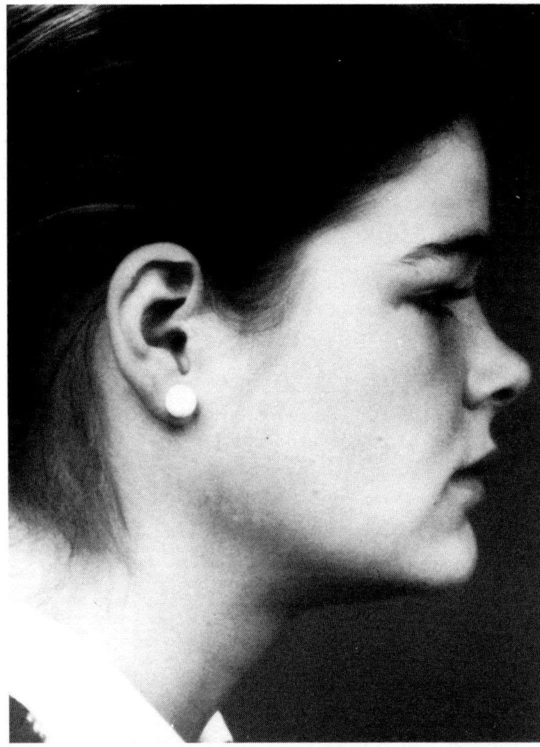
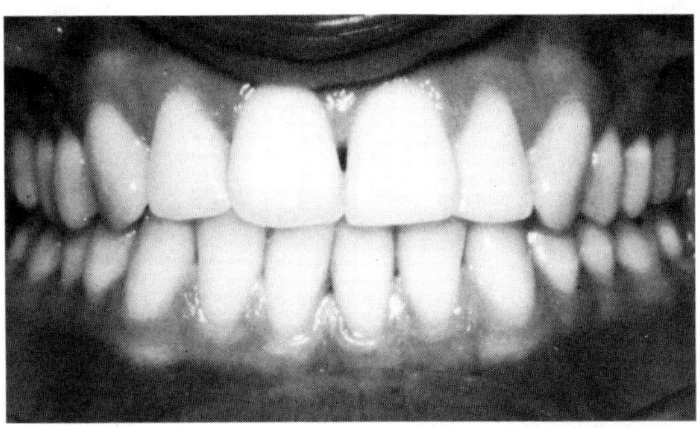
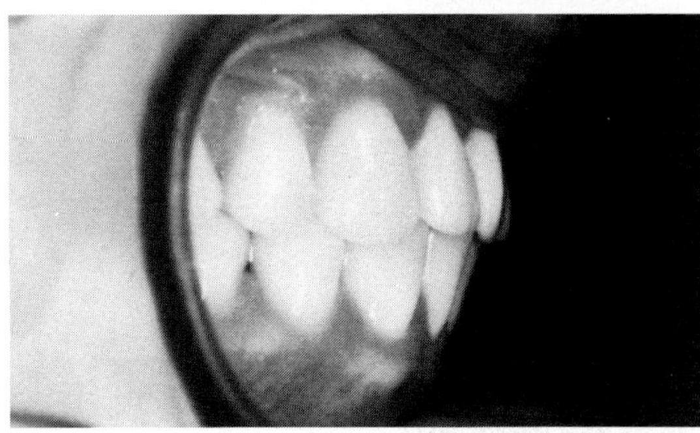
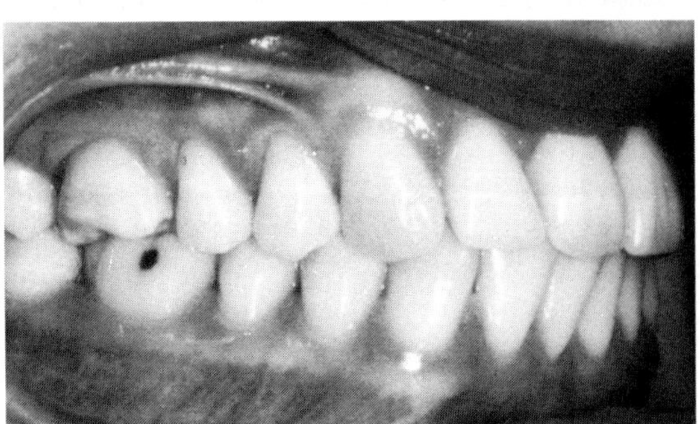
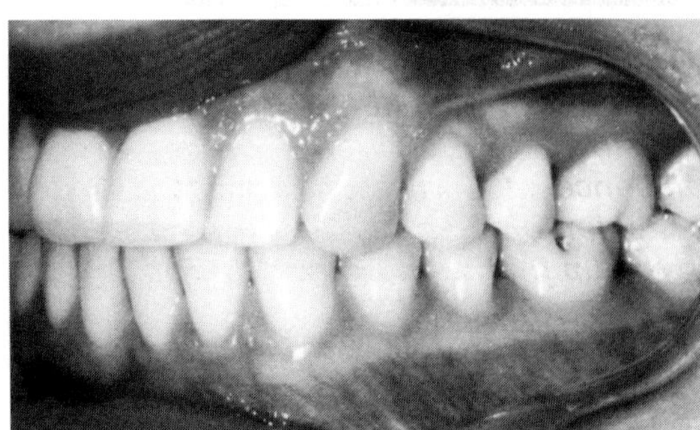

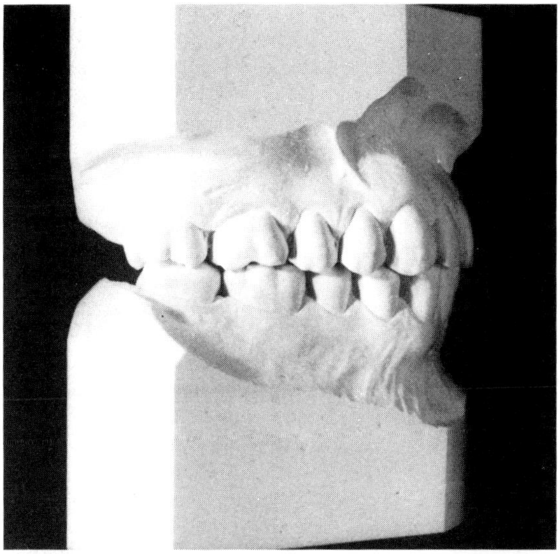

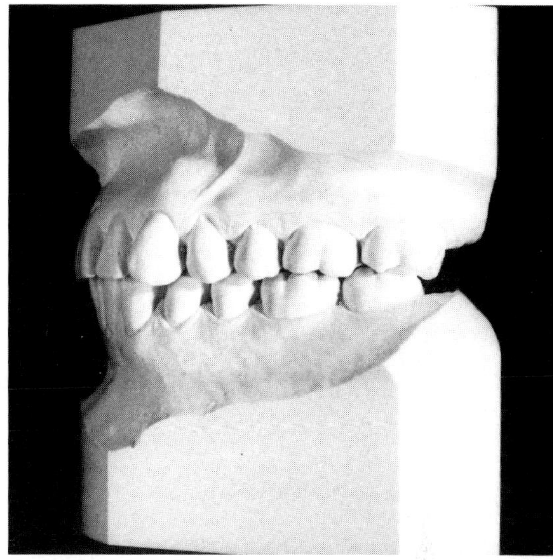

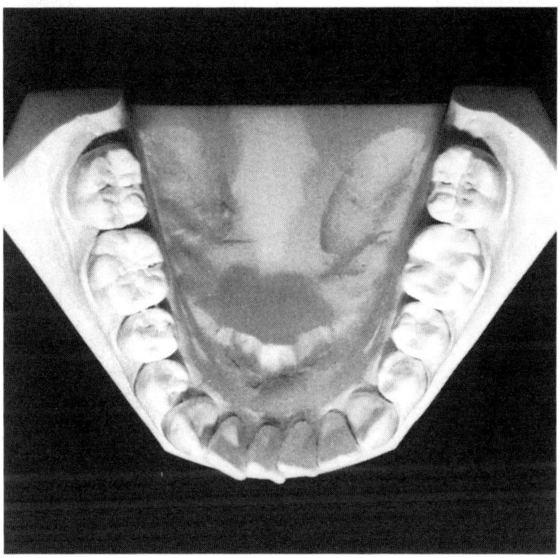

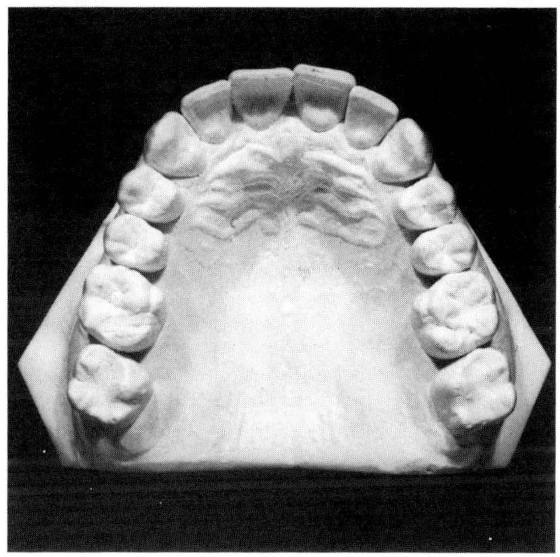

Figs 3-5 and 3-6 The adult picture at the age of 21 y, 5 mo displays mild retraction of the central papilla in the maxilla. The occlusion of the posterior teeth is optimal. The increased crowding of the mandibular incisors cannot be attributed to the presence of third molars since they were congenitally absent. It is likely that the considerable ventral growth of the mandible combined with the maturation of the lower lip musculature had contributed to this.

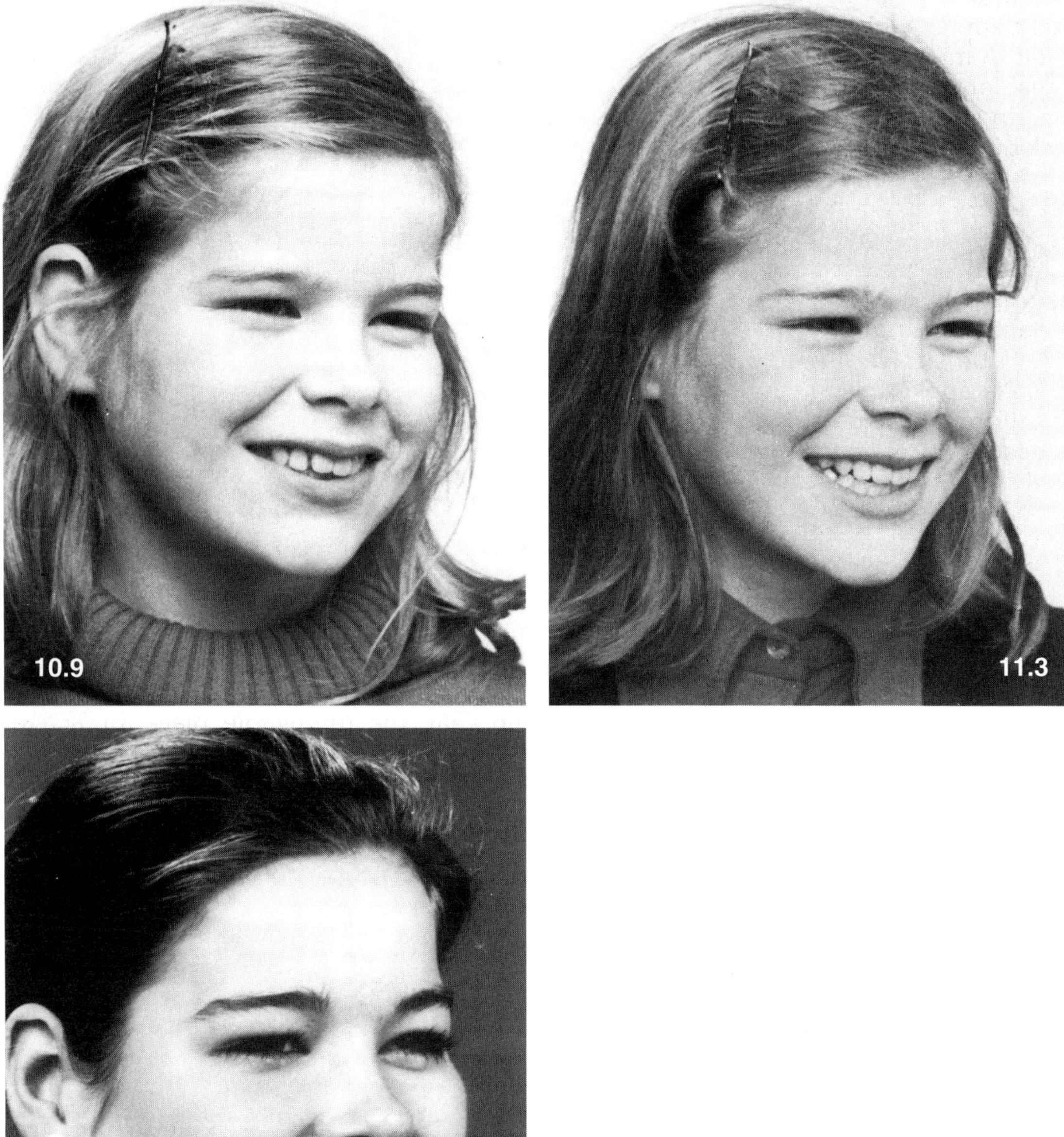

Fig 3-7 The patient's smiling face at different ages. The crowding of the mandibular incisors is barely apparent.

Whether or not irregular mandibular incisors are judged to be undesirable does not just depend on how visible they are, but also on the the way their crowding reveals itself. A mandibular central incisor that lies well lingual to the other incisors is readily considered ugly because its position makes it appear to be darker. Indeed when it is also in supraposition, a situation that often arises in these circumstances due to the lack of vertical opposition, it is thought to be particularly objectionable.

An anterior open bite is not of necessity caused by thumb- or finger-sucking, but can be caused by interposition of the tongue. Sometimes it can result from both. If tongue interposition persists, a corrected open bite will usually relapse to some degree.

A dentist seeing a child with protruding maxillary incisors and a sucking habit should ask to be shown how the sucking is done. One receives an indication of where the force is applied. It can also be ascertained if the child closes the lips entirely around the thumb or fingers. If that is the case, then a patent nasal airway is available and subsequent to treatment the patient will readily be able to achieve satisfactory lip seal if the lips are of normal length. If breathing through the nose is not easily possible, then the lips will not be fully closed around the thumb or fingers, and there will still be inadequate lip closure following treatment, even if the lips are long enough for proper closure. The upper and lower lips do not cover the labial surfaces of the maxillary incisors, so that these teeth can later move forward with a possible associated effect that diastemata can return. This phenomenon can also make its appearance if the upper and lower lips are too short to cover the labial surfaces of the teeth, regardless of nasal patency.

With good nasal patency but inadequate lip seal, the removable plate for active correction can be used, worn nights only as a retainer, to consolidate the obtained improvement until the facial skeleton and soft tissues have matured. If there is inadequate lip seal due to impeded nasal breathing, it might be better to provide splinting of the maxillary incisors and canines with a palatally fixed flexible multistranded wire (such as Twistflex). That applies also to cases in which tongue interposition persists.

The removable plate used in this case might well have worked without the labial arch wires. The use of a plate normally leads to the sucking habit being discarded, which can lead to spontaneous falling back of the incisors. The plate must of course be relieved sufficiently behind those teeth to permit them to go back. Because it is not always certain that the teeth will correct themselves, it was decided beforehand in this case to place labial arches on the plate. It might be worth noting that children compare their appliances with those of their friends, and labial arches might be thought to be the norm. Peer pressure can be used to obtain cooperation if patients think that their treatment conforms to the norm.

Finally, some patients think that the appearance of retracted interdental papillae in the incisor region is quite distressing when speaking or smiling. In this case, there was a mild retraction of the central maxillary papilla apparent at the age of 23 years. Such a development can be prevented by limiting the space available for the papilla. This can be done by timely reduction of the enamel thickness of the mesial surfaces of the central incisors and then moving those teeth together if they do not do so

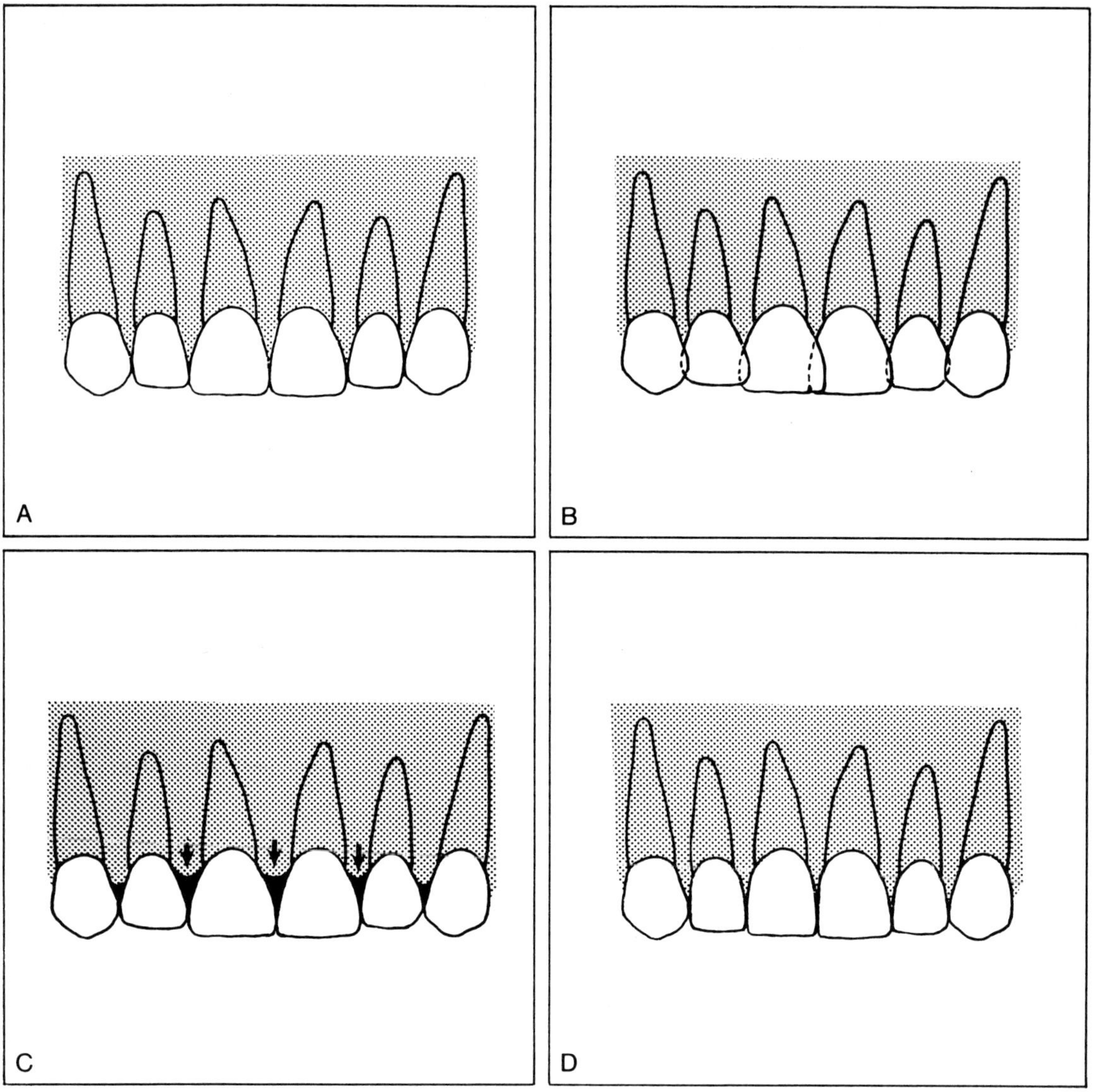

Fig 3-8 The effect of mesiodistal crown dimensions and tooth form on the shape and presence of interdental papillae.

A In a standard situation with normal crowns, the conditions are favorable for well-adapted papillae.

B Also in a situation with extrawide incisors, which are crowded and overlapping, the distances between adjacent cervical margins are small and then the interdental papillae usually fill the available space completely.

C Correction of the alignment depicted in B leads to a considerable increase in the distance between cervical margins. The papillae are then — particularly in the case of adults — usually unable to fill the space interdentally and this gives rise to ugly triangular openings between the teeth.

D With reduction of the mesiodistal crown dimensions (stripping), the distance between the cervical margins can be kept small. Moreover the associated flattening of the convex crown contours provides even more favorable conditions for the papillae to fill the spaces. This can be an important consideration, particularly for the maxillary central papilla.[33]

spontaneously. The distance between the cervical margins is made smaller and the mesial convexity of the crowns reduced. With broad triangular crown forms the distance between the adjacent cervical margins is larger and one often sees papillae retract as the patient becomes older. The danger of large interdental spaces becoming apparent is greatest when correcting rotations and overlapping of broad triangular incisors, most particularly when treating adults (Fig 3.8).

The reduction of interproximal enamel thickness should never be undertaken lightly. It is not an imaginary risk that caries could occur sooner. No more than half the enamel thickness should be removed. It is essential to polish the affected surfaces and apply fluoride after disking. The patient must be instructed in good interdental cleansing (flossing). Furthermore it is necessary to bear in mind the effect of interproximal grinding on the tooth-size relationships between opposing arches. A tooth-size discrepancy can be introduced, corrected, or made worse.[3] If there also is mandibular anterior crowding, it is obvious that one should consider to what extent compensating stripping interproximally can be performed. Finally it should be remembered that reducing the width of teeth can lead to unwished-for diastemata.

Chapter 4

Class I, lateral forced bite, crossbite from 22 to 27 inclusive

Elastics "through the bite"
Female: 16 years, 4 months to 21 years, 0 months

A girl aged 16 years, 4 months presented with asymmetry of her features, and mandibular joint troubles that became evident when her teeth were held together for a long period. She was fearful that her complaints would increase in severity. As she had the ambition to follow a career as a singer, she put much value on her outward appearance. On her left side she exhibited a crossbite of all her teeth except the central incisors. At the same time there was a lateral forced bite of 3 mm to the left. In habitual occlusion all the teeth were in contact. There were no indications of an open bite. Insofar as the circumstances indicated it, it appeared that on the basis of the cone-funnel mechanism maximal vertical contact existed.[30] The centric relation was located 1 mm dorsal to the habitual occlusion (Figs 4.1 and 4.2).

The lateral forced bite and deviant transverse occlusion that she presented are illustrated diagramatically in Figure 4.8. In such a situation, the premolars and the molars on both right and left sides have abnormal inclinations. In a unilateral crossbite without a forced occlusion, it is only the teeth on the side of the crossbite that are abnormally inclined (Fig 4.9).

The reversed transverse occlusion in this case has led to an abnormal inclination of the premolars and molars, not only on the side of the crossbite but also — even though to a limited extent — on the contralateral side. Such adaptations in inclination follow the concept of the dento-alveolar compensatory mechanism (Fig 4.10).

By providing reciprocal forces between the teeth of the maxillary and mandibular arches on the left side, using elastics "through the bite," the tooth movement required to correct the crossbite was obtained. Both their positions and their inclinations were mutually adjusted (Fig 4.11). At the same time, the lateral forced bite was eliminated. It was assumed that the transverse occlusion on the right would be left intact and that the required minor changes in position and inclination would follow spontaneously.

The patient had worn the elastics continuously apart from the time spent brushing her teeth. After four weeks, the lateral incisors and premolars had moved sufficiently and elastics now had only to be worn on the molars and canines. After another three weeks those teeth had also been corrected and the brackets and buttons could be removed. The mandibular joint troubles had vanished. Six months later, the interdigitation had become optimal under the influence of the occlusion and the

Class I, lateral forced bite, crossbite from 22 to 27 inclusive

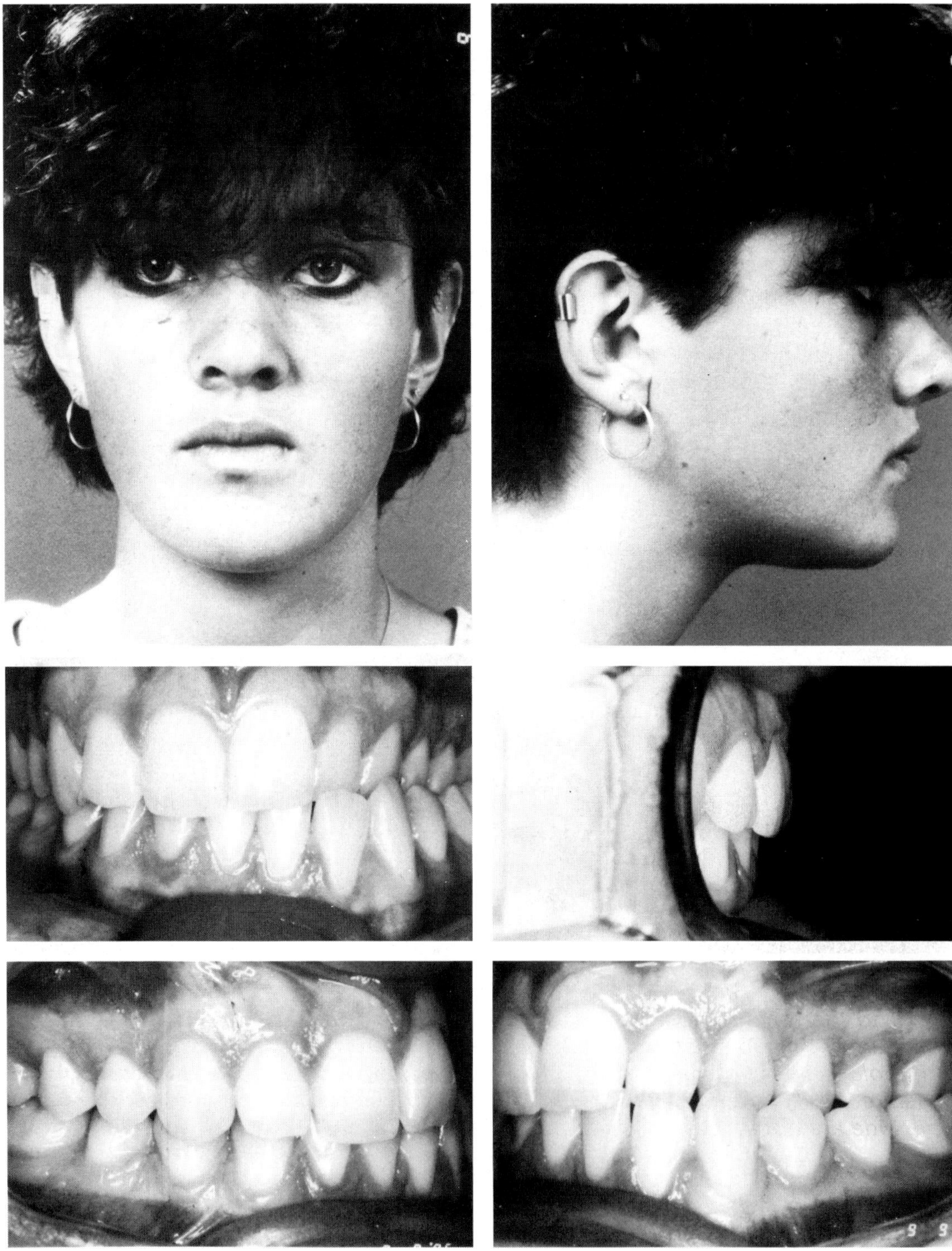

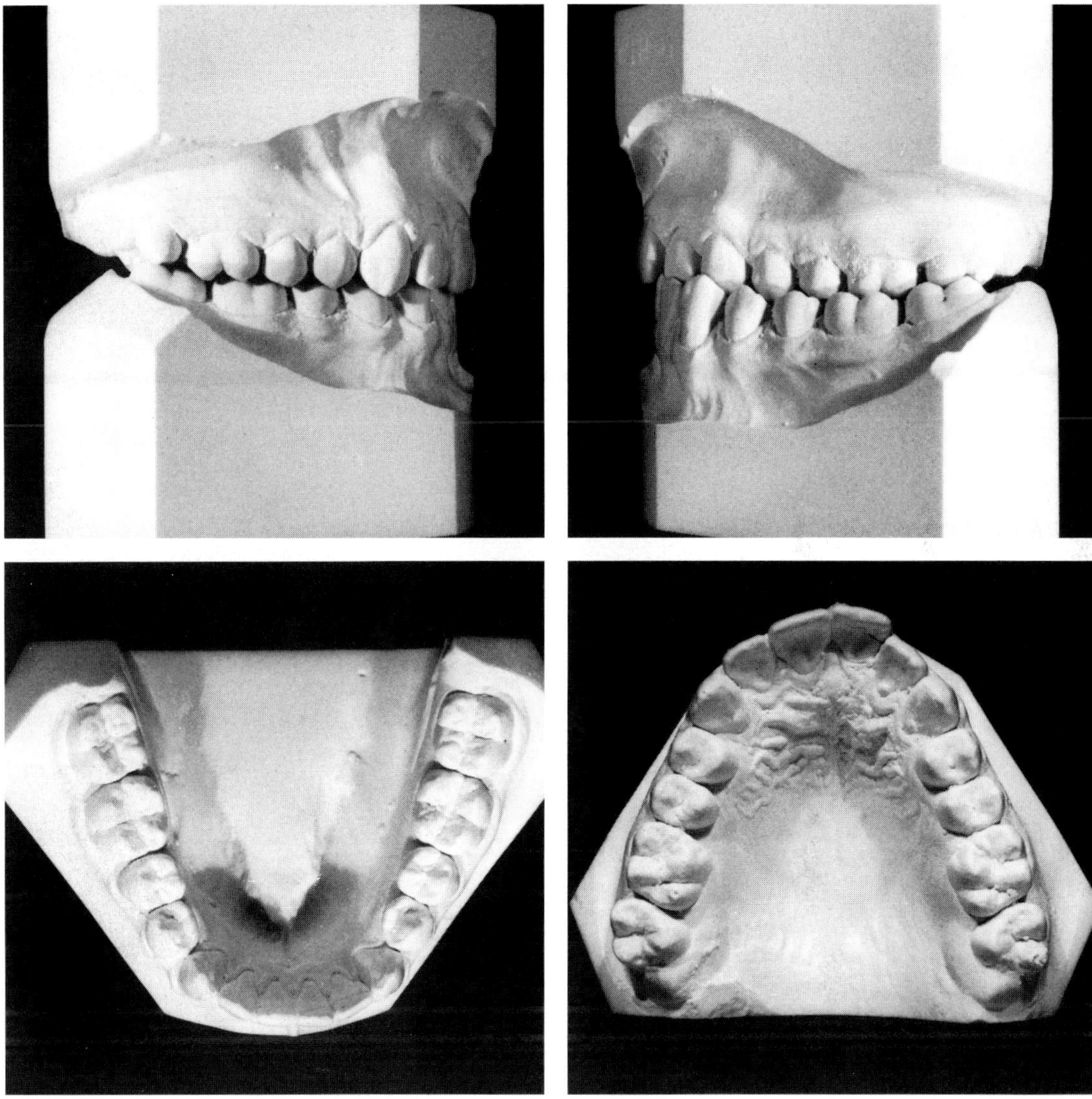

Figs 4-1 and 4-2 Girl, 16 y, 4 mo old, with a crossbite on the left from the lateral incisor to the second molar inclusive, a lateral forced bite of 3 mm to the left and a maximum retrusion of 2 mm beyond habitual occlusion was possible. The premolars and molars interdigitate fully in neutro-occlusion, although on the left it is in crossbite. The premolars and molars on the left when compared with those on the other side are tipped buccally in the mandible and palatally in the maxilla.

Class I, lateral forced bite, crossbite from 22 to 27 inclusive

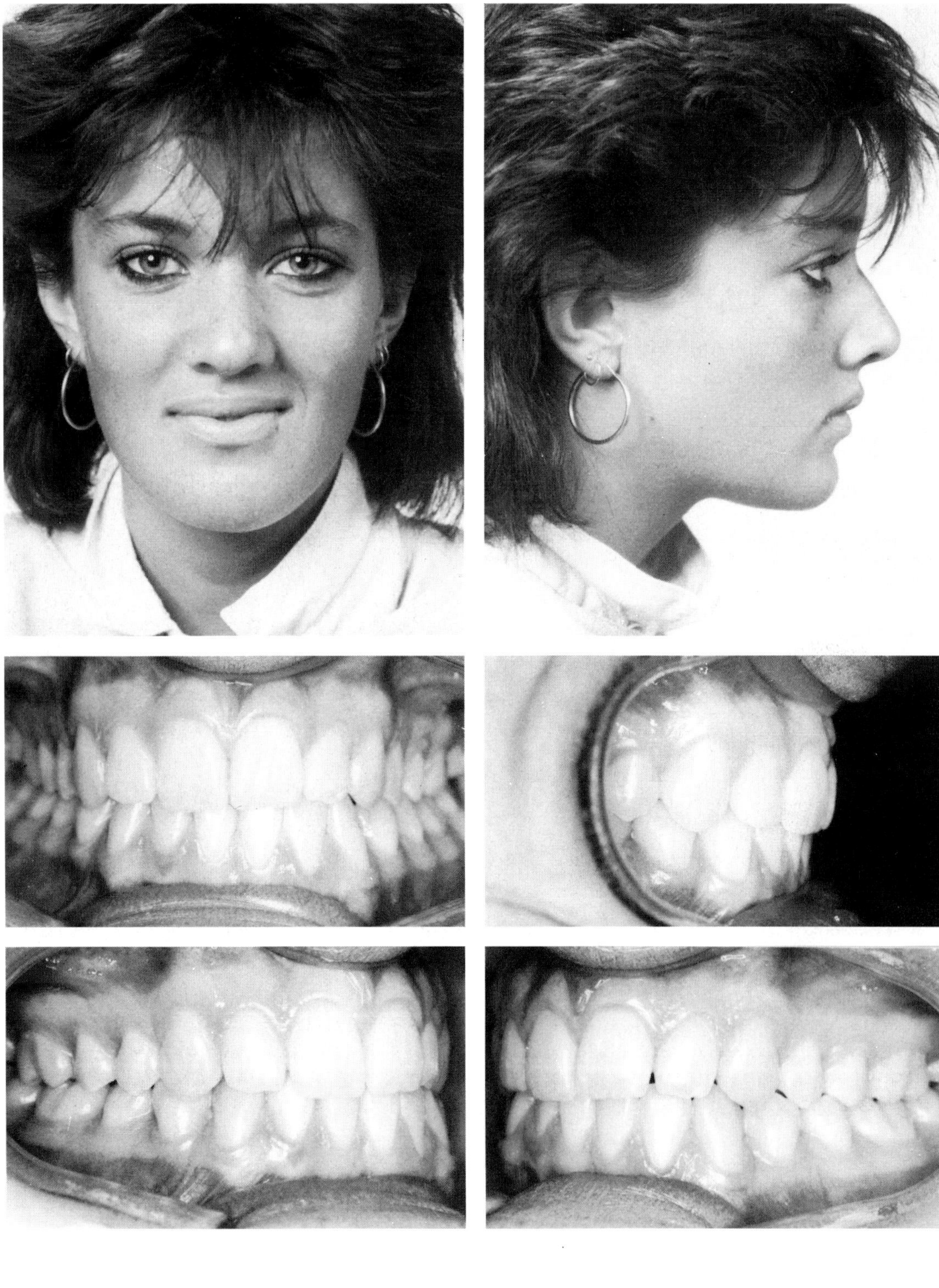

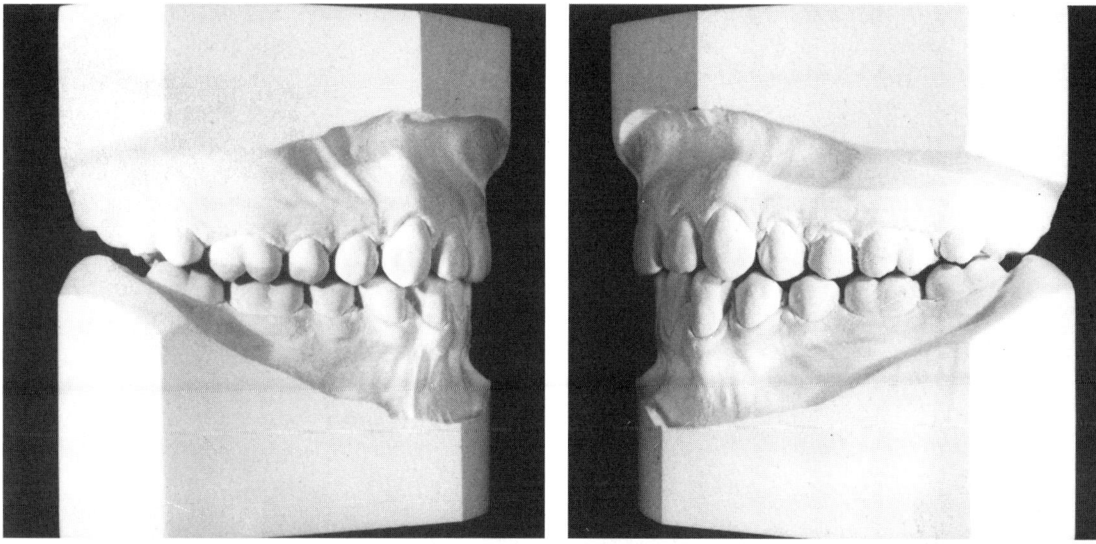

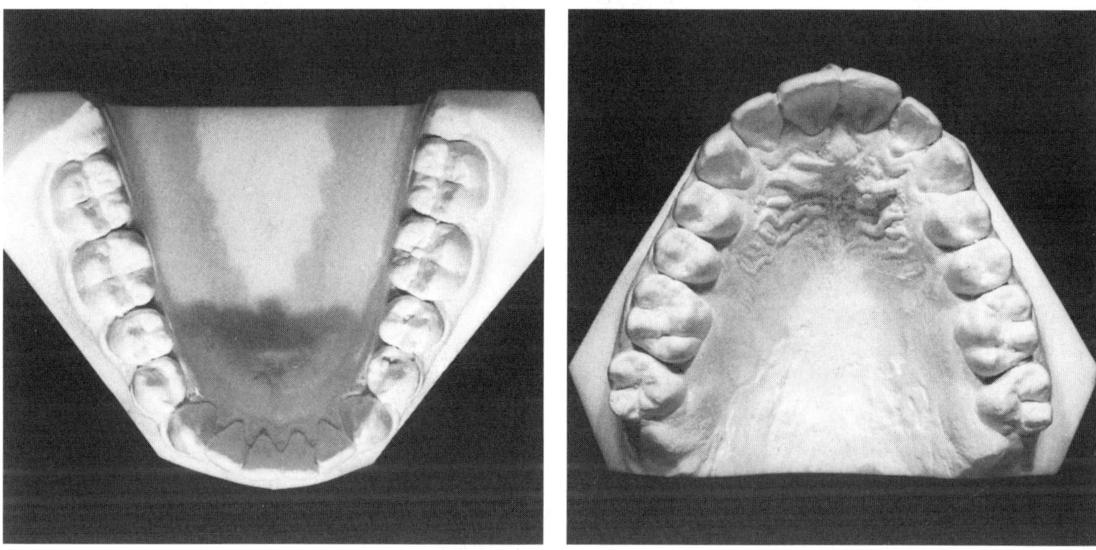

Figs 4-3 and 4-4 The records assembled at the age of 17 y, 11 mo, five months after finishing treatment, show that the crossbite has been totally eliminated. The left cheek has a fuller appearance now. The midlines of the dental arches correspond with each other. The inclination of the premolars and molars has adapted itself on the right side also and now is symmetric. The abnormal positions of the maxillary left incisors have been corrected.

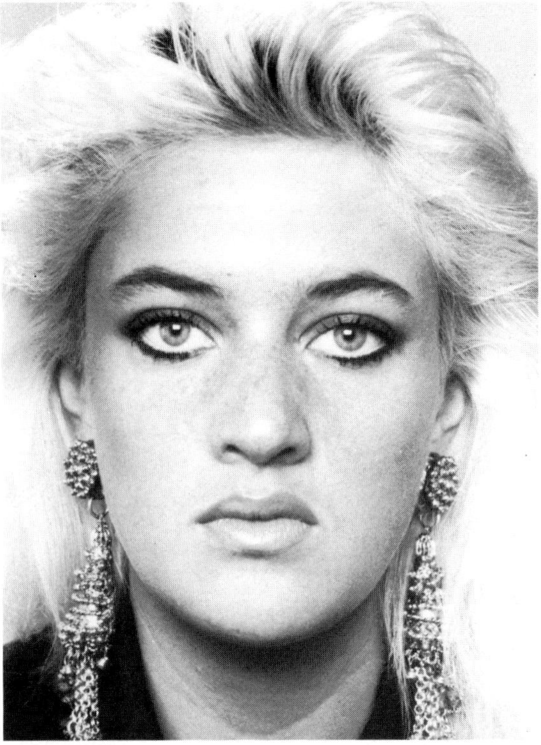
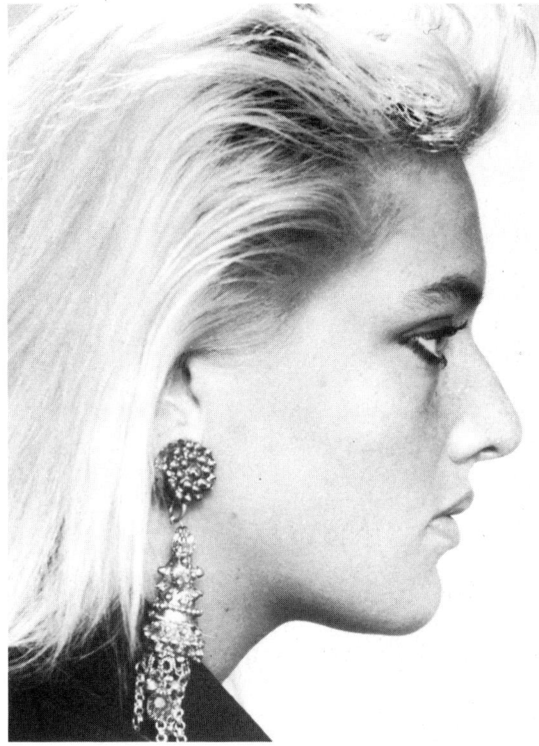
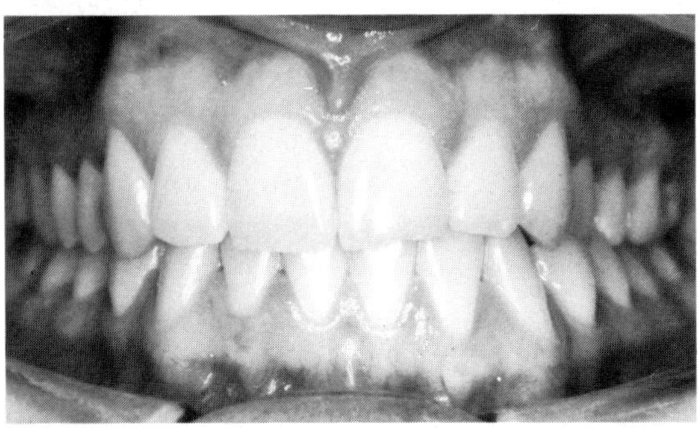
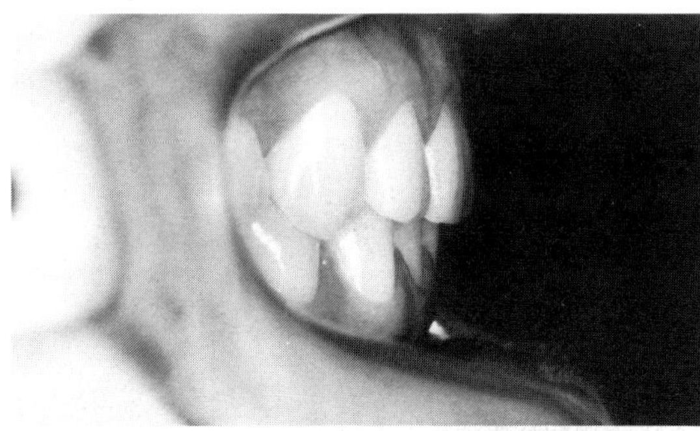
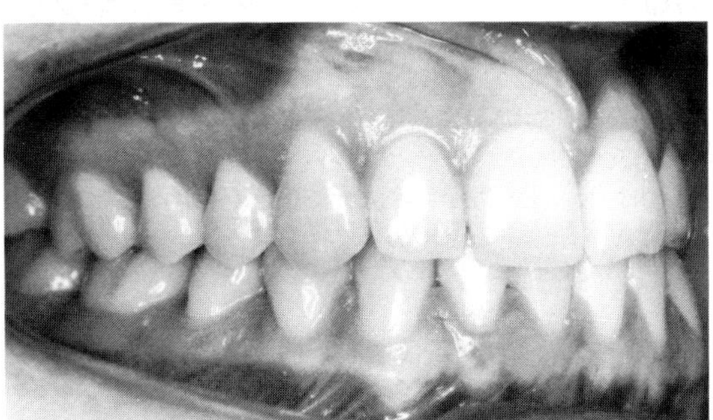
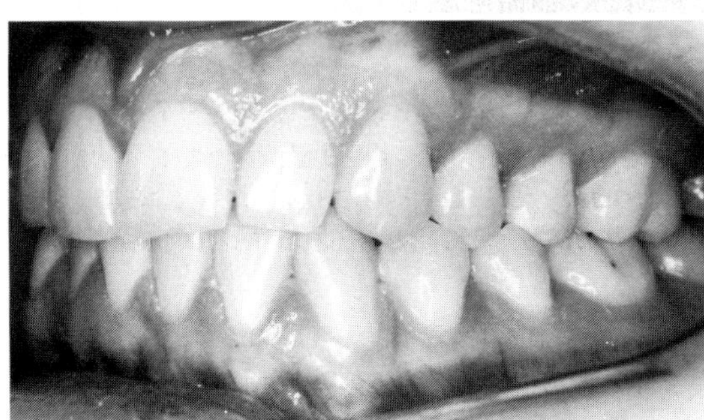

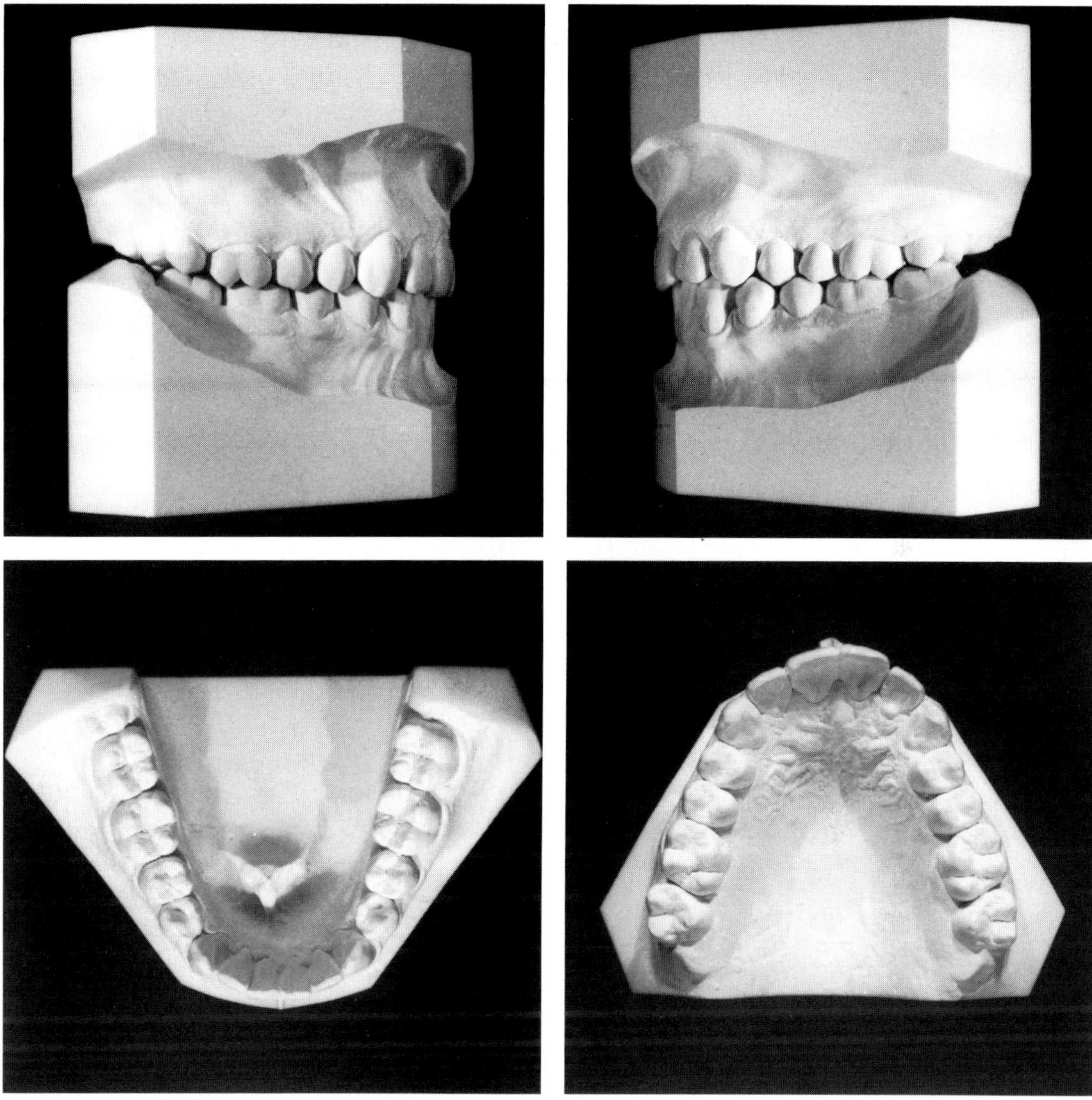

Figs 4-5 and 4-6 *At the age of 22 y, 11 mo, about 5½ years after treatment completion, the maxillary left first premolar has moved very slightly to palatal, probably due to a mild local tongue interposition, which was not observed previously or may not have existed then. Overall, the teeth occlude optimally and exhibit little change in position.*

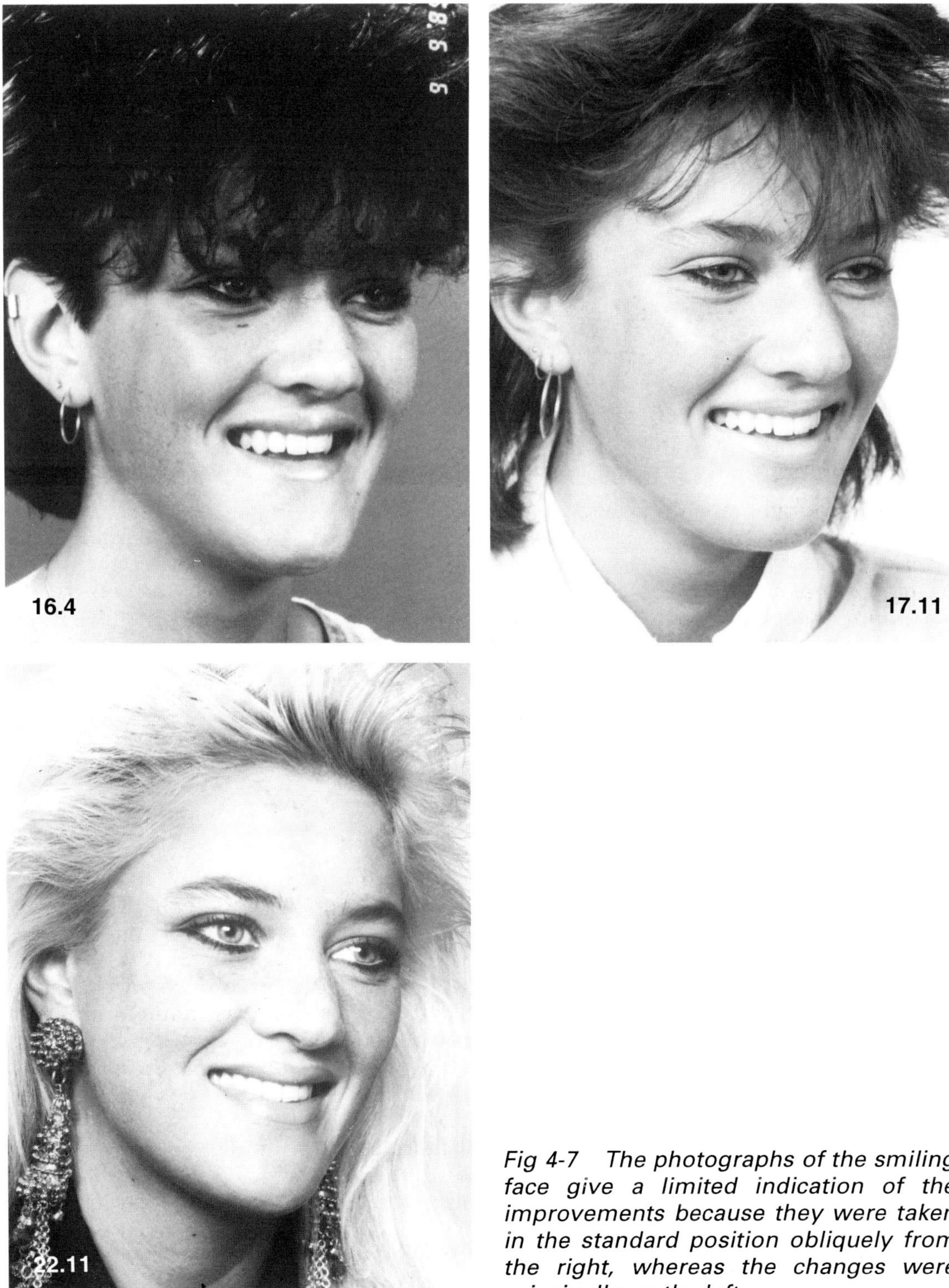

Fig 4-7 The photographs of the smiling face give a limited indication of the improvements because they were taken in the standard position obliquely from the right, whereas the changes were principally on the left.

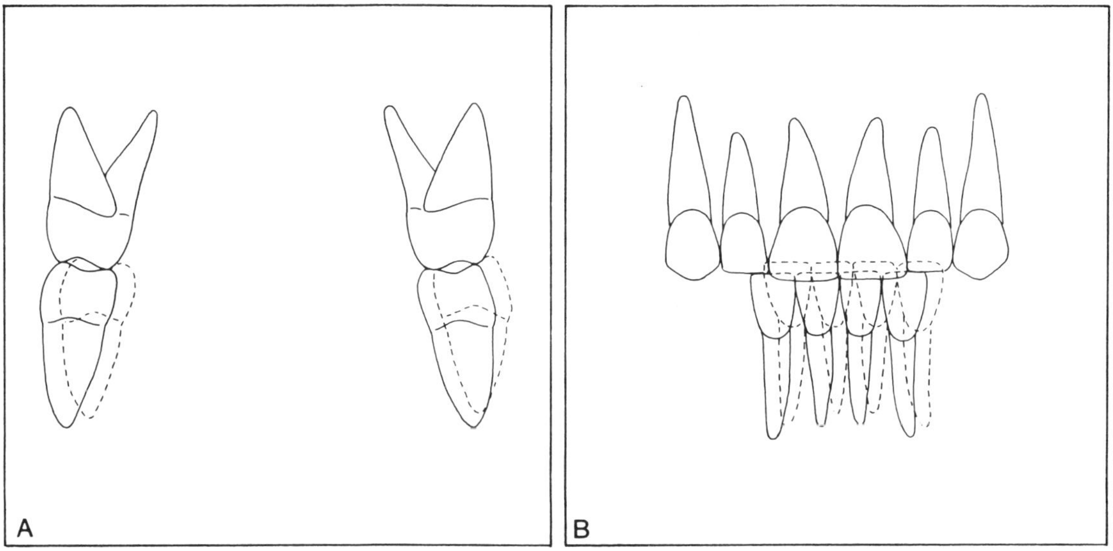

Fig 4-8 Diagrammatic illustration of a lateral forced bite. The teeth are in initial contact (continuous lines) and in maximal occlusion (broken lines) drawn from the front.

A In a normal closing movement, initial contact occurs between the posterior teeth. The maximal occlusion is more to the left with contact between the dental arches on both right and left sides. On the left side there is a reversed transverse occlusion.

B The relation of the midlines of the maxillary and mandibular arches deviates accordingly.[30]

inclination of the teeth had adapted. The depth of the bite had reduced on both sides (Figs 4.3 and 4.4). A retainer was considered unnecessary in this case on the principle that the occlusion and the normal functional conditions guaranteed stability. This assessment was only partly supported by the records taken five years later. The maxillary left first premolar had moved palatally, something that might be attributed to a slight local interposition of the tongue. This occurrence brought into question the original observations from which the diagnosis was made in which a solid interdigitation was assumed (Figs. 4.5 and 4.6). The photos of her smiling face do not give a good picture of the changes as they were taken obliquely from the right and not the left (Fig 4.7).

Crossbites can also be corrected by moving the relevant teeth relative to each other in the mandible and maxilla, but independent of each other. There must then be provision for holding the teeth out of occlusion. A removable plate with a bite plane behind the maxillary incisors is suitable. Also, a bite plane across the posterior teeth that do not need to be moved can be useful. After the errant teeth have been moved

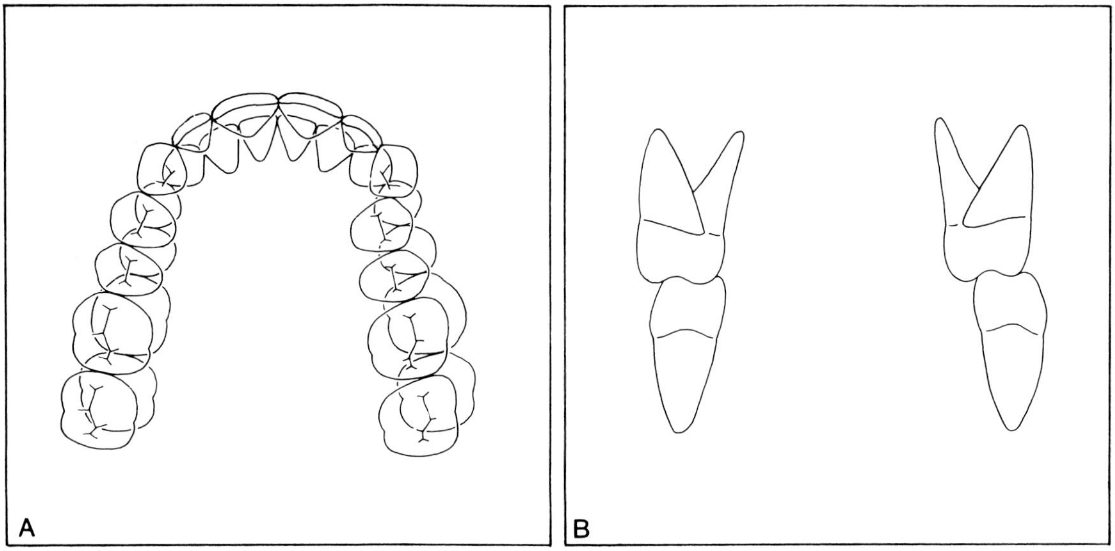

Fig 4-9 Diagrammatic illustration of a crossbite without forced bite, with a reversed transverse occlusion on one side.

A The maxillary arch crosses the mandibular one distally to the maxillary left canine (seen from cranial).

B On the right, there is normal transverse occlusion, on the left it is reversed (seen from the front).[30]

across the bite, the bite plane can be discarded and the occlusion can promote further natural correction.

When using elastics "through the bite," it is usually possible to avoid making provision for holding the teeth out of occlusion, since the elastics largely will perform that service. If, as is the case in a lateral forced bite such as this, it is desirable to perform corrections in position and inclination on the other side, it is preferable not to fix the teeth rigidly with the appliance. Otherwise spontaneous improvements on the side that is not in crossbite might not be so readily obtained.

A limitation of the use of elastics is that the success of the therapy is very much dependent on the cooperation of the patient. If the elastics are not worn the full 24 hours per day, then the teeth are quickly bitten back into their faulty positions. As a rule of thumb, if after eight weeks the crossbite has not been corrected using elastics, then another mode of therapy is required.

Furthermore, it has to be pointed out again that it will take months before the inclinations of the teeth will adapt to the changed occlusion. The necessary remodeling of the alveolar process is rather extensive and the speed with which it can be realized is limited.[31]

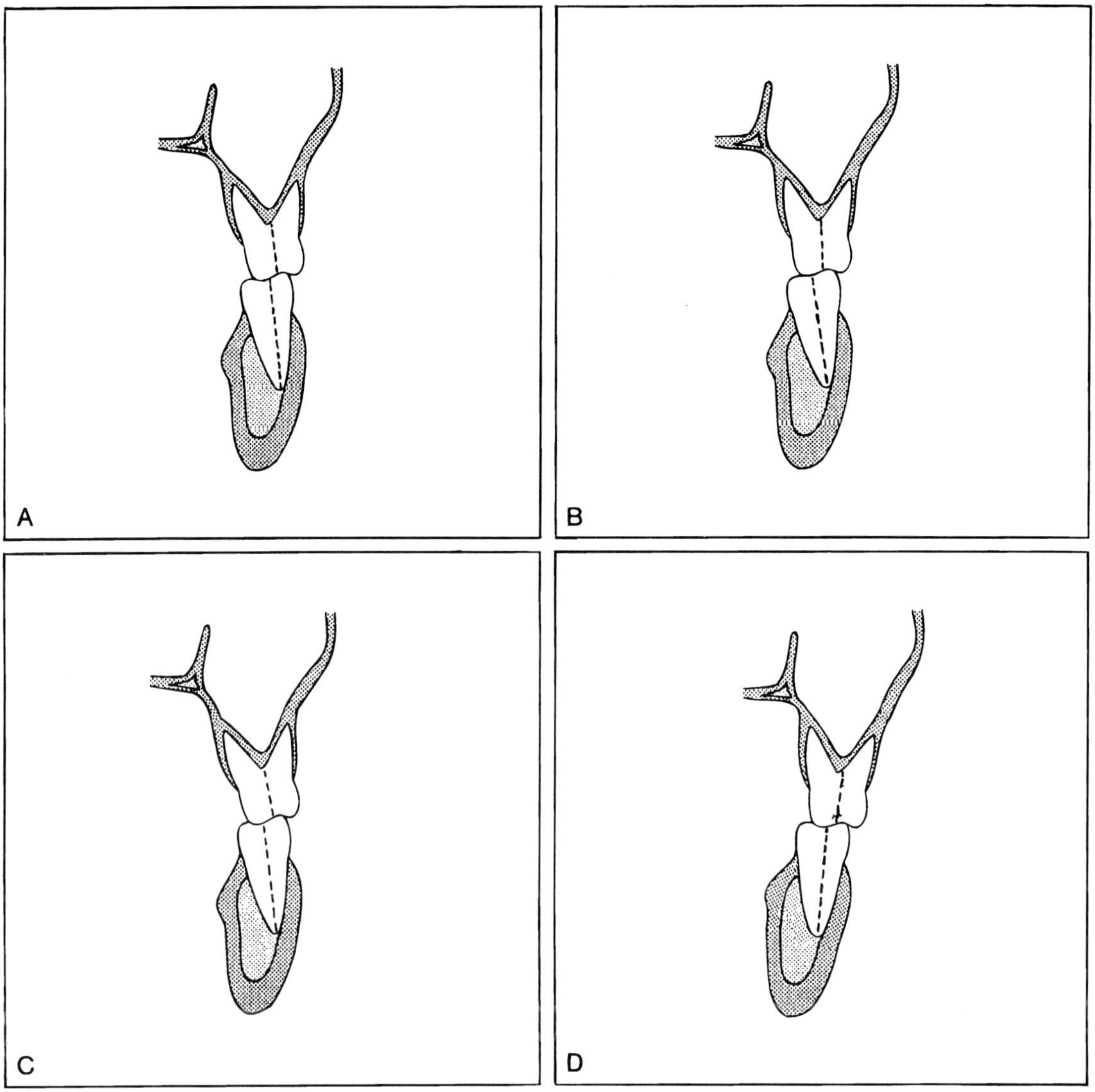

Fig 4-10 Variations in the inclination of the molars on the left, wherein differences in transverse relationships of the underlying bony structures are compensated for (dento-alveolar compensatory mechanism).

A Ideal relationship and inclinations.

B A more buccal position of the maxillary jaw structure is compensated for by a less buccal inclination of the maxillary molars.

C A pronounced palatal position of the maxillary jaw structure is compensated for by a marked buccal inclination of the maxillary molar.

D A substantially buccal position of the maxillary jaw structure is compensated for by palatal tipping of the maxillary molars and buccal tipping of the mandibular molars.[34]

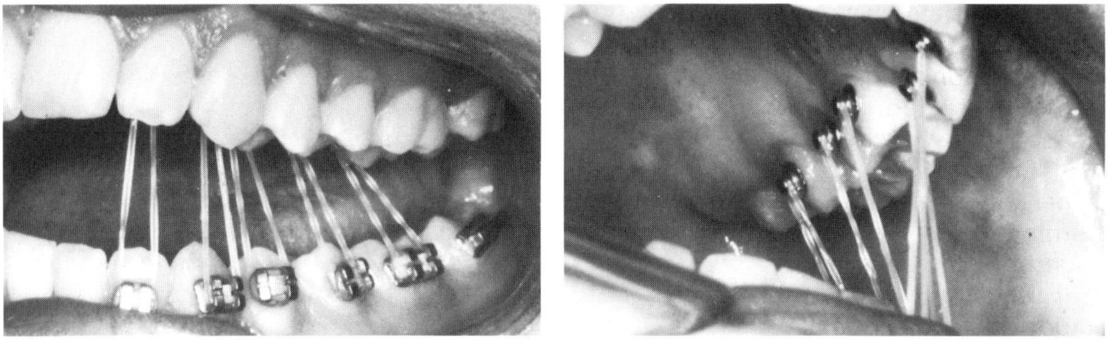

Fig 4-11 Elastics "through the bite" to reciprocally move mandibular teeth to lingual and maxillary teeth to buccal. The elastics must be worn 24 hours per day; otherwise, the teeth are bitten back into their faulty positions. Lingual buttons were attached to the maxillary teeth and brackets to the mandibular ones, the latter being chosen in case full fixed appliances might ultimately be required. The elastics were worn on the lateral incisors and premolars for four weeks, on the canines and molars for seven weeks.

In the circumstances described here (relatively narrow maxillary arch, lateral forced bite), consideration could also have been given to correcting the crossbite by means of transverse expansion of the maxillary arch. That was dismissed in this case to interfere with singing as little as possible, and also to profit as much as possible from spontaneous corrections as it can be assumed that those changes are not likely to relapse. Above all, it can be expected that through the application of intermaxillary elastics the mandibular arch would contribute more to the correction than would be the case if maxillary expansion were used.

It should be pointed out that a permanent correction of a crossbite can only be expected in cases with no tongue interposition. The majority of transverse malocclusions exhibit a narrow maxillary arch associated with open bites in the posterior region. Moving the involved teeth in such cases has no merit, since subsequently they will return largely to their original condition under the influence of the forces of the tongue and buccal musculature. Regrettably tongue interposition, especially in the posterior regions, is for all practical purposes mostly impossible to eliminate permanently. Where a crossbite with lateral tongue interposition goes together with an anterior open bite, an attempt to improve the crossbite most likely will result in an increase in the anterior open bite. If subsequently the transverse situation should relapse, then the end result will be worse than if no treatment had been undertaken.

In abnormal occlusions, the presence of partial lateral tongue interposition of a limited extent is very difficult to determine. Often it is not until afterwards that it becomes apparent that such a condition exists and that it probably was present prior to treatment. The case presented here is just such an example.

Chapter 5

Class I, marked crowding in both dental arches
Extraction of four first premolars, no appliances
Female: 10 years, 0 months to 32 years, 6 months

A girl aged just 10 years, exhibiting neutro-occlusion and neutro relation, had severe crowding in the canine-premolar regions of all quadrants. She had a round face and a mild degree of double protrusion, which meant that her mouth was situated somewhat ventrally relative to the rest of her face. All first premolars and permanent canines except that on the upper right had emerged. In the mandible, the space for the second premolars had almost completely vanished due to the premature loss of their predecessors. It was thought from the evidence of radiographs that the crowns of these premolars were hypoplastic (Fig 5.14). In the maxilla, the permanent left canine had emerged outside the dental arch and that on the right was likely to do the same. In the mandibular arch an arch length discrepancy (ALD) of —12 mm had been measured, with one of –7 mm in the maxillary arch. The midline of the mandibular arch was displaced 2 mm to the right of that of the maxilla: the overjet was 4 mm (Figs 5.1 and 5.2).

In view of the crowding in the canine-premolar regions combined with the mild double protrusion, it seemed obvious to remove a premolar from each quadrant. In the maxilla, the choice of extraction was influenced by the marked mesial angulation of the permanent canines. It could be expected that after extraction of the first premolars, the canines would spontaneously upright to distal.

The assumed inferior quality of the mandibular second premolars and the fact that the first premolars in that region had emerged favorably seemed to call for the sacrifice of the as yet unerupted second premolars. Against this was the fact that the crowns of the first premolars were small and not of optimal functional shape. Therefore extraction of the first premolars in the mandible also was preferred, bearing in mind too that the surgical removal of the second premolars could lead to a permanently undesirable effect on the bone support of the adjacent teeth. Although there was only a slight chance that the second premolars might not erupt further, it was decided to monitor this aspect by obtaining radiographs at a later stage. It was hoped that the eruption of the second premolars would lead to uprighting of the mandibular first permanent molars.

At the age of 10 years 1 month, both maxillary first premolars were extracted. Eight months later, when it was established radiographically that the mandibular second premolars had erupted further, the mandibular first premolars were removed. Subsequently the development of the dentition proceeded very well (Figs 5.3 to 5.8 and 5.14).

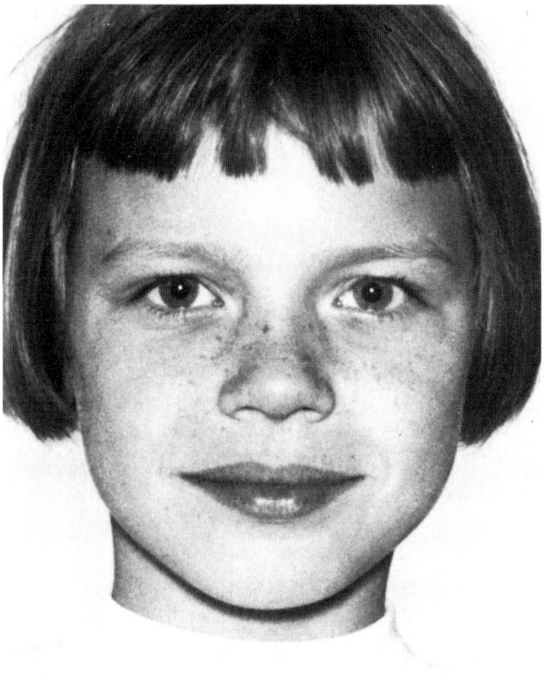

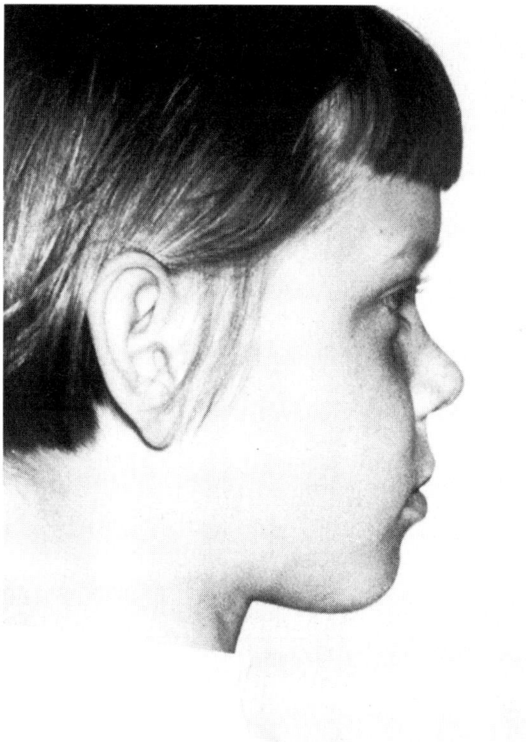

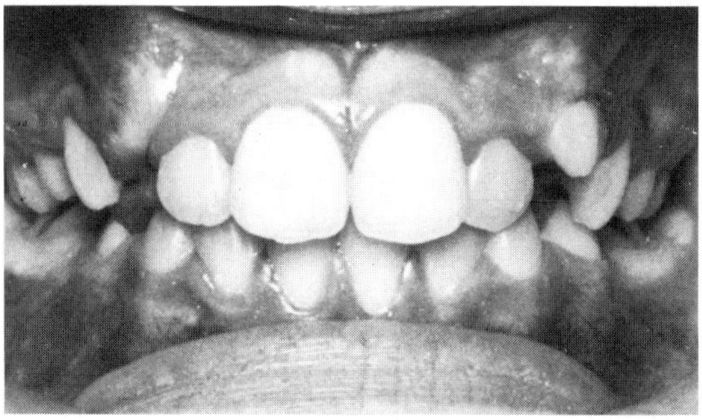

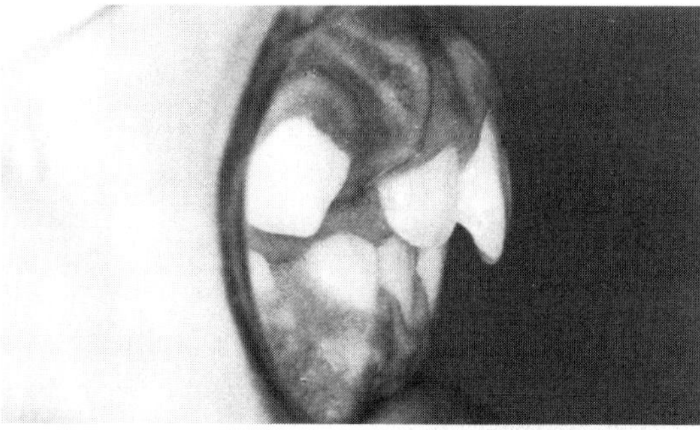

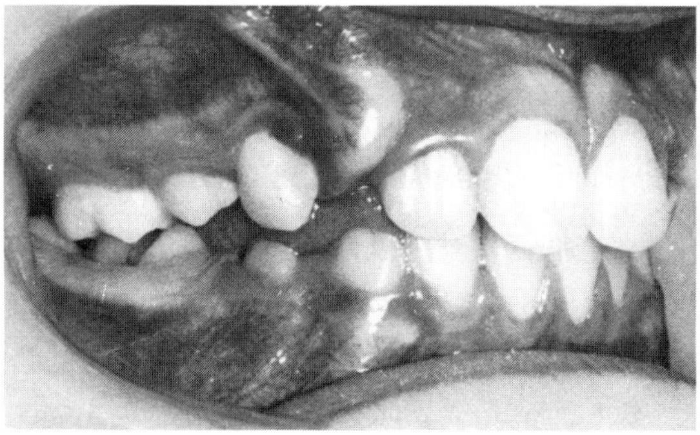

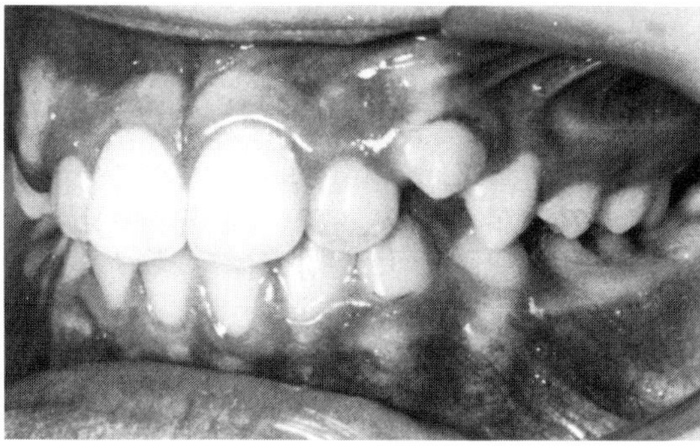

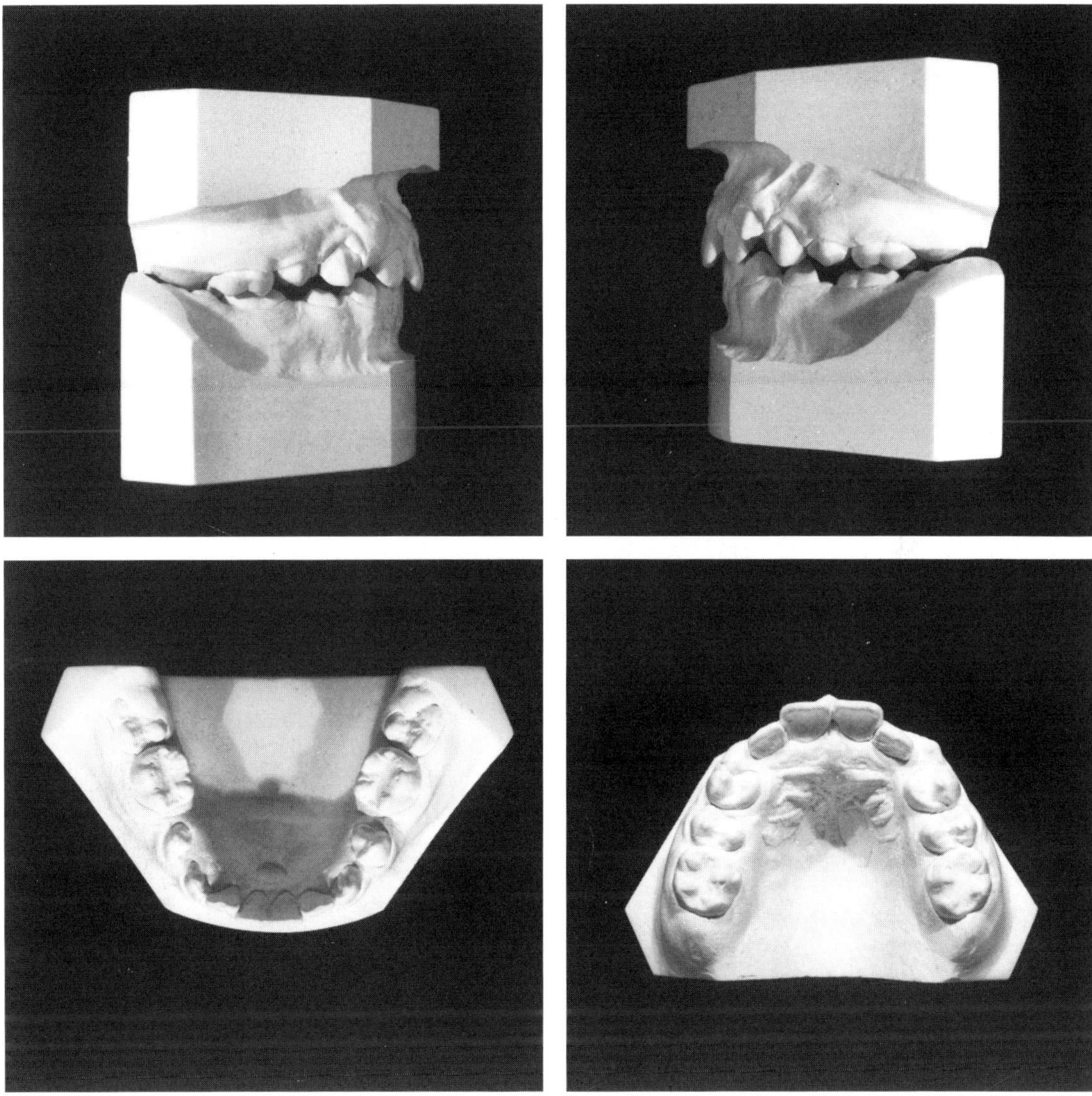

Fig 5-1 and 5-2 A girl aged 10 y, 0 mo, with class I anomaly and marked crowding. In the mandible, the crowding is in the regions of the second premolars; in the maxilla in the canine regions. Premature loss of the deciduous molars in the mandible had led to mesial migration and tipping of the first permanent molars and early emergence of the second ones. There is insufficient room for the maxillary second molars; the posterior section of the apical area is still too small for them.[31]

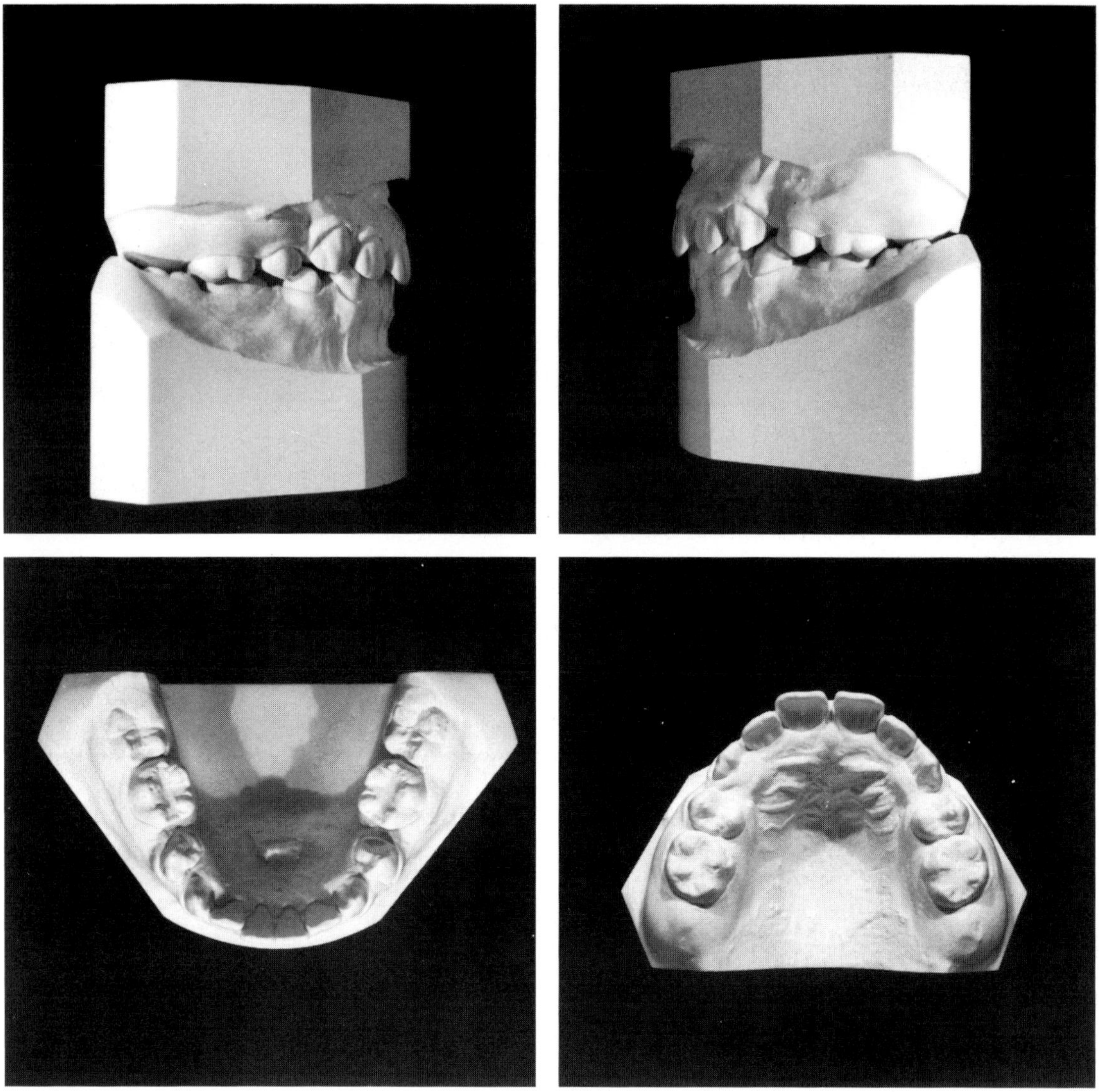

Fig 5-3 At the age of 10 y, 5 mo, four months after extraction of the maxillary first premolars, the canines in the maxilla have gone distally and palatally; they have almost filled the extraction spaces. The first premolars in the mandible were extracted at the age of 10 y, 9 mo, when it was seen that the mandibular second premolars continued to erupt.

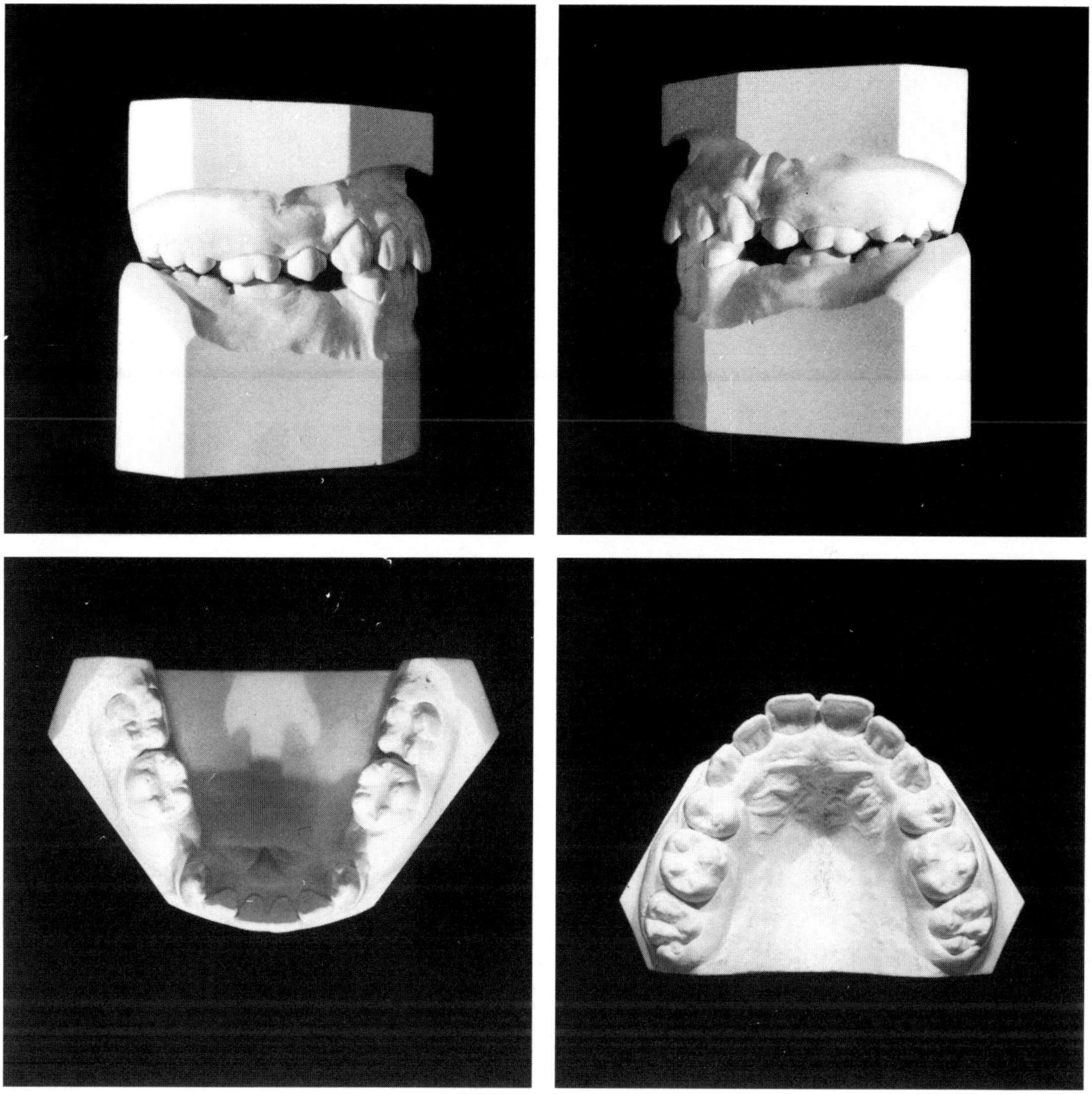

Fig 5-4 At 11 y, 1 mo, the maxillary second permanent molars have emerged and the canines are in good alignment. In the mandible, the removal of the first premolars has provided sufficient room for the second premolars to emerge.

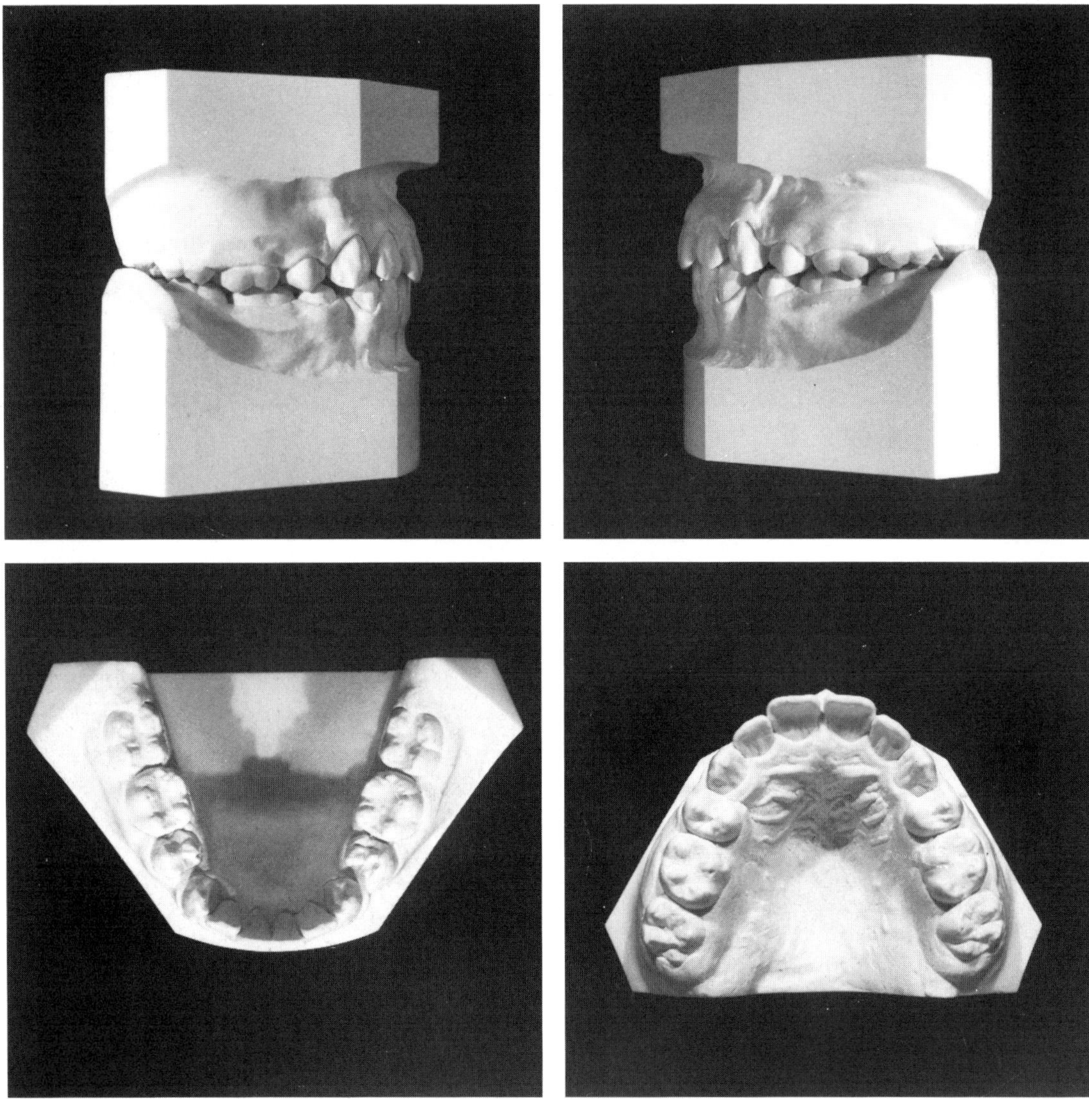

Fig 5-5 At 12 y, 6 mo, the mandibular second premolars had been present in the arch for nearly a year. Their crowns were indeed hypoplastic. Both dental arches exhibited only minor irregularities and occluded well. The mandibular first permanent molars have uprighted and have good contact with the adjacent teeth. The overjet has diminished.

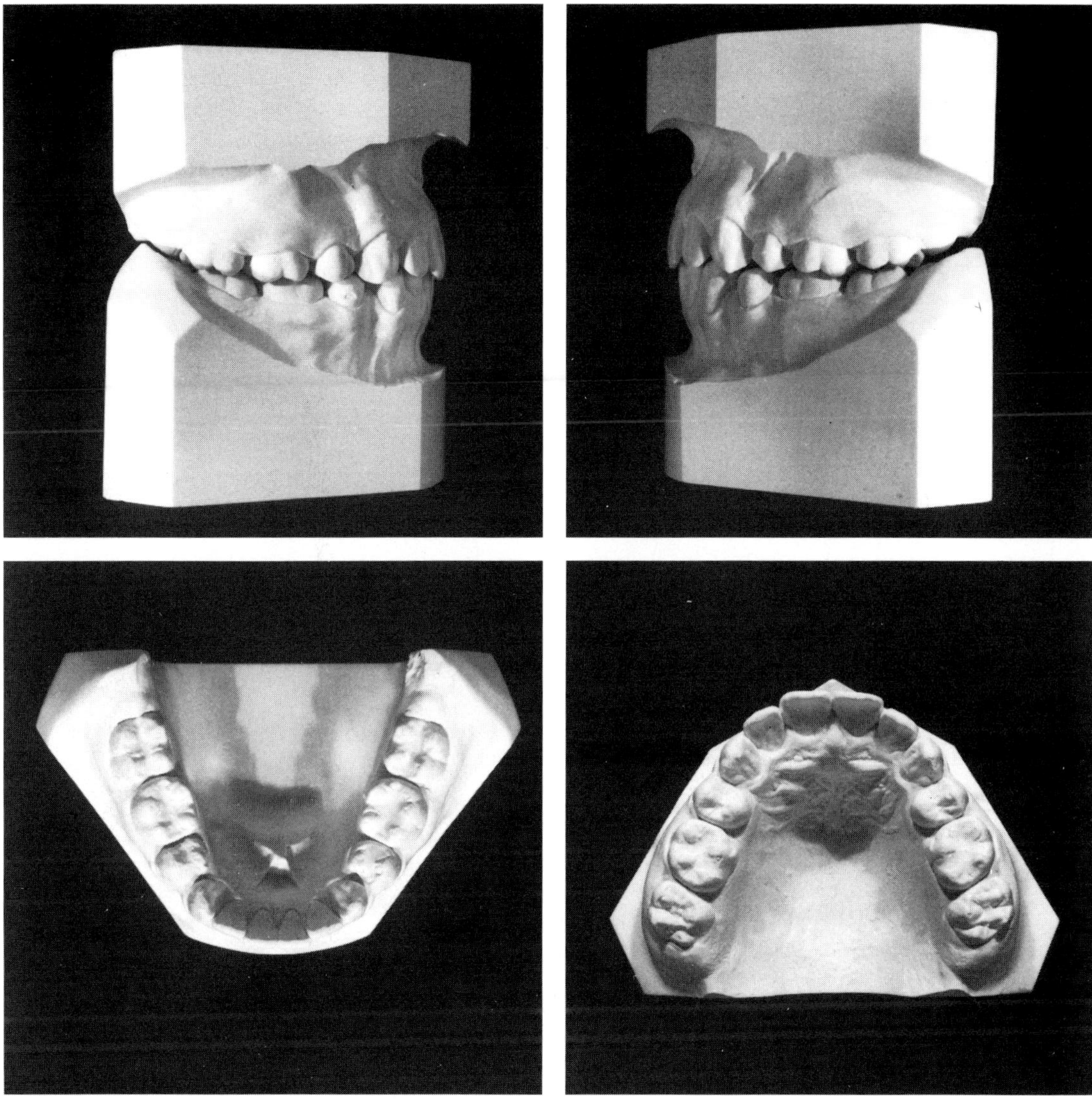

Fig 5-6 At 14 y, 11 mo, the mandibular arch is somewhat more mesially situated in relation to the maxillary arch than it was a year and a half earlier. There have been few other changes. The mandibular second premolars have been restored. The posterior section of the apical area has increased in size little and further growth in a girl of this age cannot be expected. Eventually insufficient room will probably be available for the third molars to emerge properly (see Fig 5.8).

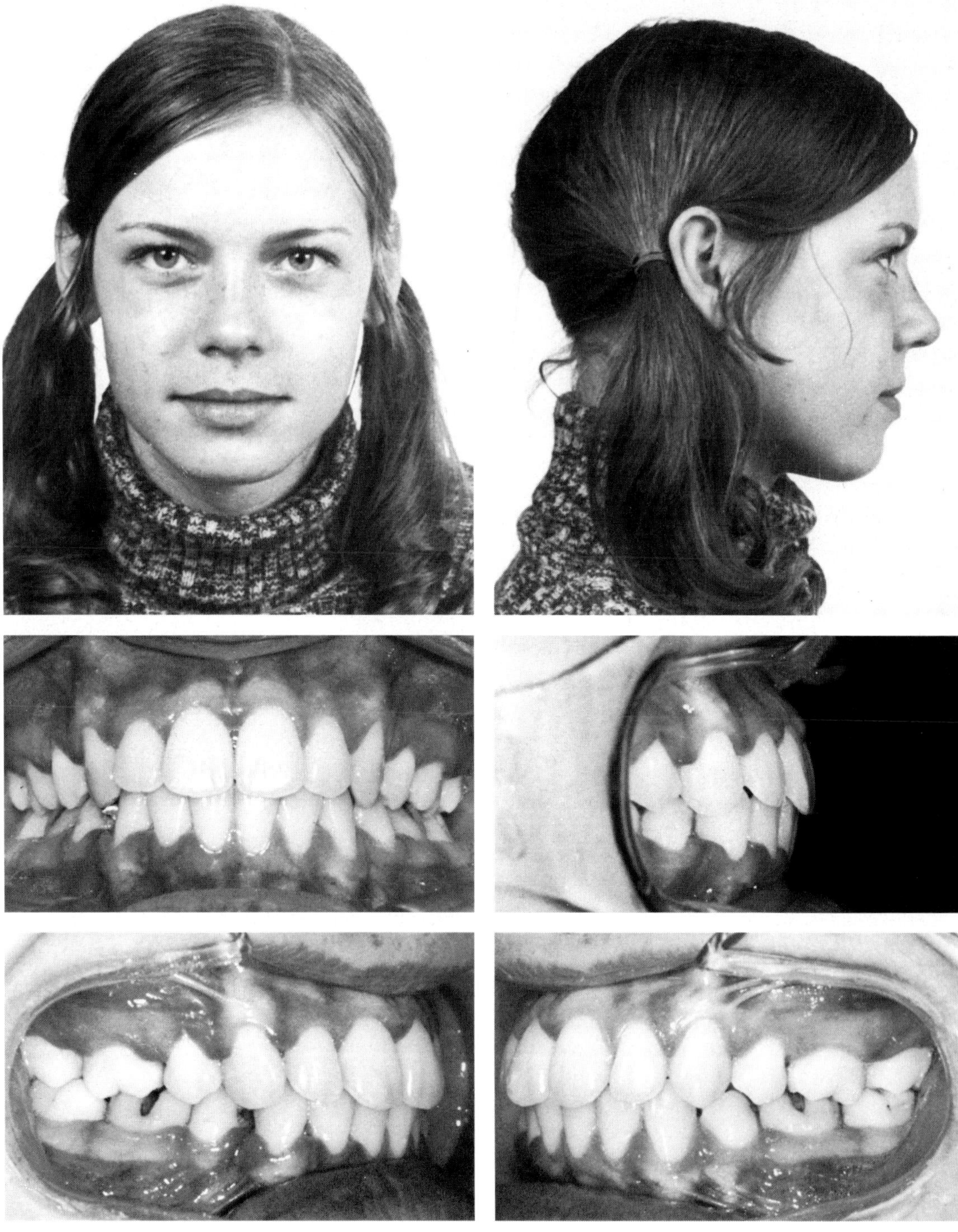

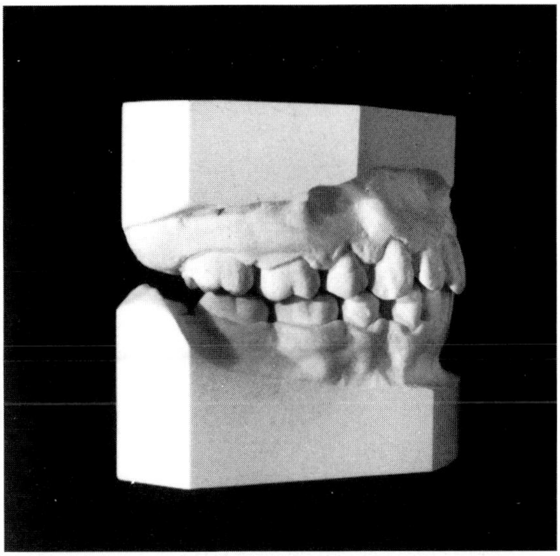

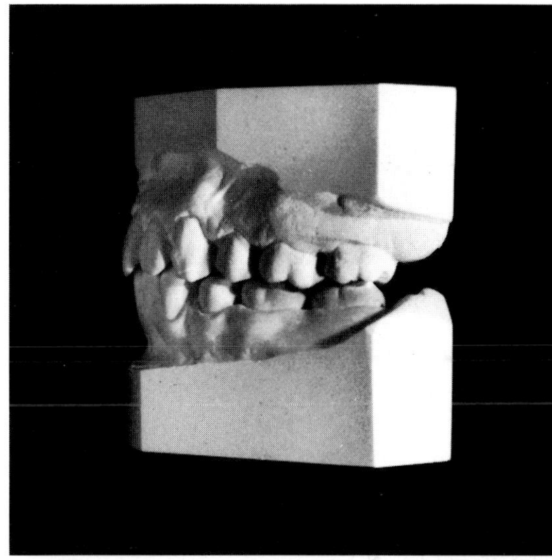

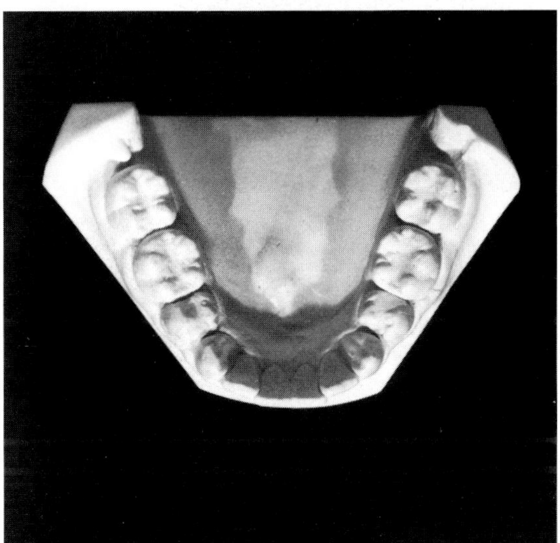

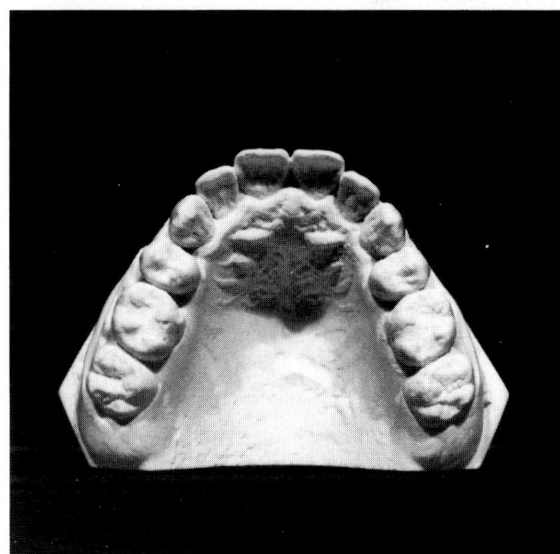

Figs 5-7 and 5-8 *At 17 y, 2 mo, facial growth has already been complete for some years. Indeed insufficient space is available for the third molars in the maxilla; the same applies for the mandibular third molars. Over the past two years, the mandibular dental arch has moved a little further mesially in relation to the maxillary one.*

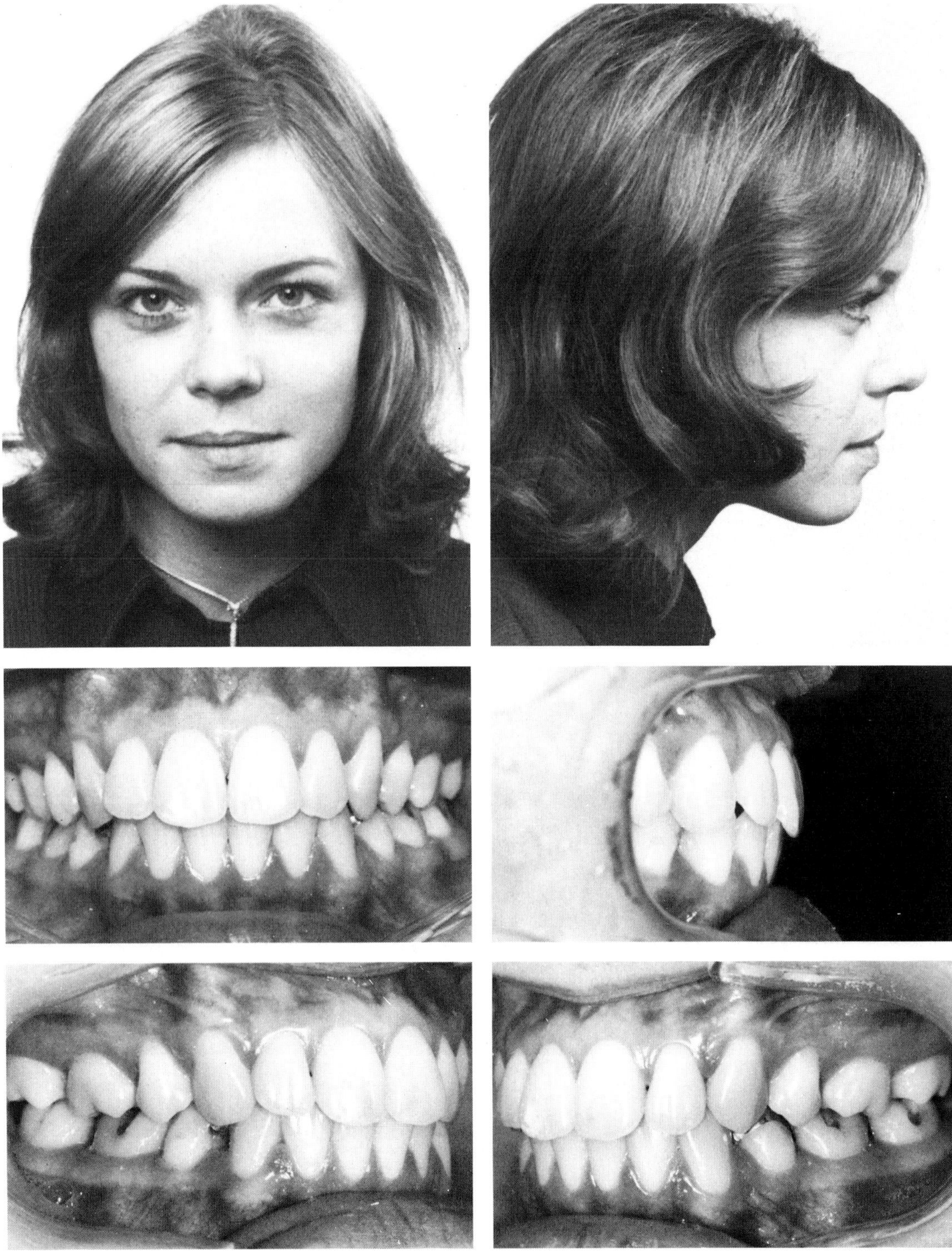

Fig 5-9 Situation at age 19 y, 2 mo.

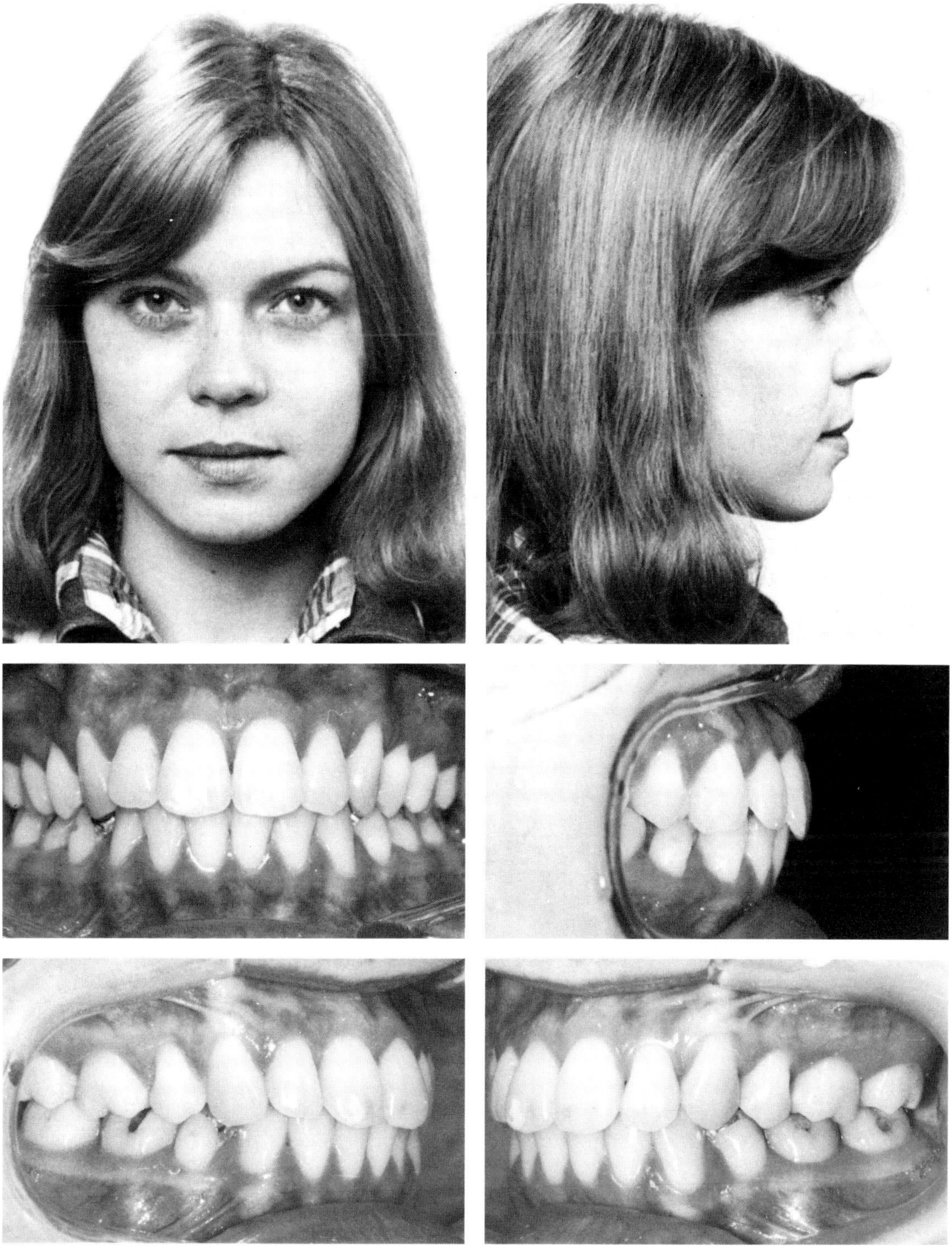

Fig 5-10 Situation at age 22 y, 7 mo.

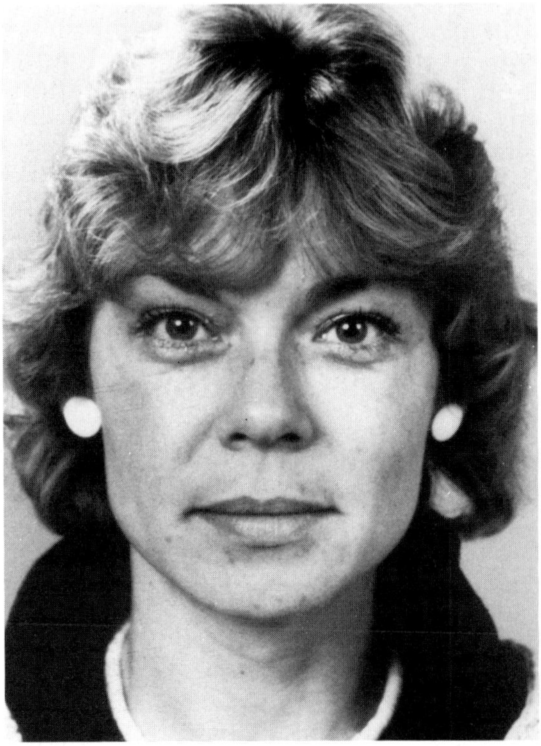

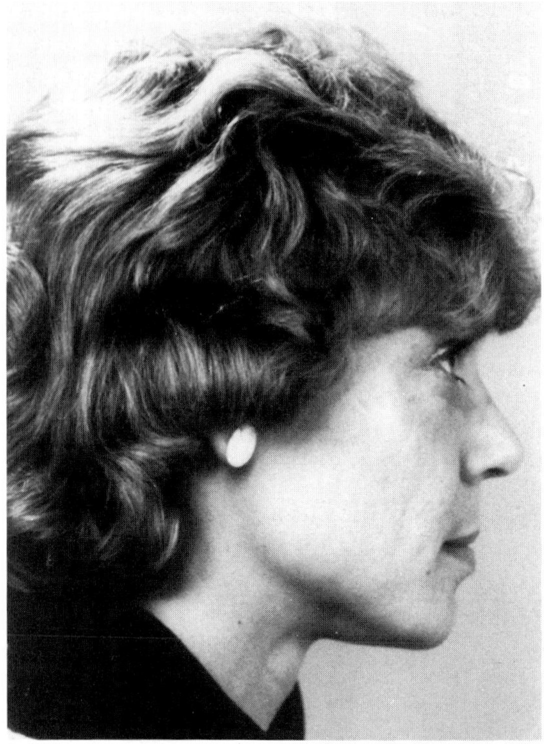

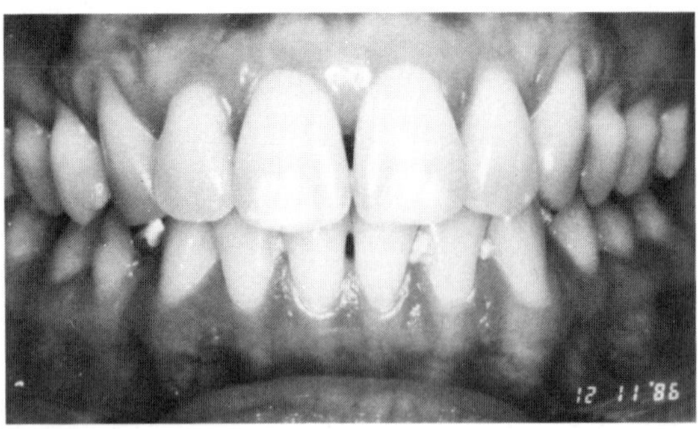
12 11 '86

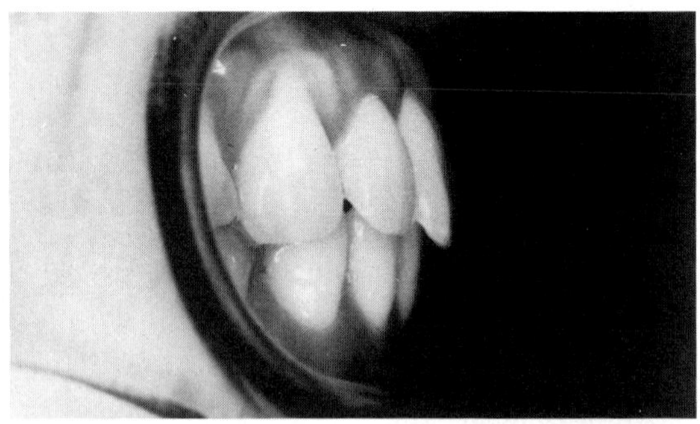

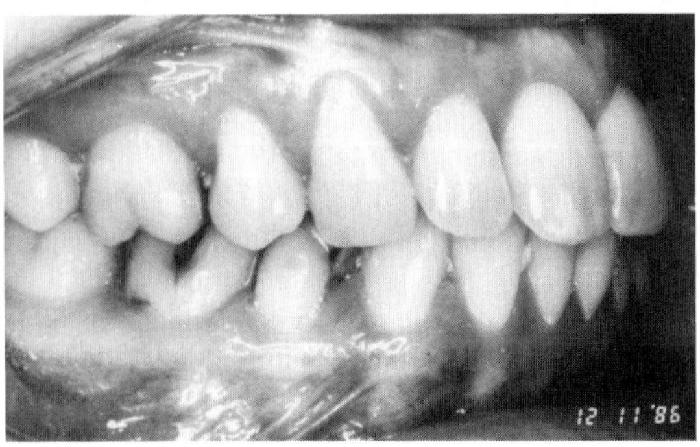
12 11 '86

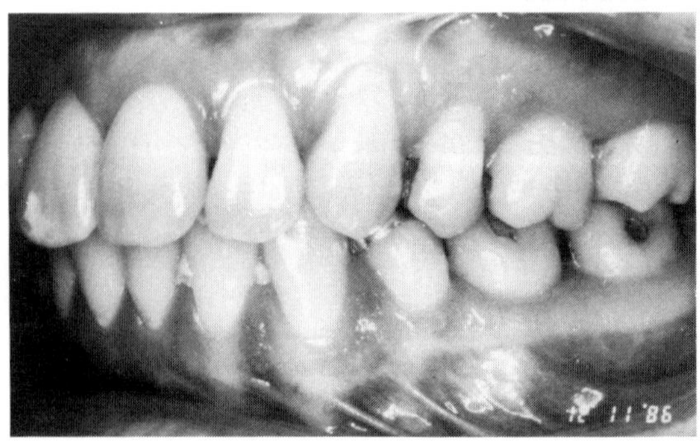
12 11 '86

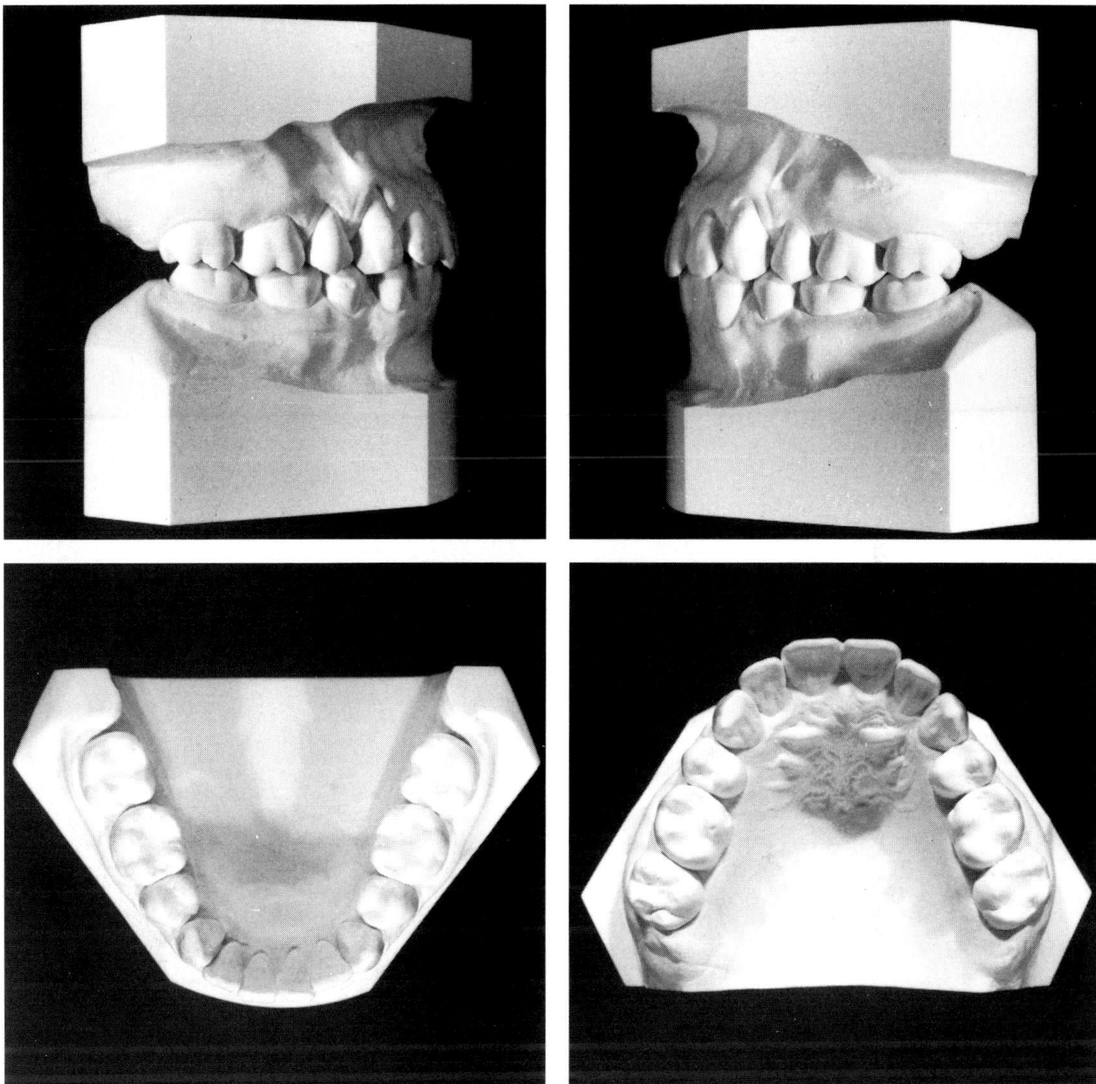

Figs 5-11 and 5-12 *At the age of 32 y, 6 mo, the teeth and face are harmonious without falling in of the region of the mouth; the nasolabial fold is well filled. The mandibular second premolars have been restored with inlays. The gingiva have receded locally with some exposure of root surfaces. The original deviation of the dental arch midlines and the excessive overjet have corrected themselves with time.*

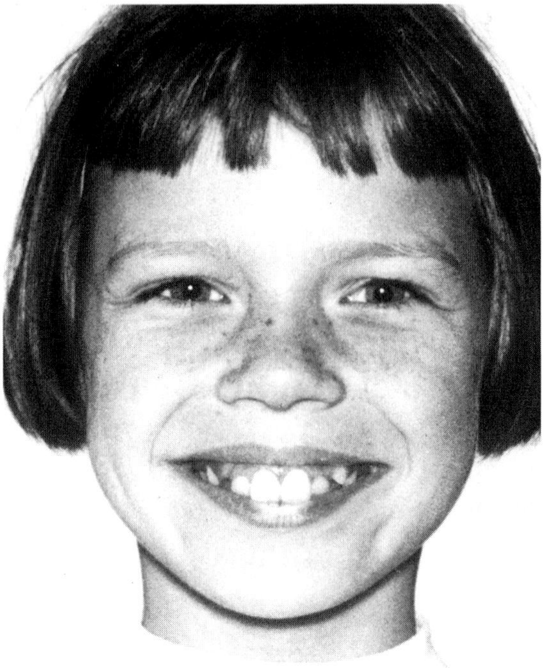

10.0

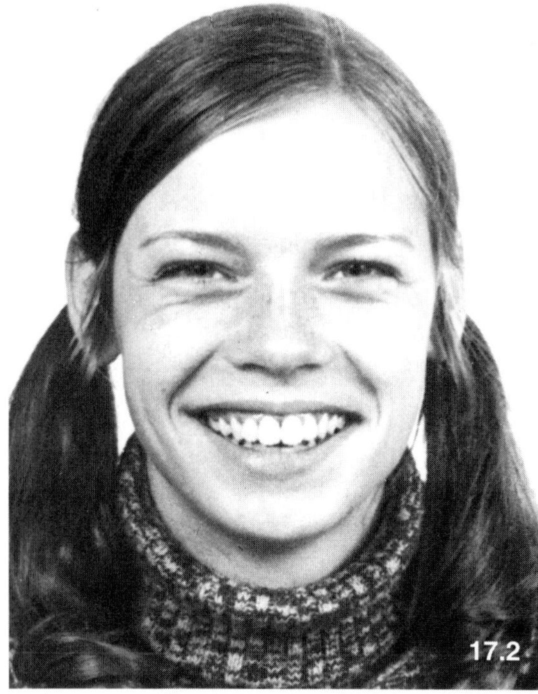

17.2

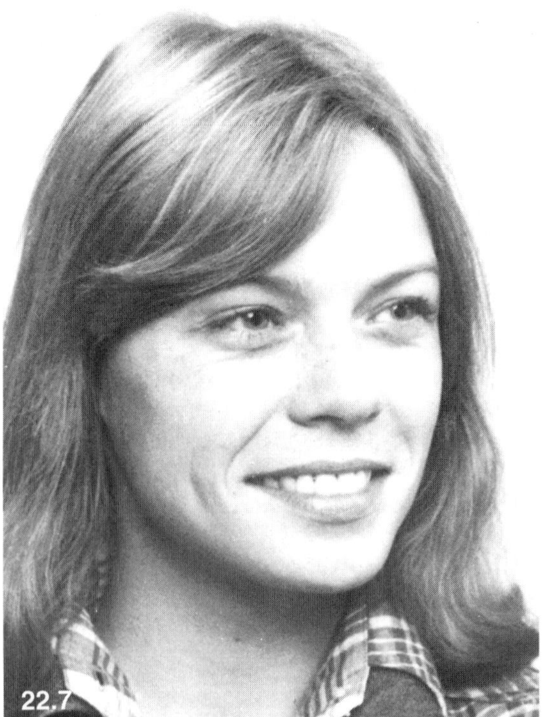

22.7

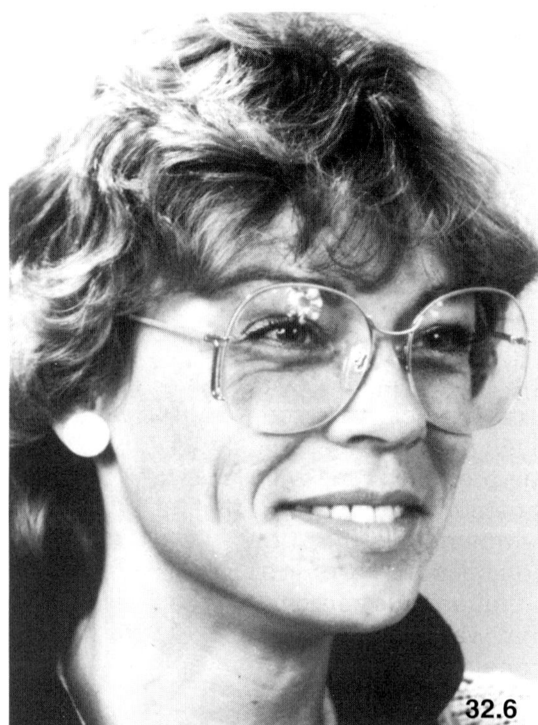

32.6

Fig 5-13 The photographs of her smiling face show a marked improvement. The high gum line is no longer evident.

The result in adulthood is satisfactory in every way (Figs 5.9 to 5.12). The initially clearly visible gums have become less apparent naturally, as a result of the lengthening of the upper lip and changes in the activity of the facial musculature (Fig 5.13). The quality of the mandibular second premolars did indeed prove to be inadequate. That applied also to the maxillary third molars, which were removed as were those in the mandible.

The case described here demonstrated unusually favorable progress. Where there is incisor crowding, a less-than-perfect result must be expected if extractions of four first premolars are performed without using appliances. With this patient, the crowding was confined to the canine-premolar regions and the maxillary and mandibular incisors were essentially in good alignment. That often is not the case and some of the extraction space must be utilized to improve the incisor alignment. It seldom occurs that it is possible by extraction of teeth in the center of the region of crowding to secure a local and direct solution to the problem.
Also when intervention takes place earlier, and deciduous canines are removed with the intention of improving the alignment of incisors, the results may leave much to be desired. It applies as much to the "serial extraction" procedure. This procedure has been developed to treat cases of marked crowding, preferably without the use of appliances. For that purpose, at particular moments in the phases of the development of the dentition the deciduous canine, first deciduous molar, and the first premolar, usually in that order, are extracted in each quadrant. Removal of the deciduous canine leads to a better alignment of the incisors and the removal of the first premolar provides adequate room for the tooth that emerges last. In the maxilla that normally is the canine, in the mandible, the second premolar. Removal of the first deciduous molar is desired to accelerate the emergence of the first premolar so that it can be removed sooner.
Favorable development such as that illustrated here can also be achieved when the crowding is located in the lateral incisor-canine region, by removing the first premolar subsequent to extracting the deciduous first molar at the same visit. If the former is located in its normal position close below the deciduous molar crown, it is easy to remove with an elevator immediately after extracting the deciduous tooth. If the dental sac does not come away with the crown, it should be removed carefully with surgical tweezers. Subsequently the canine will move into the space that has been made available in the jaw by the extraction of the premolar. If the extraction of the premolar is delayed until it has emerged, then the narrower root of the premolar is located in the place where the crown had been. The space made available by removing those narrower roots is not as great as the space that comes available by enucleation. Furthermore, the canine has erupted more in the meantime. Following simultaneous removal of the first deciduous molar and the first premolar, a canine that was located labially to the root of the lateral incisor can move to distal within the bone; the overlapping diminishes and the canine can emerge in contact with the second premolar.

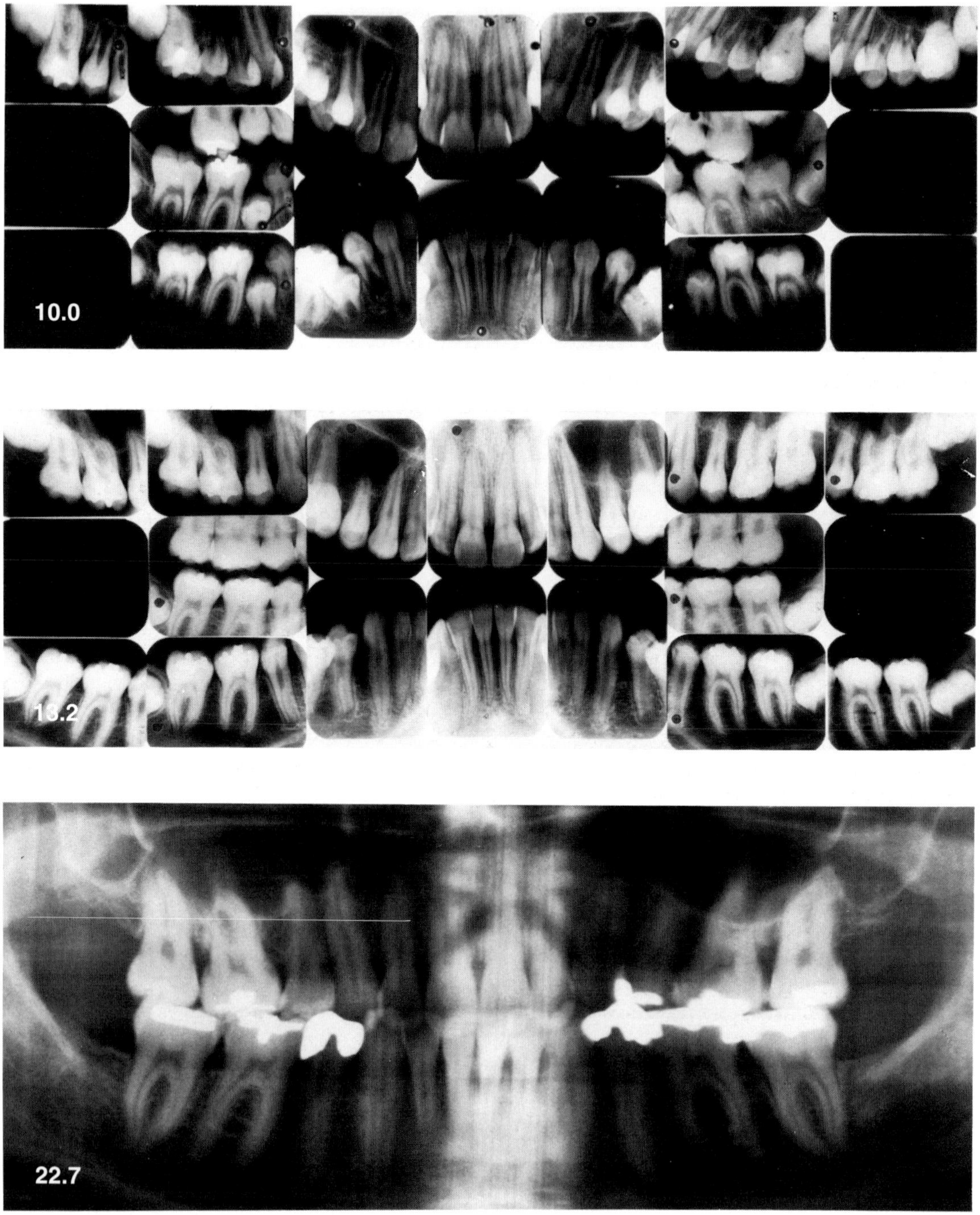

Fig 5-14 Radiographs at different ages (10 y, 0 mo, 13 years, 2 months, 22 y, 7 mo) show that the teeth have distributed themselves fairly regularly into the available space in the alveolar process. The teeth on both sides of the extraction sites show optimal angulations.

In general it can be said that extraction of first premolars in the maxilla will achieve a better result than such extractions in the mandible. This difference is largely attributed to the position in which the maxillary canine is laid down. With a small middle section of the apical area, which usually is associated in the maxilla with a dorsally positioned anterior section of the apical area, the canine is found to be markedly mesially angulated above the first premolar. In addition, the fact that the canine is the last tooth to emerge in this area of the maxilla is important. In the mandible, the premolars and permanent canine are laid down a greater distance apart than in the maxilla where the middle section of the apical area is smaller. Above all, it is usually the second premolar that is the last tooth to erupt in the second transitional period in the mandible.

If extraction therapy without the use of appliances is to be successful, the space remaining after extraction must become available for the use of the teeth for which it was intended. This calls for stringent monitoring (every two or three months) of the space with dental casts made before the extractions. It is by no means an imaginary danger that the space such as that in cases like this, can be lost by drifting from distal to such a degree that, for example, the canine no longer can fit in. The earlier the extractions are done, the more chance there is of this happening. If in the course of monitoring this appears to occur, then it will be essential to hold the space open, for example with a plate that certainly must not itself impede the eruption of the tooth in question.

Of course, other undesirable phenomena such as slow or negligible eruption, or eruption in the wrong direction or position, can be determined by such monitoring.

Because of the marked crowding there was little chance in this case that following extraction there would be so much excess space that the incisors would be able to tip lingually and no falling in of the contours of the mouth occurred. The form of her profile is also not dominated by strong growth of nose or chin, as is often seen. Particularly in a male patient, the growth of the nose and chin can be much more pronounced, with the final result much less attractive. Girls also can exhibit considerable growth, with corresponding effects overall. Such variations are difficult to forecast, and that provides another problem in establishing indications for treatment. Sometimes the profiles of the parents can suggest the outcome; however, 100% certainty is never present. The younger the child is, the more difficult it is to judge the course the growth of the profile will follow.

Following treatment in this case, the four third molars were extracted. So eight teeth had eventually been removed. In view of the relatively numerous restorations, future loss of more teeth is not unlikely — then, the extraction of the third molars might be regretted. Because the present state of the dentition is better, the situation might not arise, but the question does remain as to whether or not "automatic" removal of third molars — particularly when other teeth already have been lost — is a a sound procedure.

Chapter 6

Class II/1
Activator, positioner
Female: 9 years, 9 months to 28 years, 10 months

A girl aged 9 years 9 months was seen with a disto-occlusion of a half premolar width and an overjet of 8 mm. There was an arch length discrepancy (ALD) of +3 mm in the maxilla and –2 mm in the mandible. The shortage of space in the mandible was caused by mesial migration of the mandibular first permanent molar on the right after premature loss of the deciduous molars and movement of the incisors to the right (Figs 6.1 and 6.2). She sucked her thumb but was anxious to stop it. Although she had a clear nasal airway, she habitually held her mouth open with her lower lip between the maxillary and mandibular incisors. Most of the deciduous teeth had large cavities and some periapical abscesses were present.
It was decided to treat the anomaly with an activator and subsequently to use full fixed appliances if required. First the deciduous teeth that could not be conserved were extracted (55, 63, 64, 65, and 75). Activator therapy was initiated at the age of 10 years, 1 month. As usual, the appliance was worn only while asleep, but in the beginning to become accustomed to it she wore it additionally for one hour before going to bed. The thumb-sucking ceased simultaneously. After six months, a good sagittal relationship had been achieved and active treatment was terminated. Because the premolars and canines were not yet fully erupted, a solid interdigitation was not established, with the result that four months later some degree of disto-occlusion had returned. Insufficient room was available for the right mandibular second premolar (Figs 6.3 and 6.4). The patient was advised to return to wearing the activator at night. After three months, there was once again a neutro-occlusion, although now with solid interdigitation of the canines and premolars. To secure the slight tooth movements that were thought to be necessary, a positioner was used. For this purpose, the positioner needs to be worn every night and during the day for four hours; during the latter time it has to be actively bitten into. After a month the desired effect had been attained and for the following five months the positioner had only to be worn for retention.
At the age of 11 years, 7 months well-occluding, good dental arches blended harmoniously with the face (Figs. 6.5 and 6.6). This picture became even better in the following years, as the mandible grew further ventrally than the maxilla (Figs 6.7 to 6.14).

The case shown here illustrates well the part played by interdigitation in the maintenance of the correction of sagittal occlusion. If a solid interdigitation is not

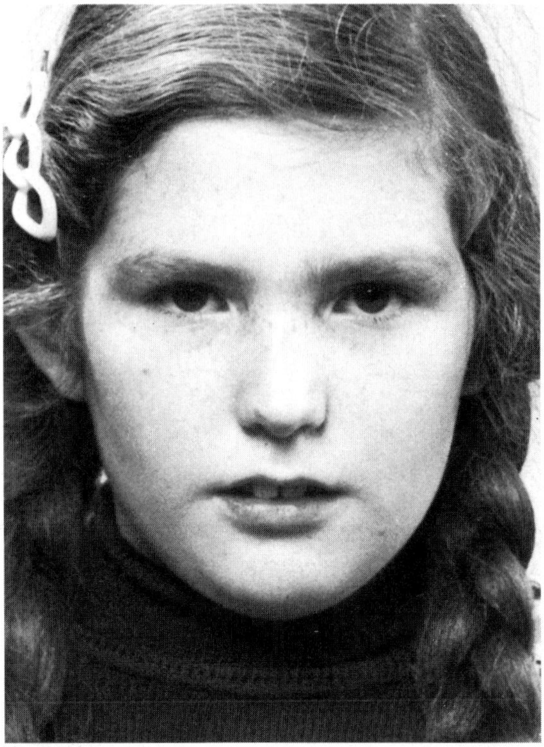

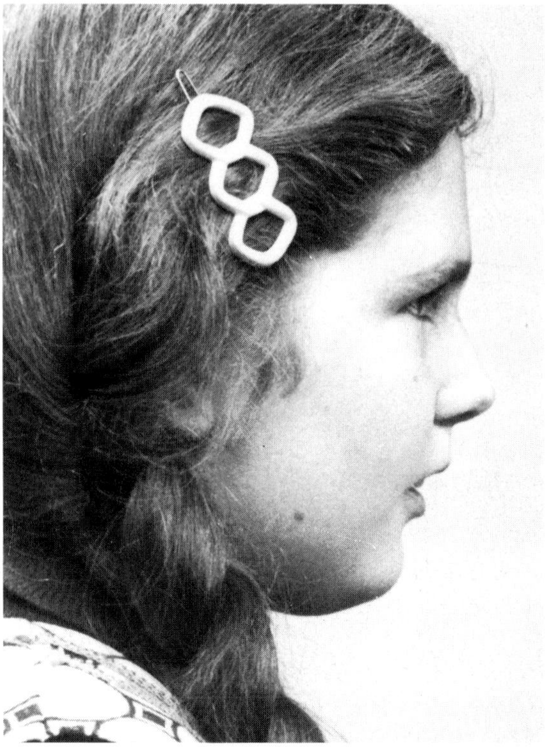

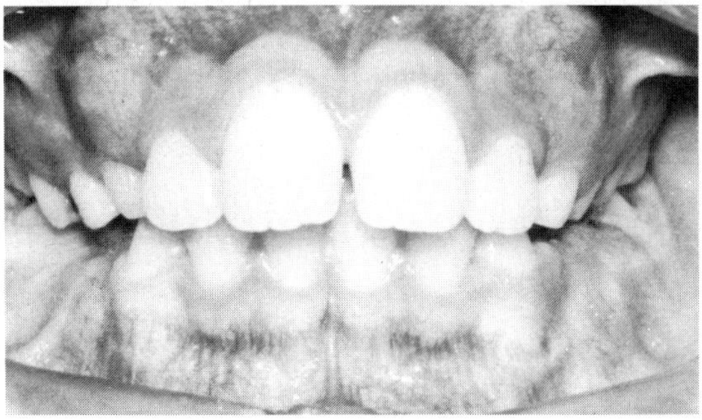

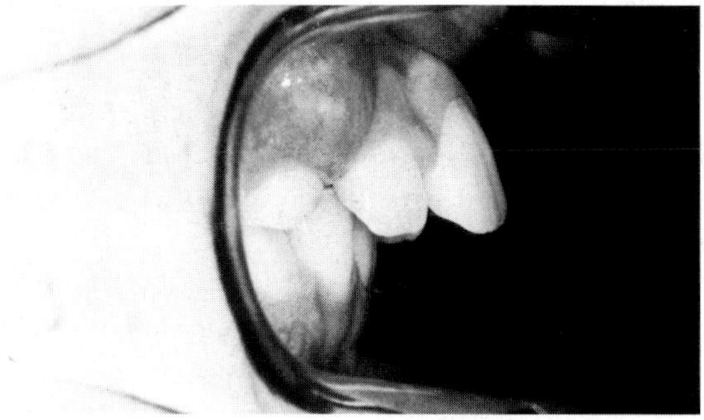

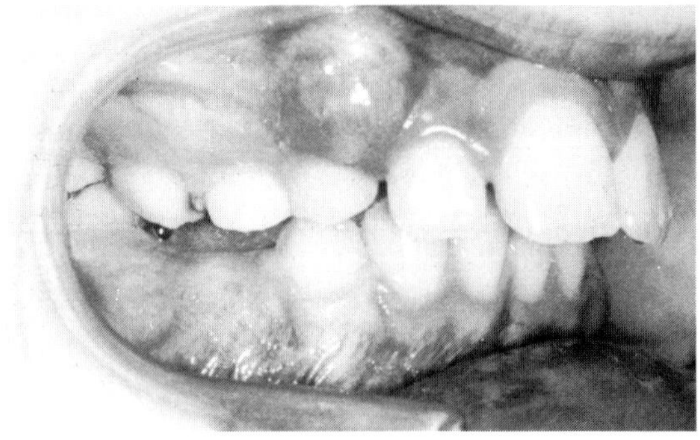

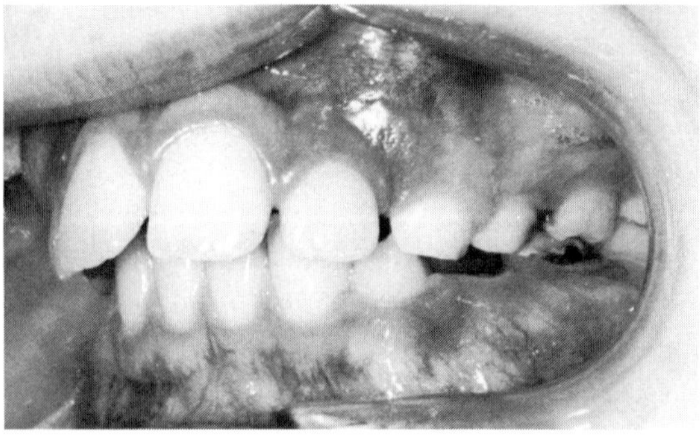

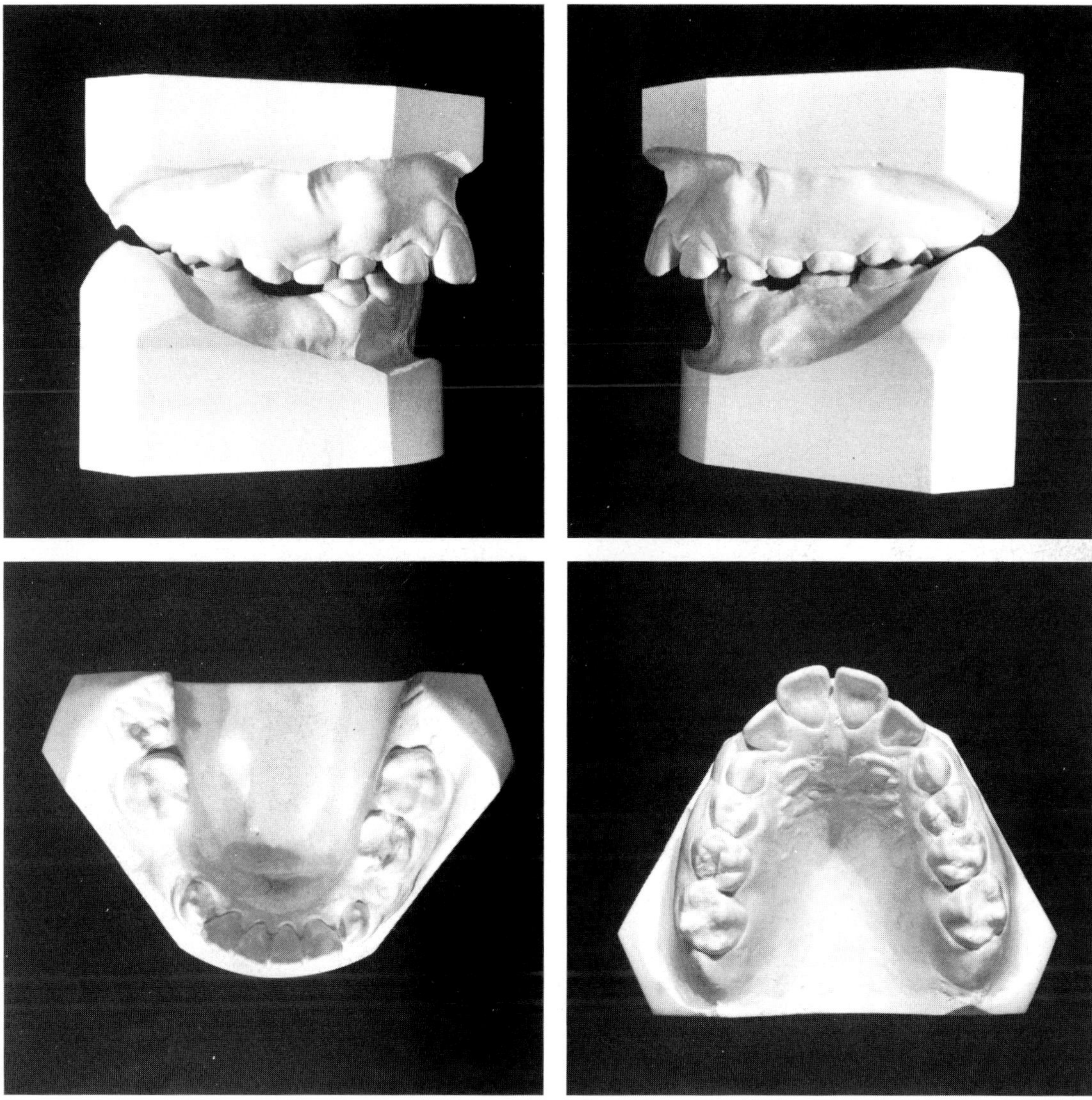

Figs 6-1 and 6-2 A girl of 9 y, 9 mo with a class II/1 anomaly (1/2 PW disto-occlusion), patent nasal airway, open lip relation, thumb-sucking habit, and a lower lip that lies behind the maxillary incisors at rest. Deciduous molars have been lost prematurely due to caries. The right mandibular first permanent molar has drifted mesially until it is blocked by the over-erupted maxillary second deciduous molar. In the mandible, there is an ALD of –2 mm; in the maxilla it is +3 mm. As a result of the premature tooth loss, the mandibular incisors have moved a little to the right. The midlines of both dental arches do not correspond.[1]

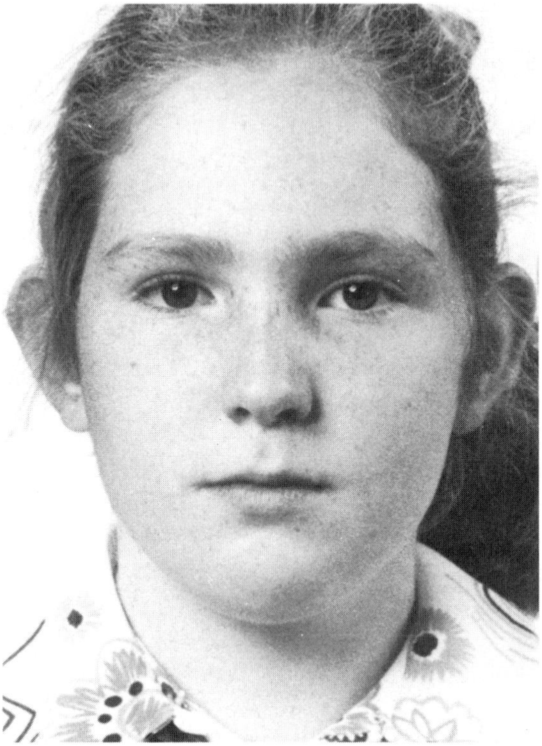

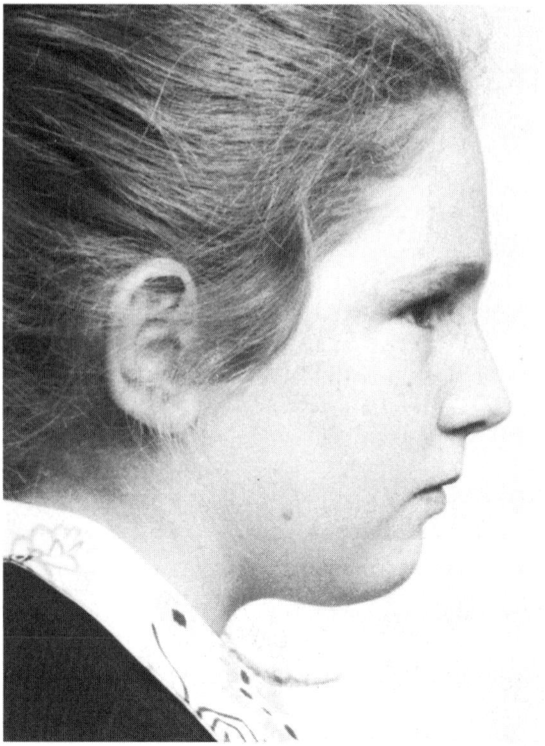

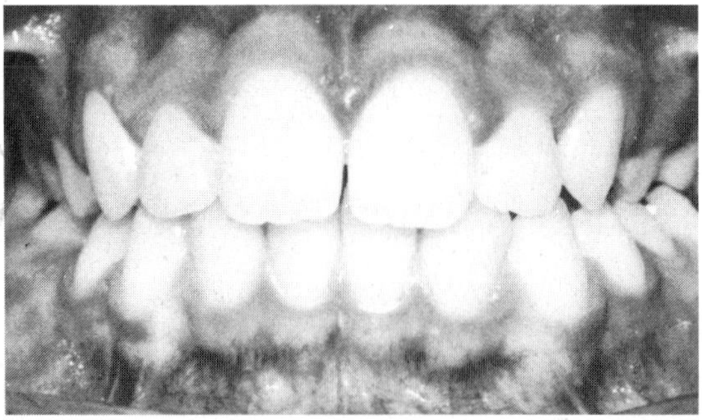

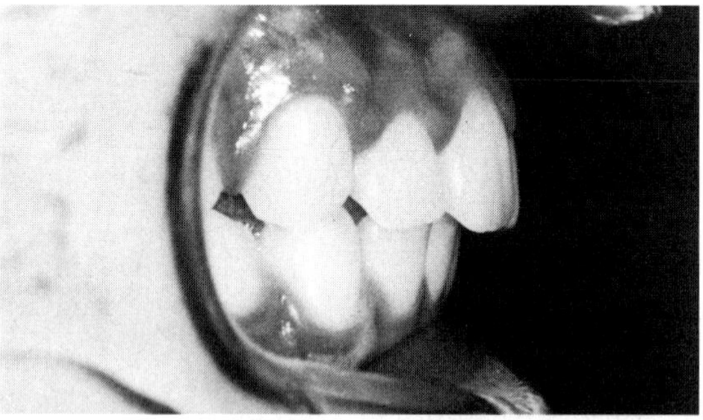

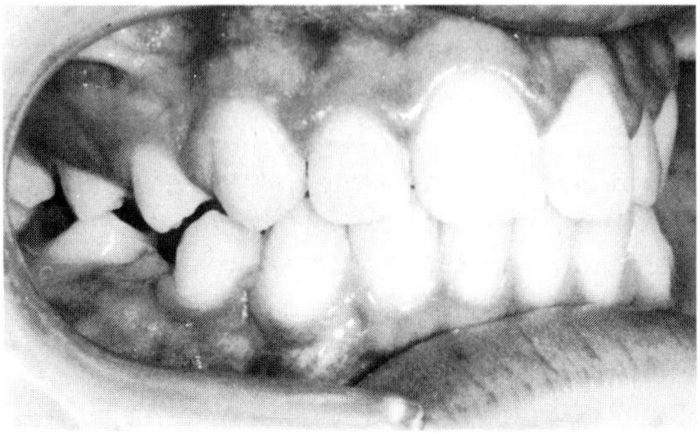

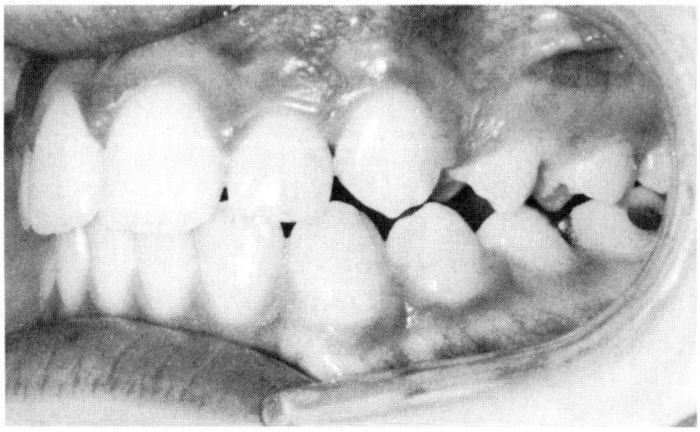

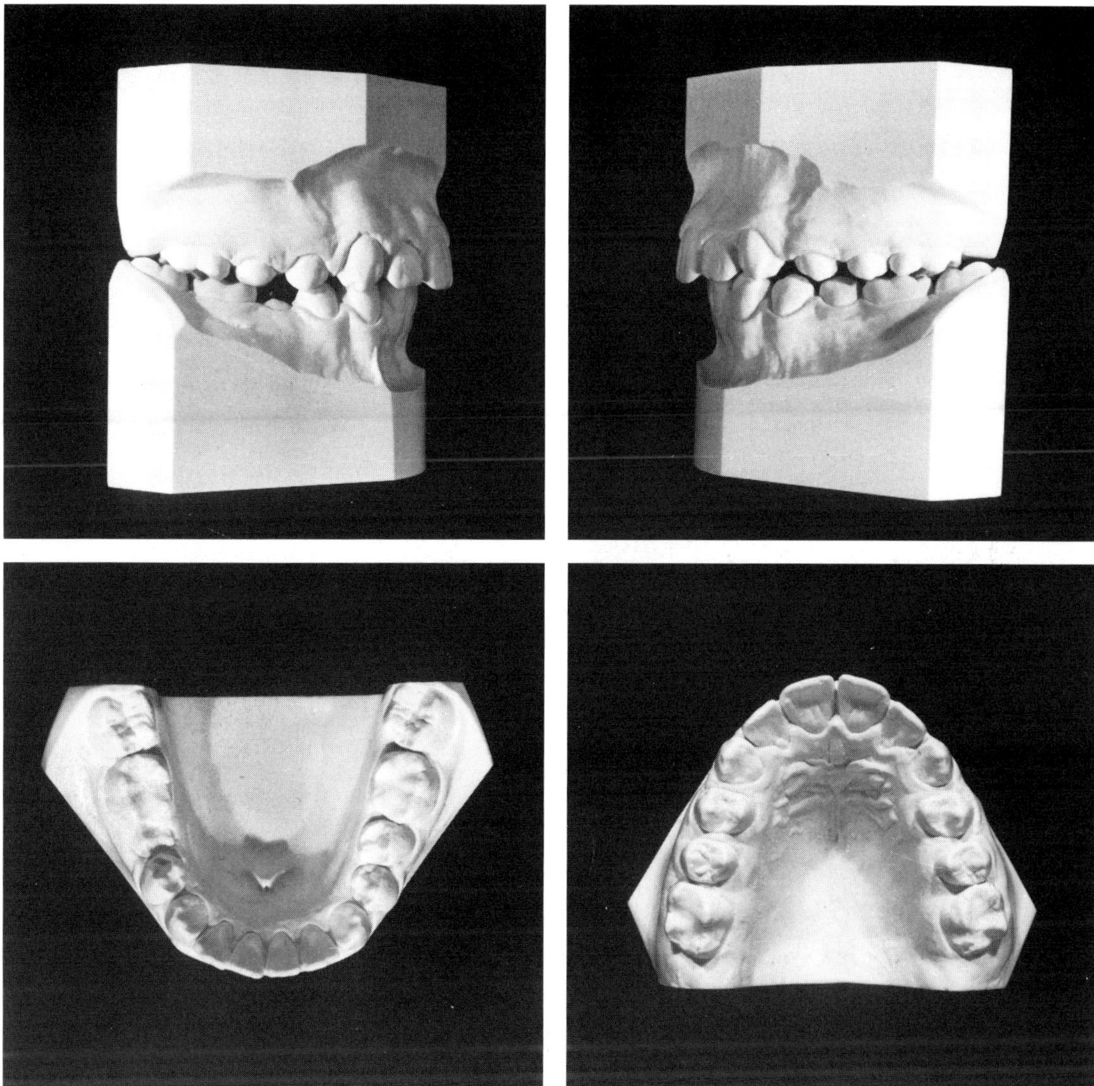

Figs 6-3 and 6-4 *After six months of activator therapy, the lower lip no longer lies behind the maxillary incisors. The mouth can be closed easily. The mandible has come ventrally in relation to the maxilla. The teeth are in neutro-occlusion. However, the premolars and canines have not yet erupted fully. There are still diastemata present in the maxilla. The mandibular right second premolar has insufficient space. The deviation between the midlines has been corrected. From lack of a solid interdigitation, the result is not stable. Four months later, there was once again a mild disto-occlusion so that activator therapy was resumed.*

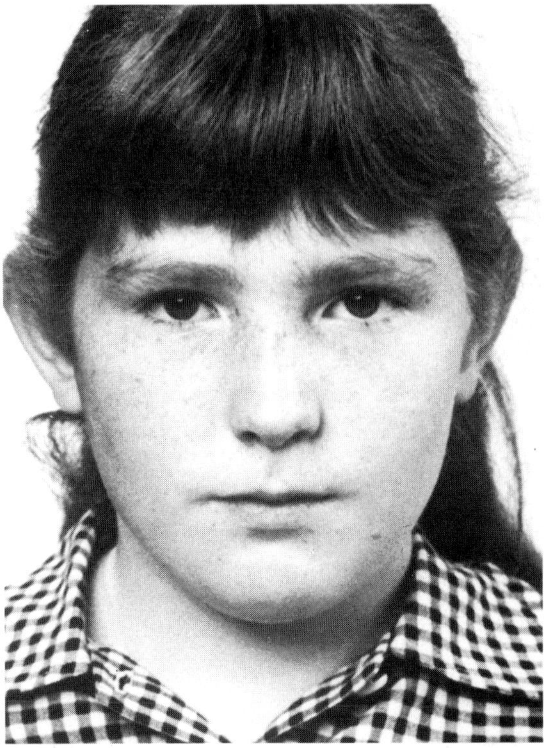

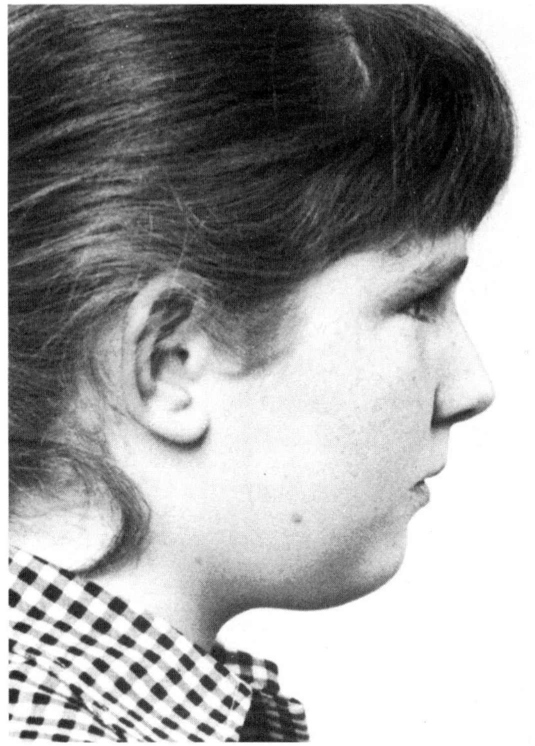

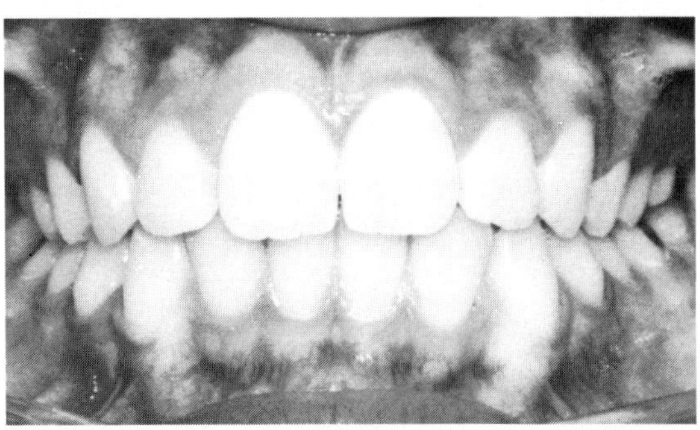

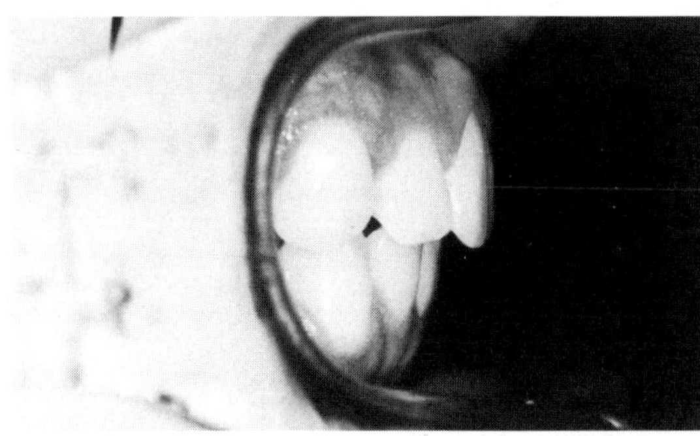

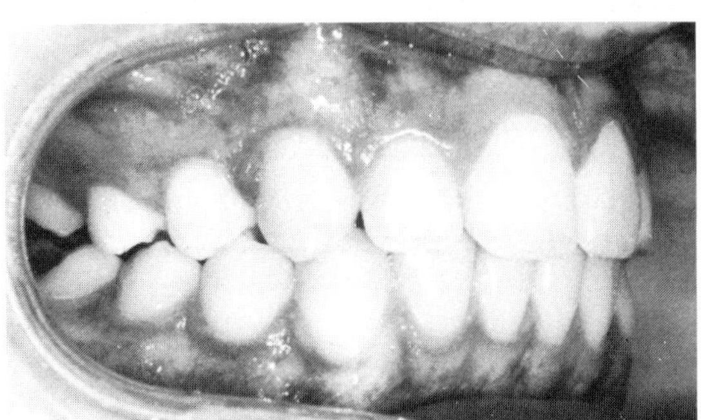

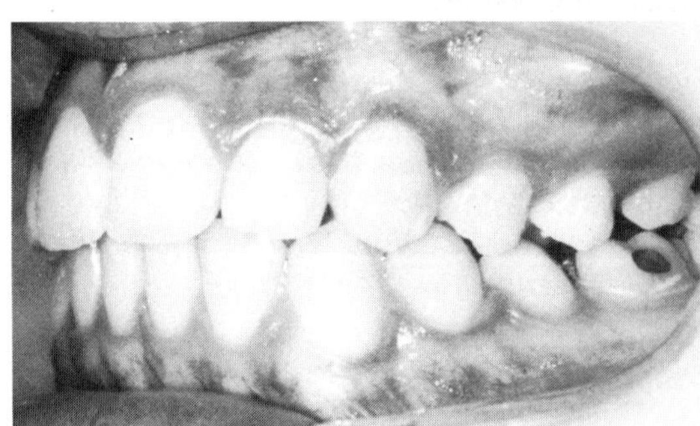

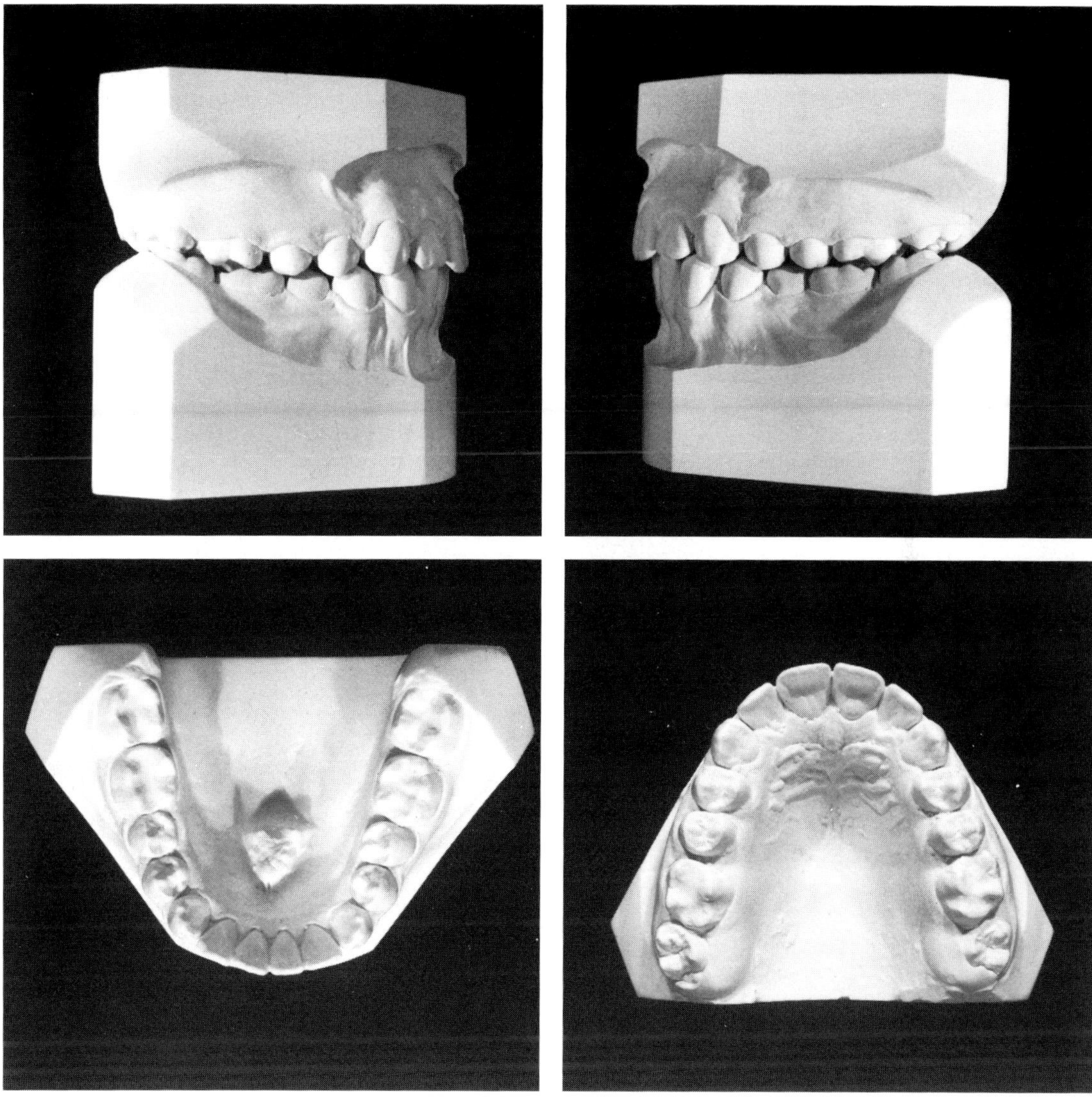

Figs 6-5 and 6-6 *At the age of 11 y, 7 mo, the desired result had been achieved; well-occluding dental arches harmoniously fitting into the face. To achieve this result, a second treatment phase of four months had been undertaken, leading to a solid interdigitation in the canine-premolar region. Note the coincidence of the midlines of both dental arches, and the good position that the mandibular right second premolar has attained in the dental arch without crowding development elsewhere.*

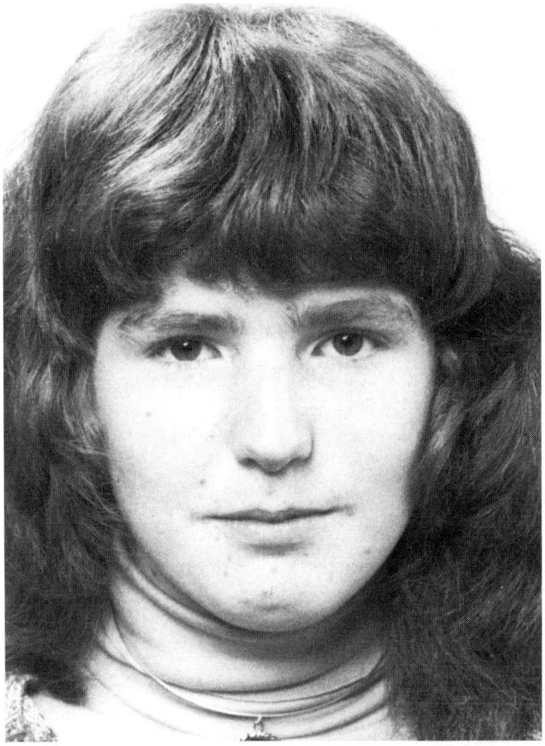

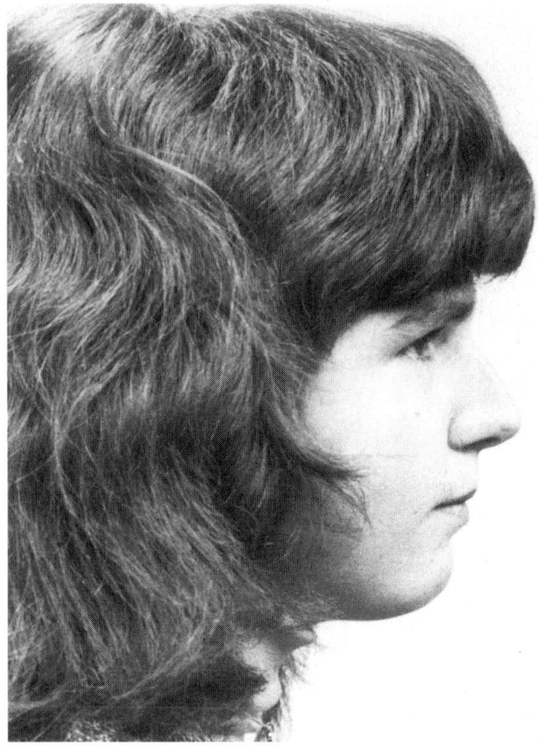

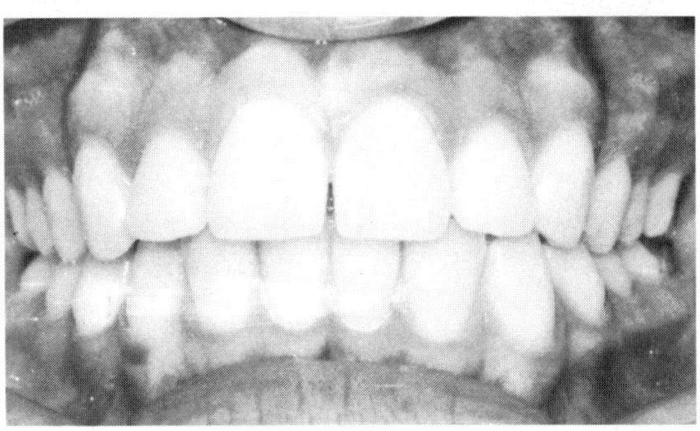

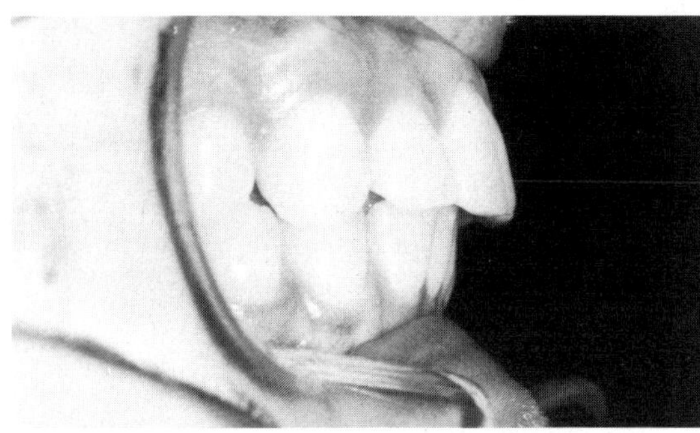

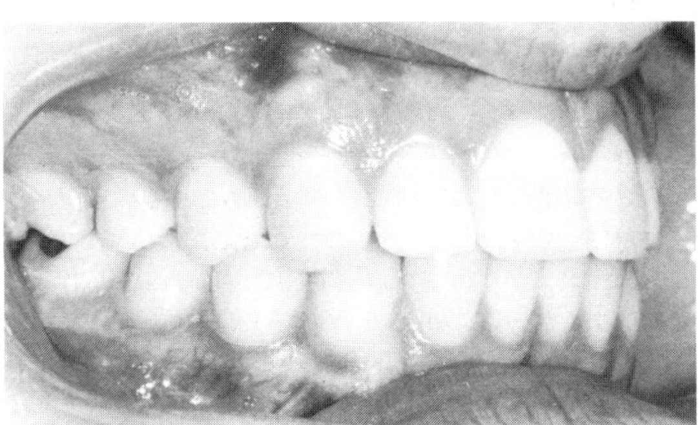

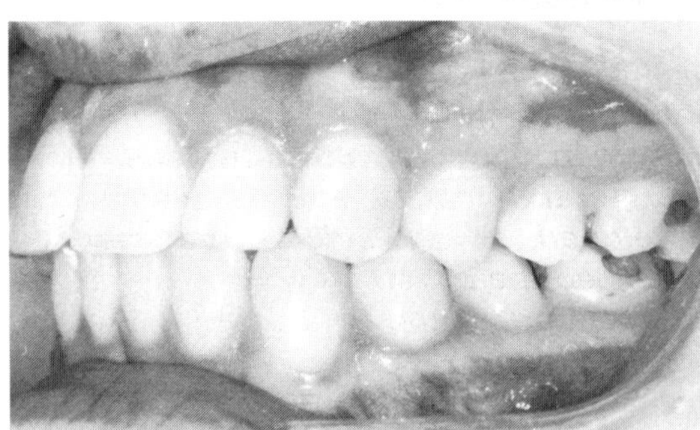

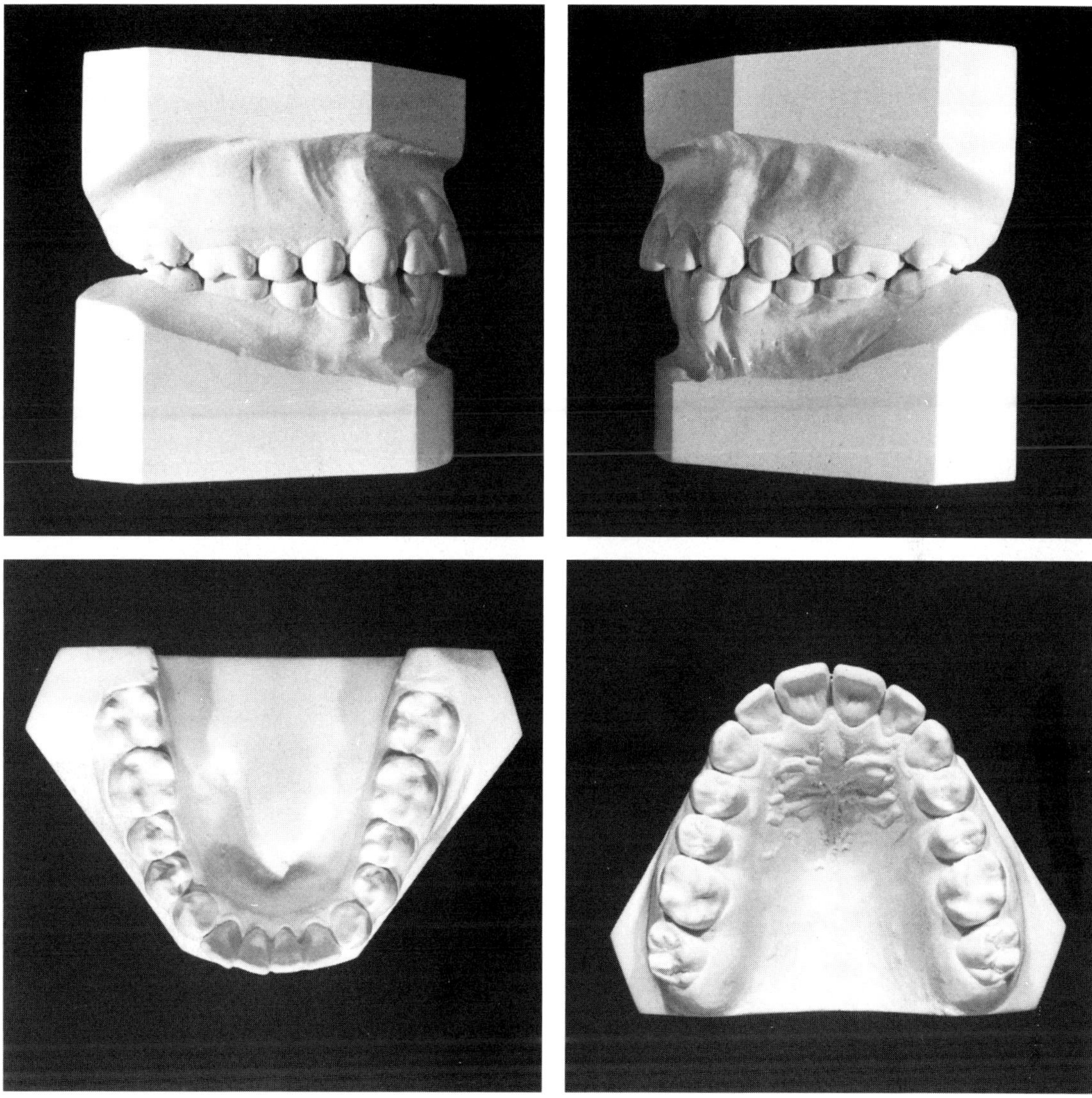

Figs 6-7 and 6-8 At the age of 14 y, 2 mo, the mandibular arch is a little further ventrally than it had been 2½ years previously. This change is associated with the coincident facial growth. Chin and nose have grown further to ventral; that applies also to the mandible as a whole. In the maxilla a mild central diastema has developed, probably due to the maxillary incisors tipping slightly labially, and this disturbed the patient. It was agreed to wait and see if it diminished spontaneously in the coming years. In addition, the mandibular right canine has moved a little lingually.

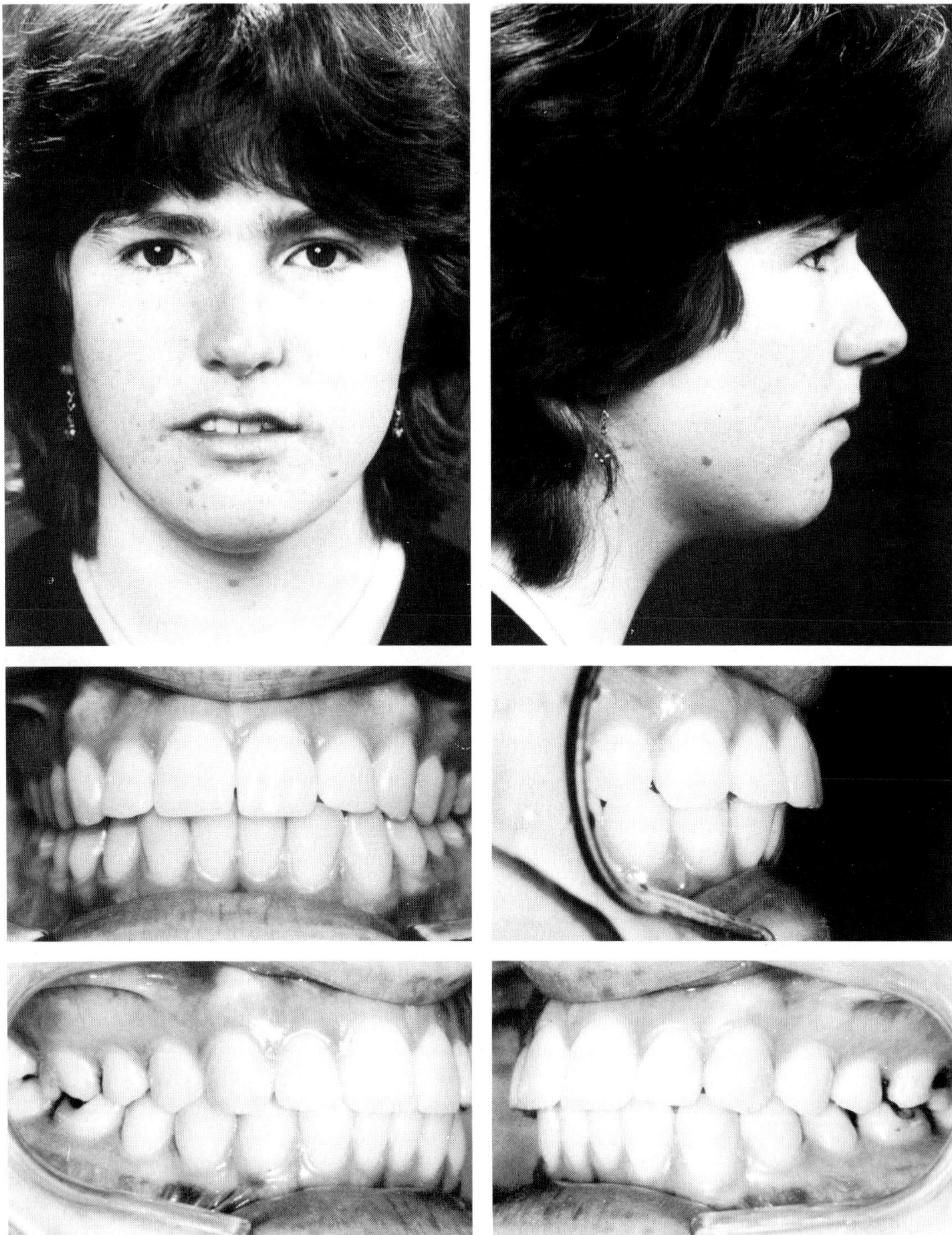

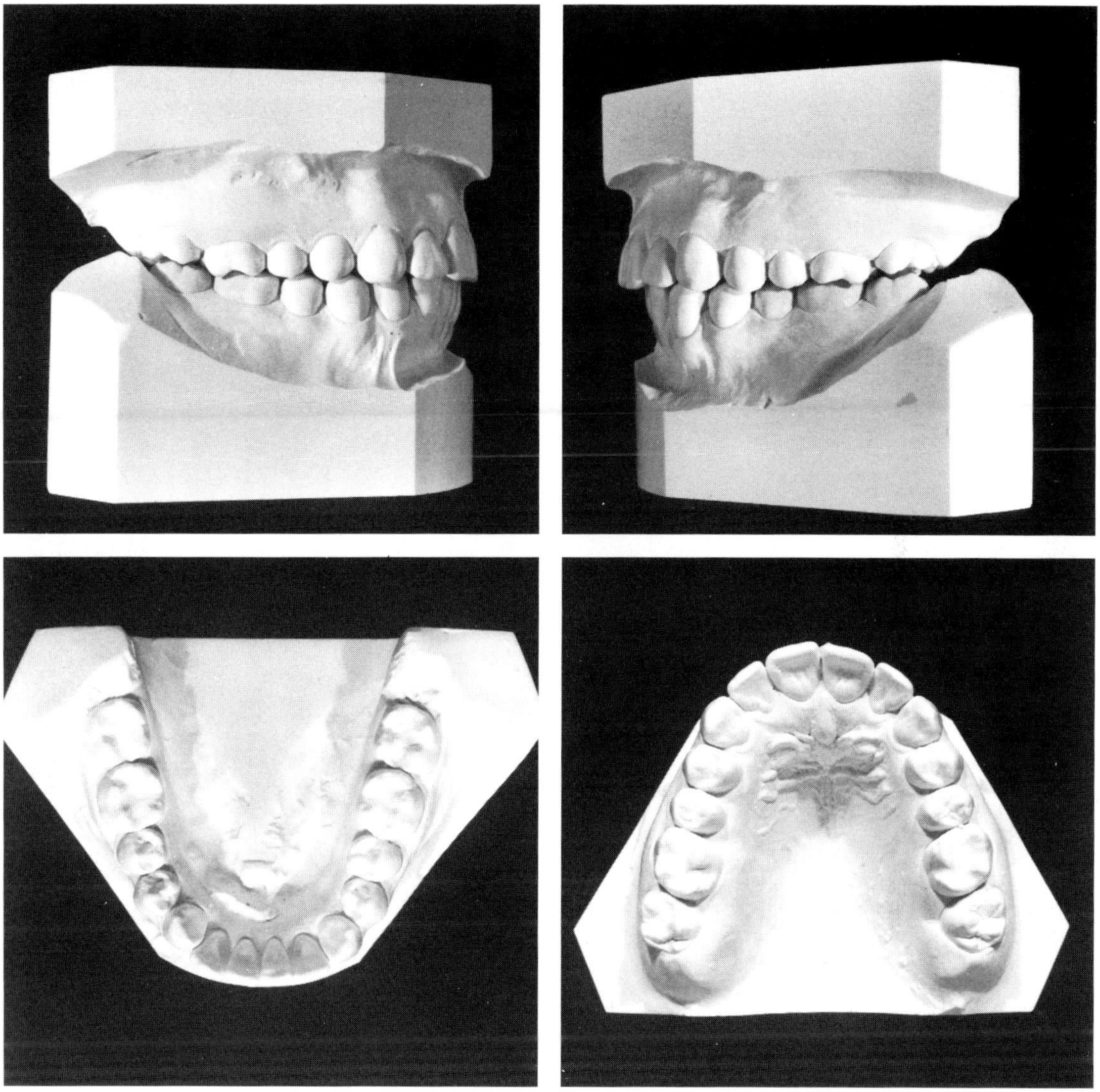

Figs 6-9 and 6-10 *At the age of 17 y, 3 mo facial growth has been complete for some years. The central diastema is gone. Further growth cannot be expected to provide sufficient space for the as yet unerupted maxillary third molars. The shortage of space can most easily be seen on the maxillary dental cast. The indication for this is the distance between the distal surface of the second molar and the dorsal limit of the tuberosity. To assess this problem, it is essential that obtained impressions should always include that area.*[36] *The space available for the mandibular third molars is not to be assessed from plaster models, but from intraoral palpation .*

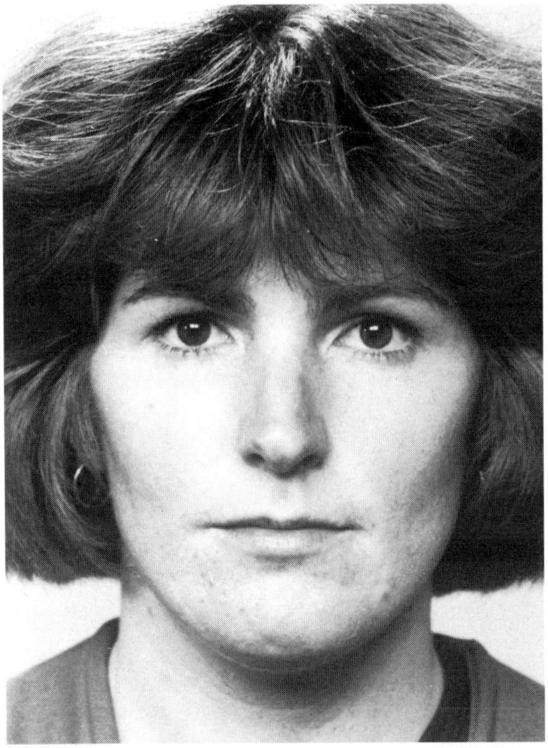

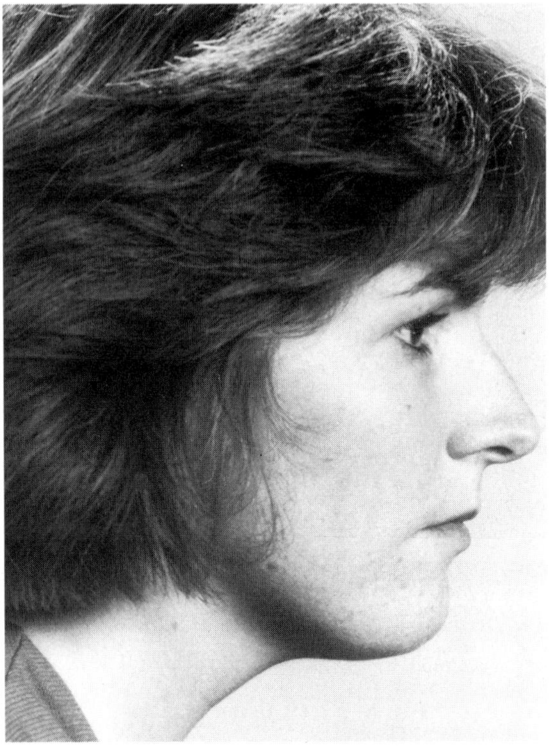

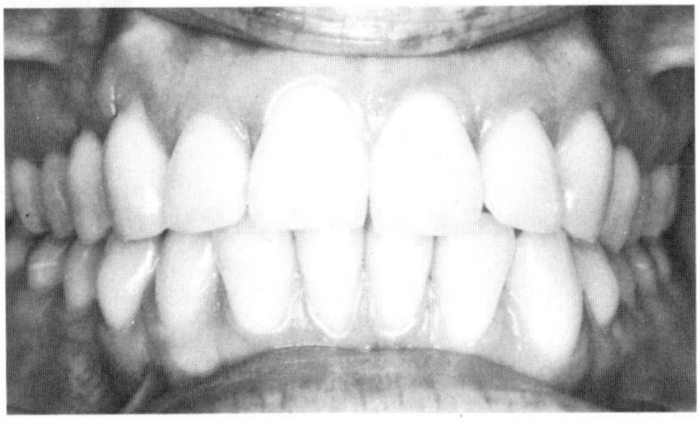

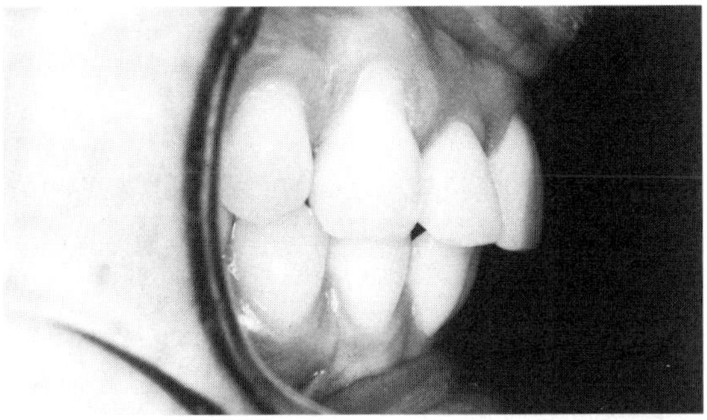

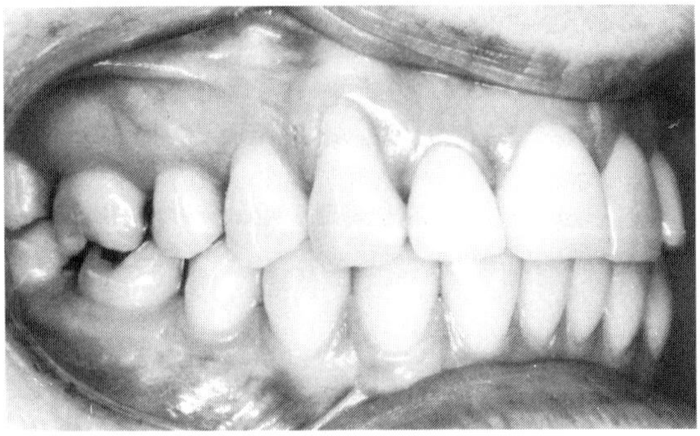

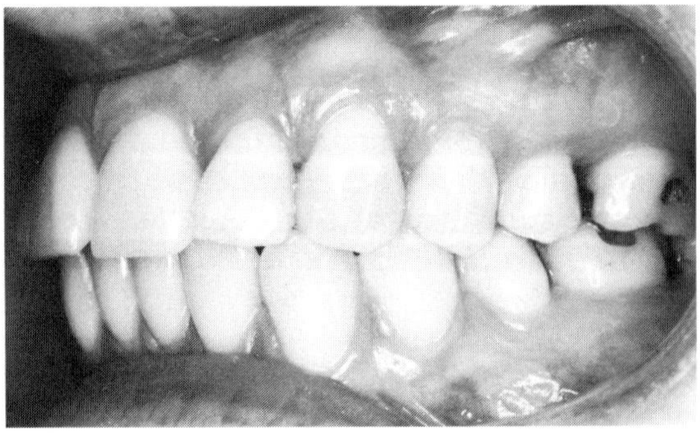

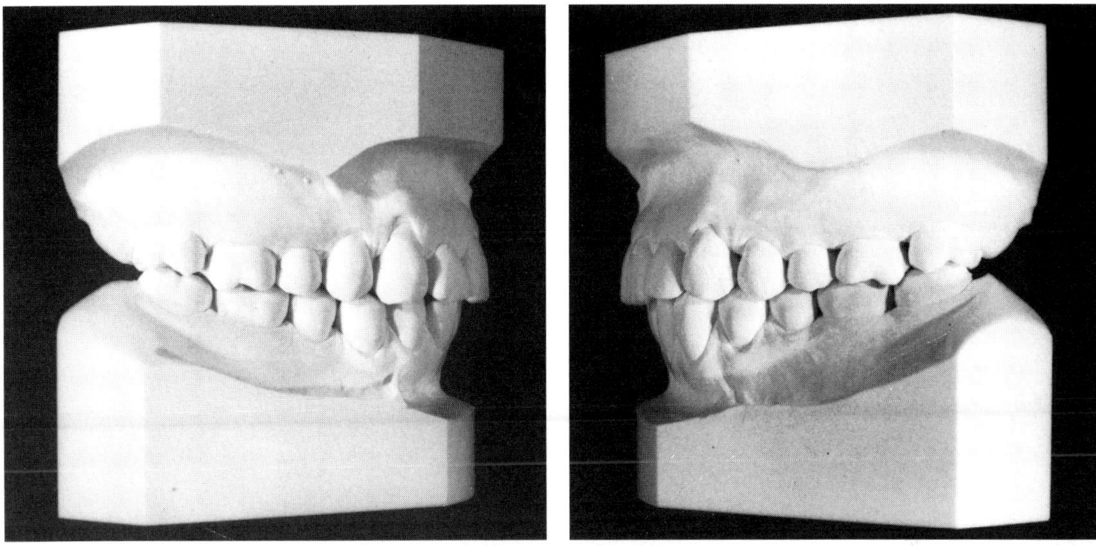

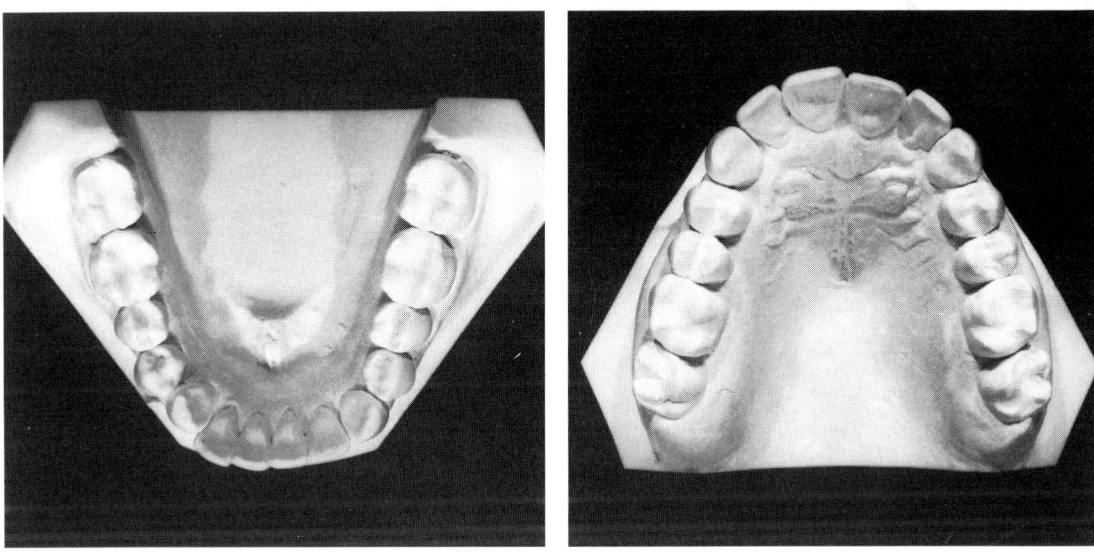

Figs 6-11 and 6-12 At the age of 28 y, 10 mo, in comparison with the records assembled six years previously but not shown here, the clinical crowns have become longer and the gingiva on the maxillary right canine have receded to such a degree that part of the root is exposed. This might be the result of excessive toothbrushing or of a disturbance in articulation; the affected tooth is markedly worn down. The mandibular right canine has rotated lingually on the distal.

Figure 6-13a

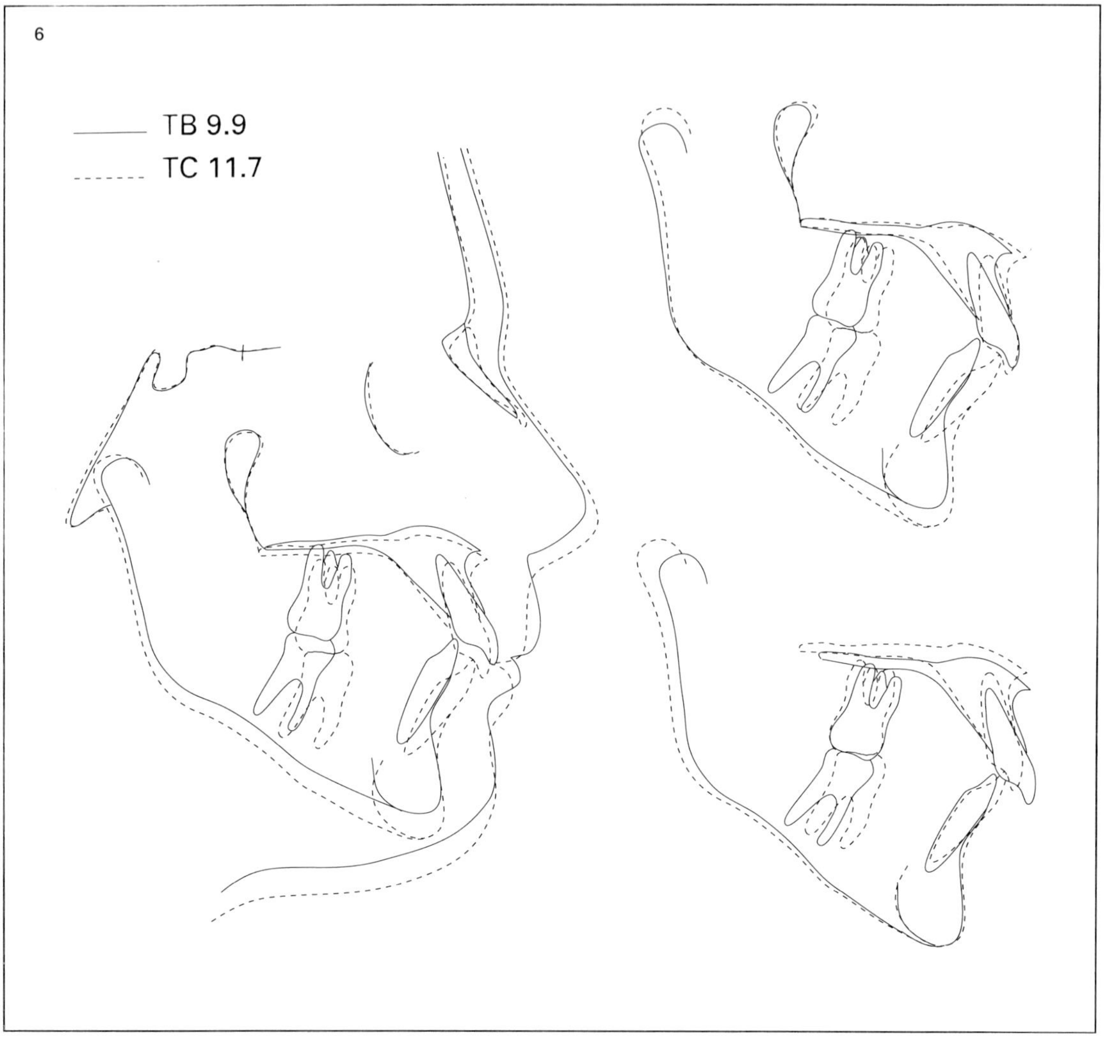

Figs 6-13a and 6-13b Superimposed tracings of cephalometric radiographs taken before treatment (TB = treatment beginning), after completion of treatment (TC = treatment completed), and 10 years thereafter (PT = post treatment). During treatment, the ventral development of the maxilla had been limited, while the mandible had grown significantly in both caudal and ventral directions. The good treatment result is primarily due to the difference in forward development of the jaws. In the years after treatment, the mandible has also come much further ventral than has the maxilla, and the maxillary incisors have tipped a little further labially. Above all there has been much growth at the condyles.

Figure 6-13b

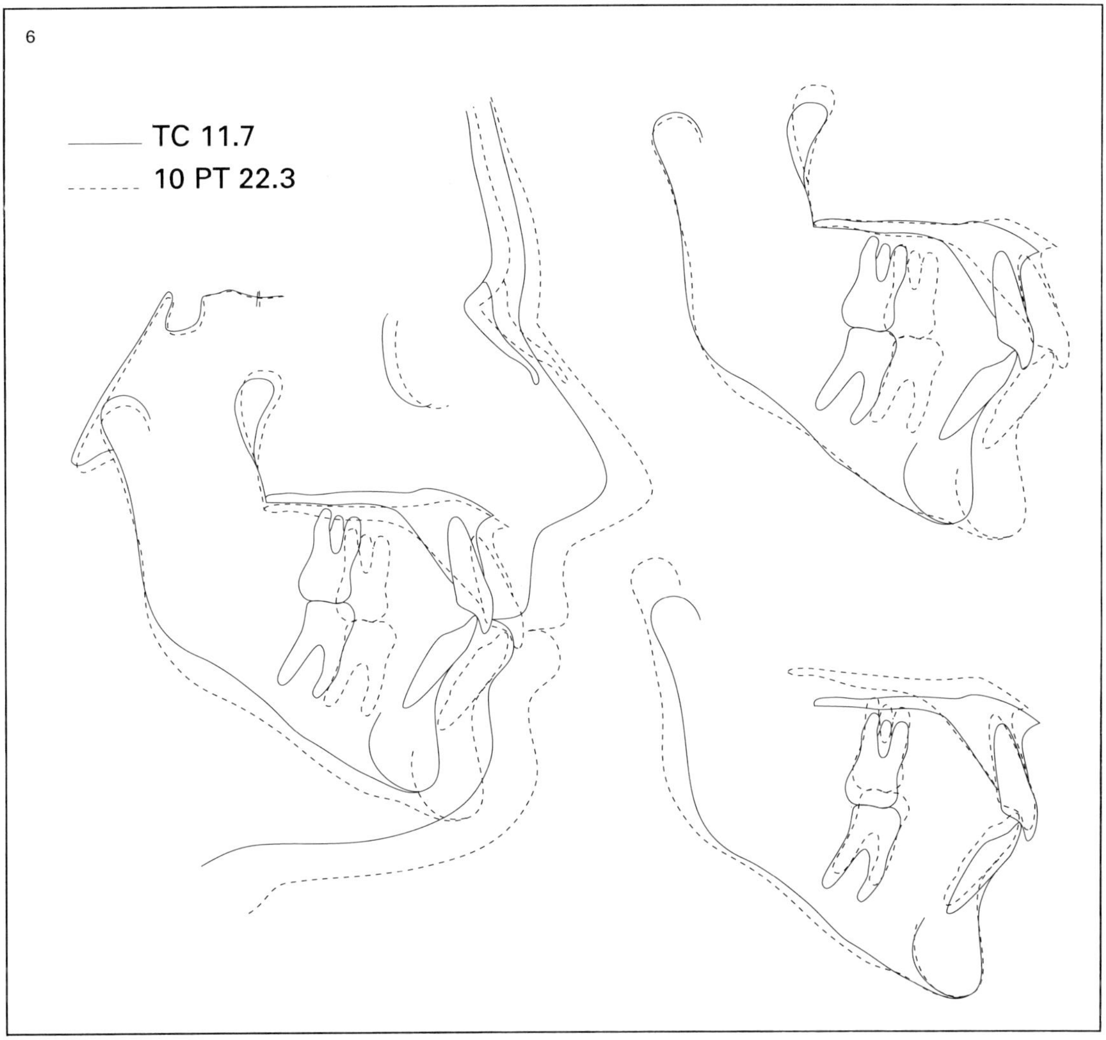

For the total survey, the tracings are superimposed on the part of the base of the skull that runs from the anterior of the sella turcica to the middle of the projections of the left and right greater wings of the sphenoid bone. The drawings that depict the changes in the maxillary complex are superimposed on the posterior of the palatal plane with the lines showing the pterygomaxillary fissure coinciding. The drawings showing mandibular changes have the chin superimposed on the lingual contour of the symphysis with the lower border of the mandibular coincident. Those methods of superimposition are applied to all such tracings in this book.

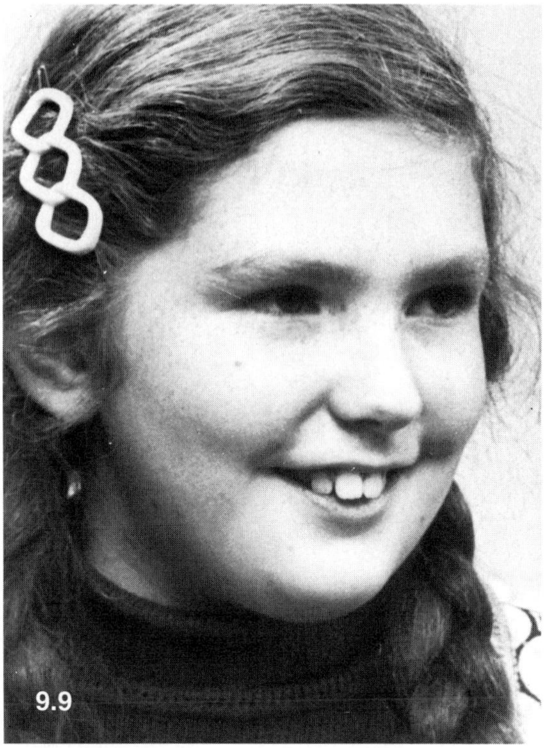

9.9

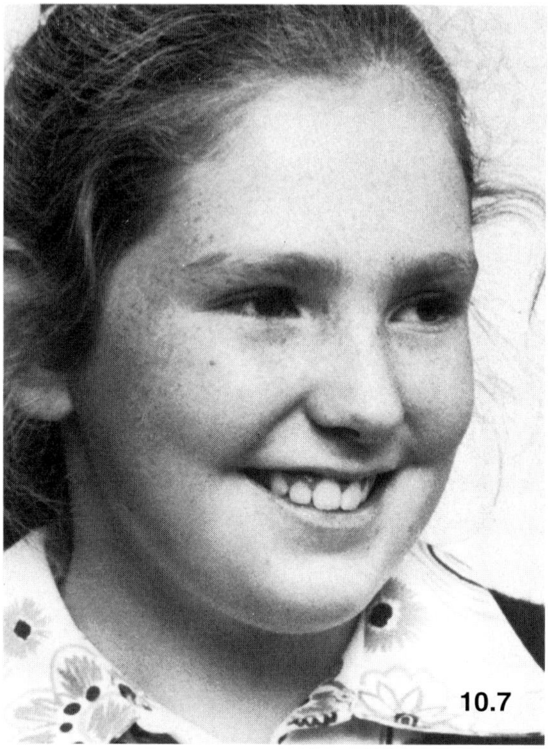

10.7

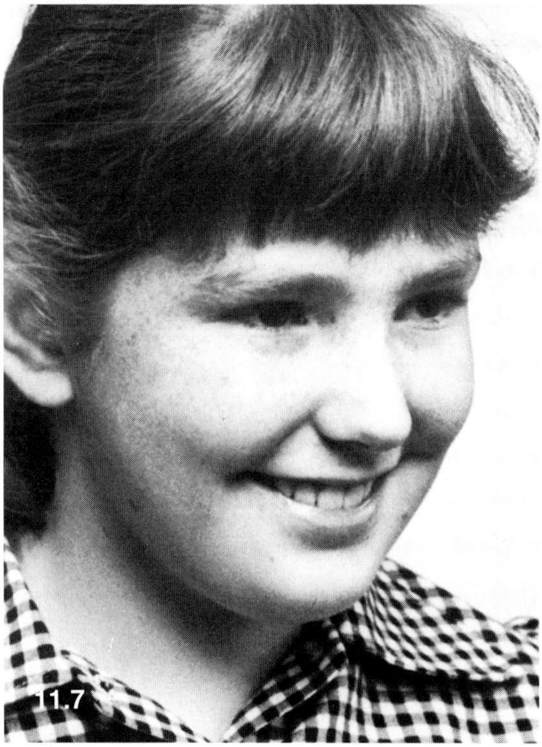

11.7

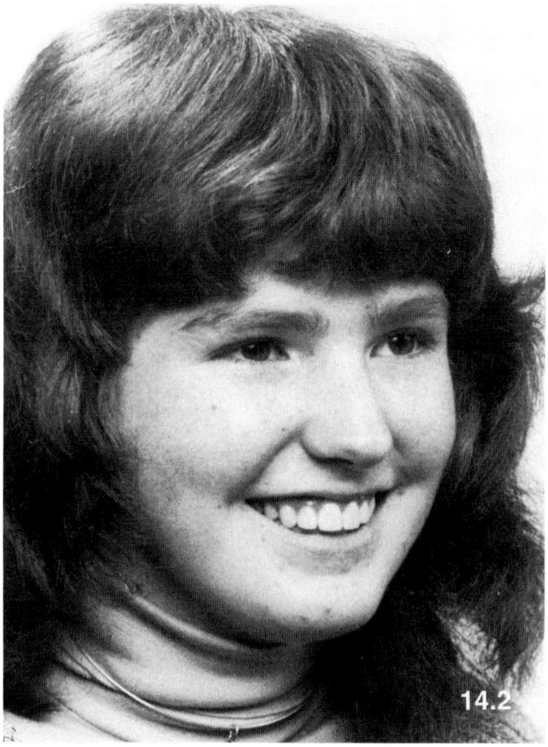

14.2

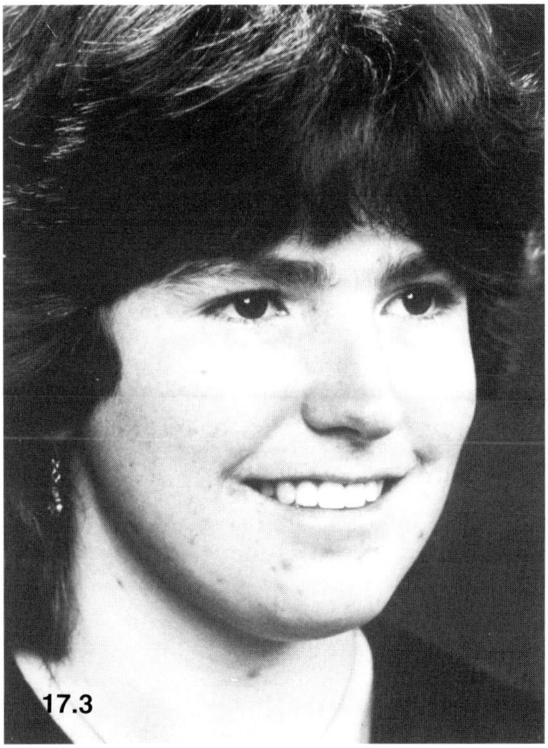

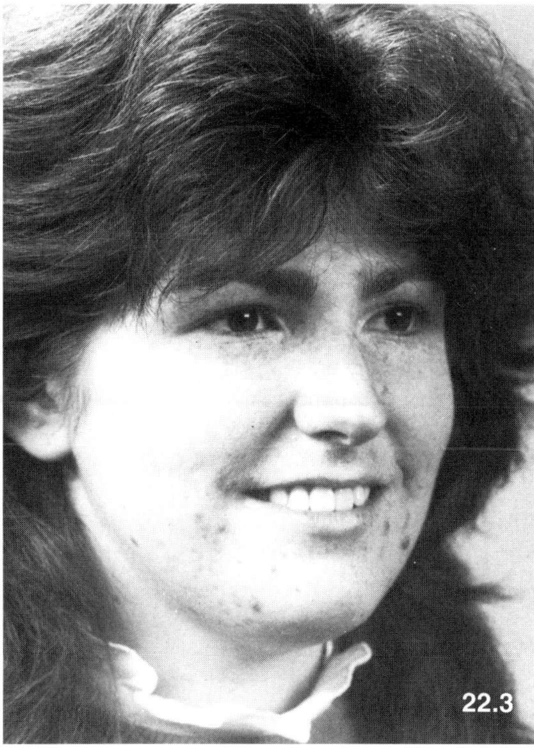

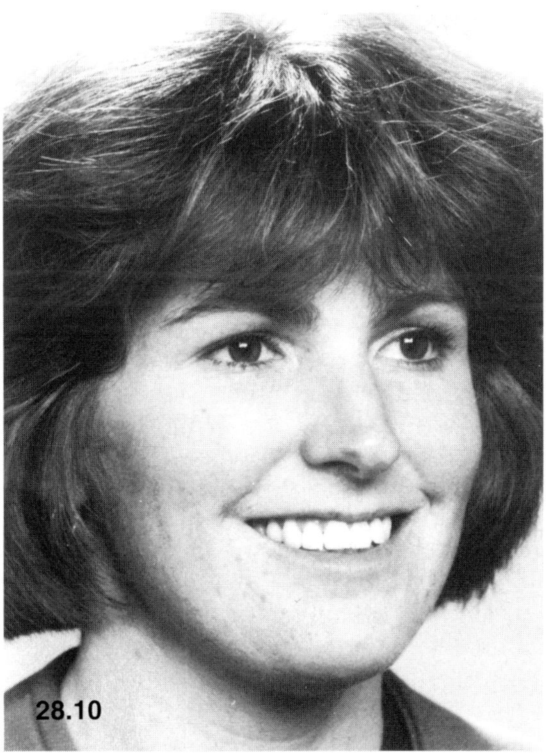

Figs 6-14a and 6-14b *Note the improvement obtained with treatment, and the increase in expressivity gained with age.*

realized following facial-orthopedic therapy through which a disto-relation has been corrected, part of the correction will be lost. Specifically that applies to treatment that is finished while deciduous molars are still present. Deciduous molars will have lost their cusps by then, and their worn occlusal surfaces no longer interdigitate in the way they did initially. Activator therapy might then be continued not to secure further improvement in the jaw relationships, but to prevent relapse. Alternatively, some relapse can be accepted temporarily if it is intended that treatment will be resumed at a later stage in the development of the dentition. The latter approach will often have preference since it is only possible to secure a well-finished result after the premolars and permanent canines are fully erupted and occlude properly.

As a rule it can be maintained that any sagittal change in occlusion, including those changes obtained by means of facial-orthopedic therapy, will only be stable if they are consolidated by solid interdigitation of the premolars and canines. If that is not the case, then a relapse of about half of the improvement obtained can be expected.

Finally, some general remarks might be made about the mode of operation and application of activators. Two frequently used types are shown in Figure 6.15.

The activator, which in principle fits loosely in the mouth and holds the mandible ventrally and caudally in relation to the maxilla, is very suitable for correction of class II/1 anomalies, in which little or no tooth movement is required in the mandibular arch nor in the lateral segments of the maxilla. It is quite possible to use the continuous labial arch to tip back the maxillary incisors, and a deep bite can also be corrected even if usually not completely.

The activator influences the growth of not only the maxillary complex but also, in both sagittal and vertical directions, that of the mandible. Every time that the patient closes his or her teeth together, whether reflexly or not, with the activator in place a force is generated ventro-caudally on the mandible and dorso-cranially on the maxilla. A similar influence is attributed to the activator when it passively (without extra muscle activity) holds the mandible more ventrally and caudally in relation to the maxilla. All this has an effect on the sutures, resulting in a retardation of the forward growth of the maxillary complex. At the same time, the growth at the mandibular condyles is likely to be temporarily accelerated. The mandible consequently comes forward in relation to the maxilla more quickly than otherwise would have been the case.

Alongwith these effects of growth, tooth movements also can be noted. In that way a part of the correction of a disto-occlusion can take place as the result of ventral displacement of the mandibular teeth.[3]

By shaping the activator correctly, it can provide for further eruption of the posterior teeth and the overjet and overbite gradually can improve. Because the activator is not worn continuously, but only for a part of the 24 hours, usually when sleeping, the patient can swallow normally for the rest of the time, with the result that the posterior teeth are stimulated by the rail mechanism to go buccally (see Fig 7.9). The maxillary incisors can be retracted with the labial arch as long as the palatal acrylic is ground away accordingly. On the other hand it might well occur that the mandibular incisors tip labially, wanted or unwanted, if these teeth are not well-capped labially with acrylic.

The activator slows down the growth of the maxillary complex and in the mandible

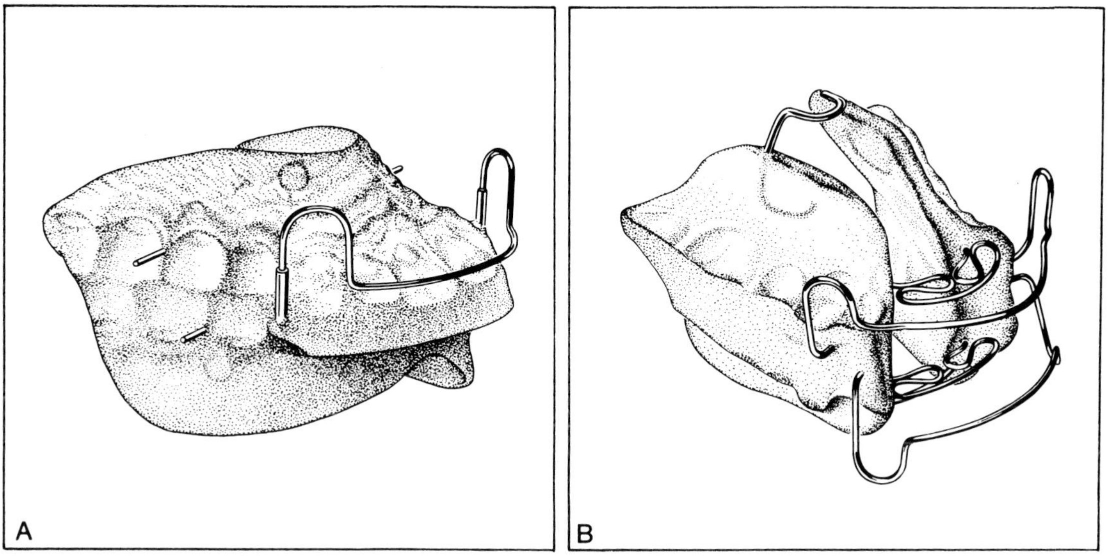

Fig 6-15 *Two frequently used activator types.*
A Activator with buccal parts ground free (model Andresen, Haupl, and Petrik).
B Open activator, which restricts speaking and breathing less than that in A.[36]

works just in the direction of its growth. On this basis, it could be expected that the effect on the mandible would be greater than that on the maxilla. However, this is not always the case as the "adaptability" of the sutures is probably greater than that of the condyles.[31]

Advantages of the activator are that it is a relatively simple appliance, causes the patient little trouble, and all improvements that are needed can be dealt with at the same time and in harmony with each other. The activator lends itself well to the treatment of class II/1 anomalies without crowding in both arches, and it can serve well as a space maintainer if deciduous molars are lost prematurely. The activator is also particularly useful for correction of class II/1 cases where it is desired to permit mesial migration of the maxillary and mandibular molars while correcting the disto-occlusion, a situation that arises when second premolars are missing. ClassII/1 anomalies with an anterior open bite caused by tongue interposition cannot be treated well with an activator. This also is true if the patient cannot easily breath through the nose, as it is then very difficult to keep the activator in place during sleep. By making a large hole in the acrylic in the center behind the incisors, that problem can sometimes be overcome.

Whenever treatment needs to begin relatively early, as is the case with class II/1 anomalies that are severe and particularly those where the lip is held between maxillary and mandibular incisors, leaving the over-erupted incisors exposed to the risk of fractures, an activator can be used. The activator does not require the molars to be sufficiently erupted to have bands fixed to them as would be necessary with headgear therapy. The banding of molars in this situation is difficult as little room is available for manipulation, the child is not as yet equal to the ordeal, and the clinical crowns are short. Consequently, molar bands fitted at an early age easily become loose. In addition the first permanent molars will readily tip distally if the second molars have not yet erupted sufficiently to provide them with distal support. The headgear then is more likely to tip the molars distally than to hold back the maxillary complex as is required.

An important advantage of the use of the activator is that the patient will try to hold the lips together over the appliance, and this helps stimulate function in upper lips that lack tone. Because activator therapy is usually used at earlier ages, when children spend more time sleeping, the appliance is worn for a relatively long time each day. Furthermore it has been suggested that the "adaptability" of younger children surpasses that of older children. Both considerations can explain how the activator can provide a marked improvement in a short time. In cases in which first permanent molars are missing and the second molars are still unavailable for banding, an activator can be very useful.

Chapter 7

Class II/1
Cervical headgear, maxillary removable plate
Female: 11 years, 7 months to 26 years, 10 months

A girl who was 11 years, 7 months old had a disto-occlusion of ½ a premolar width, a deep bite, and an overjet of 7 mm. Her facial configuration was fairly normal, although her mid-face had developed relatively far to ventral. At rest she held her lips together and no deviant functional conditions were noticed. An ALD of +1 mm was measured in the mandible, with +6 mm in the maxilla. The space in the maxillary arch was not equally disposed, with crowding anteriorly but excess space in the posterior regions that could be attributed to the persistence of the deciduous second molars, which would be succeeded by narrower premolars (Figs 7.1 and 7.2).

It was decided to provide orthodontic treatment by means of a cervical headgear and a removable plate for the maxilla. At the age of 11 years, 8 months, the maxillary first molars were banded and a cervical headgear fitted with instructions to wear it at night time plus some hours each day, in total 14 hours per day. Any mesial movement of the maxillary first permanent molars following the loss of the second deciduous molars had to be prevented. In addition, the headgear was used to rotate the banded first molars, and traction was applied to the maxillary complex through which to slow down the ventral growth of that structure. Six months later, a plate was fitted to the maxilla, the objective of which was first to move the premolars distally while simultaneously reducing the overbite. Subsequently the canines were to be retracted, followed by the incisors. The procedure followed for this will be described fully in the second half of this chapter.

After two years and one month, a satisfactory result had been achieved and active treatment was halted. The profile had improved, functional disturbances were absent, and the dental arches were in optimal occlusion, so that no retention was deemed necessary (Figs 7.3 and 7.4). A displacement of the midlines of the dental arches occurred and has increased since then, but it does not cause the patient any concern. The records collected thirteen years later support that conclusion. Apart from minor tertiary crowding in the mandibular incisors, there had been little change (Figs 7.5 and 7.6). It was apparent however from the superimposed cephalometric tracings that after treatment the maxillary and mandibular incisors had moved labially and the first permanent molars tipped mesially, which nonetheless had no deleterious effect on the profile (Figs 7.7 and 7.8).

It might be added that with the composite resins now available, the appearance of the maxillary central incisors could have been improved. In general terms it is

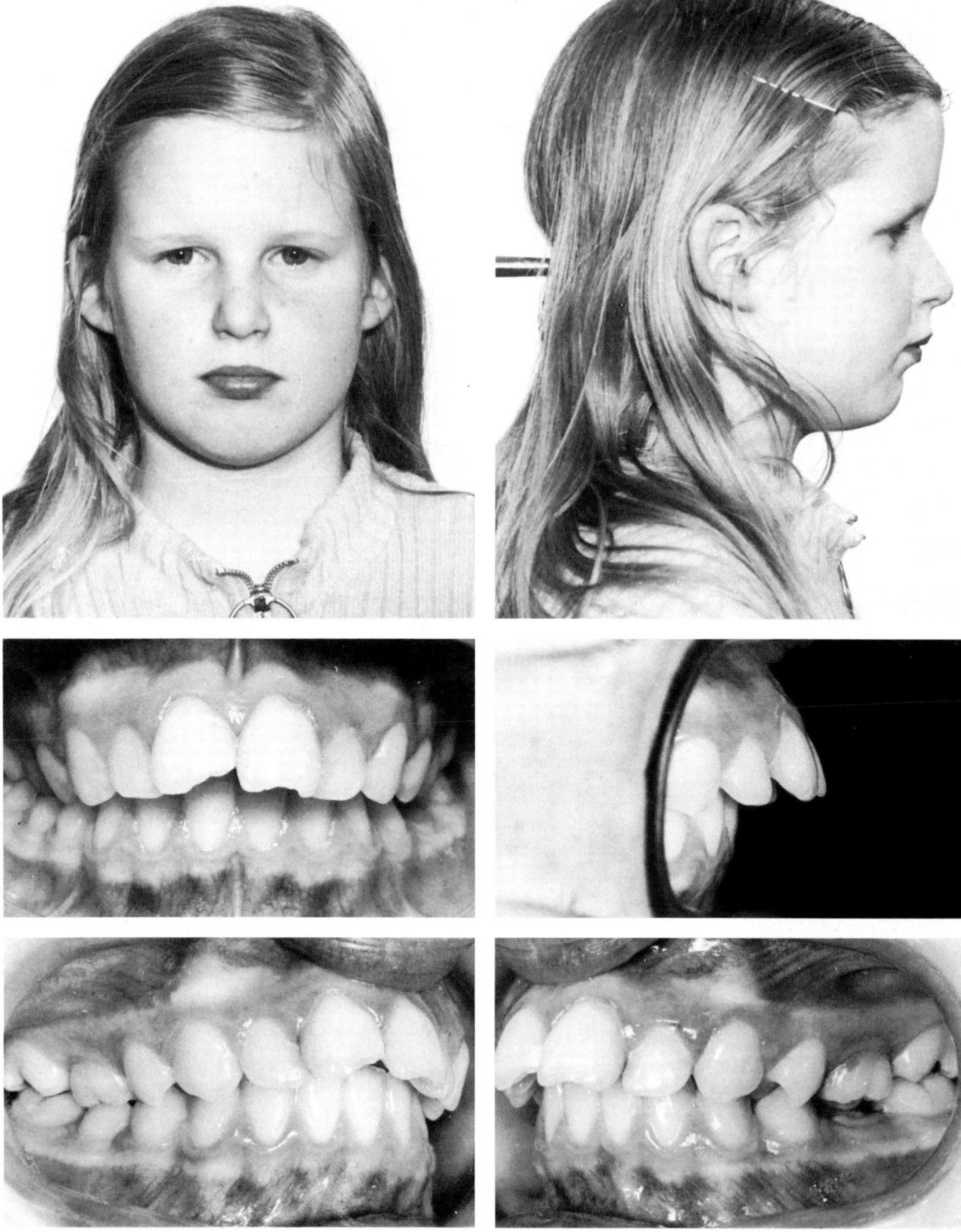

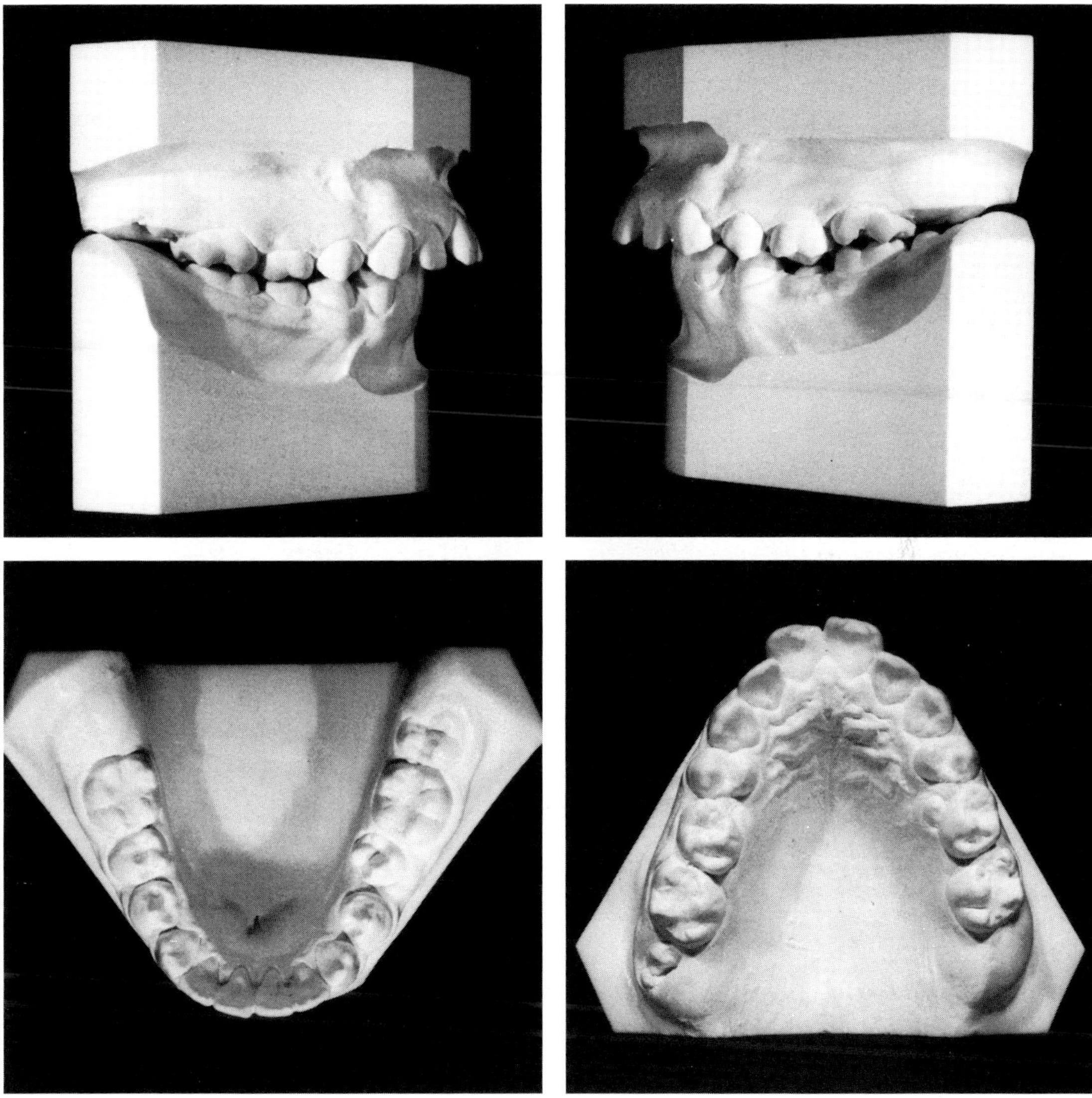

Fig 7-1 and 7-2 *A girl who was 11 y, 7 mo old had a class II/1 anomaly (½ PW), good lip seal, and normal functional conditions. Both maxillary central incisors were fractured in an accident and required endodontic treatment. The overjet is 9 mm. There is crowding in the maxillary arch in the anterior region but excess space in the posterior regions where the second deciduous molars have yet to be replaced by the narrower premolars. The mandibular arch is more or less normal.*

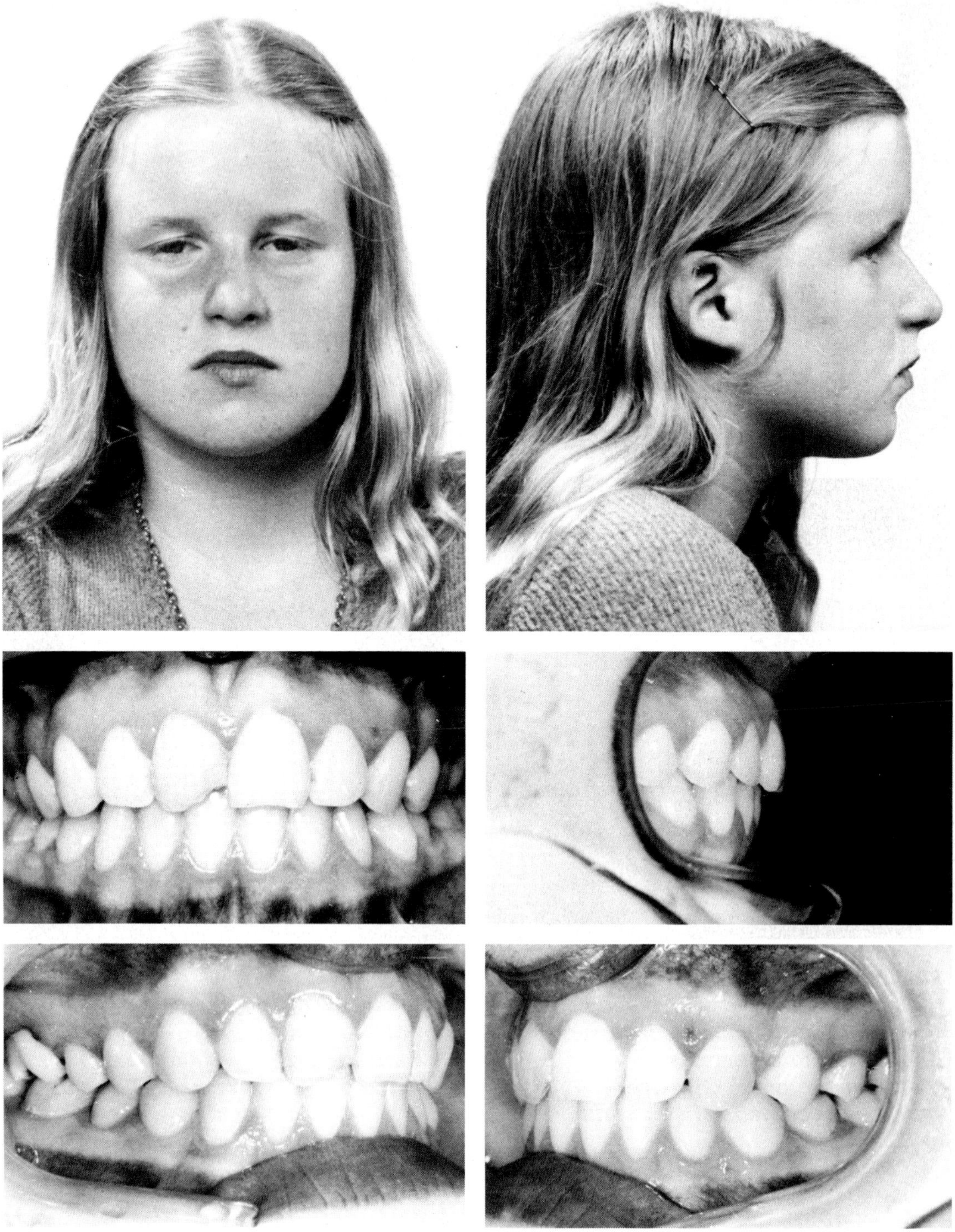

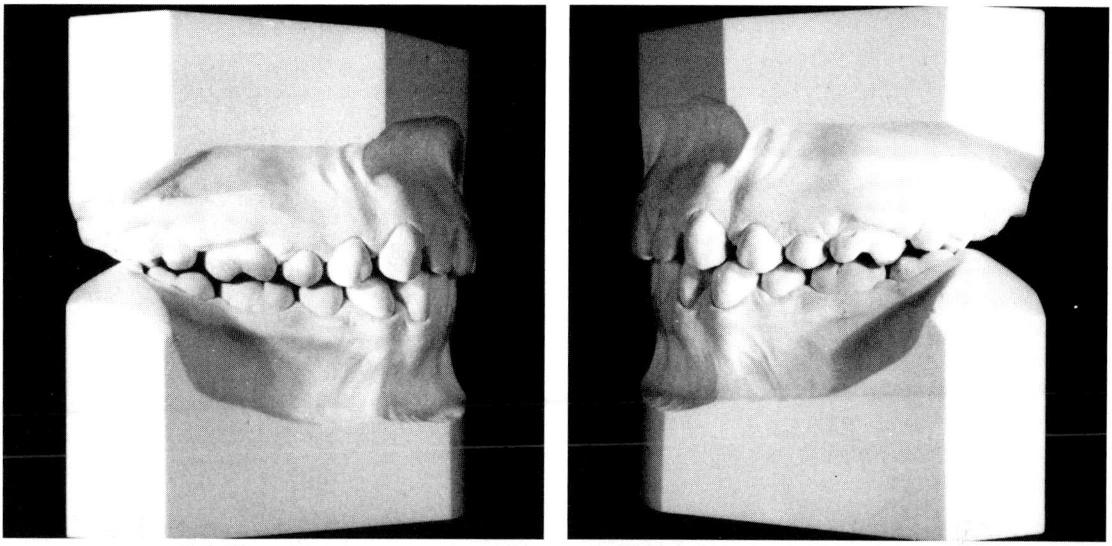

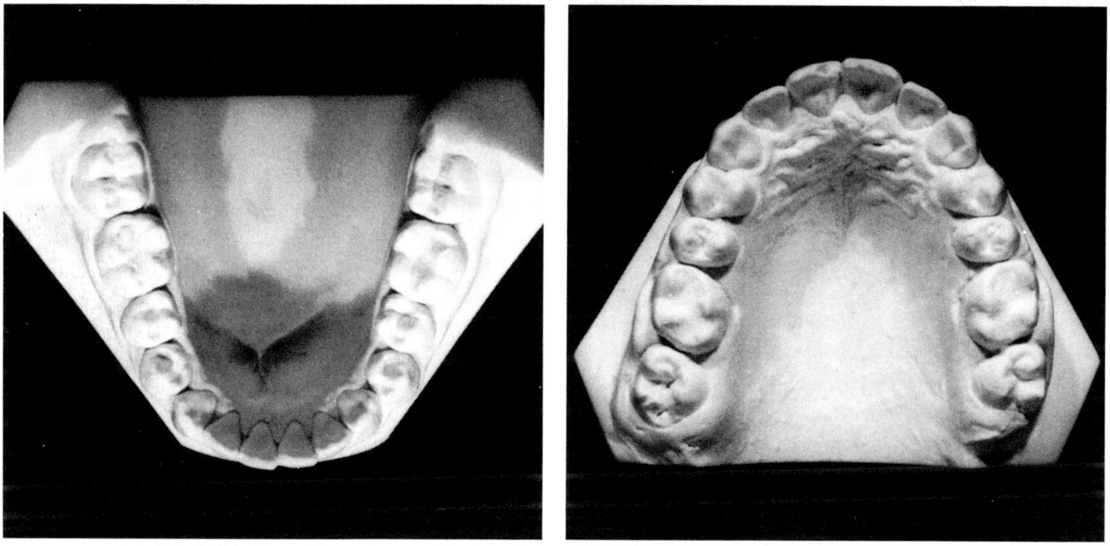

Figs 7-3 and 7-4 *At the age of 13 y, 10 mo the treatment was finished. A good result had been achieved with simple means. A solid interdigitation of the canines and premolars provides consolidation of the result of the facial-orthopedic therapy. The good interdigitation was partly realized by rotating the first permanent molars, thus reducing the amount of space they occupied in the dental arch and improving the way they occluded with their antagonists.*

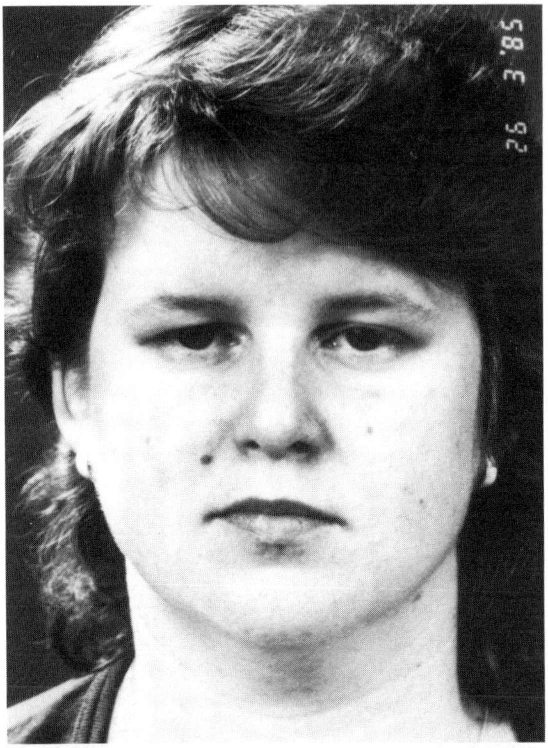

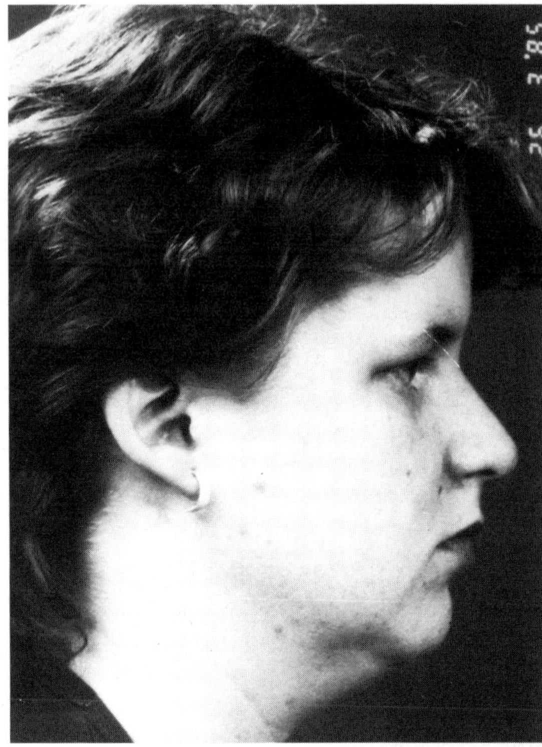

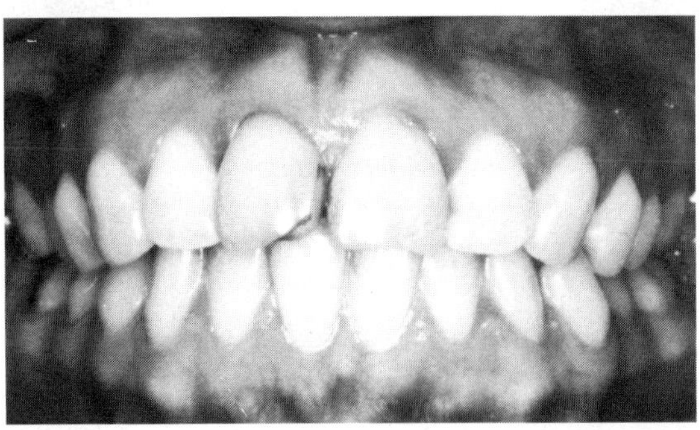

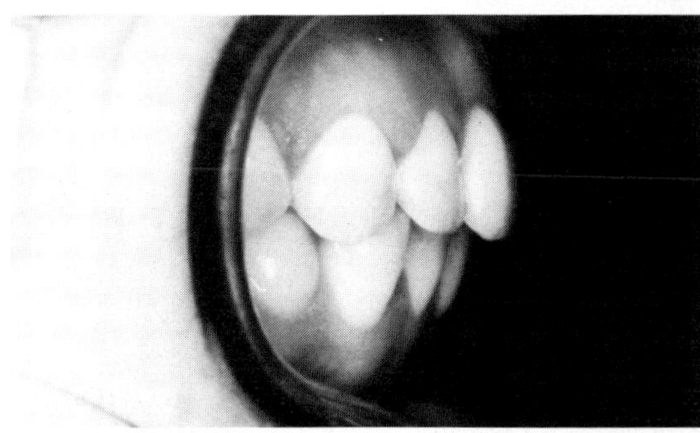

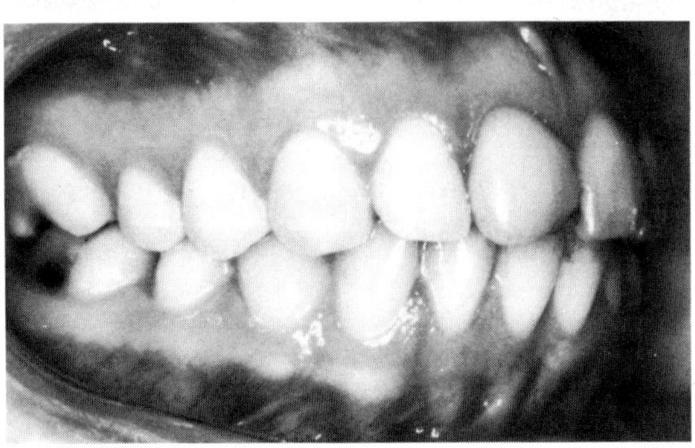

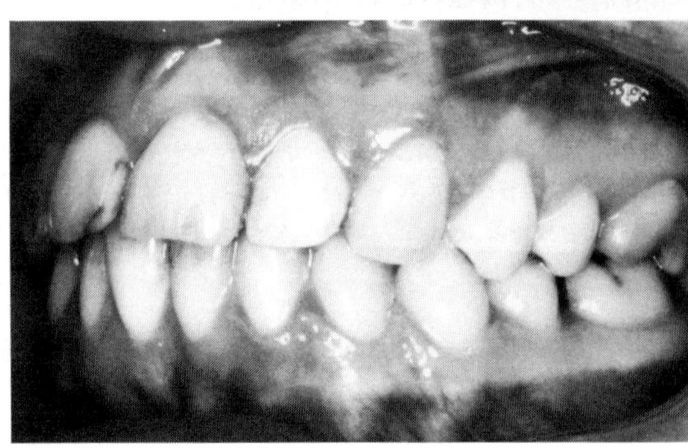

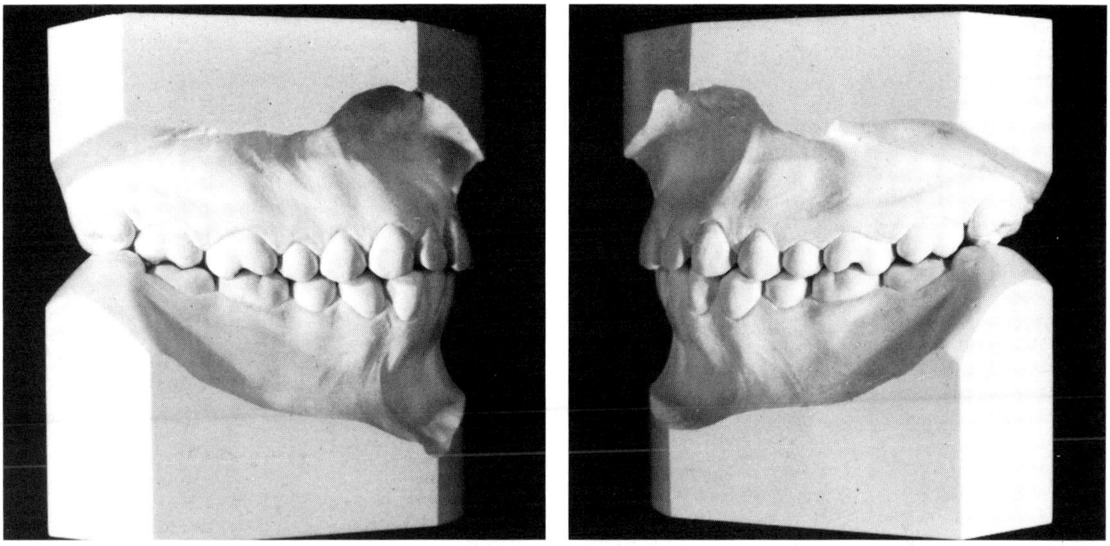

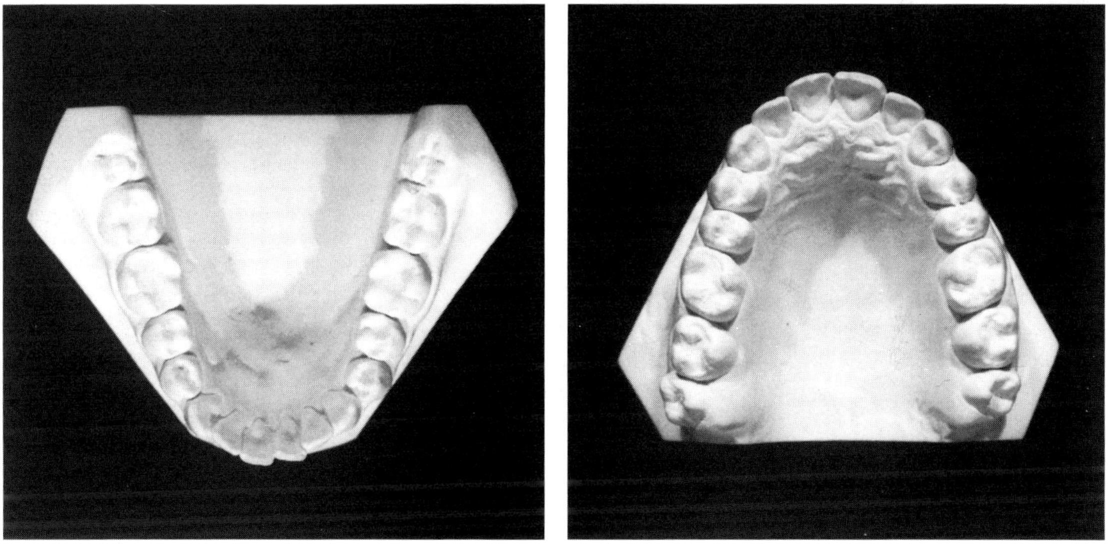

Figs 7-5 and 7-6 *At the age of 26 y, 10 mo, 13 years after treatment was finished, the result is still satisfactory. The limited crowding of the mandibular incisors is of no concern. That applies also to the inadequate restoration of the fractured mesial incisal angle of the maxillary right central incisor, although at present, a simple yet most esthetic solution would be possible with composite resins.*[25]

Figure 7-7a

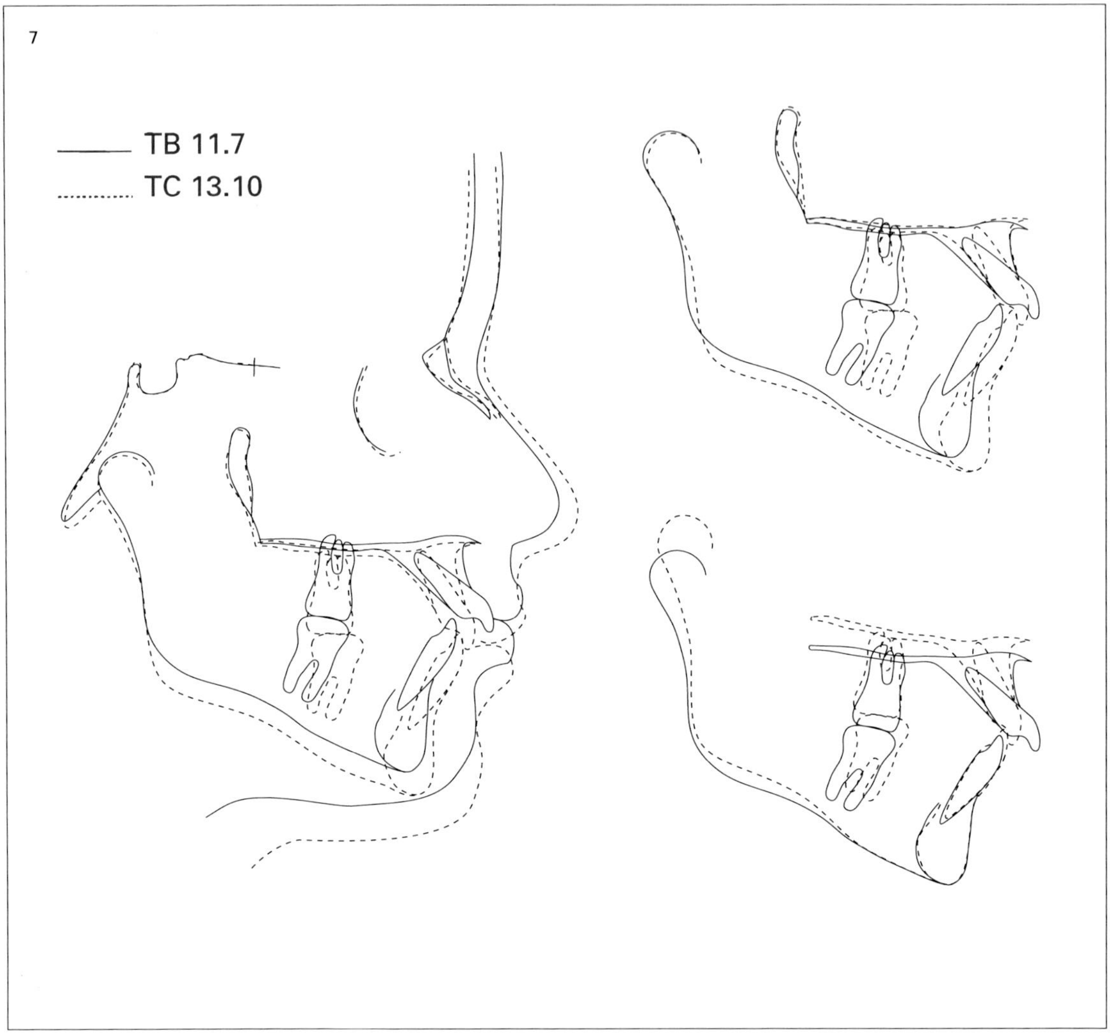

Figs 7-7a and 7-7b Superimposed cephalometric tracings of lateral headplates taken before treatment (TB), directly after treatment (TC) and 13 years after treatment (13 PT).
During treatment,the maxillary complex did not move ventrally, while the incisors were retracted. The mandible has developed to ventral, principally through condylar growth which has resulted in a notable increase in the length of the rami. The inclination of the lower border of the mandible has not become steeper. The face has grown a little since completion of treatment. The lower part of the face has increased little in height. The incisors in the maxilla have tipped forward but so have those in the mandible.

Figure 7-7b

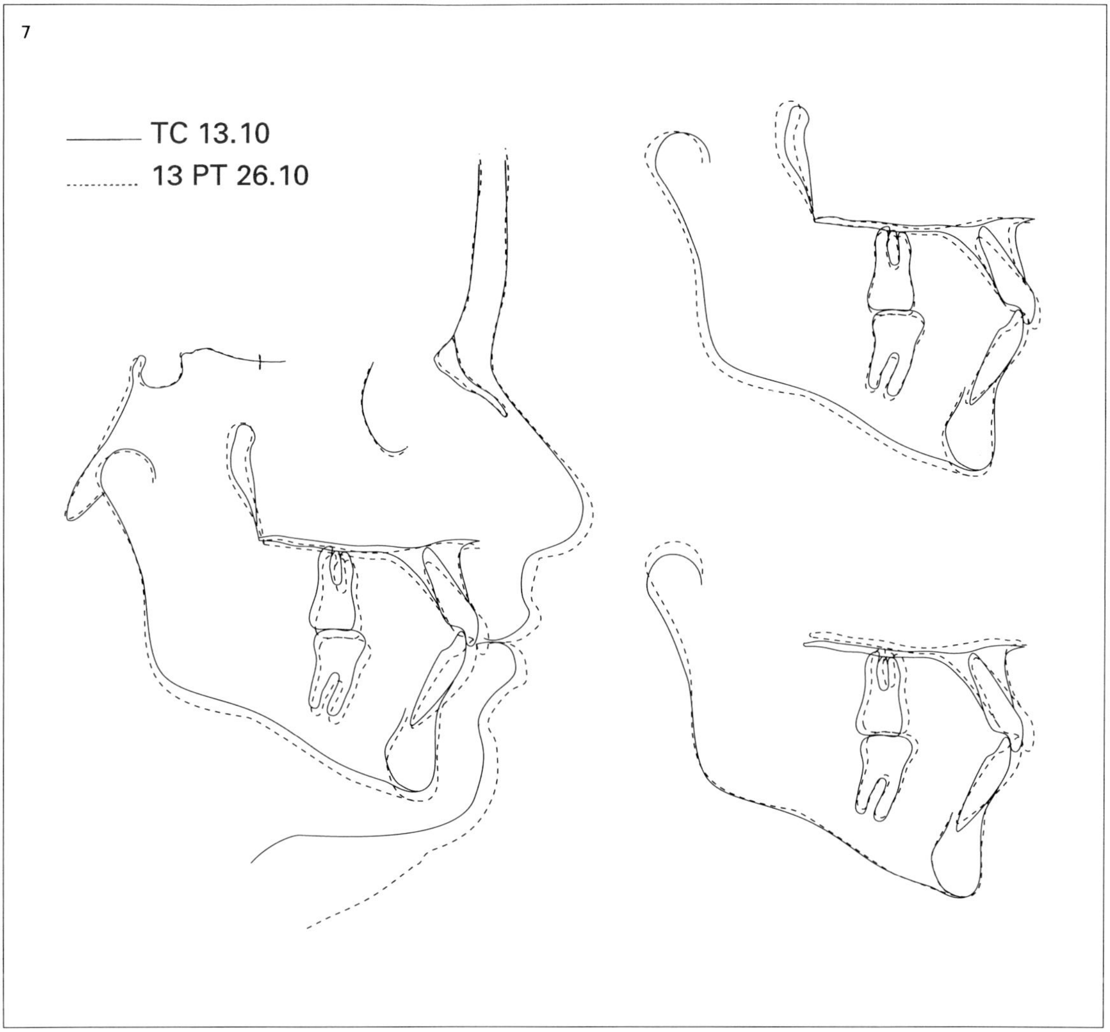

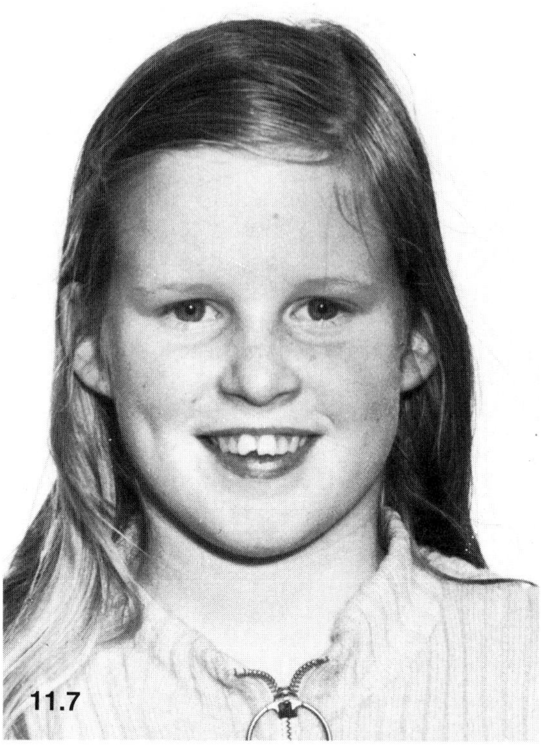

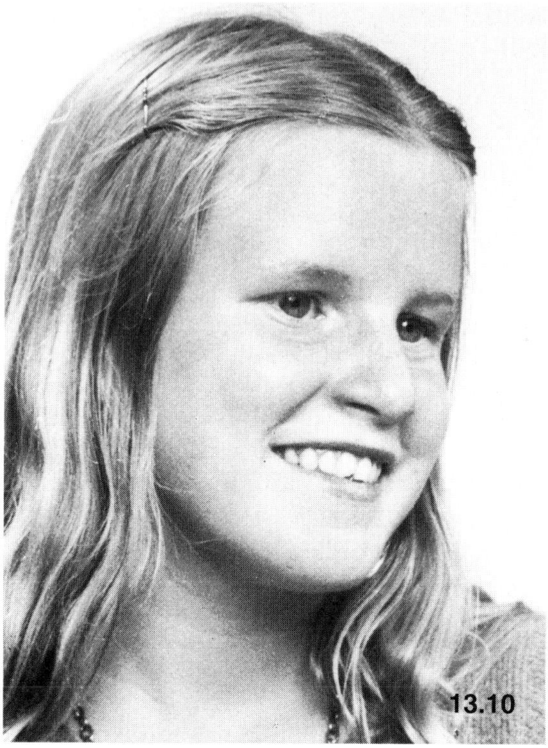

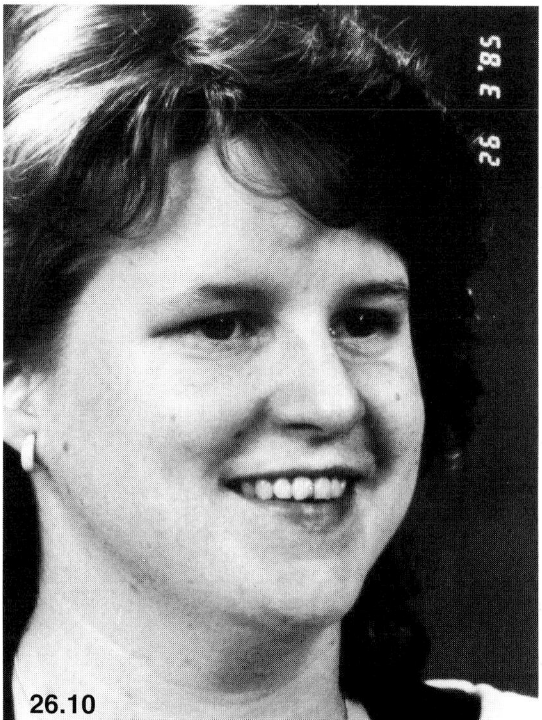

Fig 7-8 The improvements obtained and the stability of the result are evident.

sometimes possible to secure improvement just by judicious grinding of incisal edges.

The choice to treat this case with a headgear and maxillary removable plate was made because it is possible to rotate the maxillary first permanent molars and to use the space gained in the region of the premolars to improve the position of the anterior teeth. There was not only a need for the extra space to eliminate the crowding but also to permit retraction of the incisors over quite a distance. Since they were markedly inclined labially, retraction of the incisors by tipping them palatally with the labial arches of the plate was quite appropriate. If the incisors had not initially been labially inclined this could have led to their undesirable palatal inclination (see Chapter 11).

In every correction of a disto-occlusion that possesses a good transverse relationship, with vertical contact between the opposing teeth in the posterior regions, it is essential to provide conditions to allow the teeth in the maxillary arch to move buccally under the influence of the rail mechanism as the mandibular arch moves ventrally relative to the maxillary arch (Fig 7.9). If a headgear is used in combination with a plate then the design of the plate, and the periodic addition to the height of the bite plane should be in accordance with the realization of the rail mechanism.

The cervical headgear is especially suitable for correction of class II/1 anomalies with crowding in the maxilla and where it is desired to rotate the first permanent molars distally or just to hold them distally. If gaining extra space in the maxillary arch is not indicated, it has to be prevented by the wearing of a plate from the time that the headgear is fitted. Such a plate should be provided at least with wires and acrylic well adapted distal of the last molars, and with closely adapted labial arches. The plate must not hinder the realization of the rail mechanism: the premolars and molars must be free to move buccally.

In most cases a plate in the maxilla will not be fitted until the headgear treatment has already been in progress for some time. The molar occlusion will largely have been corrected. The available space can be used for moving the premolars and then the canines to distal. Simultaneously, any deep bite can be corrected with a bite plane. Because an improvement in sagittal relationship usually is not associated with a reduction of the deep bite, it has to be actively corrected. The incisors can finally be retracted with the labial arches.

Treatment of a class II/1 malocclusion with a headgear and plate will only secure a good end result if the steps to follow are carefully adhered to. In most class II/1 anomalies with a disto-occlusion of ½ PW, where the lower lip is not held behind the maxillary incisors, treatment can be delayed until some time after the beginning of the second transitional period and before the loss of the second deciduous molars. The leeway space can then be utilized in the correction of the disto-occlusion, or for the relief of an existing or impending ALD (Fig 7.10).

A headgear can be used not only to correct a disto-relation but also to preserve or even increase the available arch length. In general, it is preferable first to procure the space required in the maxillary arch, and then to fit a plate.

A headgear must be worn at least 14 hours a day, and have a clearance of 2 to 3 mm

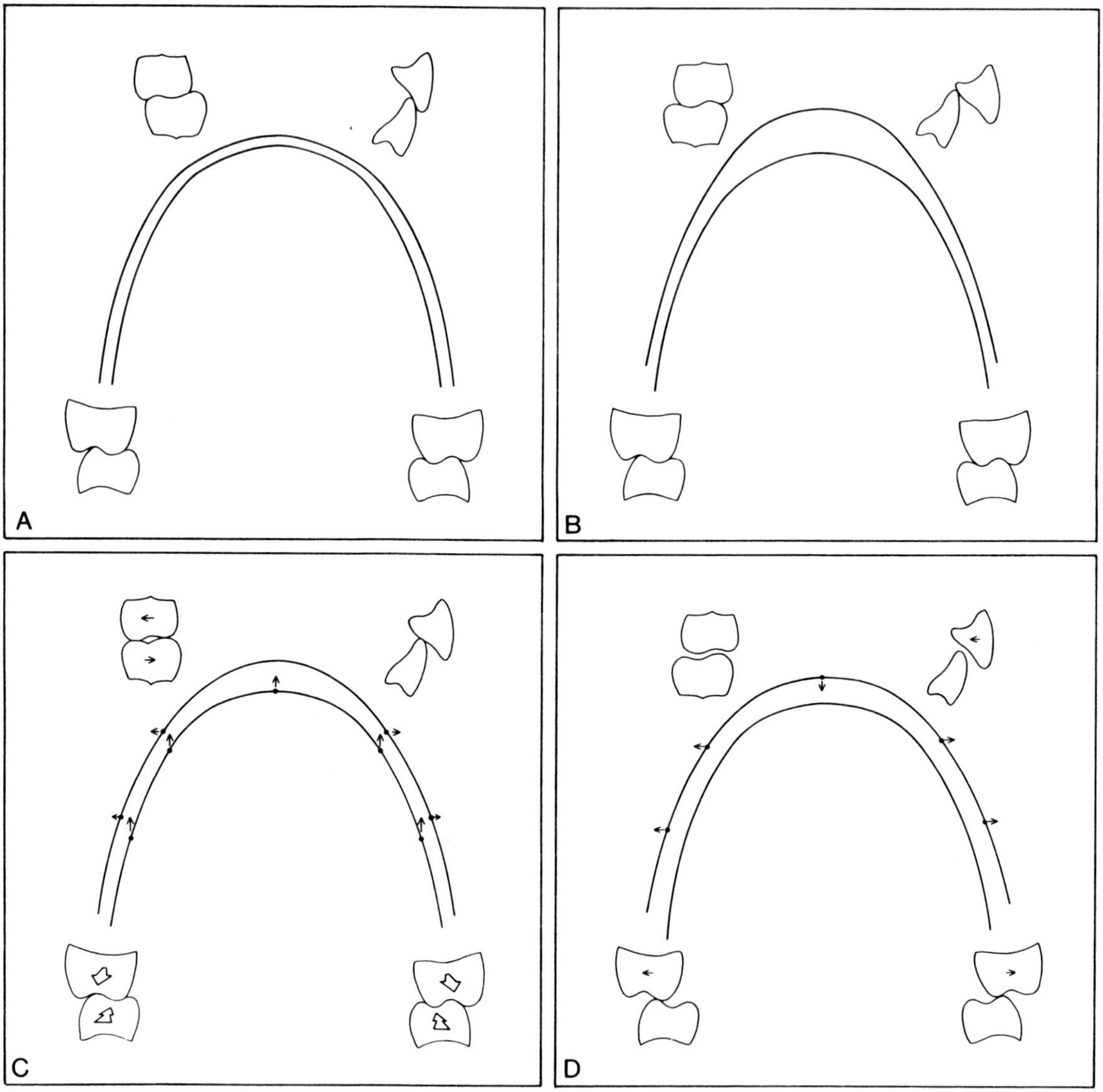

Fig 7-9 Diagrammatic depiction of the sagittal, transverse, and vertical occlusion of the mandibular and maxillary dental arches under different circumstances.

A Neutro-occlusion; normal arches, good sagittal and transverse occlusion.

B Disto-occlusion with increased overjet and overbite, labioversion of the maxillary incisors; normal mandibular arch except for the supraposition of the mandibular incisors. The posterior teeth interdigitate transversely in the normal way. The breadth of the maxillary arch is adapted to that of the mandibular one; in a case of disto-occlusion, the maxillary arch seems narrower than in neutro-occlusion.

C If the occlusion of the posterior teeth in a class II/1 anomaly is corrected, the maxillary arch becomes wider due to the teeth in the mandible contacting those of the maxilla more mesially. In headgear therapy with a changing jaw relationship, the increase in arch width is stimulated every time the teeth are closed together. In activator treatment, the latter only happens during the day, because the appliance is not worn at that time. If a headgear is combined with a biteplate, then the biteplane should be only slightly heightened so that the teeth will have regained occlusal contact soon and thus have the stimulus to move the crowns and roots to buccal. The extent to which the maxillary teeth move buccally is related to the degree by which the sagittal relationship is improved (rail mechanism).

D *Expansion of the maxillary dental arch and retraction of the incisors without simultaneously correcting the disto-occlusion lead to disturbance of the transverse interdigitation because as a rule the teeth in the mandible do not follow the increase in width of the maxillary arch.*[36]

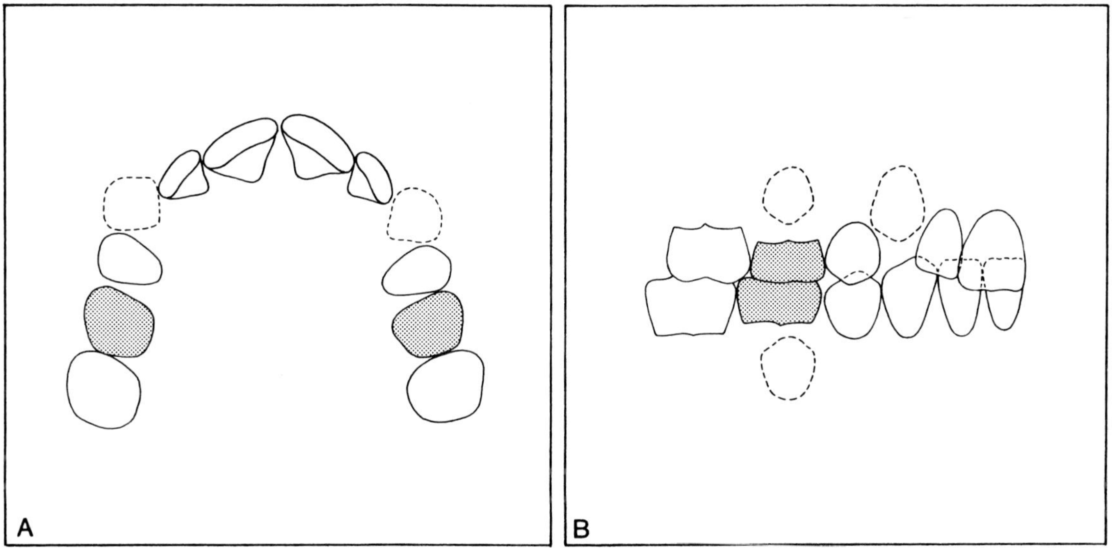

Fig 7-10 The stage of development of the dentition at which treatment with a cervical headgear preferably should begin.

A *In the maxilla, the second deciduous molars are still present and the permanent canines have not yet emerged. The second permanent molars are located in the alveolar process close to the first permanent molars and near the occlusal plane.*

B *The presence of broad second deciduous molars in both jaws provides an extra opportunity to secure a good occlusion since space becomes available, in the mandible more than in the maxilla, when they are replaced by the narrower premolars.*

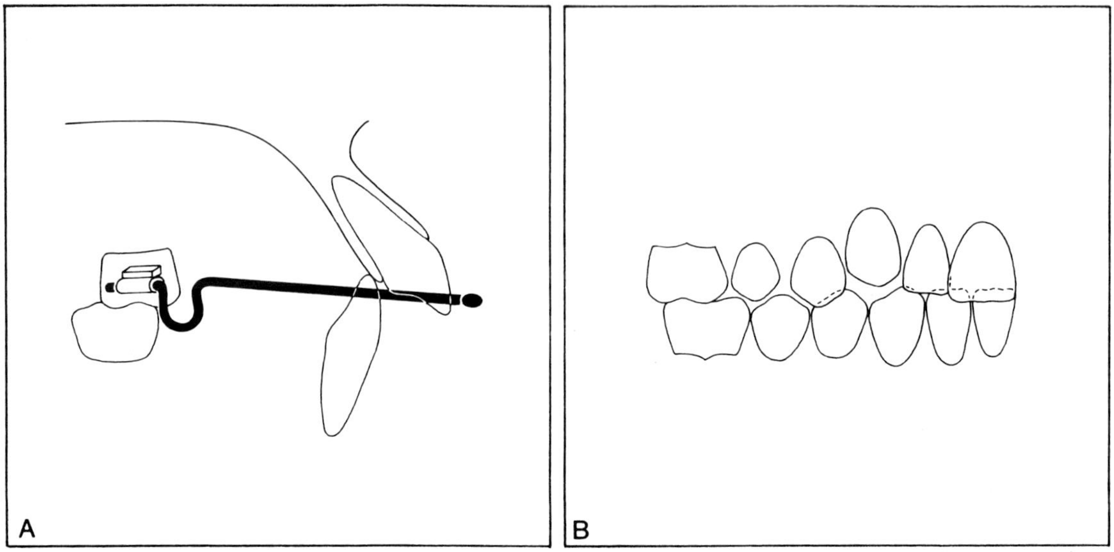

Fig 7-11 The position of a cervical headgear and its effect on the dentition.
A The headgear should have 2-to-3 mm clearance in front of the maxillary incisors and should lie between the lips a little above the level of the incisal edges.
B With the headgear it is possible simultaneously to correct the molar occlusion and procure space in the canine-premolar regions.

between it and the incisors (Fig 7.11A). If the inner arch is closer to the labial surfaces of the incisors, it will hit the teeth before the next 4- to 6-week check-up. This leads to undesired effects and discomfort for the patient. If manually heavy pressure is applied to dorsal on the junction of the inner and outer bows, and the incisors are not touched, then the inner arch is sufficiently clear of them. The inner arch should also be 2 to 3 mm clear of the buccal surfaces of the premolars. This holds the cheeks and lips away from the teeth, which together with the rail mechanism contribute to an increase in the maxillary arch perimeter. The junction of the inner and outer bows should lie between the lips just above the incisal edges when the headgear is in place with the neckstrap active.

In treatment of a class II/1 anomaly without the lower lip behind the maxillary incisors and for which the treatment is begun at the stage of the development of the dentition that is depicted in Figure 7.10, the correction of the disto-occlusion will usually be more or less complete by the end of the second transitional period (Fig 7.11B).

If, however, the lower lip does rest behind the maxillary incisors, then the molar occlusion will improve if the headgear is worn well, but the overjet will not decrease. In these cases, which frequently have spacing in the maxillary arch to begin with, a headgear should be combined with a removable plate in the maxilla from the start. That will prevent the development of excess space in the maxillary arch. Moreover, with the plate the maxillary incisors can be retracted and the diastemata closed, through which the lower lip can assume a better position and the danger of the incisors being fractured will be reduced. It is sometimes necessary to reduce the length of the inner arch of the headgear as time goes on, rather than to lengthen it, as it may otherwise hinder the change in position of the lips that will accompany the retraction of the maxillary incisors.

In addition, a "lip bumper" can be utilized on the mandibular arch, with the advantage that it keeps the lower lip away from behind the maxillary incisors.

As is apparent from the foregoing discussion, the need to combine a headgear with a maxillary plate is determined by one or more of three factors: First is the presence of sagittal contact between maxillary and mandibular incisors. In that case, successful headgear therapy will result in the mandibular incisors moving ventrally against the maxillary ones, with the result that the latter might be protruded and the lower ones retruded by the reciprocal forces generated. To prevent this and to eliminate the deep bite, a maxillary removable plate can be used. Second, a plate can be used to prevent the excess space that may develop in the maxillary arch. Third, a plate provides a means by which the teeth in the maxillary arch can be moved.

Following an increase in arch perimeter with a headgear, a spontaneous improvement often occurs in the position of the teeth that previously had inadequate space. Usually it is still required to move teeth actively. For instance, the premolars and subsequently the canines frequently must be moved distally. Ectostomatically emerged canines will not move sufficiently inward during headgear treatment, since the pressure of the labial and buccal musculature is held away from them by the inner arch of the headgear. Plates such as that illustrated in Figure 7.12 can deliver the necessary tooth movements and at the same time reduce the deep bite.

A diastema distal to the second premolar can be closed by pressure from a pig tail spring on the mesial side of the first premolar, once contact between the two premolars is established. To that end, the labial archwires have to cross the dental arch not between the premolars but occlusally of the contact point. Sufficient room is available for this procedure since the bite plane opens the bite slightly in the posterior regions. An additional advantage of the use of the bite plane to open the bite in the posterior regions is that reduction of the occlusal forces there lessens the braking effect they might have on the desired tooth movements. The labial arches and the palatal acrylic are positioned and shaped so that the distal movement of the premolars can be associated with a buccal one to arrive at a proper transverse occlusion with the mandibular teeth. To that end, the labial arches must stand clear of the buccal surface of the first premolars.

Once the premolars have been moved fully to distal,the pig tail springs that were used for that purpose should be built in with acrylic so that only the parts of the wires mesial to the first premolars are free. The free ends should be shortened, rounded, and bent in so that although they prevent mesial relapse of the premolars, they will not obstruct the distal movement of the canines into good contact with the first premolars. The palatal acrylic added at the premolars should fit well against them and thus improve the available anchorage while the canines are being retracted.

The deep bite needs to have been reduced as far as is needed before grinding away

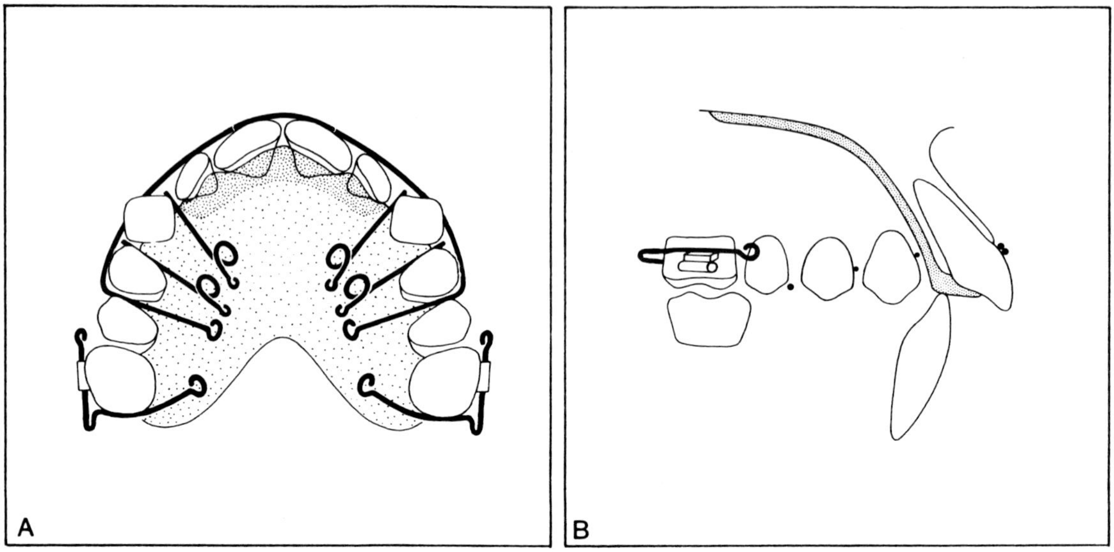

Fig 7-12 A removable plate that can be combined well with the use of a cervical headgear.

A The biteplane is supported by the palatal surfaces of the incisors and canines; those teeth are prevented from going labially by the light action of the divided labial arches. The arches also improve the retention of the plate. But they have to stand clear of the premolars to allow the rail mechanism to act. Pigtail springs are used first to move the premolars distally and then the canines. In association with those procedures, it is essential that the acrylic is trimmed away locally.

B The pigtail springs used to move the first premolars distally can also be used to move the second premolars once the premolars are in contact. To that end, the labial arches have to cross the occlusion clear of the premolars. The biteplane should be only slightly heightened. The posterior teeth must have the opportunity to be in occlusion for some time to promote the working of the rail mechanism. Only after that has occurred should the biteplane height be increased again.

the acrylic against the canines. It is undesirable to increase the height of a bite plane if it is only supported by the maxillary incisors, because the forces generated in biting will often be too great for those teeth to resist; the support from the canines in this respect is indispensable.

In the plates discussed and described here, the divided labial arches have only a limited role in retention, which is mainly obtained from wires running cervically to the headgear tubes. Those wires should lie slightly free of the buccal surface of the bands while the occlusion of the molars still needs to be improved by buccal movement or rotation. Clasps cannot be applied to other posterior teeth since the premolars still need to be moved distally and to be free to move buccally under the influence of the rail mechanism. The recommendation that the retention of a plate should involve two clasps in each quadrant thus cannot be followed in these circumstances. With careful adaptation of the clasps, the springs, and labial arches, it is still possible to obtain sufficient retention in most cases.[4]

After a plate has been processed in the laboratory it is usually too thick behind the incisors, so that when placed in position a large gap exists between the posterior teeth. For the patient, a thin biteplane is less disagreeable than a thick one, the more so as the plate has to be worn also while eating. Moreover the bite may not be opened too much because the rail mechanism may then taken out of function for too long. As the posterior teeth erupt further and meet their antagonists, the rail mechanism should be able to act so that not only the crowns but also the roots of the posterior teeth will move buccally. Only when that has been achieved may the height of the biteplane be added to again.

So in fitting the new, too thick, plate, on which often only one or two mandibular incisors bite, the acrylic in the anterior area should be ground away until the room between the opposing posterior teeth is reduced to about 1 mm. Then self-curing resin is added to the plate in the anterior area. When the resin is of a fairly thick consistency, the plate is replaced in the mouth and the patient asked to close into contact with the plate and remain still until the resin has set. Subsequently the excess is removed and ground away out of the mouth until there is a plateau behind the maxillary incisors at the level of the imprints of the six mandibular front teeth. The plateau should be made level to allow the mandibular incisors and canines to move forward without interference as the disto-occlusion becomes gradually corrected. The plateau needs to be shortened dorsally just sufficiently to leave a platform onto which the six mandibular front teeth can bite securely. While the maxillary premolars and canines are being moved distally, the plate must lie closely adapted to the palatal surfaces of the maxillary incisors. The labial arches should be slightly activated just to enhance the plate's retention, and in particular to prevent the incisors from moving labially.

Several weeks should pass between the time that occlusal contact is regained and the next increase in the height of the bite plane is performed, since the rail mechanism must have the opportunity to do its work fully. As previously stated, an interocclusal distance of 1 mm is sufficient. This can be provided if the patient bites on a thinned out cotton roll between the first permanent molars on both sides. More self-curing resin is applied, the plate placed in the mouth as before and the teeth closed with the rolls in place. After hardening, it is shaped as before.

Full support of the biteplane by the palatal surfaces of the maxillary front teeth is essential. To achieve this, it is sometimes necessary to "rebase" the plate locally. In rebasing as well as in building up the biteplane, the self-curing resin should have a certain consistency before it is used in the mouth. Collapse of the resin is prevented and inhalation of the monomer reduced. Gingiva that come into contact with the resin should be dried and lightly coated with vaseline. Quickly dipping the plate with its fresh resin into hot water will give it a smooth skin before placing it in the mouth, where it must stay until it is quite set.
With this method, it is not possible to open the bite and move the front teeth back at the same time. To open the bite, as has been explained, there must always be close contact between the front teeth and the palatal surface of the plate. Incisors should not be retracted before the deep bite is sufficiently reduced and vertical support of the posterior teeth is well established. When retracting the incisors, the acrylic must be judiciously trimmed away from behind those teeth so that they are out of contact with it. When this trimming is performed prior to establishing vertical support of the posterior teeth, the biteplane will still be active every time that the teeth are closed, which happens many times a day. For example when swallowing, the plate will be bitten on and tip while the acrylic will press the incisors to labial. Because of the tipping the plate can no longer actively open the bite, and indeed can cause irritation and hypertrophy of the gingiva and palatal mucosa. Furthermore the maxillary incisors in that situation become unduly loose and begin "jiggling."
When retracting maxillary canines, they should not be allowed to go too far buccally. For that reason, the part of the pigtail spring that lies mesial to the canine should be straight and placed so that a perpendicular to that straight part passes through the canine's center of pressure in the direction in which it should move. In addition, the labial arch, as it passes buccally of the canine, should be shaped distally in such a way as to prevent any unwanted buccal movement. The plate must be trimmed on its palatal aspect so that it offers good guidance for the translation of the canine.
After the canines have been fully retracted, they are held in place by embedding the springs that moved them in acrylic, and by surrounding their crowns palatally, mesially and distally, with acrylic (Fig 7.13A). When subsequently the incisors are retracted, the only support for the biteplane will be obtained from the canines. It is for that reason that the acrylic must accurately embrace the canine crown, especially mesially. The tipping of the plate on biting is then resisted by the vertical support from the palatal surfaces of the maxillary canines and the acrylic that lies against the mesial surface of the clinical crown.
During the retraction of the incisors it is still necessary for the labial arches to lie slightly actively against the canines to ensure that those teeth will remain in their places. The force exerted on the canines and incisors can readily be measured by sliding dental floss between the archwire and the teeth.
When the incisors are being retracted sufficient clearance should be provided also between the plate and the palatal tissues to allow rebuilding of the alveolar process, while at the same time the mandibular incisors still rest on the biteplane (Fig 7.13B). Contact with the mandibular front teeth is established by retraction of the incisors. It is often not feasible to keep the labial arches in firm contact with the canines in the last phase of retraction. If eventually it is desired to move the canines palatally, a

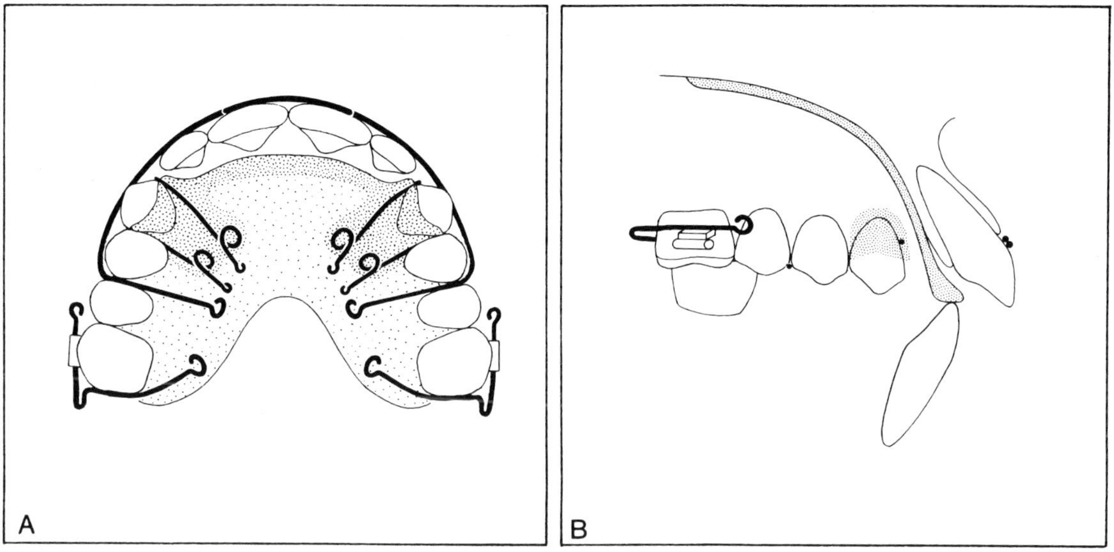

Fig 7-13 Form of the plate with which the maxillary incisors finally are retracted.
A The canines need to be thoroughly surrounded mesially, distally, and palatally by the acrylic that is added to the plate. The pigtail springs mesial to the canines must also be held rigidly against them by the acrylic. When bitten on, the plate may not tip.
B The acrylic has to be trimmed away generously at the gingival area behind the maxillary incisors to allow rebuilding of the alveolar process.

convenient method is to bend the archwires parallel back mesial to the lateral incisors so that the free ends lie against the canines to apply the required palatal pressure. At each visit, it should be checked that the inner arch of the headgear does not come into conflict with any of the parts of the plate when it is being worn and has been activated.
With good use of a cervical headgear in combination with a plate, such class II/1 anomalies for which it is suitable can be satisfactorily corrected in a relatively short time.

Chapter 8

Class II/1
Cervical headgear, maxillary removable plate, positioner
Female: 12 years, 9 months to 26 years, 1 month

This patient was a girl 12 years, 9 months old, with a mild class II/1 anomaly. Her chin was a little receded in relationship to the rest of her face. She kept her mouth open most of the time, with her lower lip touching the incisal edges of the maxillary incisors. At rest her tongue lay on the mandibular anterior teeth and between the lingual cusps of the premolars and molars on the right side. The patient had a clear nasal airway and sucked her thumb till the age of 10. Both arches showed a slight excess of space. The ALD for the mandible was +4 mm, and + 3 mm for the maxilla. The mandibular arch was well-formed but the maxillary incisors were in eversion. There was a slight disto-occlusion (Figs 8.1 and 8.2).

The patient had received orthodontic treatment previously with a maxillary removable appliance. The anomaly had subsequently returned to a great extent. This history made it difficult to determine if the tongue position had a neuromuscular origin or was adaptive.

It was decided to treat her with a cervical headgear in the first instance, and later possibly with a maxillary plate. After having worn the headgear 14 hours per day for eight months, the molar occlusion was over-corrected, but solid interdigitation had not developed. The first premolars in the maxilla were situated too far to the buccal and most of the teeth distal to them were not well positioned transversely in relationship to their antagonists. A month later, a maxillary plate was fitted, with divided labially arches to retract the maxillary incisors. Buccal springs and additions of gutta percha between the teeth and the periphery of the plate were used to correct the positions of the posterior teeth. One year and eight months later, most of the objectives had been reached, but there still was no solid interdigitation. Moreover, there was still a mild anterior open bite. It was decided to perform the final improvements with a positioner, which was worn at night and for an additional four hours during the day for one month, after which it was used for retention only when sleeping for another five months.

The records collected at the age of 15 years, 10 months show a clear improvement in profile and dentition (Figs 8.3 and 8.4). However, there is still an open bite anteriorly and no good interdigitation of the posterior teeth. In this regard, the oral photographs are more trustworthy than the photographs of the models; frequently models are finished off (and thus photographed) in a better vertical occlusion than that existing in reality in cases with a slight open bite in the posterior segments or with vaguely defined interdigitation.

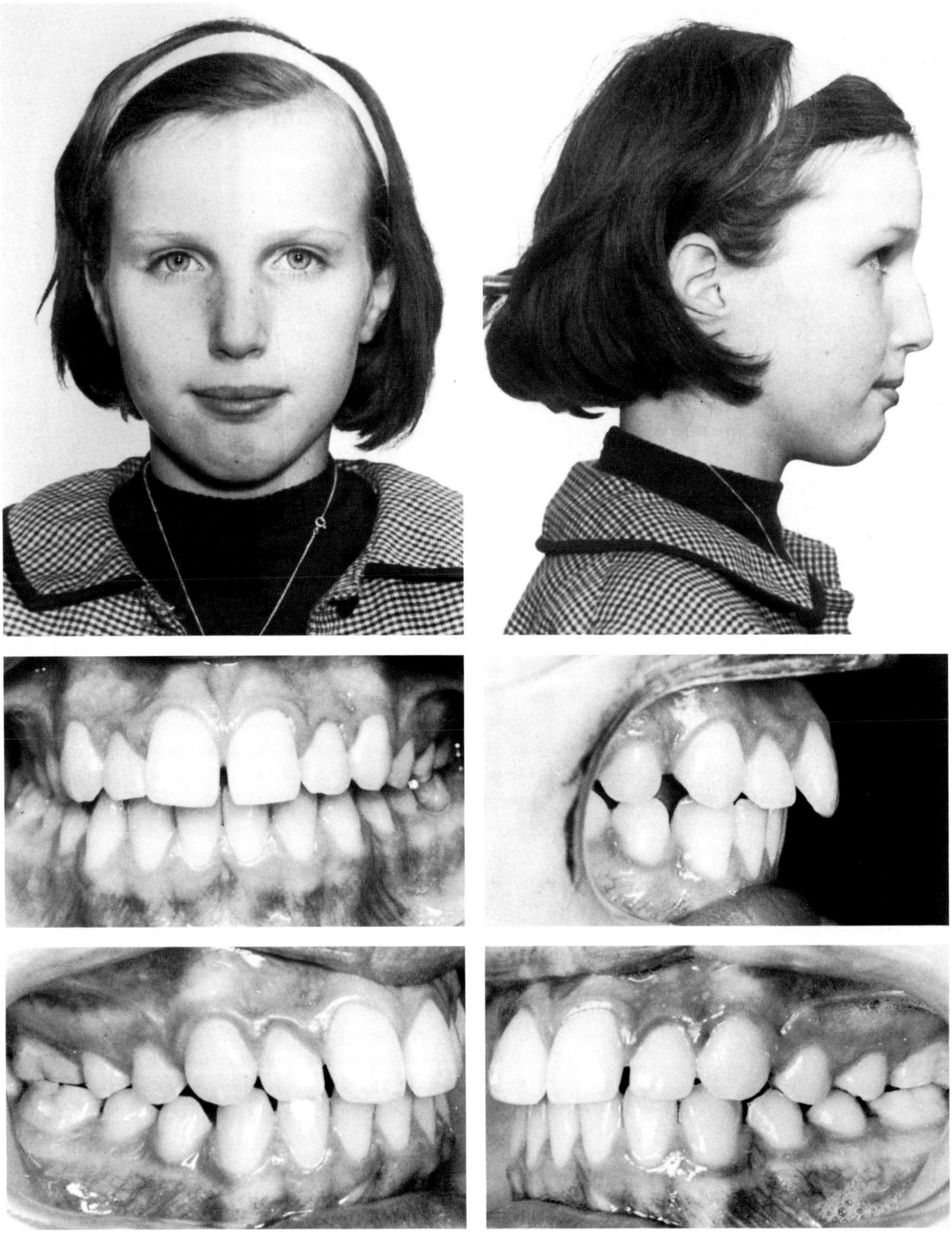

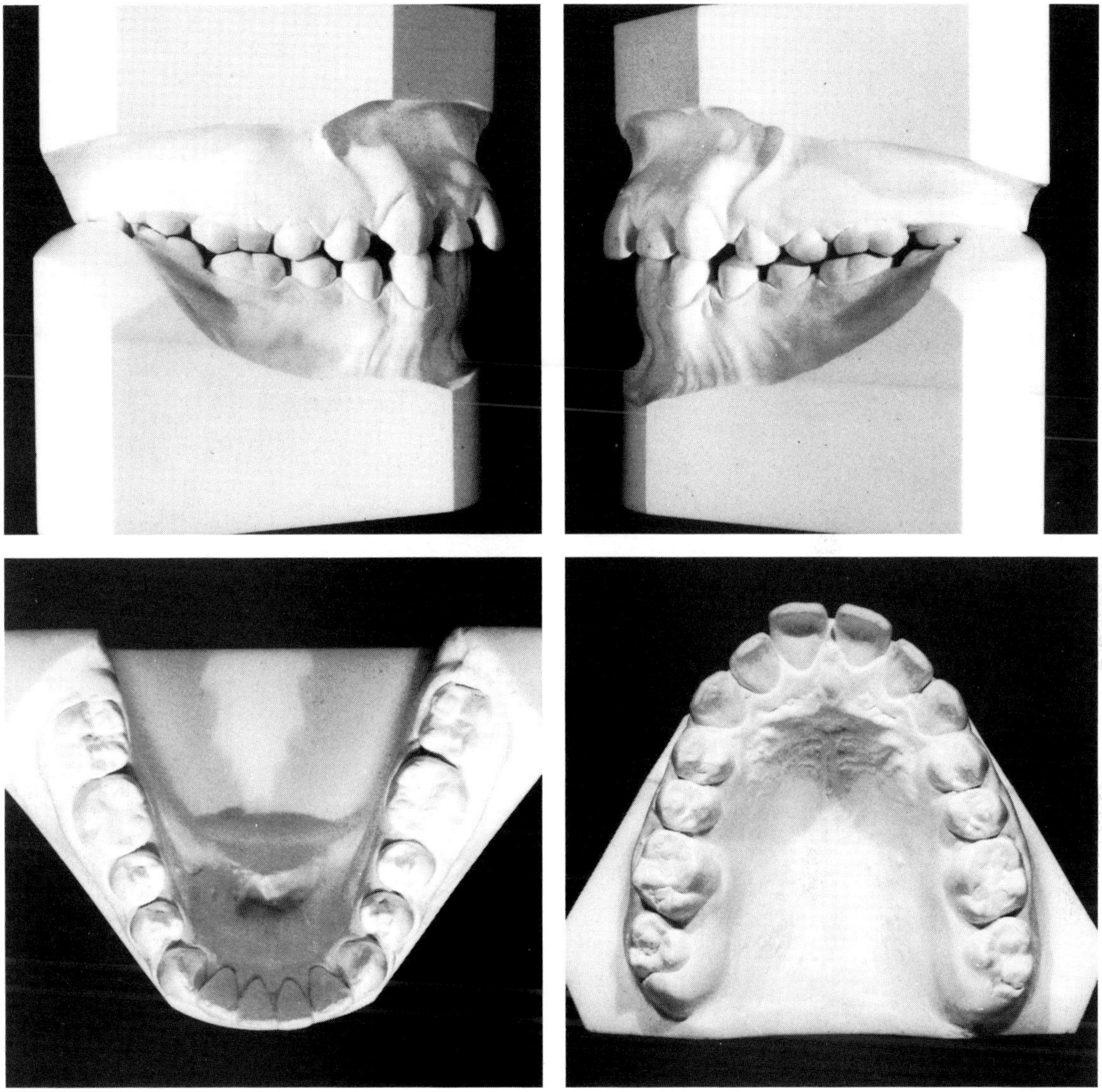

Figs 8-1 and 8-2 *A girl aged 12 y, 9 mo with a mild class II/1 anomaly. In the photographs the lips are held closed in a strained way. She habitually held her mouth open with her lower lip resting on the incisal edge of her maxillary incisors. The mandible lies more dorsally than the rest of the face. The disto-occlusion is ¼ PW; the relatively large overjet is due to the eversion of the maxillary incisors. There is an anterior open bite. On the right side, a solid interdigitation is lacking and both the maxillary premolars are positioned somewhat palatally. That applies also to the right first permanent molar, which in addition is rotated mesiopalatally.*

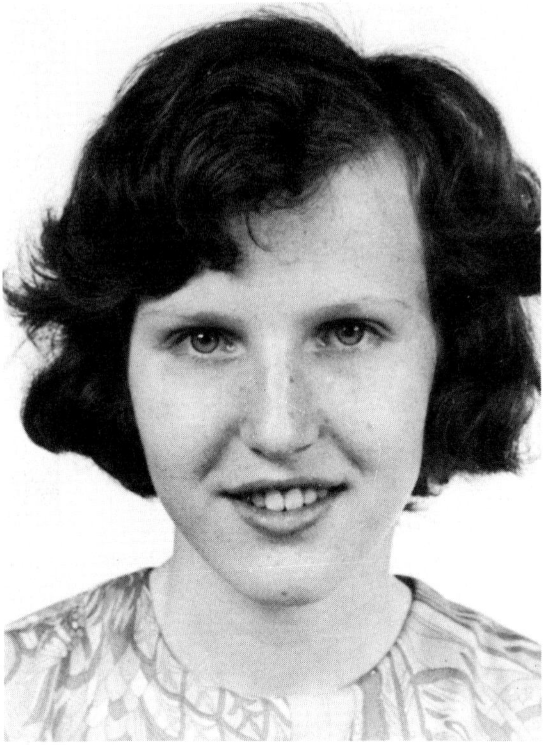

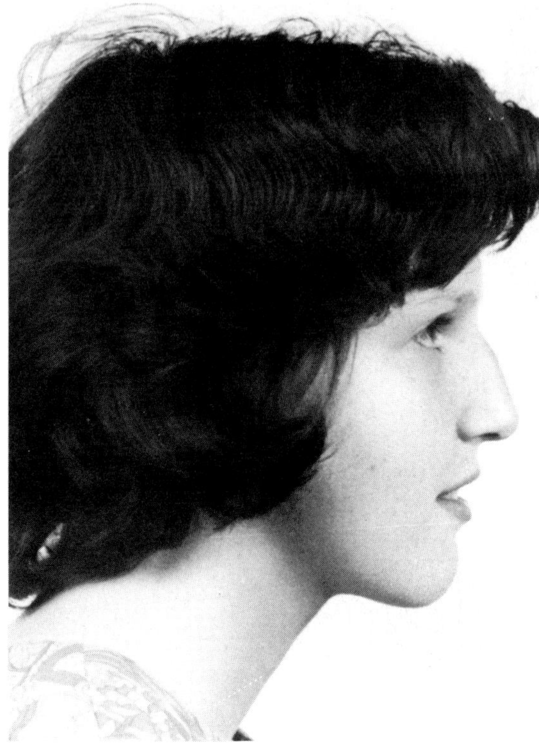

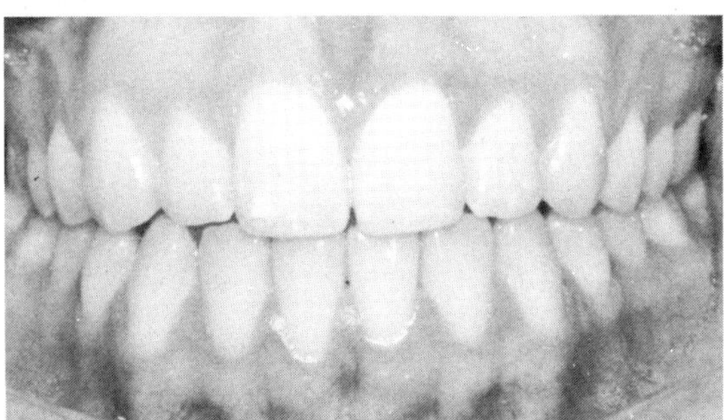

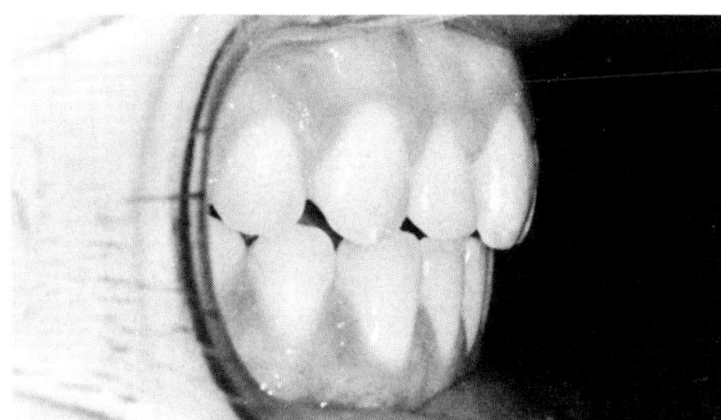

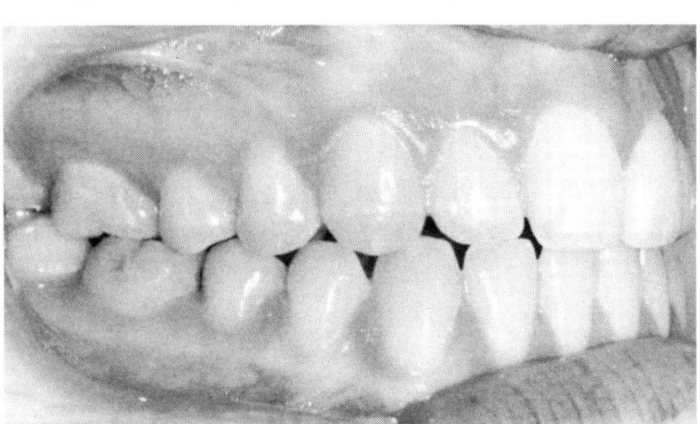

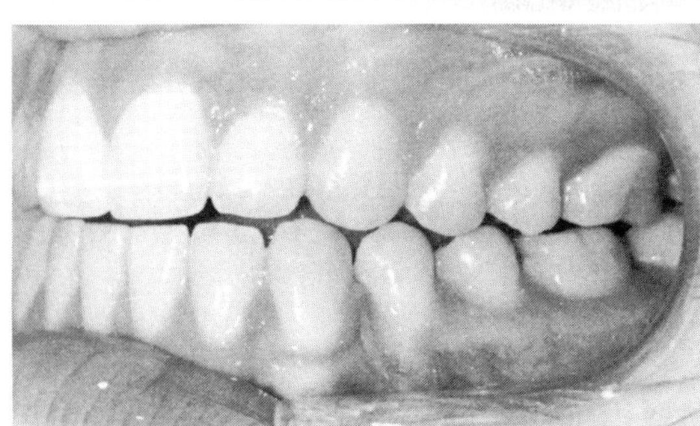

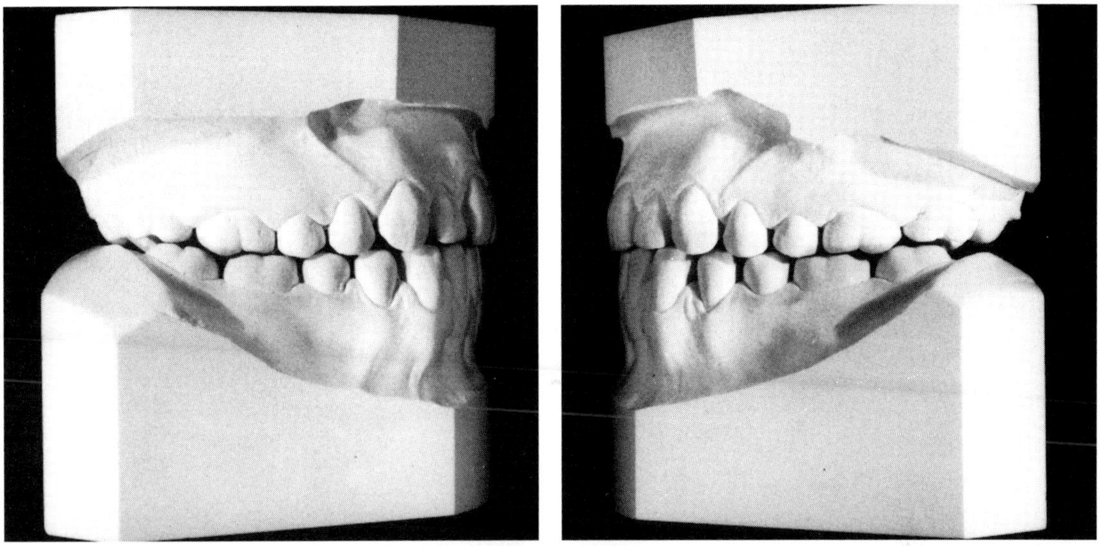

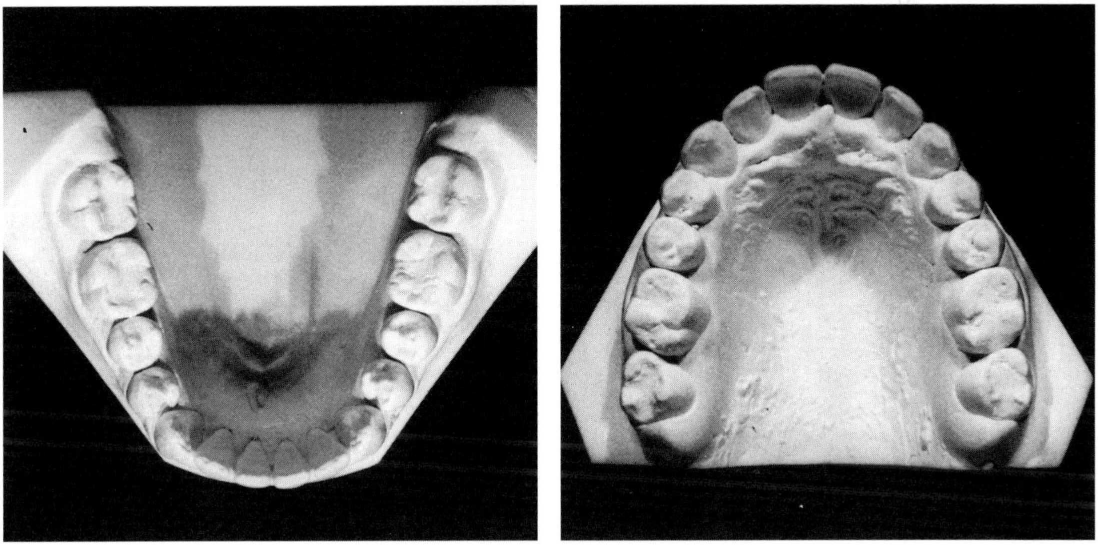

Figs 8-3 and 8-4 At the age of 15 y, 10 mo no competent lip seal was reached. The mouth was still often held open. The mandible had come relatively more ventrally, and the profile had improved. A slight anterior open bite exists and the posterior teeth do not interdigitate well. The maxillary right first permanent molar after having been rotated distally with the headgear, has returned mesially, probably because good vertical contact was lacking and excess space existed in the premolar region.

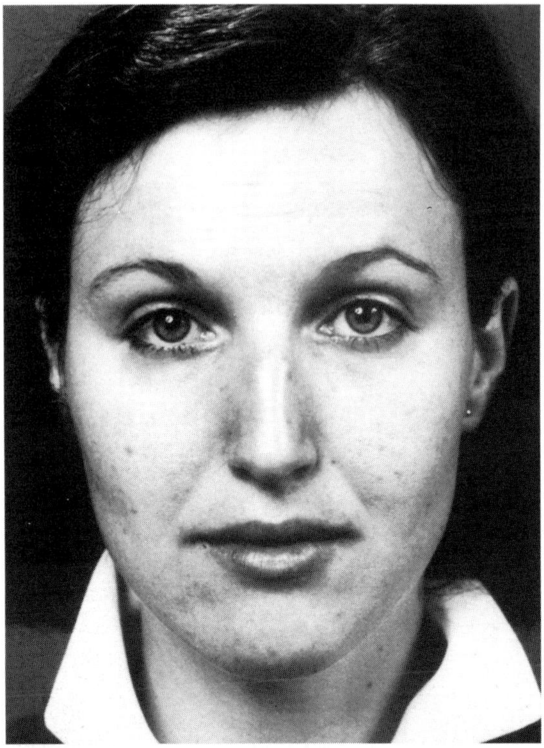

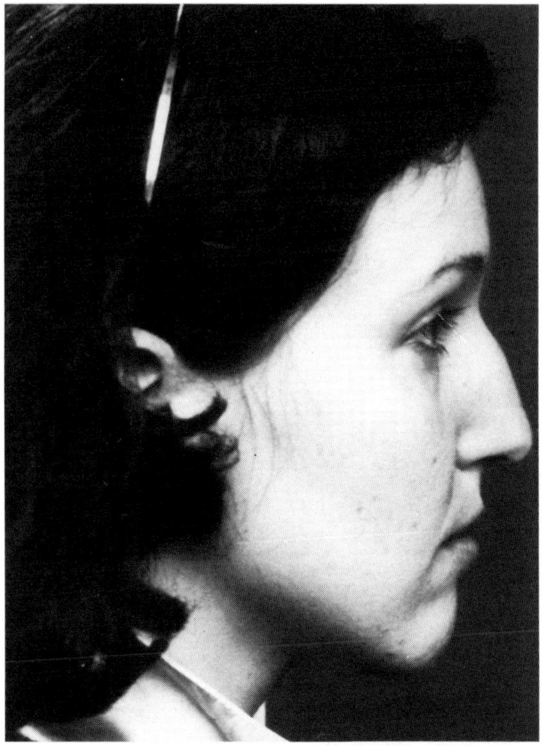

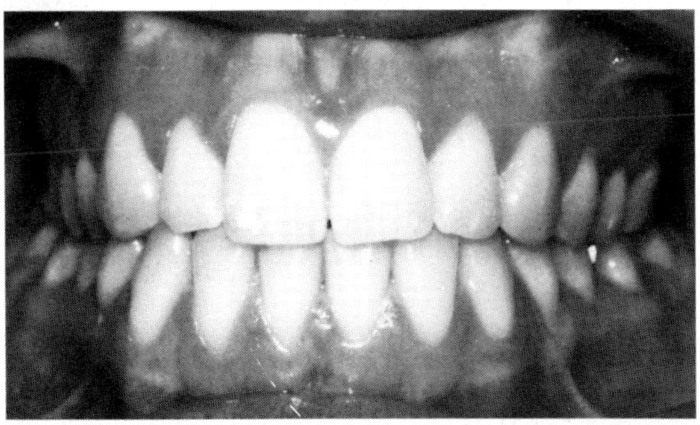

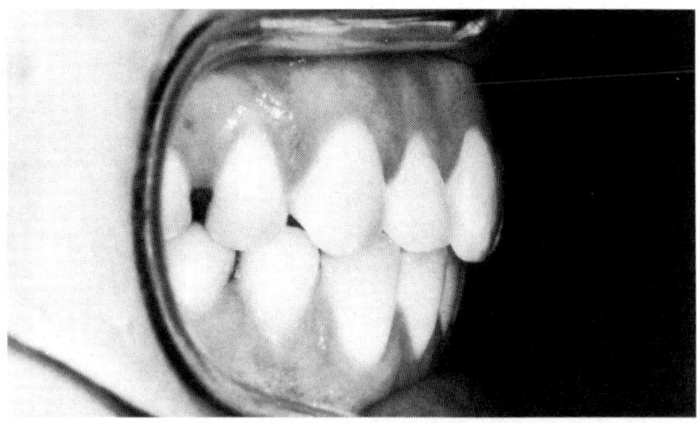

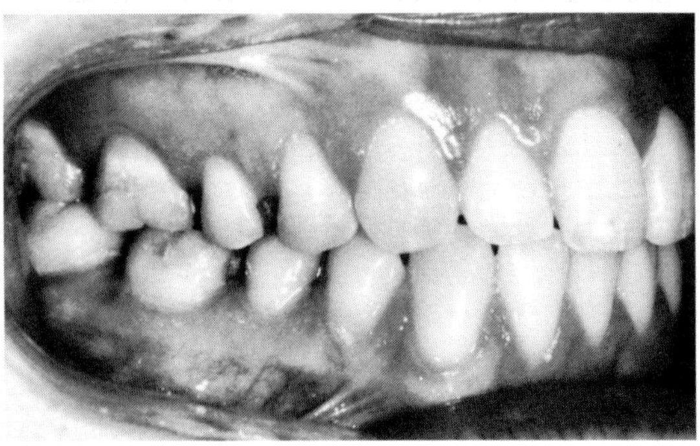

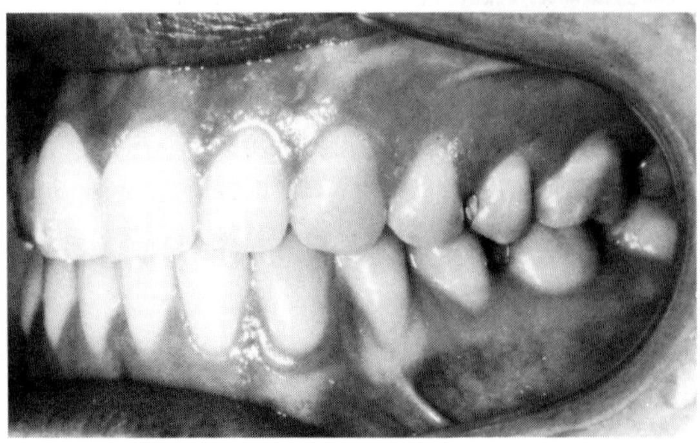

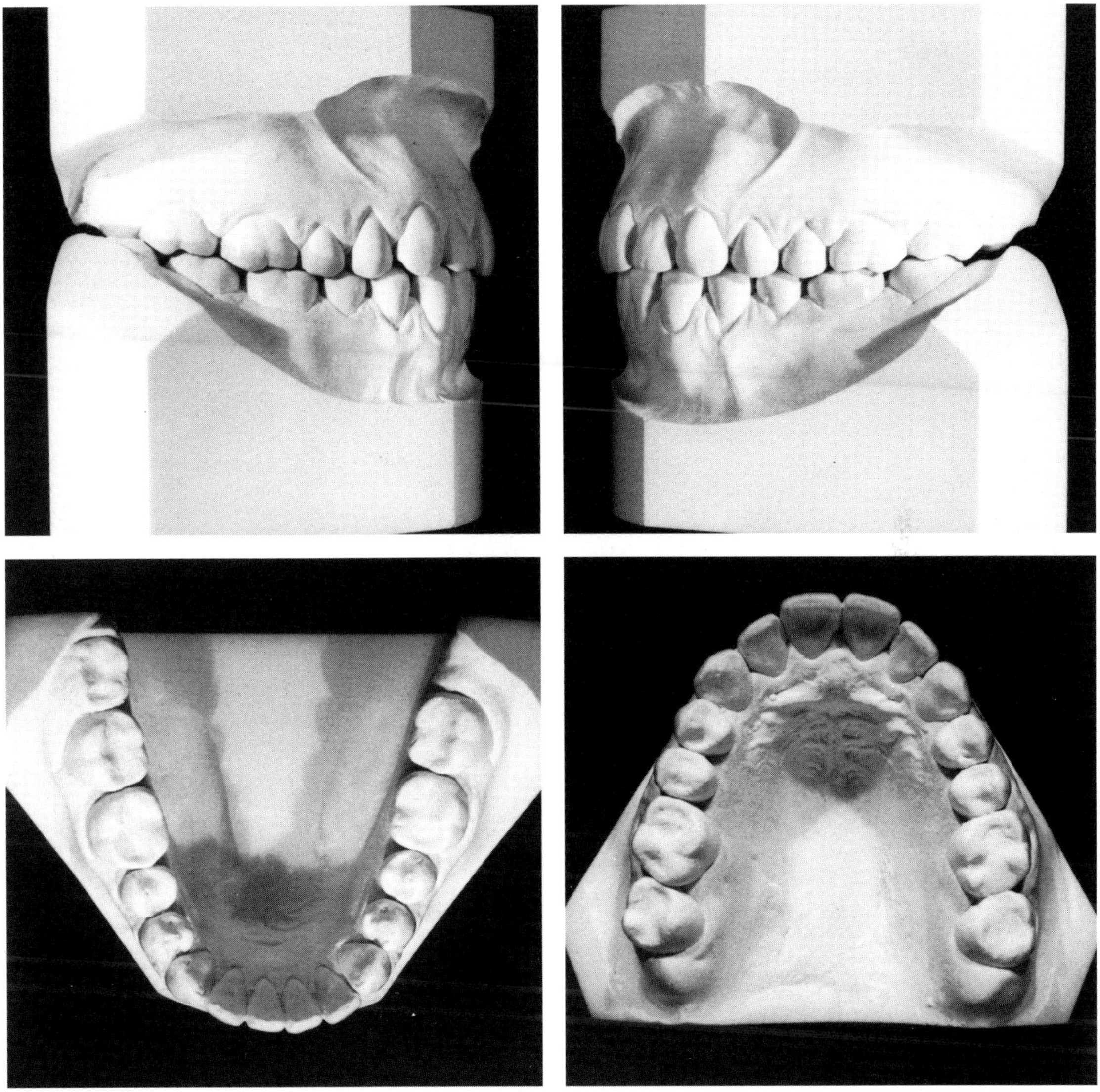

Figs 8-5 and 8-6 *At 26 y, 1 mo, the patient now holds her lips closed without difficulty. Her facial configuration is good. All teeth with the exception of the maxillary right first permanent molar are in ideal positions. Moreover they occlude perfectly. The open bite has vanished and a solid interdigitation and good articulation came about.*

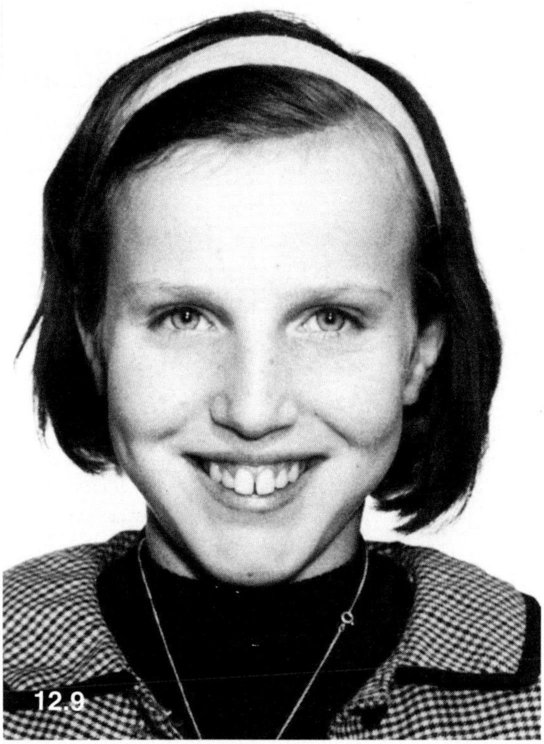

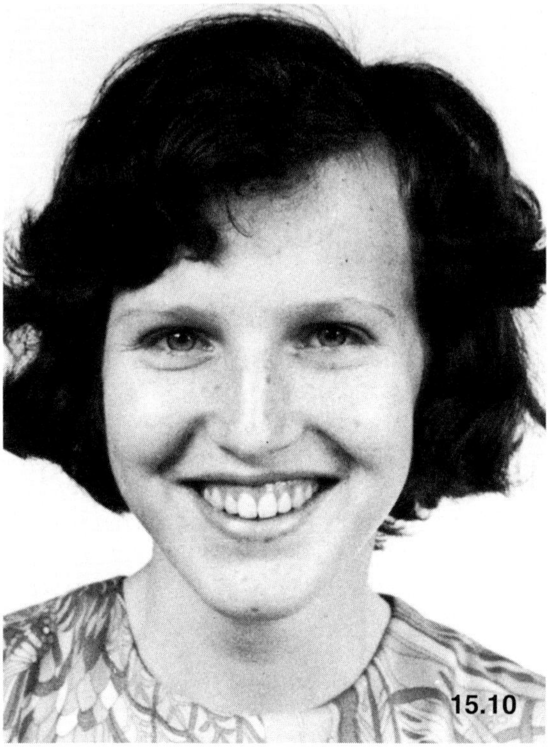

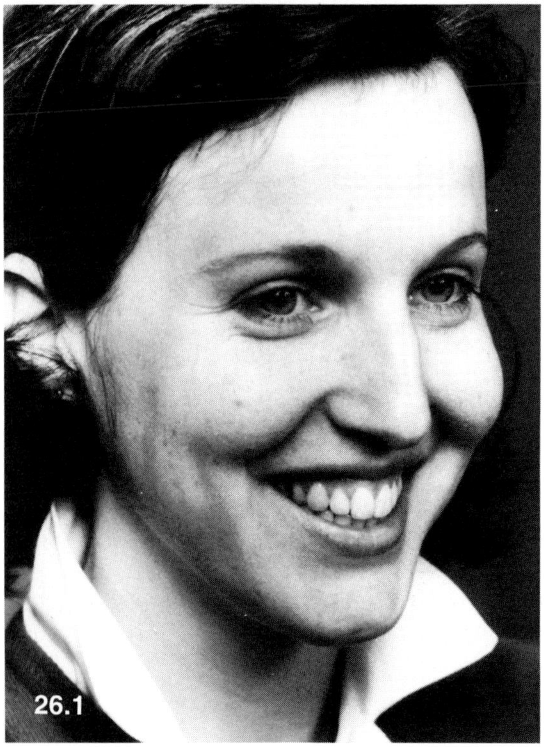

Fig 8-7 Note the improvements that occurred during treatment and the positive changes in her face and dentition that took place in the following ten years.

Two years later, the open bite appears to have closed and the posterior teeth developed fully into occlusion. This situation was maintained during the following years, as is demonstrated by the records taken at the age of 26 years (Figs 8.5 and 8.6). There was no longer any tongue interpositioning, the lips were held closed, and all the premolars and molars (except the rotated 16) occluded perfectly. During treatment, the mandible had developed ventrally more than had the maxilla. In subsequent years that tendency persisted without producing any disturbing addition to the height of the lower face, nor a deterioration of the occlusion. The photographs of the smiling face display esthetics that are in every way satisfying (Fig 8.7).

A positioner is an appliance made from rubber or other suitable flexible material, with which it is possible to secure limited minor corrections. It is made on a "set-up," in which the teeth of plaster are placed in their correct positions.[36] Mostly, after the completion of active treatment, new dental impressions have to be taken since the models made in the beginning might not have included all the permanent teeth, whose clinical crowns in any case would have lengthened in the interim. With the positioner, small diastemata can be closed, minor labiolingual movements can be achieved, and better interdigitation of the posterior teeth encouraged. Changes requiring a force and a couple to cause them, such as certain rotations, changes in angulation and application of torque, cannot be achieved with a positioner. This also applies to the reduction of a deep bite.

The positioner is usually fabricated in neutro-occlusion. If there originally was a disto-occlusion, a slight mesio-occlusion can be built into it. The positioner works as the result of deformation of the material when the teeth are bitten into it. This produces a force that induces movement of the teeth into their correct positions as dictated by the "set-up." To obtain this desired result, the patient must intermittently bite as hard as possible into the appliance for at least four hours per day for about four weeks. The appliance should be worn also while sleeping and continued to provide retention after the changes are realized.

Class II/1 anomalies with an open bite resulting from tongue interposition react differently to facial-orthopedic treatment than would be the case otherwise.[32, 36] Generally a marked increase in lower face height occurs during or after treatment, producing esthetic changes that often are thought to be unpleasing.

In the case under discussion, the tongue interposition disappeared naturally. But as well, no abnormal increase in the lower face height occurred during or after the therapy. Furthermore, the maxillary incisors had not moved labially after treatment. From the evidence it seems that the tongue interposition in this case was of a temporary nature and could have been caused by the earlier orthodontic treatment in which the plate limited the room available for the tongue and interfered with vertical contact between the incisors. Then in the course of the treatment just described, the use of a plate may well have brought about the same conditions. After the treatment, the room for the tongue seemed to have increased sufficiently by growth and ceasing to wear the appliances for the interposition to be eliminated.

The course of events shown here subsequent to treatment is by no means the rule. Unfortunately the closing of an open bite and attainment of solid interdigitation in patients with tongue interposition belongs to the world of exceptions.

Nonetheless, from this case, it should be very clear how important it is to be observant before, during, and many years after treatment. If the open bite had not diminished after treatment, then it is certain that part of the deviation would have returned. Had retreatment once more been undertaken, then some form of permanent retention would have been mandatory.[35]

Chapter 9

Class II/1
Activator, Bass plate with parietal headgear, positioner
Female: 10 years, 8 months to 25 years, 0 months

A girl who was 10 years, 8 months old presented with a class II/1 anomaly with a relatively retruded mandible and short upper lip. She could breathe through her nose easily, but kept her mouth open most of the time with her lower lip partly behind the maxillary incisors. When she smiled she displayed rather a lot of gum. There was a disto-occlusion of ½ PW, an overjet of 5 mm, eversion of the maxillary incisors and a slight excess of space in both dental arches (ALD in mandible +2 mm, in maxilla +3 mm) (Figs 9.1 and 9.2).

It was decided to treat her with an activator. After nine months, the disto-occlusion was corrected and treatment was halted (Figs 9.3 and 9.4). A little over two years later, the disto-occlusion had returned to a small degree (Figs 9.5 and 9.6) and the treatment was resumed with appliances with which the maxillary incisors could be intruded to reduce the amount of visible gingiva. For this purpose, a combination of a Bass plate and a parietal headgear was used. The headgear is anchored against the upper posterior surface of the head and is attached to the maxillary appliance in the region of the incisors with hooks into eyelets. In this way a dorso-cranial force is applied to the anterior part of the maxilla (Fig 9.15). Twelve months later, a neutro-occlusion had been realized and the maxillary incisors had been sufficiently intruded (Figs 9.7 and 9.8).

To make further corrections to individual teeth, but also with the intention of providing retention, a positioner was fitted and worn intensively for one month, and nights only for a further 17 months. The photographs and models collected ten months after the positioner had been discarded show a fine result (Figs 9.9 and 9.10). However, a certain amount of tertiary crowding had developed in the mandible. In the following years little change occurred although the tertiary crowding did increase slightly (Figs 9.11 to 9.13). The result could be described as stable. What was important for the patient was that she no longer showed so much gum when smiling as can be observed on the oblique photographs taken at different ages (Fig 9.14).

A short upper lip often leaves a large part of the gum above the maxillary anterior teeth exposed when smiling. This also occurs when a lip of adequate length is lifted up more than normal in smiling or when the maxillary anterior teeth have overerupted. Whether or not a gummy smile is considered intrusive depends on the structure, color, and form of the gingiva; the position, color, and form of the teeth; and the patient's facial form and personality. In some situations, a gummy smile is

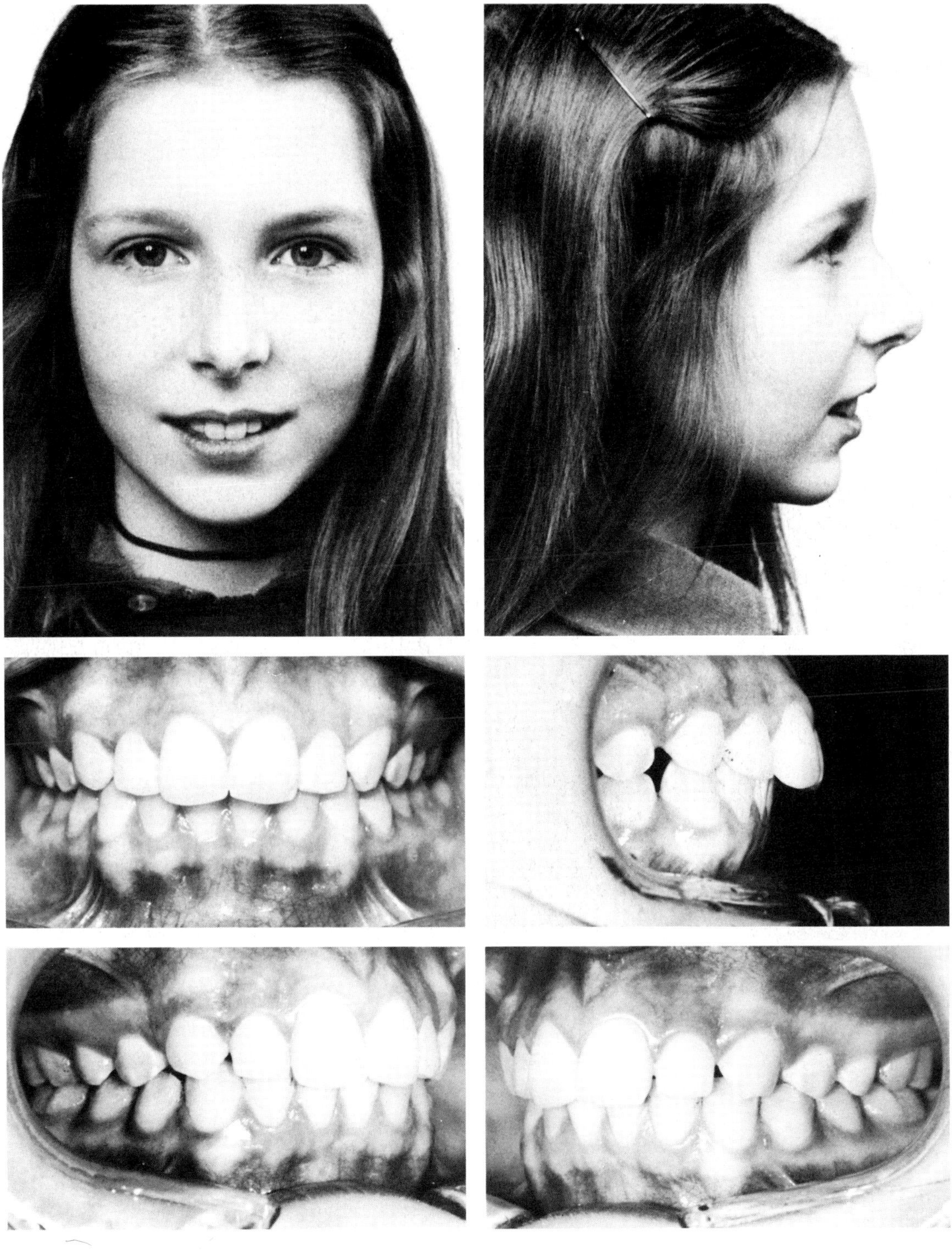

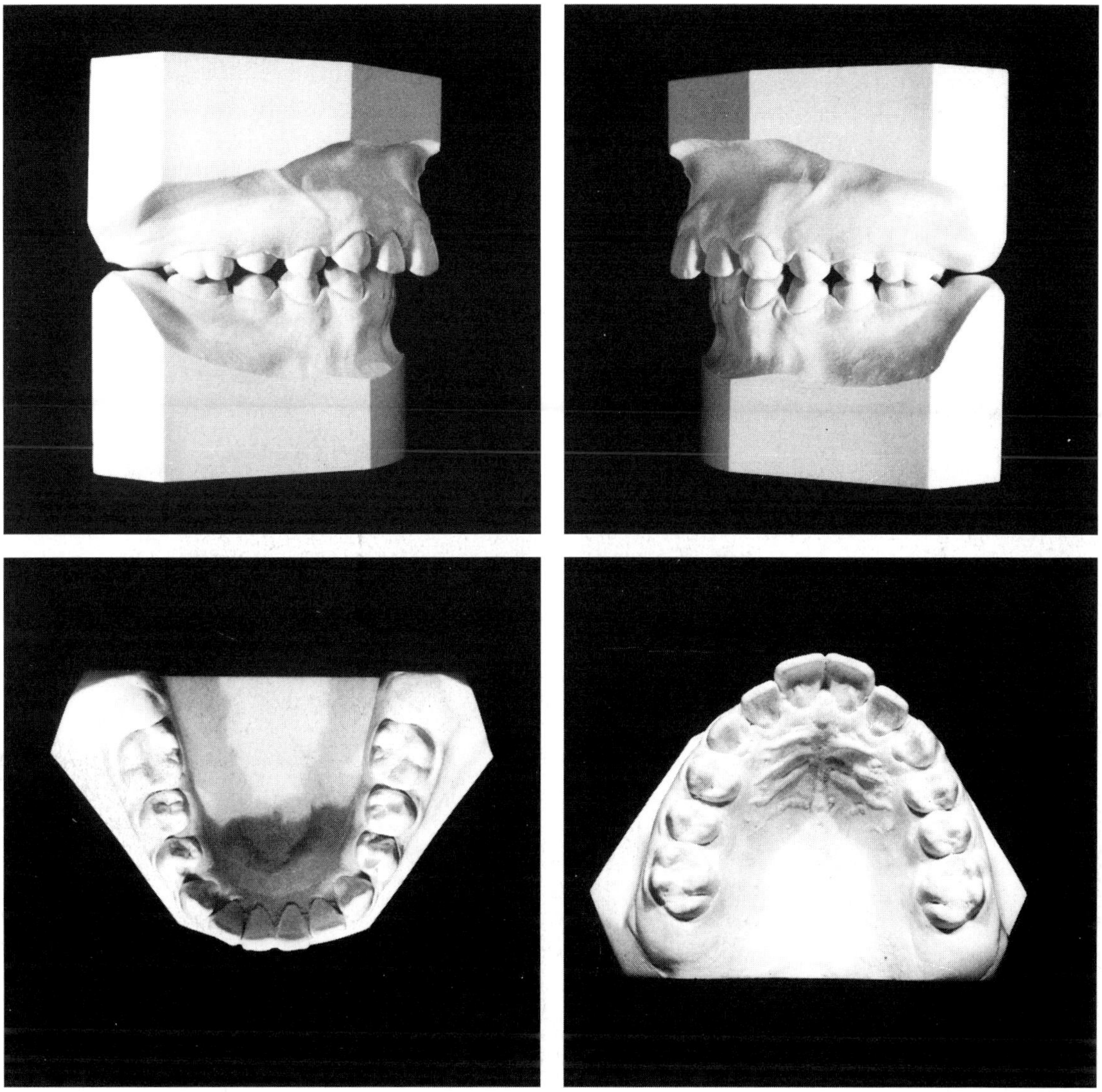

Figs 9-1 and 9-2 A girl aged 10 y, 8 mo had a class II/1 anomaly (disto-occlusion of ½ PW), a short upper lip, an open mouth, and a lower lip that lies partly behind the maxillary incisors. There is a mild excess of space in both arches. The maxillary incisors, particularly the central incisors, are everted. The overjet is 5 mm.

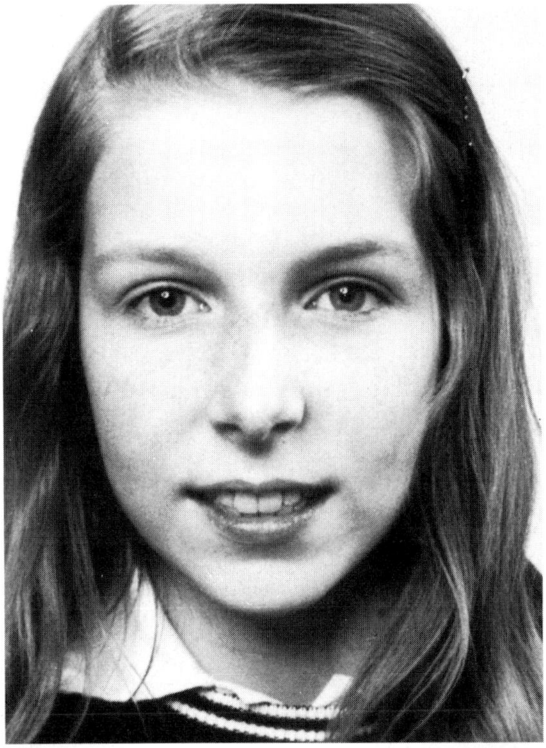
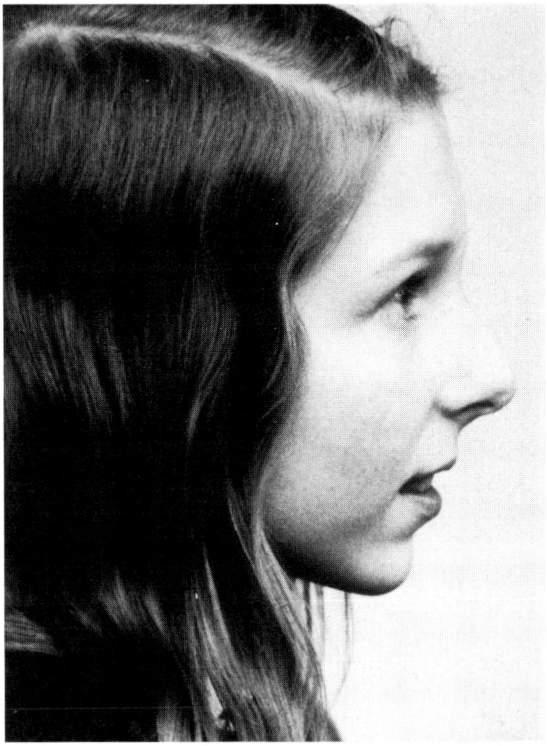
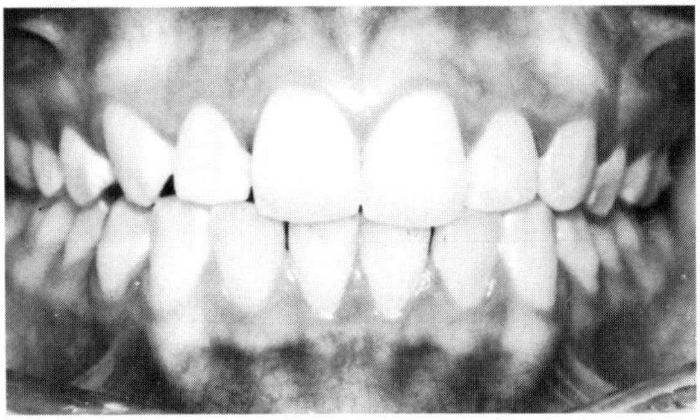
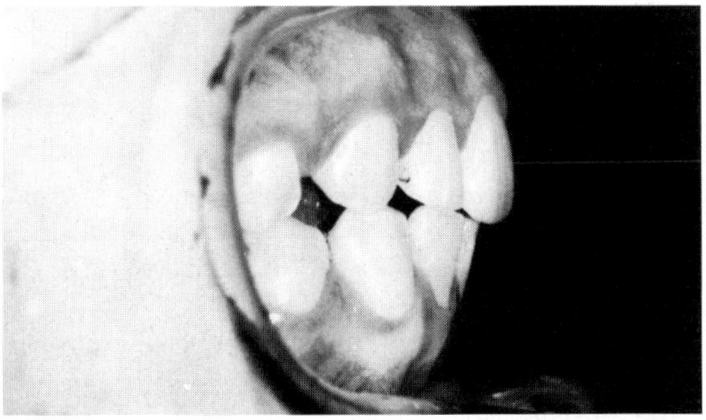
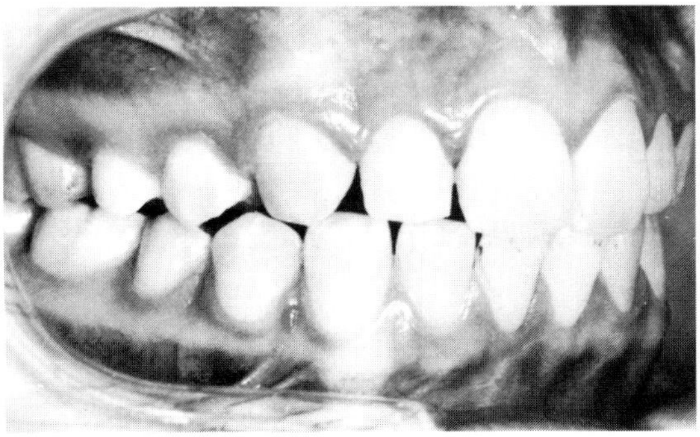
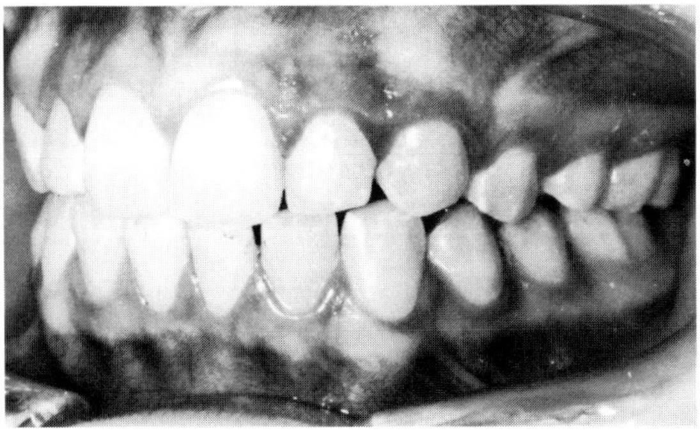

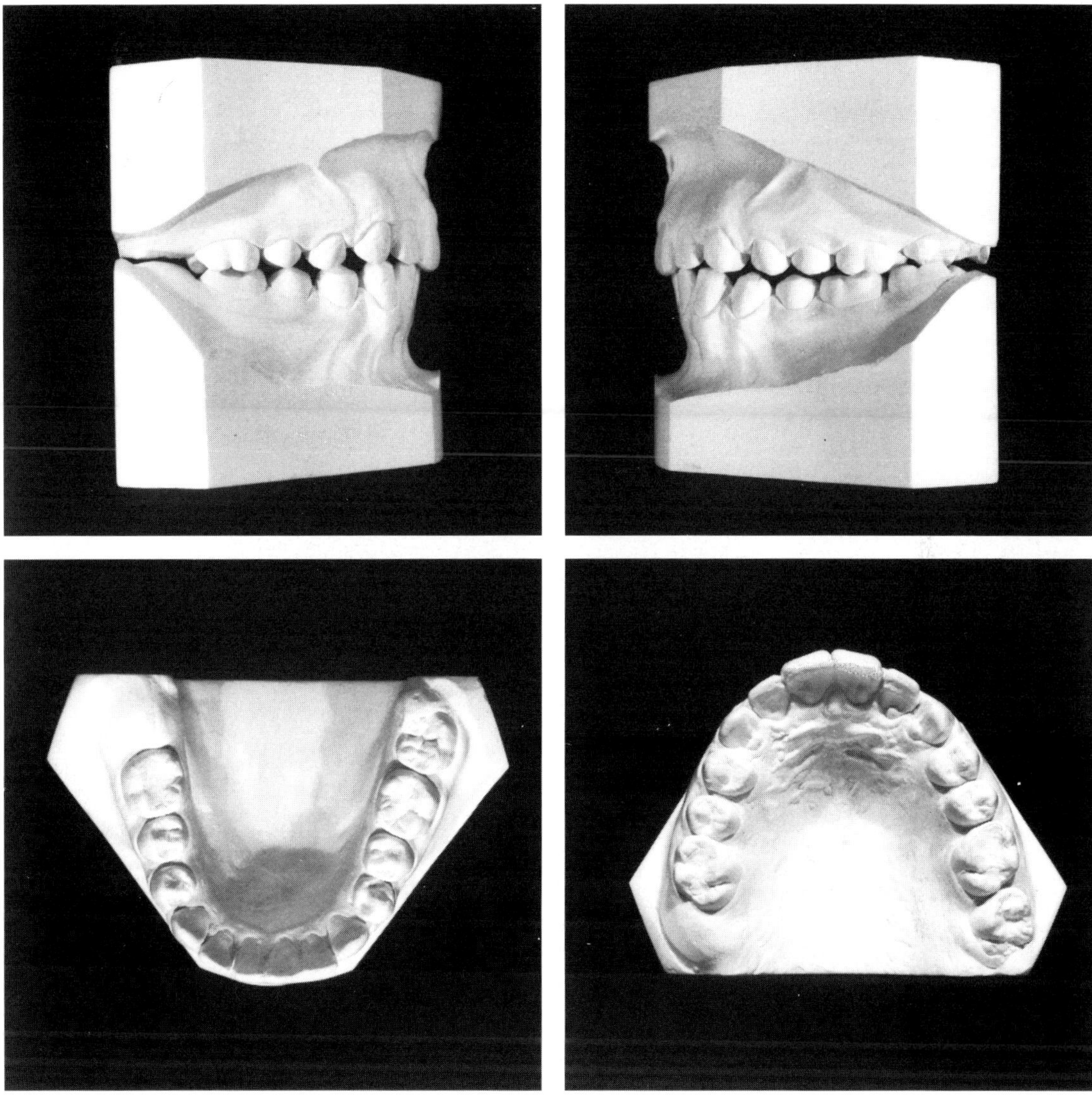

Figs 9-3 and 9-4 *At the age of 11 y, 6 mo, the disto-occlusion is corrected after nine months of activator therapy. The teeth have taken up good positions in both arches; the interdigitation leaves something to be desired. Lip seal is still not adequate and a "high gum-line" is still seen when smiling.*

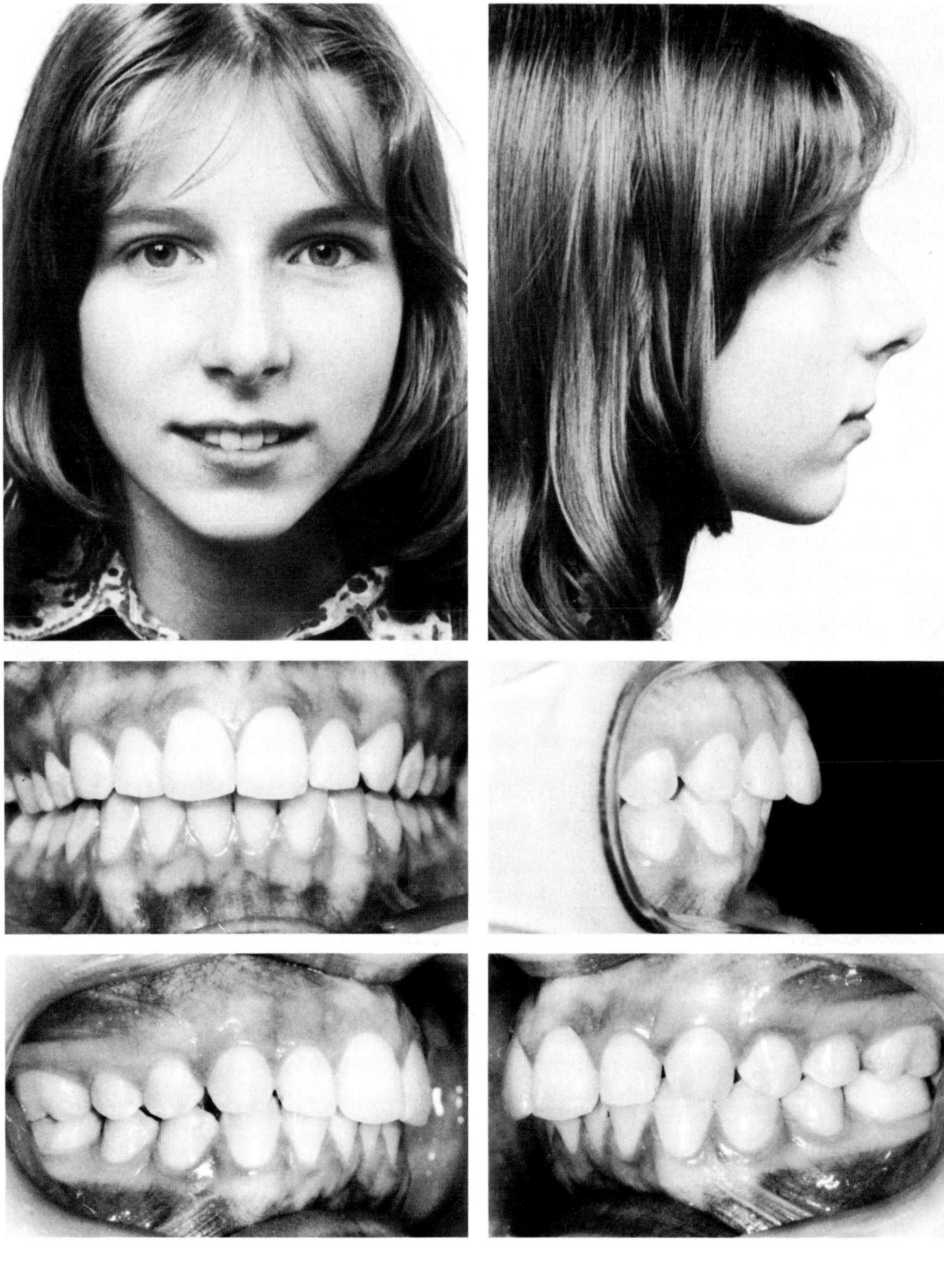

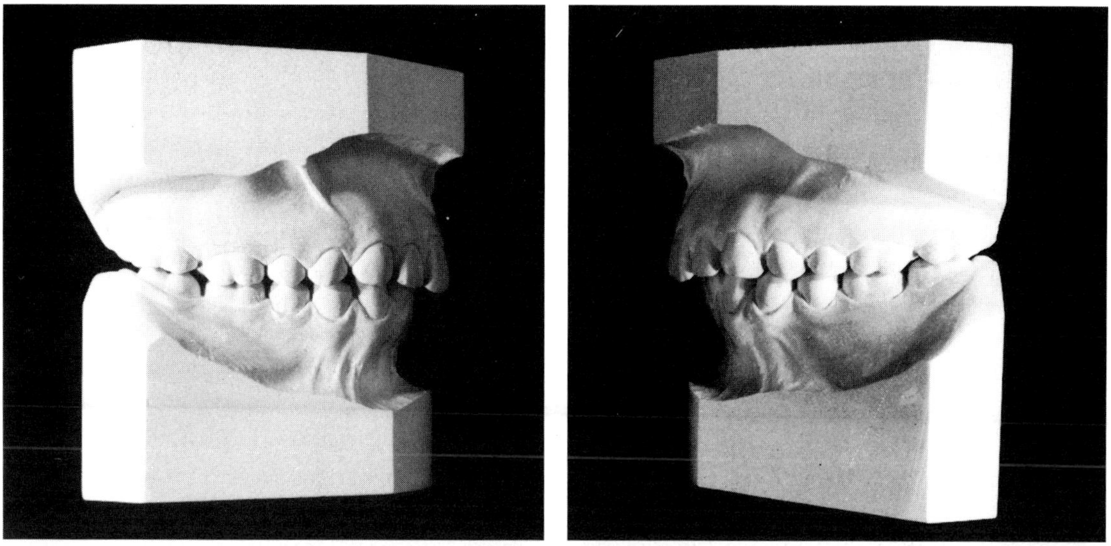

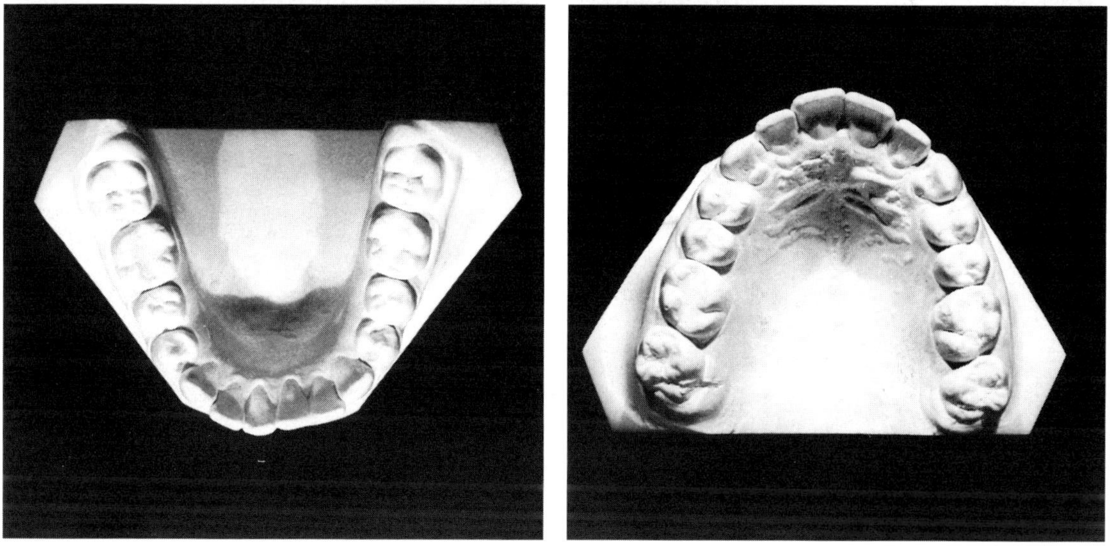

Figs 9-5 and 9-6 *At the age of 13 y, 9 mo, the disto-occlusion has returned to some extent. The upper lip is short in relationship to the rest of the face, and it cannot be expected that this relationship will change much during growth. The gum is still exposed when smiling. The maxillary and mandibular incisors now are a little irregular.*

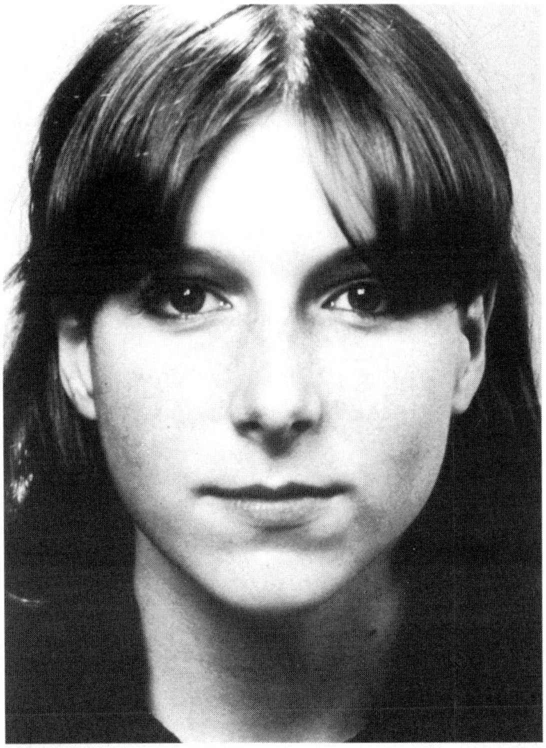
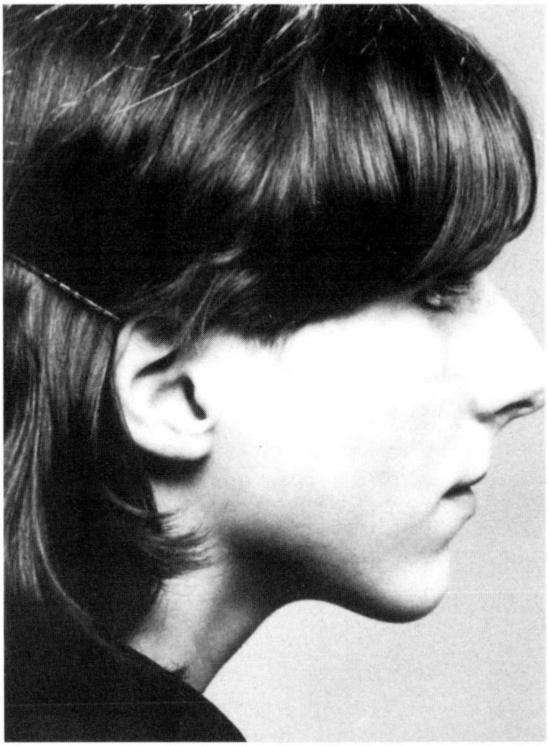
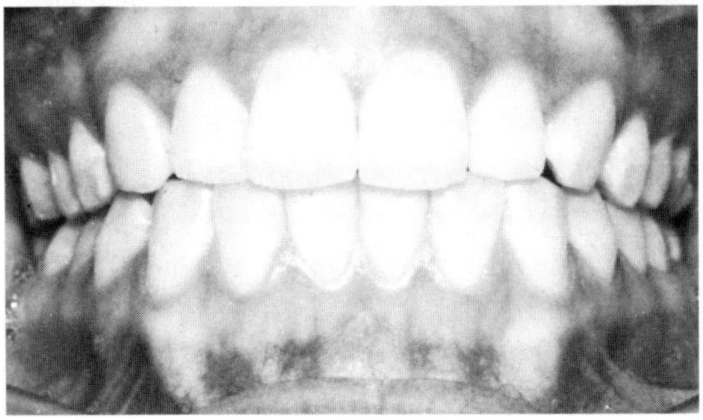
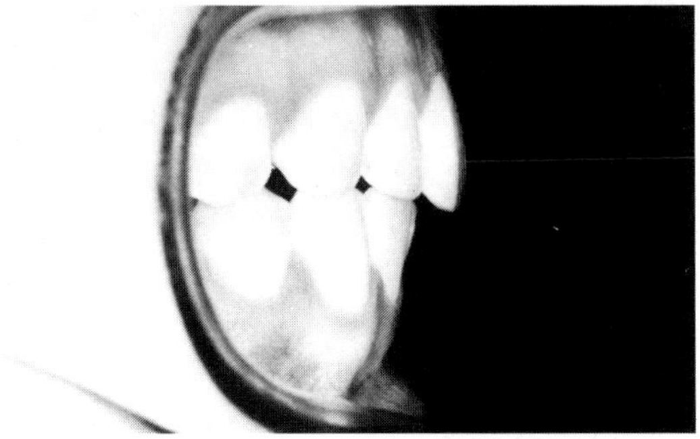
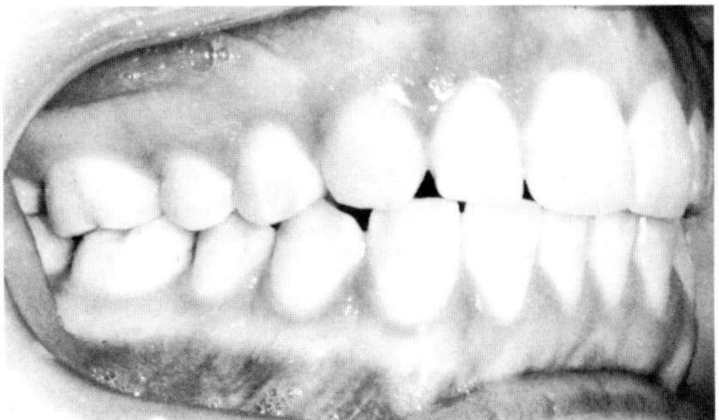
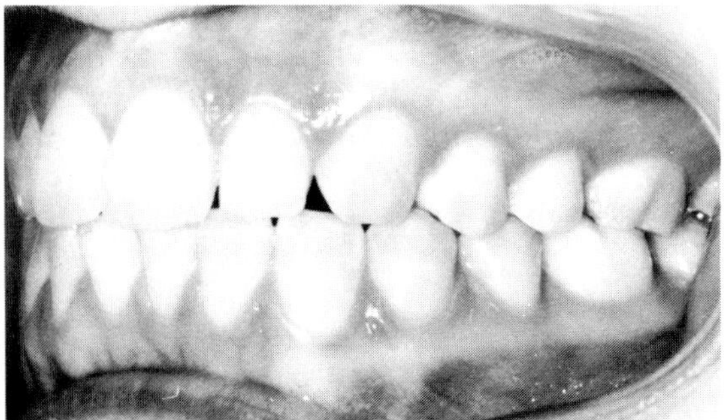

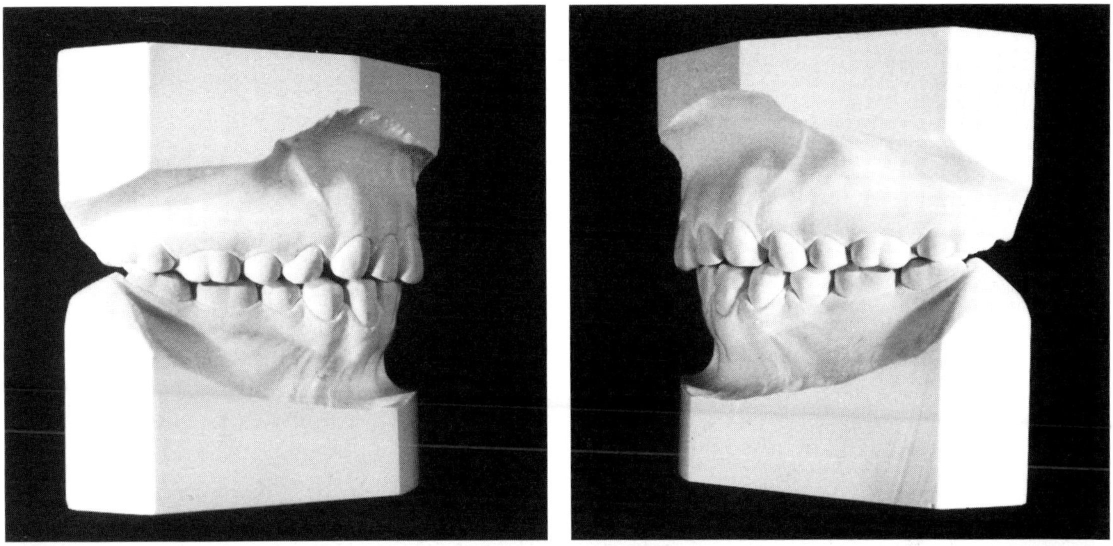

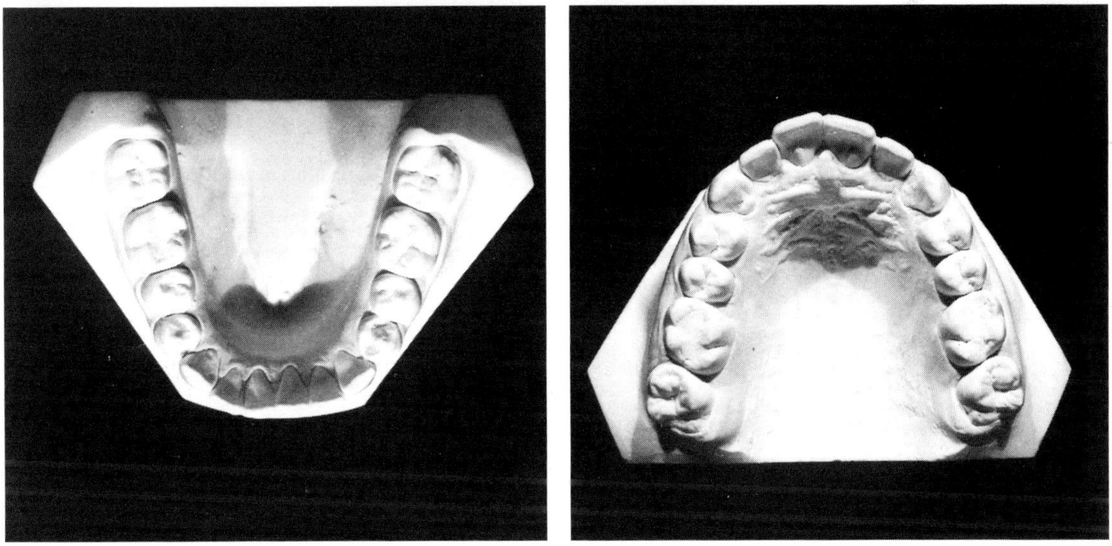

Figs 9-7 and 9-8 *By the age of 14 y, 10 mo, it has been possible to attain a neutro-occlusion and good interdigitation with a Bass plate and parietal headgear for a year. Above all, the maxillary incisors have been intruded and a competent lip seal exists.*

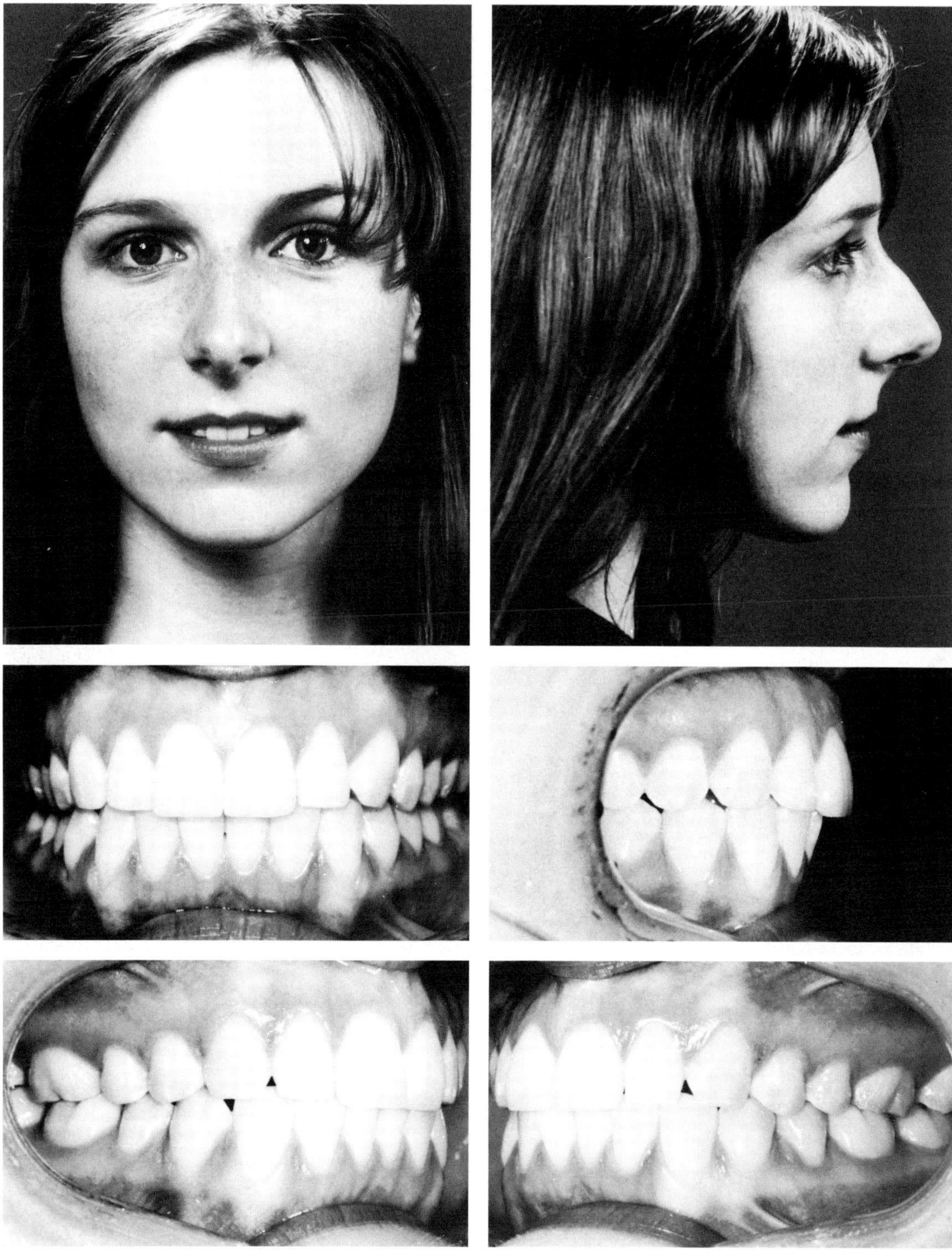

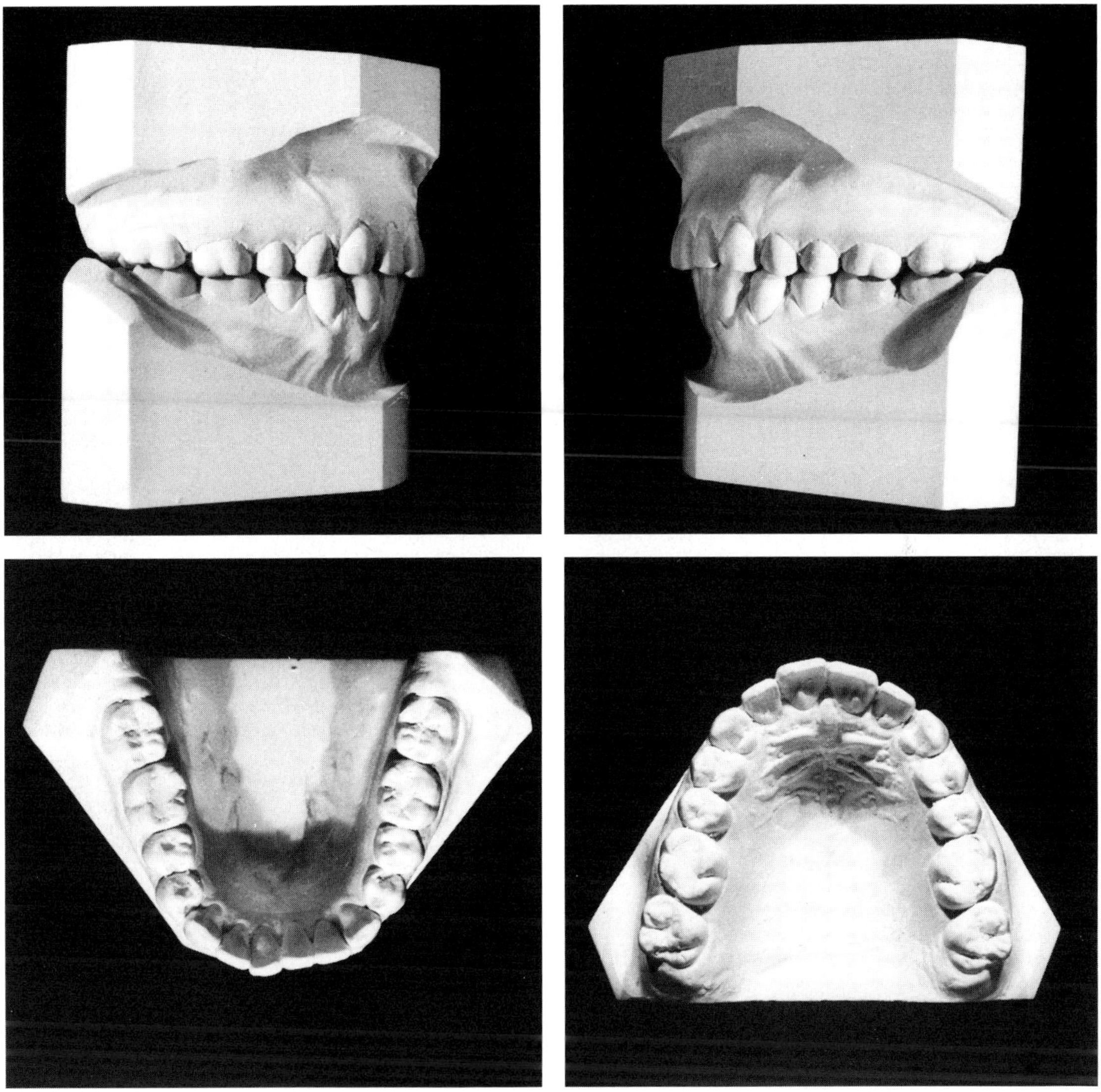

Figs 9-9 and 9-10 *At the age of 17 y, 4 mo, one year after ending retention with the positioner, the result is satisfactory.*

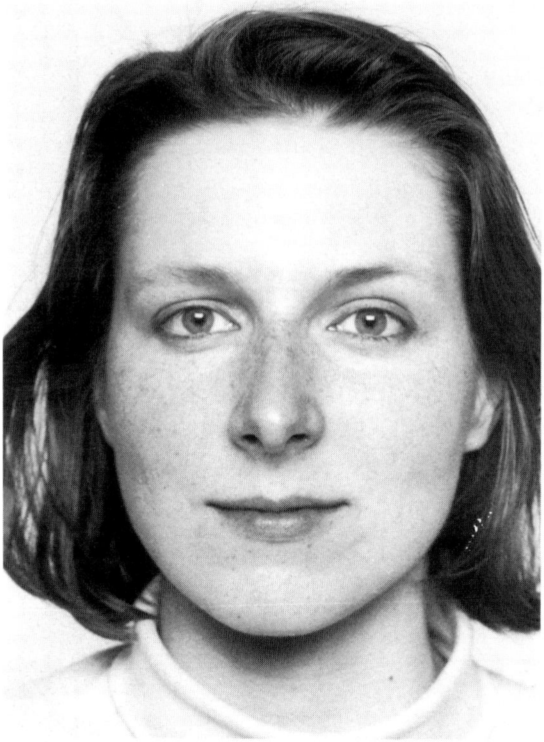
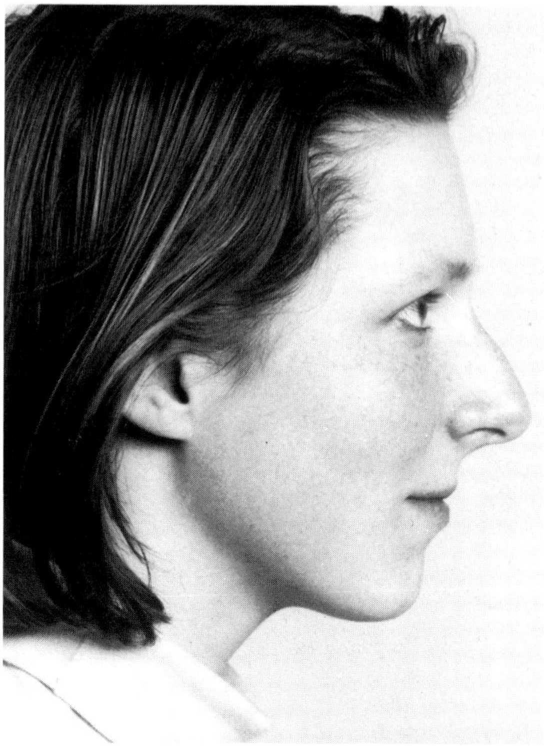
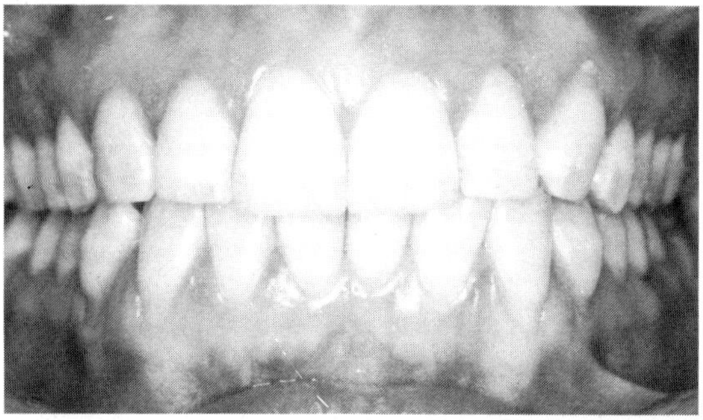
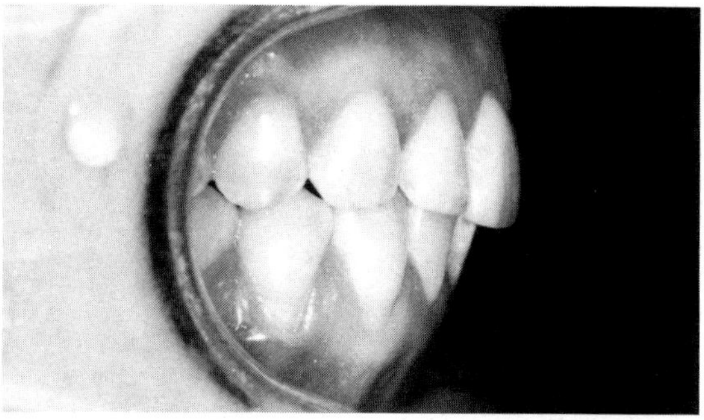
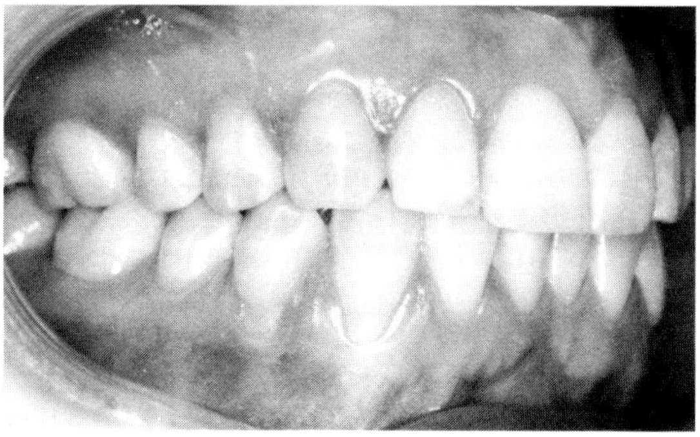
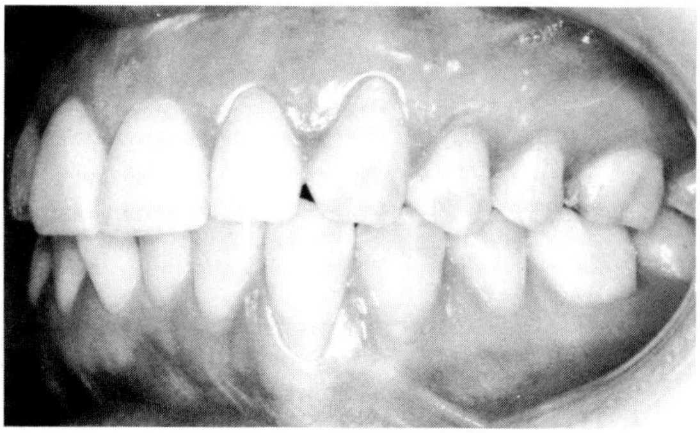

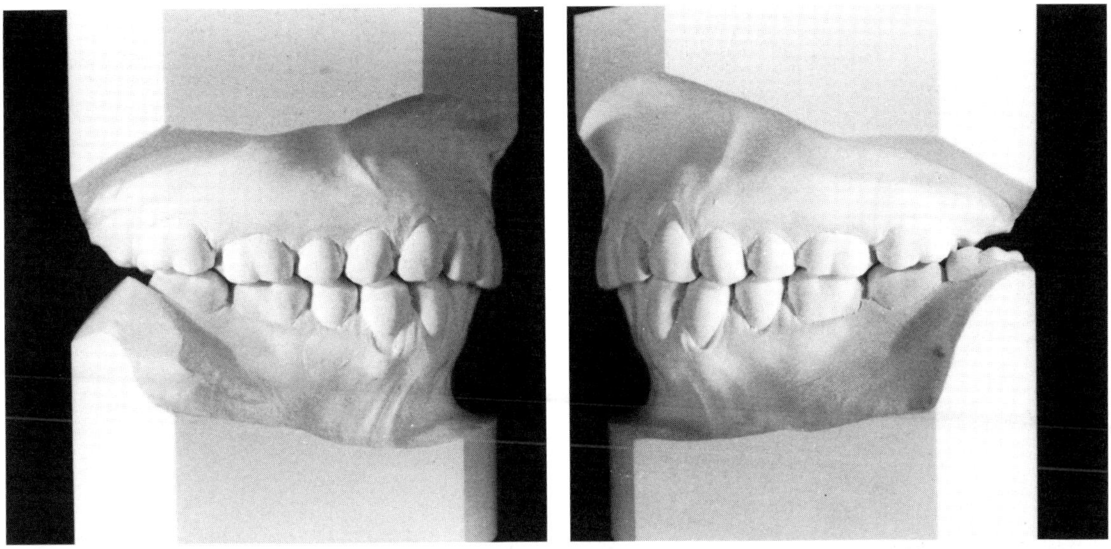

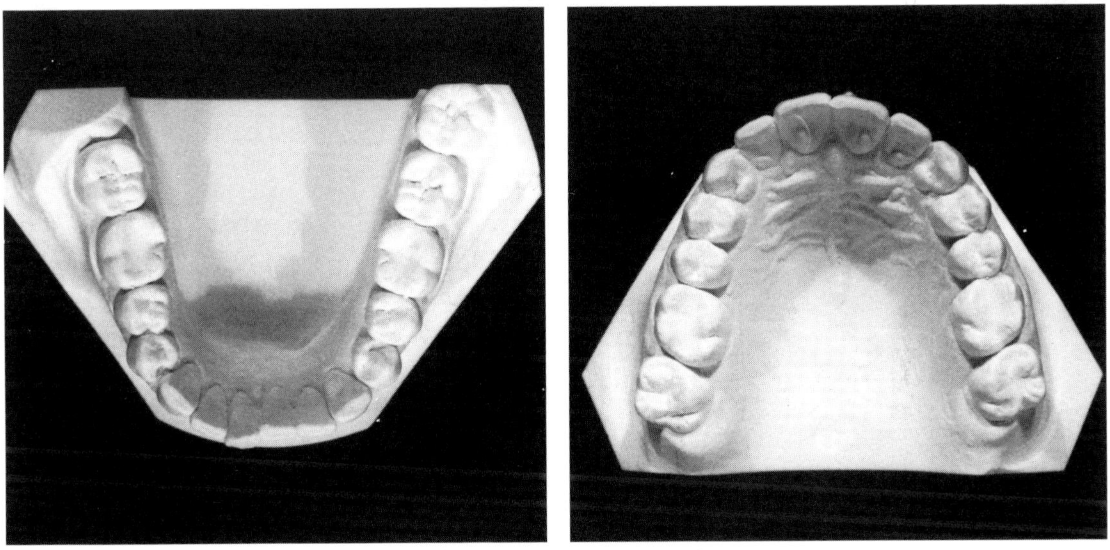

Figs 9-11 and 9-12 *At the age of 25 y in comparison with the records taken five years previously but not shown here, little has changed and it is clear that the second treatment phase has produced a permanent improvement. The maturation of the lips during which the upper lip had grown somewhat longer and thinner and the lower lip somewhat thicker, took place mainly between the ages of 17 and 20 years. This applies also to the development of tertiary crowding in the mandibular anterior region.*

Figure 9-13a

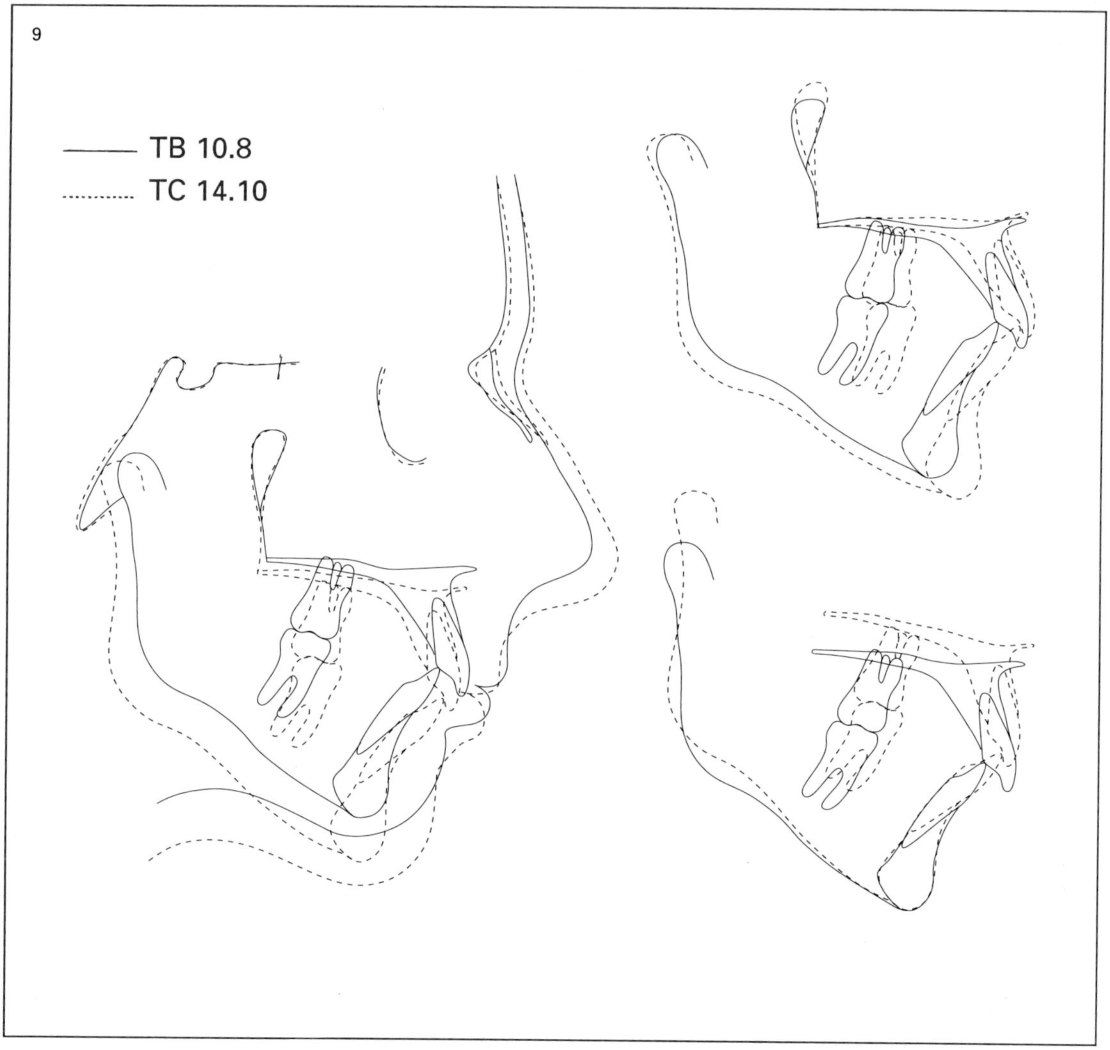

Figs 9-13a and 9-13b Superimposed tracings of cephalometric radiographs taken before treatment (TB), after treatment (TC), and a full 10 years after treatment (10PT). During treatment, the jaw relationship improved and the maxillary incisors have been intruded.

Figure 9-13b

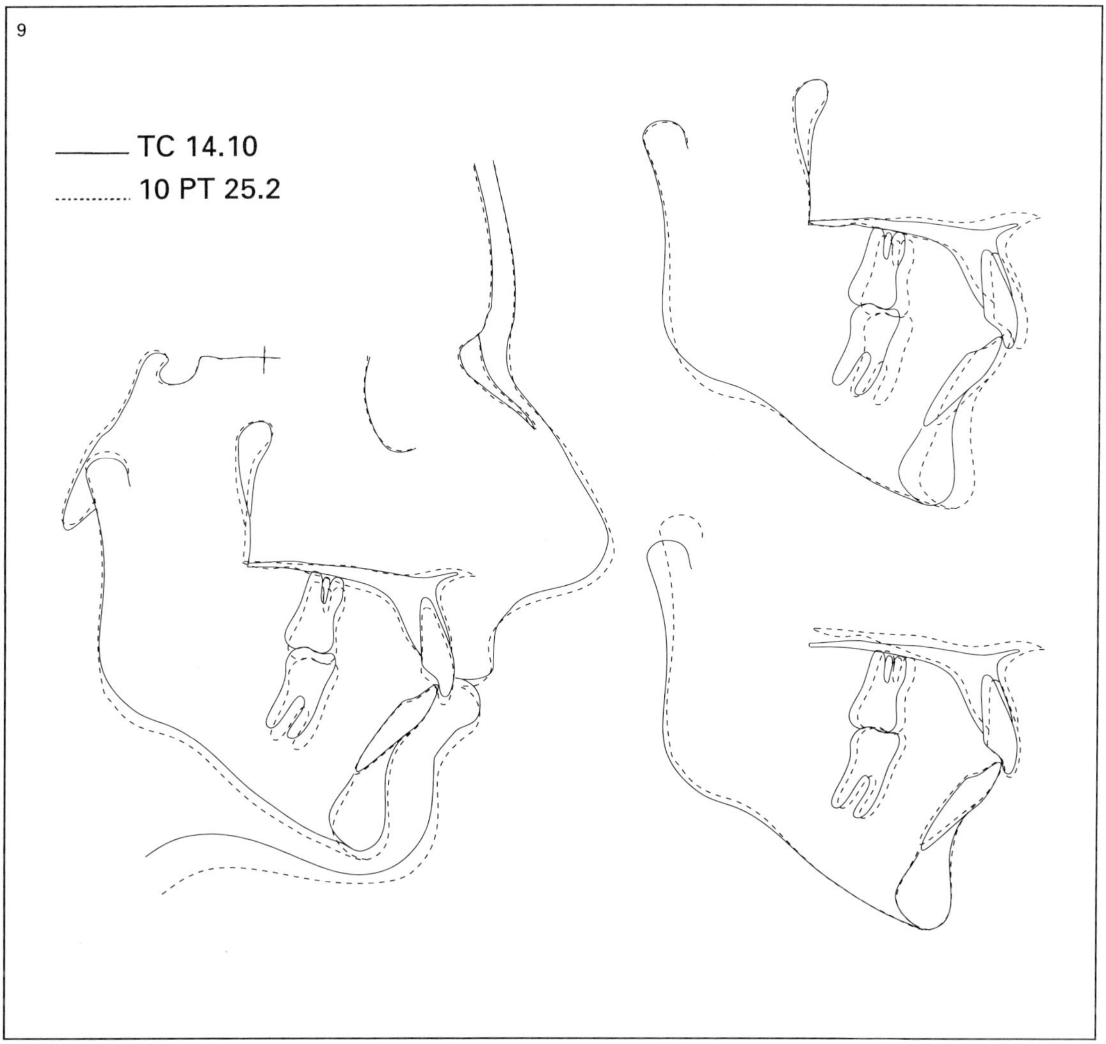

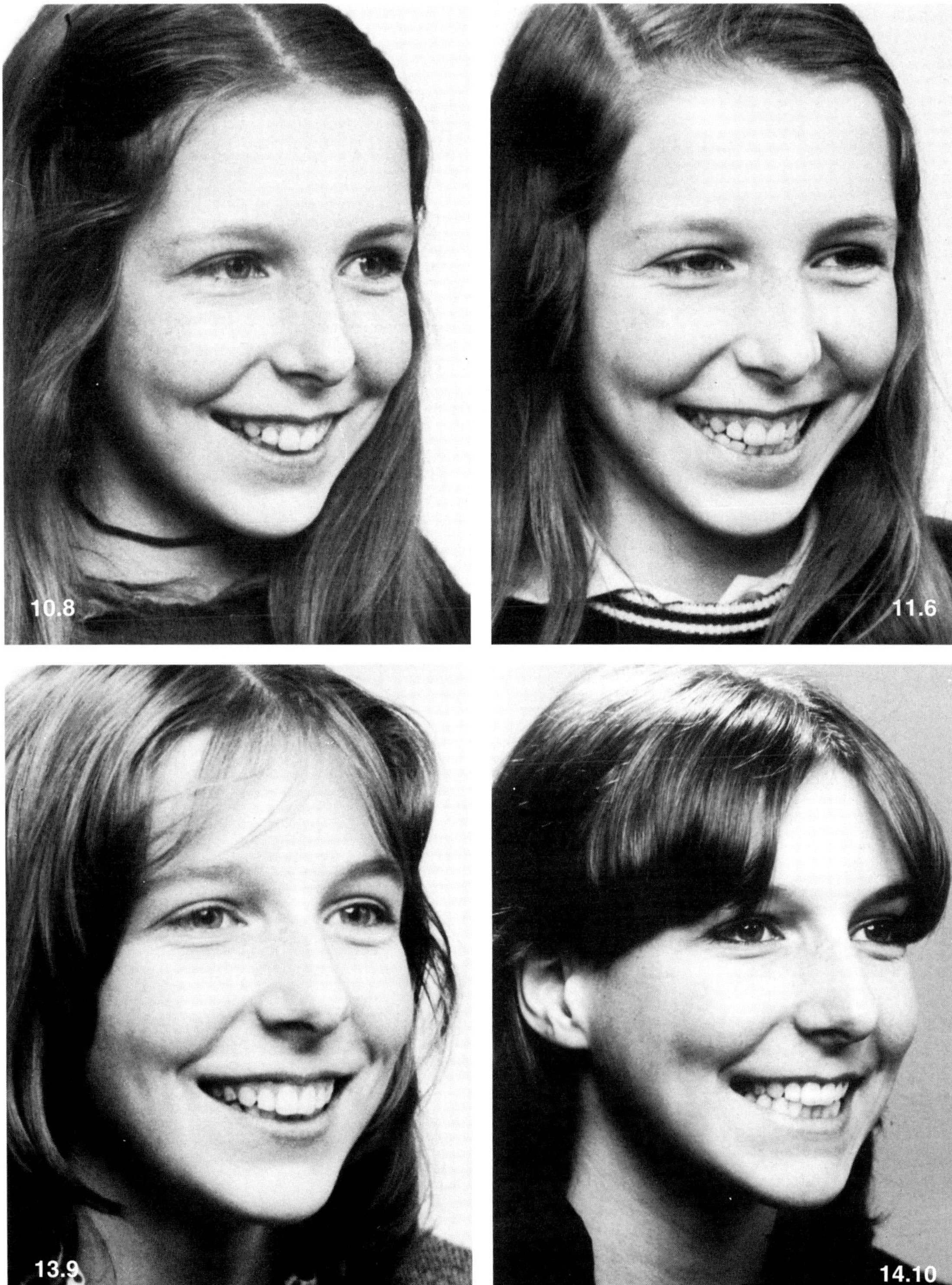
10.8
11.6
13.9
14.10

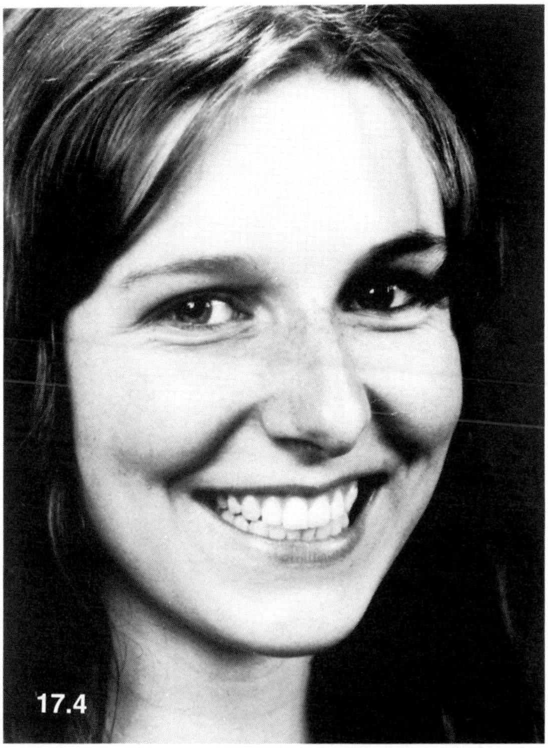

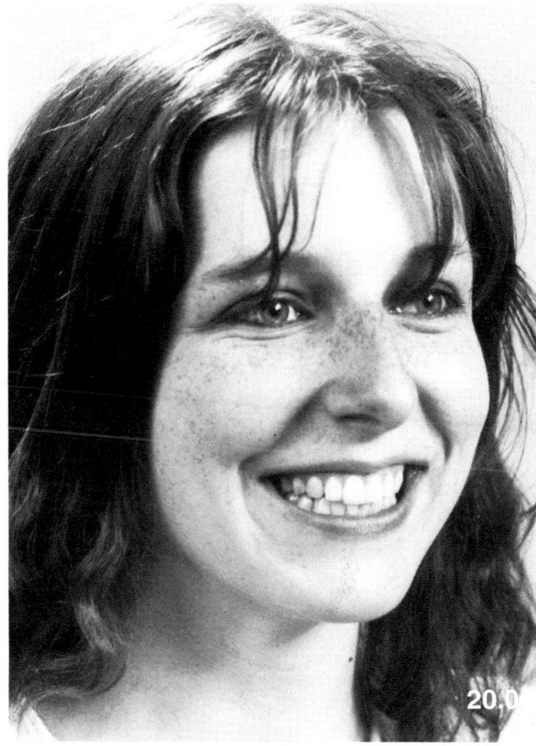

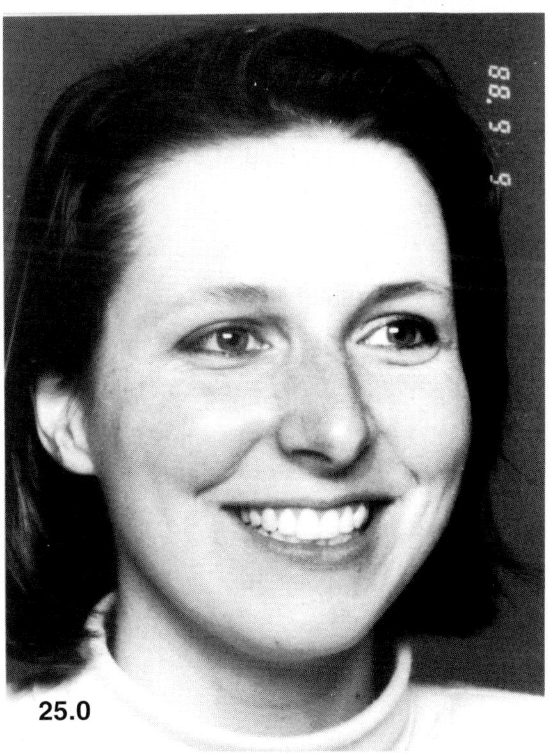

Fig 9-14a and 9-14b *Note the achieved improvements, especially the reduction of the zone of visible gingiva, which was obtained through intrusion . of the maxillary incisors over one year during the second treatment phase that began at the age of 13 y, 9 mo.*

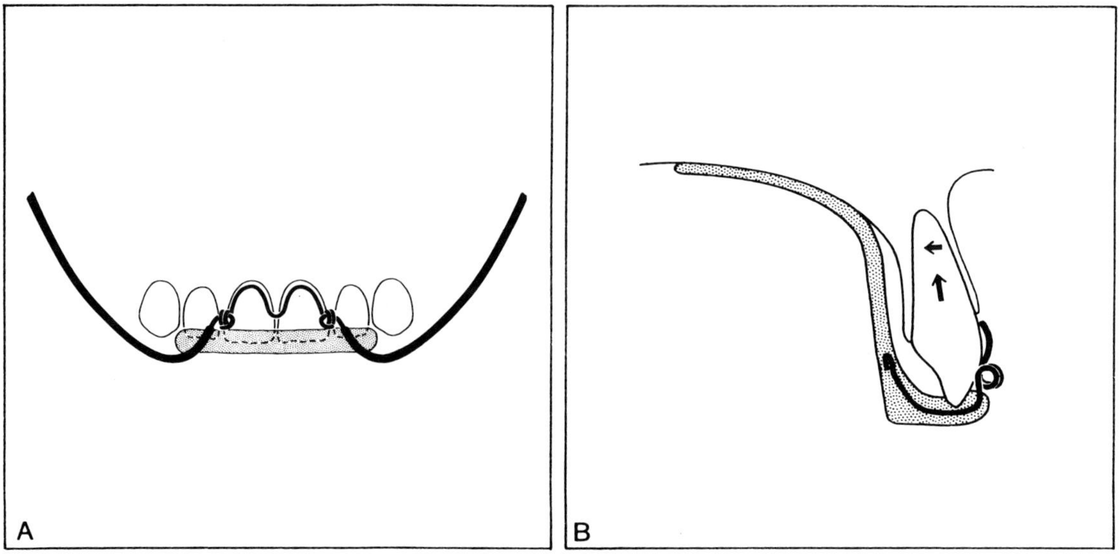

Fig 9-15 The Bass plate, with which the anterior part of the maxilla can be influenced facial-orthopedically, and the maxillary incisors intruded and, if necessary, torqued.

A The ends of the two hooks of the parietal headgear are inserted in the eyelets on either side between the central and lateral incisors. These eyelets at the same time increase the flexibility of the loops that rest against the labial surfaces of the central incisors.

B The wire, with a diameter of .6 mm, should be well-embedded in the acrylic directly after the eyelets to prevent bending that might induce unwanted reactions, and also to avoid the wire being dislodged from the acrylic by the headgear force of about 150 g.

not taken to be unpleasing; in others, it is thought to be utterly unacceptable and distressing, especially when the visible zone of gingiva is extensive.[21] In extreme cases, a satisfactory result cannot be obtained with intrusion of the maxillary incisors, and only a surgical approach can secure the desired improvement. In less serious cases, such as the one shown here, it is possible to obtain a real improvement with direct and comparatively simple orthodontic treatment.

In considering the problem of the "high gum line" one should recognize that the position of stomion relative to the incisal edges descends with age (see Fig 1.6, page 25). In addition, the movements of the upper lip decrease and over the years the upper lip is lifted up less when speaking and smiling, leading to a diminishing of the visibility of the maxillary anterior teeth and the original "high gum-line."

It is regularly found that dental and facial conditions like those originally evident in this patient, do not cause concern and treatment is not sought. The fact that in this case treatment nevertheless was undertaken displays a special facet in the assessment of the indications for orthodontic treatment. Both the patient and her parents found that her appearance did not satisfy their wishes and were prepared to put up with the burden of orthodontic treatment. Had this not been so, treatment could not have been advocated. Additionally, the necessary cooperation would most likely not have been forthcoming even if the practitioner involved thought treatment was indicated.

Despite the mild anomaly and the originally simple-seeming treatment, the course of the therapy is an illustration of a specific orthodontic problem. After a relapse, two rather simple appliances were required to achieve an acceptable result. One should ask oneself at the beginning of treatment what might go wrong, and how could it be corrected. It is also wise during treatment to keep in mind possible strategies that might be used if unforeseen circumstances arise. It is not easy to tell in advance if treatment will be simple or if it will be complicated.

Chapter 10

Class II/1
Cervical headgear, maxillary removable plate, elastics "through the bite"
Male: 10 years, 7 months to 22 years, 2 months

This boy, aged 10 years 7 months, had a class II/1 anomaly with a fairly normal profile for his age. He could breathe through his nose easily and his lips were long enough to hold them closed without strain. The disto-occlusion of ½ PW was less to be attributed to a deviant jaw relationship than to abnormal tooth positions. This showed itself among other things in the marked labioversion of the maxillary incisors with an overjet of just 4 mm. Both dental arches exhibited excess space, albeit that the mandibular right first permanent molar had migrated mesially as the result of premature loss of the adjacent second deciduous molar (Figs 10.1 and 10.2).
The treatment plan was use of a cervical headgear and a maxillary plate. In view of the excess space in the maxillary arch and the contact between the maxillary and mandibular incisors, the fitting of the plate would have to be done soon after beginning the headgear therapy.
Use of the headgear began at the age of 10 years, 9 months. Seven weeks later, the plate was fitted. At 11 years, 3 months, such an improvement in the occlusion had occurred that it was no longer necessary to wear the headgear. The plate was used first to reduce the overbite and then to retract the maxillary incisors.
At the age of 11 years, 9 months, the desired result had been achieved with a reasonable occlusion. That did not apply to the mandibular right second premolar, which shortly before had emerged lingually despite the fact that there was essentially enough room for it in the arch. When two months later it was seen that the position of this premolar had not improved, a hook was fixed to its lingual surface. The same was done to the buccal surface of the maxillary right second premolar. An elastic band was fitted "through the bite" between the two hooks and after eight weeks the mandibular right second premolar was in a good position (Figs 10.3 and 10.4).
The records obtianed two years later show, just as do those obtained ten years after treatment, a stable result (Figs 10.5 to 10.8).
From the superimposition of the cephalometric tracings, it can be seen that the mandible grew notably further ventrally than did the maxilla, while the lower face height increased only slightly. In the subsequent ten years, marked ventral development took place; the face height increased significantly also (Fig 10.9).
The oblique photographs demonstrate the obtained improvements and the considerable growth and maturity of the face (Fig 10.10).

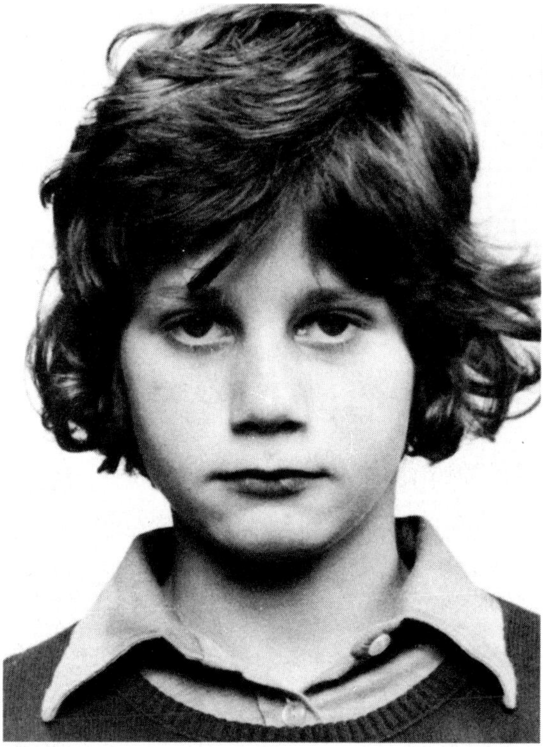

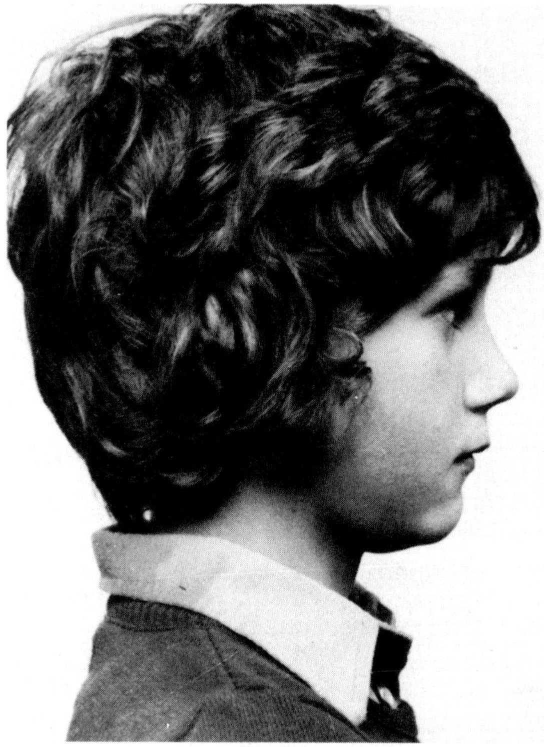

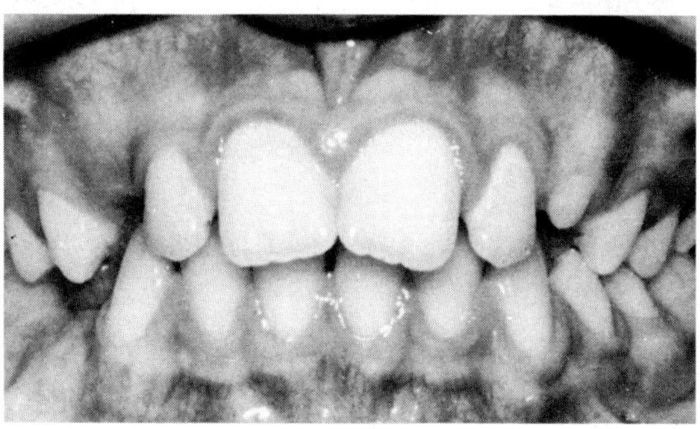

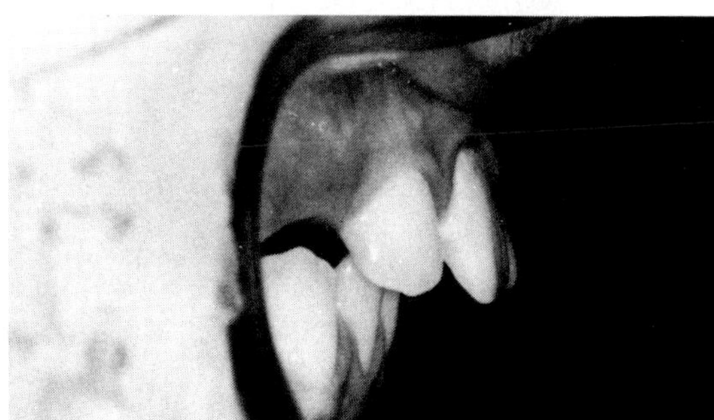

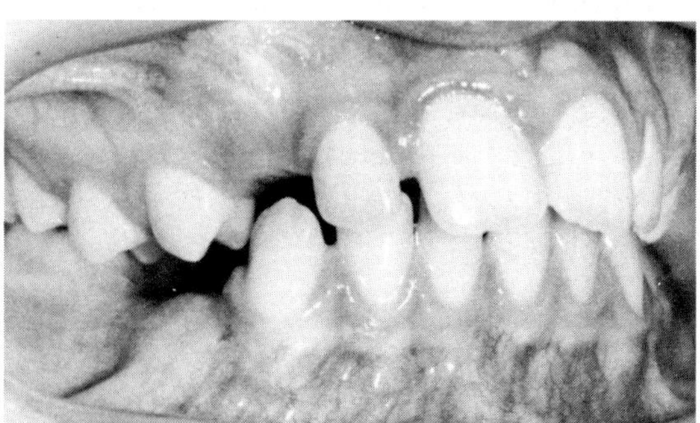

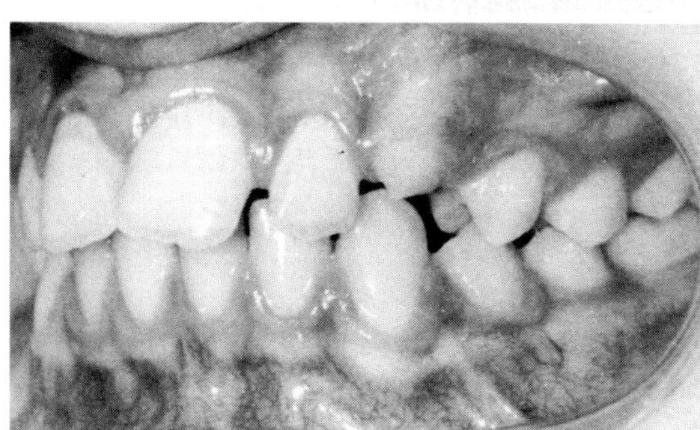

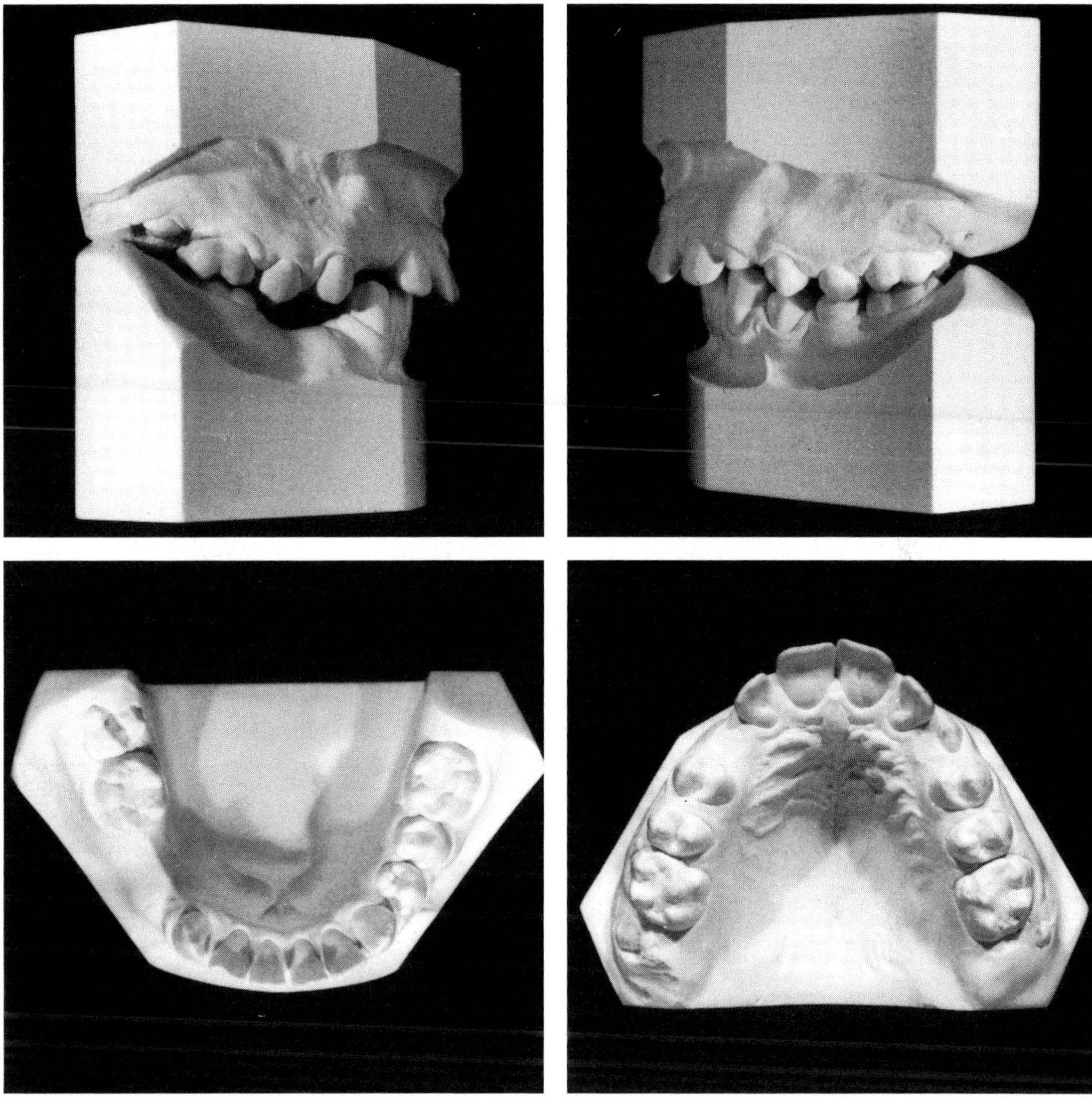

Figs 10-1 and 10-2 *A boy aged 10 y, 7 mo with a class II/1 anomaly (disto-occlusion ½ PW), a more or less normal sagittal jaw relationship and facial profile, and a shallow lower face height with lips of adequate length to secure unstrained closure. The maxillary incisors are tipped labially. Excess space is available in both dental arches despite premature loss of the mandibular right deciduous molars.*

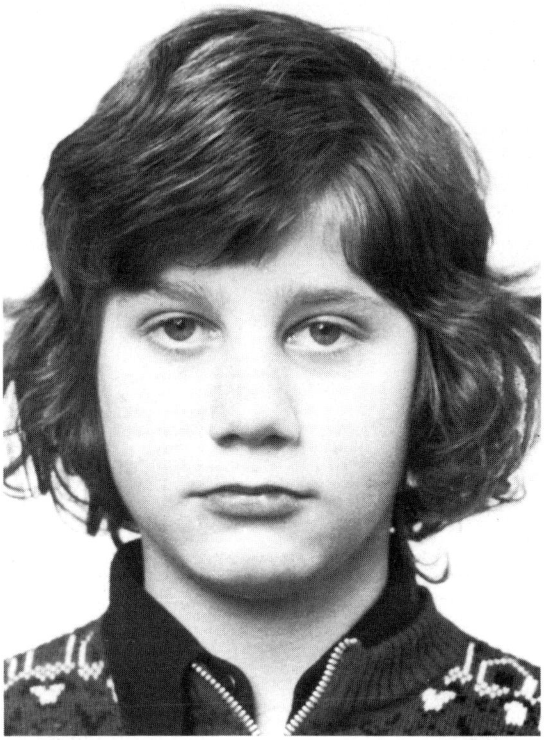
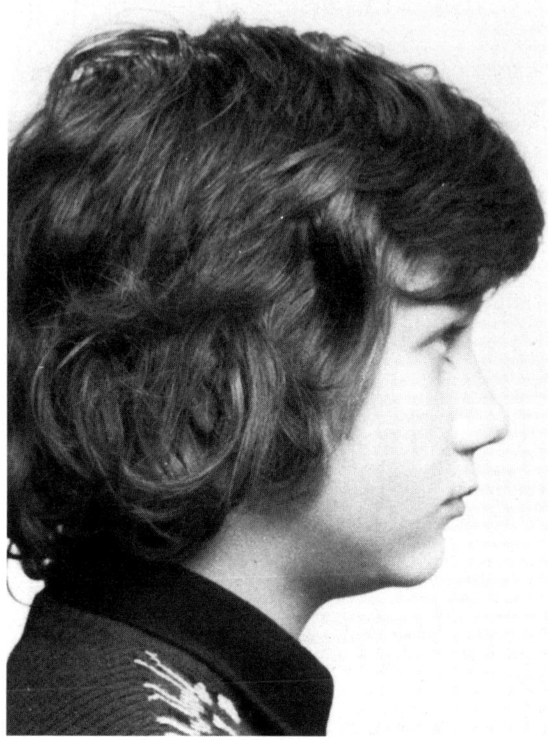
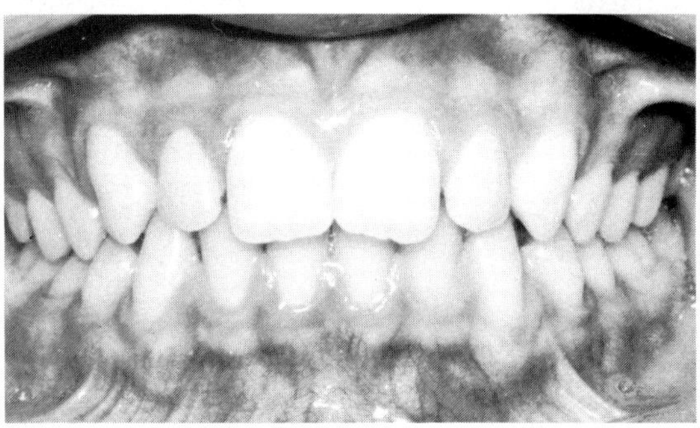
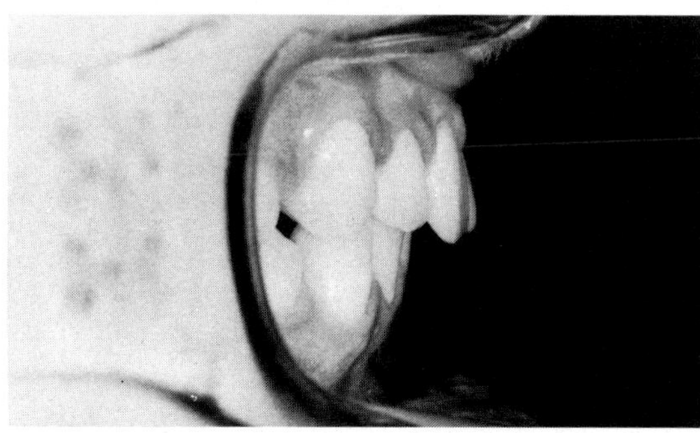
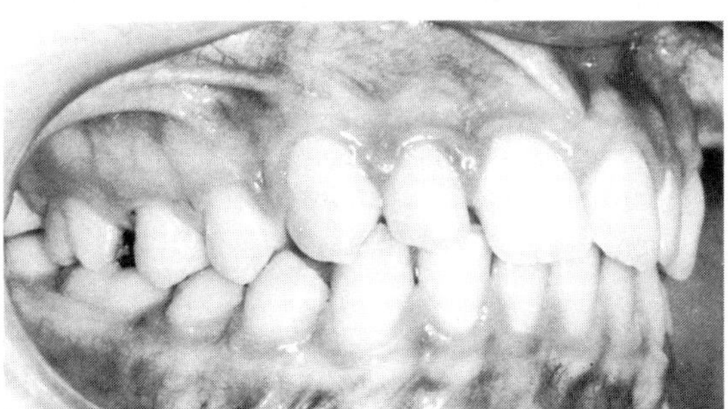
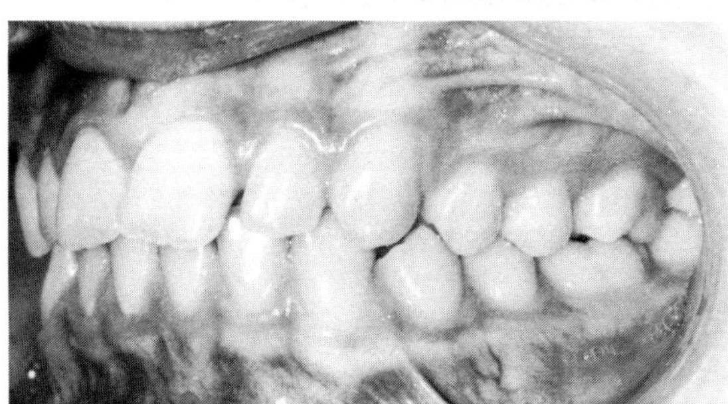

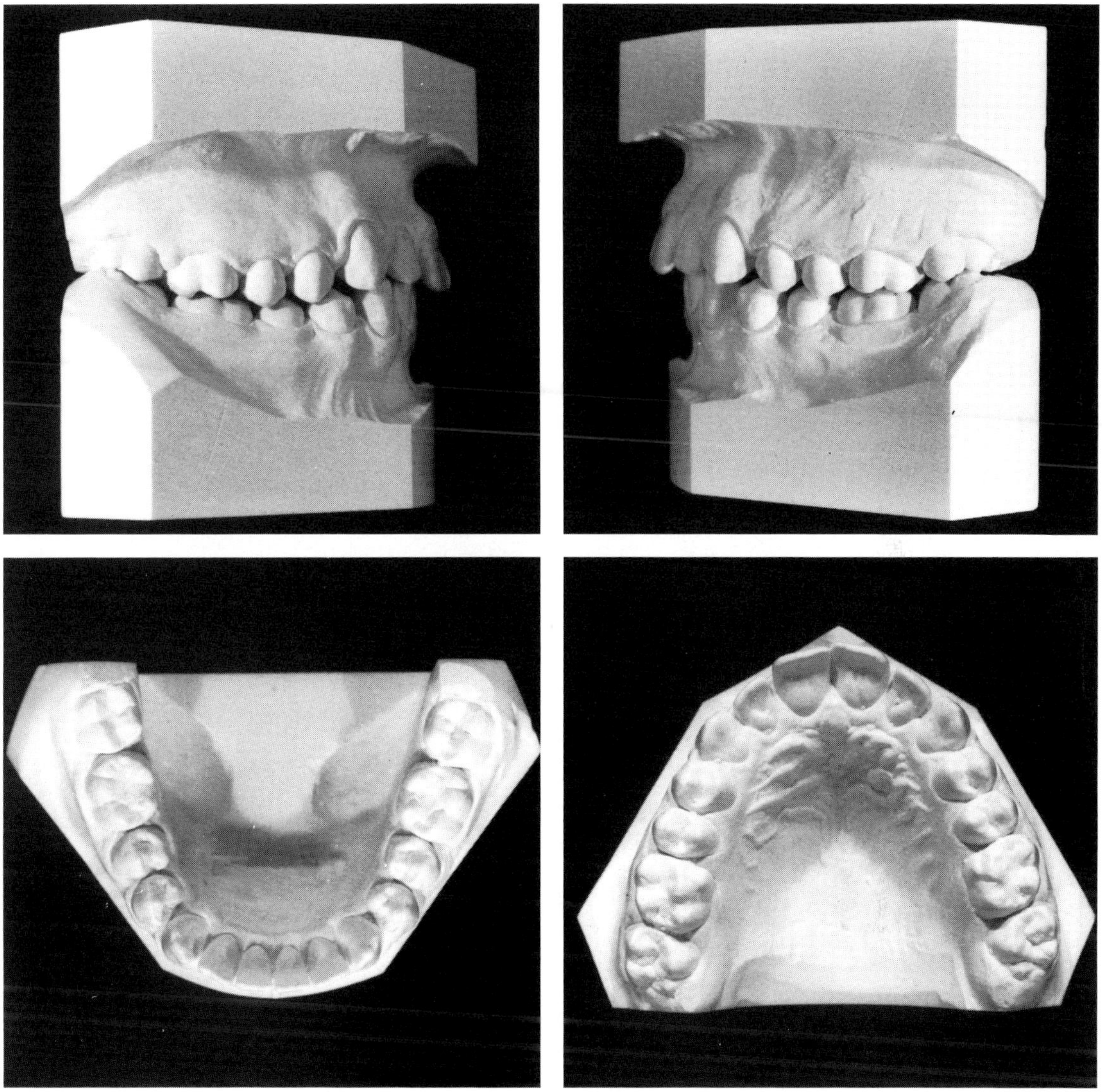

Figs 10-3 and 10-4 *At the age of 12 y, 4 mo, after treatment for about two years, a good facial configuration exists. Both dental arches are normal in form. The posterior teeth interdigitate solidly and small spaces are present between the maxillary central and lateral incisors. Angulation and vertical positions are not optimal, which can be attributed to the limitations of the appliances used.*

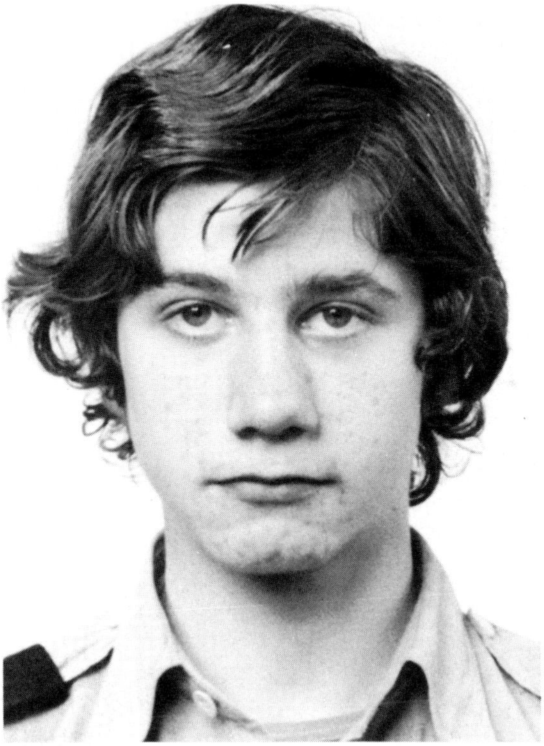
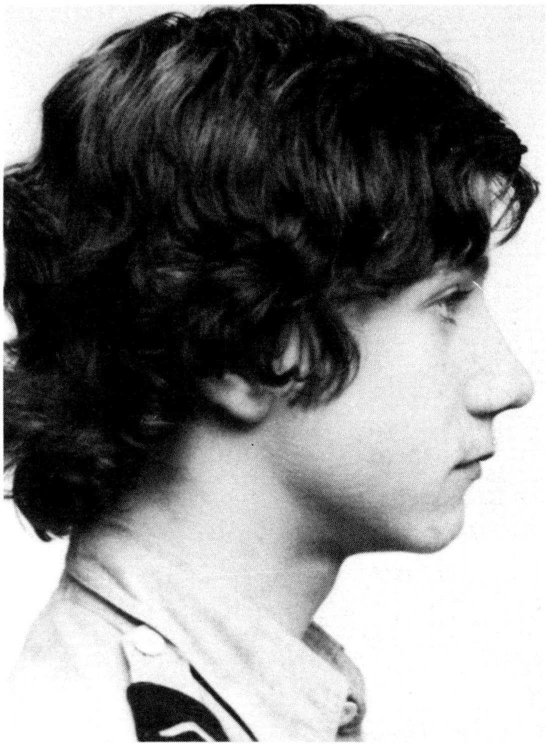
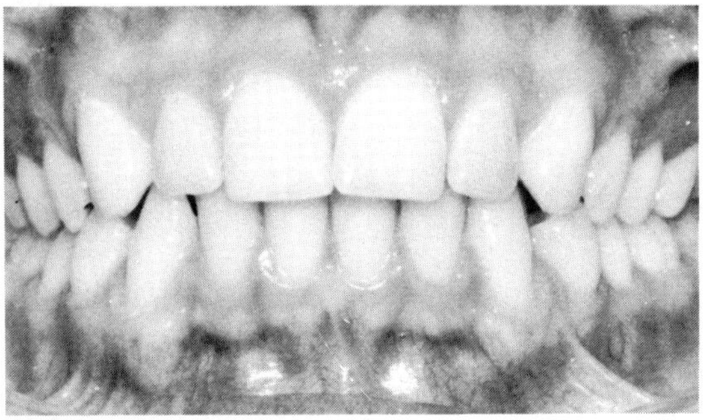
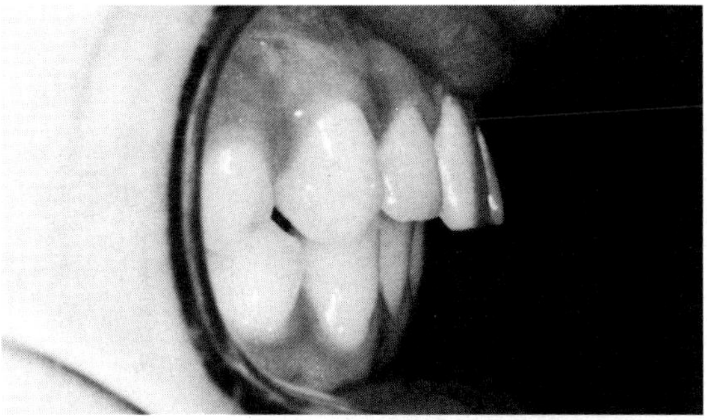
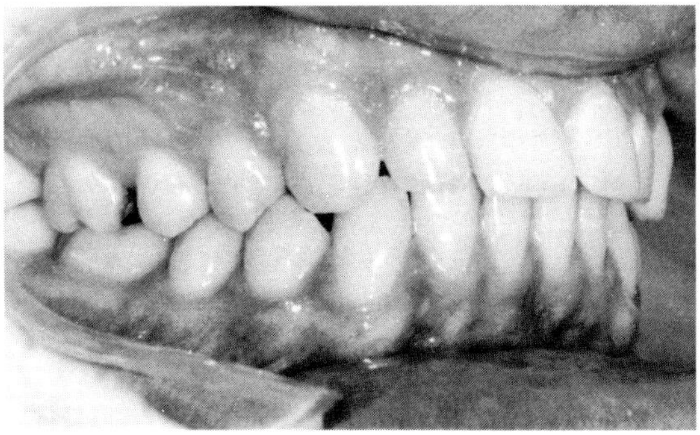
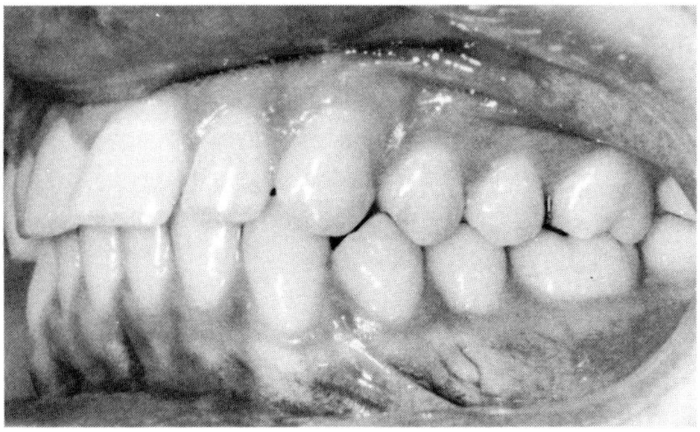

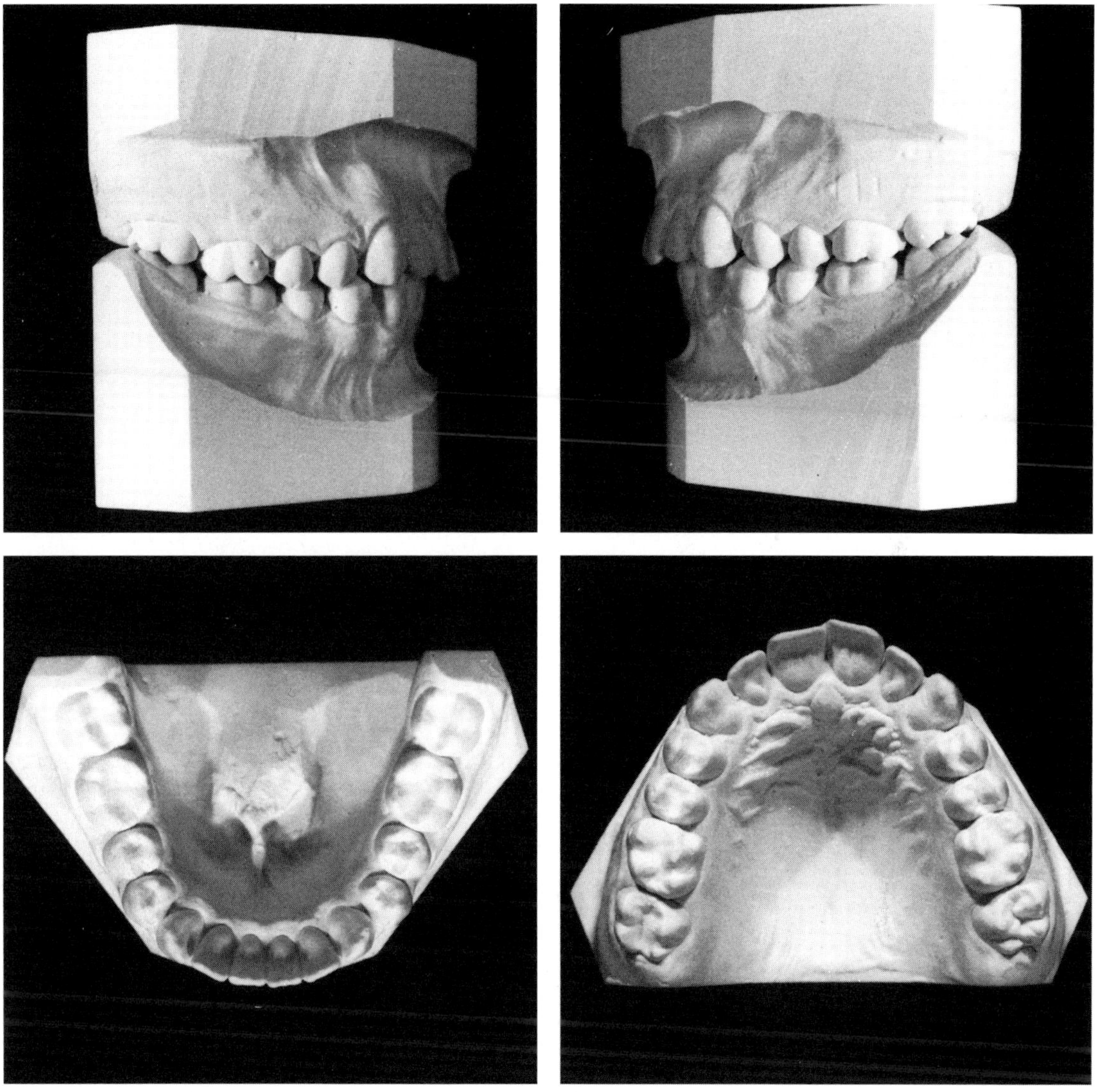

Figs 10-5 and 10-6 *At the age of 14 y, 4 mo, two years after treatment was completed, the profile has improved and the positions of the teeth are good. The spaces between the maxillary incisors have closed spontaneously. The incisal edges of the maxillary incisors have been ground to correct and improve the abnormal angles and height differences. The occlusion, inclination, and angulation of the second molars that had emerged over two years previously still need to improve. Much growth is still required in the maxillary tuberosity region to accommodate the emergence of the third molars.*

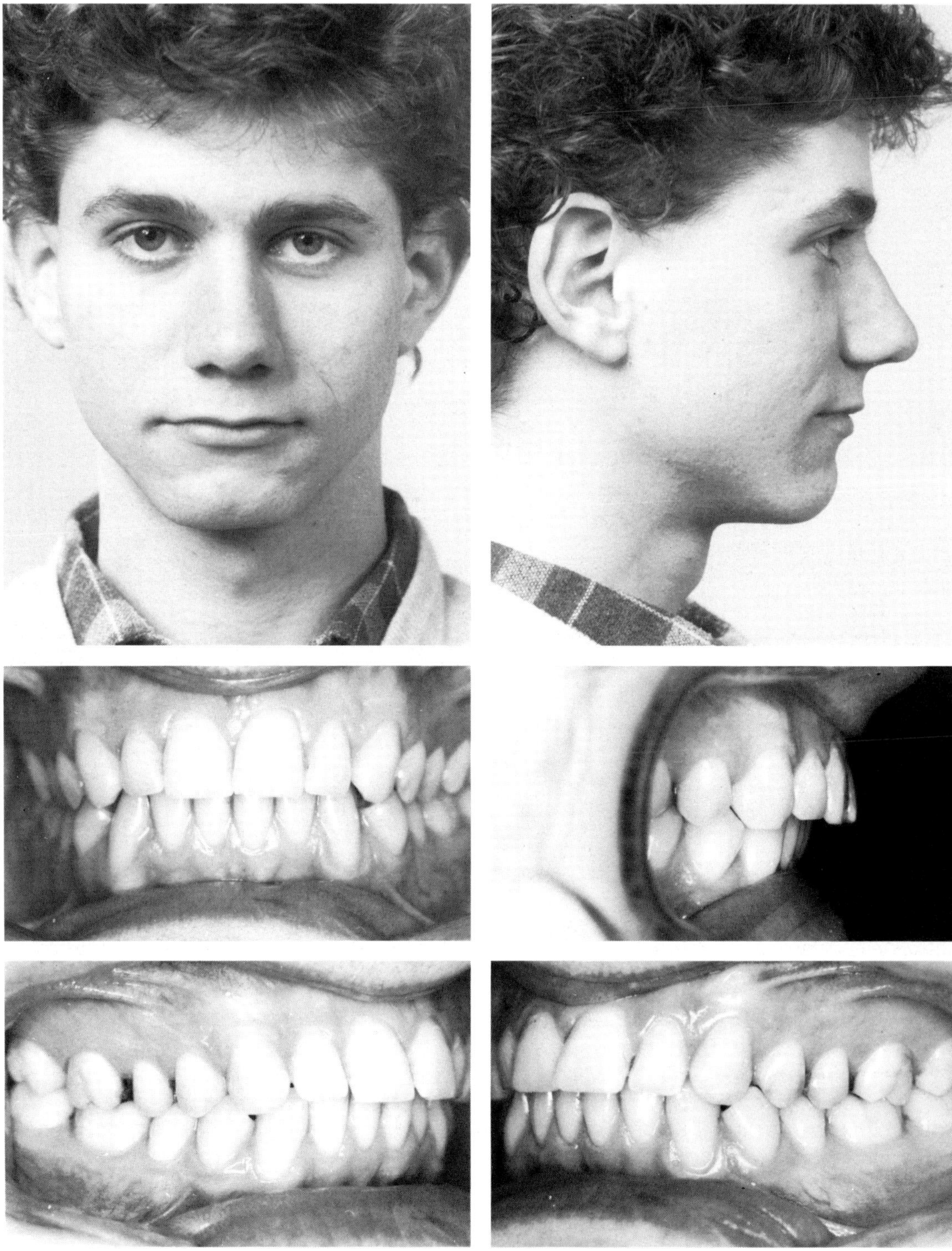

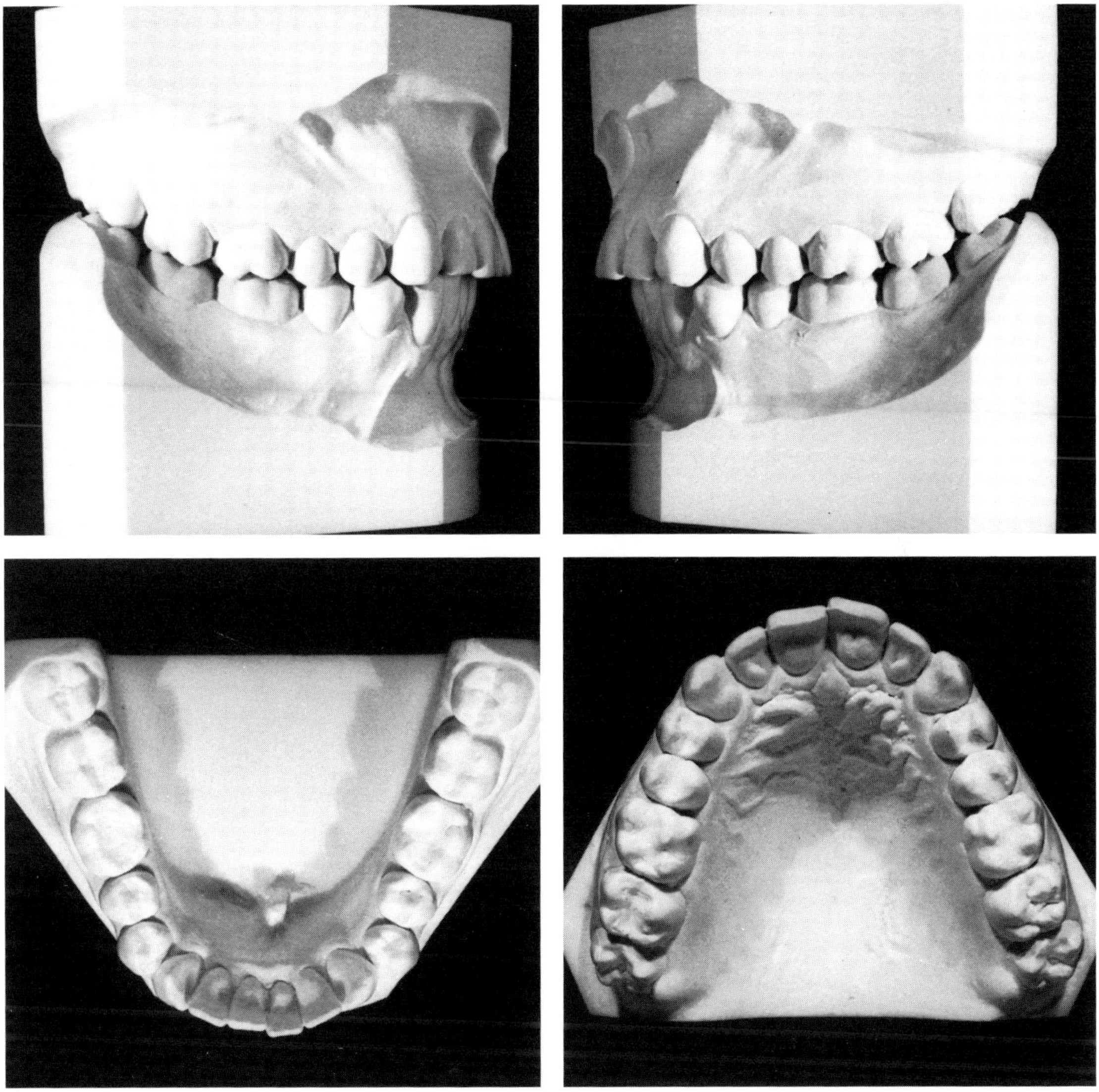

Figs 10-7 and 10-8 *Aged 22 y, 2 mo, ten years after treatment, his face is fully mature. The marked development of the lower face caudally and ventrally has been largely responsible for the improvement. Because the mandibular growth was stronger than that of the maxilla, the mandibular teeth are now relatively more mesial than those of the maxilla. The tertiary crowding now evident can be due to that, or to the further maturation of the enclosing soft tissues. Notwithstanding the stronger mandibular growth, the overjet has increased again probably because the maxillary incisors have erupted further. The increase in size of the alveolar processes was sufficient to accommodate all the third molars.*

Figure 10-9a

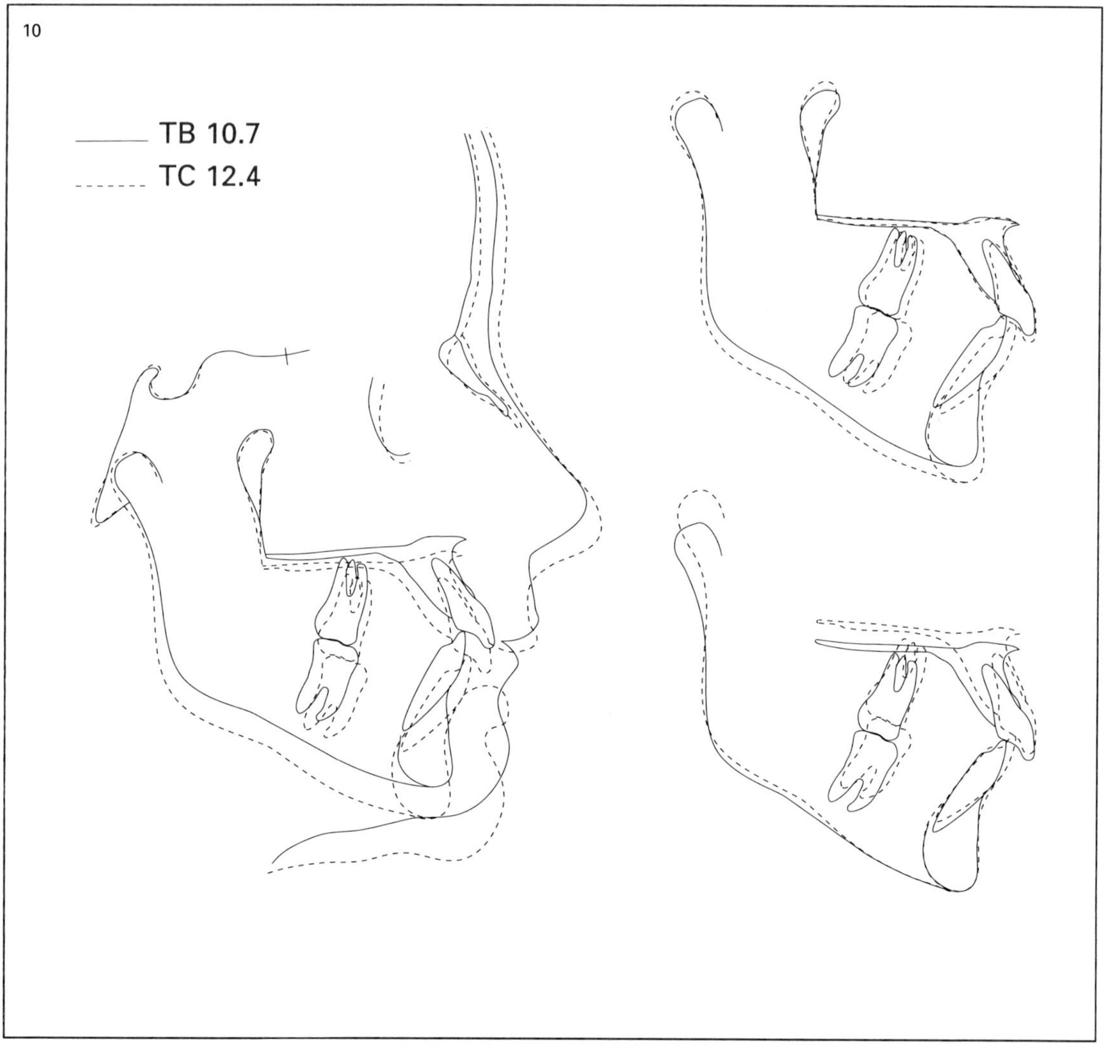

Fig 10-9 The superimposed cephalometric tracings show that the growth of the mandible during treatment was more to ventral than that of the maxilla, while the height of the lower face increased only a little. In the ten years following treatment, the marked ventral development was associated with a significant increase in face height.

Figure 10-9b

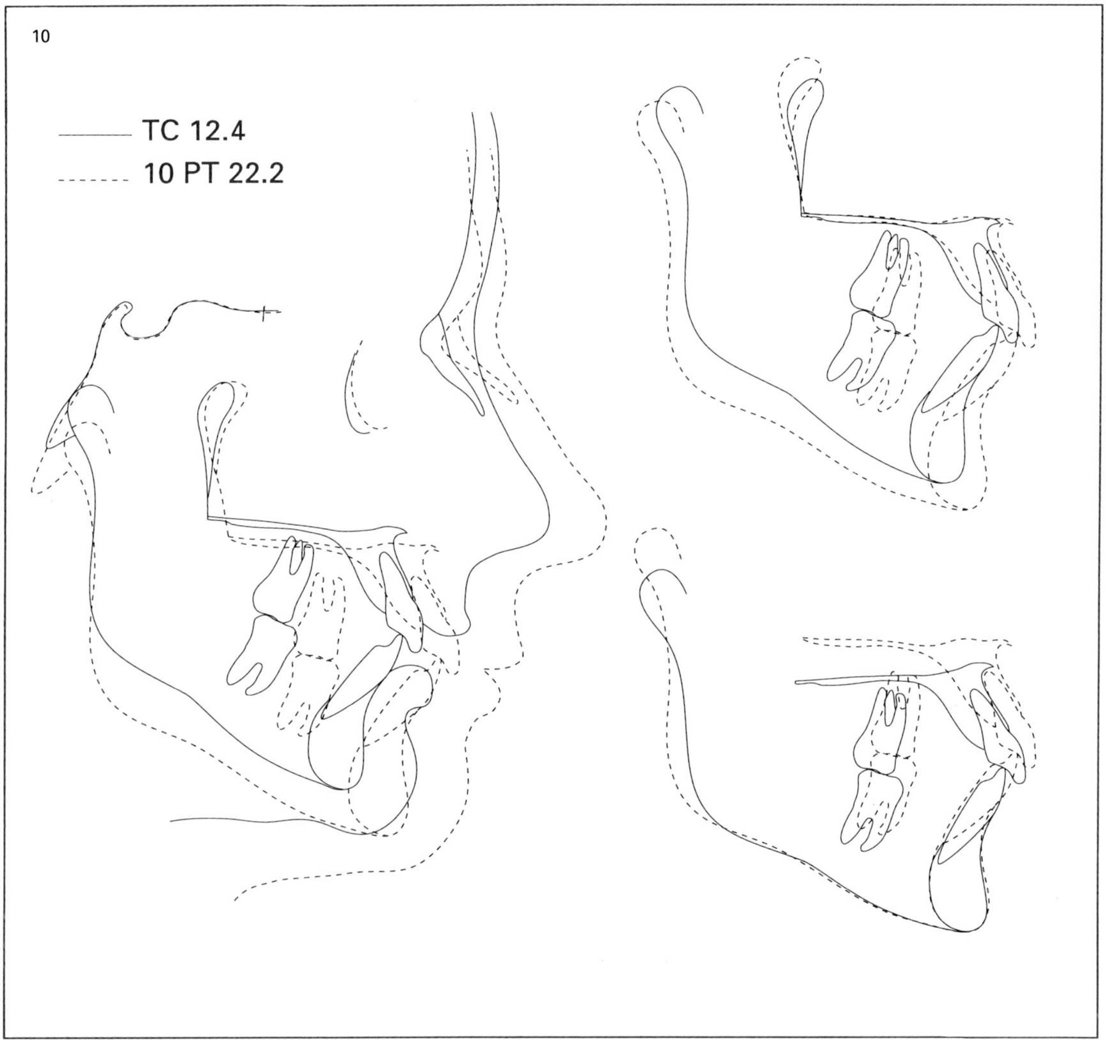

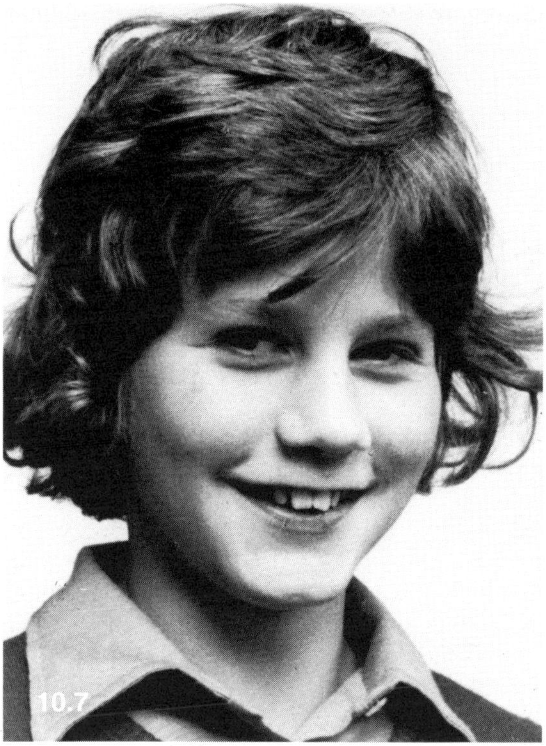
10.7

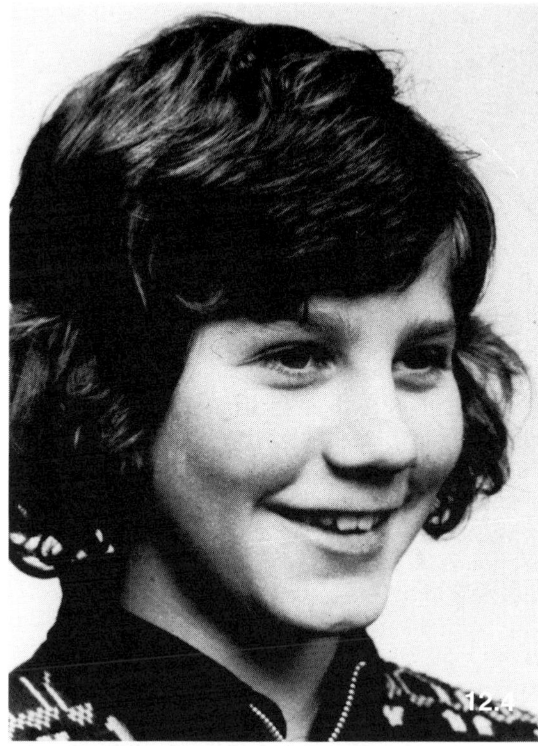
12.4

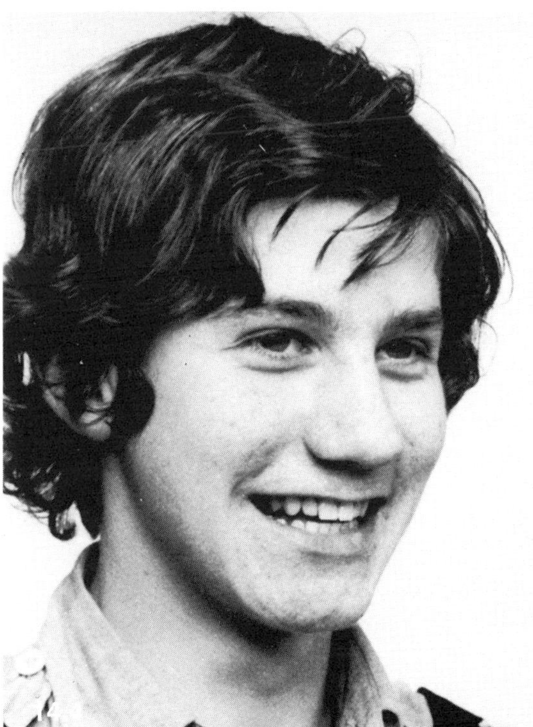

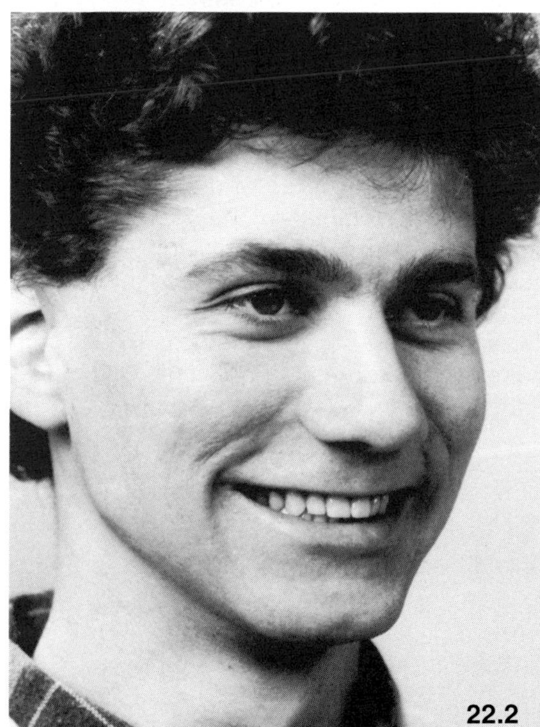
22.2

Fig 10-10 Note the improvements in dentition and facial appearance that ensued during and after treatment.

The most significant improvements during this treatment were achieved with the plate. The headgear was only needed for a short time because the growth pattern was favorable for the correction of the disto-occlusion. The extra space made it easy to tip the maxillary incisors back. Because the four maxillary incisors were not irregular either vertically or horizontally, it was possible to get a good result just with a removable plate carrying divided labial arches such as those described in chapter 7. Retention was not thought necessary since normal functional conditions were present.

In dental arches with excess space, usually no lasting unfavorable effect results from premature loss of mandibular deciduous molars since the antagonist, usually the maxillary second deciduous molar, can over-erupt. That is probably what happened in this case. Even with a shortage of space for a mandibular second premolar, such a tooth can often manage still to emerge into the arch by pushing adjacent teeth aside. An example of this is seen in chapter 6 (see Figs 6.4 and 6.6, pages 81 and 83). If a mandibular second premolar does indeed erupt in endo-occlusion with its antagonist, it is impossible for it to come into acceptable occlusion without intervention. An elastic band "through the bite" can correct the situation and incidentally help to increase the space in the arch. It is necessary to watch that the maxillary tooth to which the elastic is attached cannot be displaced, unless of course the latter is wished for. It is also necessary to take into account that teeth elsewhere in the mandibular quadrant may become displaced.

Considering the stage of development of the dentition, treatment for this patient was begun relatively late. The fact that jaw growth continues in boys for a long time generally offers adequate opportunity for improvements in jaw relationships. The question then is as to whether the necessary cooperation can be obtained, particularly as puberty occurs during this period. On the other hand, it often happens that such patients are easy to talk with, and if they understand how things stand, are quite cooperative and well motivated.

Chapter 11

Class II/1

Cervical headgear, maxillary removable plate, mandibular "lip bumper"
Male: 11 years, 1 month to 31 years, 3 months

A boy aged 11 years, 1 month had a class II/1 anomaly with a marked ventral development of the mid-face, a retruded chin, and consequently an increased step between upper and lower lips. He could easily breathe through his nose and at rest his lower lip was held partly behind the maxillary central incisors. If in considering the molar relationships, the mesial drift of the mandibular first permanent molars due to premature loss of the deciduous molars was allowed for, there was a disto-occlusion of 1 PW. The ALD in the mandible was –4 mm; in the maxilla, –2 mm. Both maxillary central incisors, of which the left one had been fractured a year previously, were positioned more labially than the lateral incisors, with an overjet of 8 mm. The pronounced discrepancy in the jaw relationship, demonstrated also by the great antero-posterior distance between the anterior sections of the apical areas in both jaws (clearly to be assessed from the dental casts) indicated that the class II/1 anomaly was of skeletal origin (Figs 11.1 and 11.2).
It was decided to treat the problem with a cervical headgear, a plate in the maxilla, and a "lip bumper" on the mandibular arch (Fig 11.12). Originally it was intended subsequently to fit full fixed appliances, but the patient later was not prepared to accept them. For this reason, the situation arose in which a pronounced anomaly had to be treated with simple appliances, although it was clear that it was not possible to obtain a perfect result with such means.
The headgear treatment was begun at the age of 11 years, 4 months. Two months later, the maxillary plate was added. Five months later, the mandibular first permanent molars were banded and a lip bumper fitted. After a treatment of two years and two months, all appliances were removed. A good occlusion of the posterior teeth and solid interdigitation of the canines and premolars was obtained, although the maxillary canines and incisors were too upright. Crowding in the mandible still existed and most of the interproximal contacts between the mandibular anterior teeth were unsatisfactory (Fig 11.3). To finish, a retainer was fitted for the maxilla, with a continuous labial arch to provide rigid fixation for the maxillary incisors, and a biteplane to control the overbite. Further retention of the plate was provided by two three-quarter clasps embracing the first molars from the distal. The plate was ground free of the premolars palatally, and after three months worn only at night. The total retention time was one year and five months. The models made subsequently show little had changed in the maxillary arch, and that the overbite had not increased. The occlusion in the posterior regions had remained stable, because of the solid interdigitation. In the mandibular arch, the right central incisor had moved slightly to lingual (Fig 11.4).
Two years after ending retention, at the age of 17 years, the patient still has a convex profile. The maxillary right lateral and the left central incisors have moved a little

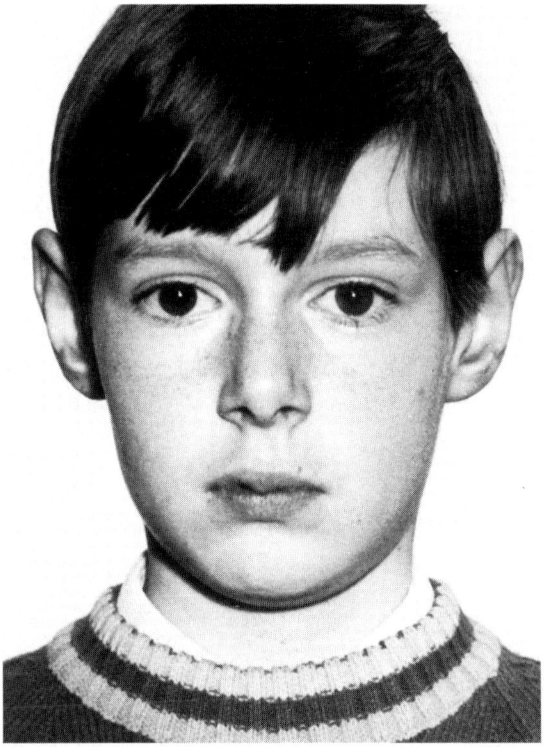

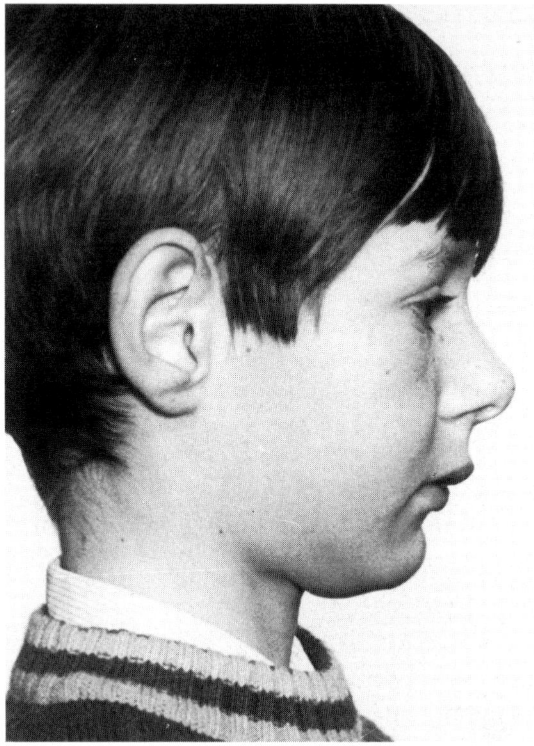

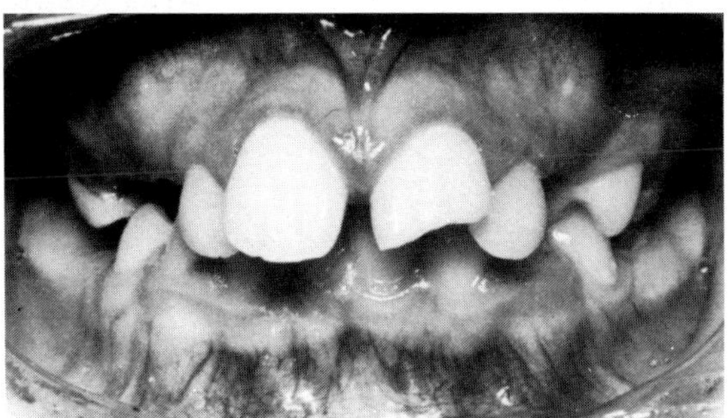

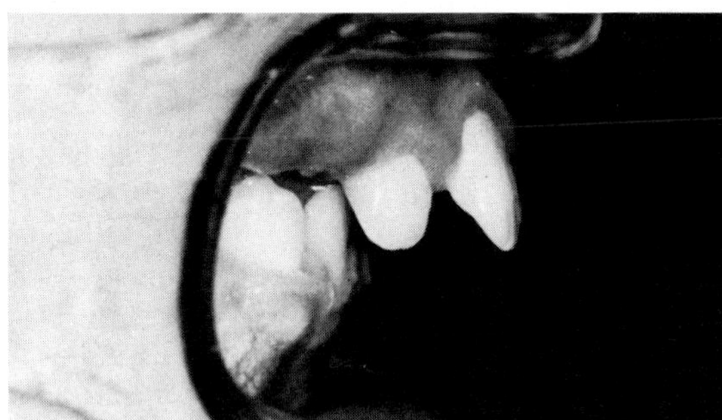

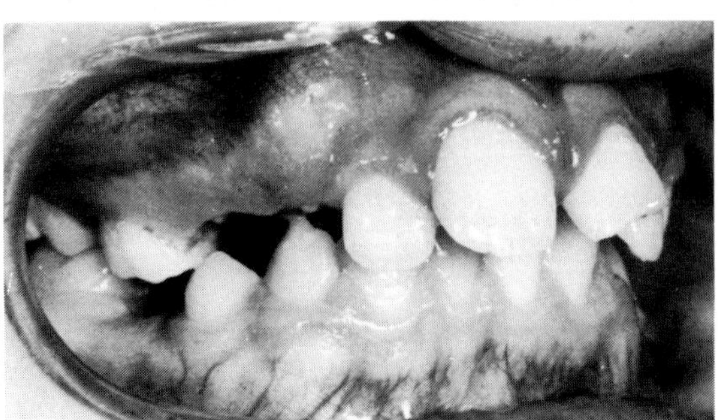

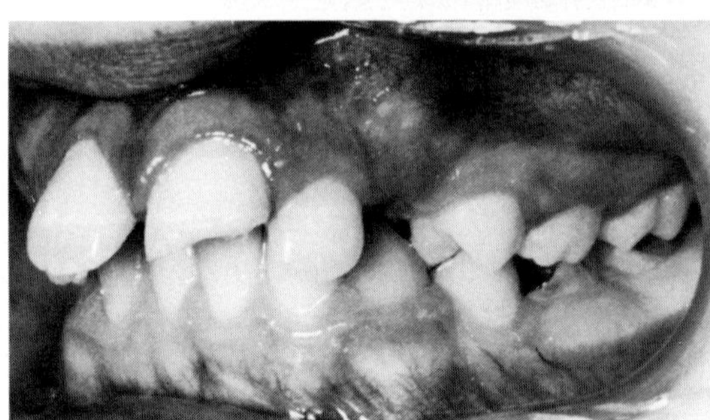

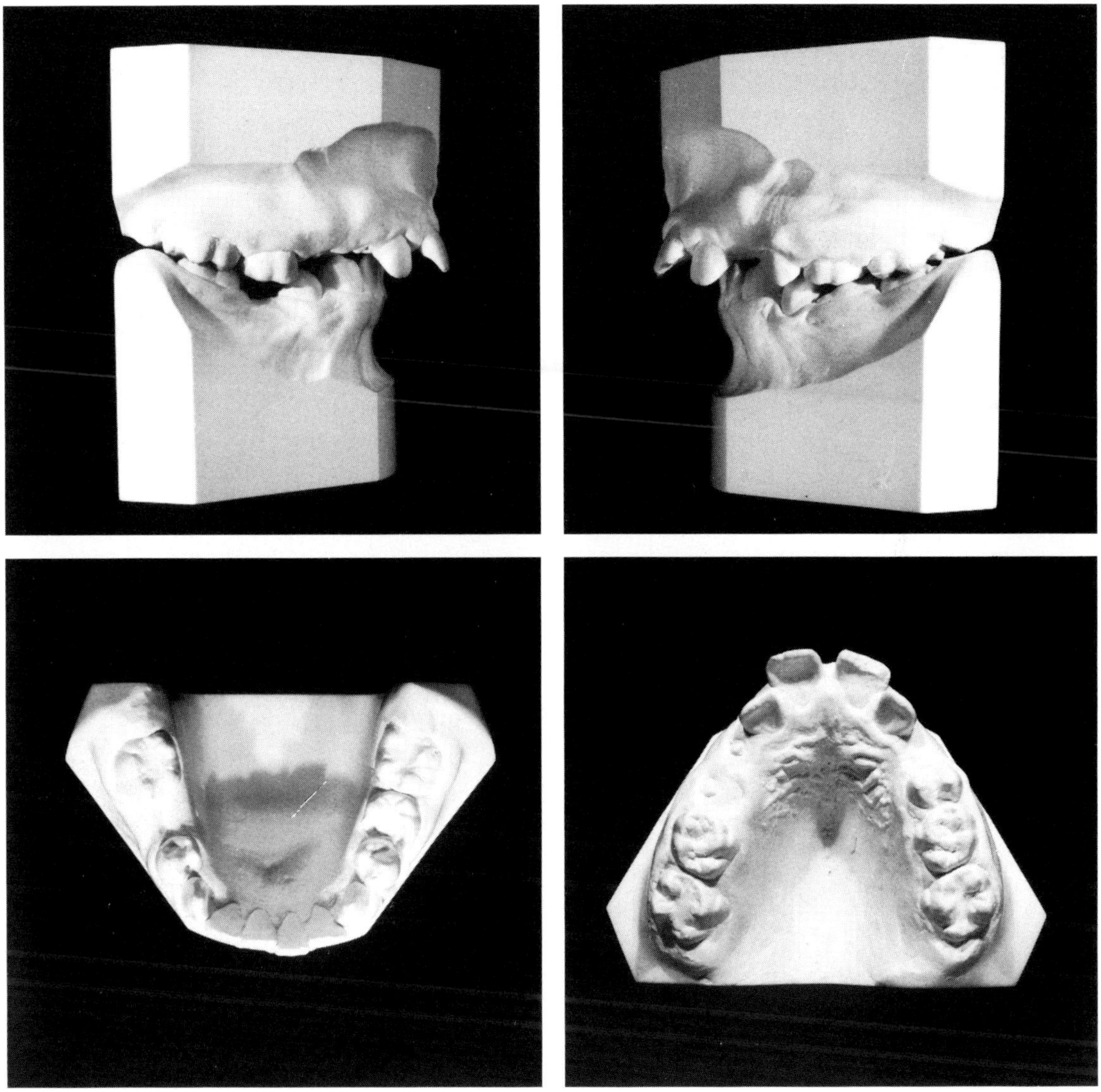

Figs 11-1 and 11-2 A boy of 11 y, 1 mo with marked ventral development of the mid-face, a receding chin, and a class II/1 anomaly. The disto-occlusion (1 PW) is attributable to the pronounced sagittal deviation between the jaws. This deviation can be seen well on the dental casts where the labial surface of the alveolar process at the height of the apices lies far further forward on the maxilla than on the mandible. Mild crowding exists in both arches. On the right the over-eruption of the maxillary second deciduous molar has blocked the mesial drifting of the mandibular first permanent molar that was occurring after the early loss of the mandibular right second deciduous molar.

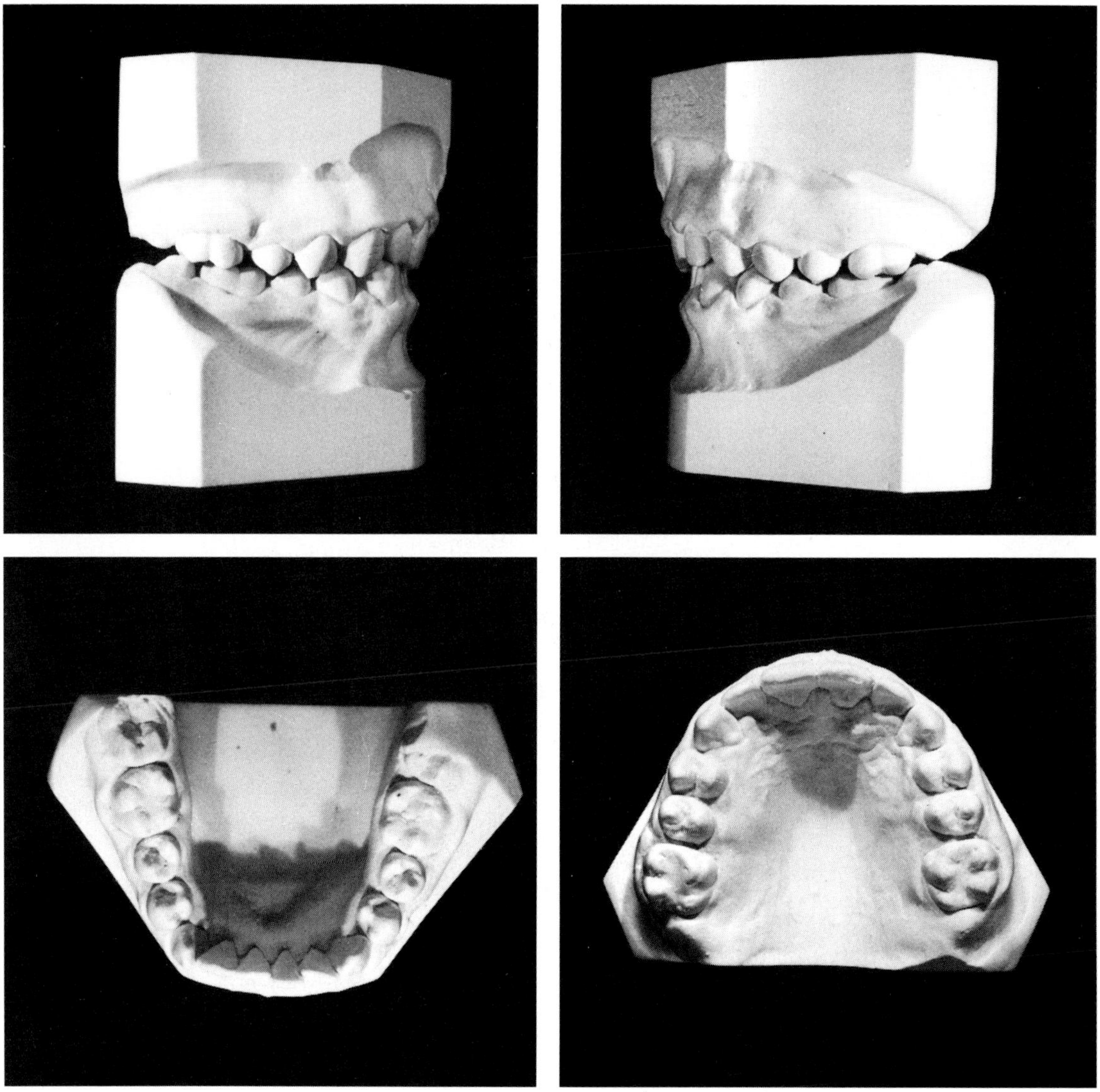

Fig 11-3 At the age of 13 y, 6 mo, after two years of treatment with a cervical headgear, a maxillary plate, and a mandibular lip bumper, neutro-occlusion has been achieved with solid interdigitation of canines and premolars. The form of both arches is good. However, the maxillary incisors are rather too steeply positioned and crowding prevails in the mandibular arch with associated poor interproximal contacts. With a good occlusion of canines and premolars it is clear that the mandibular incisors cannot be well aligned if the maxillary ones are too steeply inclined, unless there is a tooth size discrepancy with a relative shortage of tooth material for the mandibular incisors.

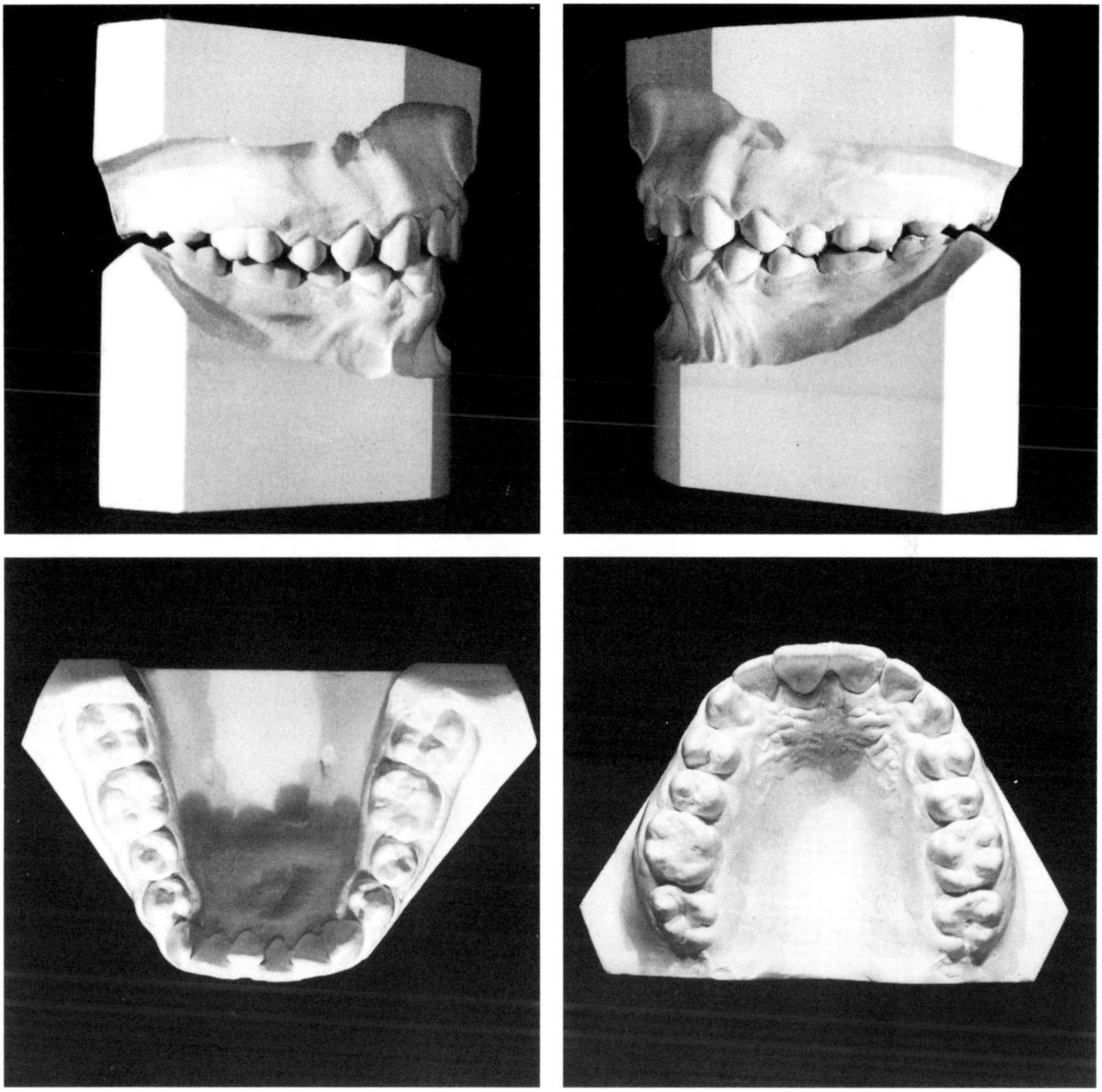

Fig 11-4 At the age of 14 y, 11 mo, after nearly 1½ years of retention with a maxillary plate, there is still a good occlusion in the posterior regions. Due to the presence of the retainer the bite has not deepened, and the alignment of the maxillary incisors has changed little. The crowding in the mandible has increased; the right mandibular central incisor has moved lingually. Dorsally the maxillary tuberosities have grown sufficiently for the second permanent molars to emerge well.

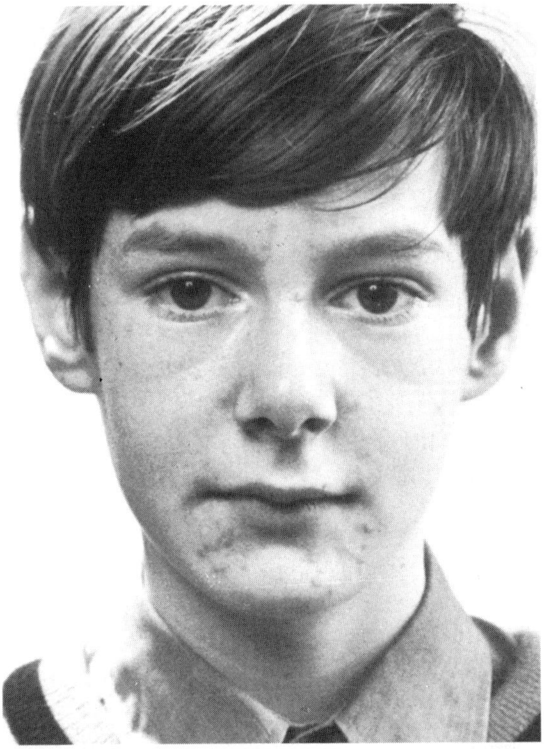
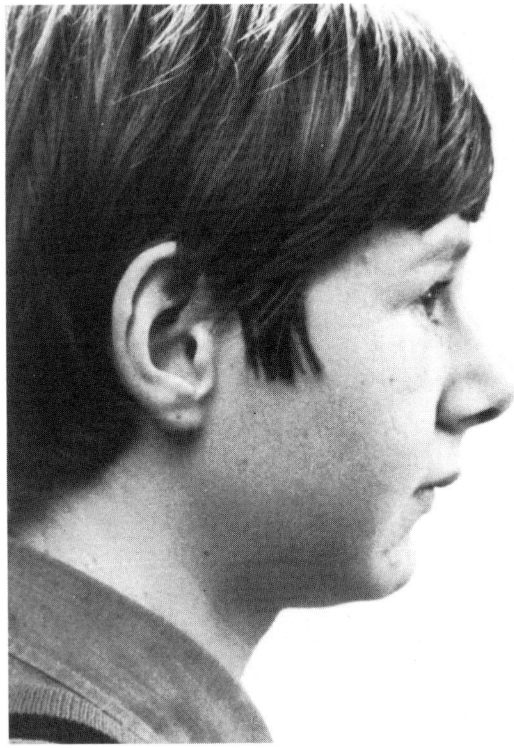
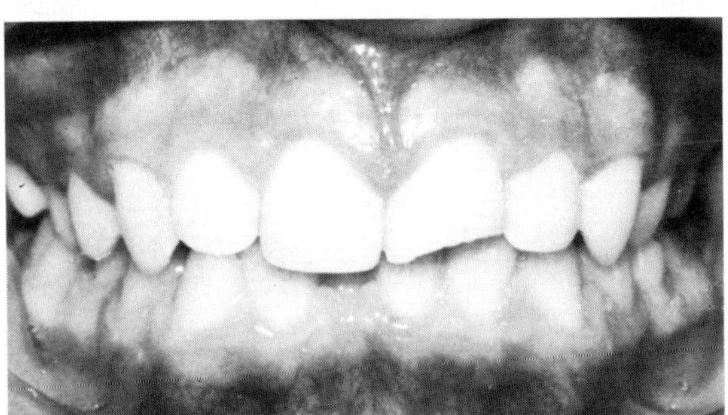
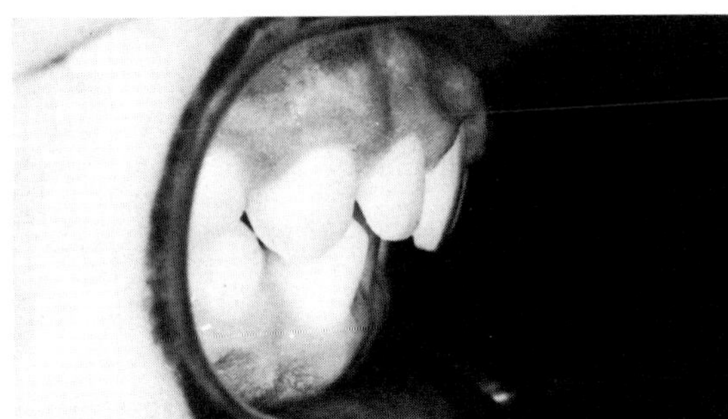
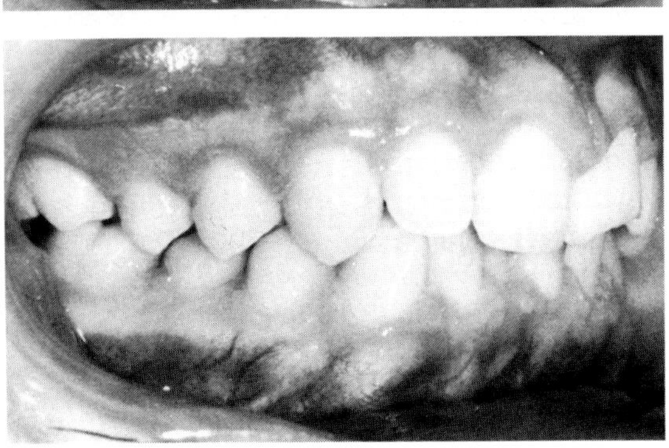
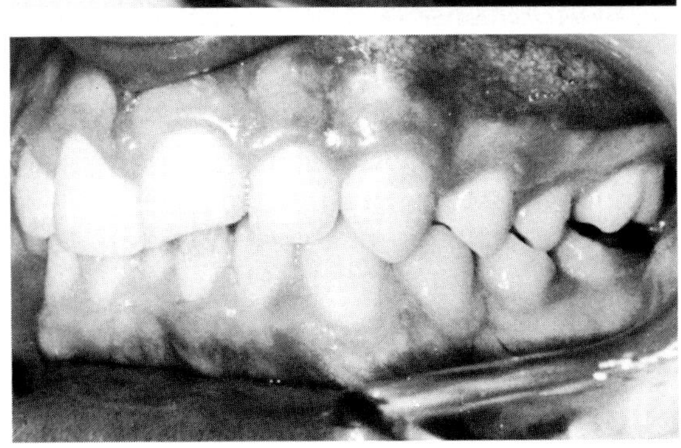

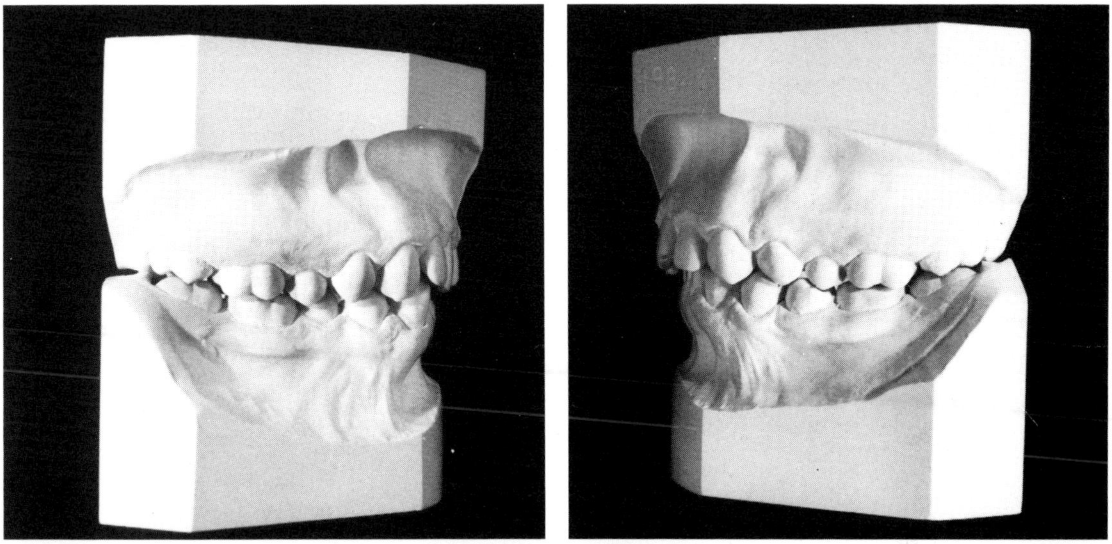

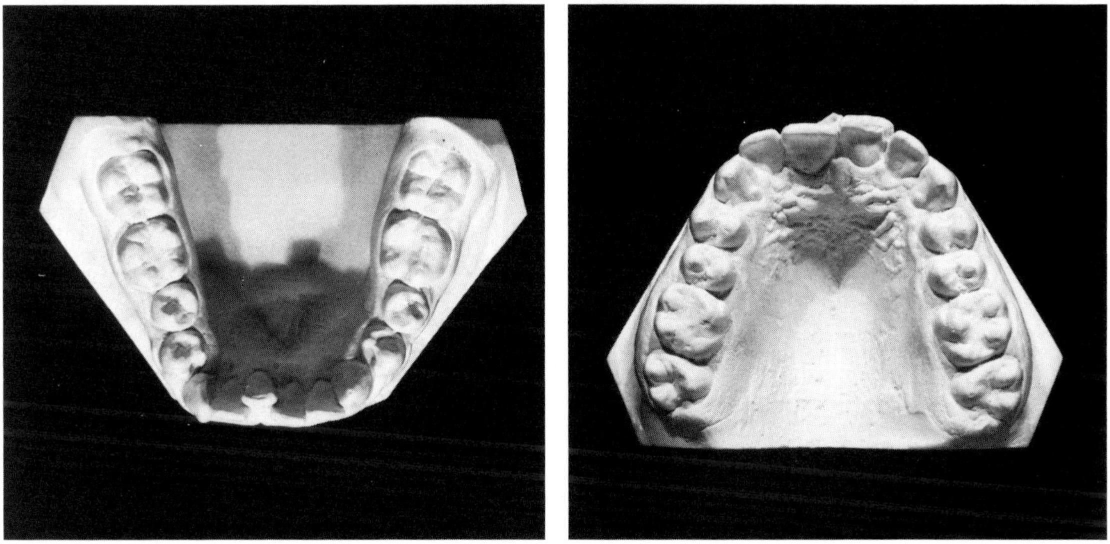

Figs 11-5 and 11-6 At the age of 17 y, 2 mo, the patient's appearance is still characteristic of a class II/1 anomaly, despite the fact that there is a stable neutro-occlusion. The bite has deepened and in the maxilla the right lateral and left central incisors have gone labially. In the mandible, the anterior crowding has increased further and the interproximal contacts have become worse. The right canine has slipped further forward past the lateral incisor, and the central incisor has moved more to lingual.

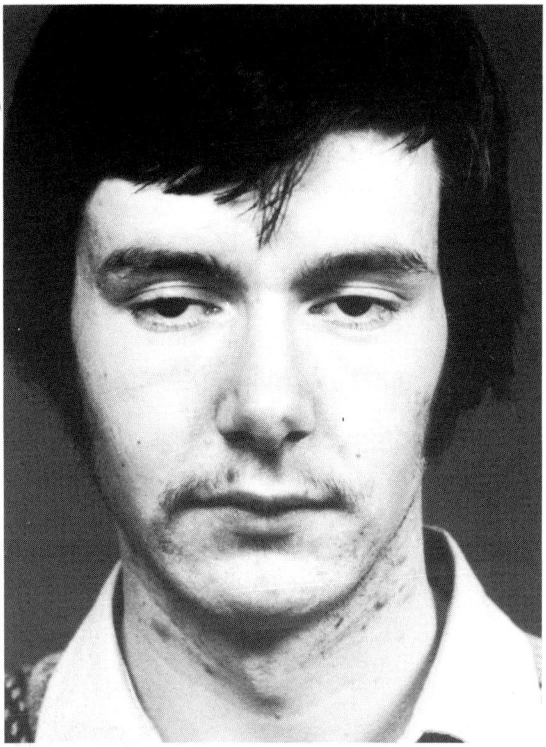

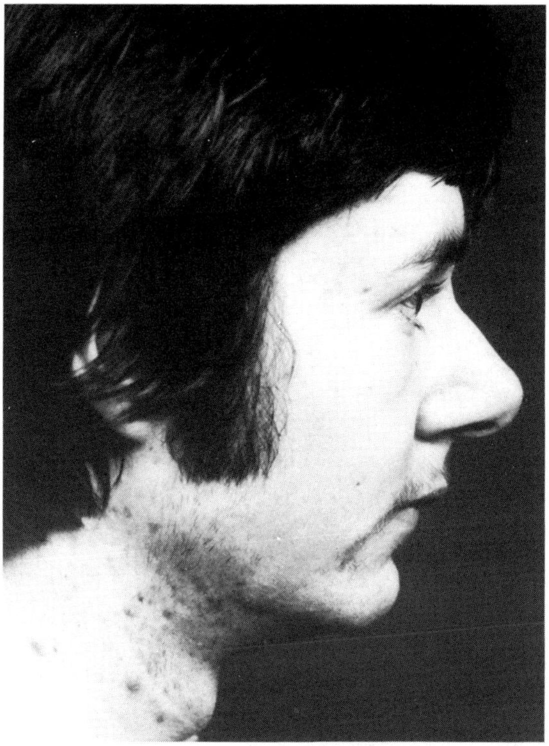

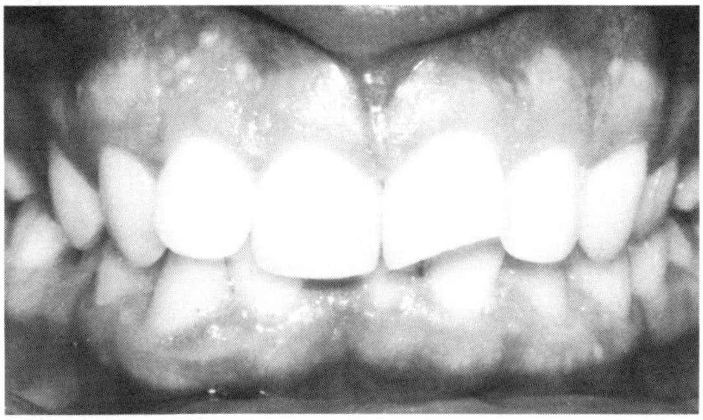

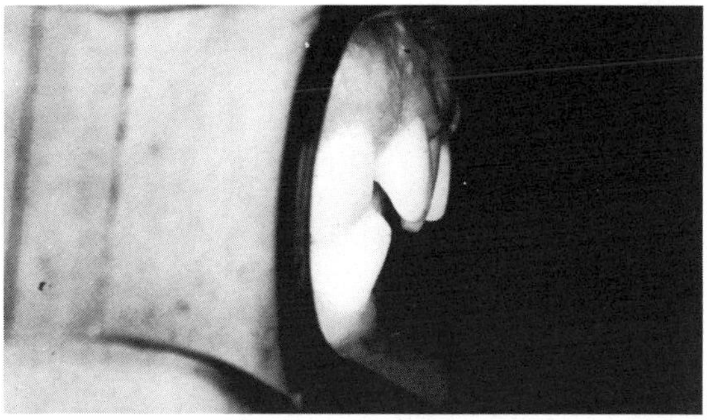

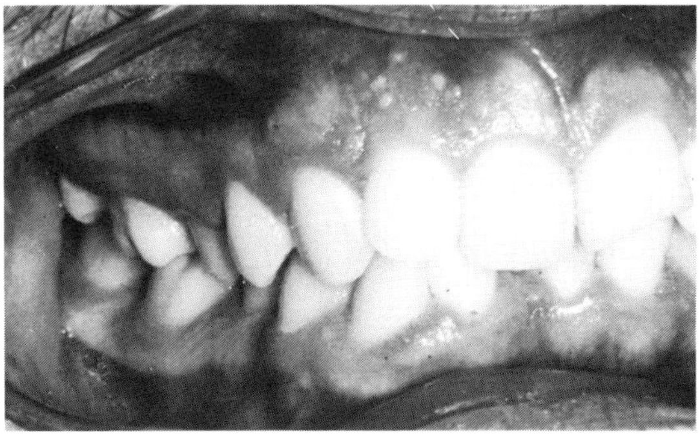

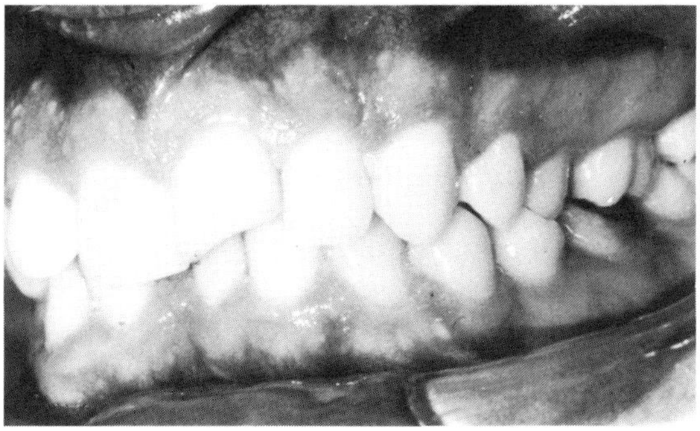

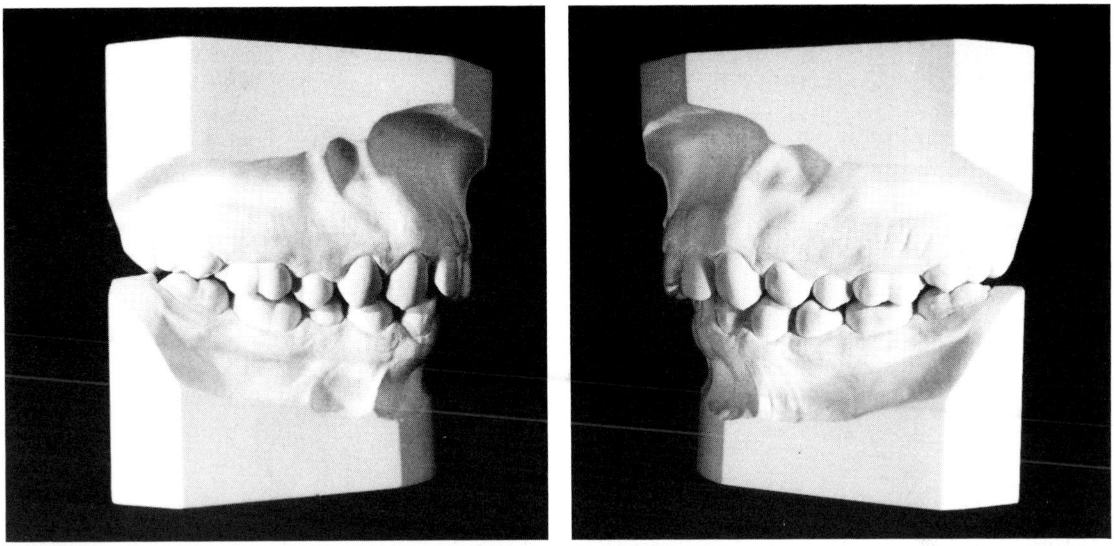

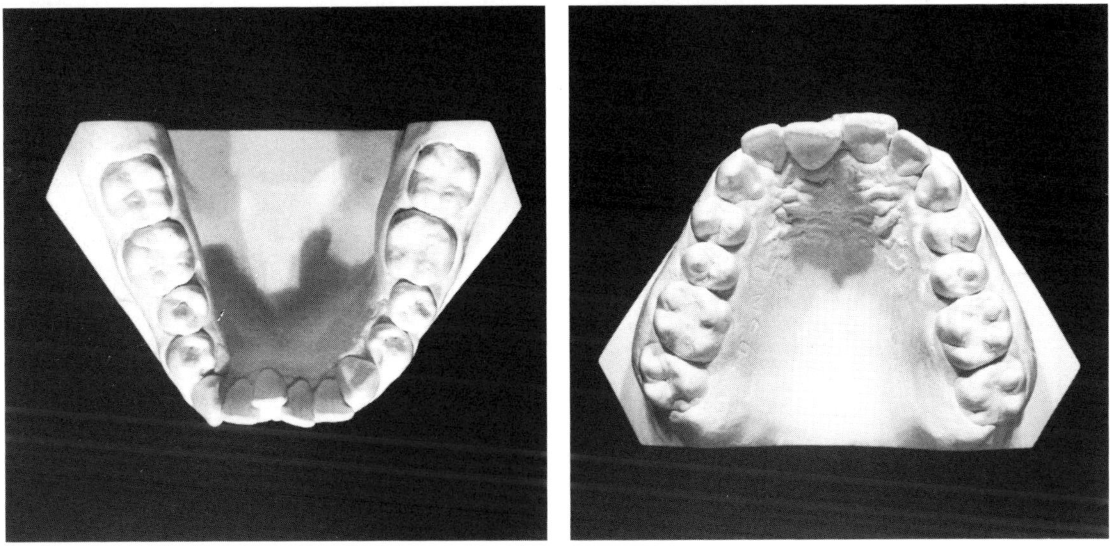

Figs 11-7 and 11-8 *At the age of 20 y, 10 mo the patient's face is clearly different in size and configuration from what it was 3½ years earlier. The nose has become much larger and the chin has become more prominent. The dentition now lies further back in relationship to the perioral tissues. The profile has become straighter. The irregularities in the position of the incisors of both jaws have increased. As the result of asymmetric movement of the teeth, the midlines of both dental arches no longer coincide.*

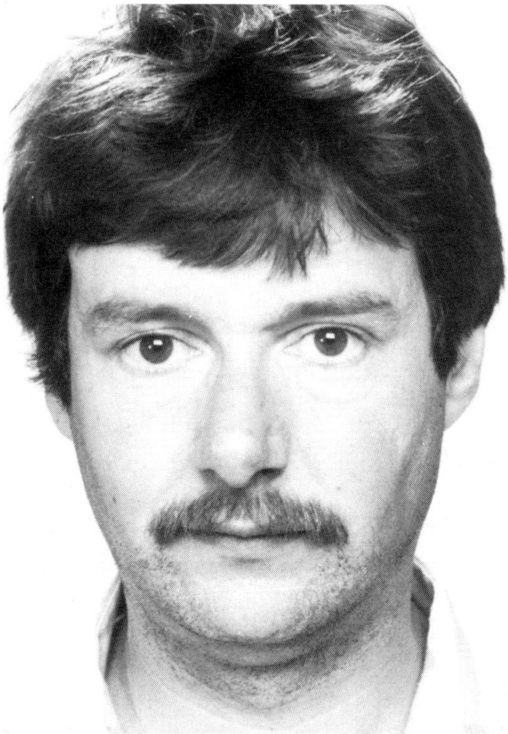

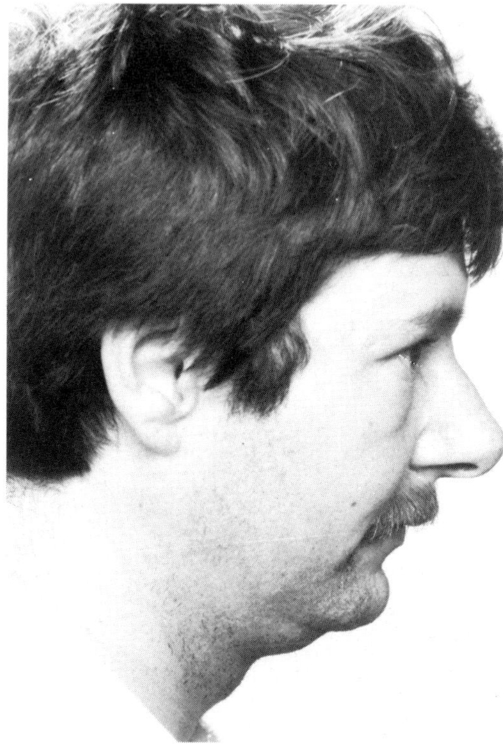

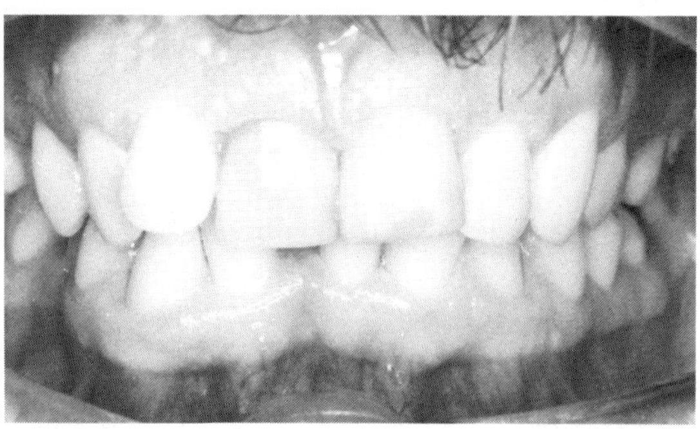

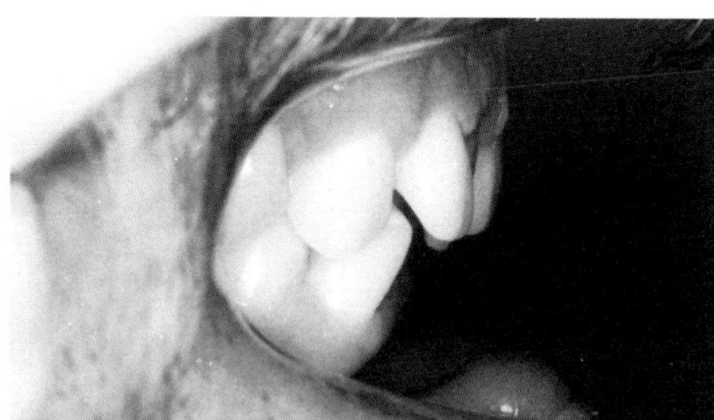

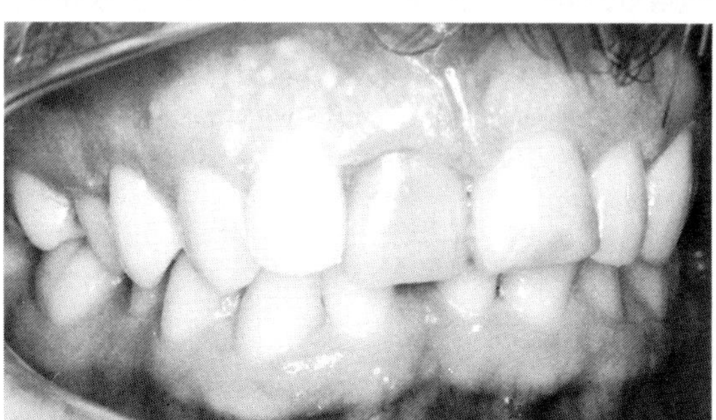

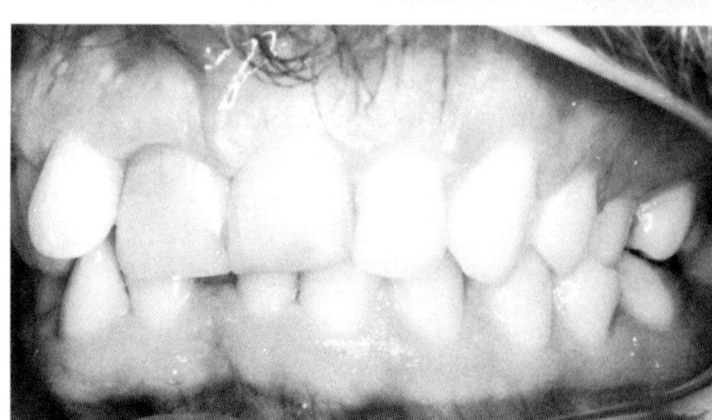

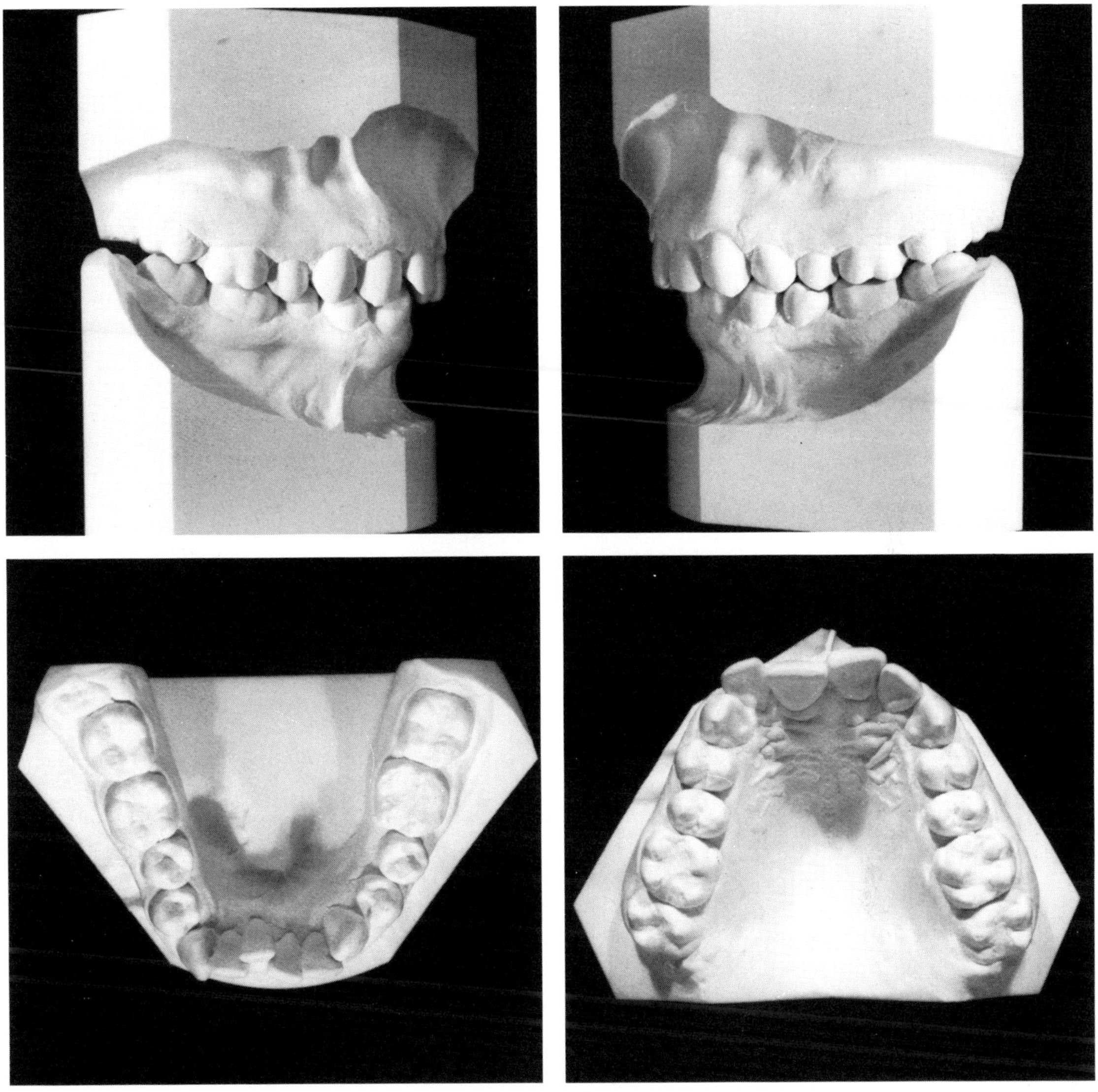

Figs 11-9 and 11-10 *At the age of 31 y, 3 mo, the face is now fuller and the dentition less obvious than ten years previously. The occlusion in the posterior regions has barely changed. The crowding in maxilla and mandible has increased. In both jaws the right central incisor has moved further to lingual.*

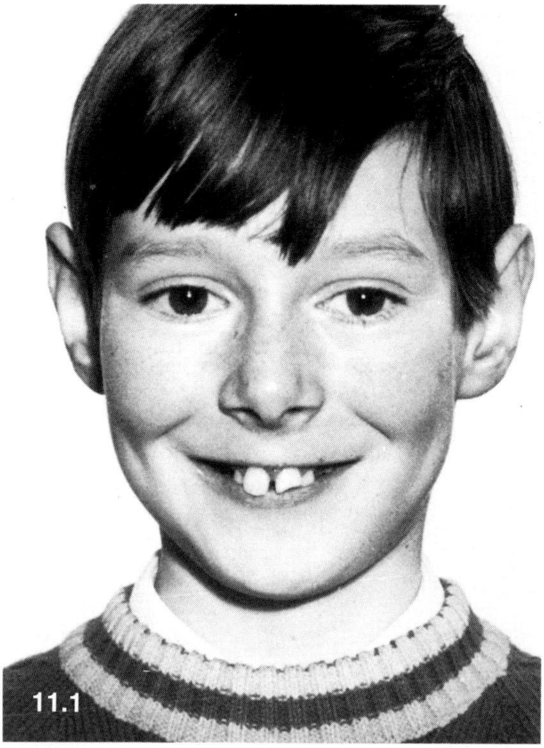

11.1

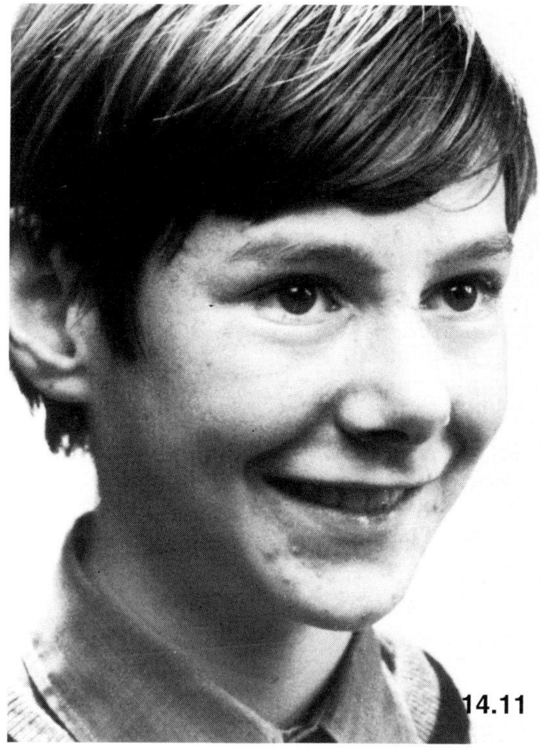

14.11

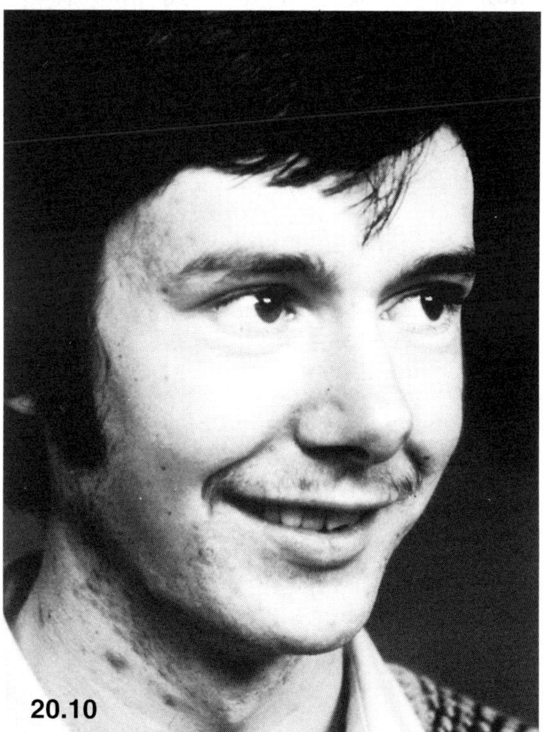

20.10

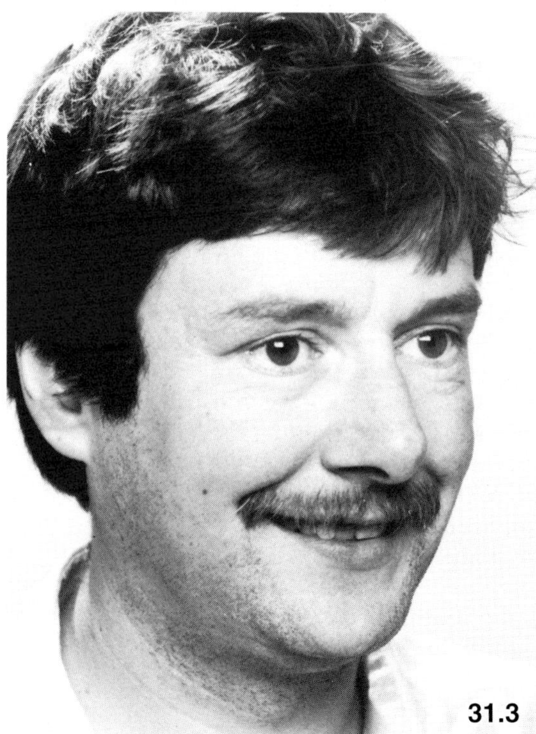

31.3

Fig 11-11 Note the changes that have occurred as the result of treatment and growth.

labially. The crowding of the mandibular incisors and the depth of bite have increased (Figs 11.5 and 11.6). These unfavorable developments continued in the following three years (Figs 11.7 and 11.8).
It is striking how strongly the face still grew after the age of 17. The nose has become much larger and the chin has clearly developed to ventral. Such late facial growth is regularly seen in young men. Girls complete their growth earlier, and generally have achieved adulthood well before their seventeenth birthdays.
At the age of 31 years, the crowding in the anterior regions of both arches has increased further (Figs.11.9 to 11.11).

In class II/1 anomalies with a large sagittal deviation in jaw relationship, it is as a rule impossible to secure a satisfactory result with only simple appliances. Besides, it is seldom possible to obtain good interproximal contacts in the mandibular arch without the use of fixed appliances. Indeed a lip bumper can lead to an increase in dental arch length through its action in holding the vestibular musculature away from the teeth. Under the influence of the tongue, the teeth can move further buccally than would have been possible if the pressure of the lips and cheeks had remained active against them. However, good interproximal contacts in the anterior region are seldom established, and at removal of the lip bumper, the position of the teeth can deteriorate. The elimination of the influence of the perioral musculature also has the disadvantage that the spontaneous corrections of tooth alignment that can occur because space became available, are guided from lingual only, without the effects of vestibular forces. So a lip bumper works well insofar as increasing available arch length is concerned; on the other hand, functional components that might encourage natural corrections are partly taken out of action. Other indesirable effects may be involved occasionally, such as tipping the mandibular first permanent molars to distal, and rotating them or moving them lingually by injudicious bends in the appliance. These changes occur at the cost of proper interproximal contacts with the second permanent molars, particularly when these teeth have not emerged yet.
In cases with a large overjet and little labial tipping of the maxillary incisors, it is not possible to retract the incisors sufficiently while maintaining good axial inclinations if just a plate is used. Fixed appliances are essential to torque the incisor apices palatally as the crowns are retracted and to move the canine apices distally in a similar way. If the sagittal discrepancy is small, as was true in case 10, or if a significant improvement in the overjet can be expected from mandibular growth, then these limitations are not applicable and a good result can be achieved. If not, then either the incisors become too steeply positioned or the overjet is insufficiently reduced. Steeply inclined maxillary incisors provide problems after treatment. The incisors generally erupt further, which results in a deeper bite, and the mandibular incisors that already were unable to assume good alignment become even more crowded. If the lower lip covers the maxillary incisors excessively, subsequent to treatment a "cover bite" can develop (see chapter 35).
From the previous description, it might seem that in situations comparable with this case that it often is not possible to achieve a good result with simple means. The use of fixed appliances is demanded in such cases and even then it is not certain that the obtained result will be permanent.

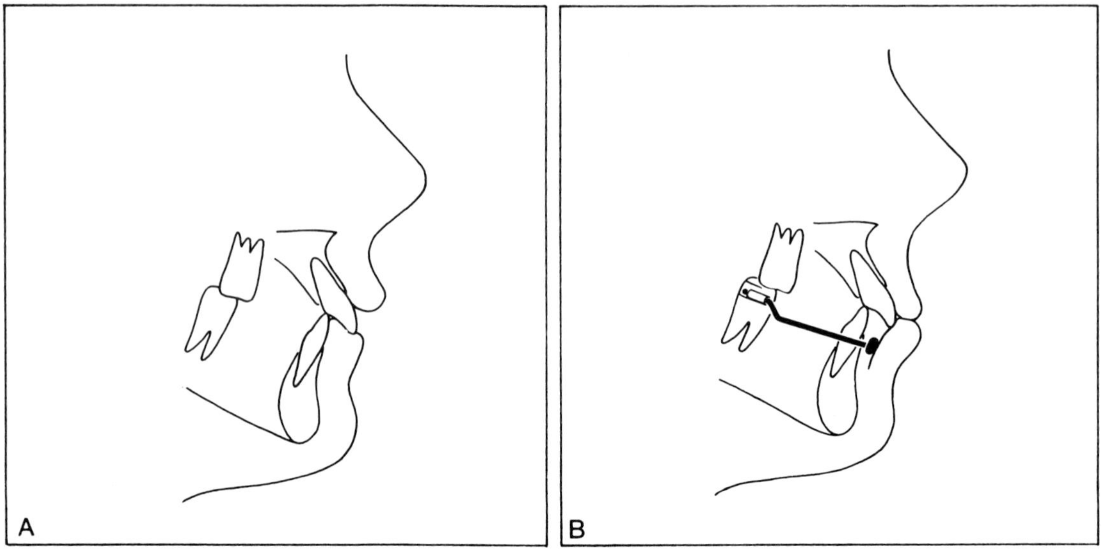

Fig 11-12 Lip bumpers can be utilized to change the position of the lips and to increase the room available in the dental arch.
A If the lower lip lies behind the maxillary incisors and the mandibular incisors are in inversion as a consequence, a lip bumper can improve both situations simultaneously.
B The lip bumper is removable, and is fitted into tubes (.045 inch = 1.2 mm approx.) that are attached to bands cemented to the mandibular first permanent molars. The lip bumper should lie about 2 to 3 mm clear of the alveolar process.[36]

When fixed appliances are used and the apices of the maxillary incisors are moved to palatal, this by no means implies that the profile will always have been notably improved. As the result of the movement to palatal of the apices, the upper lip in the region of the nose will also have fallen back. The nose will then appear to have increased in size; above all, the patient's mouth can look like that of a person with badly constructed false teeth.
The overall conclusion might be that in situations such as this, everything must be done that can be done to eliminate the excessive overjet early with facial-orthopedic means that restrict the ventral development of the maxillary structures and have a favorable effect on mandibular growth. In that respect, boys have better chances. If they indeed profit from a marked mandibular growth then it might be possible to procure in addition sufficient retraction of the maxillary incisors with labial arches on a plate, if those arches are carefully applied to the cervical of the incisor crowns and cautiously activated. Sagittal contact can be attained without causing the incisors to stand too steeply, the more so if the mandibular incisors are either well angulated or in mild eversion.

Chapter 12

Class II/1
Extraction deciduous canines, cervical headgear, lingual arch, maxillary removable plate, positioner
Male: 8 years, 2 months to 25 years, 2 months

A boy aged 8 years, 2 months exhibited a mild class II/1 anomaly with crowding in mandibular and maxillary anterior regions. Oral functions were normal and unstrained mouth closure was routine. The maxillary right lateral deciduous incisor had been lost early and the mandibular permanent lateral incisor on the left had emerged lingually. The disto-occlusion was ½ PW (a little more on the left than on the right) and the midlines of the dental arches did not coincide. Moyers' mixed dentition analysis indicated a lack of space of 4 mm in the mandible and 6 mm in the maxilla. The narrow maxillary lateral incisors pointed to an anterior TSD with relatively too much tooth material in the mandibular anterior teeth (Figs 12.1 and 12.2).

It was decided that in the first instance the asymmetric development of the dentition in the anterior regions of both jaws would be corrected by removal of the maxillary left and mandibular right deciduous canines. The intention was that the incisors should drift toward the extraction spaces to reduce the deviation of the midlines (Figs 12.15 and 12.16). Six months later, the other two deciduous canines were removed. At a later stage a lingual arch would be placed on the mandibular arch to maintain the extra arch length that would become available in the posterior regions upon exfoliation of the deciduous molars. The lingual arch would serve not only to maintain the arch length for the benefit of the permanent mandibular canines that still were to emerge, but also to correct the linguo-position of the mandibular left lateral incisor.

In the treatment plan, the possibility of reducing the mesiodistal diameter of the mandibular incisors (stripping) was left open since there seemed likely to be an excess of tooth material in the mandibular incisors relative to the maxillary ones after emergence of the mandibular permanent canines. With a cervical headgear, an asymmetric type if required, the disto-occlusion would be corrected and space provided for the permanent canines in the maxilla. This space would be gained in part by the distopalatal rotation of the maxillary first permanent molars.

The subsequent treatment was begun three years after the extraction of the deciduous canines, which had resulted in the expected improvements (Fig 12.3). All the deciduous teeth except the second deciduous molars had been replaced by their successors, although the permanent canines had emerged only a short time previously. The lingual arch was fitted, then a month later the cervical headgear was installed. The models made at the age of 11 years, 10 months show an intermediate

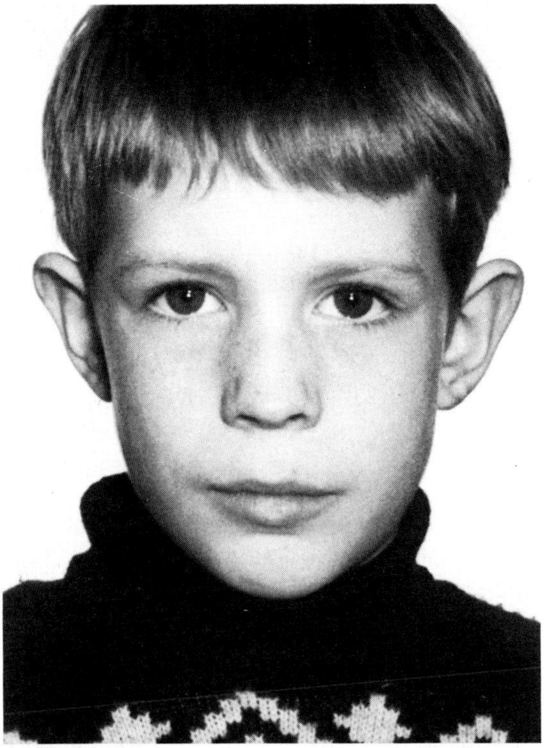

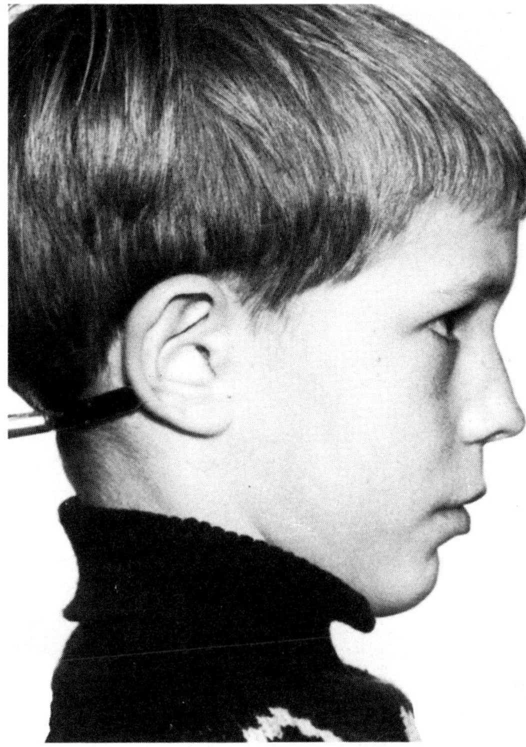

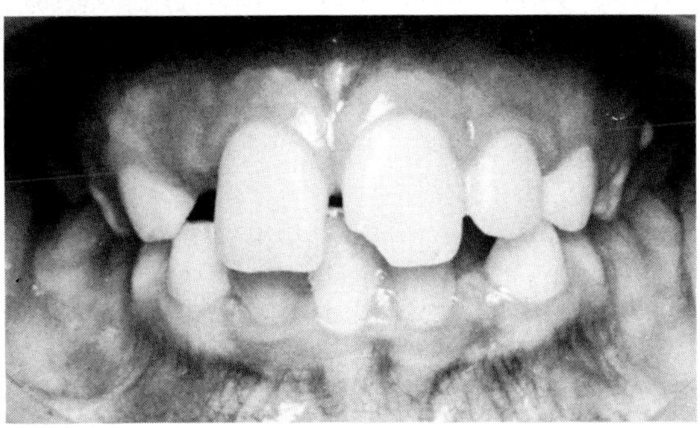

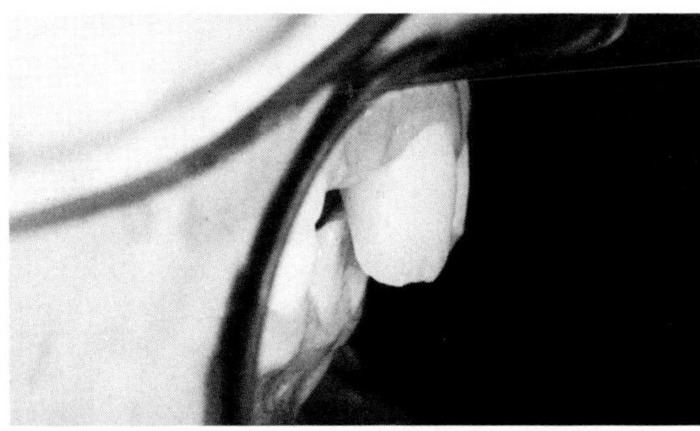

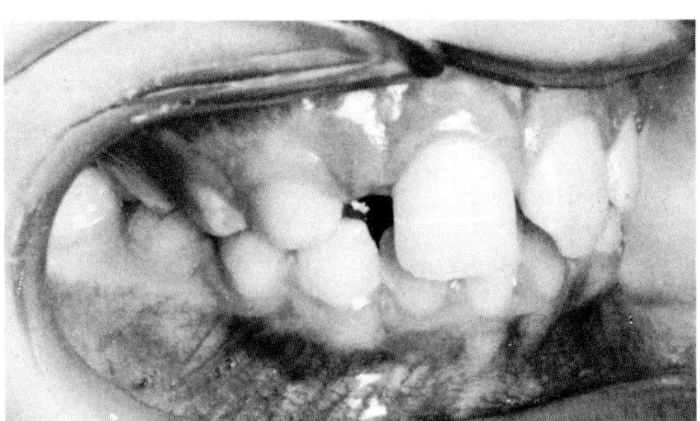

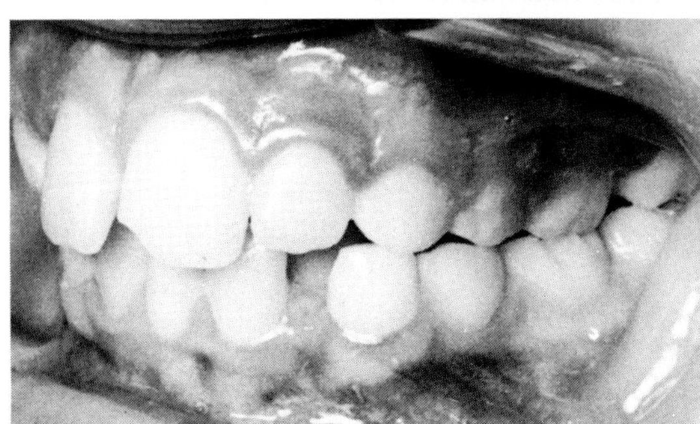

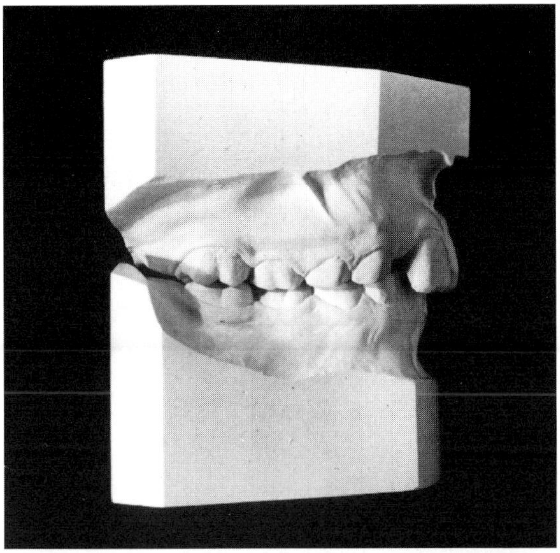
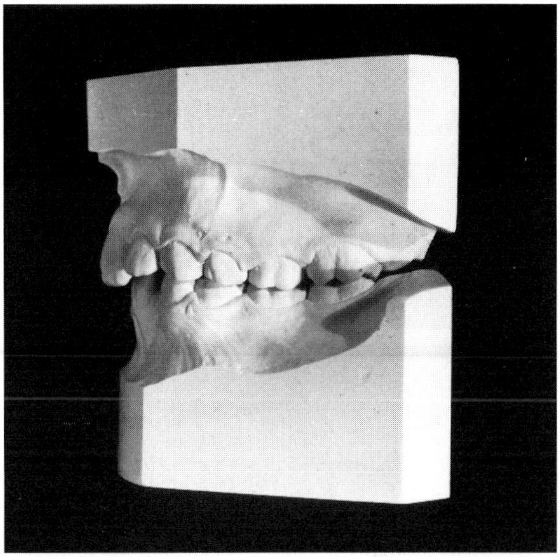
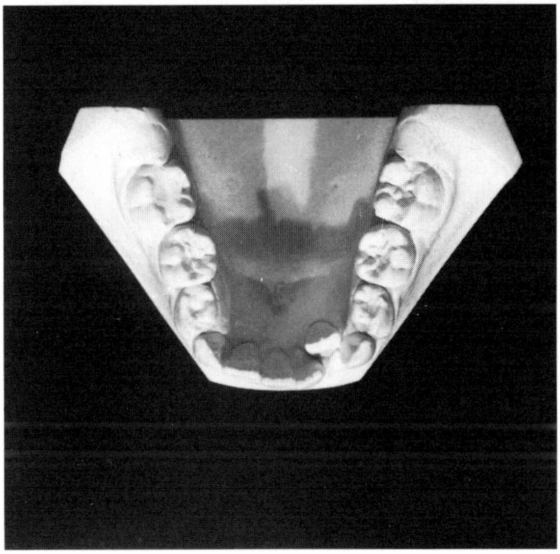
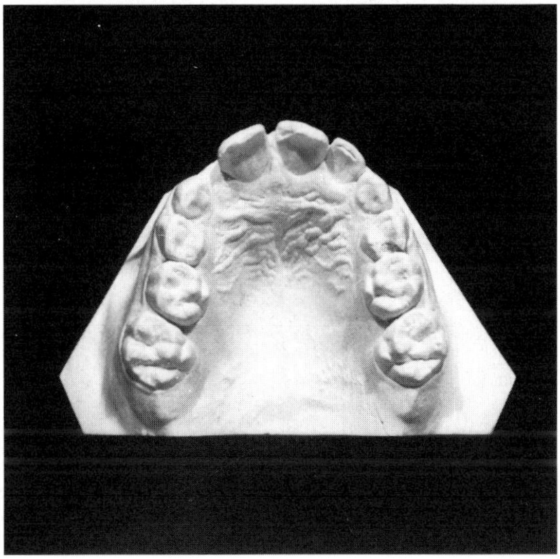

Figs 12-1 and 12-2 *A boy aged 8 yr, 2 mo with a moderate class II/1 anomaly (disto-occlusion of ½ PW), a slightly receding chin, normal function, and competent lip seal. The mandibular and maxillary anterior regions exhibit crowding, which is concentrated on the mandibular left lateral incisor that is in linguo-position and on the maxillary right lateral incisor, which has insufficient room in which to emerge. The predecessor of the latter exfoliated due to resorption of its root before the emergence of the maxillary right central incisor. In the maxilla, the midline of the dental arch deviates to the right; in the mandible, to the left. The midline discrepancy is quite obvious.*

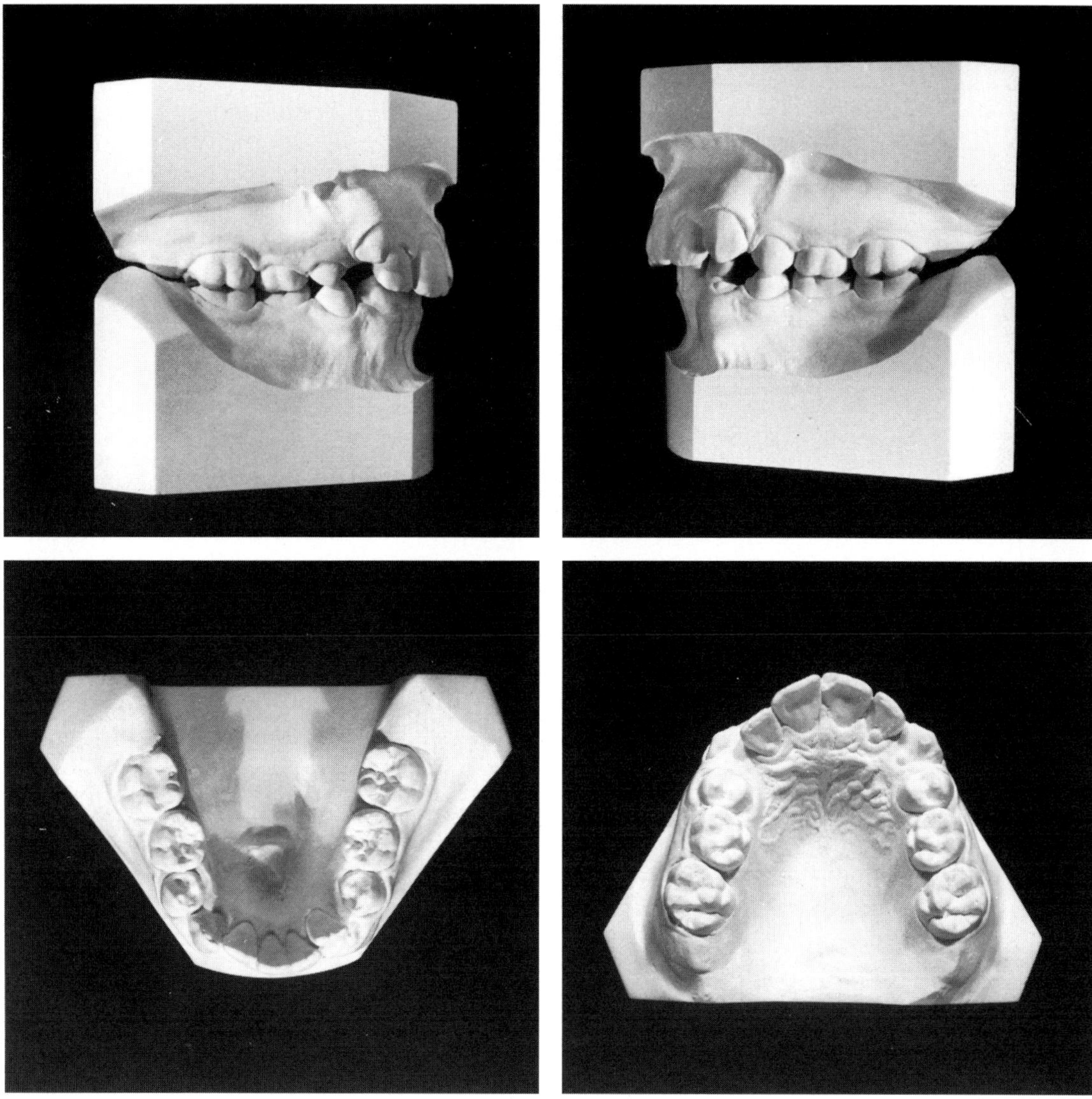

Fig 12-3 At the age of 11 y, 3 mo, three years after extraction of the deciduous canines, the maxillary and mandibular incisors have been for some time in better positions and the deviation in the arch midlines has largely been corrected, particularly in the maxilla. Since there has not been any active treatment in the meantime, the molar occlusion has barely changed.

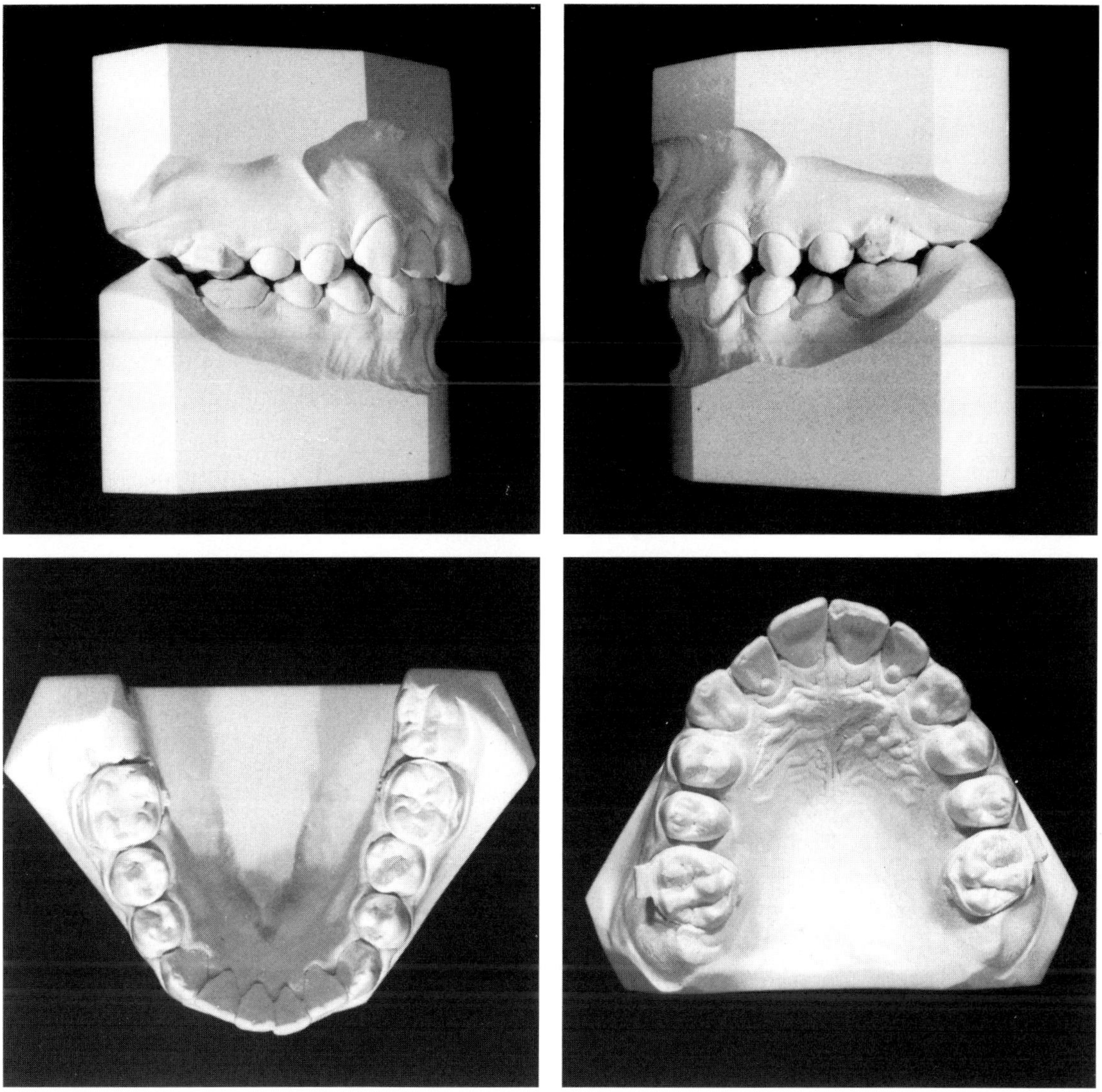

Fig 12-4 At the age of 11 y, 10 mo after six months of treatment with a cervical headgear and a lingual arch, the disto-occlusion has been entirely corrected on the right and almost corrected on the left. In the mandible, mesial migration of the first permanent molars after exfoliation of the deciduous second molars has been prevented. Moreover, in the mandible on the left more room has been obtained for the permanent canine and the lateral incisor has moved labially. In the maxillary arch more than enough space has been obtained, partly due to the first permanent molars having been rotated distopalatally (still not enough on the left). The canines have drifted to distal and palatal.

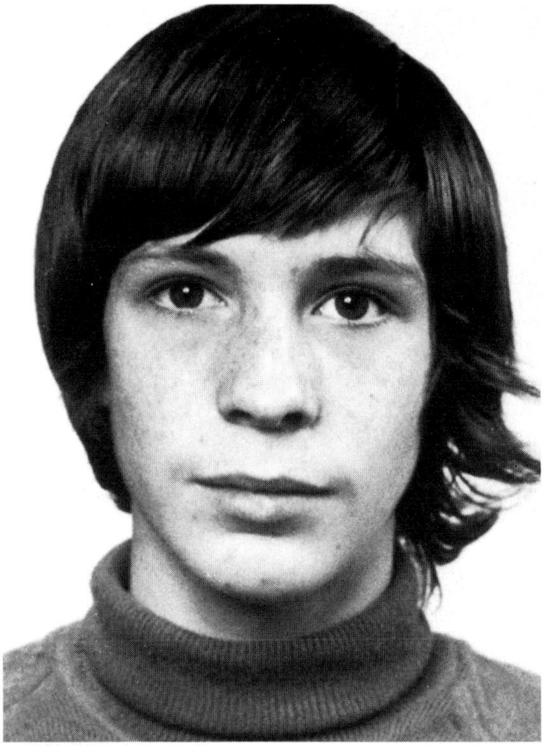
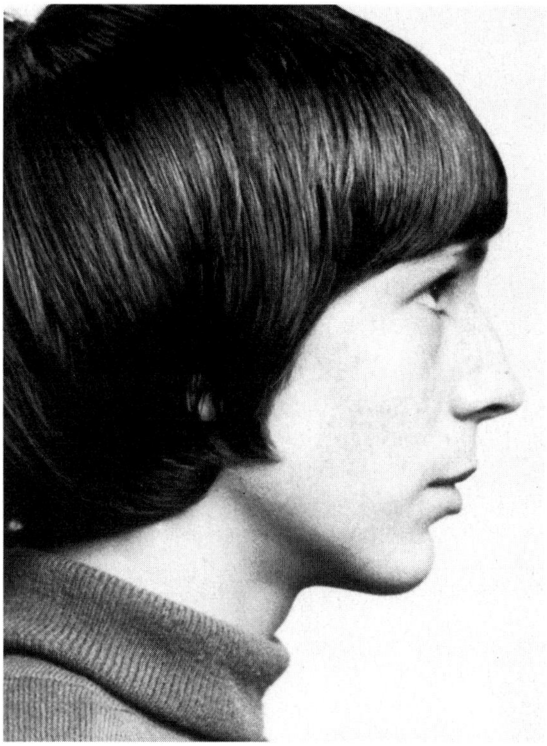
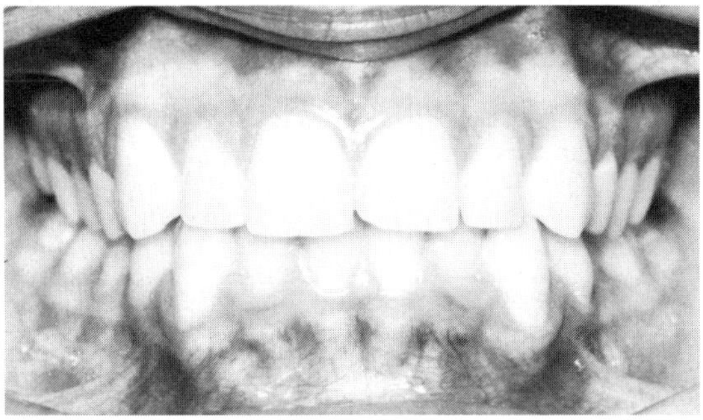
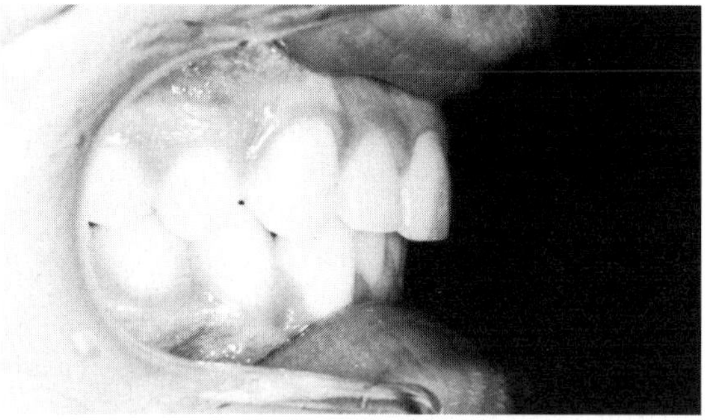
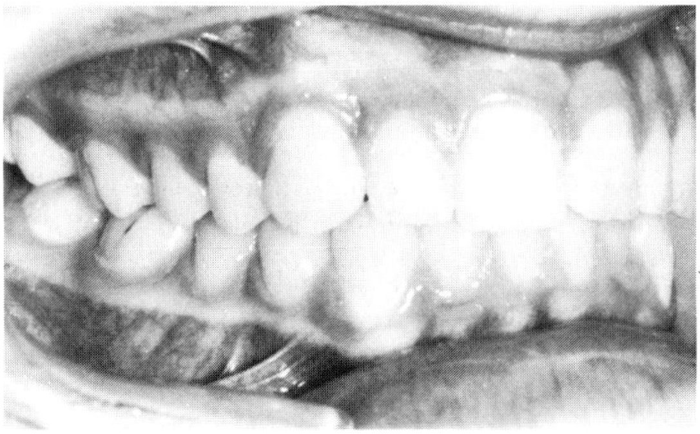
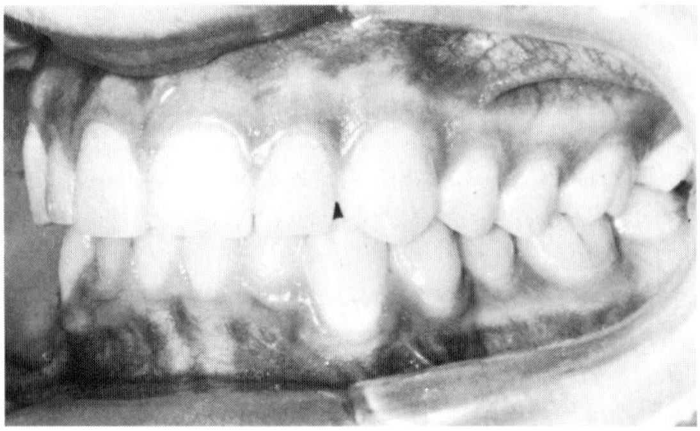

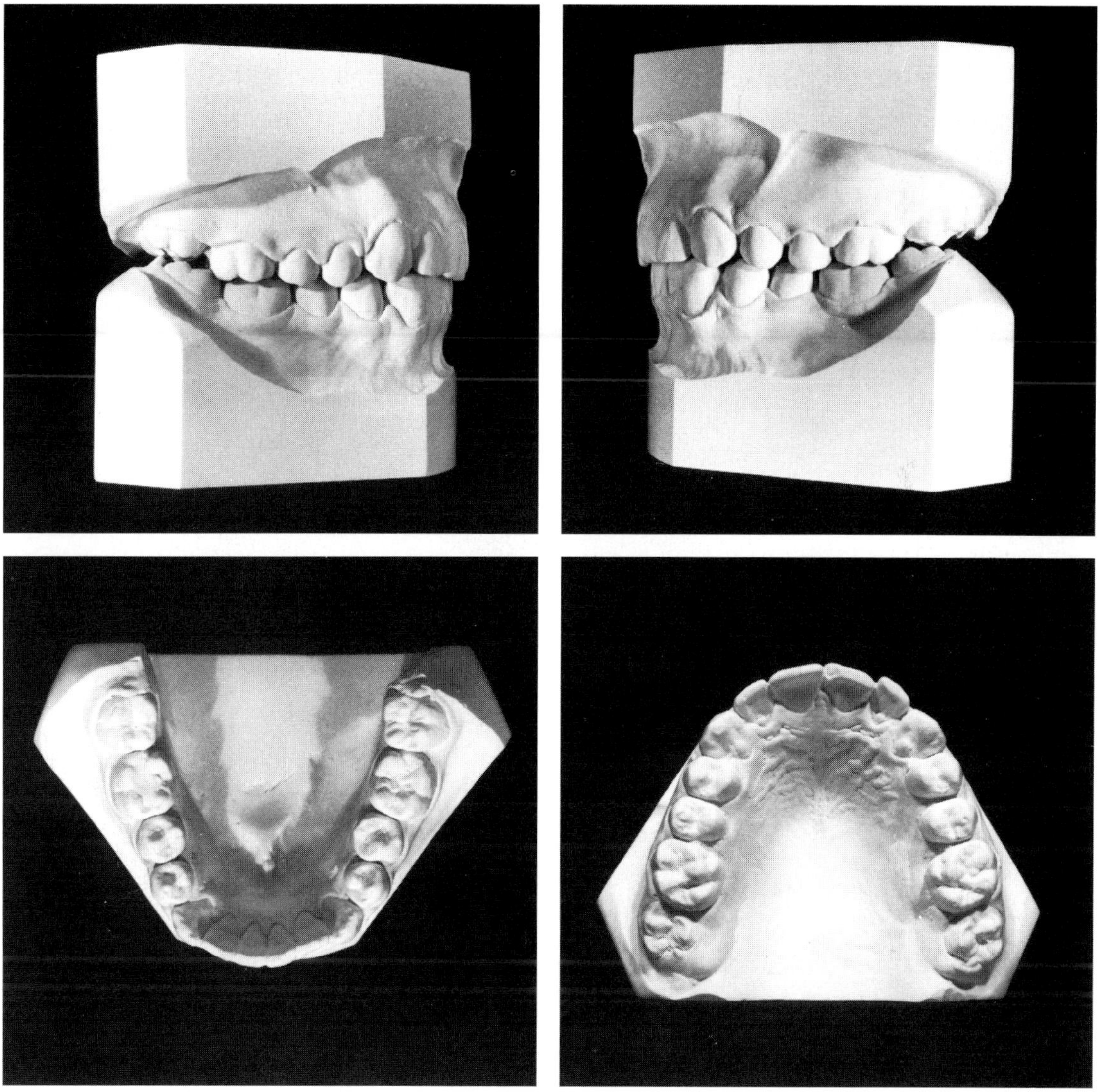

Figs 12-5 and 12-6 *At the age of 15 y, 2 mo after an active treatment period of two years and three months with simple appliances, followed by a retention period of one year and nine months with a positioner, a good result has been obtained. The midlines of both arches now correspond. There is a good occlusion with solid interdigitation of canines and premolars. The fractured maxillary left central incisor has been ground incisally and the crown of the right central ground shorter to match it.*

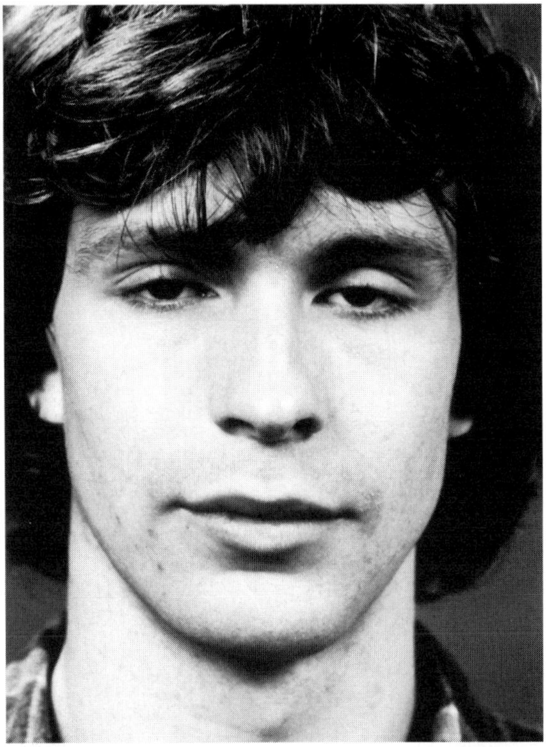
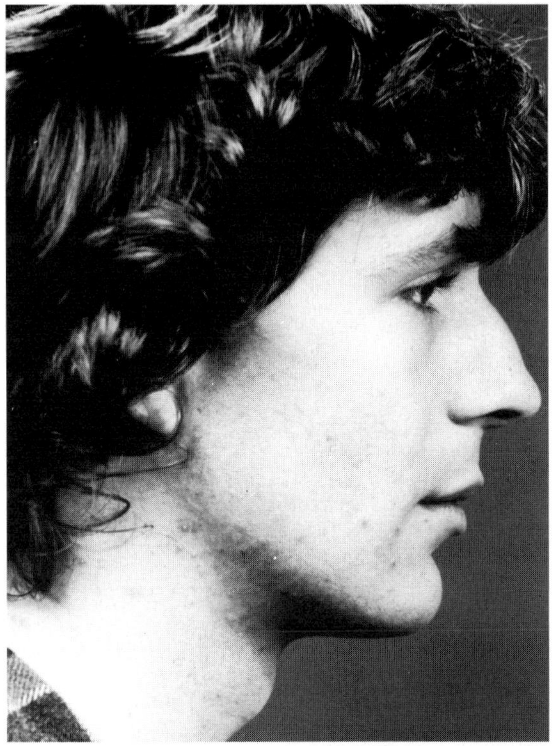
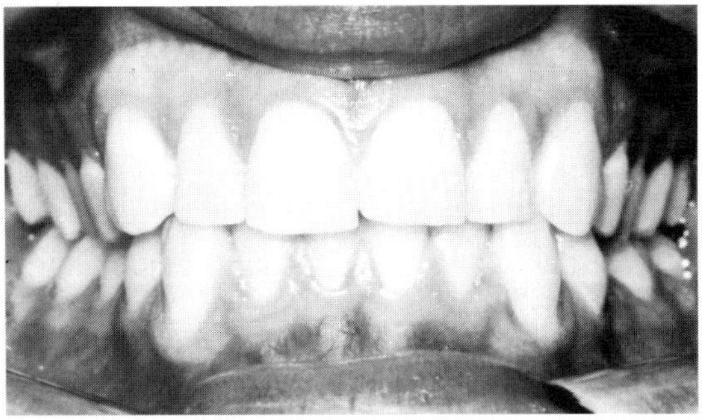
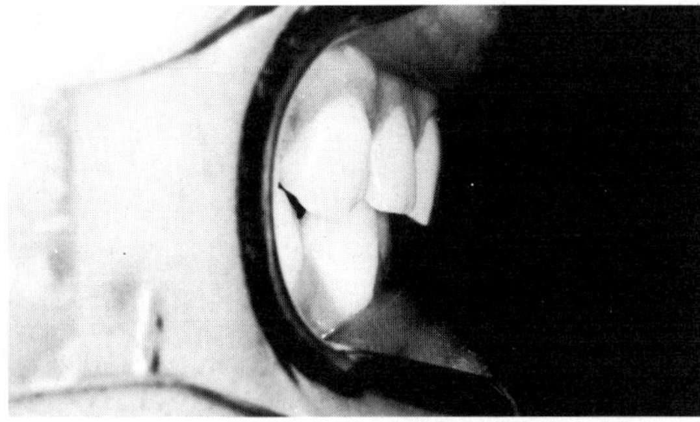
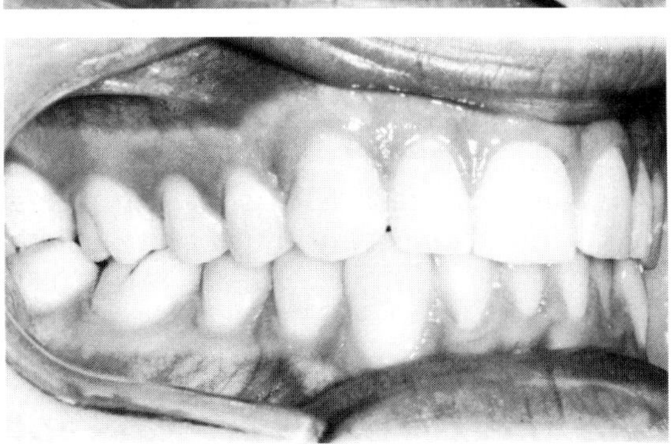
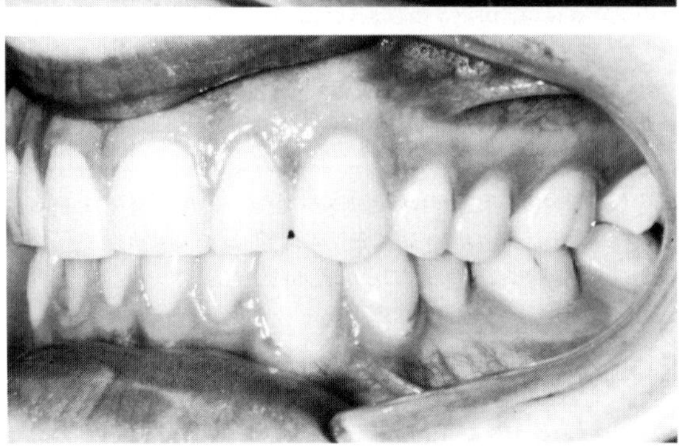

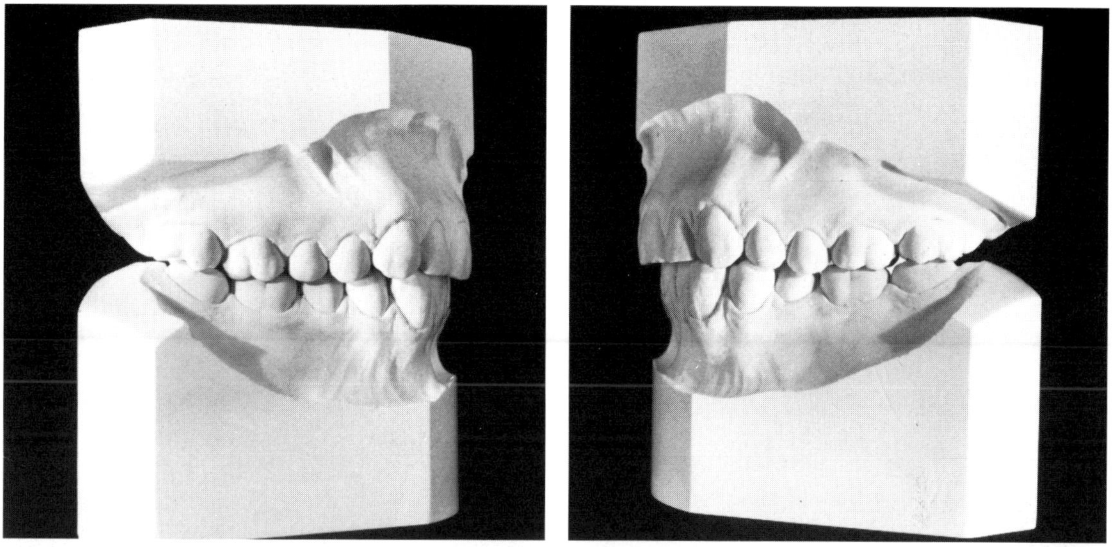

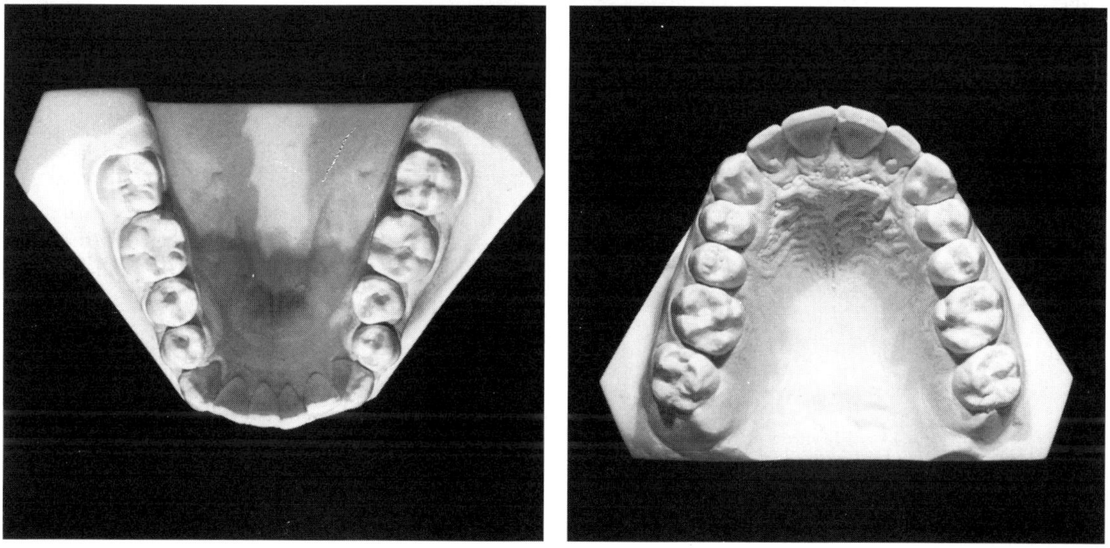

Figs 12-7 and 12-8 *Now aged 20 y, 2 mo the face has developed further. The nose is larger and the chin is more prominent. Changes in the dentition are limited mainly to the occurrence of slight tertiary crowding in the mandible, in the anterior region and in the left premolar region. The mandibular left lateral incisor has moved lingually again a little way toward its original position. Apart from the maxillary right third molar, the third molars were congenitally absent.*

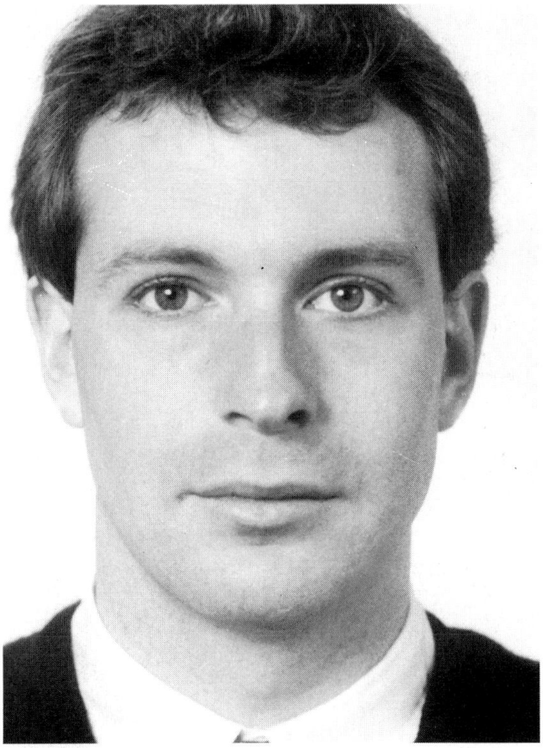

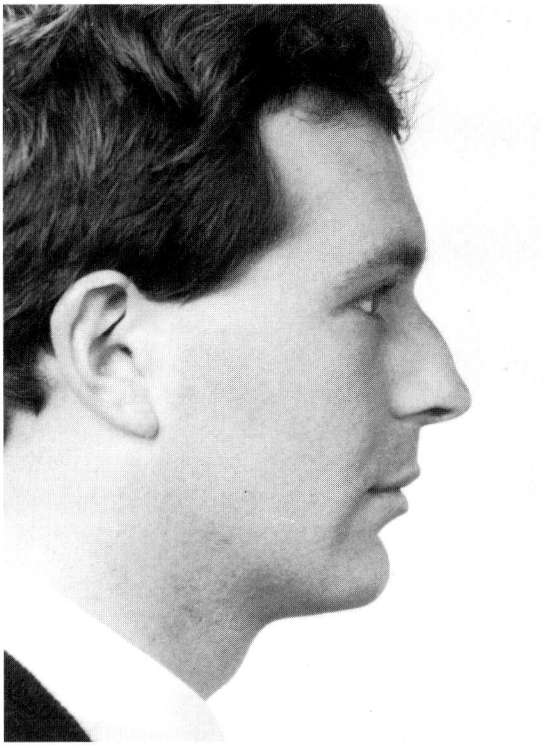

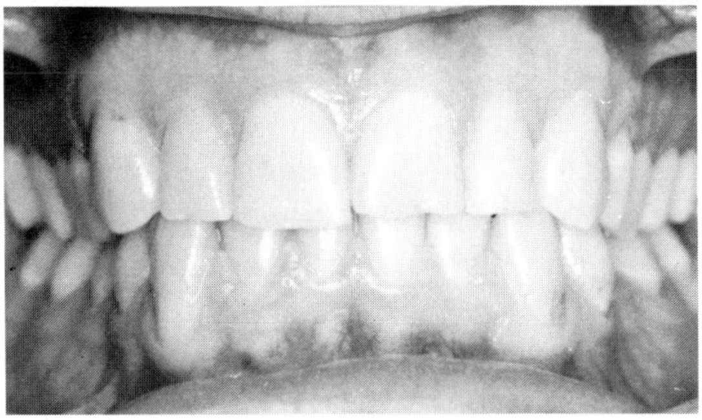

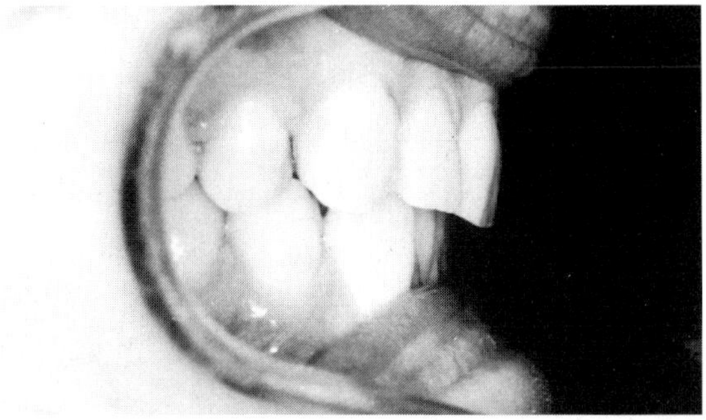

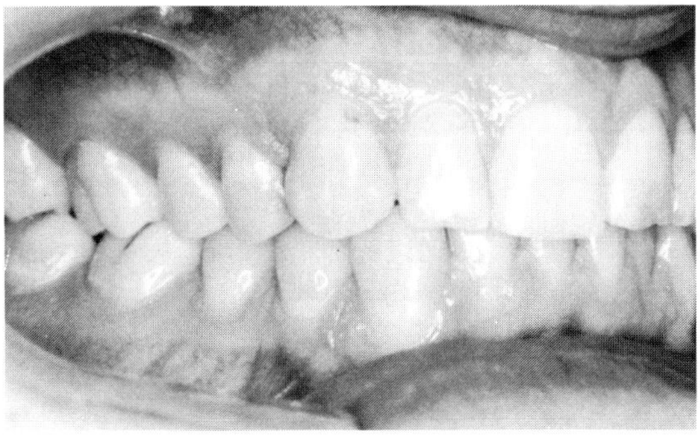

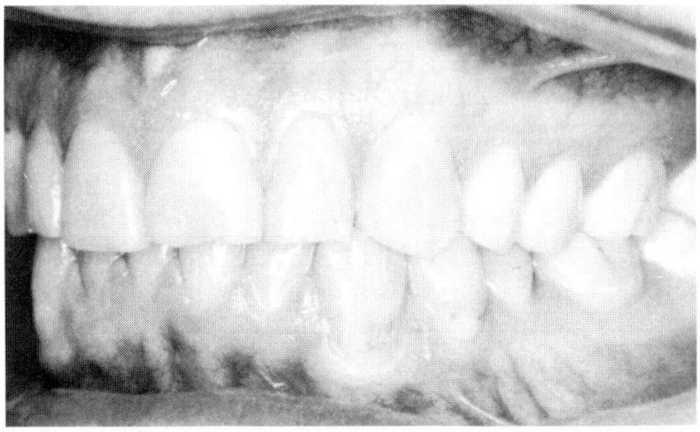

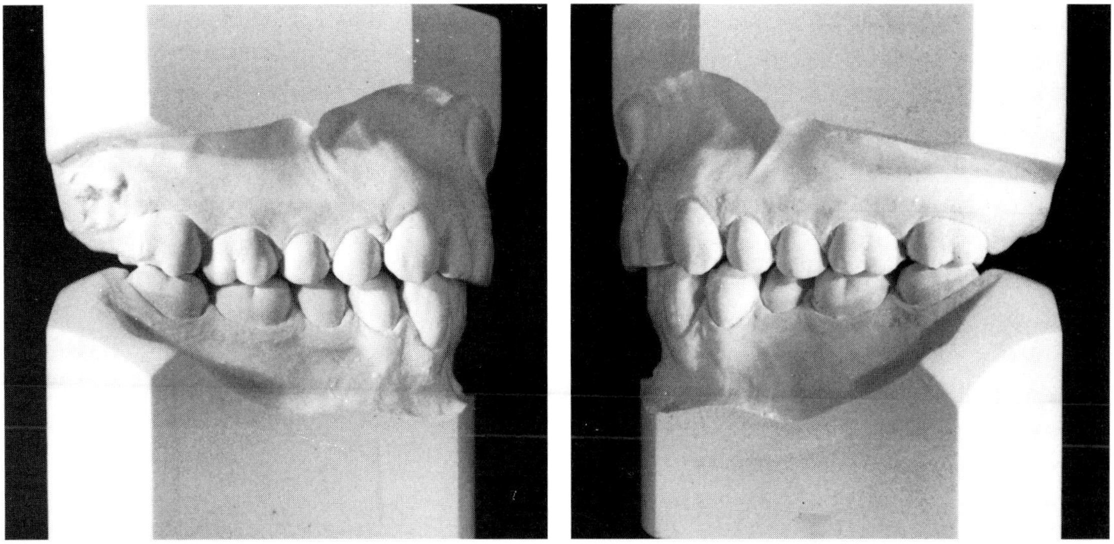

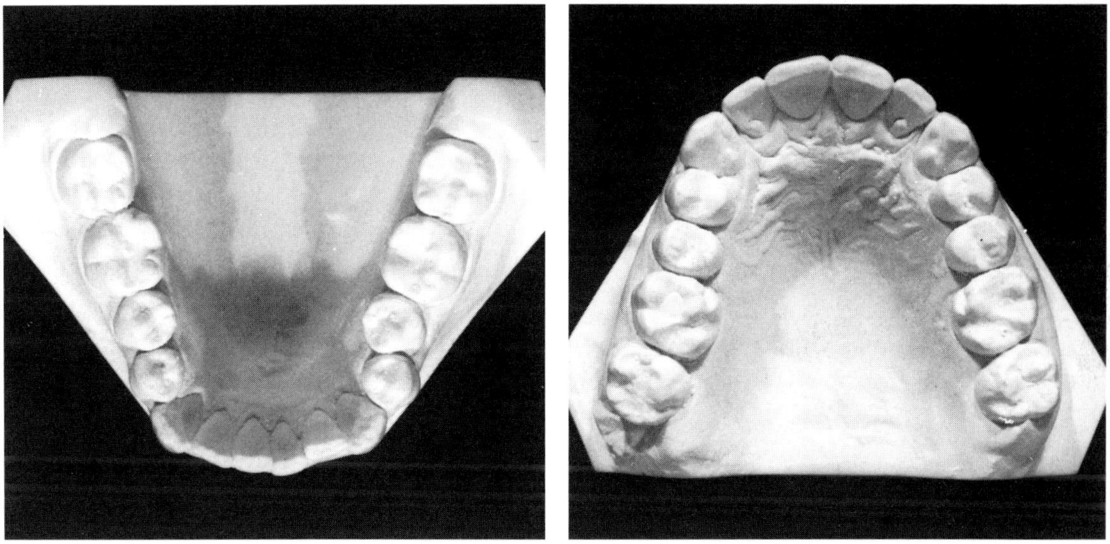

Figs 12-9 and 12-10 *Aged 25 y, 2 mo the patient's face is harmonious. The crowding on the left of the mandible has increased a little. The solid interdigitation and the normal functional conditions justify the suggestion that this result will remain essentially stable.*

The right maxillary third molar had emerged about a year previously. Its presence had prevented the roots of the adjacent second molar going to distal and improving the latter's angulation and occlusion. On the left where both third molars were absent, the position of the maxillary second permanent molar could still improve. This difference incidentally, could be seen at an earlier time (see Fig 12.8).

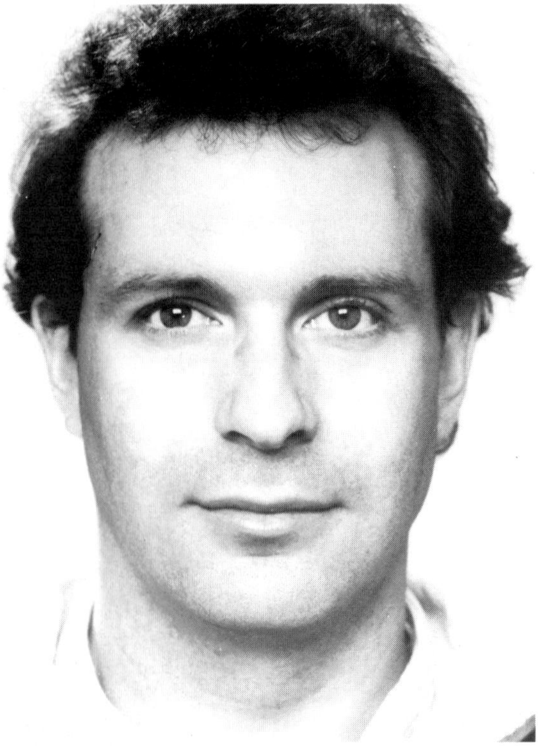
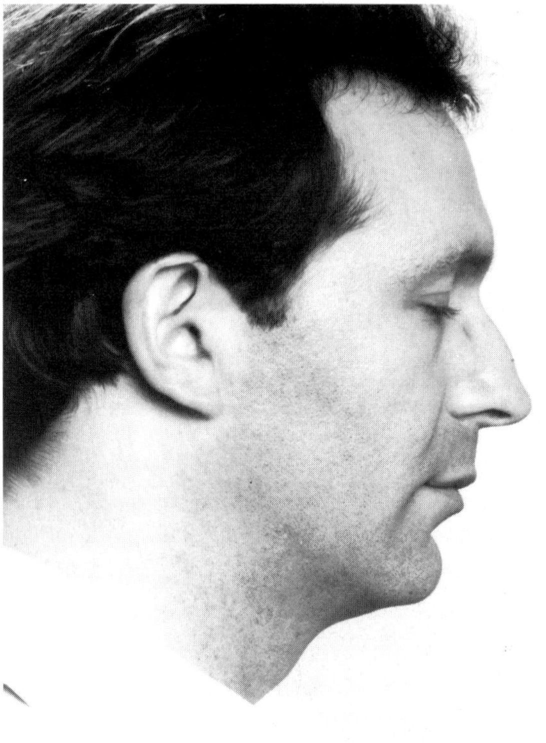
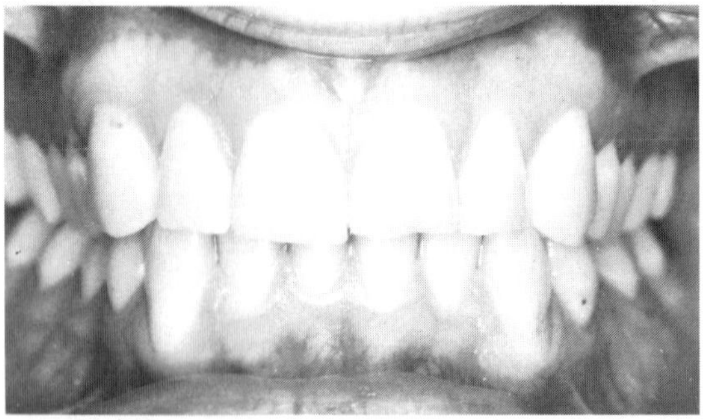
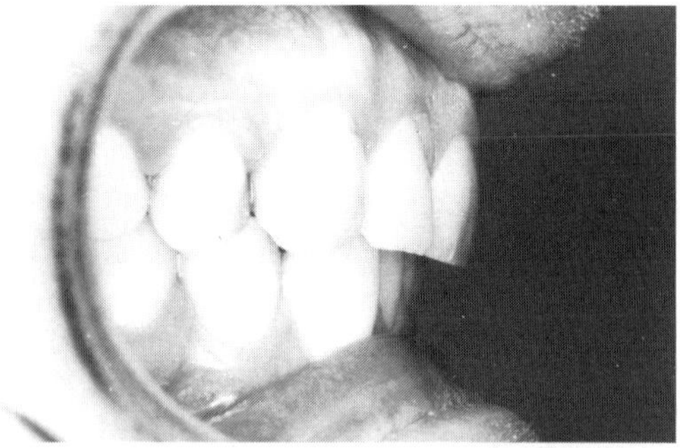
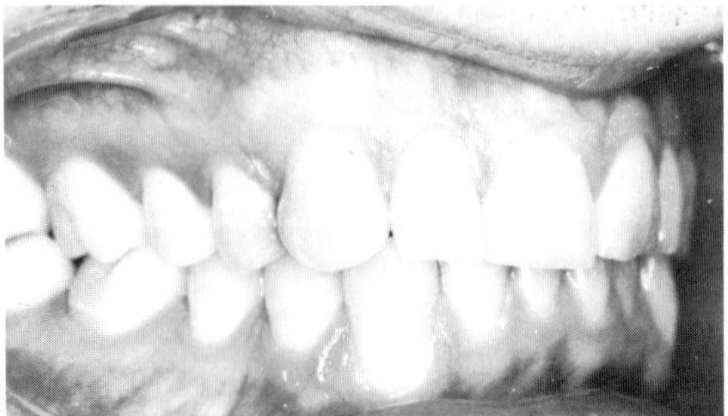
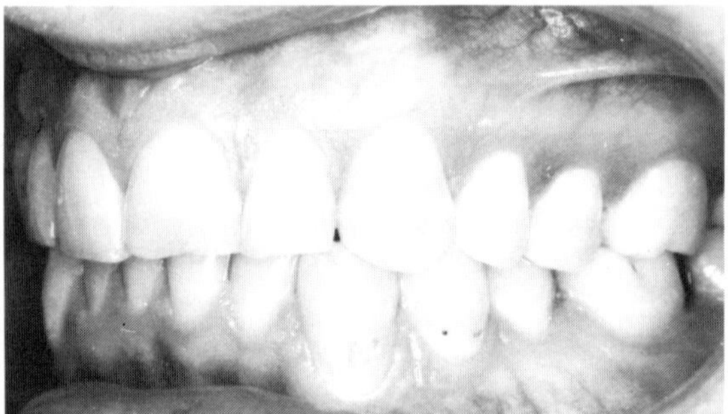

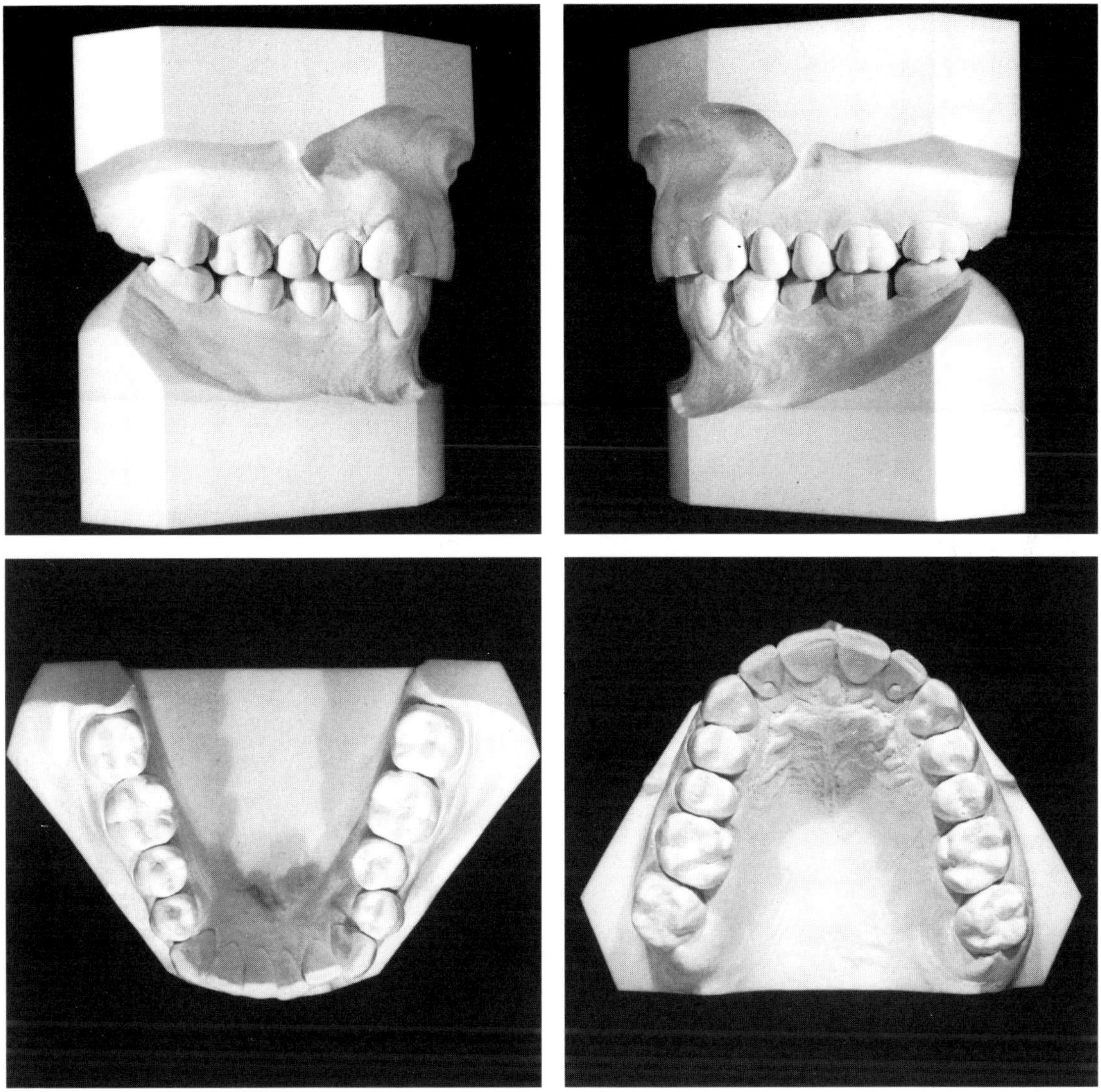

Figs 12-11 and 12-12 *At the age of 30 y, 6 mo, the situation has changed little in comparison with five years earlier. The maxillary right third molar had been extracted in the meantime and the angulation and occlusion of the adjacent second molar had improved.*

Figure 12-13a

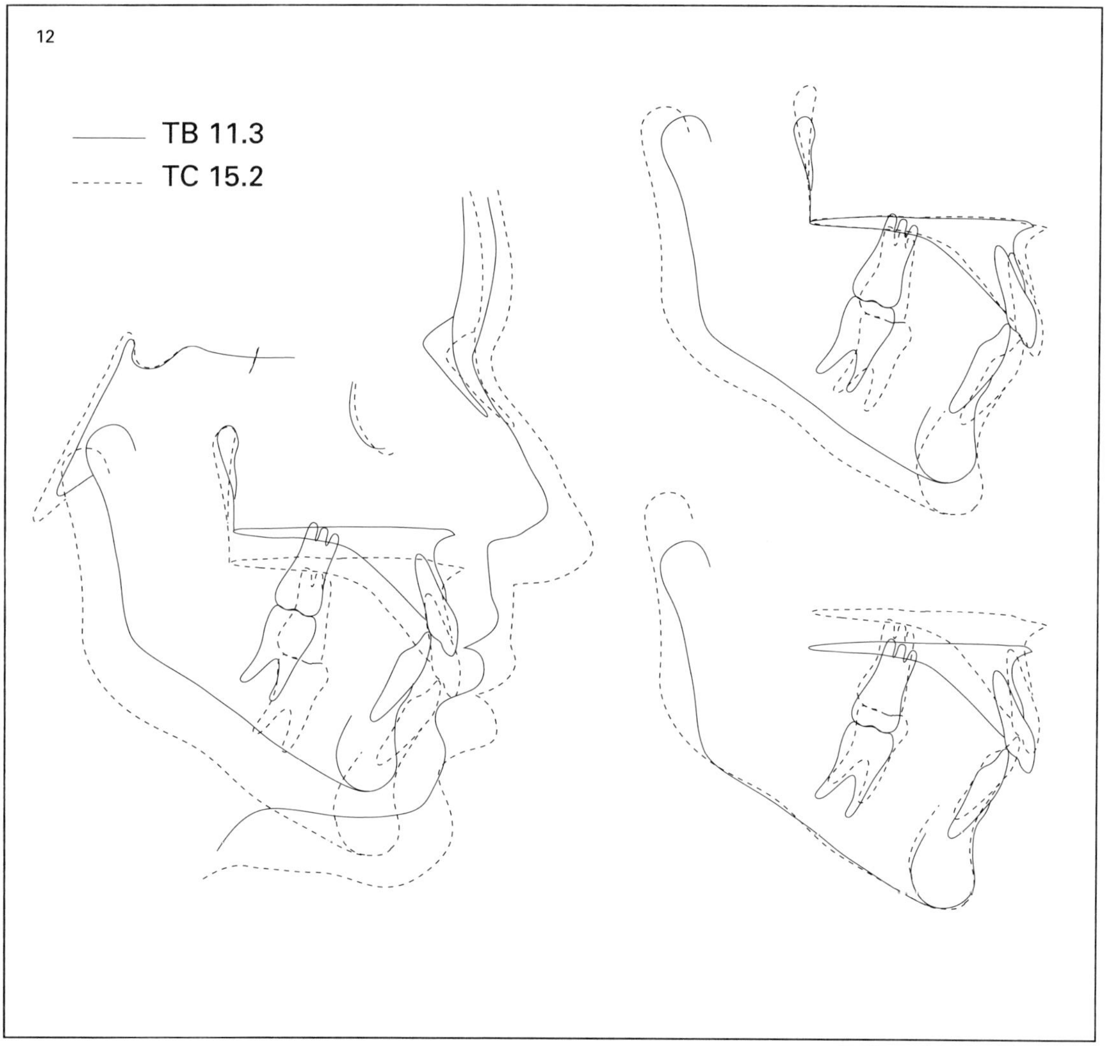

Figs 12-13a and 12-13b Superimposition of cephalometric tracings shows that both during treatment and after it, more ventral growth had taken place in the mandible than in the midfacial complex.

Figure 12-13b

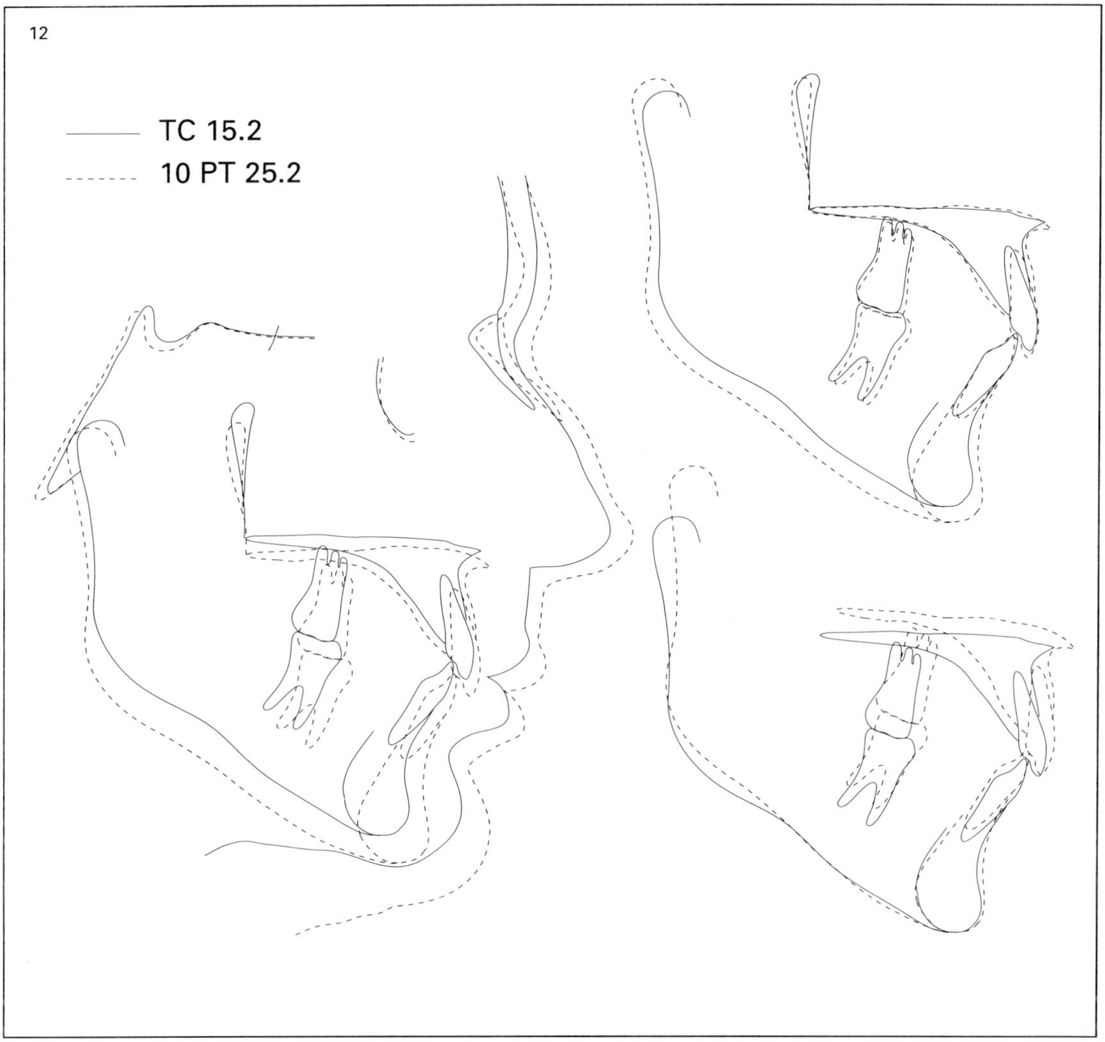

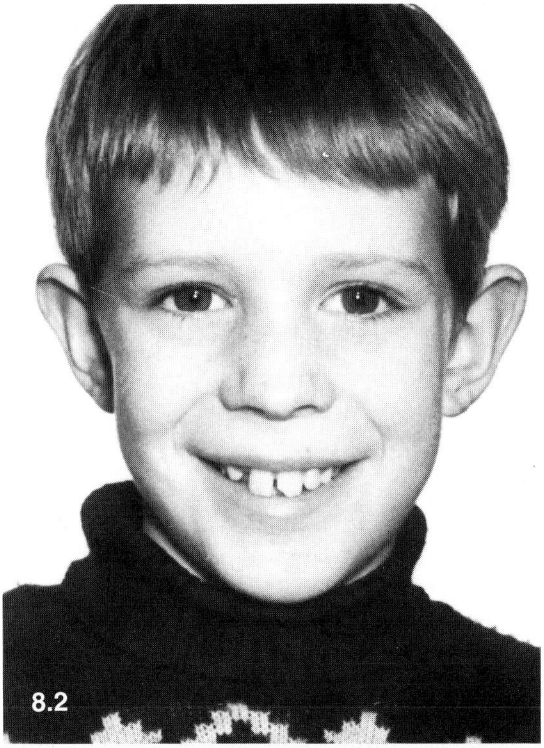

8.2

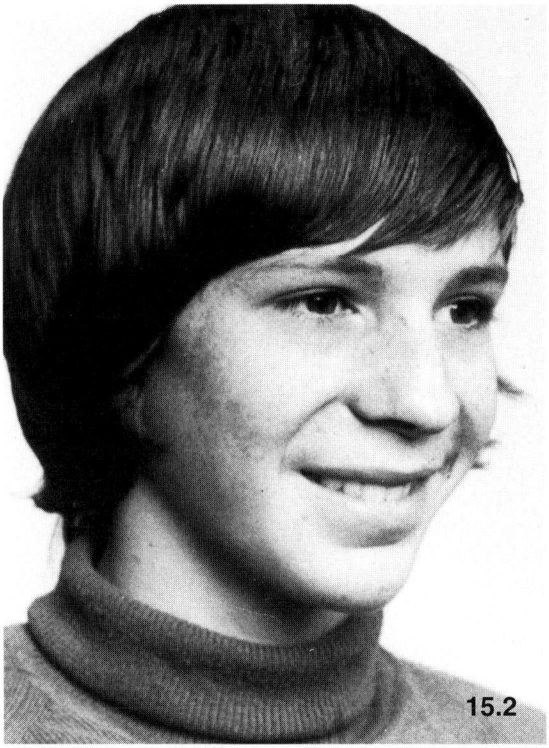

15.2

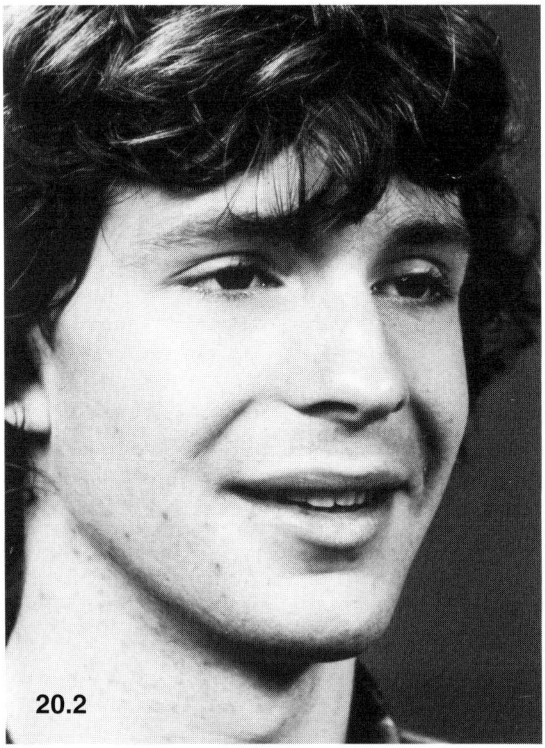

20.2

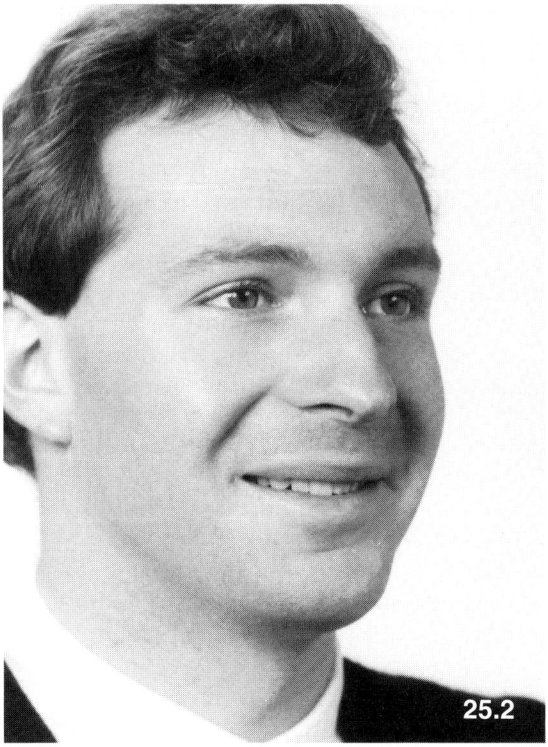

25.2

Fig 12-14 Note the improvements in dentition and facial configuration during and after treatment.

stage in the treatment (Fig 12.4). The mesiodistal diameters of the mandibular anterior teeth could be reduced by 1 ½ mm (stripped). With that procedure, the TSD was corrected and more space was obtained in the mandibular arch. Moreover, a consequence of the broader contact areas created by the stripping was that better resistance to undesired tooth movements (tertiary crowding) was provided than was available with the original, more rounded approximal contours.

The lingual arch prevented lingual tipping of the mandibular incisors. To further reduce the depth of the bite and to obtain some individual tooth movements, a maxillary plate was inserted at the age of 13 years, 4 months. Four months later after two years and three months of active treatment, all appliances were removed. To secure improvements in details of the tooth alignment and to obtain better matching of the occluding surfaces of the dental arches, a positioner was provided. This was worn intensively for a month, and then for another year and eight months at night only for retention. The result was in every way satisfactory (Figs 12.5 and 12.6).

Five years later, the face had developed further and the dental situation had changed little (Figs 12.7 and 12.8). This also applied to the situations at the ages of 25 and 30 years (Figs.12.9 to 12.12).

Superimposition of cephalometric tracings gives an impression of the growth and changes that occurred during and after treatment. This patient gives further evidence of the fact that boys can exhibit significant facial growth after the age of 15 years (Fig 12.13). This phenomenon is illustrated also by the oblique photographs of his smiling face at different ages (Fig 12.14).

Deviations in the midlines of the dental arches and asymmetric occlusions are difficult to correct, particularly if attempted in a late stage of treatment when most other corrections have been completed. In such cases it is worthwhile to consider early the application of simple measures to take advantage of "spontaneous" improvements, or to make later treatment easier. Asymmetric extraction of deciduous canines can be used for that purpose where appropriate, but have to be followed by orthodontic treatment subsequently, especially in cases with lack of space. As in the case described, this might not be until some years later. Cervical headgear, where necessary an asymmetric type, is very appropriate for obtaining more space in the maxilla in class II/1 anomalies. If the occlusion is neutral, a lip bumper or .045" arch can be used in the maxilla; however, this can provide an asymmetric effect only with difficulty, if at all.

It is useful to compare the advantages and disadvantages of lingual arches and lip bumpers before making a choice. In the previous chapter some of the characteristics of lip bumpers were described. Hereunder those of lingual arches will be enlarged upon.

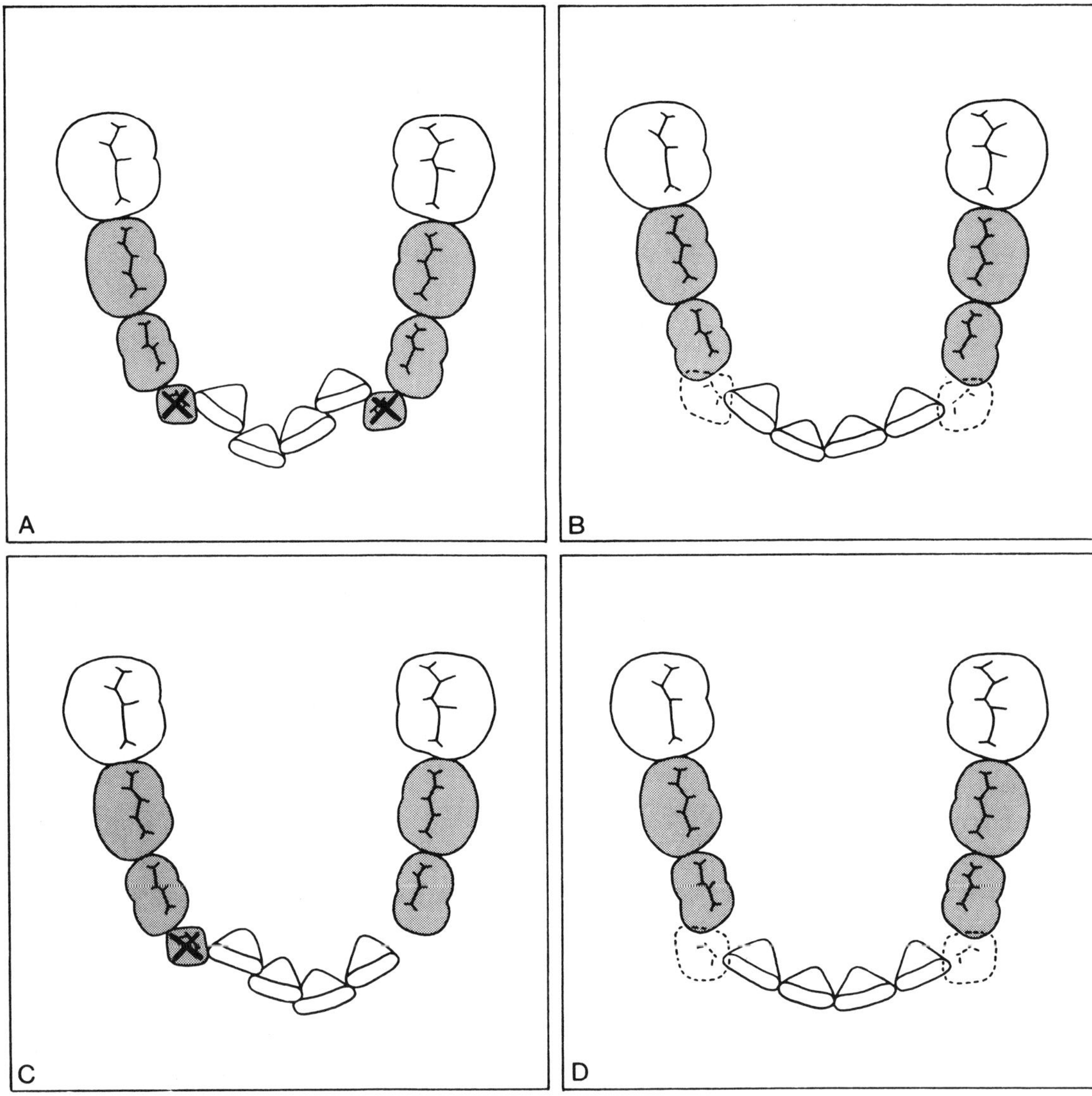

Fig 12-15 Spontaneous improvements in the alignment of permanent incisors after extraction of deciduous canines in the mandible.

A Timely extraction of deciduous canines in crowding cases leads to an improvement in the position of the permanent incisors. Where there is an asymmetric disposition of the mandibular incisors it should be decided if it would help to extract first the deciduous canine on the least crowded side.

B Subsequently insufficient space remains for the permanent canines; moreover, the mandibular incisors may have tipped lingually.

C When due to premature root resorption a deciduous canine has been lost on one side, extraction of the deciduous canine on the other side will lead to an improvement in the position of the mandibular incisors.

D The deviation of the dental arch midline will be reduced; the remaining space available for the permanent canines will be too small.[33]

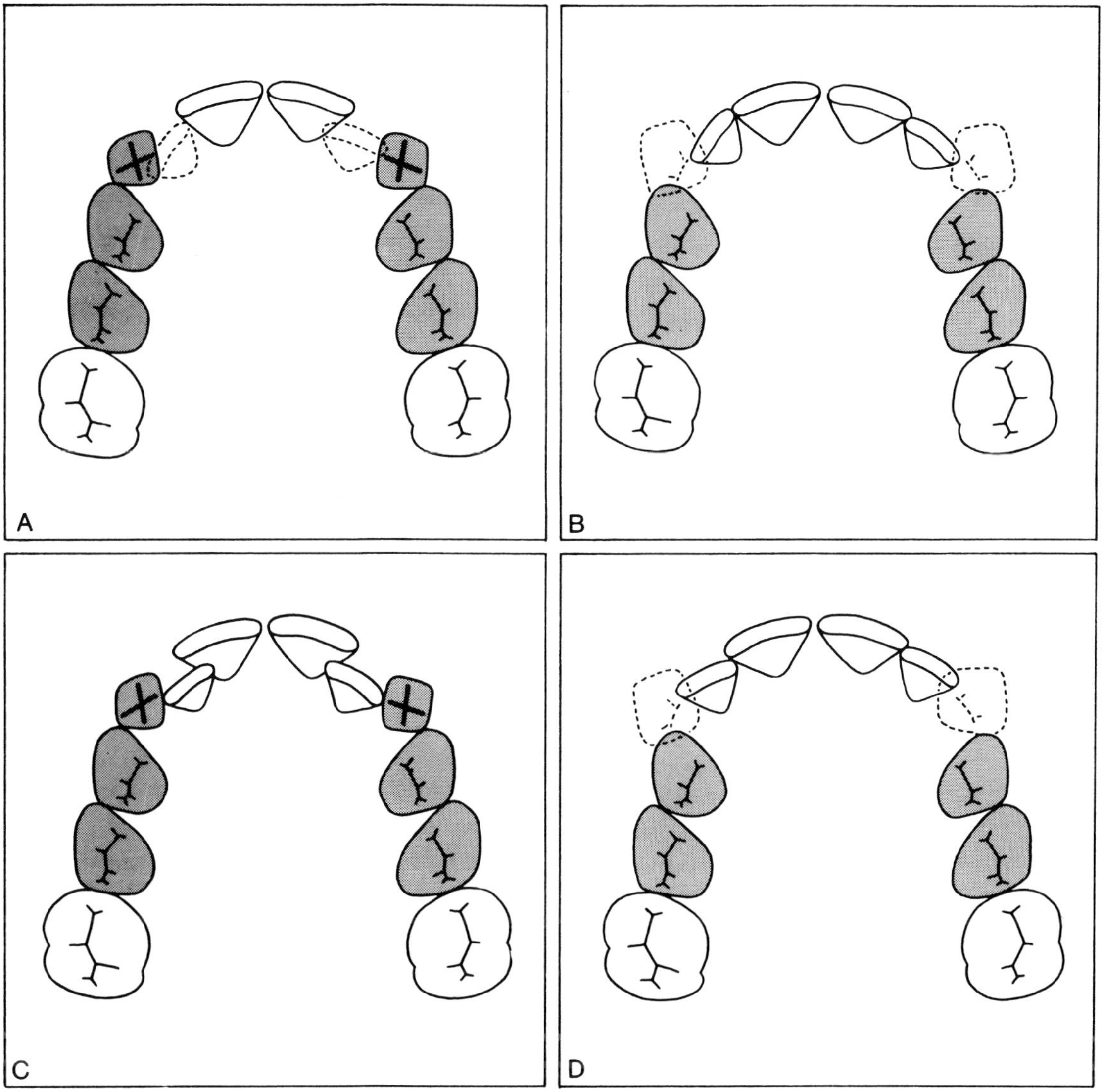

Fig 12-16 Spontaneous improvements in the alignment of permanent incisors after extraction of deciduous canines in the maxilla.

A The permanent lateral incisors in a case of serious crowding can emerge in a better position if the deciduous canines are removed at the correct time.

B Subsequently insufficient space remains for the permanent canines. During the intertransitional period, space should be created for the canines to emerge in a good position.

C Extraction of the deciduous canines after emergence of the lateral incisors can still lead to an improvement in the position of the maxillary incisors.

D The improvements, which usually are less than those when extractions were done earlier, are obtained at the cost of the space remaining for the permanent canines to emerge into.[33]

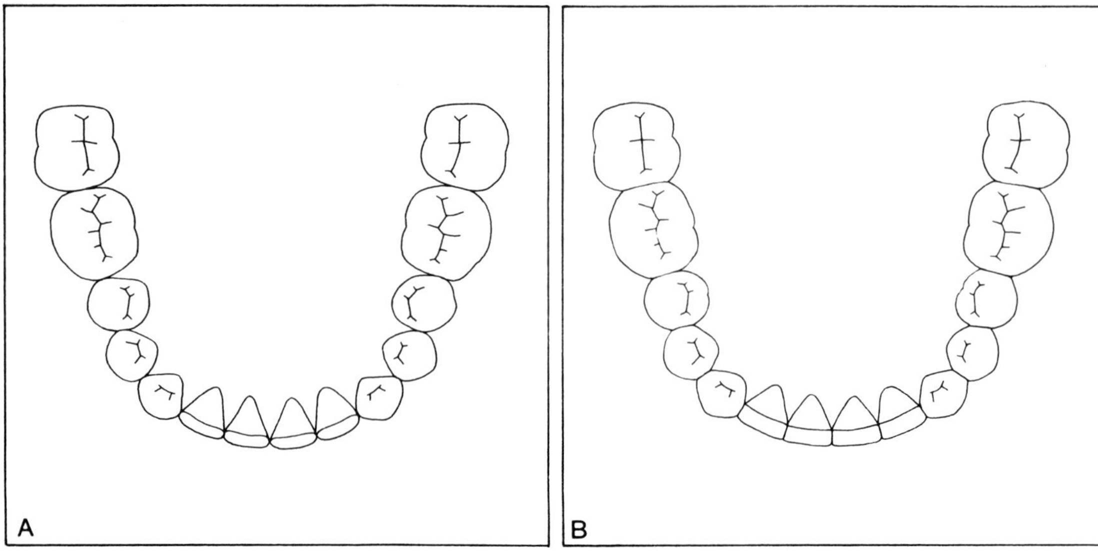

Fig 12-17
The appearance of the interproximal surfaces is important for the stability of the mandibular anterior teeth, both in regard to prevention of tertiary crowding and the retention of alignment after orthodontic treatment.
A Good mutual support between teeth reduces the chance that they will begin to overlap each other.
B Flat contact areas reinforce the effect of the so-called "Roman arch" and in this way enhance its stability.[31]

Lingual arches are fitted, just as are lip bumpers, mostly to the first permanent molars. However, there are greater difficulties with possible damage to the periodontal structures and in keeping adjacent teeth clean than where a lip bumper is fitted. The construction of a lingual arch is not "gingiva friendly." The appliance cannot be removed by the patient, which makes good oral hygiene difficult. In addition, activation is troublesome. The inclination of the molars to which the lingual arch is fixed can be changed by it (torqued). Although lingual arches do not interfere with the cheek and lip musculature, they nevertheless influence the result of the pressure on the teeth exerted by those soft tissues. The presence of the lingual arch lying against the lingual surfaces of the teeth prevents them from moving lingually. Similarly the teeth are shielded to some degree from the pressure of the tongue.
An advantage of the lingual arch is that teeth can be moved to the labial and buccal and can be prevented from moving to the lingual. These two aspects were decisive in the choice of appliance for this case. Another useful feature of the lingual arch is its ability to prevent the mesial migration of mandibular first permanent molars during

the second transitional period. It will also prevent lingual tipping of the mandibular anterior teeth if for example, during cervical headgear therapy, the mandibular incisors are contacting the maxillary ones. Those aspects were applicable to this patient as well.

The controlled movement of individual teeth into a good position remains difficult with a lingual arch, even using auxiliary springs soldered to it. Three-dimensional control such as can be obtained with full fixed appliances is not possible with a lingual arch. This is particularly important in treating the mandibular anterior teeth because optimal interproximal contacts and good inclination are essential for stability of the result. In this case it would have been possible to move the apex of the mandibular left lateral incisor to labial if a fixed appliance had been used. With the lingual arch any movement of that nature was insufficient. The later partial relapse of that tooth to lingual can largely be blamed on this inadequacy.

Very occasionally in a situation such as that described here, one is confronted with the option of extracting the mandibular left lateral incisor. Such an option should be dismissed out of hand. Indeed a good mandibular arch will usually develop although the deviant midline will be displaced even further.The patient is unlikely to notice that. The initial impact will be one of marked improvement. Because of the excess of room, the mandibular incisors will fall back with consequent increase in overjet and overbite. If after a number of years an attempt is made to correct the increased deviation, more problems arise. This is not just because of the greater size of the anomaly, but also due to the TSD resulting from the extraction, there now being relatively too much tooth material in the maxilla. As a result it is not possible to get good interdigitation unless a tooth is extracted from the maxilla. The problems with symmetry increase and treatment with fixed appliances is indicated. Even then a reasonable occlusion with a stable end-result will seldom be obtained, unless teeth are extracted also on the other side. The good effect obtained in the short term is in the long term very costly.

In conclusion, it might be reiterated that in cases with a TSD with relatively too much tooth material in the mandibular anterior teeth combined with crowding, those teeth might be made narrower. The flatter interproximal surfaces that result will enhance the likelihood of the improved alignment being stable (Fig. 12.17). Apart from that it has to be mentioned that stripping must be done strictly according to the rules to avoid increasing the risk of interproximal caries, and in some cases to avoid actually causing a TSD to develop.

Chapter 13

Class II/1, scissorbite right side

Cervical headgear, lingual arch, maxillary removable plate, activator
Male: 11 years, 11 months to 24 years 2 months

A boy of 11 years, 11 months had a somewhat round face with a prominent mid-face and receding chin. He could easily breathe through his nose but kept his mouth open. He had a pronounced distorelation; the overjet was 7 mm. Excess space was available in both dental arches despite the early loss of mandibular deciduous teeth. A complete scissorbite existed on the right side. A TSD could be expected since the maxillary lateral incisors were narrower than those in the mandible (Figs 13.1 and 13.2).

It was decided both to correct the distorelation and decrease somewhat the maxillary arch width with a cervical headgear. Moreover, a maxillary plate would be fitted to open the bite to enable transverse changes to be procured. The mandibular arch would be widened with a lingual arch and the mandibular right first permanent molar tipped back and torqued buccolingually. An elastic "through the bite" between maxillary and mandibular first permanent molars on that side would be used as required.

The headgear and removable plate were fitted at the age of 12 years 2 months. With a flexible three-quarter clasp on the maxillary right first permanent molar and a buccal spring from mesial onto both deciduous molars, those three teeth were moved palatally. In the process, a biteplane was used that was sufficiently high to avoid interference by the opposing teeth with that movement. In addition, the inner arch of the headgear was narrowed so that it operated to compress the maxillary arch somewhat. Four months later, the lingual arch was fitted and removed again after five months. At the same time, use of the maxillary plate was terminated because a reasonable result had been achieved and also because the appliance had been repaired many times. At the age of 12 years 11 months, a good transverse occlusion had been obtained and it was decided to continue treatment with the cervical headgear only. A year later, a good sagittal relation was attained, so continuing to wear the headgear but only during sleep was advised.

Six months later, at the age of 14 years, 5 months, the maxillary first premolars and the mandibular second premolars had emerged. On the upper right the premolars had erupted too far buccally. A new plate was made to move those teeth palatally and make some other corrections at the same time. At 15 years, 1 month, an activator was used and worn for seven months as a retainer, but advantage was taken also of its capacity to guide the growth that was taking place. The result

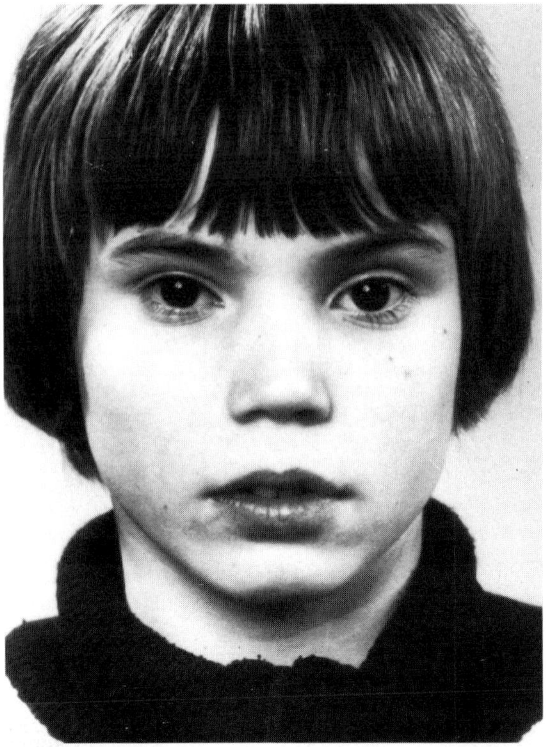
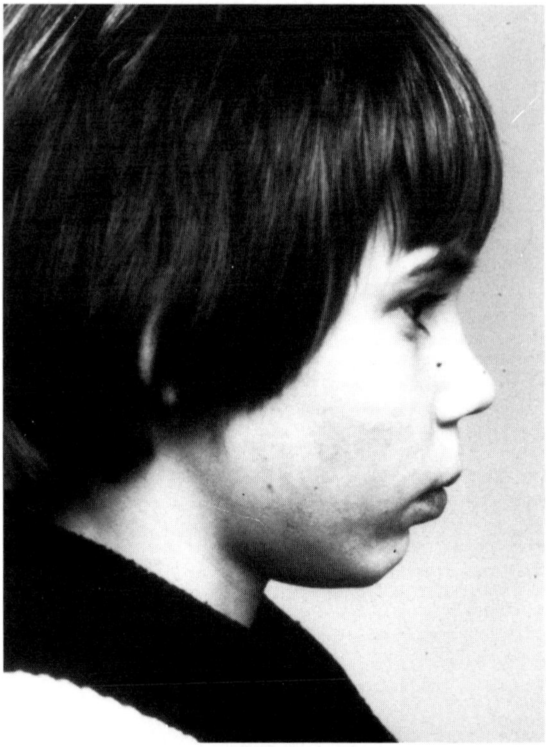
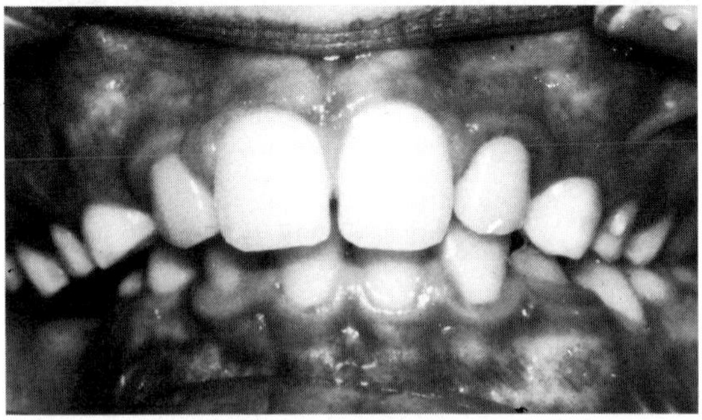
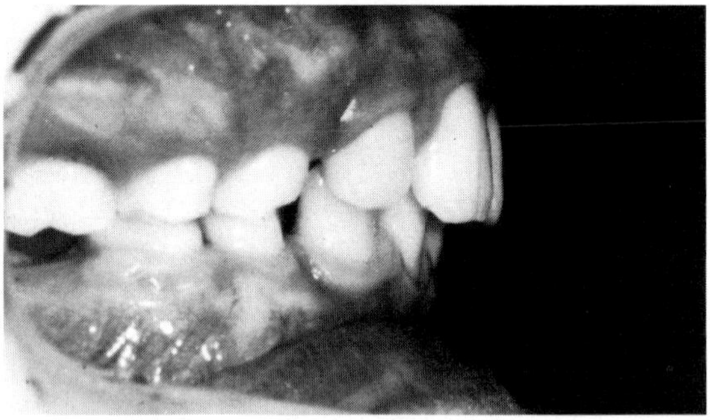
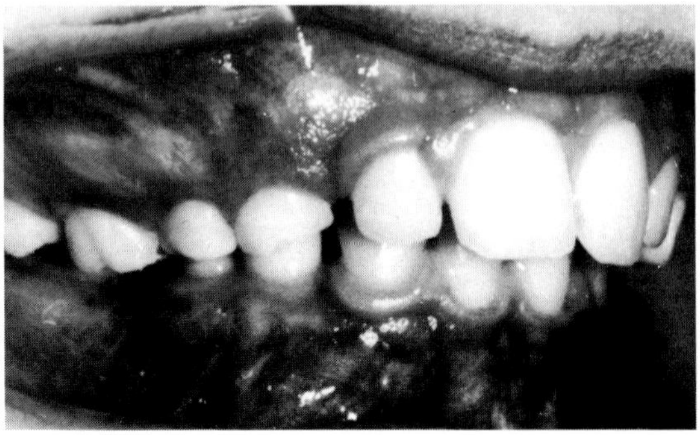
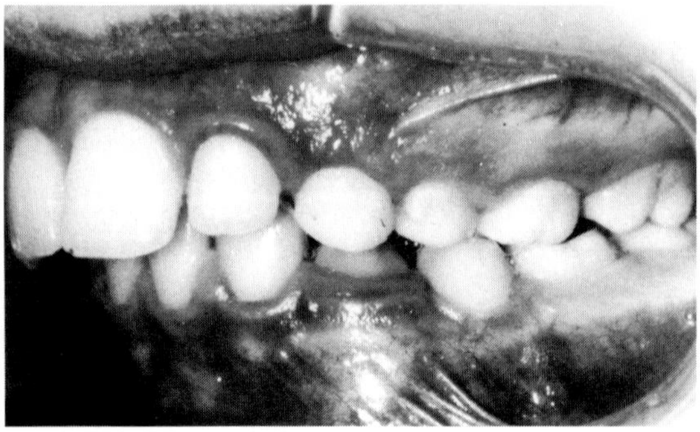

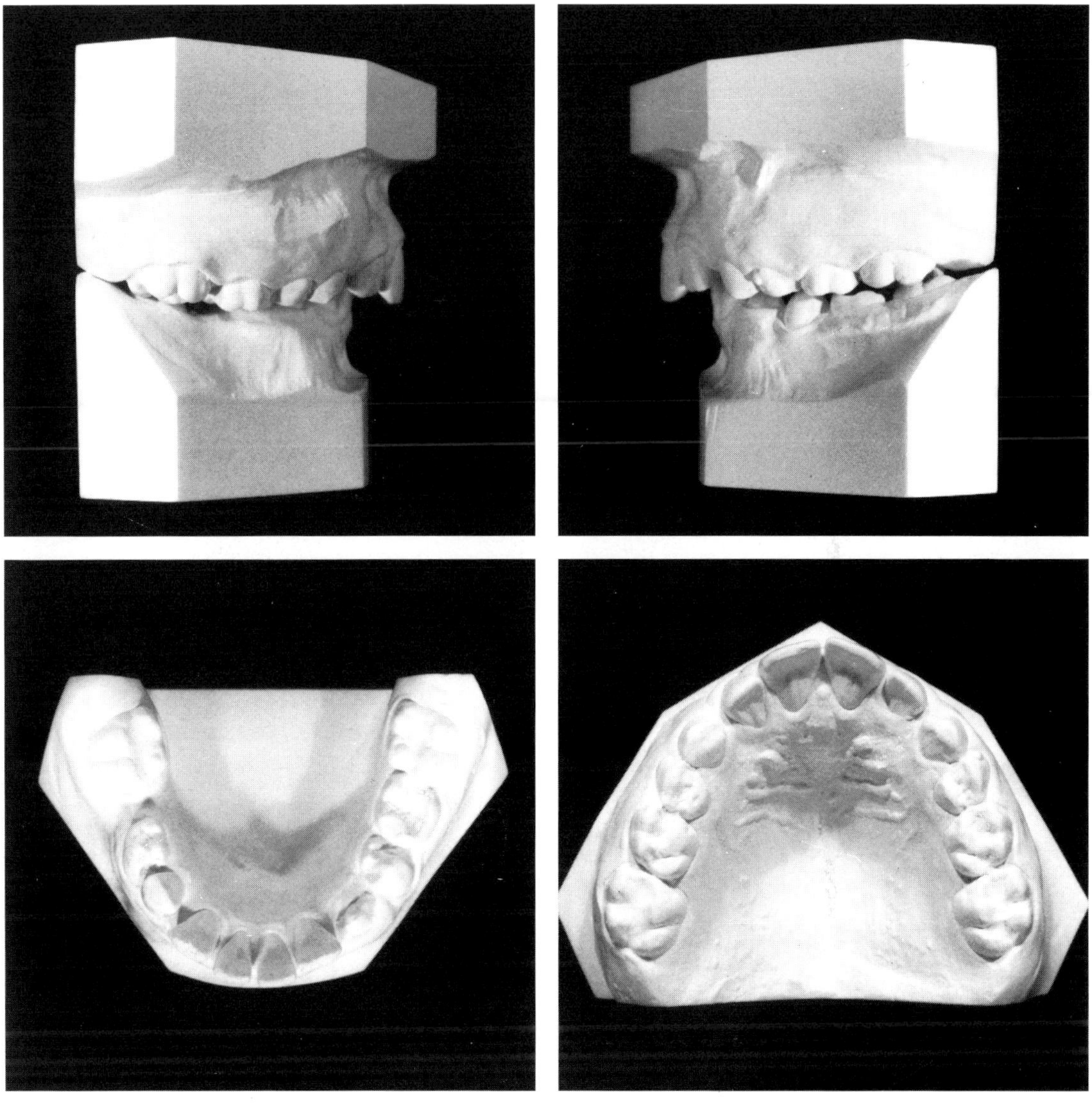

Fig 13-1 and 13-2 A boy aged 11 y, 11 mo with a class II/1 anomaly (disto-occlusion 1 PW), a large deviation in sagittal jaw relationships and complete scissorbite on the right. The mandibular right first permanent molar had tipped lingually and mesially after the early loss of the adjacent second deciduous molar. Nevertheless there is still sufficient space in the mandibular arch. The maxillary arch is fairly broad. The mandibular incisors are in labioversion; those in the maxilla are steeply inclined. The maxillary lateral incisors are narrower than those in the mandible, which may indicate a TSD.

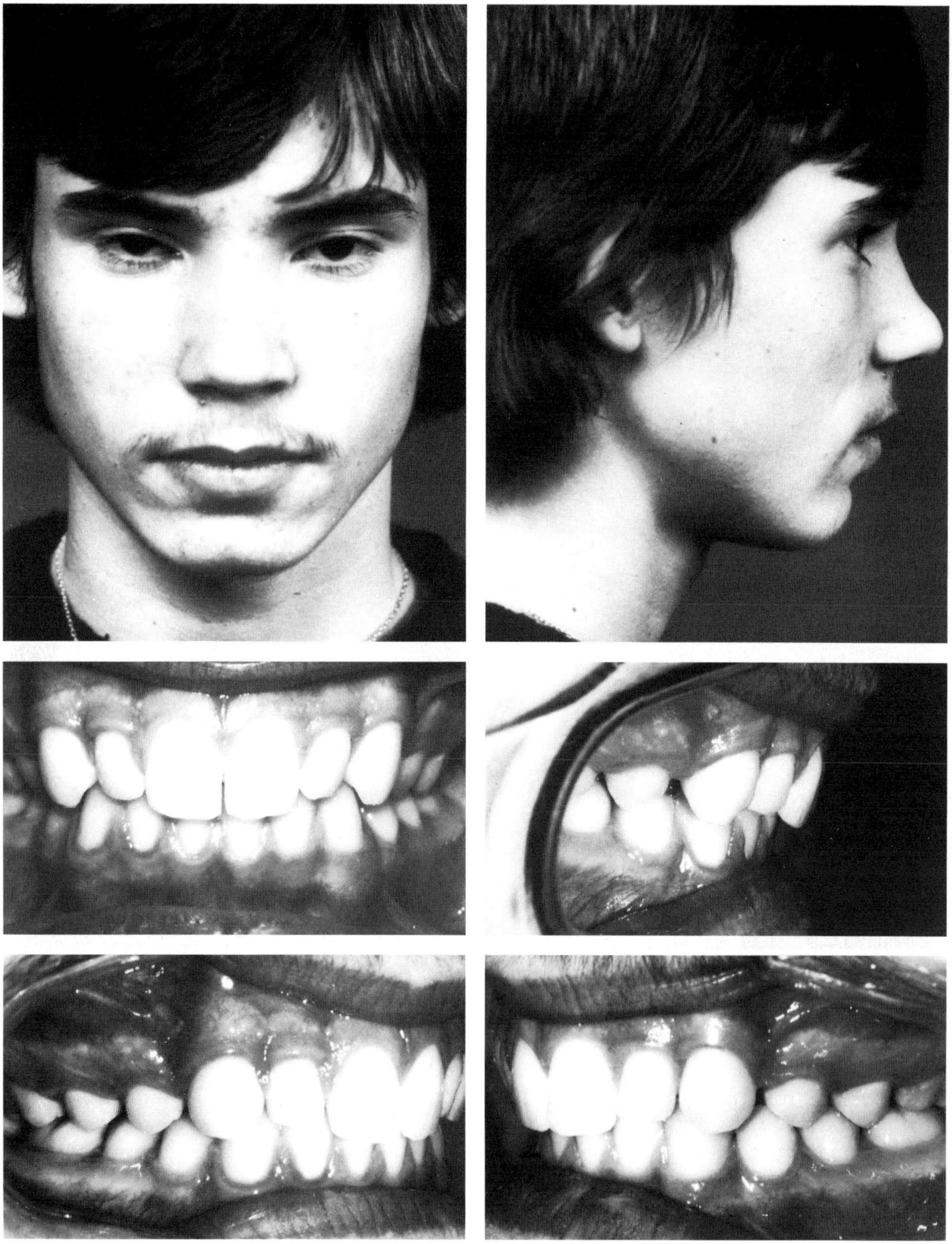

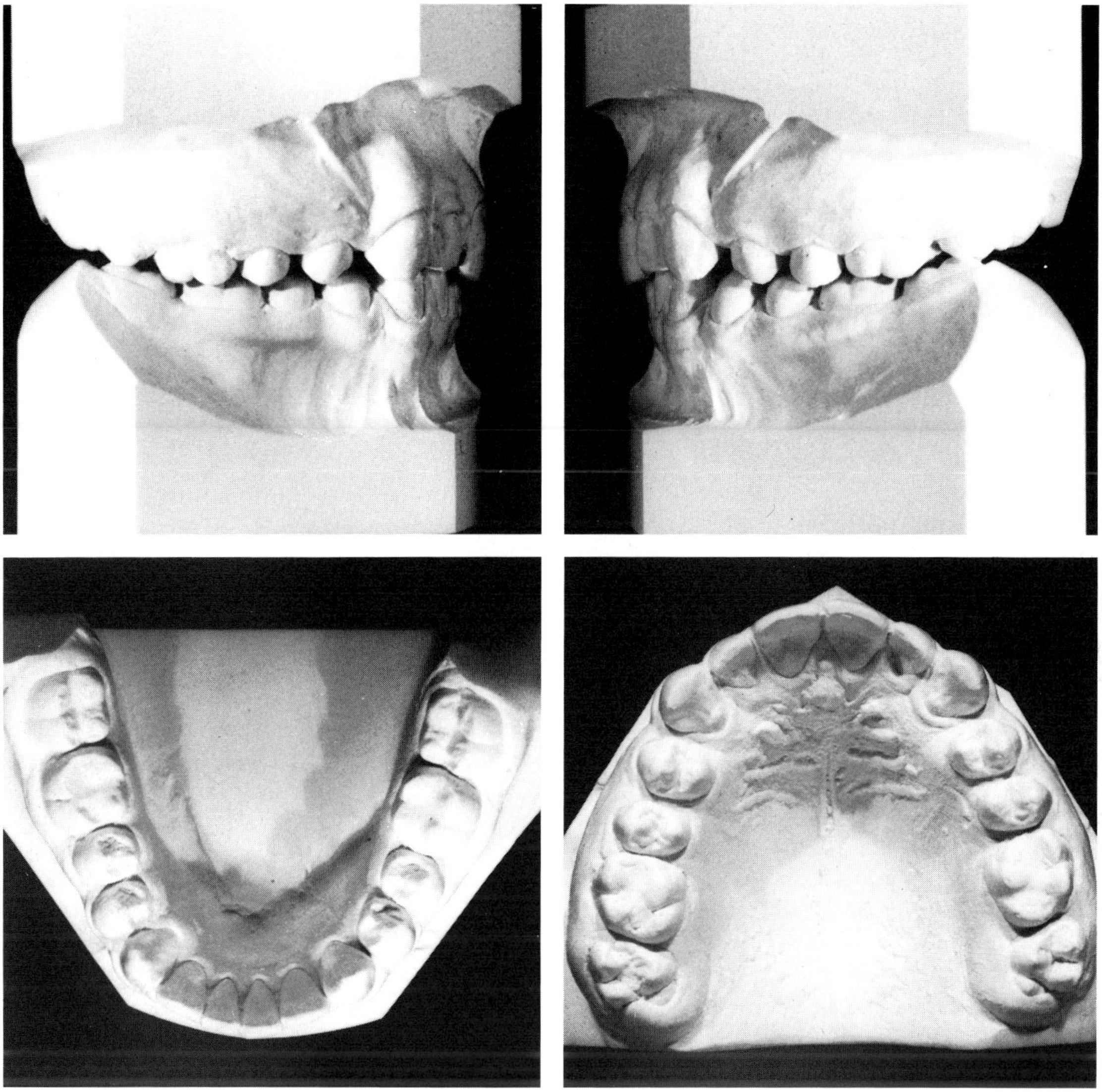

Figs 13-3 and 13-4 *At the age of 15 y, 8 mo, a harmonious facial appearance with competent lip seal exists. The midlines of the dental arches coincide and the posterior teeth occlude well transversally. The maxillary second premolars and lateral incisors are relatively too narrow to occlude properly without diastemata. A TSD exists in the incisor as well as in the premolar regions with relative deficiency of tooth material in the maxilla. The maxillary incisors are steeply inclined. The apices of the maxillary canines are located too far mesially. Above all, their crowns are, in comparison with those of the incisors, decidedly prominent labially.*

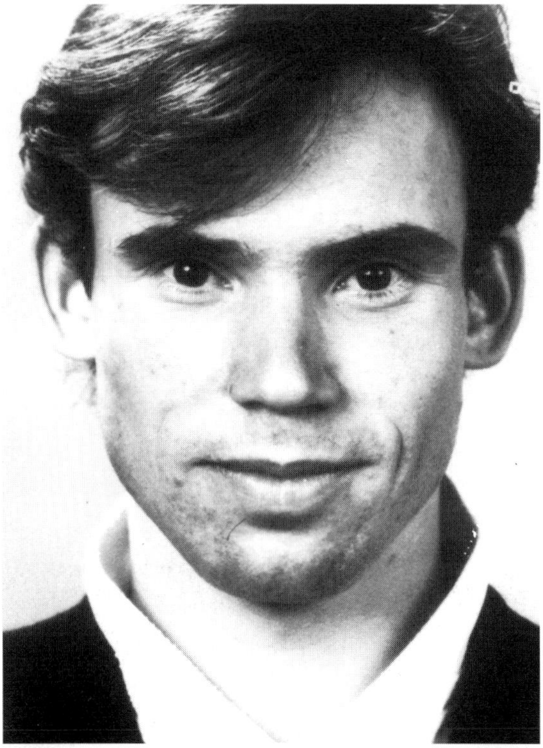

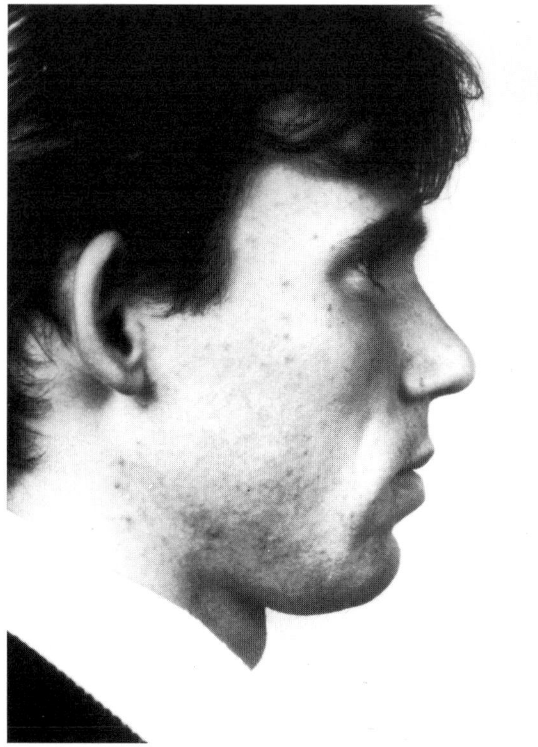

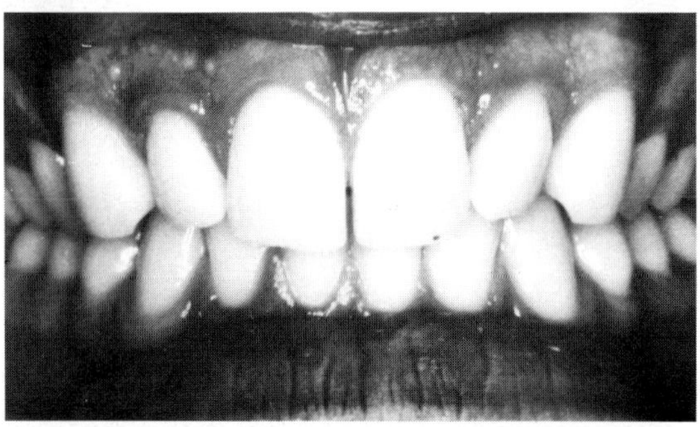

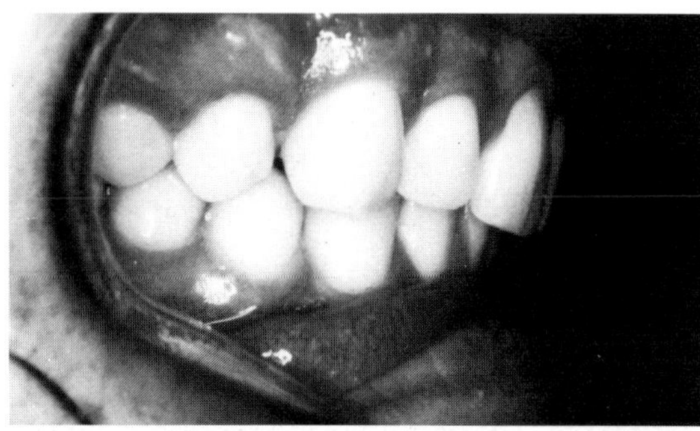

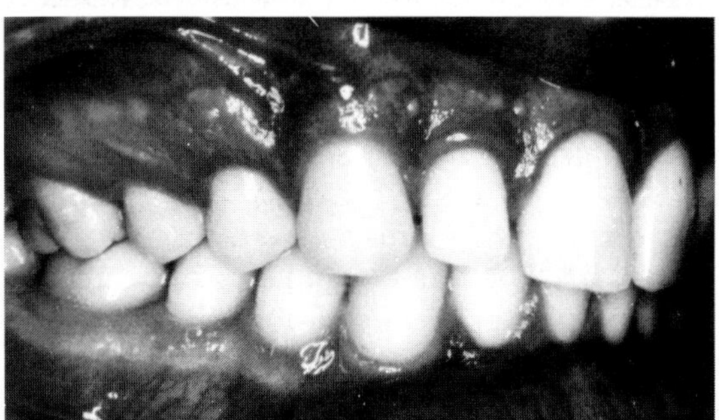

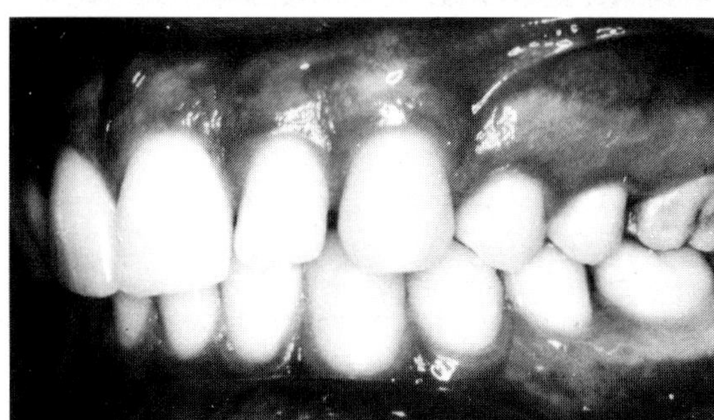

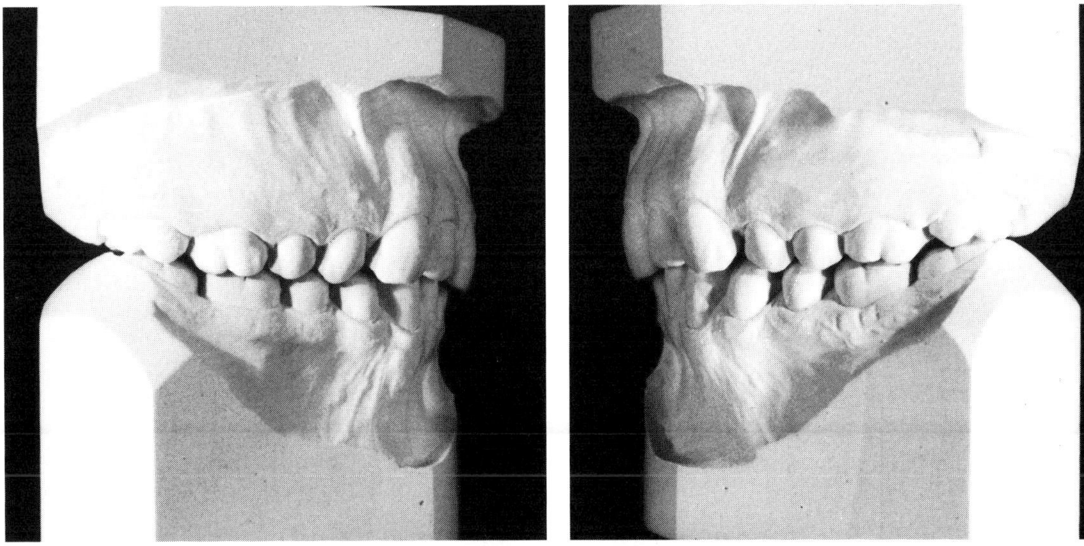

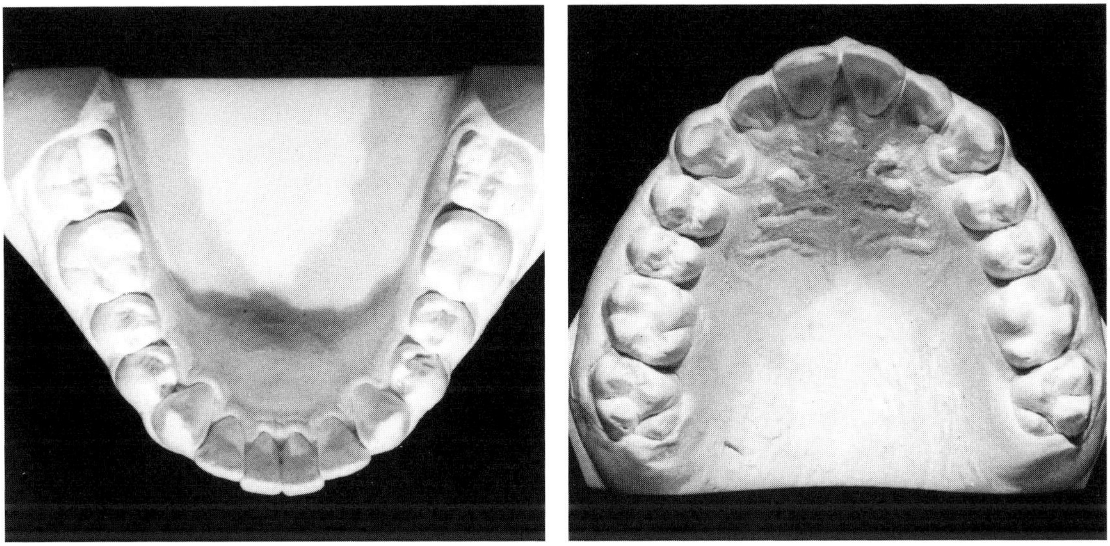

Figs 13-5 and 13-6 *At the age of 20 y, 9 mo, the face is that of an adult. The mandible has come forward, the chin is more prominent. The dentition shows some noticeable changes in comparison with five years previously. The canines have worn down markedly and the mandibular canines have fallen more lingually than the maxillary ones have. In the posterior regions the occlusion has changed as the diastemata in the maxilla have closed to the mesial. Apart from that, the mandibular arch has taken up a more ventral relationship with the maxillary arch. The various factors involved have led to the first premolars occluding more mesially and the molars occluding less mesially than before. The maxillary incisors are now less steeply inclined.*

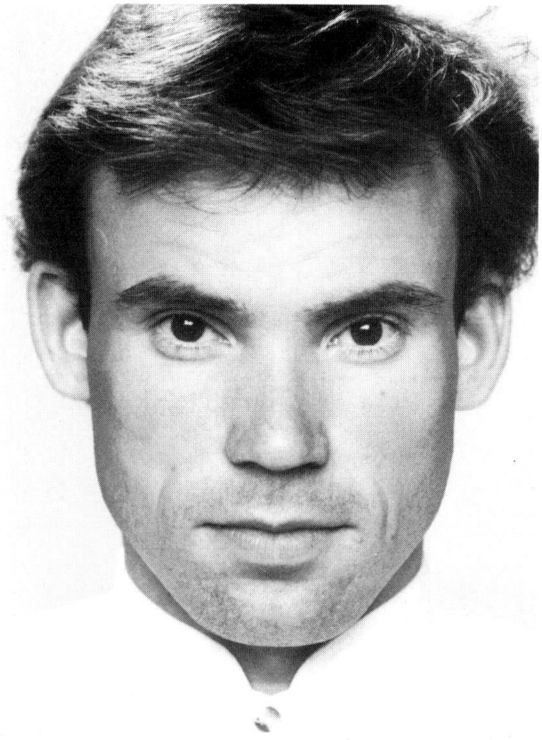

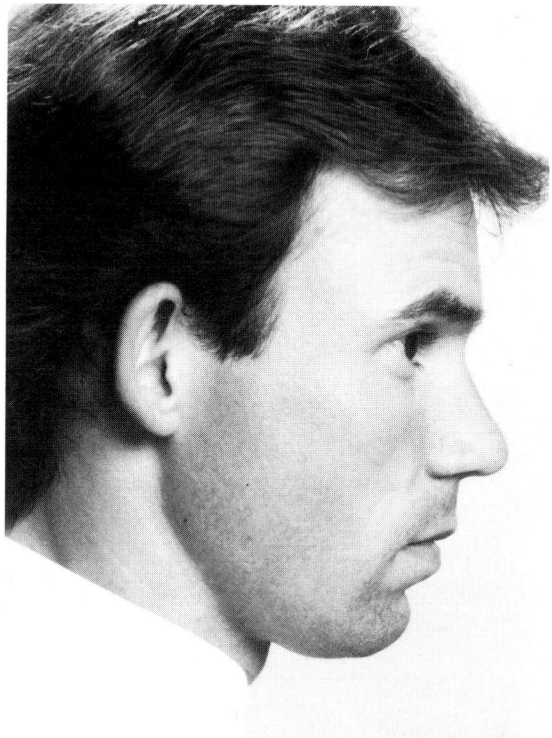

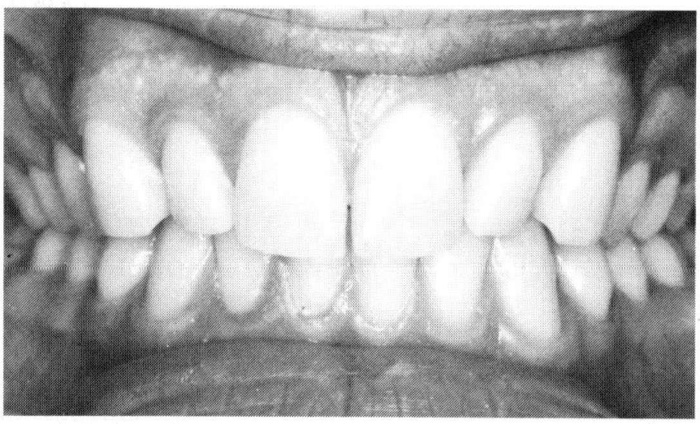

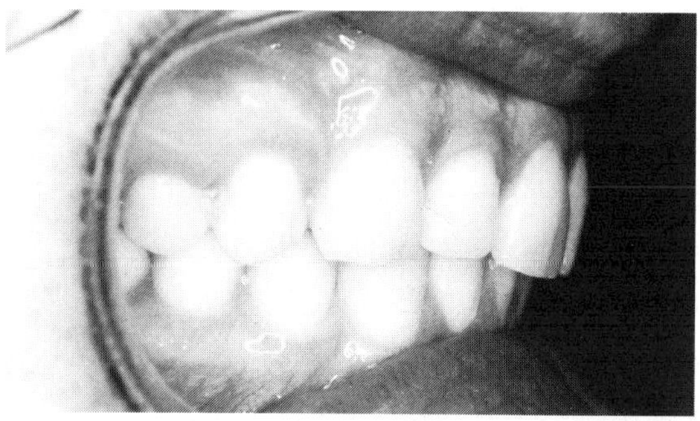

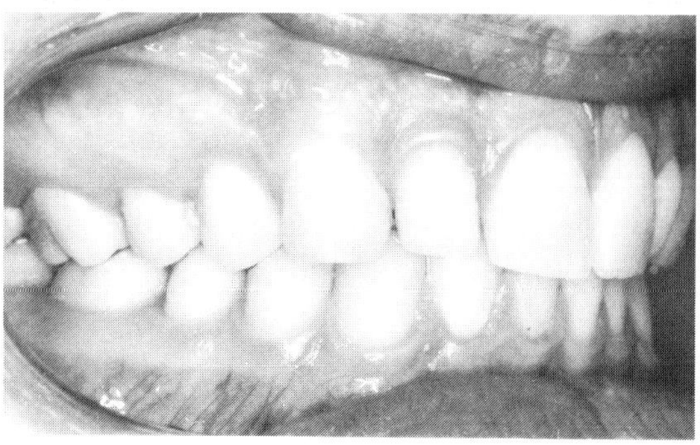

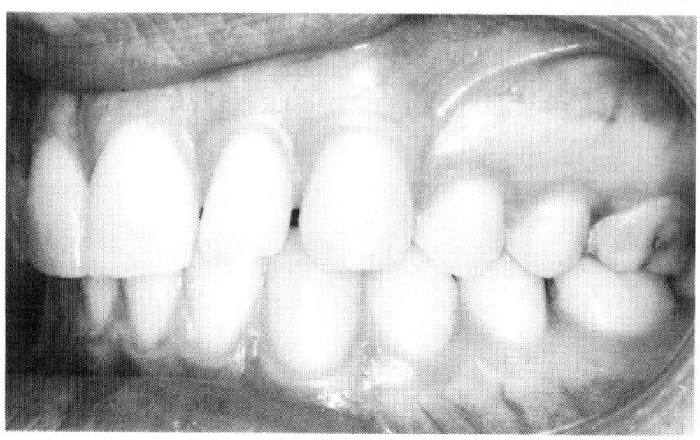

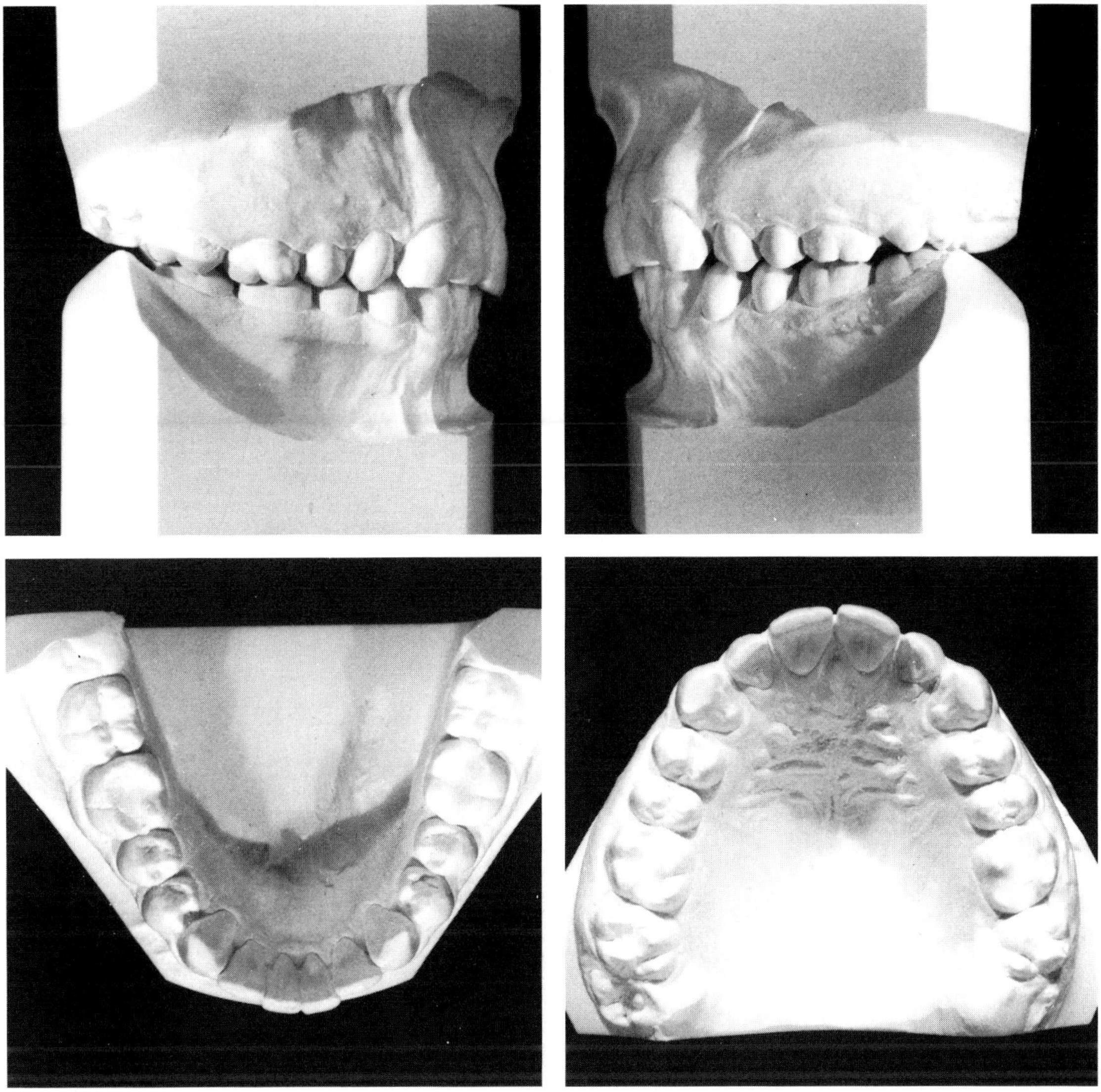

Figs 13-7 and 13-8 Aged 24 y, 2 mo, 8½ years after the conclusion of retention, little has changed. In the meantime three third molars have partially emerged. Insufficient room is available for them to complete eruption and to arrive into good positions. It already can be seen on the models made earlier (see Fig 13.6:20 y, 9 mo; Fig 13.4:15 y, 8 mo) that there would be insufficient room for those teeth. The mandibular left third molar is impacted. It was recommended that all third molars be removed.

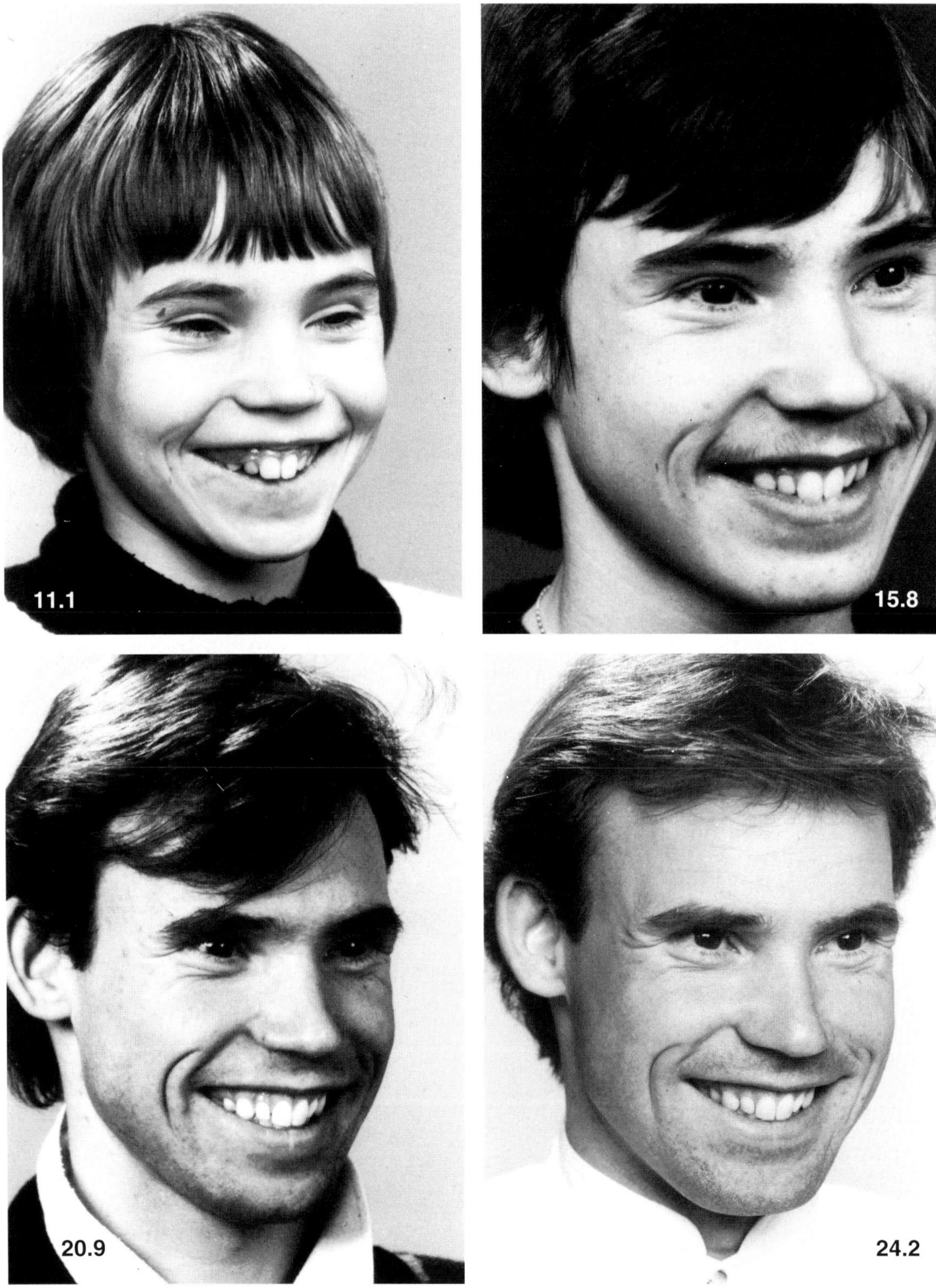

11.1 15.8 20.9 24.2

Fig 13-9 Note the growth and maturation of the face that occurred after the age of 15 y, 0 mo.

obtained at that time was rewarding, particularly considering the simple appliances being used. The face no longer showed class II/1 characteristics and the dental arches fitted well. Indeed, the maxillary incisors were somewhat steeply inclined, and the canines too perpendicularly angulated. There was not only a TSD in the anterior teeth but also in the posterior teeth because the maxillary premolars, as well as the laterals, had rather small crowns (Figs 13.3 and 13.4).

Five years later, the face had developed further and matured. The maxillary canines were somewhat less dominant. They had moved slightly palatally, this being possible due to the mandibular canines having moved lingually. In addition, the canines had worn down significantly. With further growth, the mandibular arch had moved forward somewhat in relationship to the maxillary arch. The effect of this on the occlusion has been strongly influenced by the closing to the mesial of the spaces in the maxillary posterior segments (Figs 13.5 and 13.6).

Three and a half years later at the age of 24 years, 2 months, this picture had changed very little (Figs 13.7 and 13.8). The oblique photographs provide a good indication of the changes that had ensued due to growth and treatment (Fig 13.9).

A scissorbite can be quite disturbing for a patient, certainly when it is bilateral ("telescope" bite). A scissorbite occurs almost exclusively in class II/1 anomalies, which is connected with the form of the dental arches. Usually the involved teeth in the mandible are tipped lingually and those in the maxilla to the buccal. They can overerupt, since they are not opposed by the teeth in the other arch. However the mandibular teeth unlike those in the maxilla usually do not come to be in supraposition since they are held back by the tongue.

Correction of a scissorbite is only possible if the bite is so far opened at all times that buccolingual movement of the teeth is not obstructed by the occlusion. Depending on the position and inclination of the teeth concerned, the tooth movement has to take place more in one jaw than the other, or both equally. In the latter case, the obvious course of action is to use the reciprocal force of elastics through the bite with clearance of the bite with a plate with a biteplane, or with an occlusal overlay on the good side (Fig 13.10). To make palatal movement possible, the acrylic must be ground away appropriately. If such movement is not desired, the acrylic is left intact and the elastic force will not displace the maxillary teeth and consequently only the mandibular teeth will be moved transversely. It is most important that the plates used in such treatment are worn at all times, so also during eating. Even during tooth brushing, when the patient must remove the plate, he or she should try to keep their jaws apart to avoid any chance that the teeth might be bitten back to the original malpositions.

A scissorbite of a maxillary first permanent molar can originate from the early loss of the corresponding mandibular second deciduous molar in a class II/1 anomaly before the emergence of the adjacent mandibular first permanent molar. That is very likely what happened in the case just described. Subsequently, other teeth can develop a scissorbite.

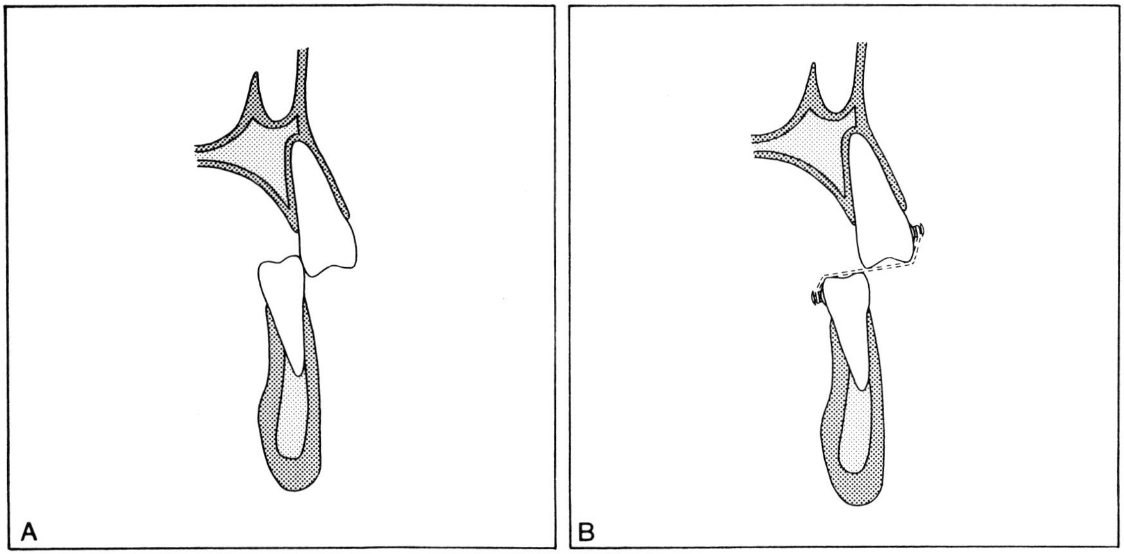

Fig 13-10 A coronal section of two premolars in scissorbite.

A The maxillary tooth has over-erupted into supraposition; the mandibular tooth normally does not, since it is held back by the tongue.

B Reciprocal movement with an elastic "through the bite" is particularly useful when both teeth need to be tipped. During this process, the mutual interference of the teeth has to be eliminated by opening the bite by means of a removable plate with a bite plane or an occlusal overlay. If the acrylic of the plate is removed adjacent to the maxillary tooth, that tooth can move palatally. If the change in transverse occlusion is only required from movement of the mandibular tooth, then the maxillary tooth can be held in its place by leaving the plate intact against it.[33]

A scissorbite is easier to correct if the disto-occlusion is corrected simultaneously, because the wider part of the mandibular arch is brought forward and the buccolingual discrepancy becomes smaller.

An anterior TSD that depends on relatively narrow maxillary lateral incisors being present as in this case does not always need to be compensated for by stripping the mandibular anterior teeth as was described in the previous case. In the absence of sagittal contact between the incisors, stripping is only sensible if prevention or relief of mandibular incisor crowding is the objective. Stripping is contraindicated in situations where the maxillary incisors are steeply inclined. Reduction of the width of mandibular incisors that are well-aligned will lead to them tipping backward. The bite will deepen and the maxillary incisors will become more steeply inclined. In such a

situation, it is better to accept the spacing in the maxillary arch, as in this case, or subsequently to build up the width of the maxillary teeth with composite resin.
Finally it might be remarked that, as in this case, the limitations inherent in the use of simple appliances will be seen in the end result. It would have been possible to improve the angulation of the maxillary canines, to torque palatally the apices of the maxillary incisors, and to finish up with a less deep bite, if fixed appliances had been utilized.

Chapter 14

Class II/1
Cervical headgear, brackets 12, 11, 21 and 22, slicing 55, 65, 75, and 85
Female: 10 years, 8 months to 29 years, 0 months

A girl aged 10 years, 8 months presented with a well-formed face with a slightly receding chin, an exaggerated plica mentalis, and normal function. She had a class II/1 anomaly (¾ PW disto-occlusion) with crowding in the mandibular and maxillary anterior regions. The four second deciduous molars present were the last remaining of her deciduous teeth; as usual they had greater mesiodistal dimensions that their successors, especially in the mandible. Their broad crowns offered a possibility for correction of the anterior crowding. Estimation of the ALD indicated discrepancies of +2 mm in the mandible and –2 mm in the maxilla. Considering the degree of disto-occlusion, the overjet of 5 mm was small; this aspect could be attributed to the crowding in the anterior region combined with a lack of labio-version of the maxillary incisors (Figs 14.1 and 14.2).

The treatment plan was to use a cervical headgear and later to use a partial fixed appliance on the maxillary arch. It was assumed that mesial slicing of the mandibular second deciduous molars would be sufficient to deal with the mandibular arch. The cervical headgear was fitted at the age of 10 years, 9 months. At the same visit, the mesial convexity of the second deciduous molars in the mandibular and maxillary arches was ground away (Fig 14.19). With headgear therapy and mesial slicing, the maxillary first premolars migrated distally and room became available for the permanent canines. Simultaneously with the reduction of the disto-occlusion, the width of the maxillary arch increased mainly due to the action of the rail mechanism. The result of the changes was the appearance of diastemata in the maxillary anterior region. In the mandible, the first premolars also drifted distally until they contacted the now flat mesial surfaces of the deciduous second molars which, after the slicing, were about the same crown width as their successors. As a result, the mandibular canines could move distally, enabling the lateral incisors to come properly into the dental arch under the influence of tongue pressure.

At the age of 12 years, 10 months, edgewise brackets (.022" × .028" slots) were placed on the four maxillary incisors and a .0175" twistflex archwire was fitted (Figs 14.13 to 14.18). Two months later, this arch wire was replaced with a solid rectangular .019" × .026" stainless steel arch to retract the maxillary incisors and at the same time keep their axial inclinations under control. For that purpose the archwire had torque installed and stops were soldered to it 4 mm in front of molar tubes. Before soldering on the stops, a section of open coil spring (.010" × .030")

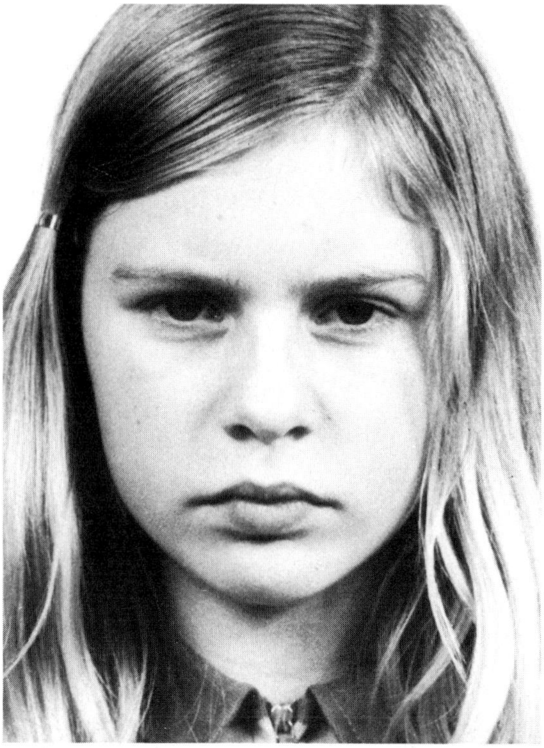

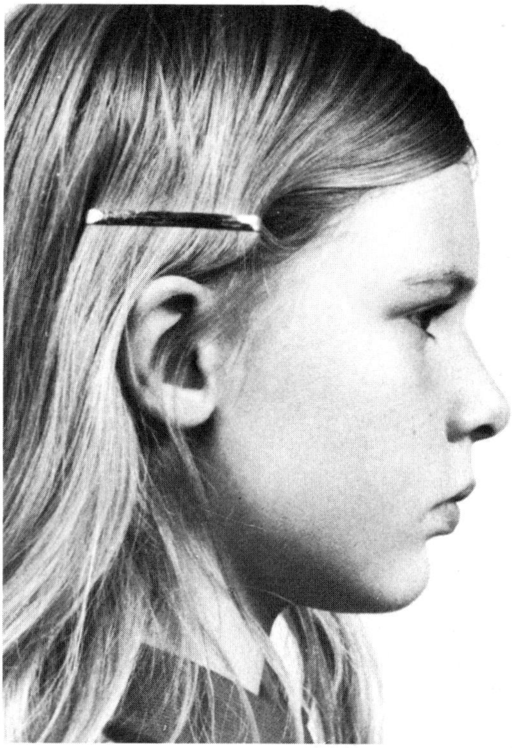

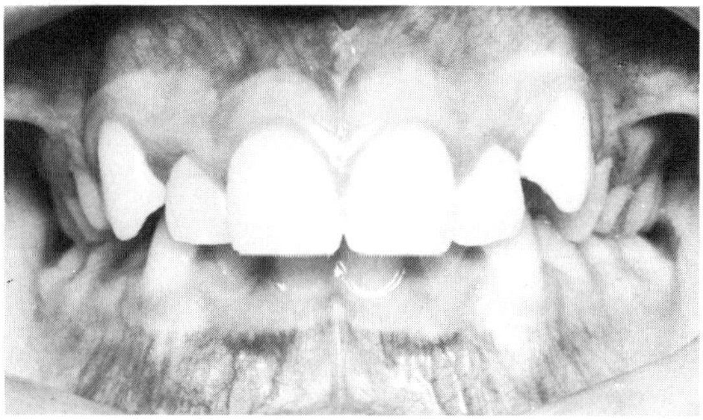

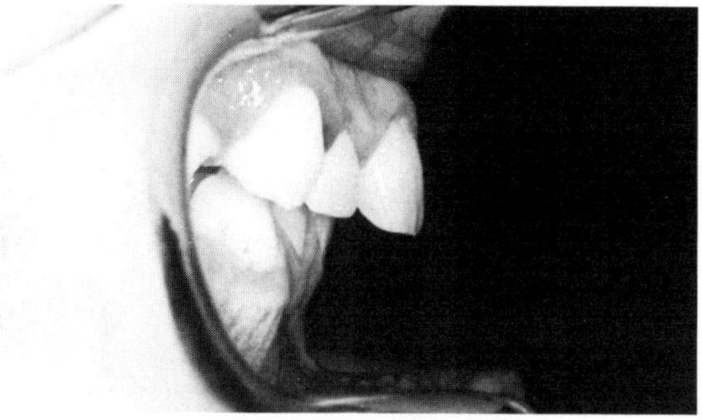

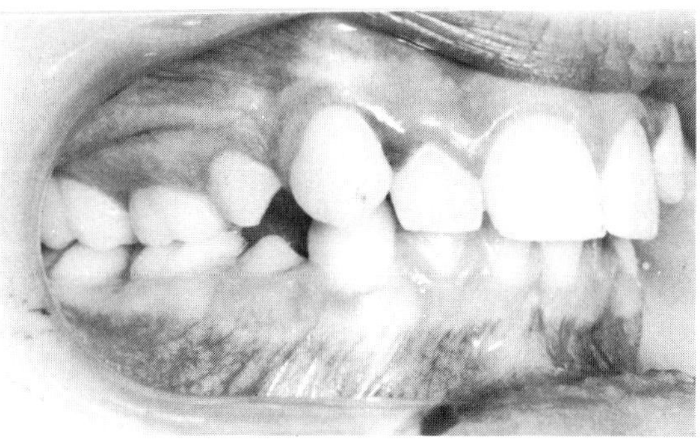

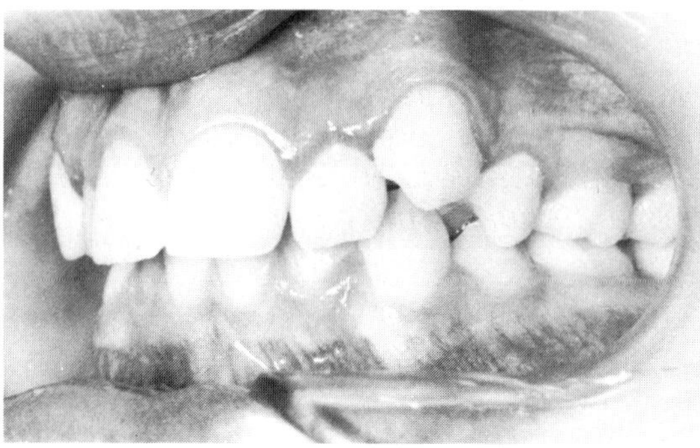

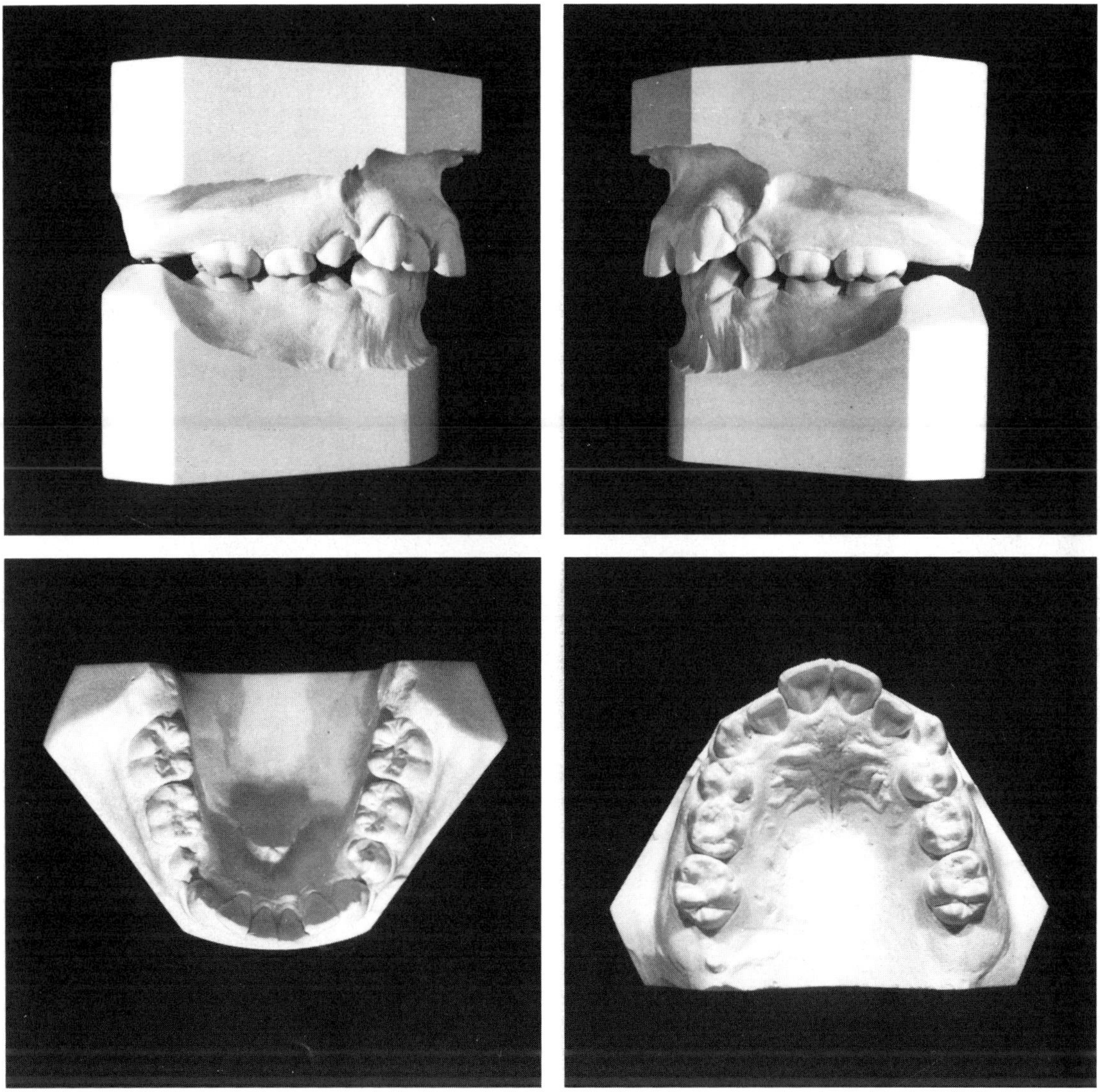

Figs 14-1 and 14-2 A girl of 10 y, 8 mo with a class II/1 anomaly (¾ PW disto-occlusion), a receding chin and a competent lip seal. A short time previously the maxillary first premolars and the maxillary canines had emerged. All second deciduous molars are still present. In both jaws, the lateral incisors are located a little too far lingually; the central incisors have normal inclinations.

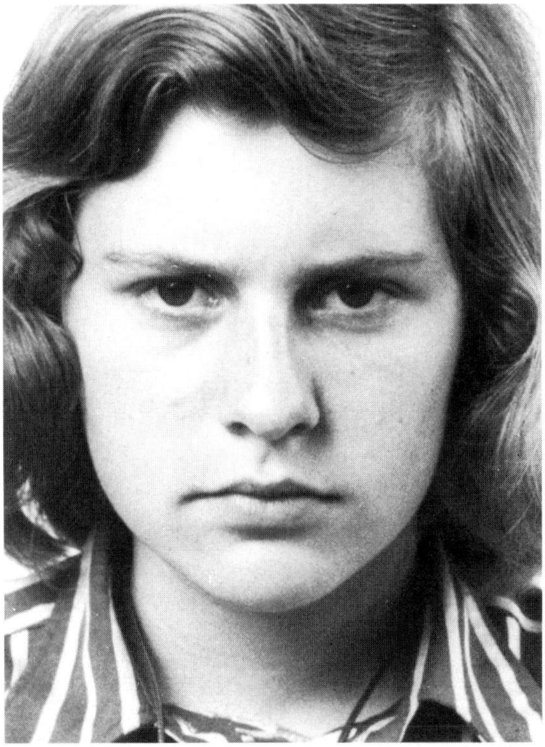
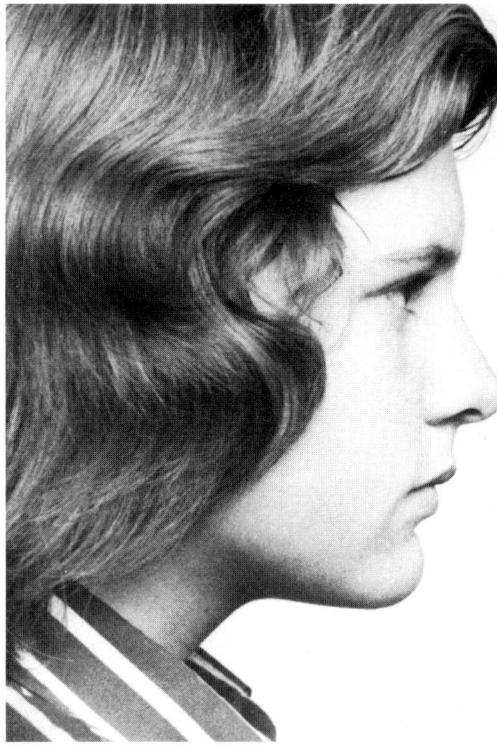
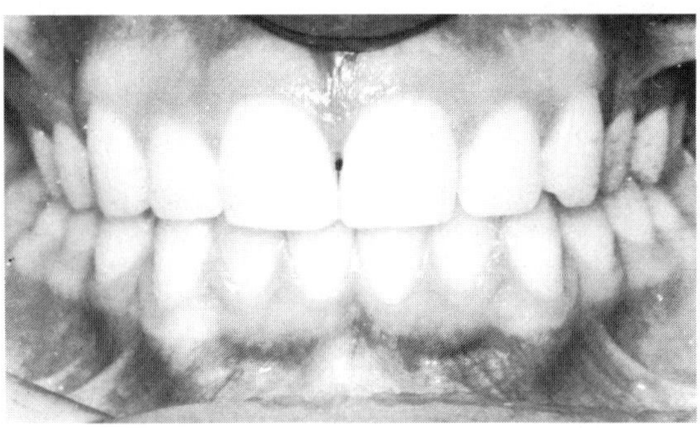
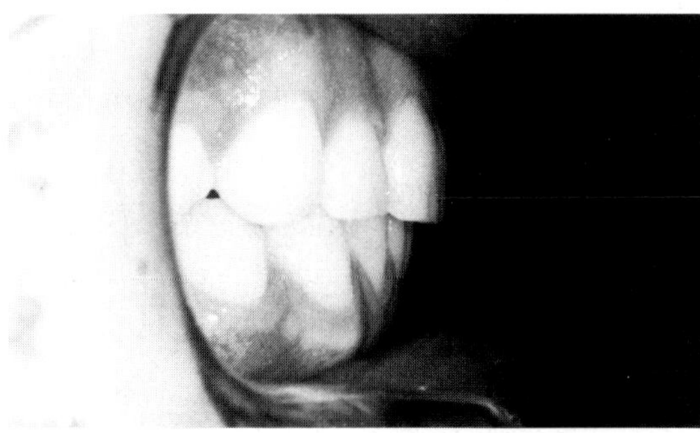
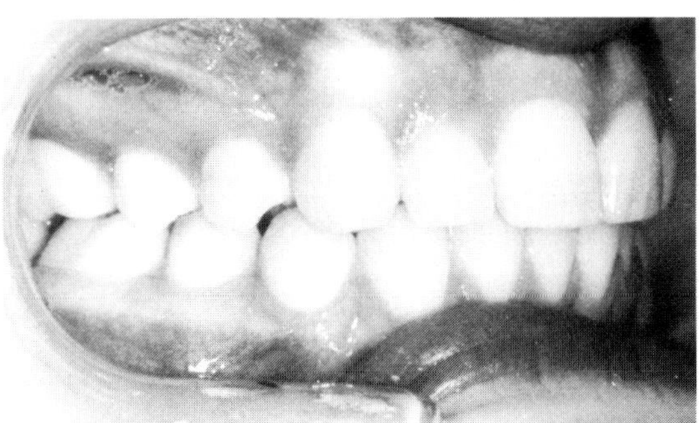
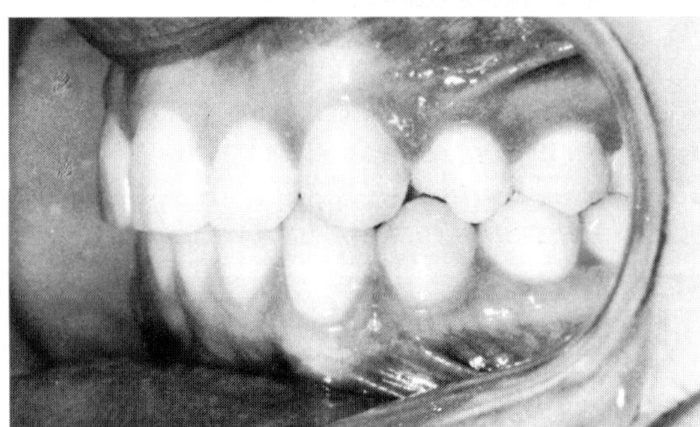

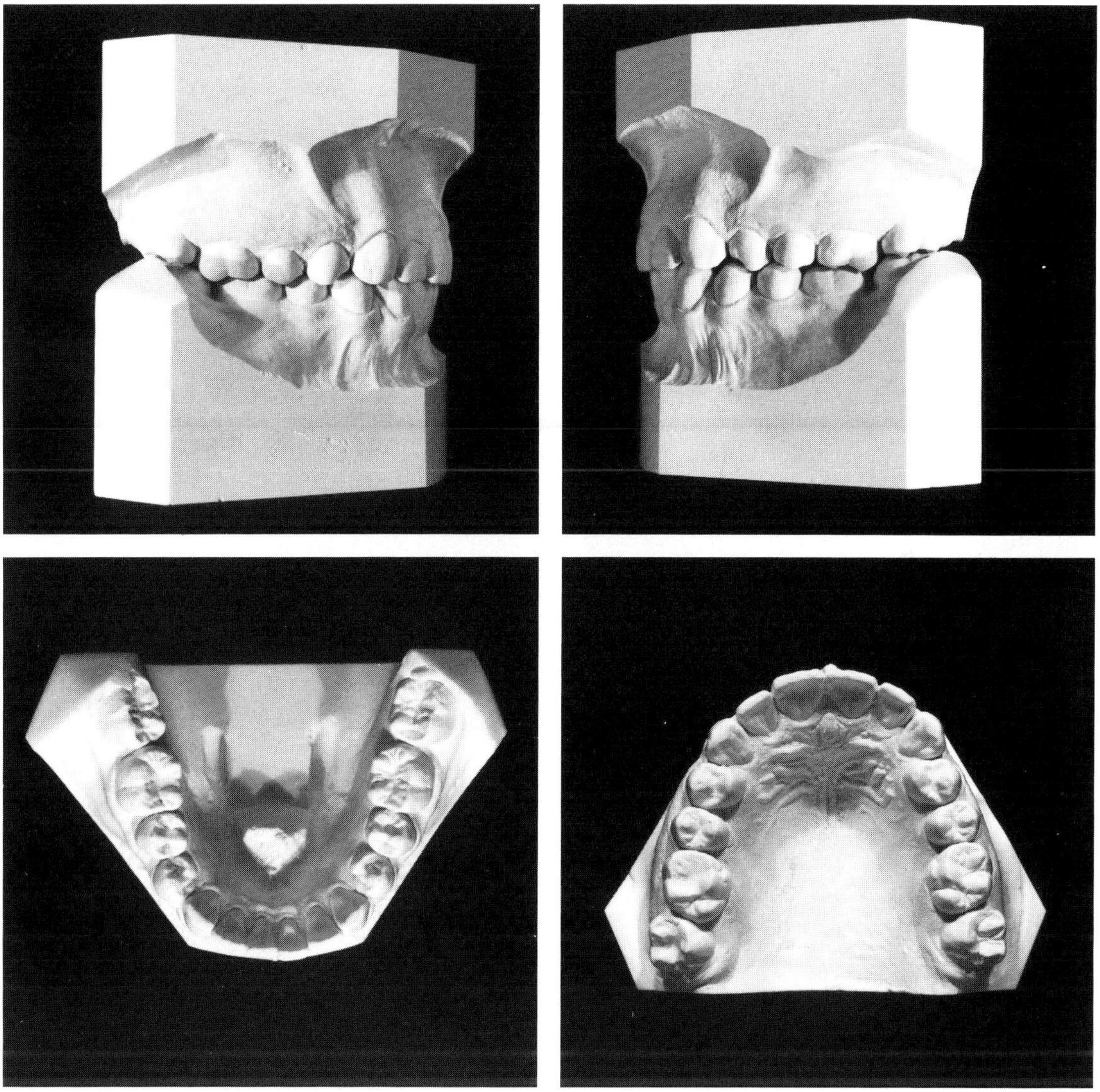

Figs 14-3 and 14-4 *At the age of 13 y, 0 mo, at the conclusion of treatment, there is a nice profile and a nearly ideal dentition. Also the position and inclination of the maxillary incisors, the alignment of the mandibular incisors, and the occlusion up to and including the first permanent molars leaves little to be desired. In the maxilla, insufficient space is available for the second permanent molars, which are positioned in buccoversion. On the basis of the space already available for them at the beginning of treatment (see Fig 14-2), it might be assumed that two y later they would have been well-placed in the dental arch. In the mandible, the right second molar is rotated mesiolingually. It might be emphasized that the disappearance of the mandibular incisor crowding and the correction of the lingual position of the lateral incisors after the slicing of the mandibular second deciduous molars occurred without the use of any appliances.*

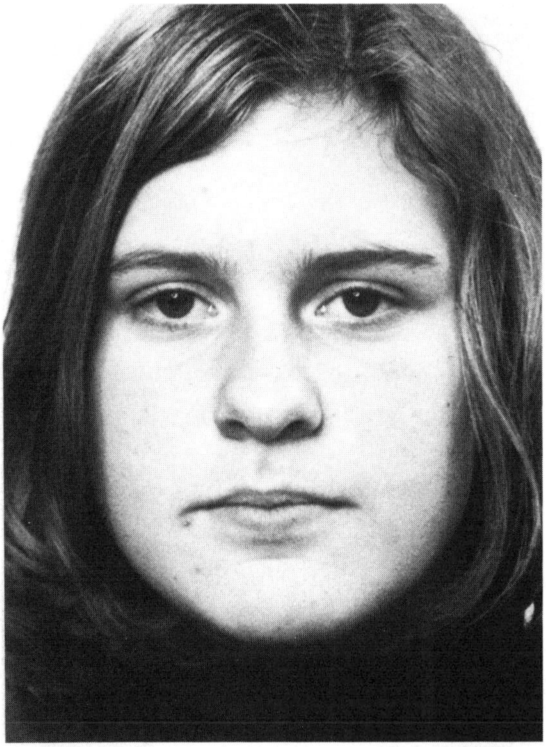

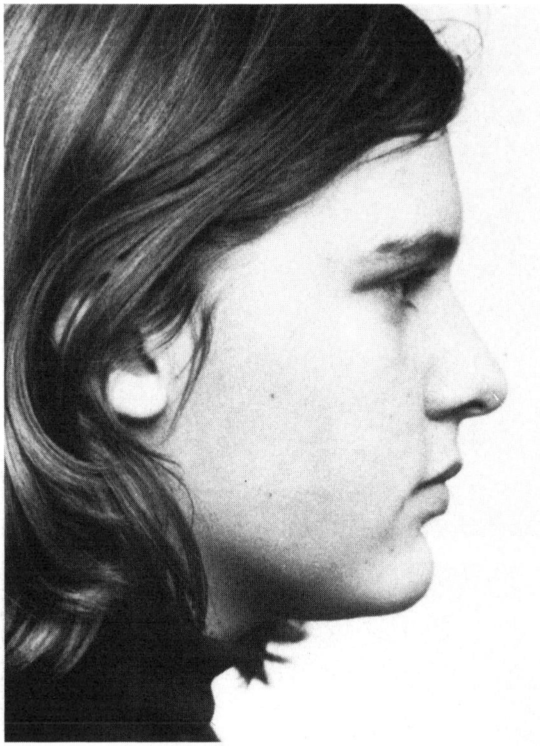

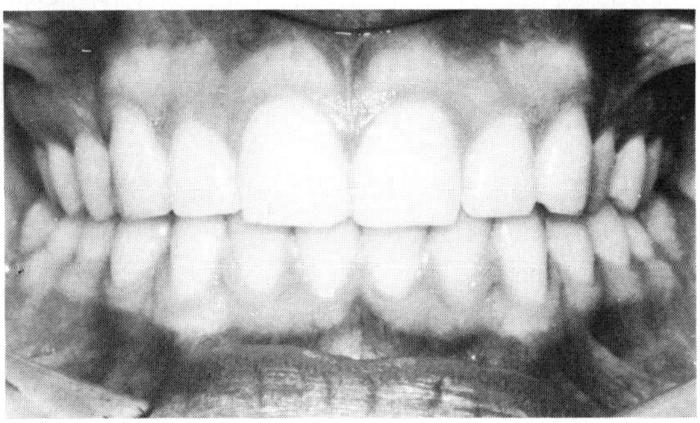

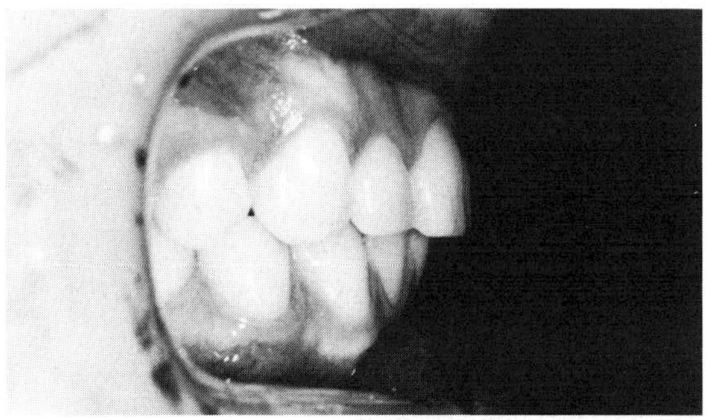

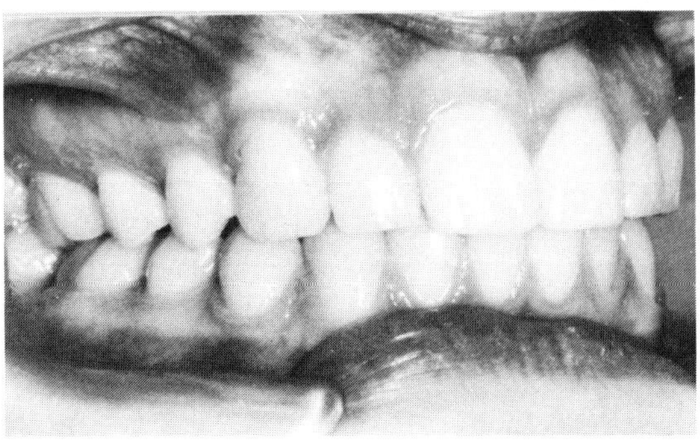

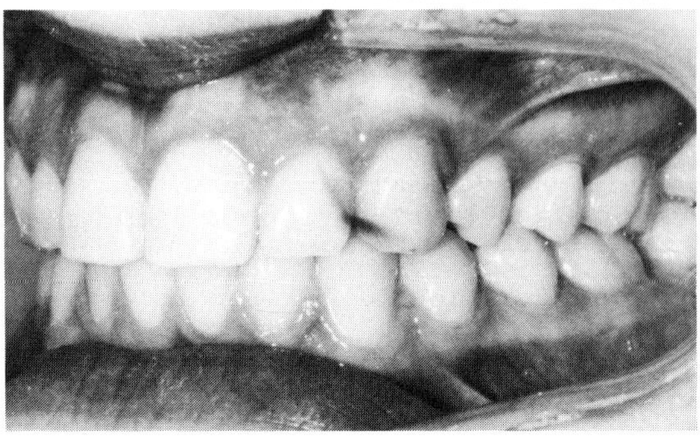

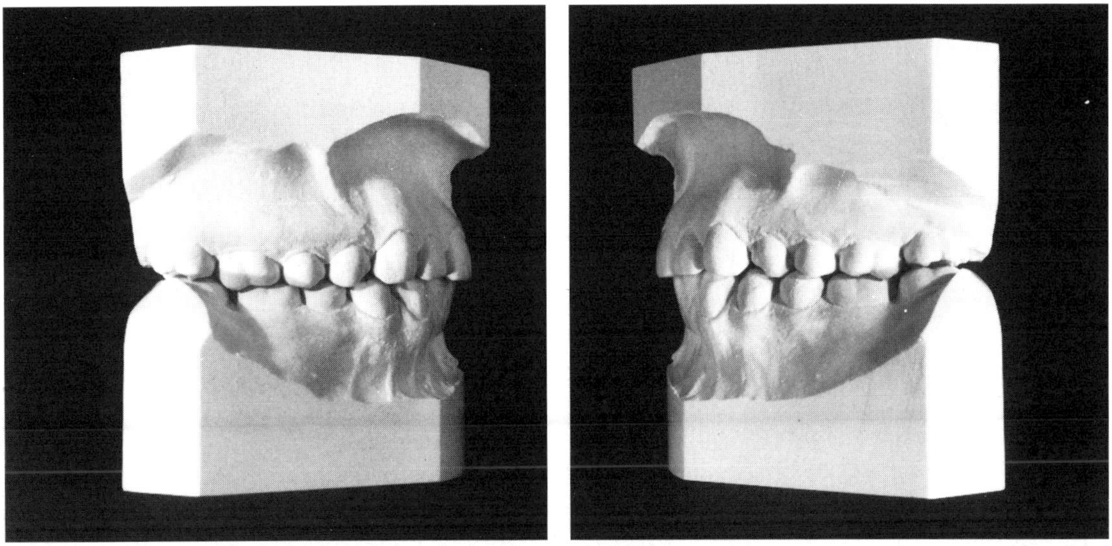

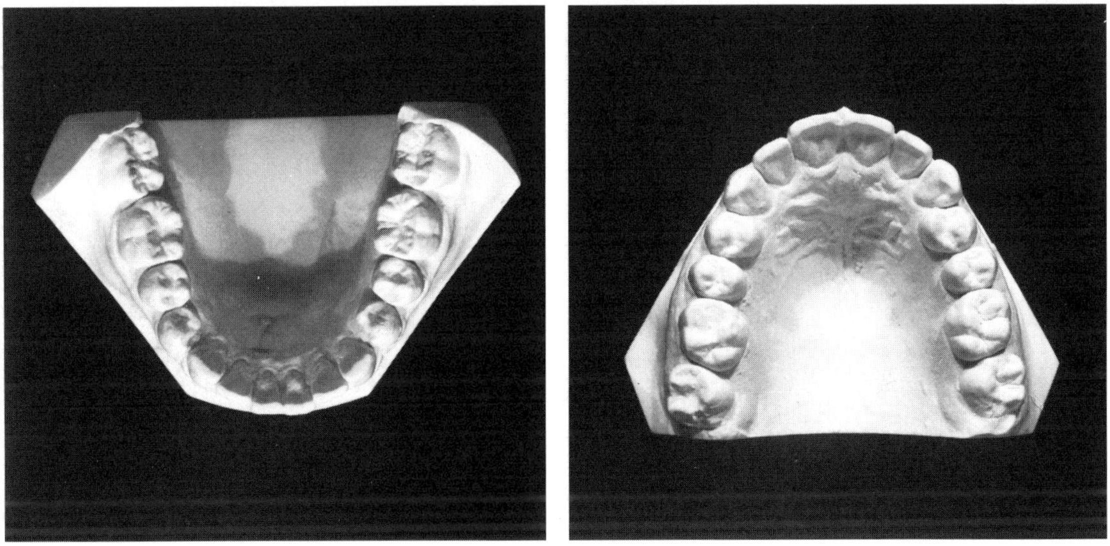

Figs 14-5 and 14-6 *At the age of 15 y, 0 mo, the face has changed little in comparison with two years earlier. The dental conditions are likewise almost the same. The mandibular right second molar has indeed uprighted itself and rotated into a better position. This movement is associated with more space becoming available through the growth of the mandible. That also applies to both the maxillary second molars, which are positioned more palatally than two years earlier. However, they still do not occlude well.*

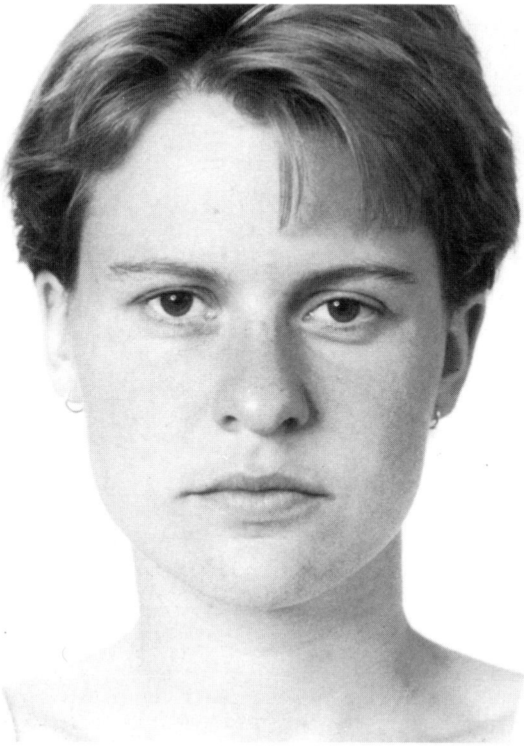

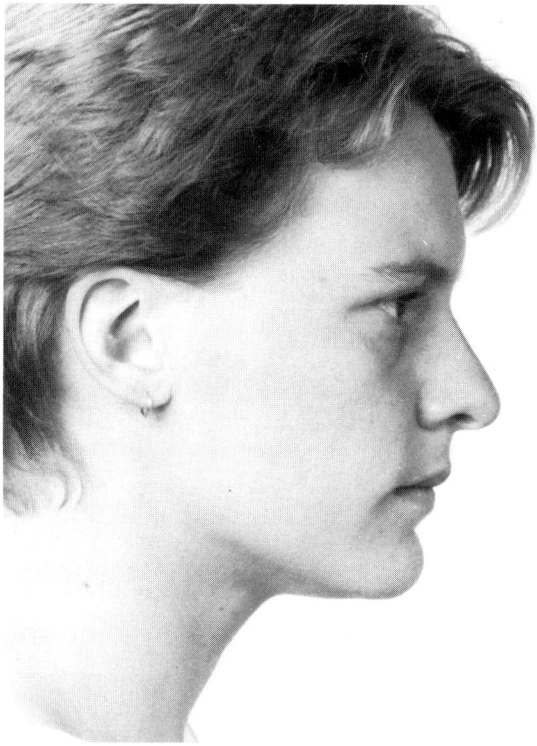

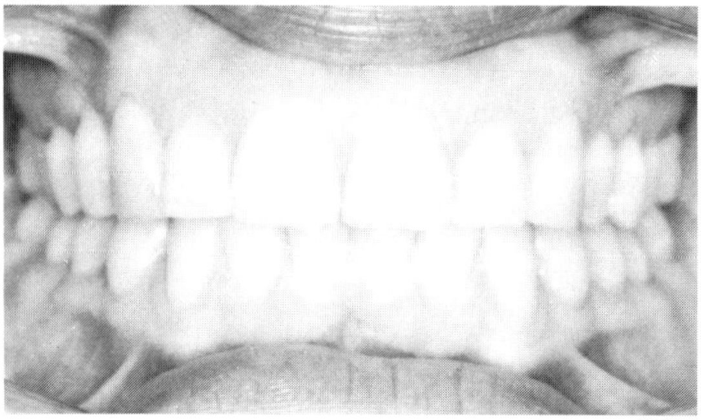

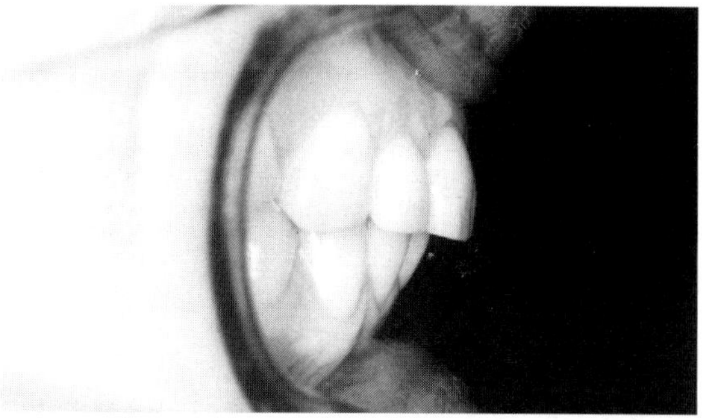

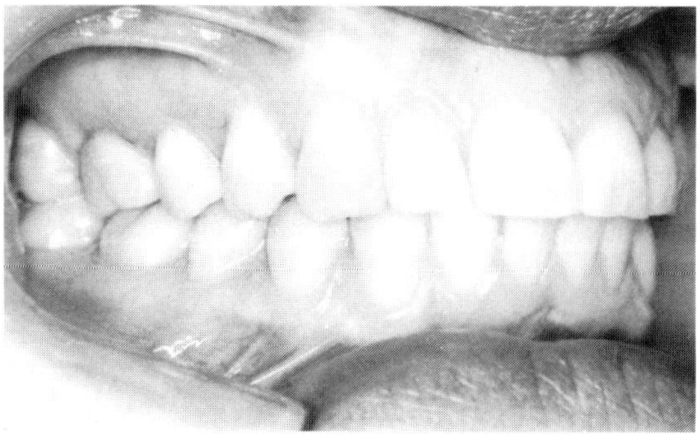

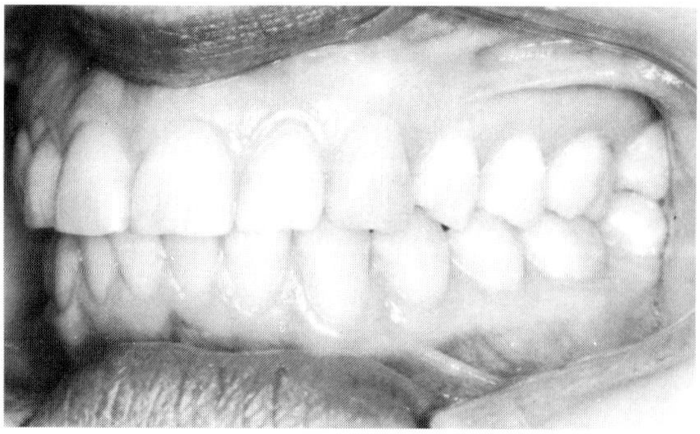

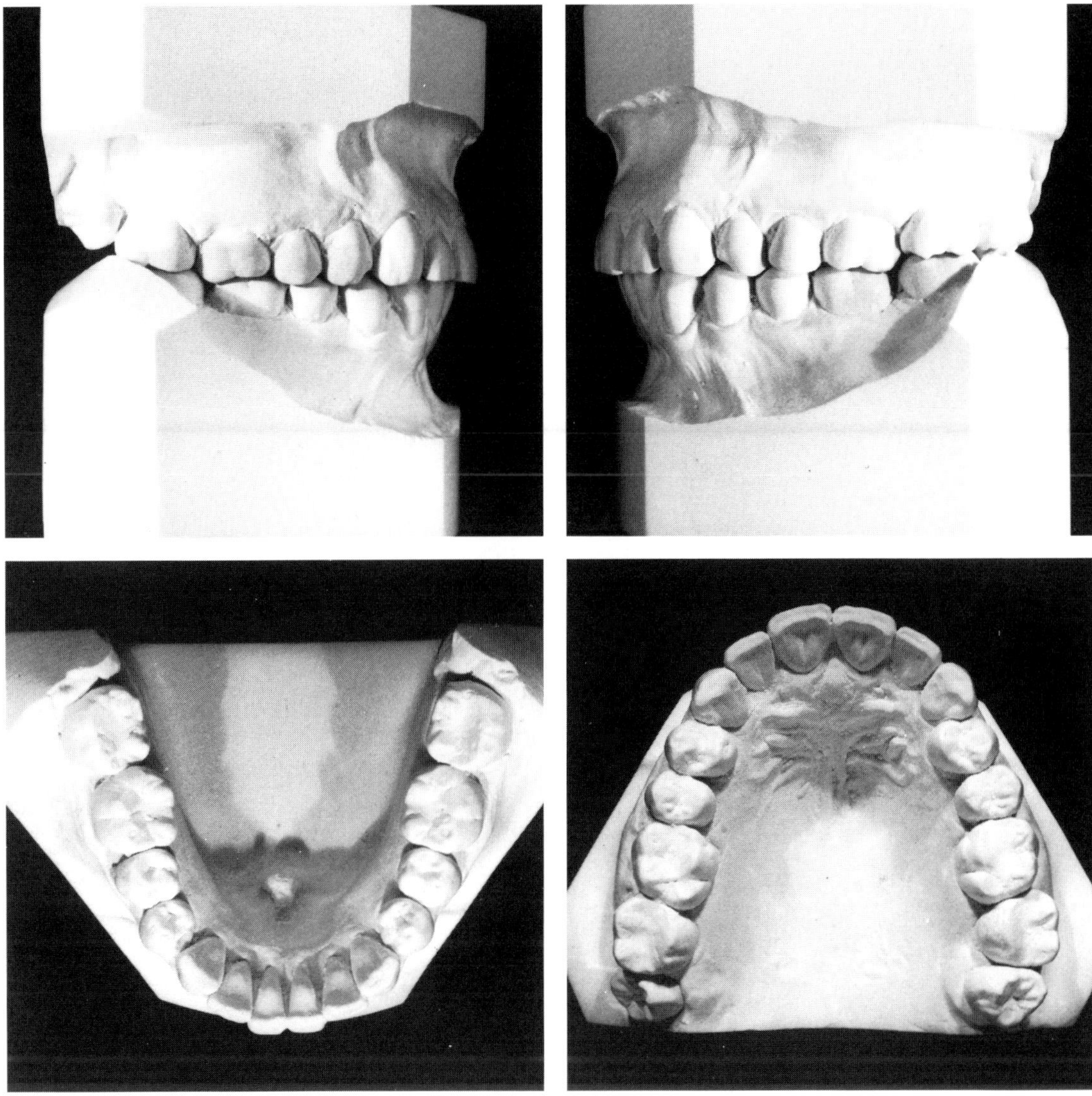

Figs 14-7 and 14-8 The result is still very acceptable at the age of 26 y, 2 mo, thirteen years after treatment; a nearly ideal dentition in a harmonious face. Tertiary crowding has developed in the mandibular anterior region, with the canines displaced slightly to the lingual and the central incisors to the labial. The third molars in the mandible are impacted, and those in the maxilla have erupted in abnormal positions due to lack of space.

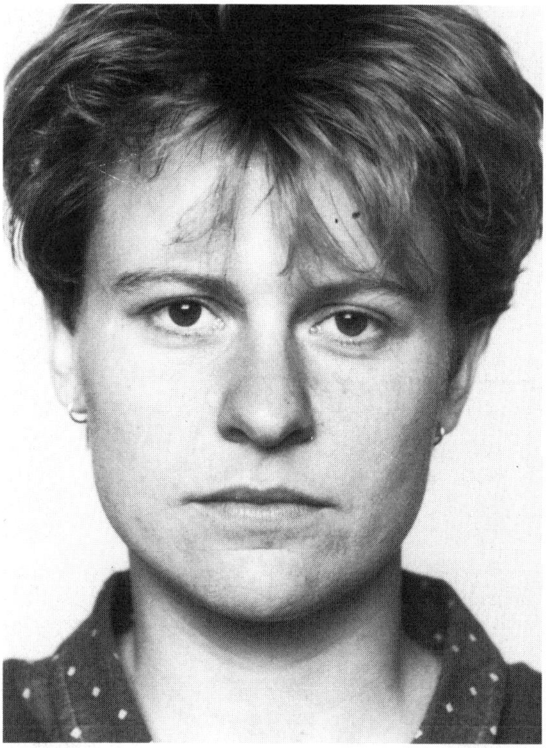

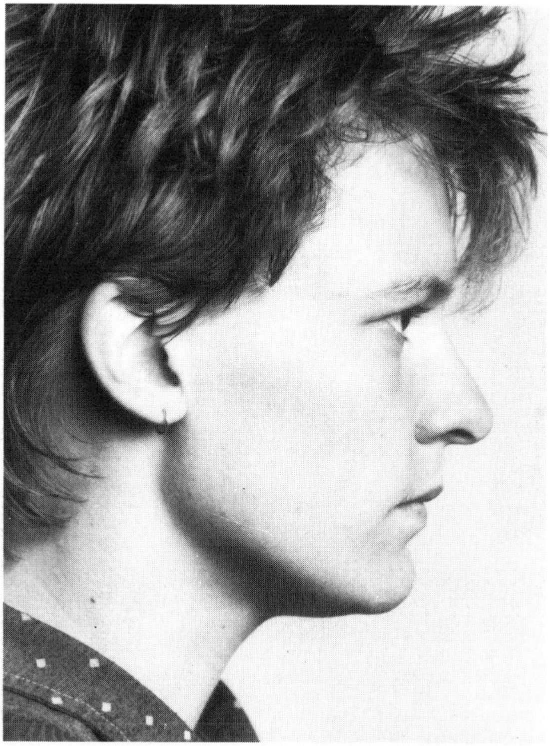

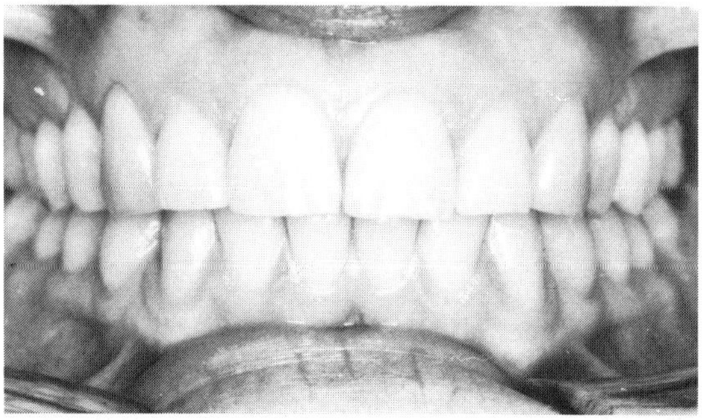

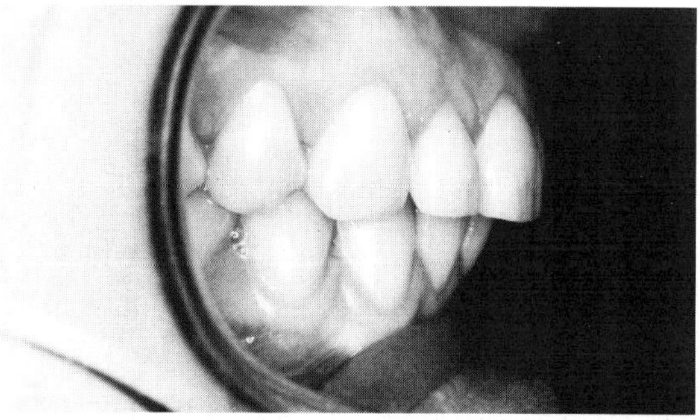

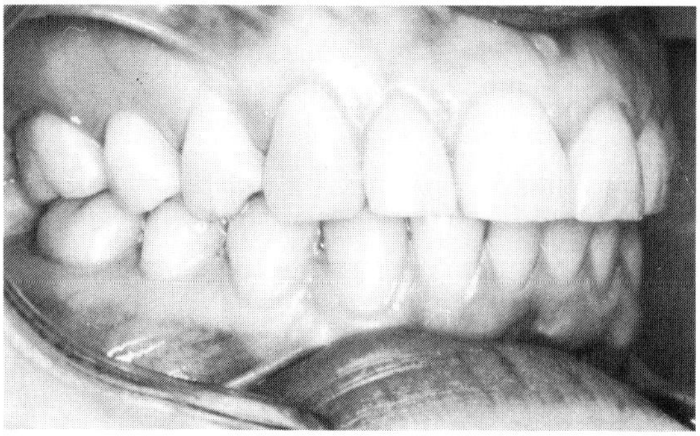

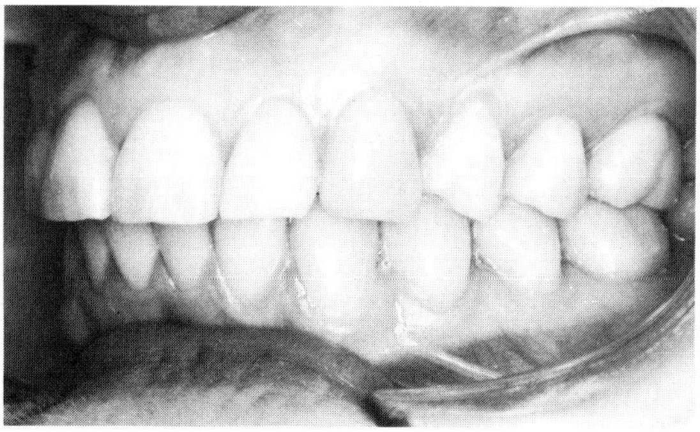

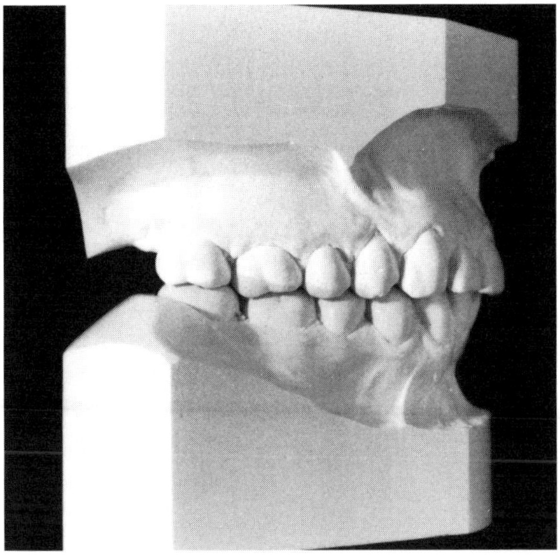
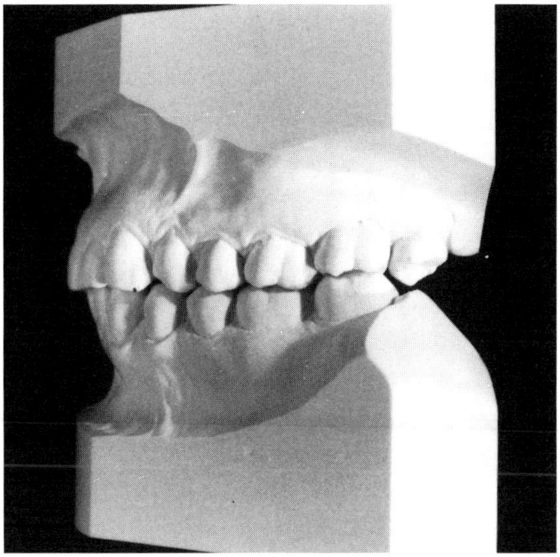
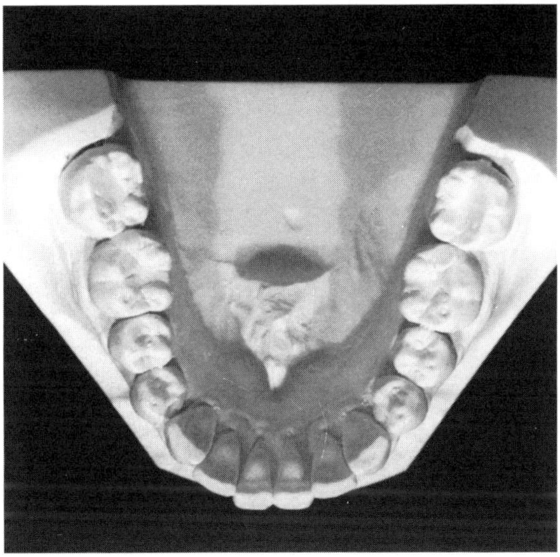
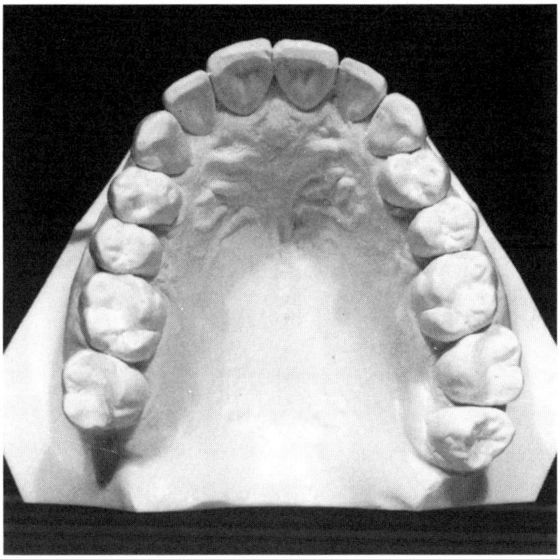

Figs 14-9 and 14-10 *At the age of 29 yr, 0 mo, the face and dentition have changed only slightly. In comparing the occlusal photographs with the previous ones, the effect on the position of second molars of third molars that are impacted or emerge into a crowded arch becomes obvious. Well over 2½ years previously, the third molars were removed, with the exception of the maxillary left molar. After extraction of the maxillary right third molar, the second molar could move to palatal and its roots tip to distal in the space that previously was occupied by the third molar. Also the mandibular second molar could improve somewhat in position in which case the cone-funnel mechanism probably has been instrumental. The right second molars now occlude fully. This is not the case on the left side, where the maxillary second molar could not improve its position.*

Figure 14-11a

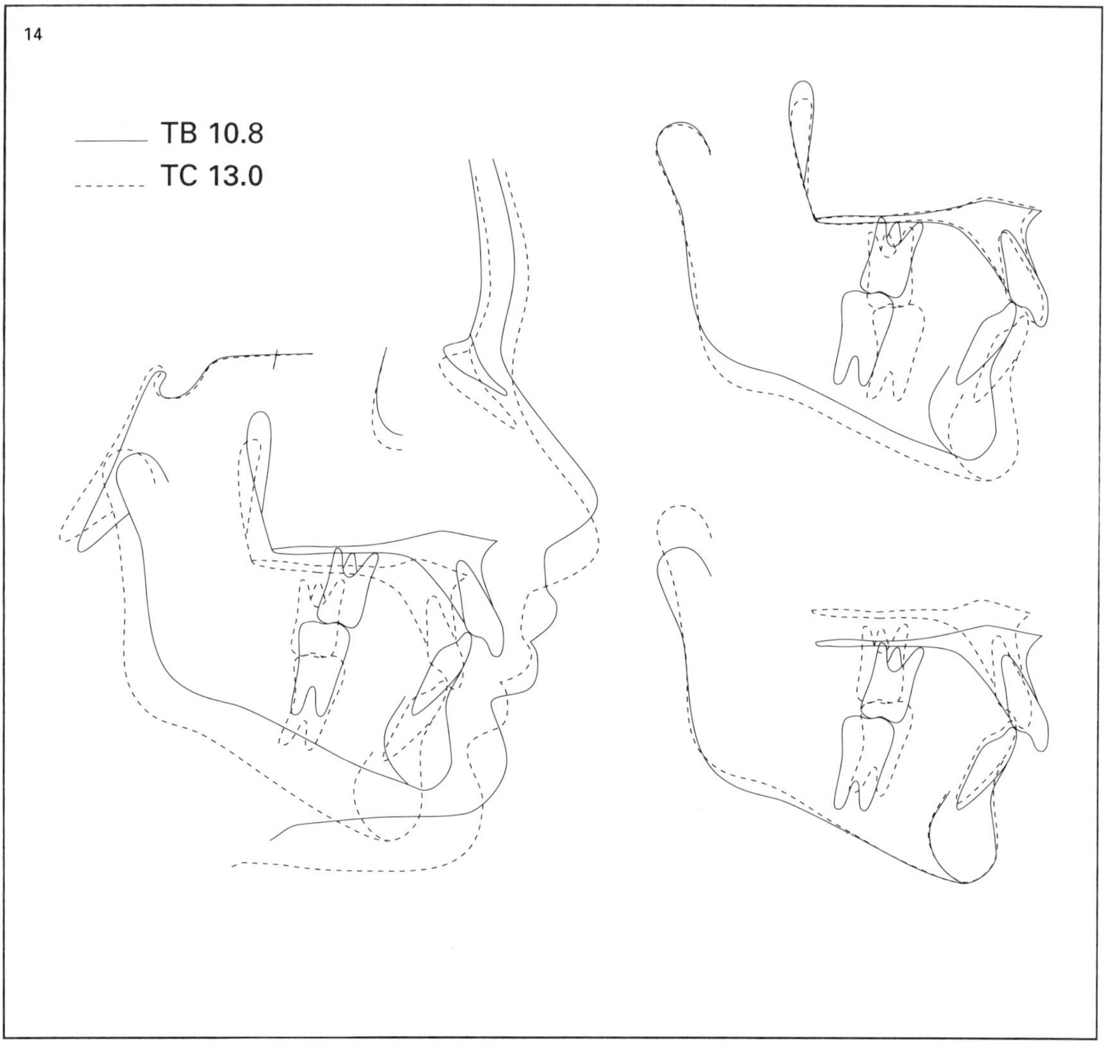

Fig 14-11 Superimposition of cephalometric tracings show that during treatment, the mandibular length increased notably while the forward development of the maxillary complex was retarded. The distance between the posterior surface of the maxilla and the first permanent molar has not increased. Little or no growth has taken place in the region of the maxillary tuberosities. The first molars have indeed erupted further vertically. The vertical development of the ramus has kept pace with that. The face height has increased noticeably.
After treatment, the face has continued to develop markedly to ventral while the height barely increased. In addition the incisors in both jaws have tipped more labially.

Figure 14-11b

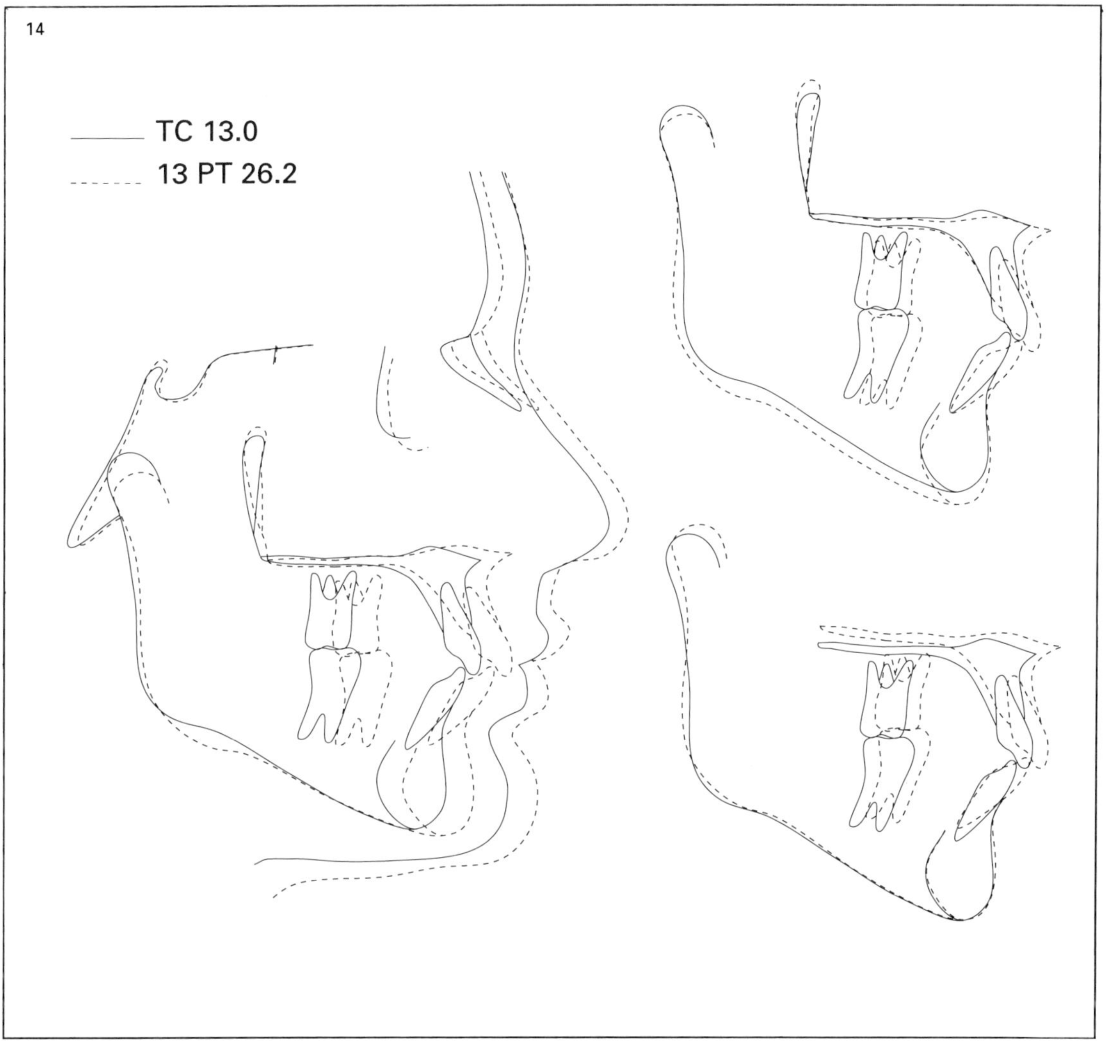

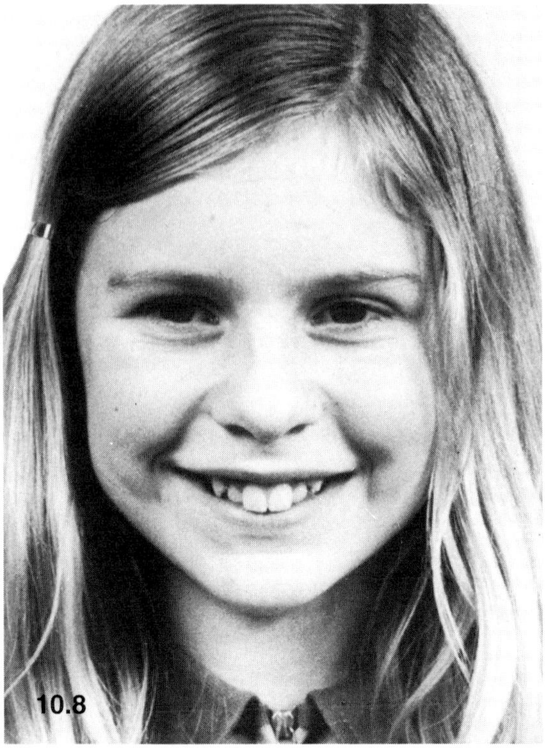
10.8

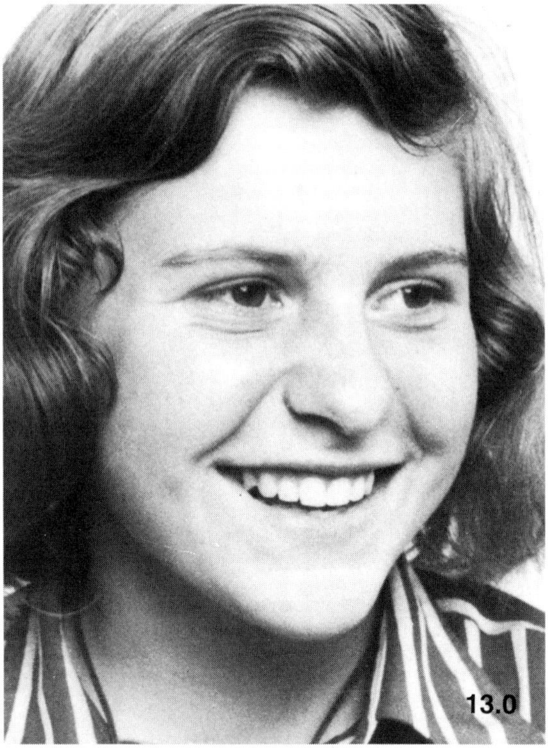
13.0

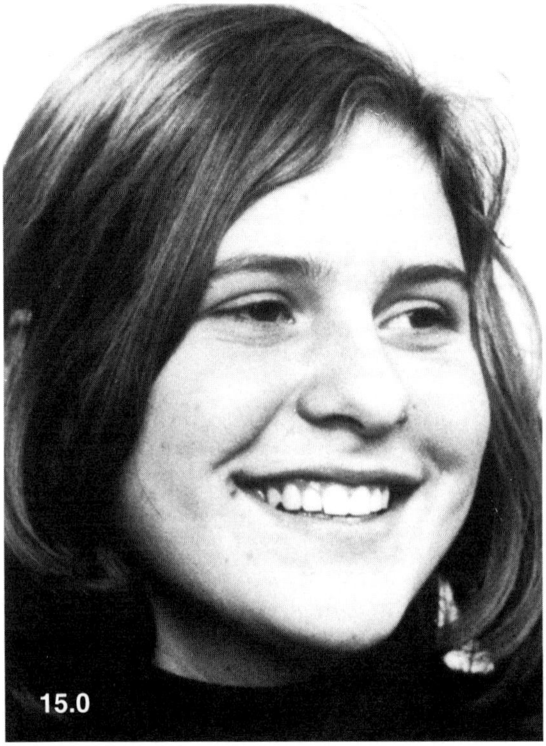
15.0

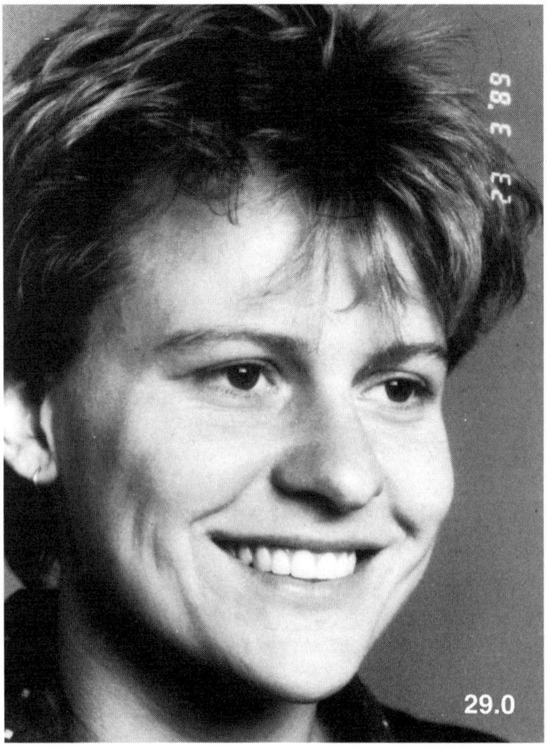
23 3 '89
29.0

Fig 14-12 The face of this girl changed little after the age of 15 years. Just the soft tissues show some gain in maturity. This picture is representative of the normal facial development of women.

6mm long was placed on each side of the archwire. Those springs sufficed to place a slight distal force on the maxillary incisors. They were activated by tying thin soft stainless steel ligatures (.010") from the distal of the molar tubes to two turns round the archwire in front of the anterior end of the coil springs, which compressed the coils when the ligature was shortened.

In this situation continuing, use of the headgear is imperative because otherwise the space will close from the distal. At subsequent visits, the retraction of the maxillary incisors was reactivated by compressing the coils that had opened up, until they were almost closed again. This action was repeated until all spaces had closed. Then the coil springs were removed and the archwire tied firmly back to the molar tubes with a ligature to the stops themselves, to keep the diastemata closed. In addition, a light intrusive force was applied to the incisors by the archwire. By allowing the wire to rest against the buccal surfaces of the canines, those teeth were nudged a little to palatal.

When all the anticipated changes had been realized, the headgear, which had been worn 14 hours per day, was not used. The fixed appliance was left in place another four months to consolidate the improvements that had been attained in the maxillary arch. A specific retainer was not considered to be required. Treatment was concluded at the age of 13 years, 0 months. The profile was harmonious and the dental arches were well-formed. They occluded optimally with a solid interdigitation of the canines and premolars. Only the position of the second permanent molars left something to be desired. In the maxilla these were too far to buccal. In the mandible the right second permanent molar was tipped too far to lingual and was rotated (Figs 14.3 and 14.4). These anomalous positions of second molars are symptoms of crowding in the posterior sections of the apical areas.

Two years after treatment (15 years, 0 months), the result appeared to be stable. Indeed, more room had been provided for the second molars; those in the maxilla had moved palatally, while the mandibular right second molar had uprighted and lost its rotation (Figs 14.5 and 14.6). Thirteen years after treatment, there were few changes to be seen except for minor movement of the mandibular anterior teeth. The maxillary third molars had emerged distally. It was suggested that the impacted mandibular third molars be removed, and to avoid problems of over-eruption that the maxillary ones also be extracted. This was done a short time later, with the exception of the maxillary left third molar (Figs 14.7 and 14.8).

The records at the age of 29 years are provided because they show the effect of extraction of a third molar on the position of the second molar in locally crowded situations. It seems that after extraction on the right side some changes did occur. The second molars in both the mandible and maxilla had the opportunity to re-align on the right side, but not on the maxillary left side. In the maxilla, due to the crowding in the posterior section of the apical area, the presence of the third molar had previously impeded the adequate movement of the second molar to palatal and of its apices to the distal. By the age of 29 years, those movements had occurred on the right side but not on the left side (Figs 14.9 and 14.10).

It can be seen from the superimposed tracings that favorable mandibular growth had taken place during the headgear therapy, while the forward development of the maxilla had been reduced (Fig 14.11). It is also obvious that, during that time, the posterior sections of the apical area in the maxilla had not increased in size. A dorsal traction applied to the maxillary complex does not only affect the sutures, but also the amount of bone formed on the dorsal aspect of the maxillary tuberosity. Part of the observed crowding of second and third molars can be ascribed to this reduced bone formation and part to the fact that use of a headgear limits the mesial migration of the molars, which takes place under natural conditions.

The photographs of the smiling patient present changes that have occurred during and after treatment (Fig 14.12). It can also be seen that other factors, such as hairstyle, can change the impression given by a face. This girl did not grow significantly beyond the age of 15 years. Of course,there are signs of maturity in the soft tissues.

The appliances used differ essentially from those used in the class II/1 anomalies described previously. For this patient,extra auxiliaries were used (four brackets and archwires), which made it possible to exercise three-dimensional control over the maxillary incisors. This control is required for an optimal result in cases with a large disto-relation, even when the incisors are excessively labially inclined. The same applies in cases where the maxillary incisors require retrusion but where their inclination may only be altered slightly if at all. It is only in situations where the disto-relation is small and the incisors are in fairly marked labioversion that it is possible to get a good result with nothing more than a removable plate. Such a case was described in Chapter 10.

The limitations imposed on treatment without three-dimensional control over the movement of the maxillary incisors in class II/1 anomalies can also be expressed in relationship to the size of the overjet and overbite, and to the growth-dependent improvement in the jaw relationship that might be expected.

If facial-orthopedic therapy does not secure sufficient correction of the disto-relation because growth is inadequate, or if cooperation is not good enough or if the reaction of the dentofacial complex is not as favorable as was hoped for, then an improvement of the overjet depends almost entirely on what tooth movements can be performed. Sometimes it is possible to bring the mandibular incisors forward permanently. But if retraction of the maxillary incisors has to provide the major contribution to the reduction of an overjet, the prognosis with use of a removable appliance is unfavorable because the inclination of the incisors becomes steeper the more they are retracted. Even with very careful activation of accurately fitting labial arches, the incisors will tip, with the point of rotation approximately halfway down the part of the tooth root that is invested in the alveolar process. Large overjets where only little change in incisor inclination would be acceptable can seldom be dealt with satisfactorily without fixed appliances. It also has to be realized that not only torque is required but also intrusion of the incisors, which emphasises the indications for the use of fixed appliances.

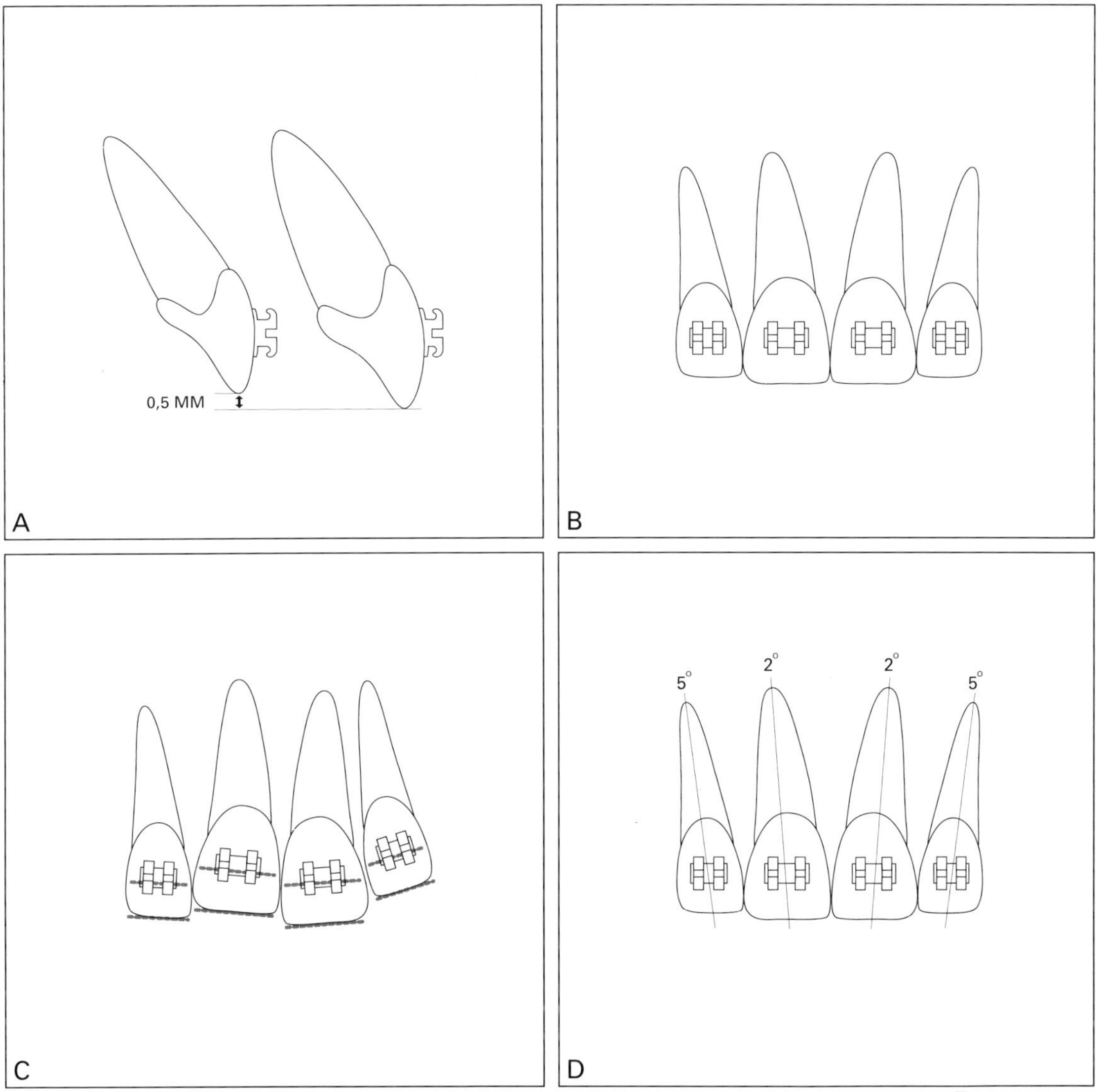

Fig 14-13 Guidelines for the location of brackets with built-in angulation, torque, and compensatory base-thickness on maxillary incisors.

A The bracket base must fit well against the labial surface. On a central incisor, the bracket slot should lie 0.5 mm further from the incisal edge than on a lateral incisor. With normal inclinations, the bracket slots should run parallel to the occlusal plane.

B Mesiodistally the bracket must be placed in the middle of the tooth.

C With normal crown forms, the interior edges of the bracket slots should be parallel to the incisal edges of the incisors. Depending on the manufacturer of the brackets, the edges of the bases may or may not be parallel to the slots.

D On maxillary incisors, the bracket slots should not be perpendicular to the long axes of the teeth, but diverge from them slightly; for central incisors by 2 degrees and for laterals by 5 degrees.

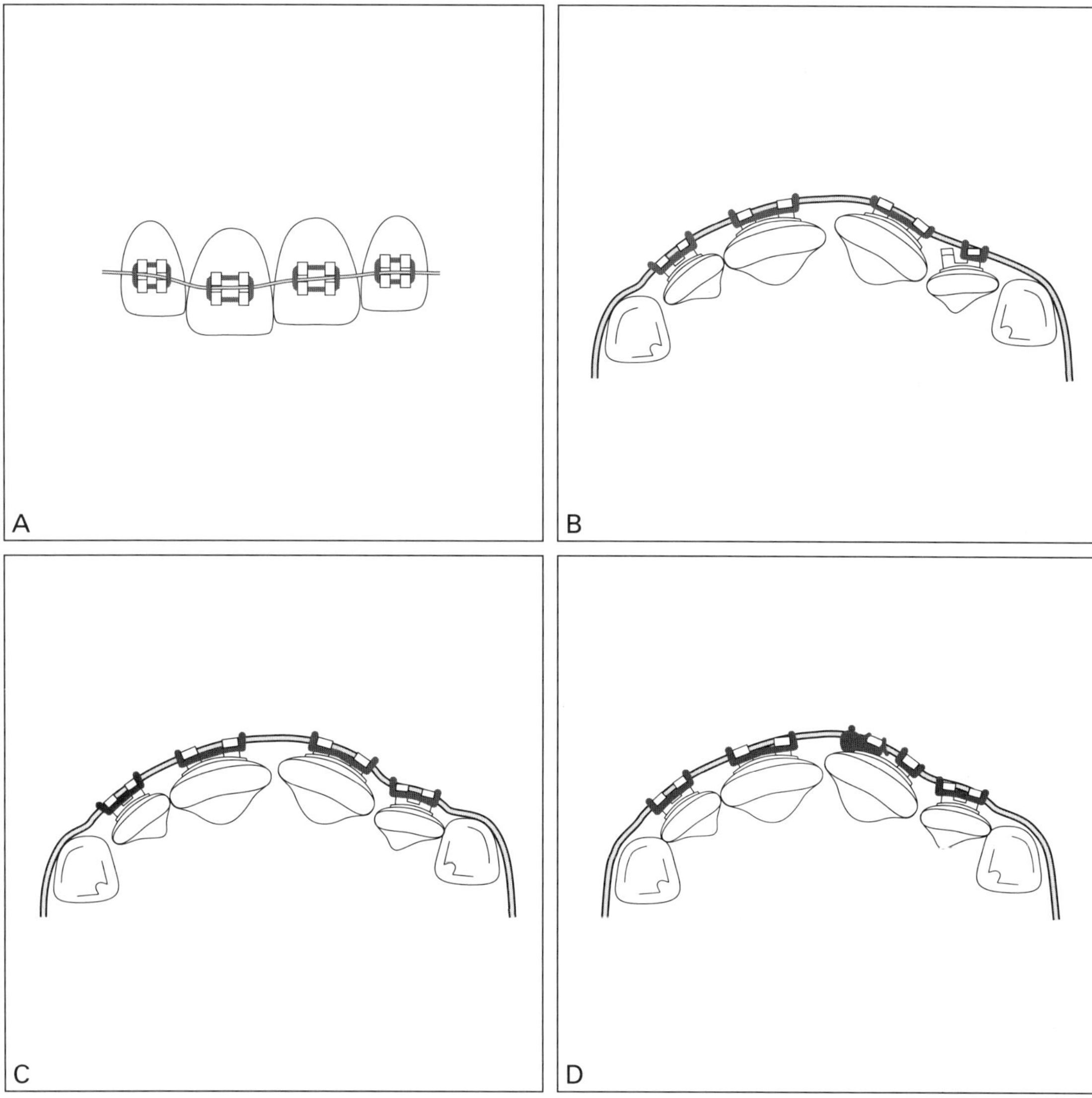
A
B
C
D

Fig 14-14 Correction of maxillary incisor positions with .022" x .028" edgewise brackets and a .0175" twistflex arch.

A The supple horseshoe-shaped archwire, which must be adapted to the form of the dental arch, is bent up behind the molar tubes to prevent the forward movement of the incisors. The archwire can be fastened in the bracket slots with soft 0.010" stainless steel ligatures or elastic rings if the irregularity of the teeth is minor. Where the irregularity is marked, a thinner .015" twistflex archwire should be used first.

B With rotations, it is possible to avoid an excessive force by initially using only the bracket wing that lies close to the archwire, as is shown here with the left lateral incisor.

C At a later visit, when some tooth movement has occurred, the bracket can be fully tied to the archwire.

D Teeth such as the left central incisor can be rotated better and further with rotation wedges. When maxillary incisors are moved with partial fixed appliances before the permanent canines have emerged, the latter might be displaced within the alveolar process and become impacted. Moreover the roots of the lateral incisors might be severely resorbed. If a partial fixed appliance is used early, something which really only is justified for severe rotations (see chapter 22), then those risks should be considered.

Furthermore, rotations and other irregularities in tooth alignment can only be corrected if sufficient space is available and the occlusion does not inhibit the improvements. The previous limitations also apply to treatment involving removable appliances.

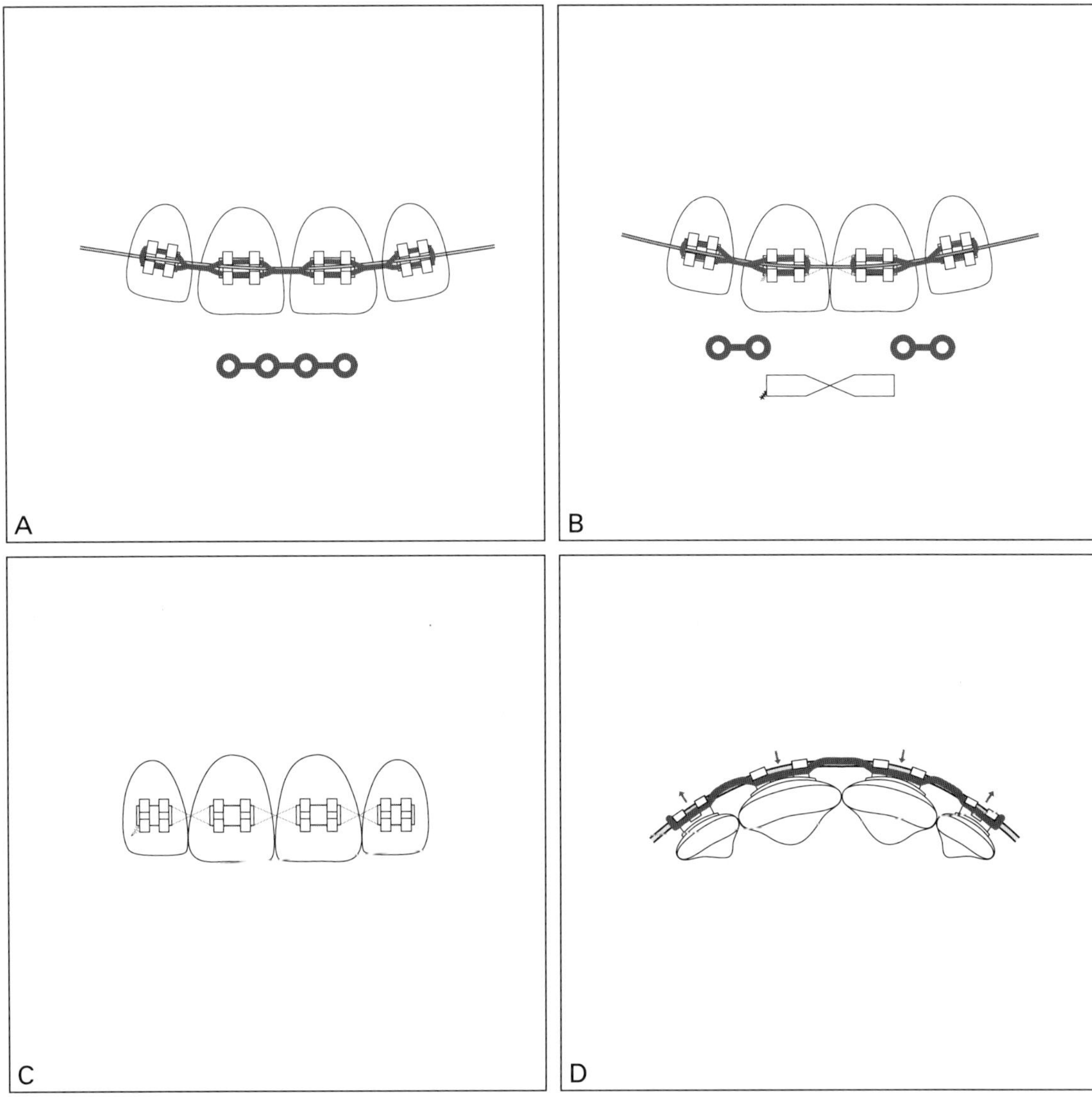
A
B
C
D

Fig 14-15 Closing diastemata between incisors.

A An "elastic chain" is used to pull the teeth together along the archwire over which the brackets can freely slide.

B When contact between neighboring teeth is established, that correction is maintained by tying a soft stainless steel .008" ligature between the brackets as illustrated. The pigtail made when twisting the ends of the ligature must be tucked out of the way, under the archwire, to prevent irritating the lips or having it broken while toothbrushing. The elastic chain is only used where diastemata are to be closed.

C Once all the spaces have been closed, the teeth are held together with a .008" ligature wire laced across the four teeth.

D When an elastic chain is used across a curved arch segment, flattening of that curve has to be expected. To prevent unwished-for flattening of the maxillary anterior teeth, the use of an elastic chain should be dispensed with once all the spaces have closed.

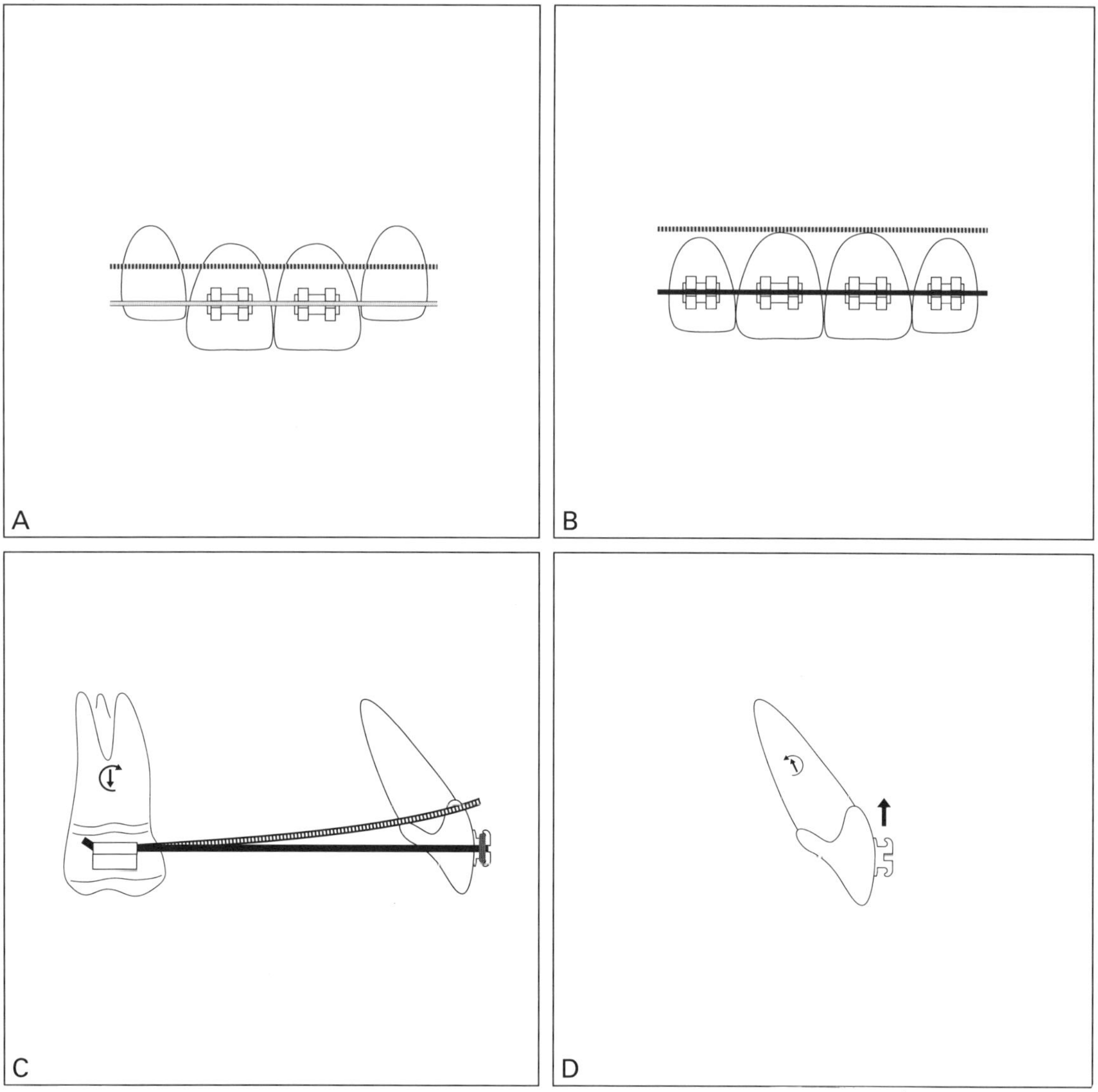
A
B
C
D

Fig 14-16 The intrusion of maxillary incisors.

A If central incisors are in supraposition, they can be intruded with a .016" x .022" braided archwire. A maximum force of 30 to 50 g may be applied to each incisor. If the lateral incisors also need to be intruded, they should only be included in the system later (the archwire is drawn in its passive position with broken lines).

B For simultaneous intrusion of the four maxillary incisors, it is also possible to use a stainless steel .019" x .026" solid archwire with which a force of 30 to 50 g on each tooth can be exerted, as generally is the case if the archwire in its passive configuration lies approximately 4 mm above the bracket slots.

C The reactive force that acts on the first permanent molars has the effect of extruding and tipping them distally. If the force used is so large that the molars indeed do tip, then the archwire no longer has the desired effect on the incisors.

D Because the intrusive force on the incisors is directed vertically and is applied to the teeth in front of their center of resistance, a couple is developed, which tends to rotate the incisors in the sagittal plane. The incisal edges will move labially while the root apices move palatally (see Fig 19-11 page 324).

In all these situations, the archwire has to be passive buccolingually in the molar tubes, and the distal end needs to be bent up to prevent the incisors from moving labially.

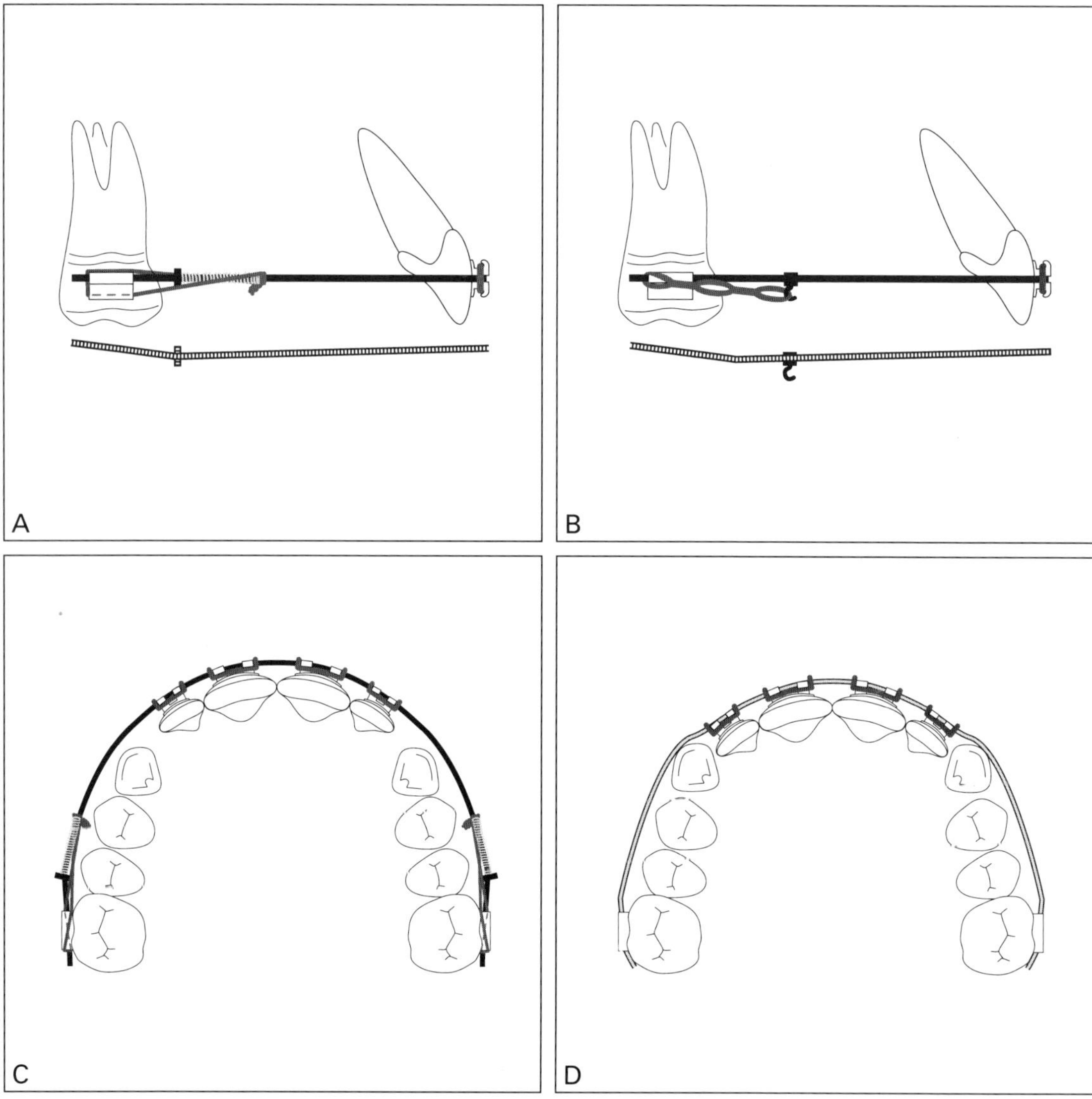
A
B
C
D

Fig 14-17 The retraction of maxillary incisors.

A After closing the spaces between the incisors, the four teeth ligated together can be retracted as a unit with a .019" × .026" archwire to which a small distal-acting force is applied. This can be done for example, first by placing on the archwire on each side a section of open coil spring (.010" –.030") about 6-to-8 mm long and then soldering or clamping stops on the archwire sufficiently mesial to the molar tubes to allow for the distal movement of the incisors. Once the archwire has been fastened in place, the coil springs are compressed by about 1 or 2 mm with soft (.010") stainless steel ligatures that run from the distal of the molar tubes to in front of the coil springs where the ligatures are wound twice around the archwire and then twisted together. At subsequent visits, the coil springs that have opened up are compressed again by pulling them almost closed with the ligatures, the ends of which are wound tighter with needle forceps or the like.

B The distally directed force can also be produced by "elastic chains" stretched between hooks designed to be fitted to the archwire and the ends of the archwire that protrude distally through the molar tubes.

With these approaches, excessive activation has to be avoided, as otherwise after space closure has occurred the canines and premolars will be pushed out of the dental arch. Moreover undesirable mesial movements of the first molars have to be avoided.

C A reactive force is exerted on the buccal of the maxillary first permanent molars that tends to tip them to mesial and rotate them mesiopalatally. The tipping and rotation should be countered by bending the part of the archwire distal to the molar stops. This part should run cranially and palatally as shown in the drawings. These compensatory activations are shown both in this figure and in A and B separately. The width of the archwire needs to be such that no unwanted transverse movements of the molars will ensue.

D The situation after the incisors have been fully retracted. By allowing the archwire to lie against the buccal surfaces of the canines, those teeth can be moved palatally. The archwire needs to be bent up distal to the molar tubes to prevent forward relapse of the incisors.

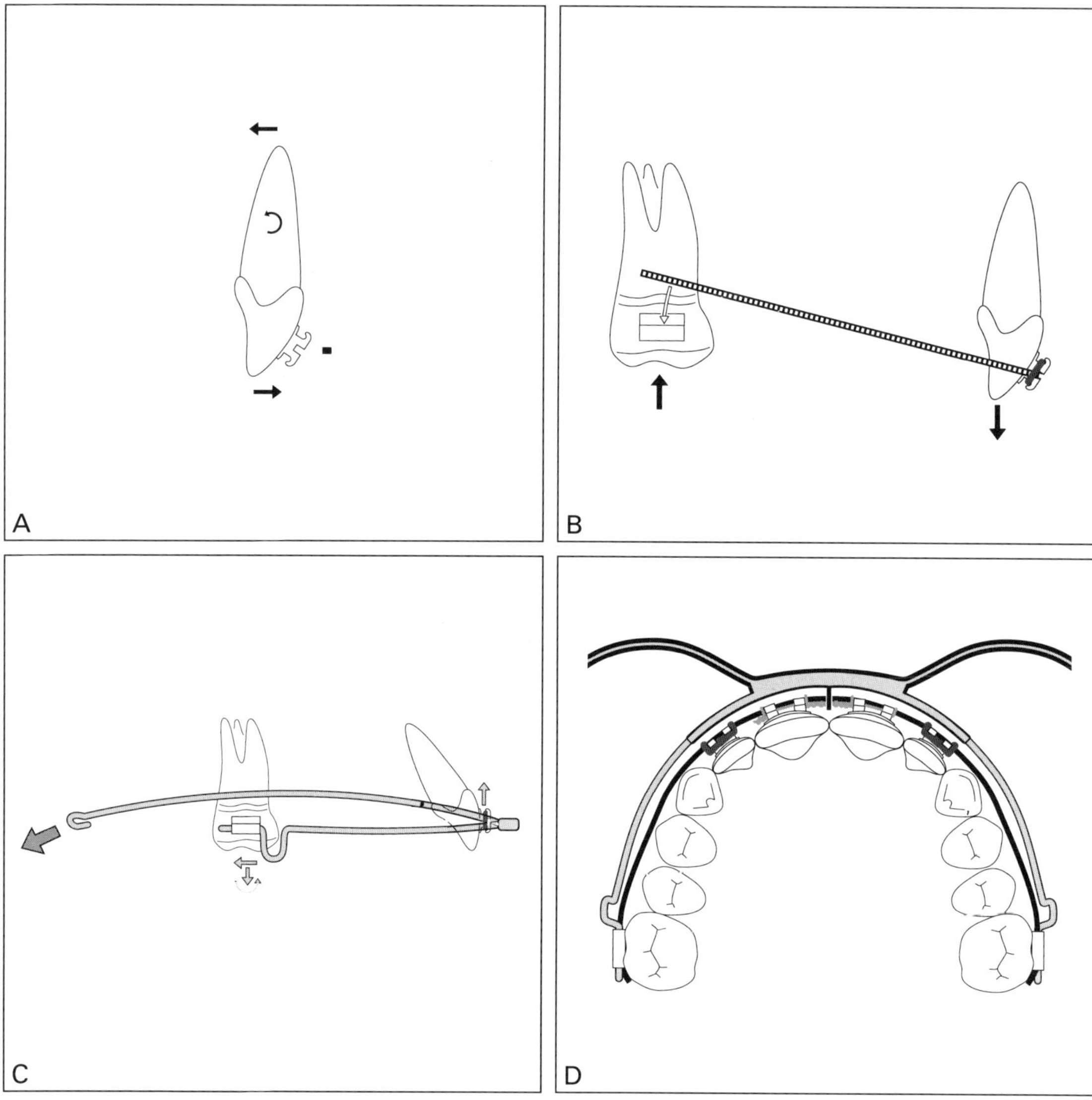
A
B
C
D

Fig 14-18 Torquing and intruding maxillary incisors.

A Where maxillary incisors are steeply inclined, an archwire without torque, when engaged in the molar tubes, will exert a palatally directed force on the root apex (lingual root torque) and a labially directed force on the crown (labial crown torque) of each incisor. If the latter is counteracted by for example tying back the archwire to the molar tubes, then the root apices will move palatally.

B An archwire with lingual root torque will also have an extruding effect on the incisors and an intrusive and buccally tipping effect on the anchor molars. The effects on the molars originate in the application of the intrusive force buccally to the center of resistance and in the spreading out of an arch with torque applied in front.

C A cervical headgear with a Kahn spur can oppose extrusion and even cause intrusion of the incisors. In addition, the torque is enhanced since the intrusive force is applied ventral to the center of resistance. The archwire that is in the brackets must also have an intrusive and torquing effect. The intrusive force must not be too great since the force from the Kahn spur will be added to that of the archwire (see also Fig. 19.10, page 322).

D The creation of a central diastema and mesiodistal tipping of the central incisors can be prevented by strongly twisting a steel ligature (.012") between the brackets of those central incisors.

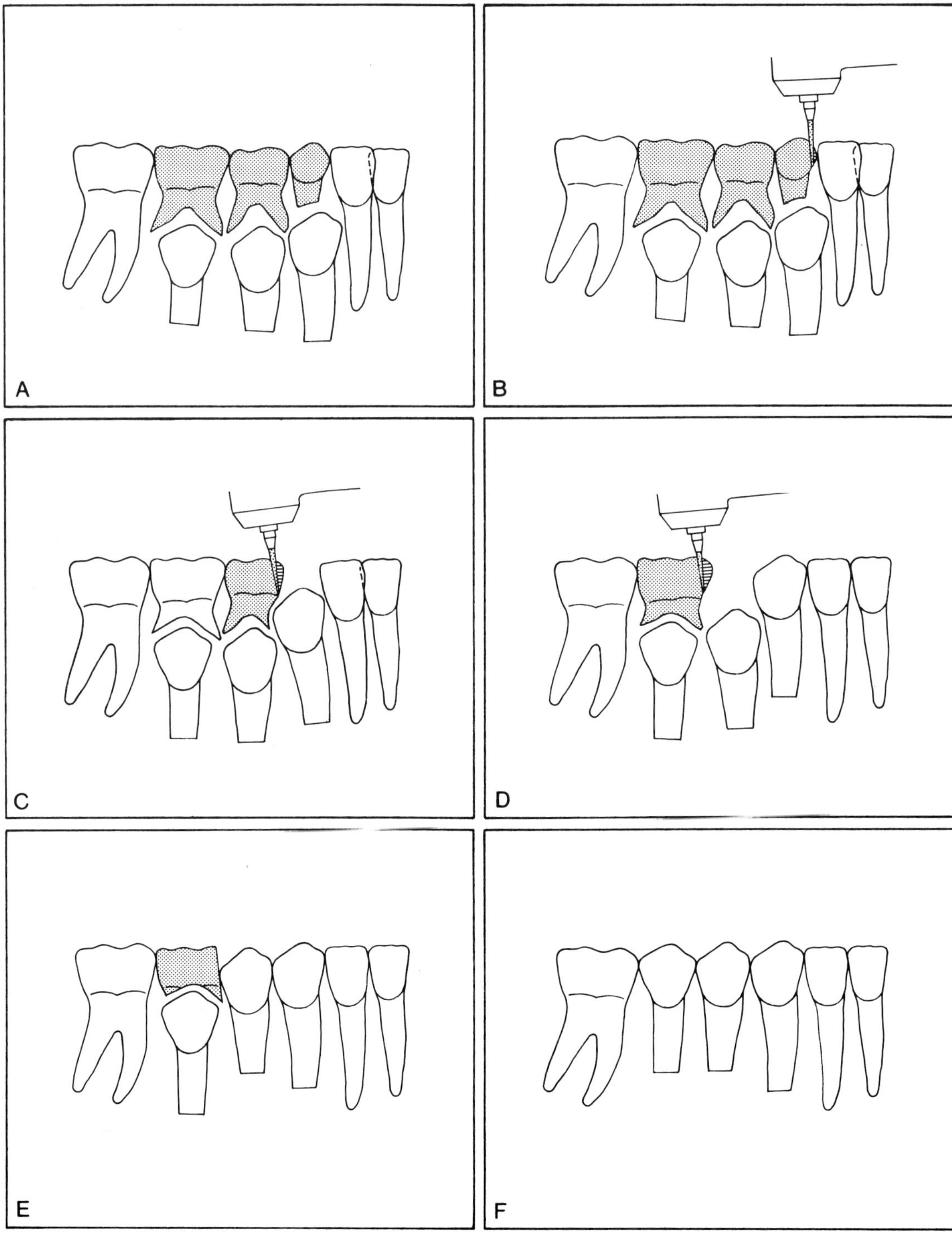
A
B
C
D
E
F

Fig 14-19 The slicing procedure, to be performed to benefit from the difference in crown width between the deciduous molars and their successors to prevent or even correct crowding.[36]

Providing brackets on the maxillary incisors is not at all difficult with current procedures. The appropriate use of partial fixed appliances is really not so simple (anchorage problems, detailed positioning of the incisors), but it can provide a remarkable improvement in the finished result. In the treatment dealt with in the following chapters this will frequently come into consideration. The technique of three dimensional control of the movement of maxillary incisors with brackets and preformed archwires will be clarified in Figures 14.13 to 14.18.
The procedure of slicing, which was used in this case, is illustrated in Figure 14.19. By grinding away part of the mesial contours of particular deciduous teeth, and taking advantage of the extra room provided when the deciduous teeth exfoliate, it is often possible to prevent or correct crowding in the dental arches. The difference in mesiodistal crown diameters of corresponding posterior deciduous and permanent teeth is greater in the mandible than in the maxilla. The effect of slicing is therefore also greater in the mandible so it is more often indicated there. The benefits of slicing are seen best with mandibular second deciduous molars. These teeth show the most width difference in relationship to their successors, and also have the largest mesial convexity available for slicing.
The fact that the headgear was chosen in this case to treat the disto-relation is associated with the fact that crowding existed in the maxillary arch. As previously mentioned, arch length can be gained with careful use of the headgear, partly by rotating the anchor molars. That would not have been possible with an activator, for example. At the same time, it had already been forecast that in view of the limited eversion of the maxillary incisors, it was very likely that a partial fixed appliance would be needed later. For this reason, double molar tubes were used on the molar bands (one for the headgear and one for the probable archwires for a fixed appliance), which simplified the eventual provision of the partial fixed appliance.
Through continuing to check up on patients sometimes changes from treatment are observed years later. This is illustrated here by the situation involving the third molars. In this regard it might also be pointed out that if the last tooth in the dental arch has no antagonist it can over-erupt. Lack of an antagonist can be due to agenesis, extraction, or impaction. Although over-eruption does not always occur, it is always wise to follow up this situation with possible problems at the distal end of the dental arch in mind. Such problems can be eliminated or prevented. It is mostly in orthodontic treatment where extractions were performed in one arch only that such problems can arise. Finally, judging whether or not there is good or bad occlusal contact in the far posterior part of the mouth is often troublesome. In doubtful cases, the solution is to prepare dental casts; it is then easy to examine that region from all angles.

Chapter 15

Class II/1 subdivision

Cervical headgear, brackets 12, 11, 21 and 22, maxillary removable retainer
Male: 8 years, 0 months to 24 years 0 months

A boy aged 8 years, 0 months with a normal facial configuration for that age even if his chin was receding, exhibited a class II/1 subdivision anomaly. He had a competent lip seal and functionally all was normal; however, his lower lip covered approximately half of the labial surfaces of the maxillary incisors. The maxillary incisors were steeply inclined; the bite was deep and the overjet was 4 mm. Mandibular deciduous molars had been lost early. Three premolars had already emerged. The arch length discrepancy in the maxilla was +2 mm and in the mandible –1 mm (Figs 15.1 and 15.2).

It was decided to await further development of the dentition and at a later stage to undertake treatment with a cervical headgear, supplemented later on with partial fixed appliance on the maxillary incisors. Six months later, the maxillary lateral incisors were inclined similarly to the central incisors and were in the arch alongside them. A year after that, the maxillary left lateral incisor had moved more palatally under the influence of the canine erupting adjacent to it. The maxillary permanent canines and first premolars had emerged (Fig 15.3). It was decided to slice the mesial of the mandibular right second deciduous molar and to anticipate development of the dentition, taking into consideration the fact that the level of cooperation in treatment would as yet not be adequate.

Active treatment was started at the age of 10 years 10 months, by fitting a cervical headgear (Fig 15.4). This appliance was not worn enough and every four or five months had to be replaced due to fractures. After six months, the headgear was made asymmetric to procure a greater effect on the right side. The outer arm on the left side was shortened for that purpose, so that the loop to which the elastic neckstrap was hooked lay at the level of the molar tube. The outer bow on the right had its leg bent slightly outward (see Fig 24.7, page 404). Both modifications lead to more traction being applied to the first permanent molar on the right than on the left. The right molar does indeed suffer loading to palatal at the same time, and this cannot just be countered by making the inner arch wider without there being other effects on the dental arch.[26] After some time, the headgear was left out for two months to give the right first molar, which had displaced palatally as described, the opportunity to return to the buccal. This applied also to its antagonist, which had been moved lingually by occlusal interaction. The development of the mandibular arch was so favorable that treatment of it was considered unnecessary.

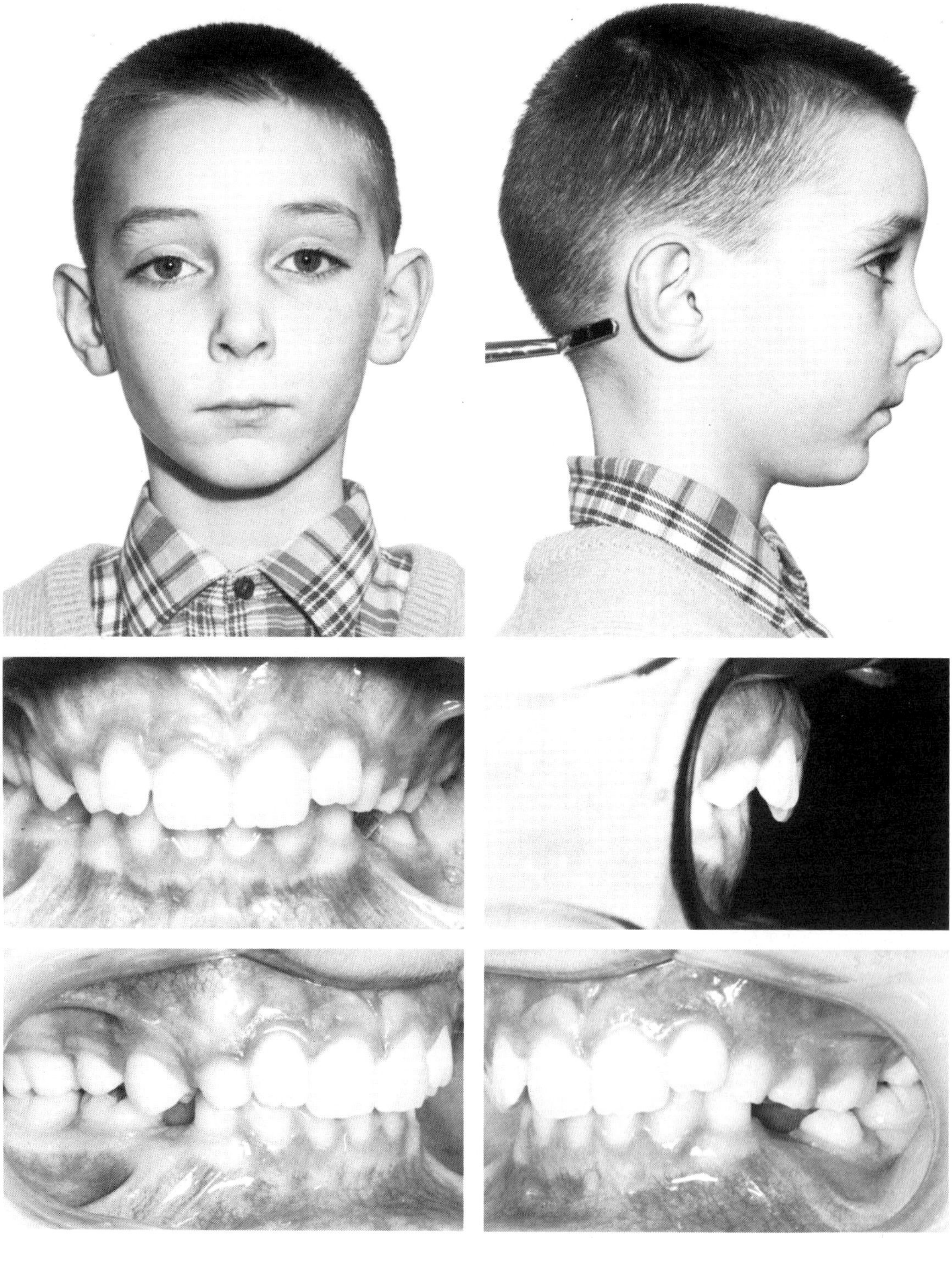

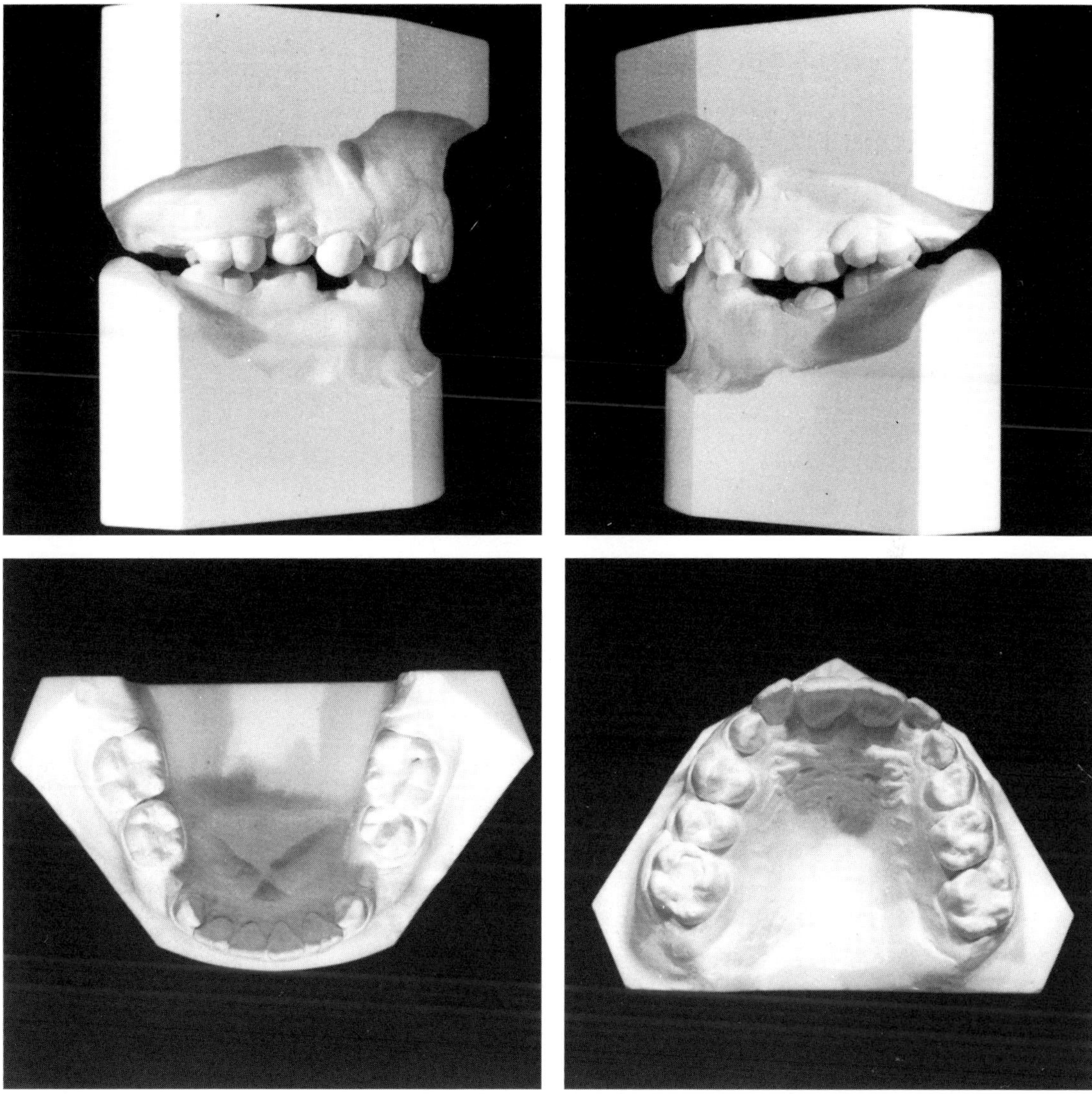

Figs 15-1 and 15-2 A boy of 8 y, 0 mo with class II/1 subdivision (disto-occlusion R: 1 PW, L: ½ PW); a deviation of the dental arch midlines; and steep inclination of the maxillary central incisors, which have half their labial surfaces covered by the lower lip. Both dental arches are of normal form. Deciduous molars have been lost in the mandible. Three premolars have already emerged, which is very early.

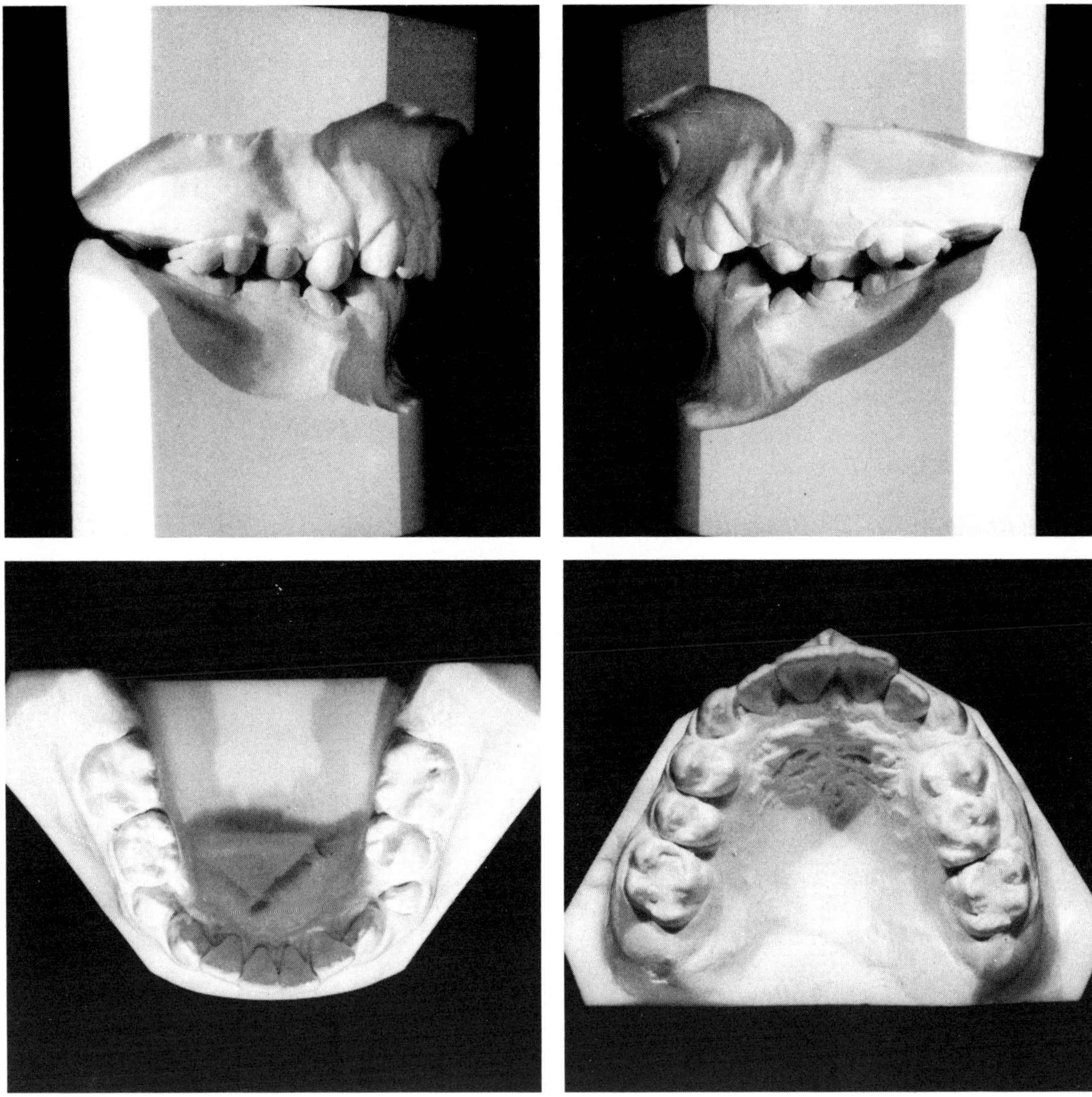

Fig 15-3 At the age of 9 yr, 6 mo, the maxillary permanent canines and the mandibular first premolars have emerged a short time previously. The maxillary left lateral incisor was displaced palatally by the erupting permanent canine. Of the deciduous teeth, only the maxillary left and the mandibular right second deciduous molars remain. Mild crowding exists in both maxillary canine regions, but more notably in the mandibular premolar regions where space has diminished because of premature loss of deciduous teeth. It was decided to slice the mesial of the mandibular right second deciduous molar and await further development of the dentition. It was thought that cooperation in active treatment at this time would be inadequate.

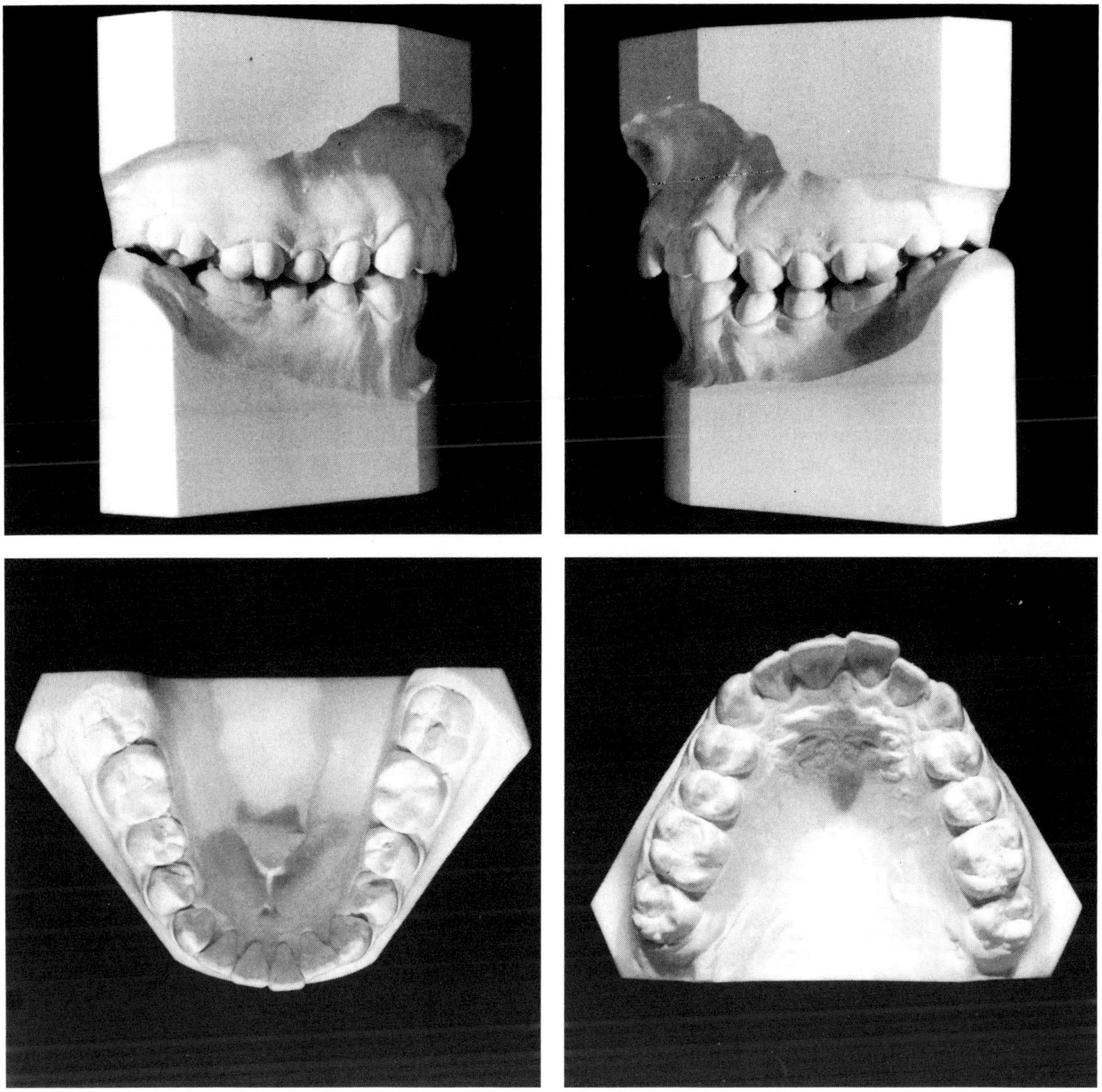

Fig 15-4 *At the age of 10 y, 10 mo active treatment was begun. All permanent teeth except for the third molars had emerged. In the mandible more or less sufficient room developed for the premolars without the crowding increasing in the anterior region. The development in the maxillary arch has also been favorable where more space has become available for the right canine.*

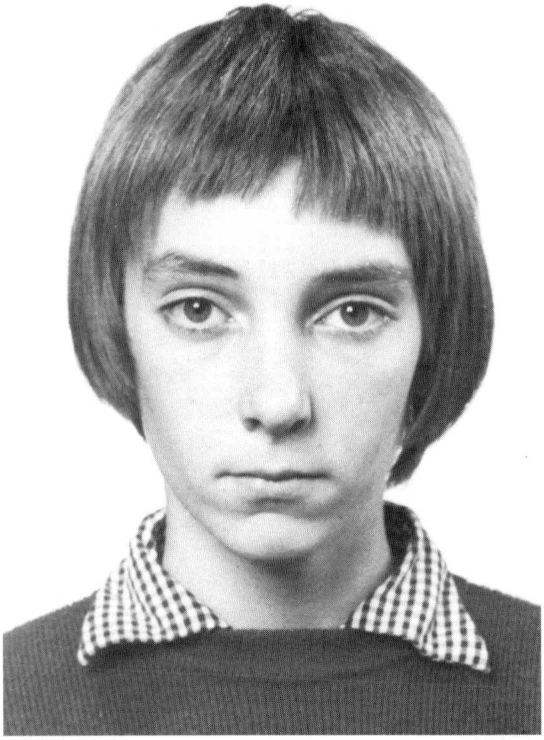

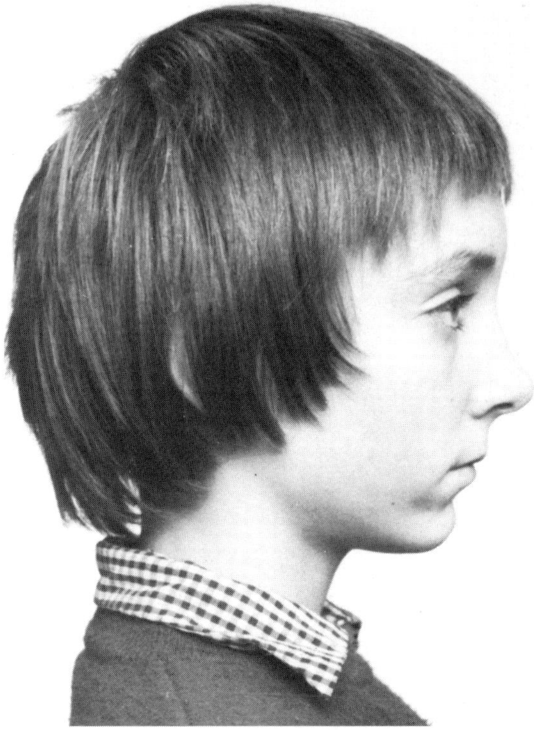

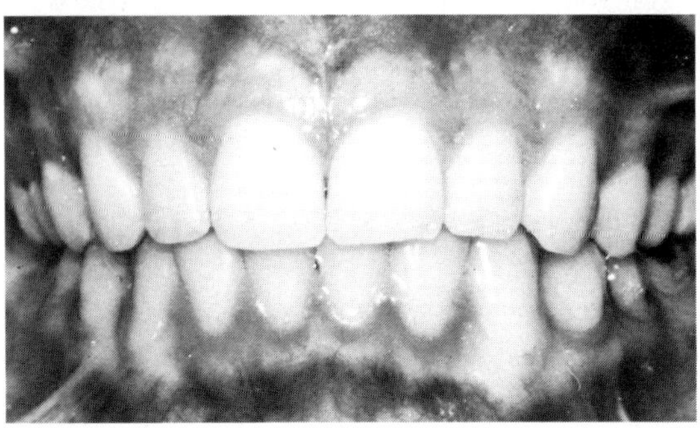

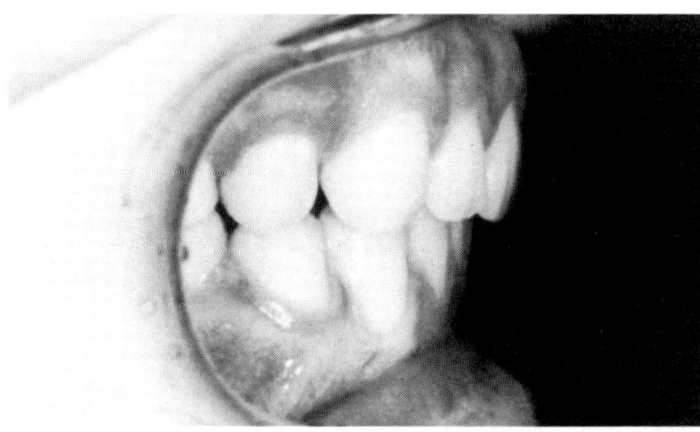

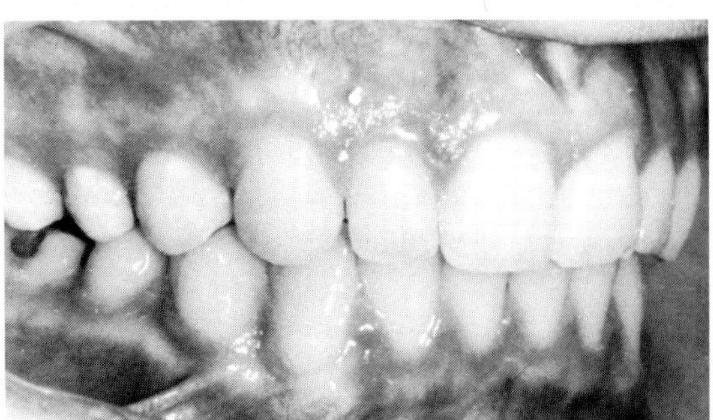

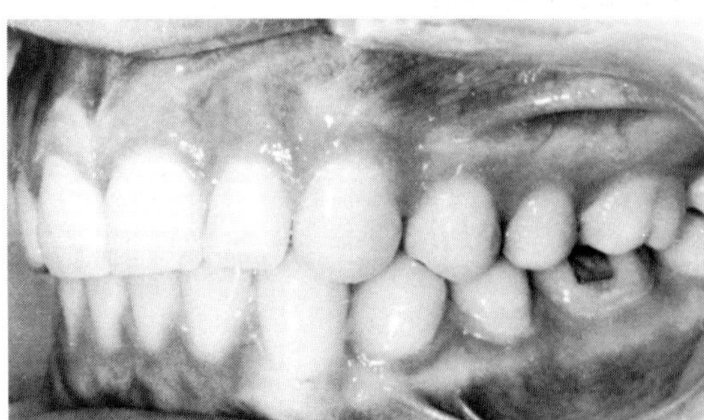

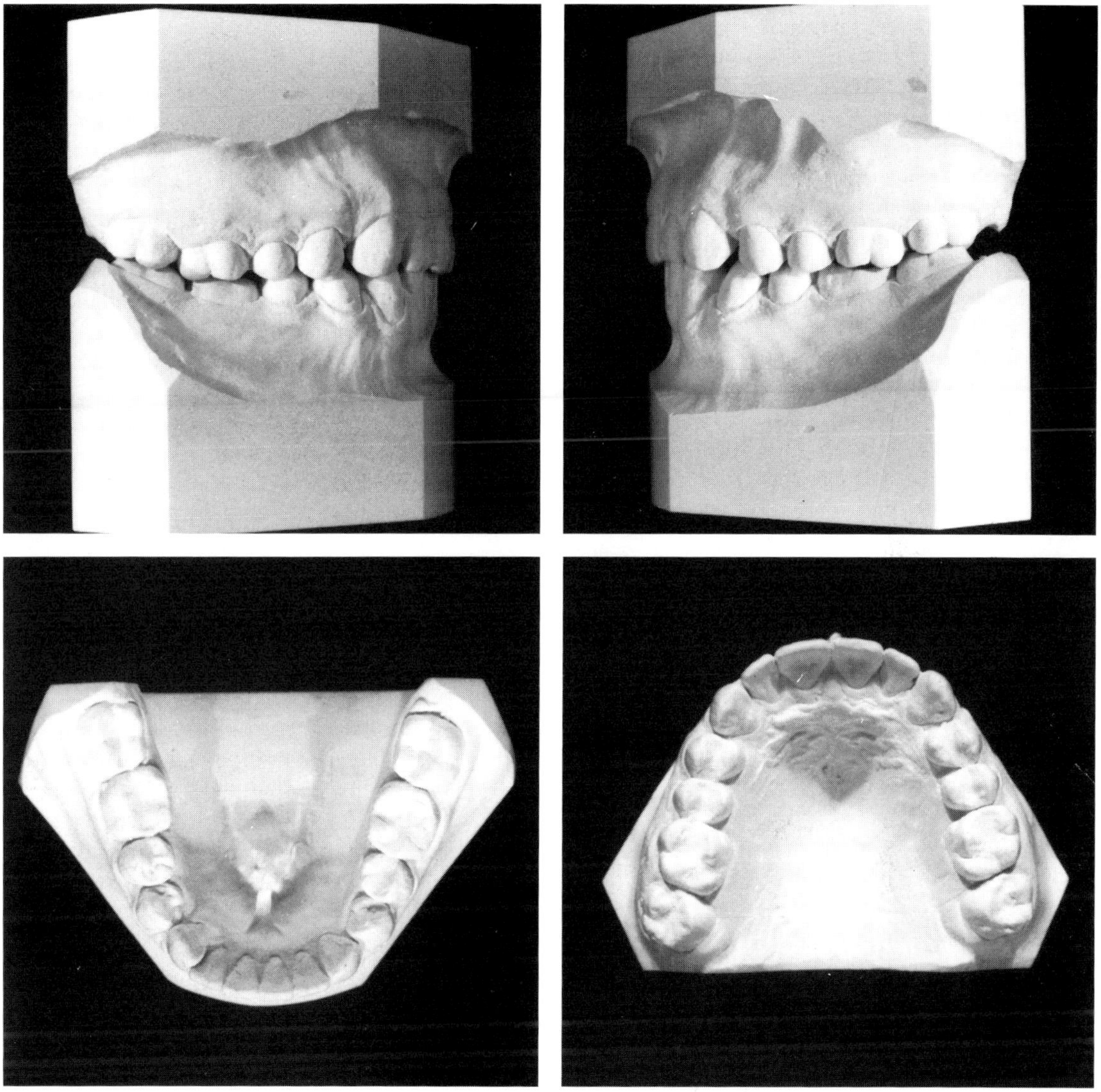

Figs 15-5 and 15-6 *At the age of 13 y, 10 mo, a good result has been achieved with a harmonious face and well-aligned dentition. The spontaneous correction of the midline deviation in the mandibular arch and other improvements are striking. Sufficient space has become available in the mandible for the right first and second premolars and the left first premolar without crowding appearing elsewhere. A good occlusion has been established with solid interdigitation of the premolars. Stomion is now lower in its level with respect to the maxillary incisors through impeding the eruption of these teeth and intruding them, so that they no longer are excessively overlapped by the lower lip.*

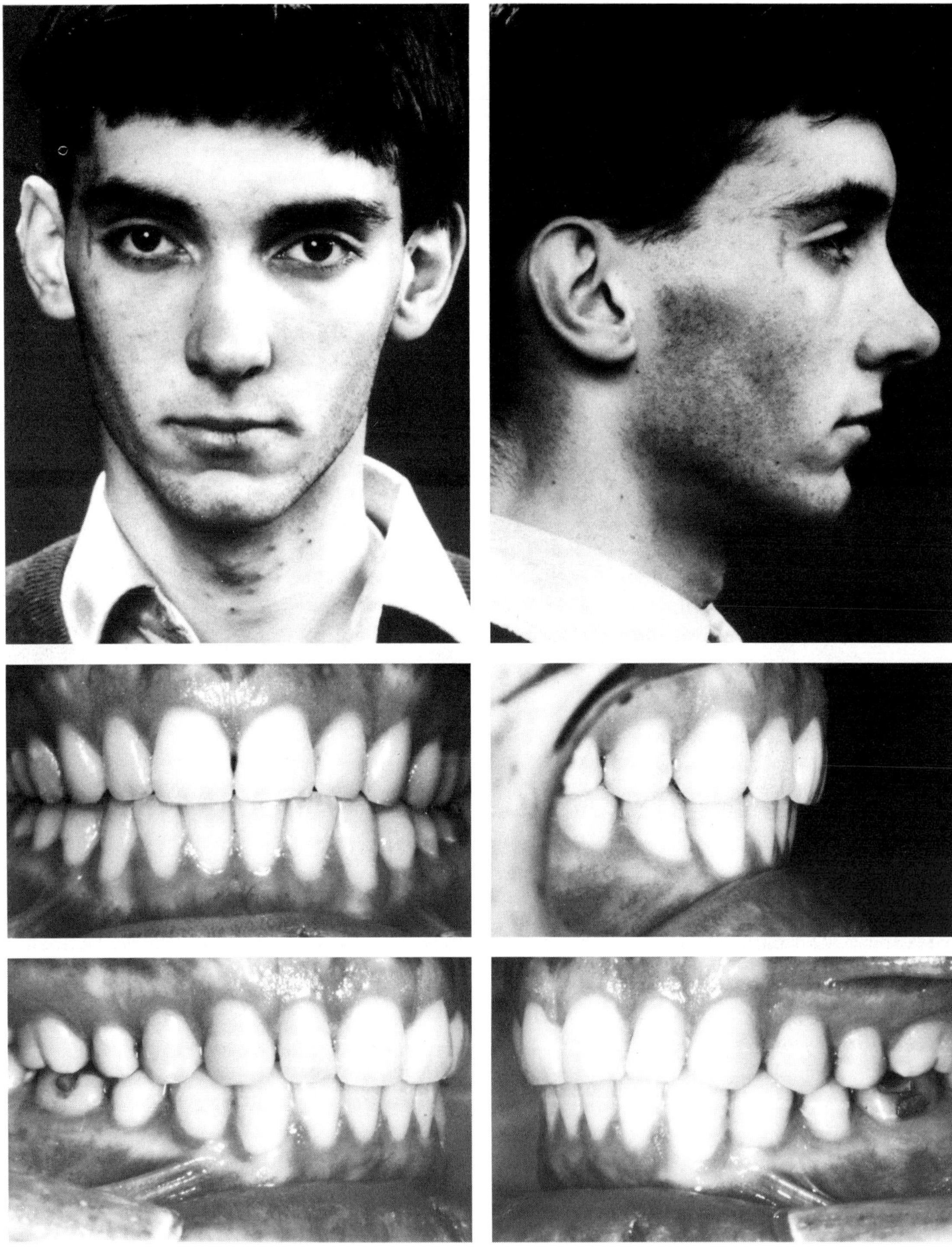

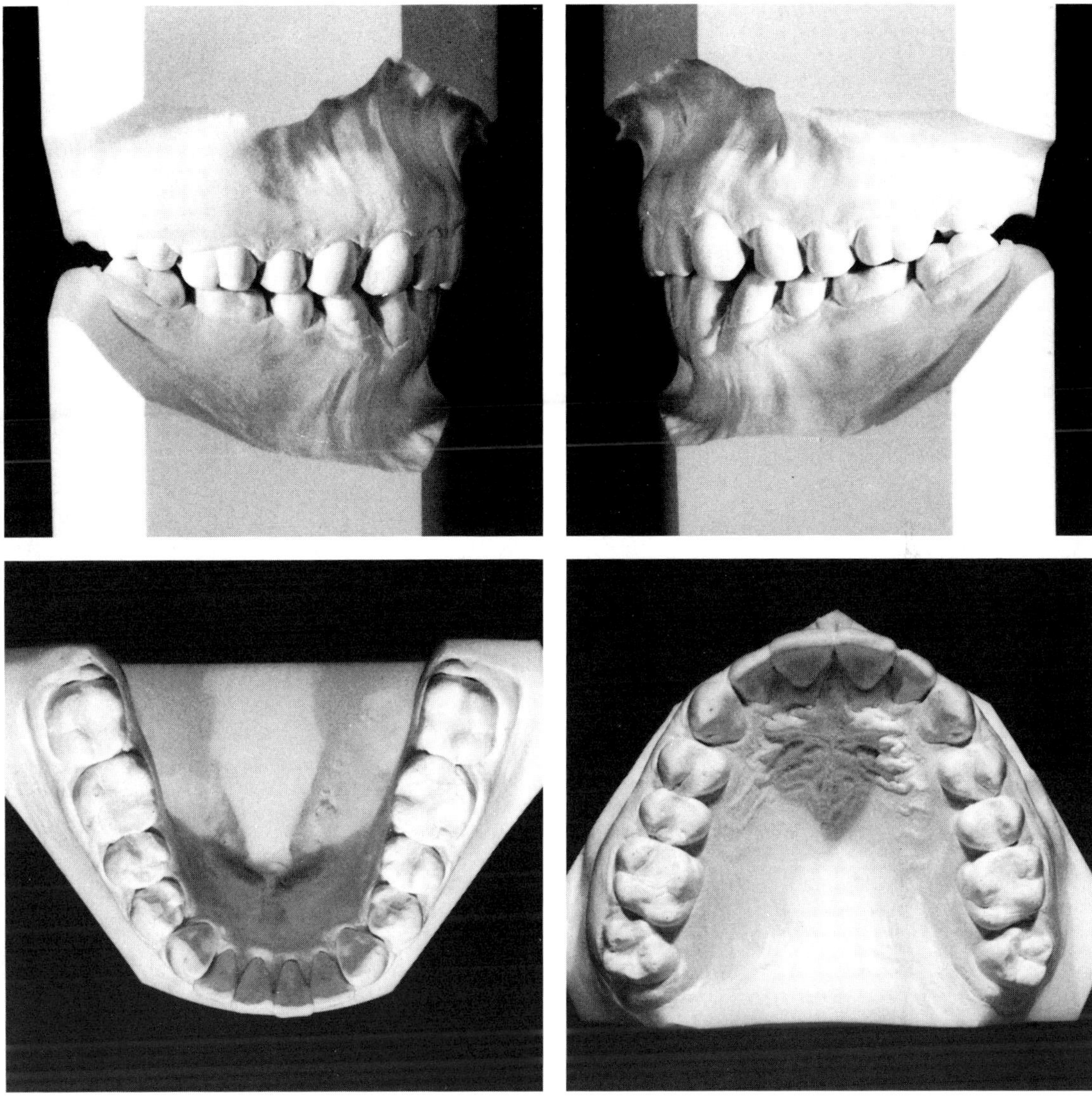

Figs 15-7 and 15-8 Aged 19 y, 0 mo, five years after treatment, the result appears to be stable. Since the mandible has grown more ventrally than the maxilla, the occlusion is relatively more mesial. Further changes, if any, have been small.

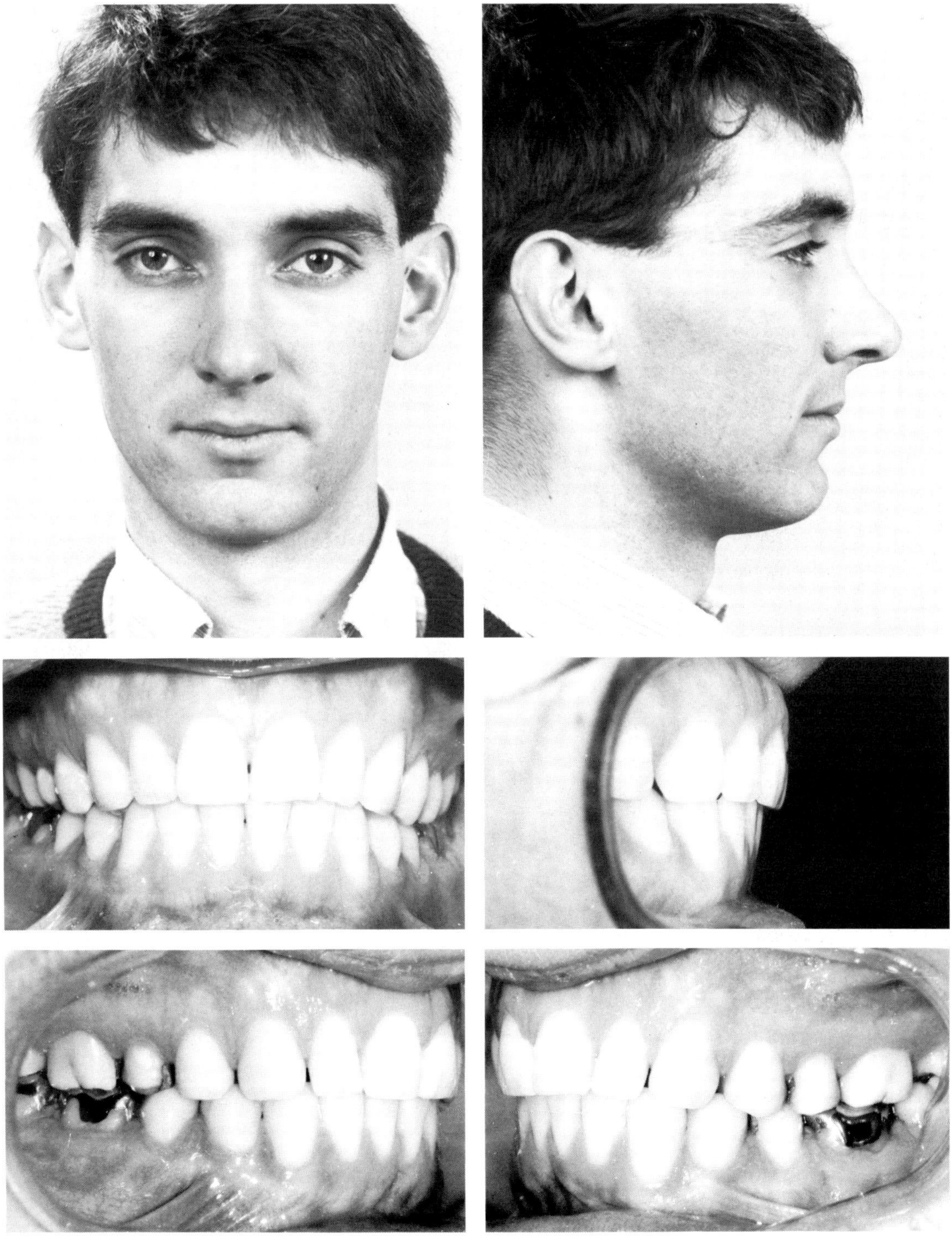

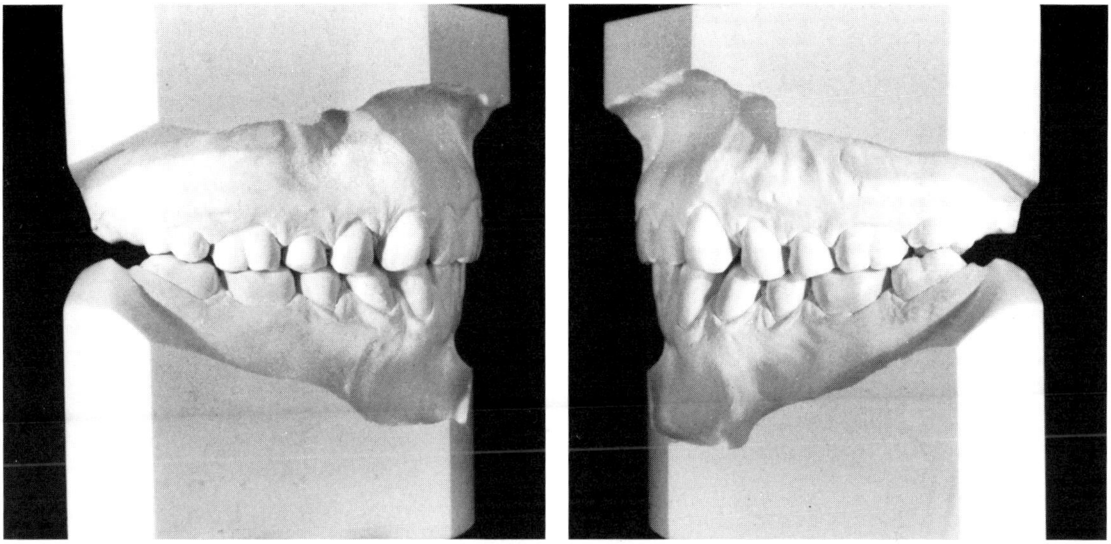

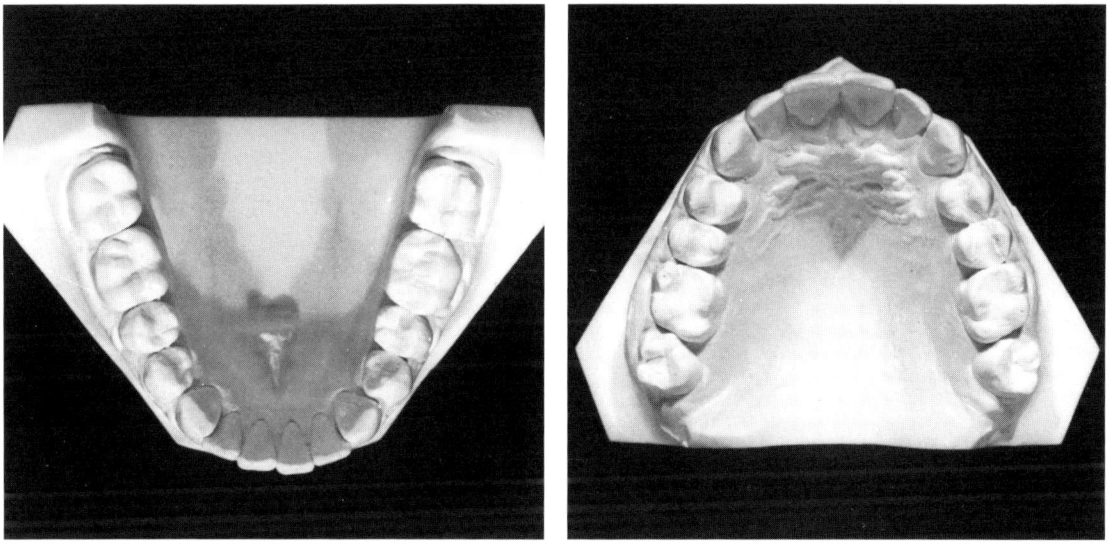

Figs 15-9 and 15-10 Aged 24 y, 0 mo, ten years after treatment, the patient's face has developed further. The mandible has grown slightly more to ventral and the chin prominence has increased. A minor change in the mandibular incisor alignment has occurred but it is barely noticeable.

Figure 15-11a

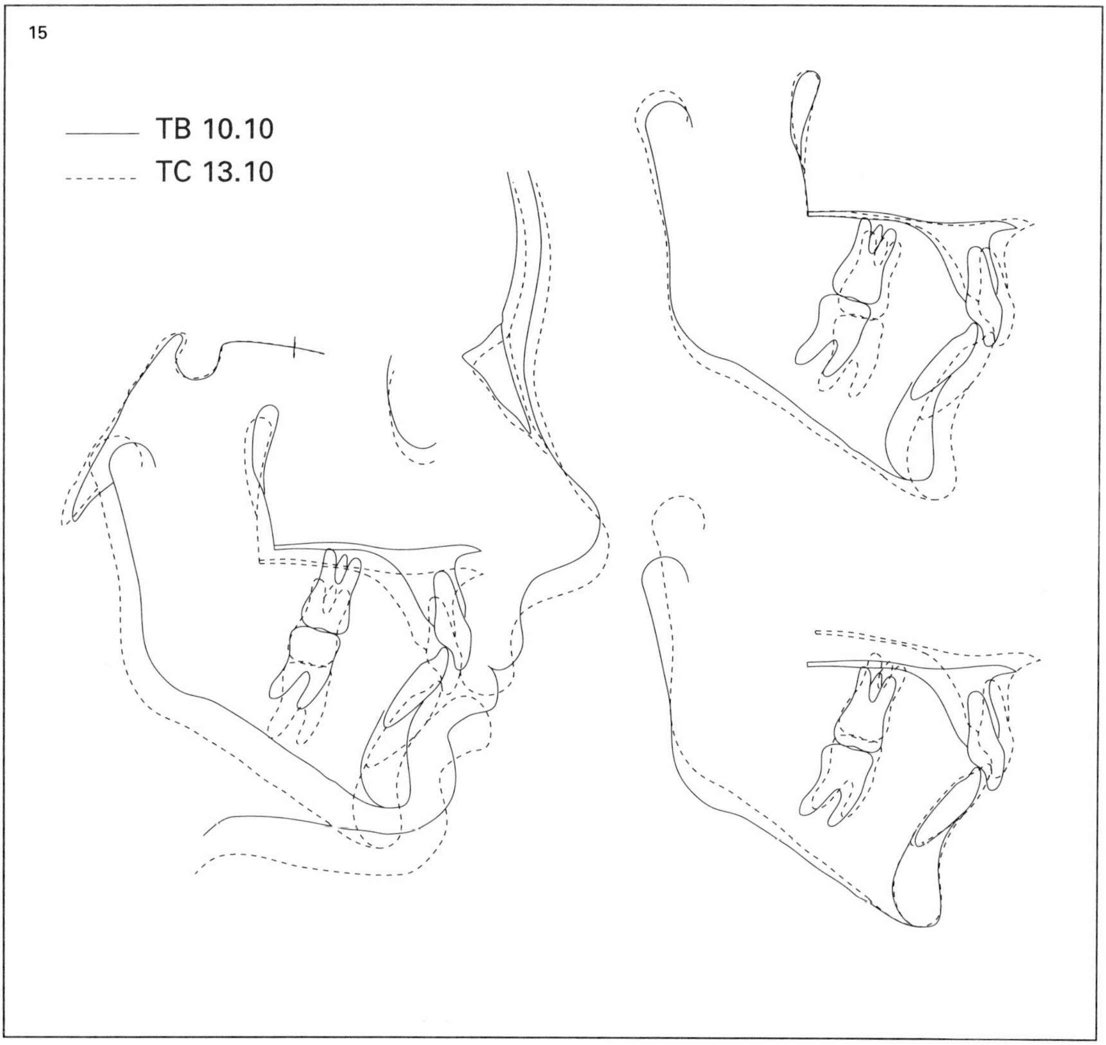

Fig 15-11 Superimposition of cephalometric tracings shows that during treatment the mandible has grown noticeably while the development of the maxilla has been reduced. The increase in height of the face occurred mostly in the mid-face. The maxillary incisors have become less overlapped by the lower lip than prior to treatment. This improvement is principally to be attributed to the inhibition of the eruption of the incisors and their intrusion.
The face, including the lower third, continued to grow noticeably both vertically and ventrally after treatment.

Figure 15-11b

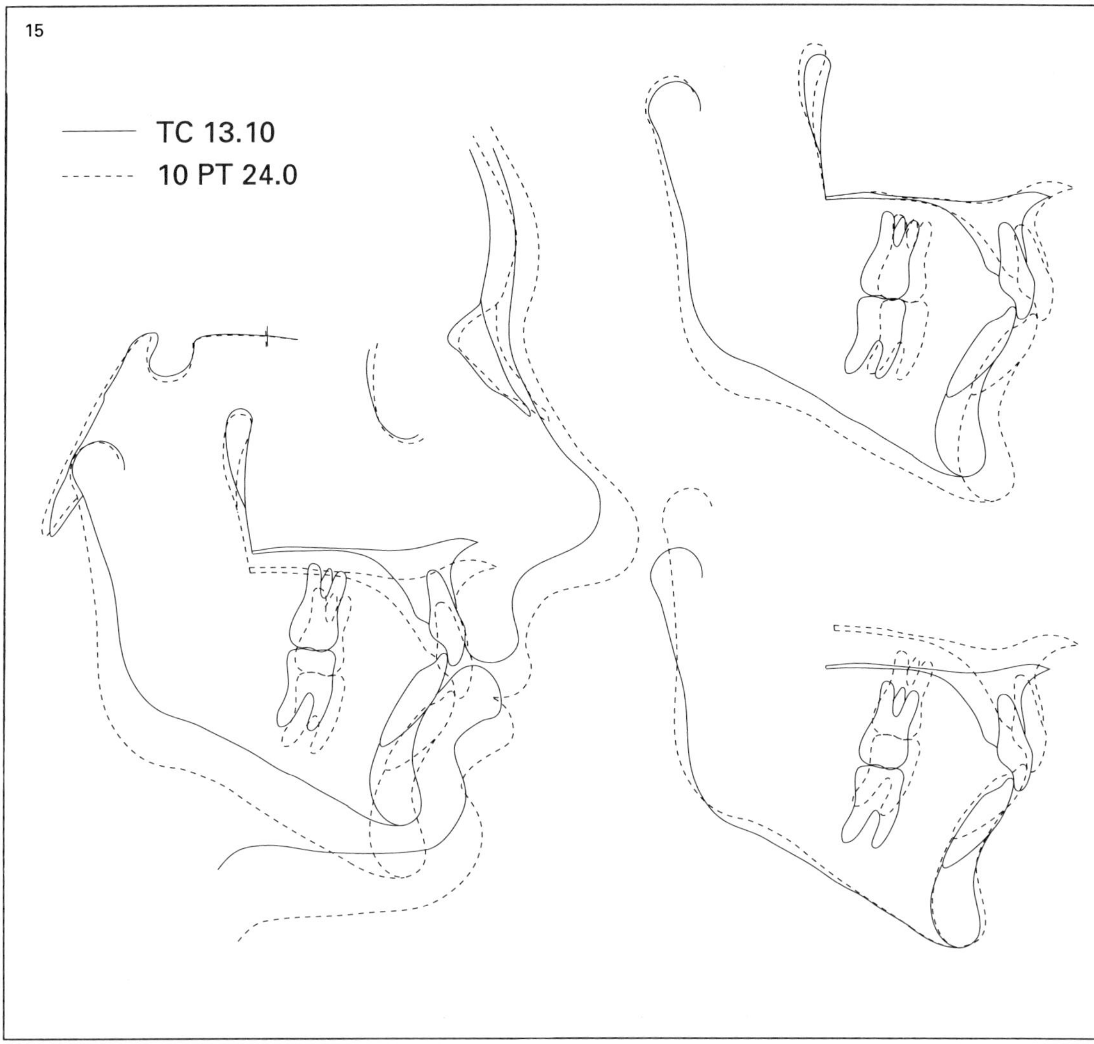

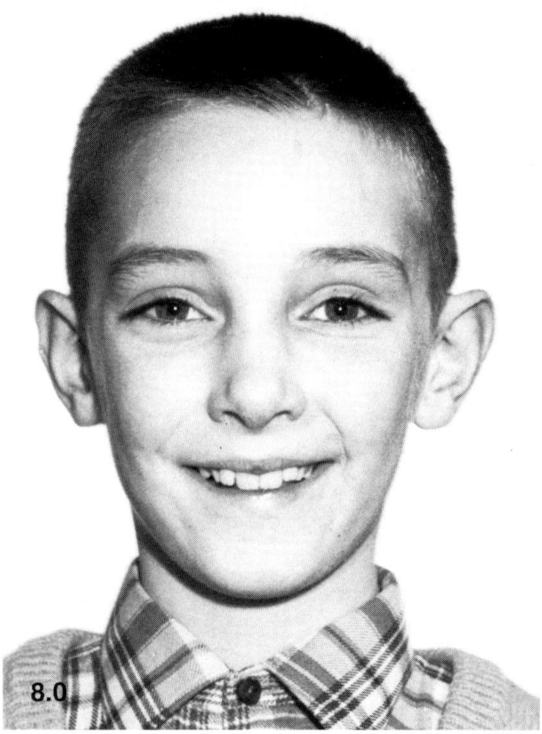
8.0

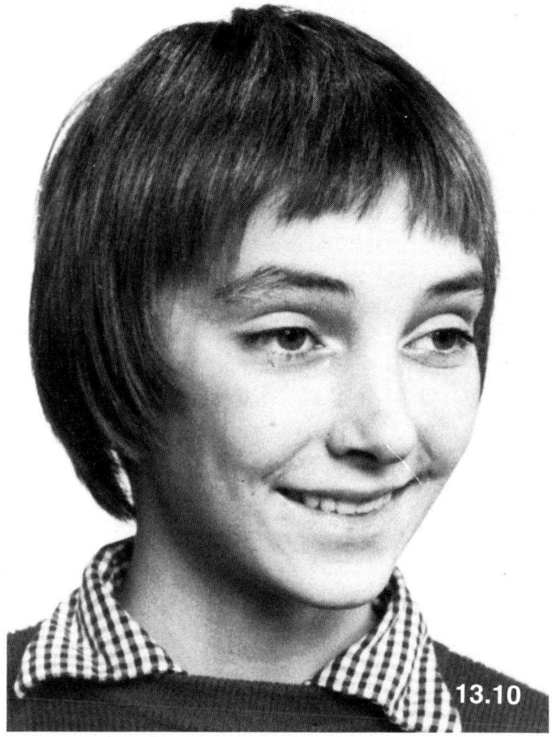
13.10

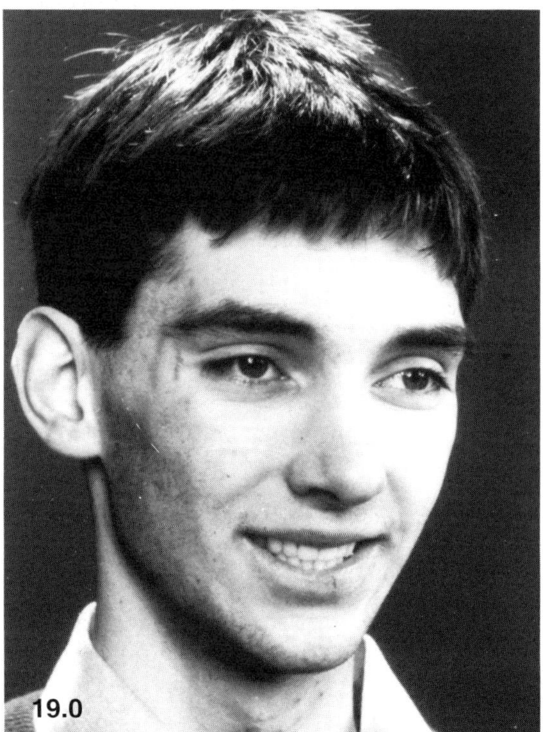
19.0

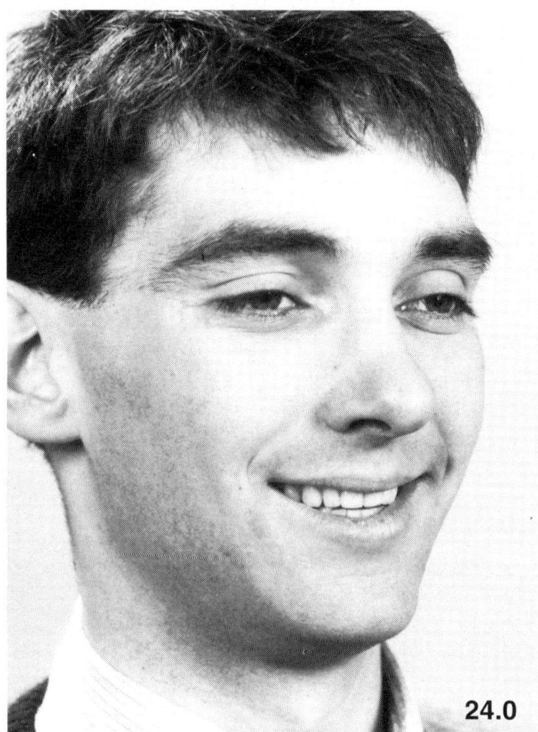
24.0

Fig 15-12 Great changes have taken place during growth and treatment. The maturation in facial expression is clear.

By the age of 13 years 0 months, the occlusion was slightly over-corrected on both sides. Then brackets (.022" × .028") were placed on the four maxillary incisors, and first a .0175" twistflex archwire followed by a .019" × .026" rectangular solid one, was inserted. It was no longer necessary to wear the headgear. Four months later, the appliances were removed and a maxillary removable plate provided for retention. That appliance was worn day and night for three months, then nights only for three months, gradually reducing the time it was worn until finally one night a week. The achieved result was satisfying (Figs 15.5 and 15.6).
In the five years after treatment, the face developed further so that the mandible grew relatively more to ventral than did the maxilla. This led to a more mesial occlusion of the dental arches, particularly on the left (Figs 15.7 and 15.8). During the subsequent five years, the forward mandibular growth persisted and the chin prominence increased. Ten years after treatment, a harmonious facial appearance and good-looking, well-established dentition were present. The teeth have been somewhat worn down by bruxism. The mandibular joints function normally and cause no complaints (Figs 15.9 and 15.10).
Superimposition of the cephalometric tracings shows vertical growth of the face during the treatment period, but also that the lower facial height did not contribute significantly to that increase. Consequently, the lowering of stomion is mainly to be attributed to impeding the eruption of the maxillary incisors and their active intrusion. Subsequent to treatment, there still was noticeable growth of the face both vertically and to ventral, including growth in the lower facial third (Fig 15.11).
The photographs of the smiling face show the changes that came about due to treatment and growth. They also show that facial growth in boys continues for a long time, even until the age of nineteen years or more (Fig 15.12).

Premature loss of deciduous teeth in the mandible does not always lead to problems in the permanent dentition. There are many factors involved.[30, 33] It is enough to make the point here that second premolars in the mandibular arch often are able to regain the space they need for a place in the arch. Generally that occurs when space exists elsewhere in the dental arch and some room in the jaw is available between the not-yet-emerged second permanent molars and the first molars. In addition, the occlusion must permit some tooth movement and the second premolars must emerge centrally between the adjacent teeth. In this case, this process did occur with regard to the mandibular left first premolar. As a rule, the situation is quite different in the maxilla, where emerging second premolars usually are not able to regain the space they need. Should second deciduous molars be lost prematurely in the maxilla, consideration has to be given to remedial action. In such a case a length of orthodontic wire of an appropriate size can be bonded to adjacent teeth with composite resin to act as a space maintainer. Such a loss in the mandible calls for no more than observation of the situation, certainly if it appears that later orthodontic treatment will be required in any case.

Put simply, the effects of premature loss of second deciduous molars can be looked at as follows. In 50% of cases, this loss leads to such limited reduction of space that it has no effect on the development of the dentition. The other 50% of cases exhibit a negative effect; but in half of these cases the loss of space is eventually regained spontaneously, while in three-fifths of the remaining 25% a need for orthodontic treatment already exists for other reasons than lack of space. So of the original cases, only 10% remain for whom it would have been better to take preventive measures against a permanent disturbance of development of the dentition. This is apparent mostly in the maxilla, when second deciduous molars have been lost prematurely.

One of the reasons why there was such a long delay before initiating treatment in this case was the great difference in times of emergence of the premolars. At the age of 7 years, the maxillary right premolars had already emerged, while those on the left were still located high in the alveolar process. Two years later, the maxillary left first premolar had indeed emerged, but the adjacent second premolar did not emerge until eight months later. A similar situation was seen in the mandible, with the left second premolar present in the mouth at age 7 years but that on the right emerging at the age of 10 years, 2 months. It was to be expected that if treatment began early it would involve an inordinately long treatment time. On fitting the headgear it was expected that active treatment would not take longer than a year and a half. The fact that it took one year more might be ascribed to lack of good cooperation.

Symmetric headgears do not always work in the same way on both sides. Perhaps this is due to some patients sleeping for long periods on one side. When there is an asymmetric occlusion, it is recommended first to use a symmetric headgear because it is easier to become accustomed to it. It is also advantageous to see what effects it will have. If the desired effect does not appear, or if an incorrect asymmetric one appears, then the facebow of the headgear can be modified accordingly.

Asymmetric headgears are more troublesome for patients than symmetric ones. The molar to which the greater force is applied soon becomes mobile and sensitive. When pressure is applied to the long outer bow, the inner arch easily slips out of the molar tube on the other side. This last discomfort can generally be overcome simply if the part of the inner arch that fits into the pertinent tube is given a slight bend transversely with strong triple-beaked pliers so that the wire wedges against the buccal wall of the tube.

Because of the difference in lengths of the two legs of the facebow, the molar on the side of the long arm will experience a greater extrusive force. Moreover, that molar would be under pressure to palatal. Movement in that direction can be prevented with a well-fitting plate that will oppose any palatal change in the position of the molar. A disadvantage of the use of a plate is that it can also prevent distal movement of the molar and the passive drifting of the second premolar that would follow it.

In cases with a solid interdigitation of the posterior teeth, it is also possible that the occlusion blocks the palatal movement of the molar, although it is also possible for both antagonist molars to move lingually as occurred in this patient. After leaving the headgear out for two months, both molars were back to normal and the use of the headgear could be resumed.

Undesired movement of the more heavily loaded molar can usually be corrected to some extent when the headgear is replaced with a symmetric one, as has to be done once the occlusion is similar on both sides. It is also possible at a later stage to use a plate with a spring activated to move the molar buccally. Clearly it is important to keep the effects of any appliance under very critical surveillance and, where necessary, to institute corrections if untoward reactions are seen.

In this case, brackets were placed on the maxillary incisors in the final phase of treatment to torque and intrude those incisors. The latter was necessary because during the treatment only a limited increase in height of the lower face took place and consequently stomion did not descend sufficiently.

This patient was indeed supplied with a retainer, primarily because it was desirable to prevent an increase in overbite as further facial growth occurred. With the girl discussed in the previous chapter that was not required because there was little growth to be expected after treatment and there was no need to fear that excessive overlapping of the incisors by the lower lip would occur.

Finally if the development of the mandibular arch had been less favorable, it would have been necessary to use full fixed appliances to secure a good result for this patient.

Chapter 16

Class II/1, excessive maxillary arch width
Cervical headgear, brackets 12, 11, 21, and 22
Male: 13 years, 0 months to 30 years, 1 month

A boy aged 13 years, 0 months displayed a class II/1 anomaly with deviant buccolingual occlusion and a high gum-line. He had been treated for six years with a removable maxillary plate incorporating a continuous labial arch and an expansion screw. By turning the screw, the maxillary arch was widened and at the same time the incisors were retracted. Nothing had been done during this time to correct the anomalous sagittal jaw relationship, with the result that the maxillary dental arch was now too broad in relationship to the mandibular dental arch. The boy often held his jaw in a more ventral position in which the arches matched better ("Sunday bite"). The anterior open bite probably was due to the use of the plate. There was inadequate room in the fourth quadrant to accommodate the second premolar. It was likely that no consideration had been given to that situation in the previous treatment (Figs 16.1 and 16.2).

It was decided still to attempt to correct the sagittal jaw relationship using extra-oral traction. A cervical headgear was fitted at the age of 13 years, 2 months to be worn 16 hours per day to obtain the desired facial-orthopedic effect. After 7 months, brackets (.022" × .028") were placed on the four maxillary incisors and a .019" × .026" archwire was fitted to torque, retract, and intrude those incisors. At the age of 14 years, 8 months after a treatment time of 18 months, all appliances were removed. Retention was not thought to be necessary since a solid interdigitation of the posterior teeth had been established and no extreme malposition of teeth had existed originally. During treatment, the face and particularly the mandible experienced a marked adolescent growth spurt, giving rise to rapid improvement. Central relationship and habitual occlusion now corresponded. The anterior open bite had more or less gone, although the occlusion and alignment of the teeth still showed some shortcomings. The same could be said about the standard of oral hygiene (Figs 16.3 and 16.4).

Five years later ,the face had grown further. The mandible had come still farther ventrally with the mandibular arch occluding a little more mesially as a result. The maxillary incisors were a little less steeply inclined but there was now a central diastema, which the patient did not like. It was decided to wait and see if spontaneous closure would occur. Tertiary crowding had developed in the anterior mandibular region (Figs 16.5 and 16.6).

Fifteen years after treatment, the central diastema was practically closed. The tertiary

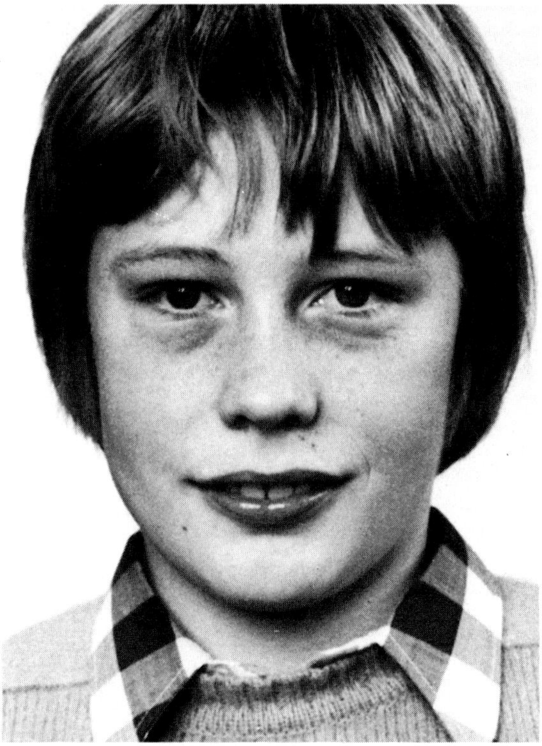

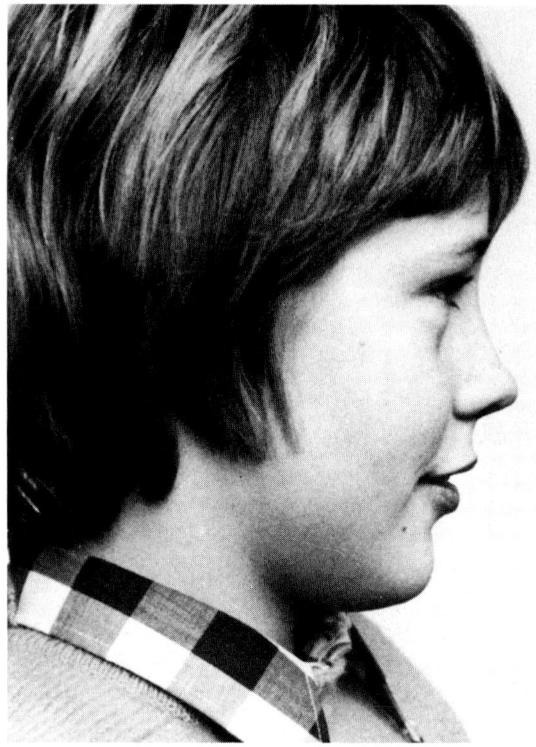

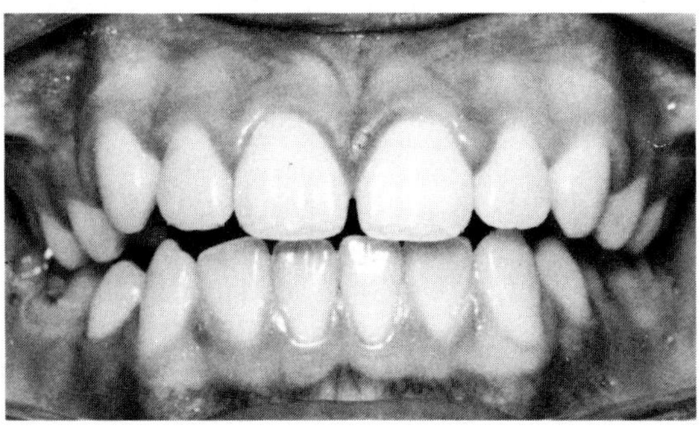

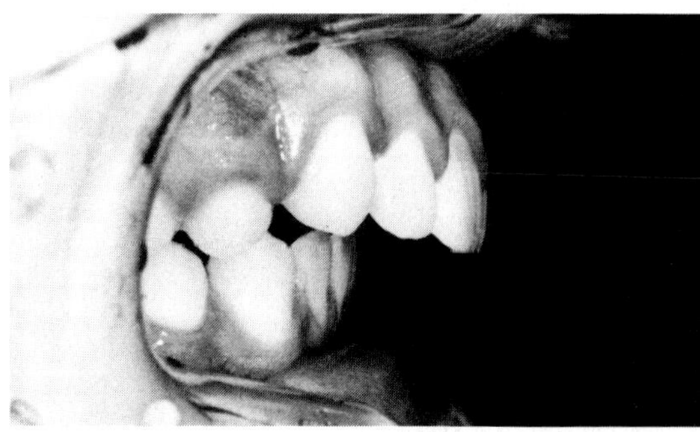

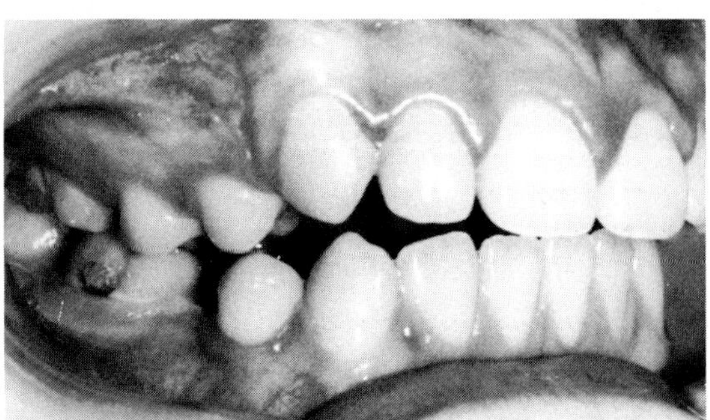

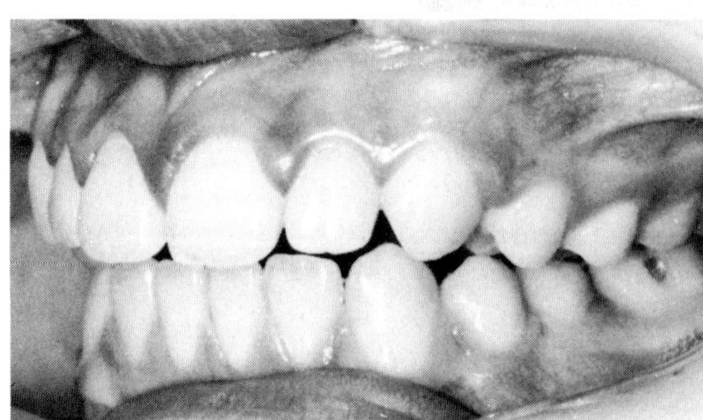

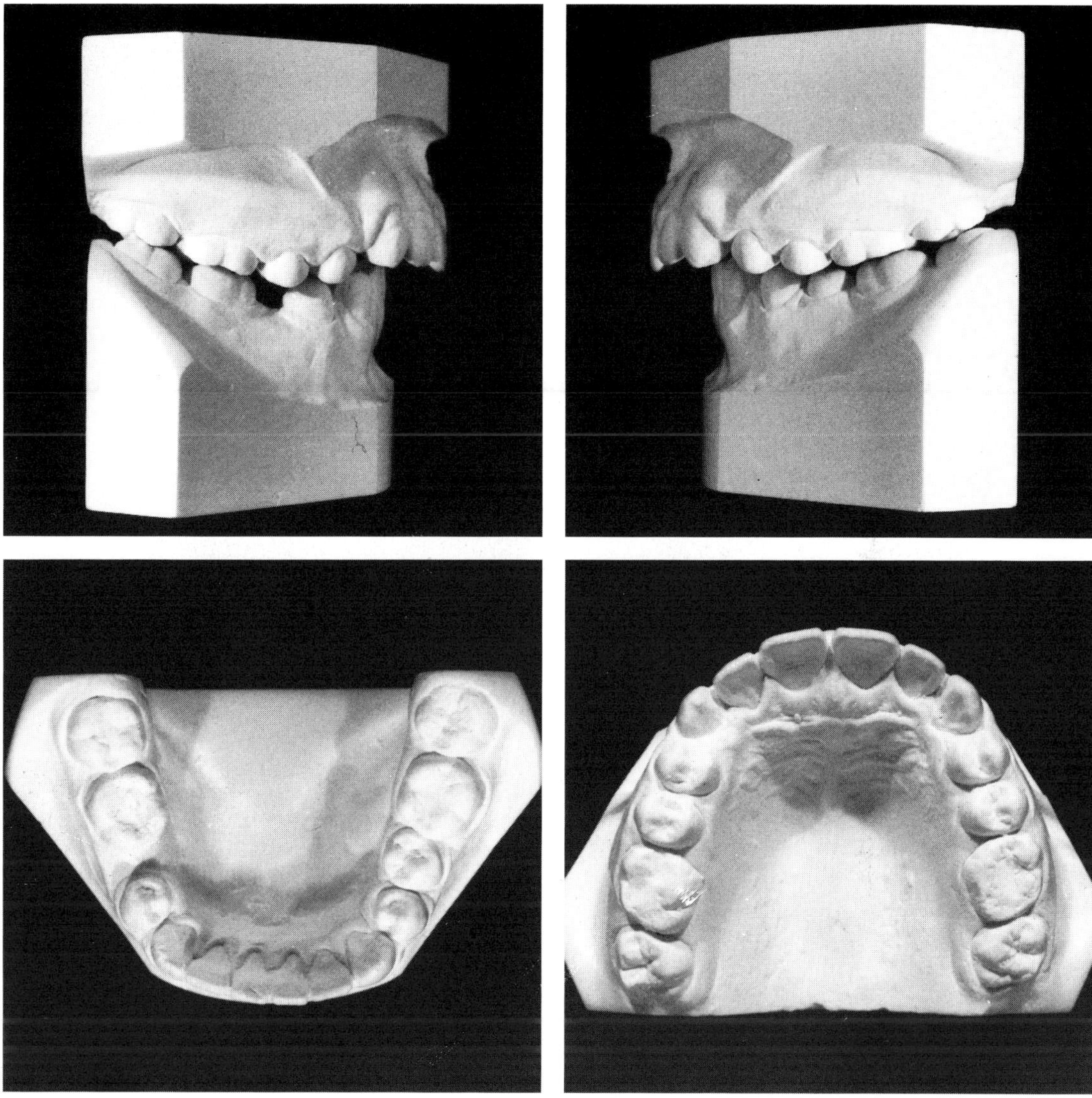

Figs 16-1 and 16-2 A boy of 13 y, 0 mo who already had been under treatment for six years with a removable maxillary expansion plate. He deliberately held his mandible forward as the dental arches then fitted together better and his appearance was improved ("Sunday bite"). Only the lateral oral view of the incisors and the oblique photographs in Figure 16-10 were obtained with the mandible in central relationship and display the sagittal overbite of 12 mm. The oral photographs as well as the facial ones were otherwise obtained with the jaw in the "Sunday bite" posture. The dental casts show how the maxillary arch is excessively broad. The maxillary premolars are outside those of the mandibular arch. There is insufficient room for the mandibular right second premolar.

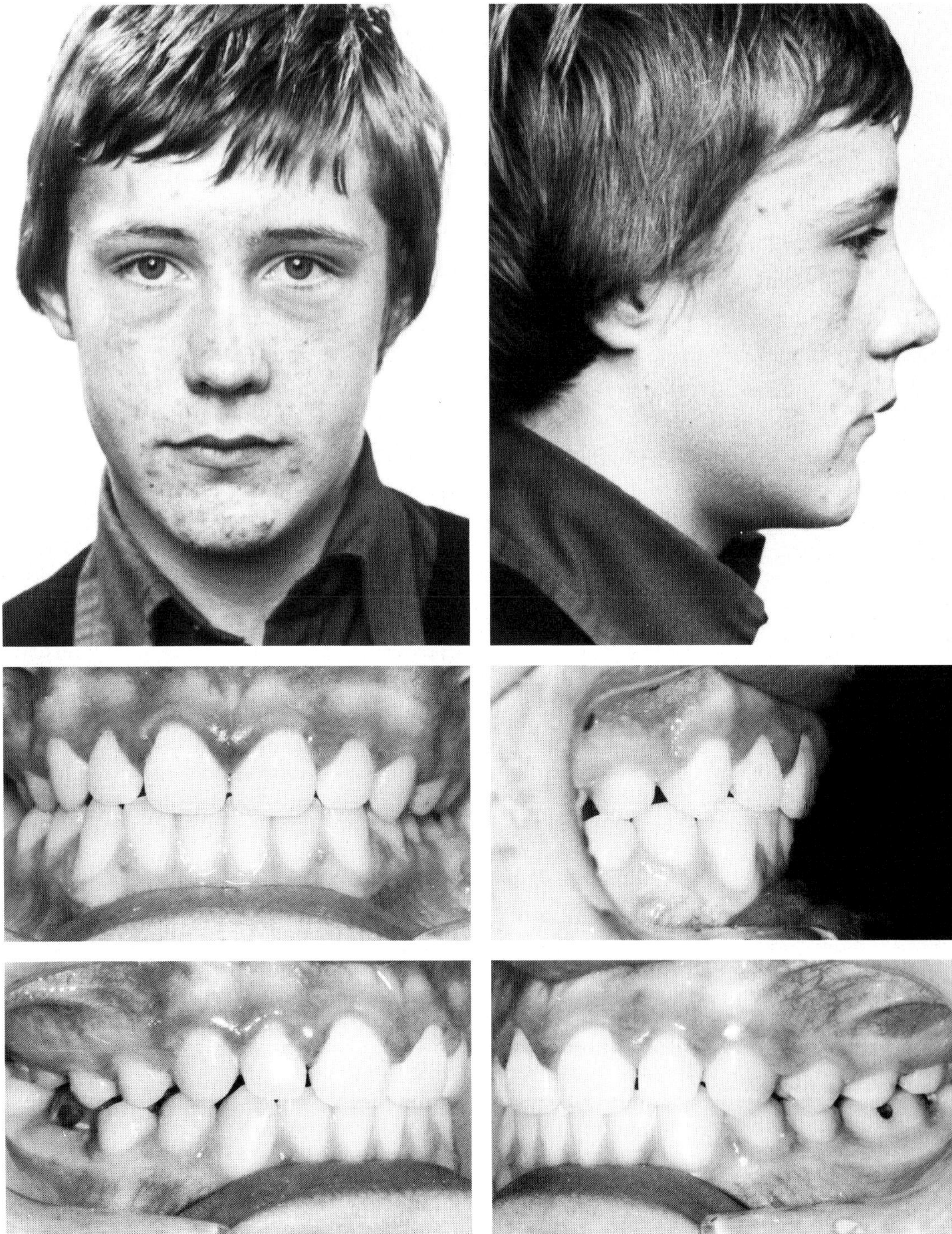

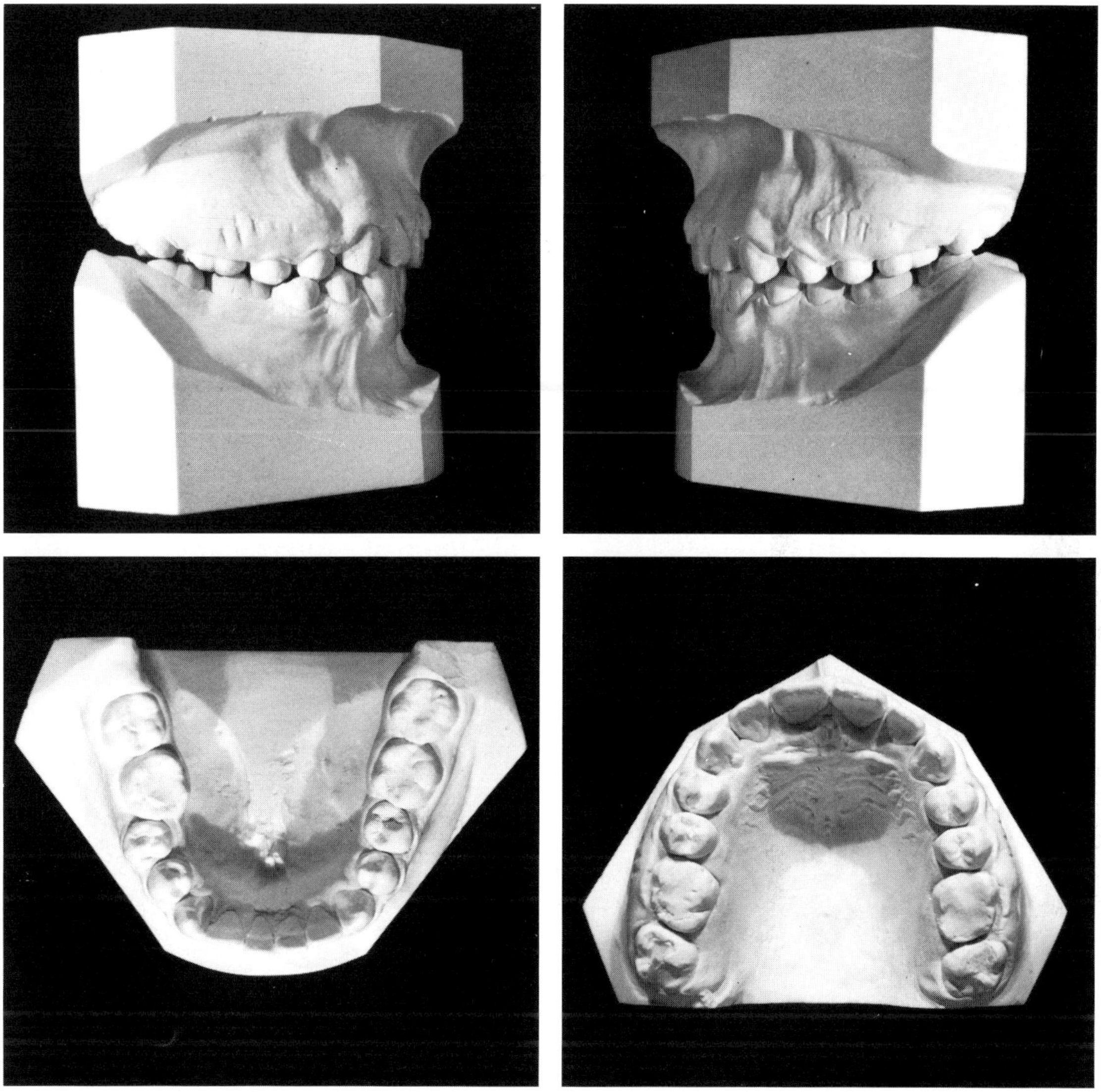

Figs 16-3 and 16-4 At the age of 14 y, 8 mo the central and habitual occlusions correspond. The mandible has developed remarkably to ventral. There is now a good occlusion in sagittal and transverse directions with solid interdigitation of canines and premolars. The maxillary incisors are too steeply inclined. The mandibular right second premolar has emerged in the interim and in so doing has displaced the first permanent molar somewhat to lingual. The mandibular right second premolar is in exo-occlusion.

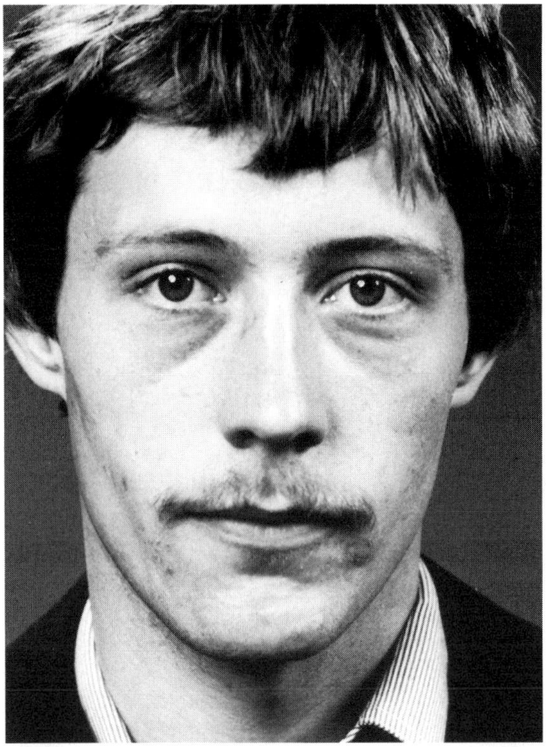

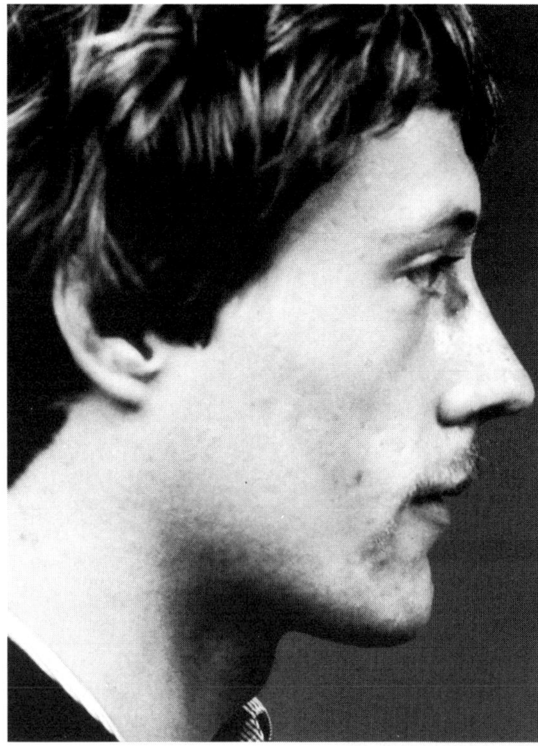

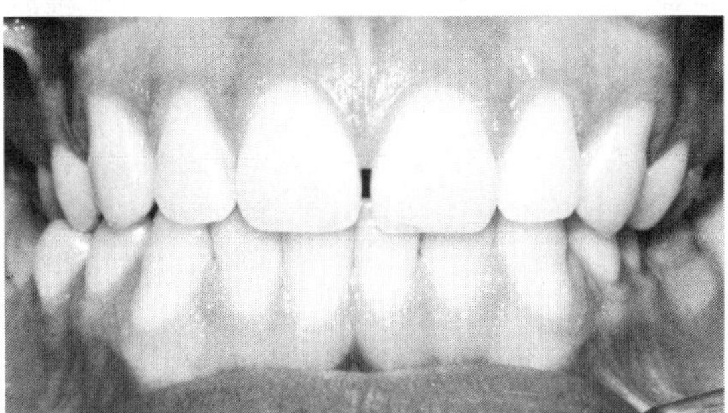

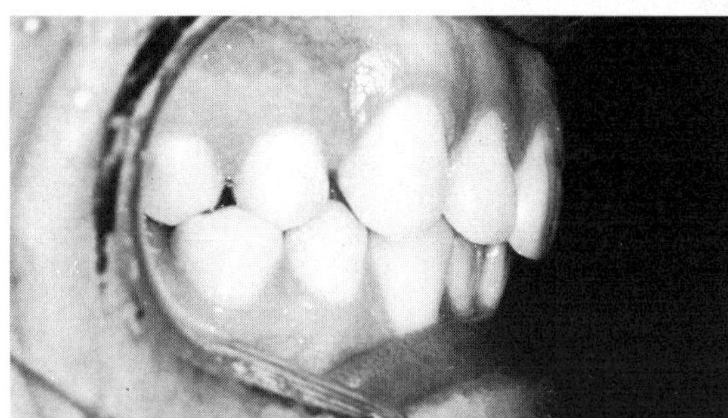

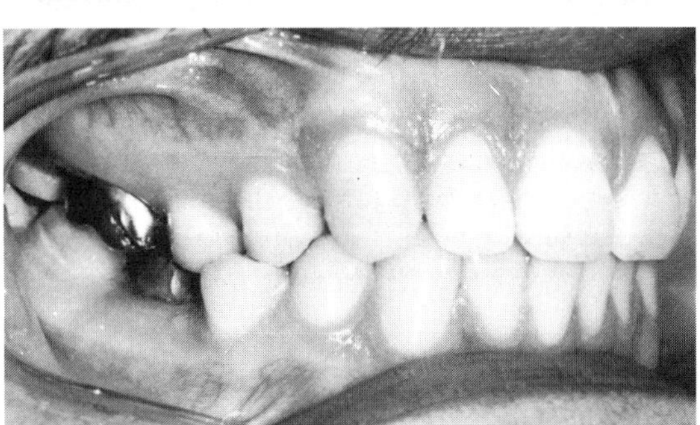

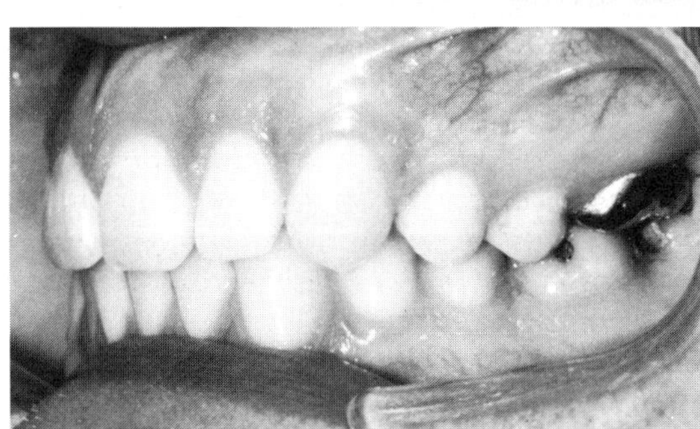

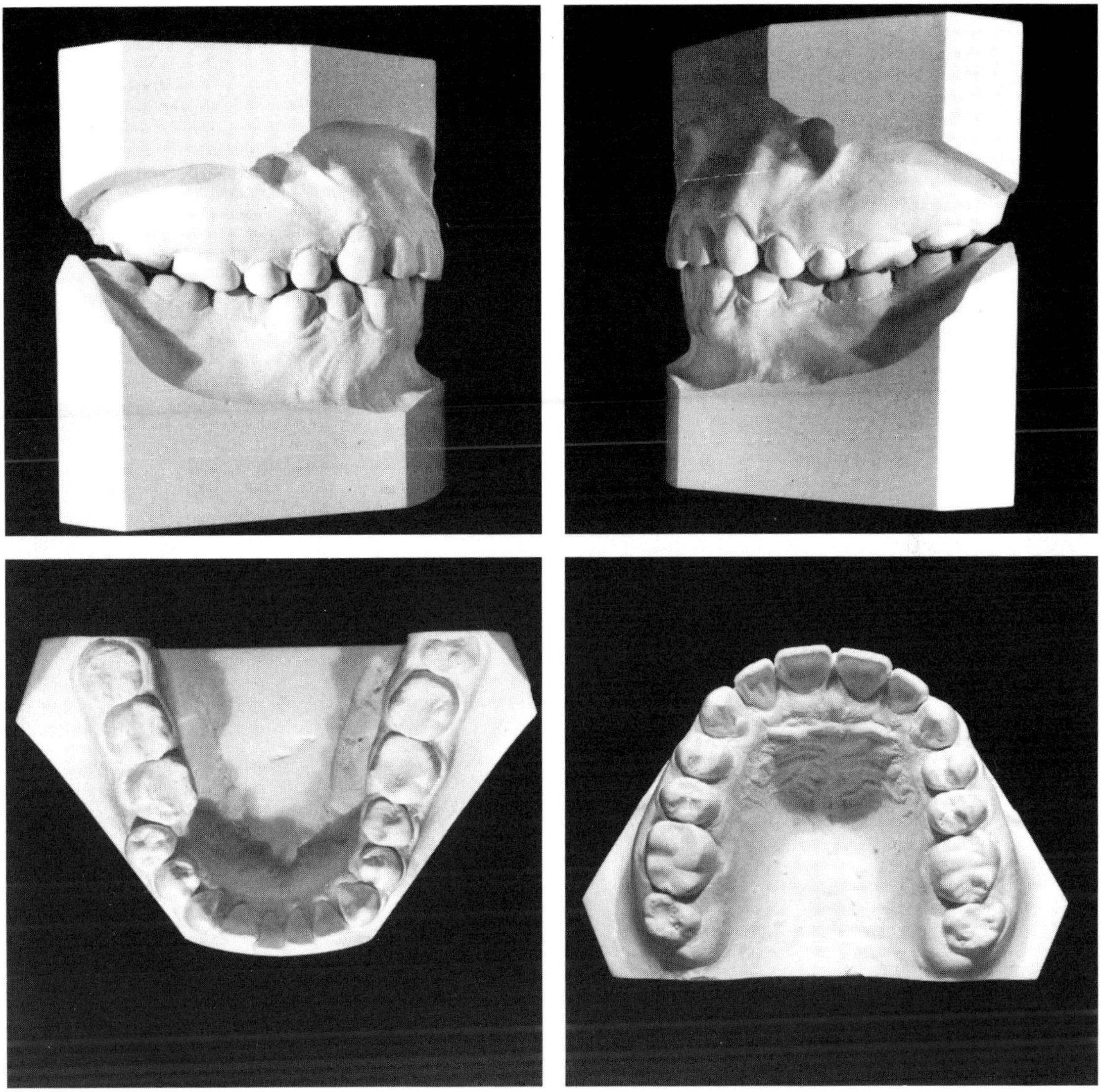

Figs 16-5 and 16-6 *At the age of 19 y, 9 mo, five years after treatment, the patient's face has developed further and matured. The chin prominence has grown and the profile is good. The occlusion has changed little. The late growth changes of the mandible leading to the mesial displacement of the mandibular arch are likely to have played a part in the maxillary incisors becoming less steeply inclined, the appearance of a central diastema, and the development of tertiary crowding in the mandibular incisors.*

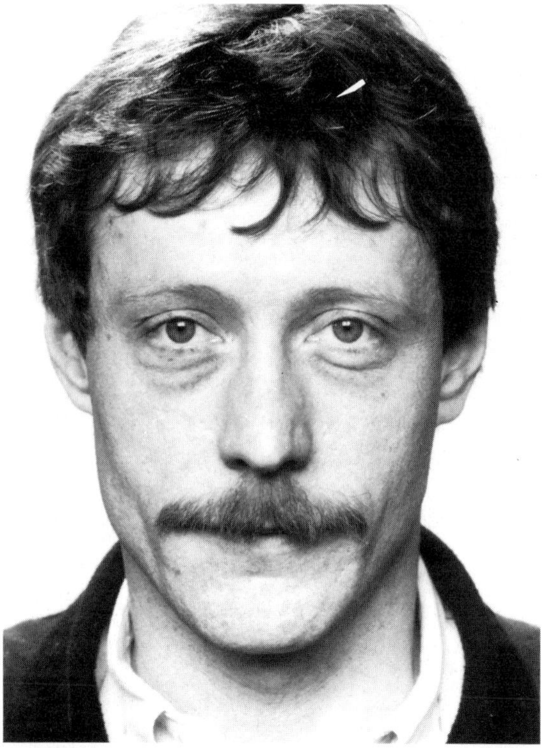

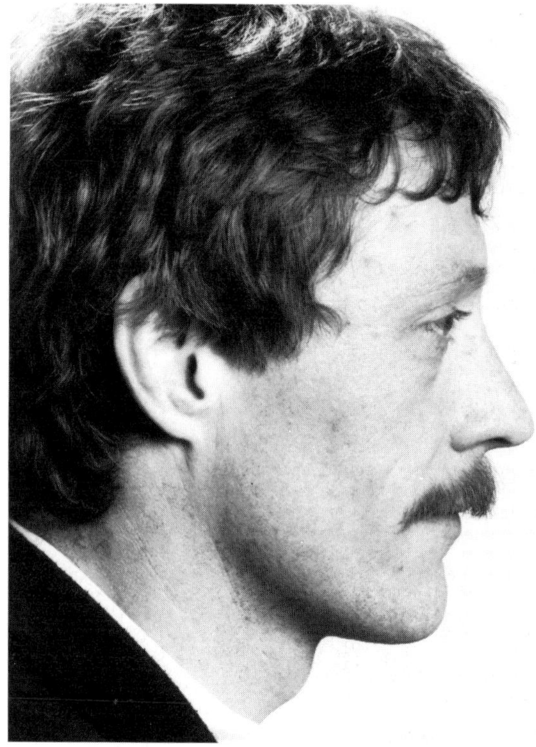

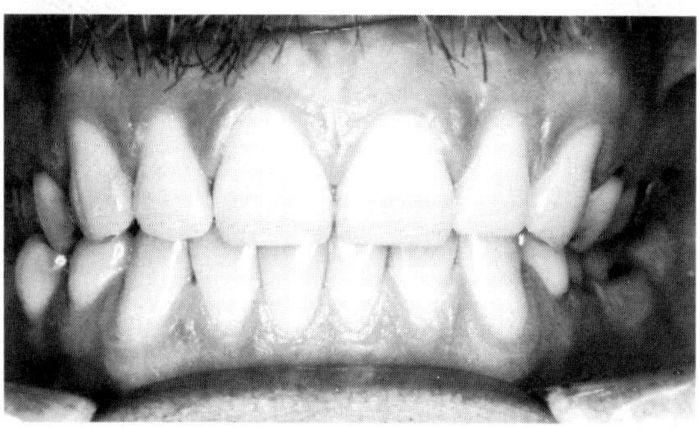

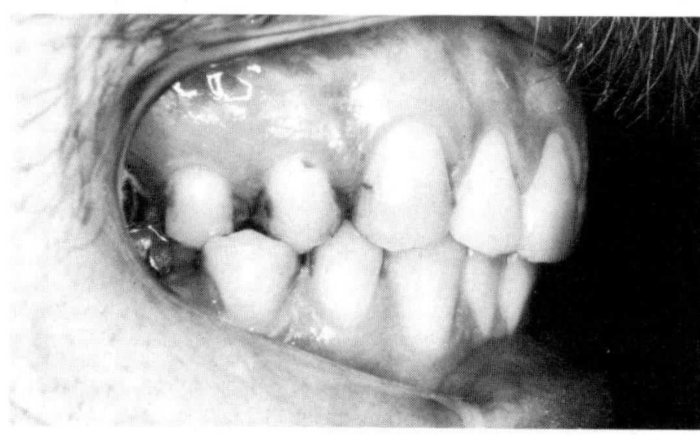

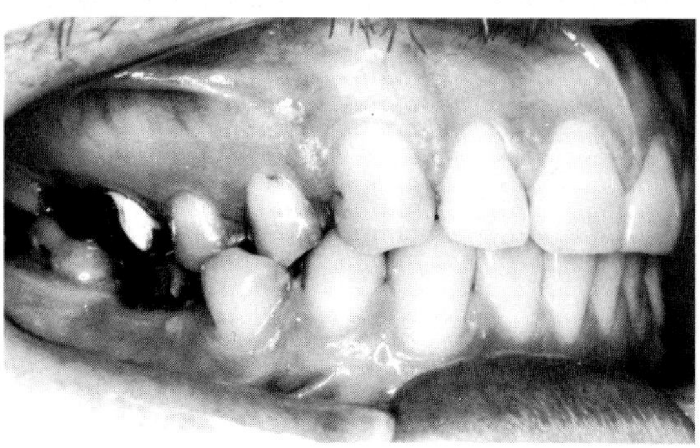

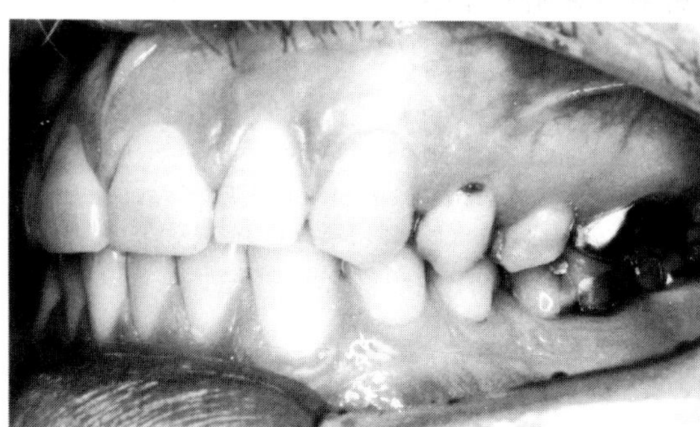

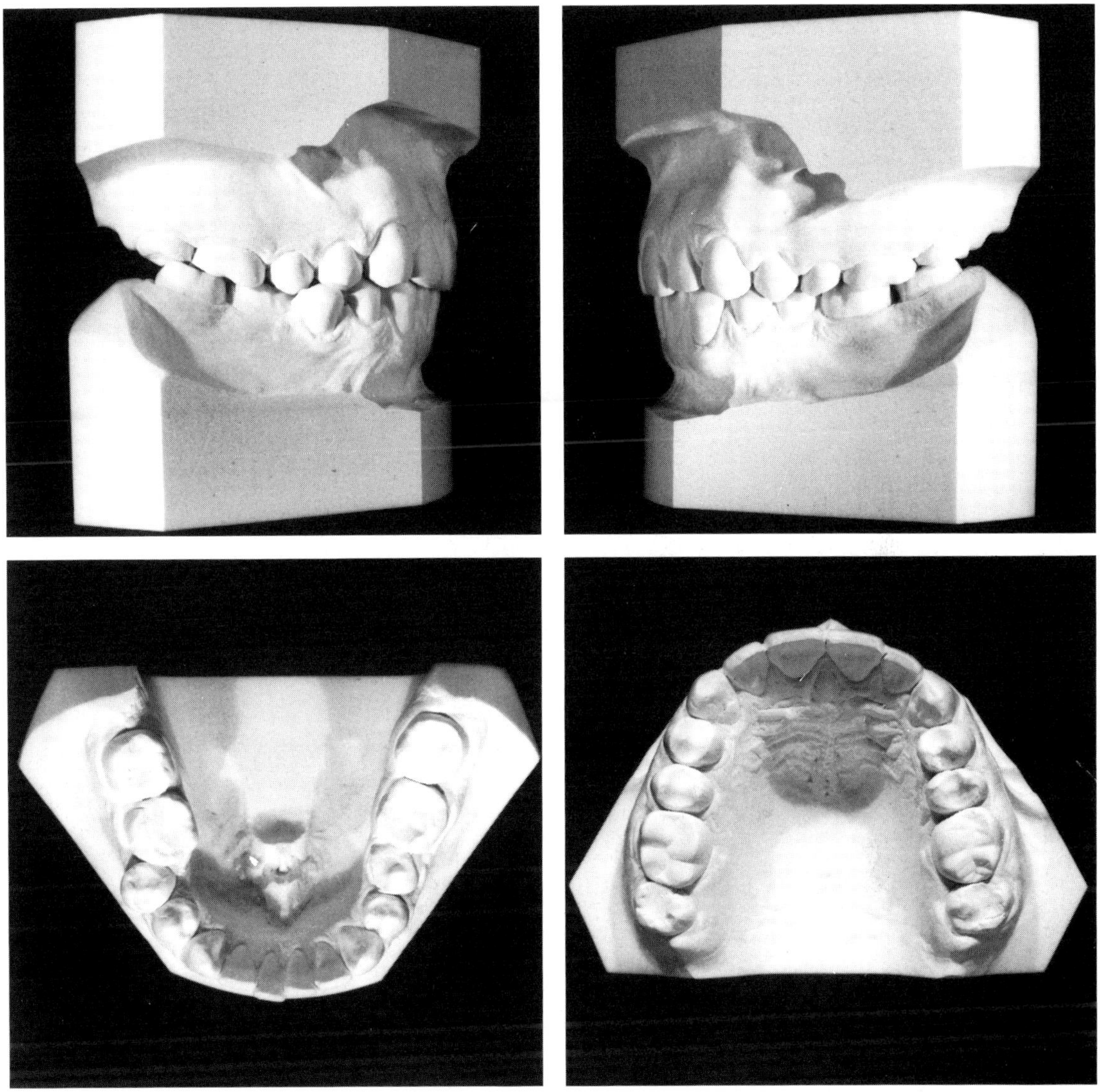

Figs 16-7 and 16-8 *At the age of 30 y, 1 mo, fifteen years after treatment, the face has still altered a little compared with the situation ten years previously. The chin has come forward more. The alignment of the posterior teeth has not changed visibly. The third molars have indeed been removed. The central diastema has more or less closed again. The tertiary crowding in the mandibular incisors has increased but is not considered objectionable.*

Figure 16-9a

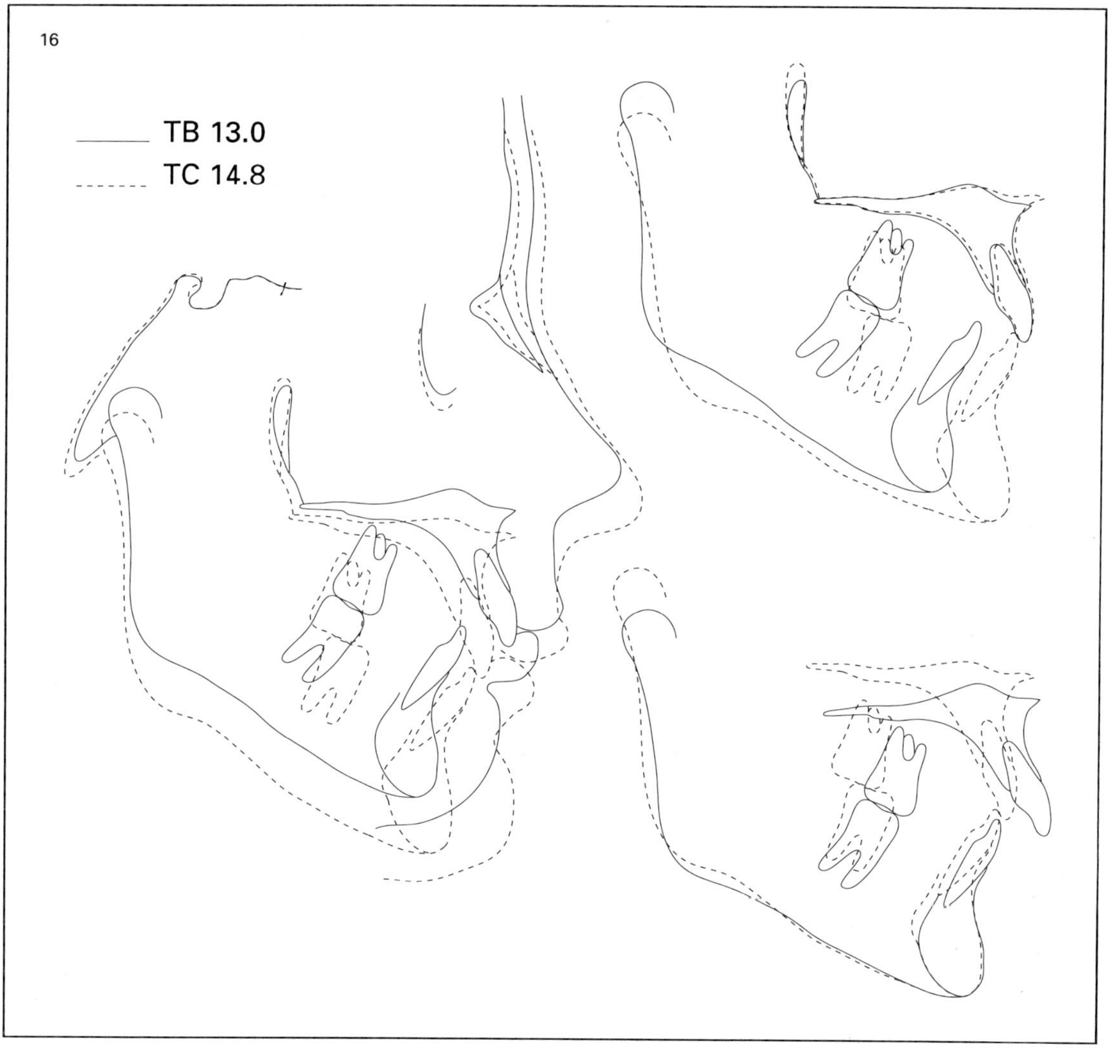

Fig 16-9 From the superimposition of the cephalometric tracings, the remarkable growth that occurred during the treatment is evident. It is probable that the treatment coincided with the period of the adolescent growth spurt affecting the mandible. The mandible exhibited an exceptional increase in length. The development of the maxilla to ventral was more or less totally halted. Through the combination of these aspects of change it was possible for the pronounced disto-relation to be corrected in a relatively short time.
Growth after treatment was limited.

Figure 16-9b

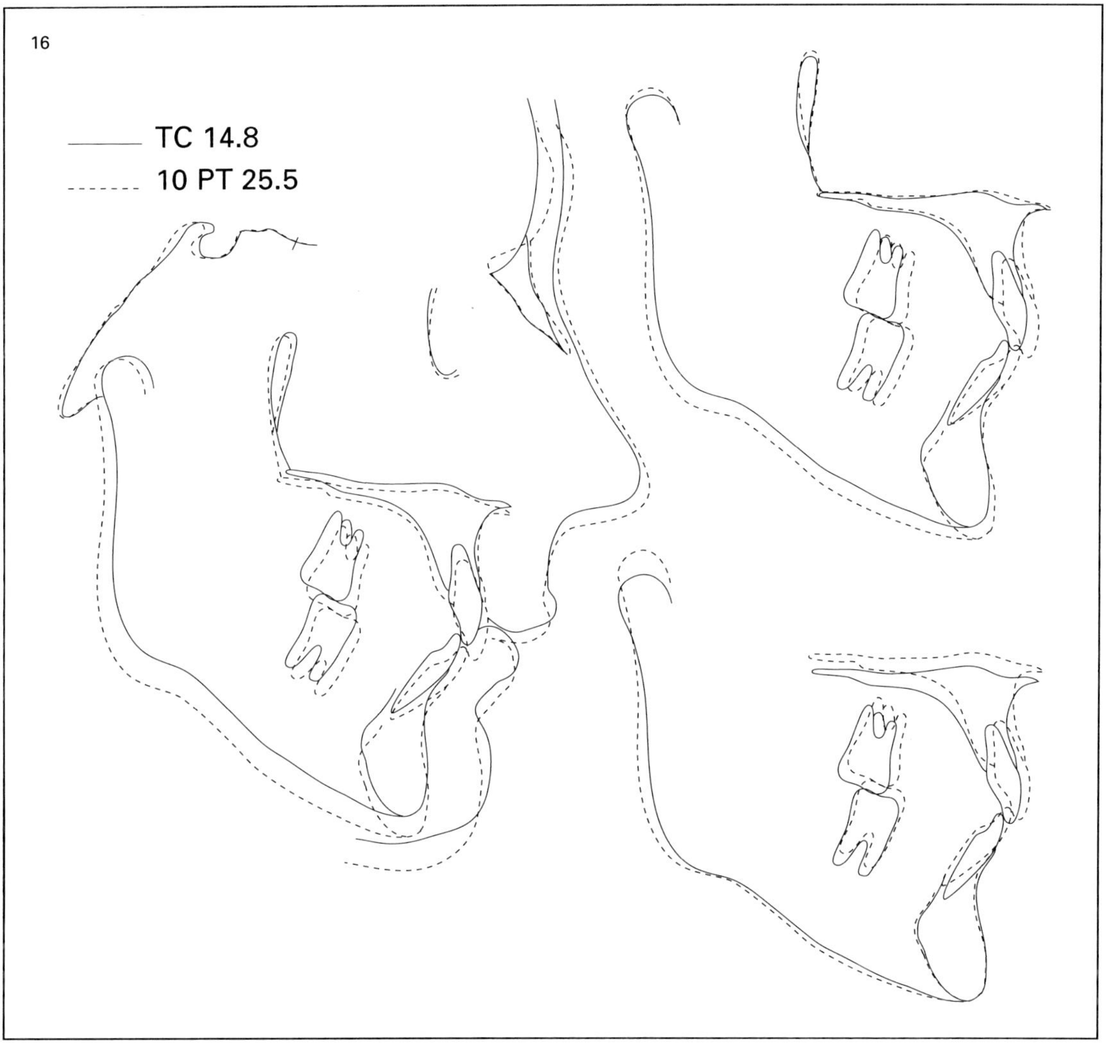

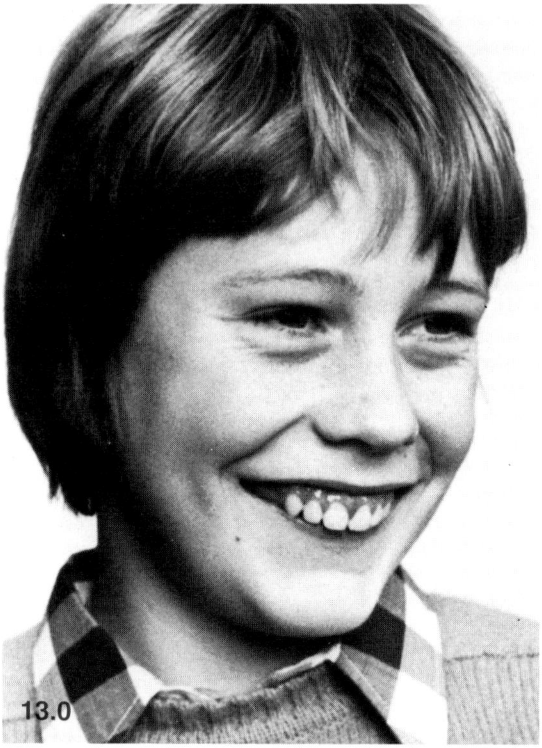
13.0

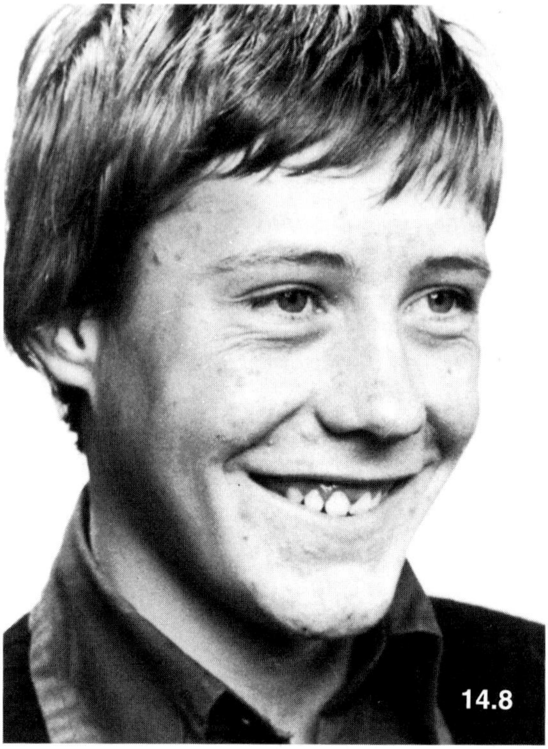
14.8

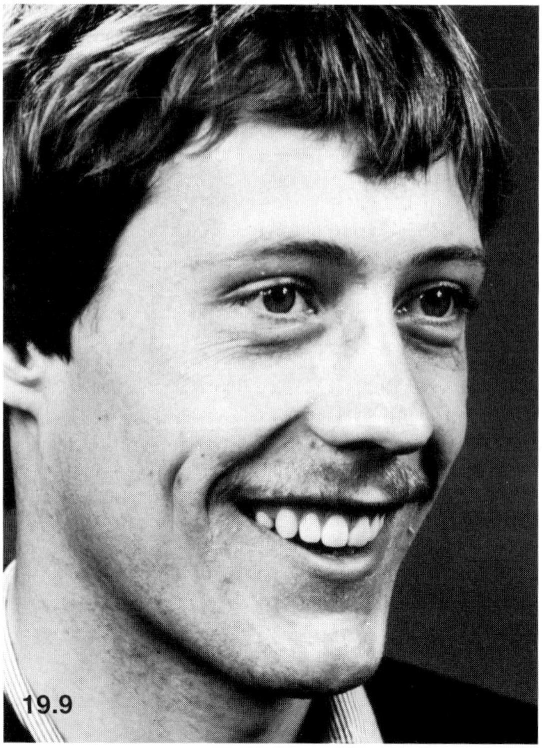
19.9

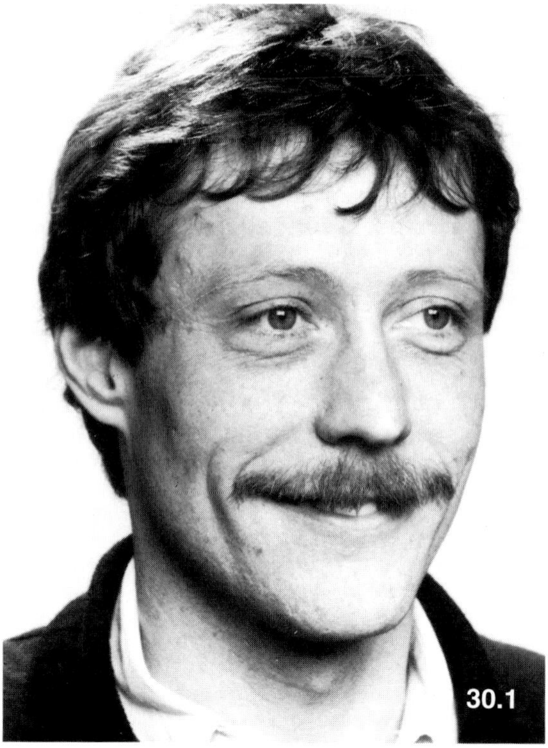
30.1

Fig 16-10 Note the pronounced disto-relation and high gum-line prior to treatment. Through the intrusion of the maxillary incisors and the increase of height of the lower face, the degree of exposure of the gingival mucosa was reduced. The increase in lower face height continued with resultant improvement subsequent to treatment.

crowding in the mandibular incisors had increased but this was not considered disturbing since there were no rotations or vertical irregularities (Figs 16.7 and 16.8).
Superimposition of the cephalometric tracings shows the pronounced facial growth that had taken place during treatment. It can clearly be seen that the reduction in the ventral growth of the maxilla allowed the mandible to overtake it in its forward growth. The maxillary molars had been extruded, in contrast to the maxillary upper incisors. The growth that has taken place since treatment has brought about considerable improvement in the patient's appearance (Fig 16.9).
The oblique photographs show how marked the initial sagittal anomaly in the jaw relationship was, and how the high gum line was reduced (Fig 16.10).

The maxillary dental arch was made much too broad by the treatment with expansion plates (see Fig 7.9D, page 108). There was no sense in trying to adapt the mandibular arch to that width because the mandibular basal bone with its thick cortical plates and relatively narrow apical area does not permit permanent displacement of the roots to buccal. It might have been possible in this case to achieve the required changes in a short time with activator/headgear combination therapy. However, when the revised treatment was undertaken, combined treatment had not been introduced, and either headgear or activator was used exclusively. The use of the headgear was chosen because it would give more freedom for the dentition to return to a state of equilibrium.
Out of consideration for the long duration of the treatment that had already taken place, and the caries susceptibility of the dentition, the use of full fixed appliances was rejected. With such appliances it would have been possible to move the mandibular right second premolar into its correct position and to align the mandibular incisors so that they had good interproximal contacts. Above all, it would have been possible to secure a better improvement in the steep inclination of the maxillary incisors. Even with the partial fixed appliance, a better result should have been achieved if it had been used longer. Seeing that there would have been an extra burden imposed by the use of full fixed appliances, also with a great chance that tertiary crowding still would have followed unless permanent retention plates were installed, that approach was put aside.
In this type of case, the possibility of surgical intervention should be considered, certainly if the sagittal discrepancy is great.[28] Whenever a patient is using a "Sunday bite" and achieving a neutro-occlusion in which the arches fit well together, an obvious thought would be to perform a mandibular osteotomy through which the body of the mandible as a whole is brought ventrally (Fig 16.11). Surgical corrections may as a rule be done only after the completion of facial growth. In this case it would have been necessary to wait a number of years. Of course there are also other more

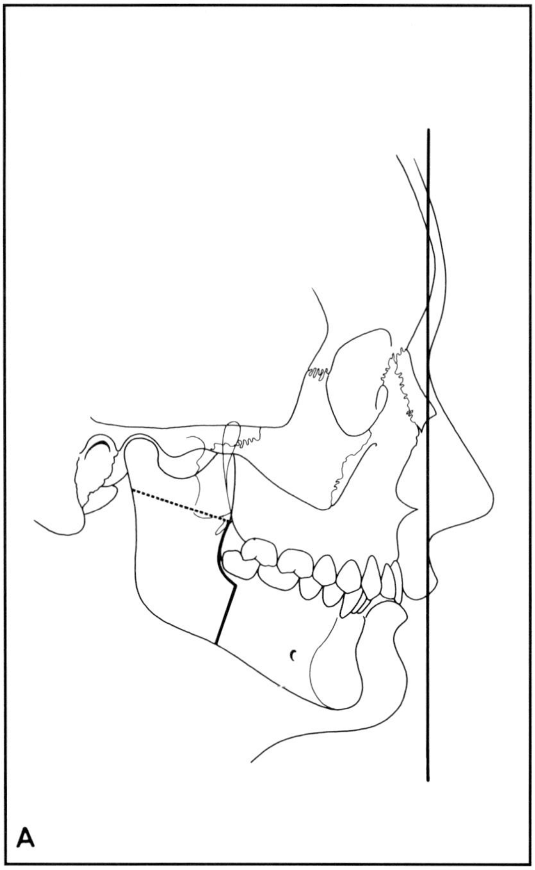

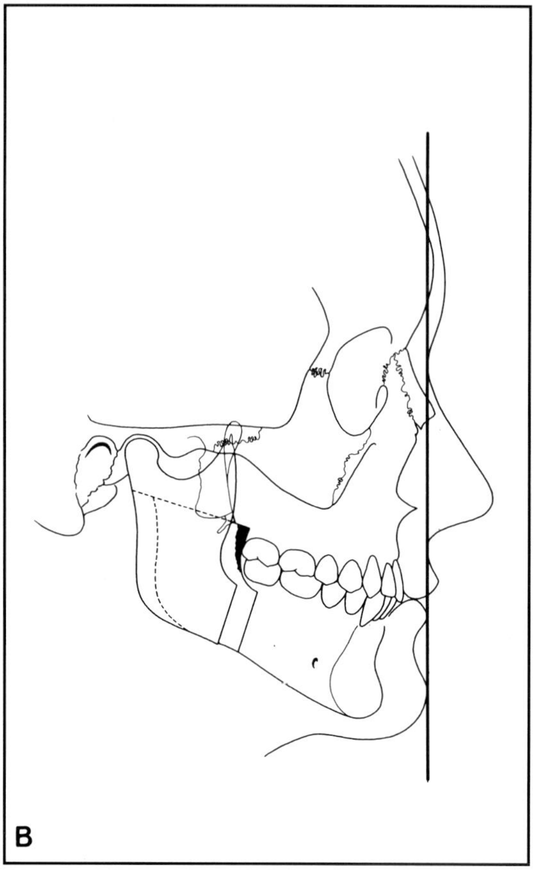

Fig 16-11 Osteotomy of the mandible according to Obwegeser-Dal Pont, for a class II/1 anomaly with mandibular retrognathy (sagittal-split osteotomy).

A The lingual cortical plate of the mandibular ramus is sawn through caudal to the mandibular condyle and the coronoid process. From the buccal, the body of the mandible is sawn ventral to the angle of the mandible until the cortical plate has been cut through. After that, the intervening part is split away sagittally along the interior of the buccal cortical plate.

B Subsequently the body of the mandible is displaced ventrally and fixed to the ramus with steel ligatures or other means. The sharp point on the ventral of the ramus is made round. Intermaxillary fixation is essential.[37]

weighty considerations involved in such treatment, the consequences of which need to be taken into account.

In conclusion, the foregoing treatment with expansion of the maxillary arch is a typical example of incorrect treatment planning and inadequate observation of its consequences. The first aspect has already been commented on. Regarding the observation, four points should be added.

In the first place, after six years of expansion, an even broader maxillary arch might have been expected. It is then questionable as to whether the screw in the plate was always active or whether the patient was wearing it well. If the potential for expansion with the plate was not being utilized, then why was the plate worn so long? If the patient had not worn it well, was there any purpose in keeping up the pretense for six years? It is, incidentally, important to realize that expansion screws sometimes will turn themselves back during use as the plate segments flex, so that lack of change cannot always be blamed on poor patient cooperation.

Second, it should be pointed out that to undertake treatment in the manner described brings with it a clear danger of the patient suffering "treatment fatigue." The fact that the patient under discussion was still prepared to undertake new treatment and indeed obviously did cooperate very well in its execution, could be considered to be rather exceptional.

Third, if the patient had been a girl of the same age, facial growth would have been more or less complete and headgear therapy would not have had the potential to secure the improvements noted in the boy. To obtain a good result, a girl would have had to undergone surgery with the risks that are involved in that. It would also have been likely that orthodontic treatment before and after surgery would have been required.

Fourth a long-continued habit of adopting a "Sunday bite" can have unfavorable consequences for the temporomandibular joints.

Chapter 17

Class II/1 subdivision, lateral tongue-interposition
Asymmetric cervical headgear, brackets 12, 11, 21, and 22, maxillary removable retainer
Male 14 years, 7 months to 32 years, 5 months

A boy aged 14 years, 7 months exhibited a class II/1 subdivision anomaly with neutro-occlusion on the right and a disto-occlusion of ½ PW (premolar width) on the left. The tongue at rest lay between the lingual cusps of the maxillary and mandibular molars on the left side. There were no other abnormal functional conditions. There was excess space in the maxillary arch (ALD: + 3 mm). The maxillary first permanent molars had abnormal crown forms and did not occlude well. Indeed, the maxillary first permanent molar on the left was in endo-occlusion and the mandibular first and second molars on that side were rotated. The middle of the dental arch in the maxilla was displaced to the right with respect to that of the mandible. Because of the narrowness of the maxillary lateral incisors a tooth-size discrepancy (TSD) of 1.5mm existed (Figs 17.1 and 17.2).

Because of the age of the patient, it was decided to commence treatment immediately and to fit an asymmetric cervical headgear. It was not considered sensible to correct the position of the maxillary left first molar since it was probable that such a correction would relapse as a consequence of the tongue interposition and the somewhat triangular form of the crown. Consideration of course had to be given to the possible development by the asymmetric headgear of a force to palatal on the left molar, which might cause that molar to move still further inward. Following achievement of neutro-occlusion on the left side, brackets were to be placed on the maxillary incisors to close the diastemata and to correct other irregularities.

At the age of 14 years, 8 months, a cervical headgear was fitted that had the right hand outer leg shortened and the one on the left bent outward. After nine months, both the disto-occlusion on the left side and the discrepancy between the arch midlines had been eliminated. Consequently the asymmetric headgear was replaced with a normal one. Two months later, brackets were placed on the maxillary incisors and a .0175" twistflex arch was fitted. This was replaced after some time with a solid .019" × .026" archwire. Four months later, the required corrections of the maxillary anteriors had been obtained so that the brackets could be taken off and a removable maxillary retainer provided. The maxillary first permanent molar on the left was still in endo-occlusion and the maxillary right second premolar was a little too far to palatal. The positions of these teeth were corrected with springs on the retainer. The plate was worn for eight months continuously and then for two more months only at night.

By the age of 16 years 10 months, a satisfactory result had been achieved with good

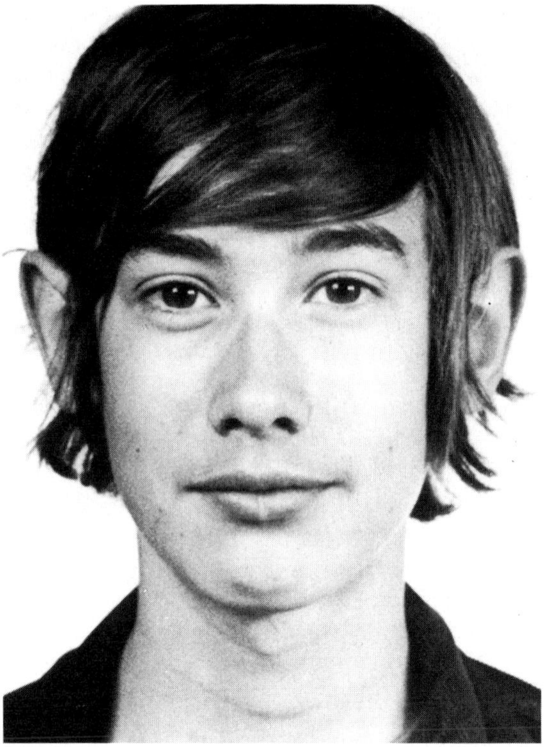

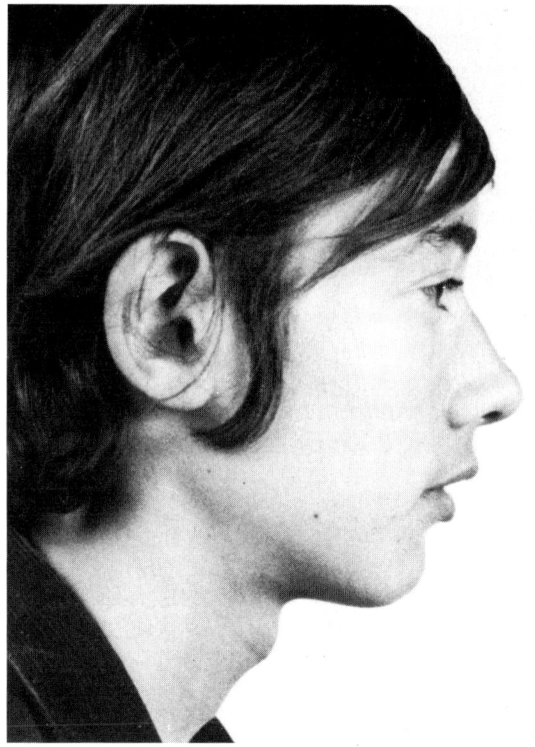

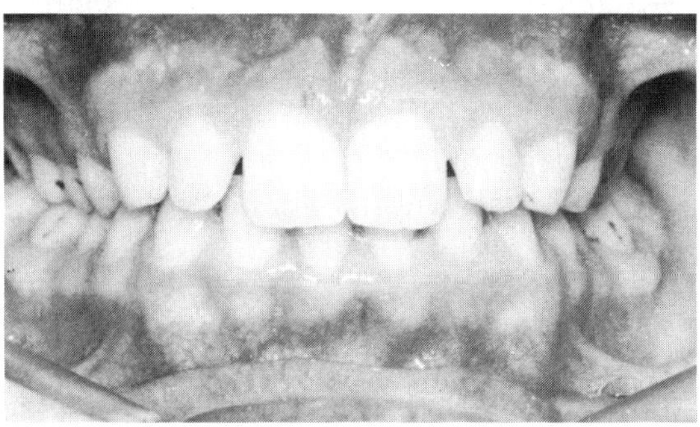

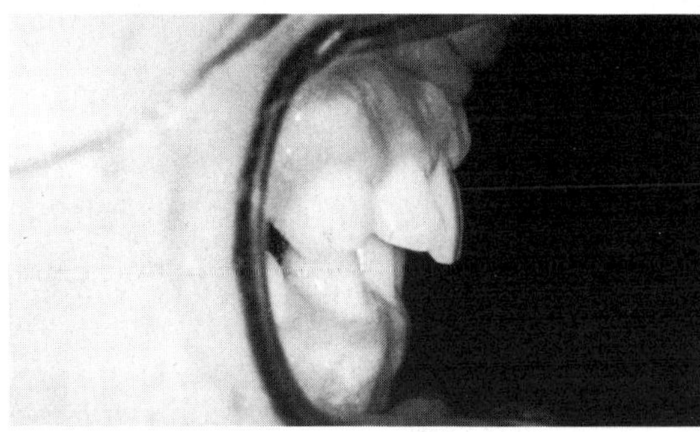

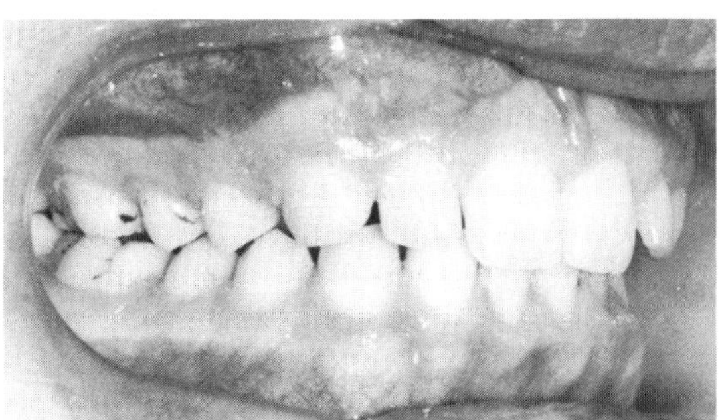

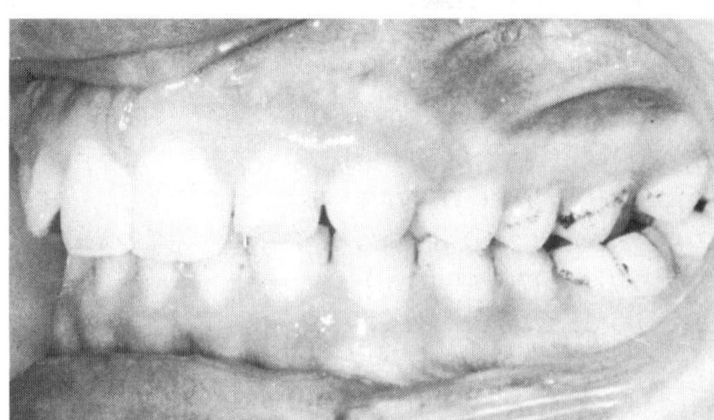

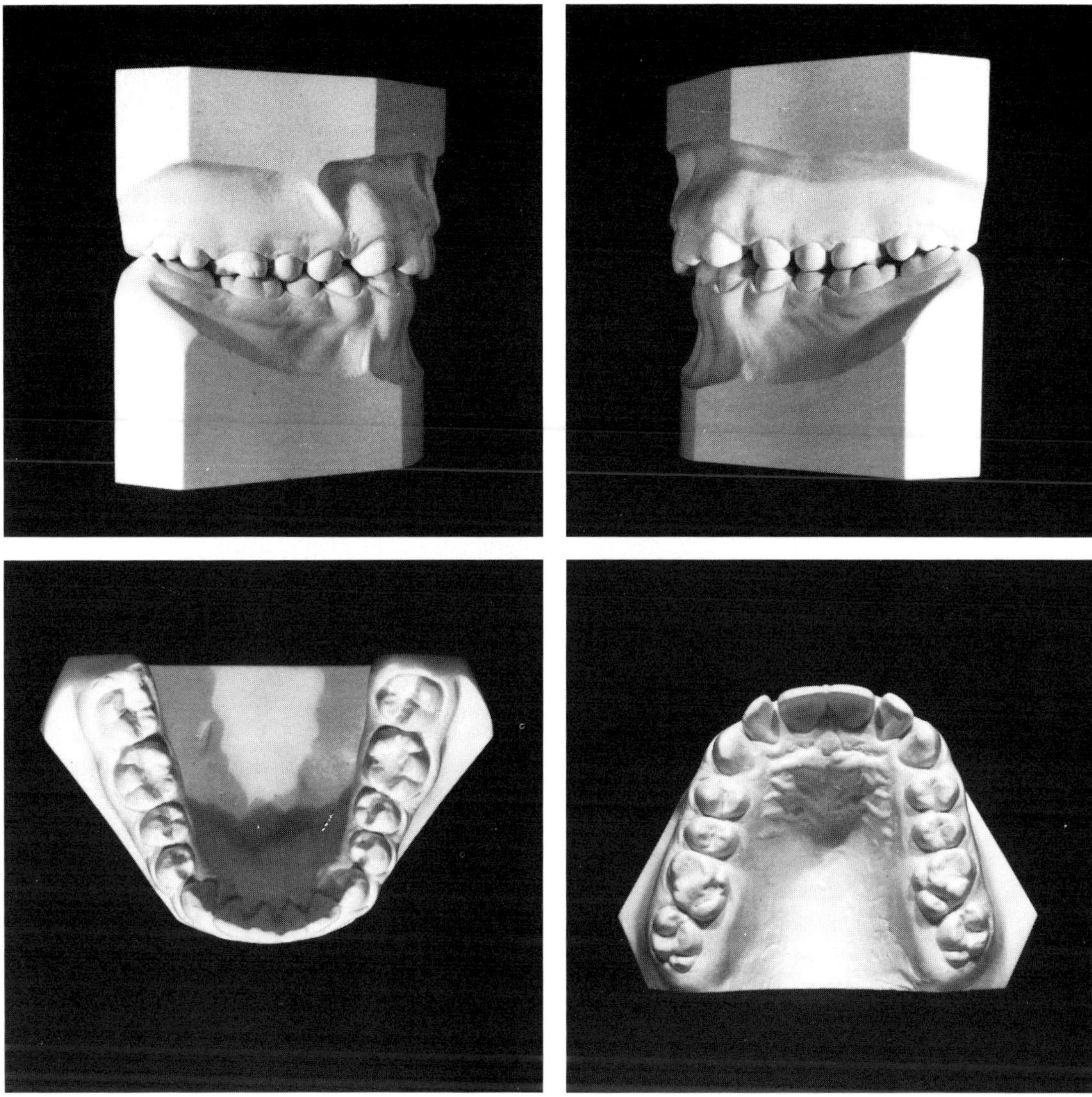

Fig 17-1 and 17-2 A boy of 14 y, 7 mo with class II/1-subdivision anomaly. The face is well-formed. The mandibular left first and second molars are rotated. There is an anterior TSD, with narrow maxillary lateral incisors, that are in labioversion. The maxillary first permanent molars have abnormal crown forms. The buccal surface runs at an angle toward the distopalatal from the mesiobuccal cusp. The crown is more triangular than rhomboid, especially on the left. That tooth is rotated and is in endo-occlusion. Its antagonist is rotated in the dental arch. In the intraoral photographs, the molars on the left can be seen not to occlude well; there is no solid interdigitation. The same applies to the first molars on the right. Furthermore, all the teeth in the posterior segments have shallow cusp heights.

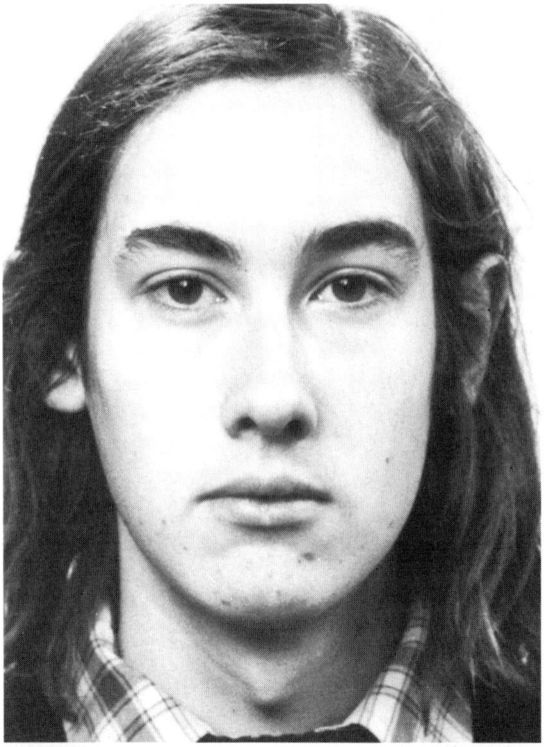
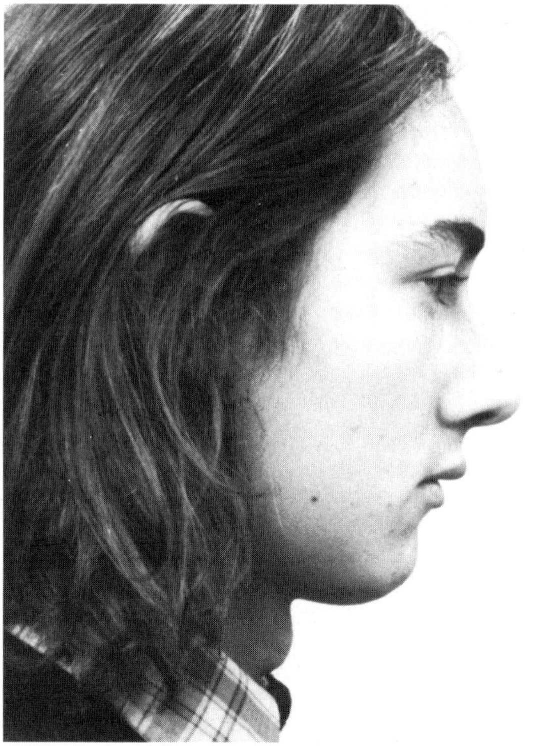
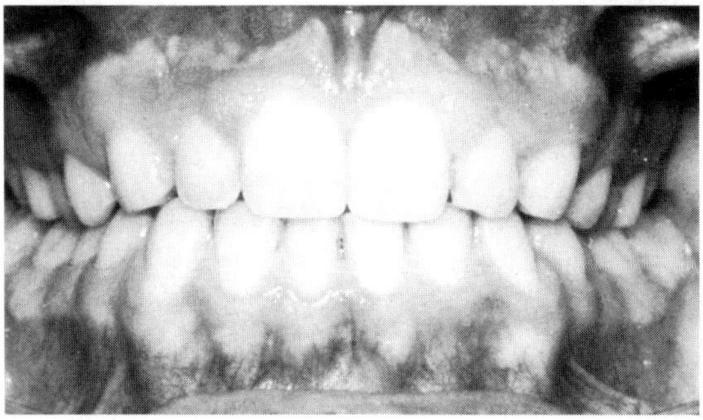
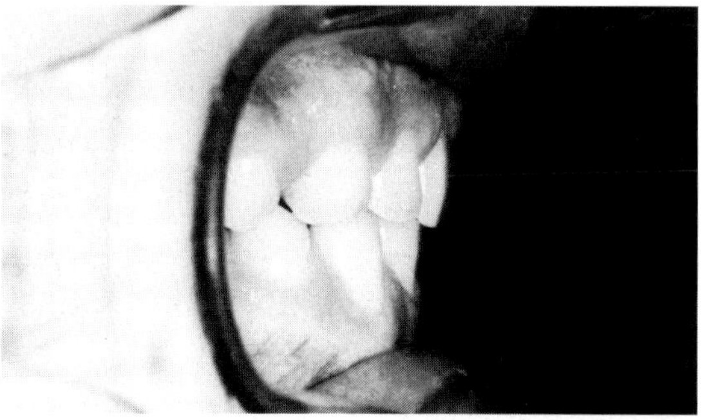
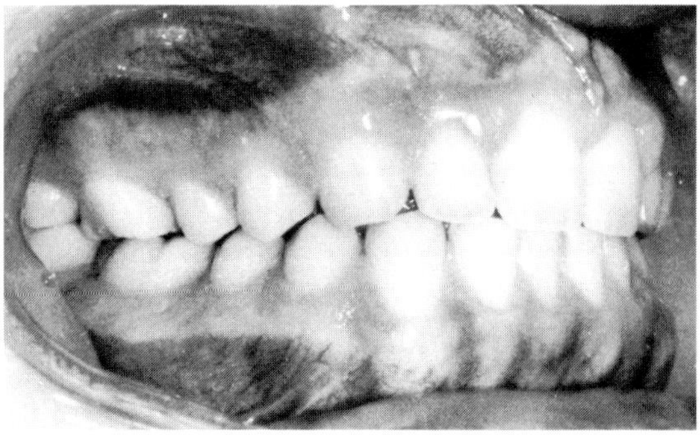
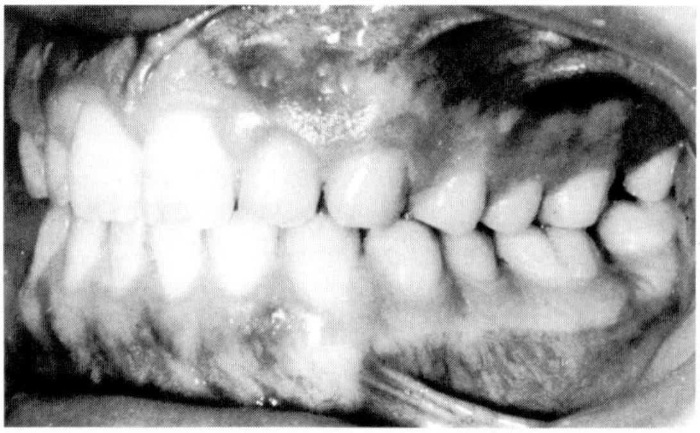

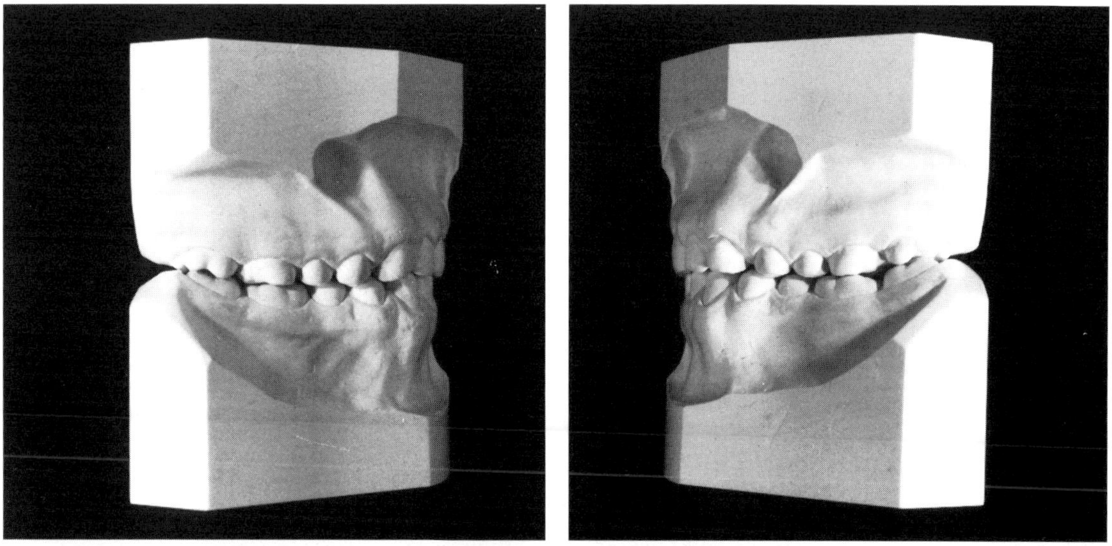

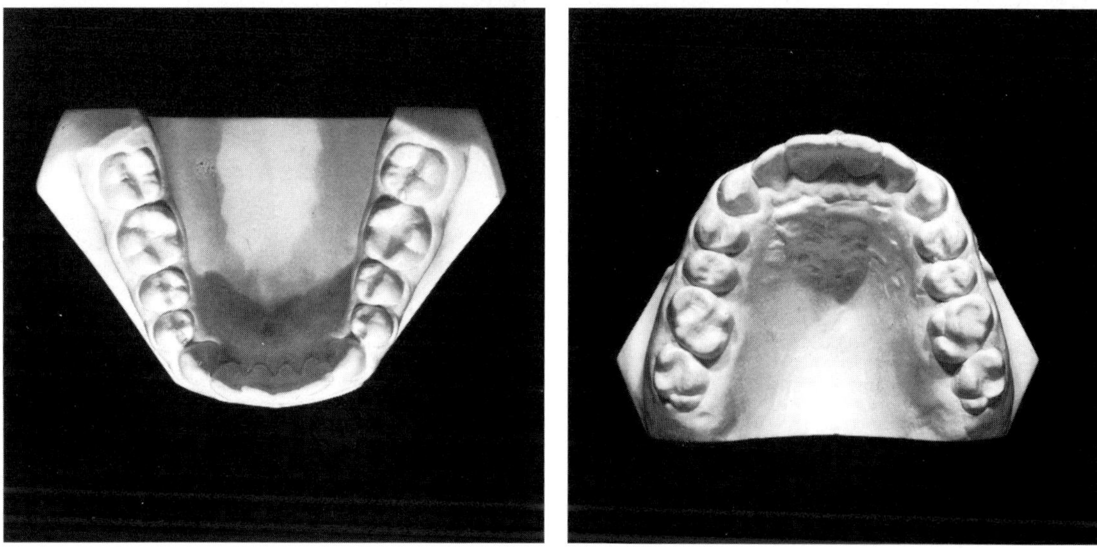

Figs 17-3 and 17-4 At the age of 16 y, 10 mo after active treatment for 16 months and a period of 10 months retention, the dentition is fine. Both dental arches and their midlines match well. No definite interdigitation has developed because of shallow cusp heights. This has been exaccerbated on the left by tongue interposition. In the mandibular anteriors, the distal surface of the right central incisor has gone a little to lingual. The posterior section of the apical area in the maxilla is small and it is not certain if sufficient room will become available for the third molars.

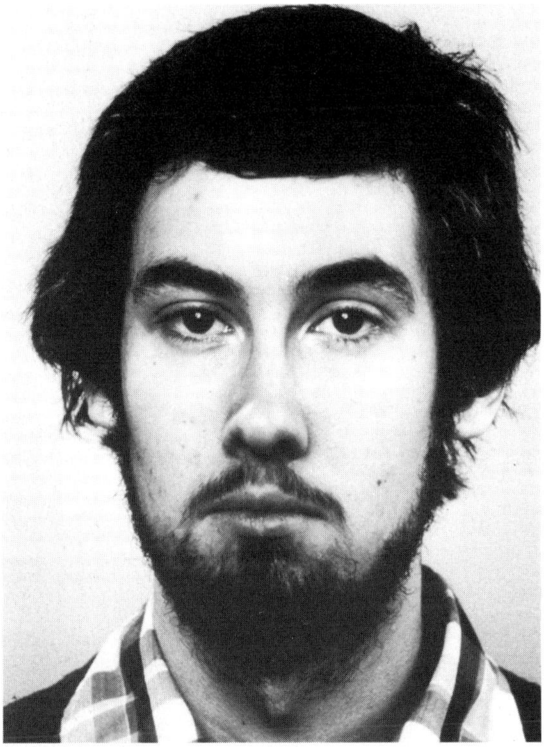
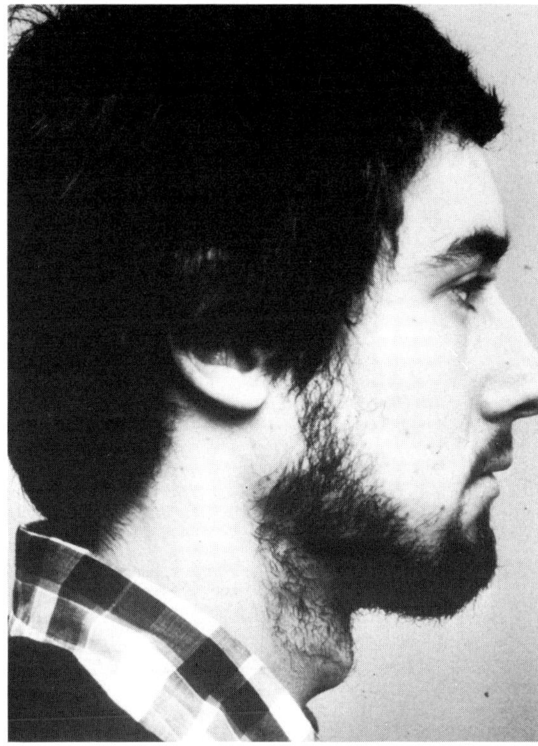
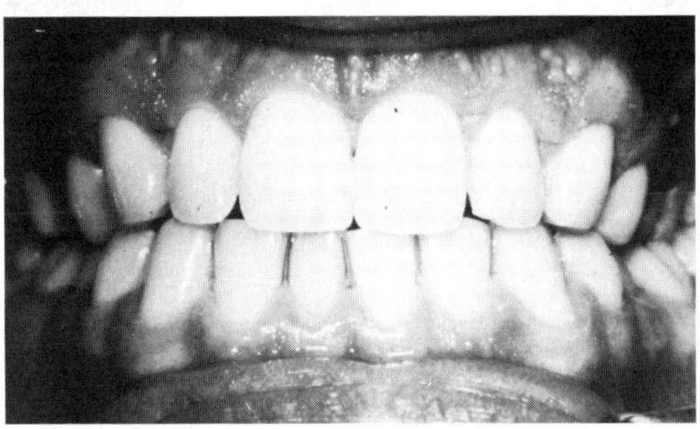
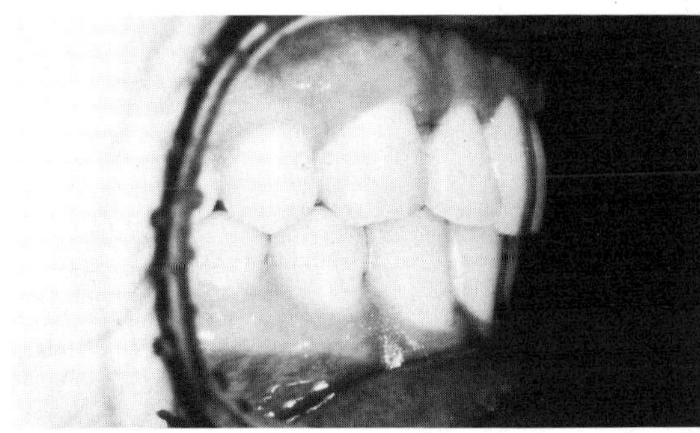
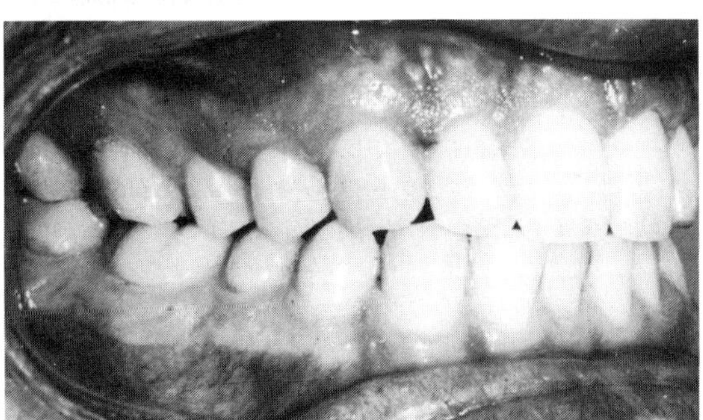
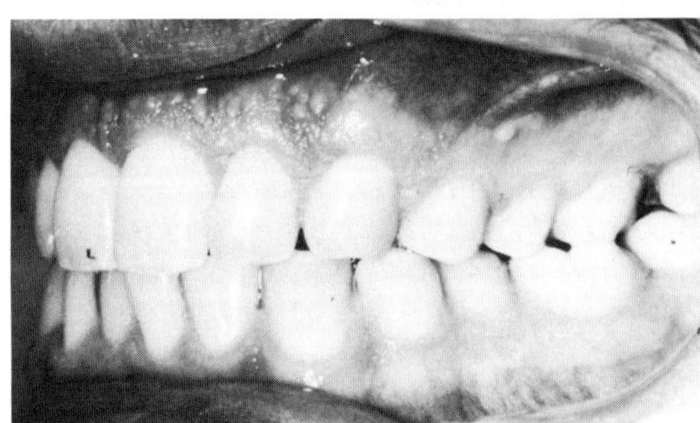

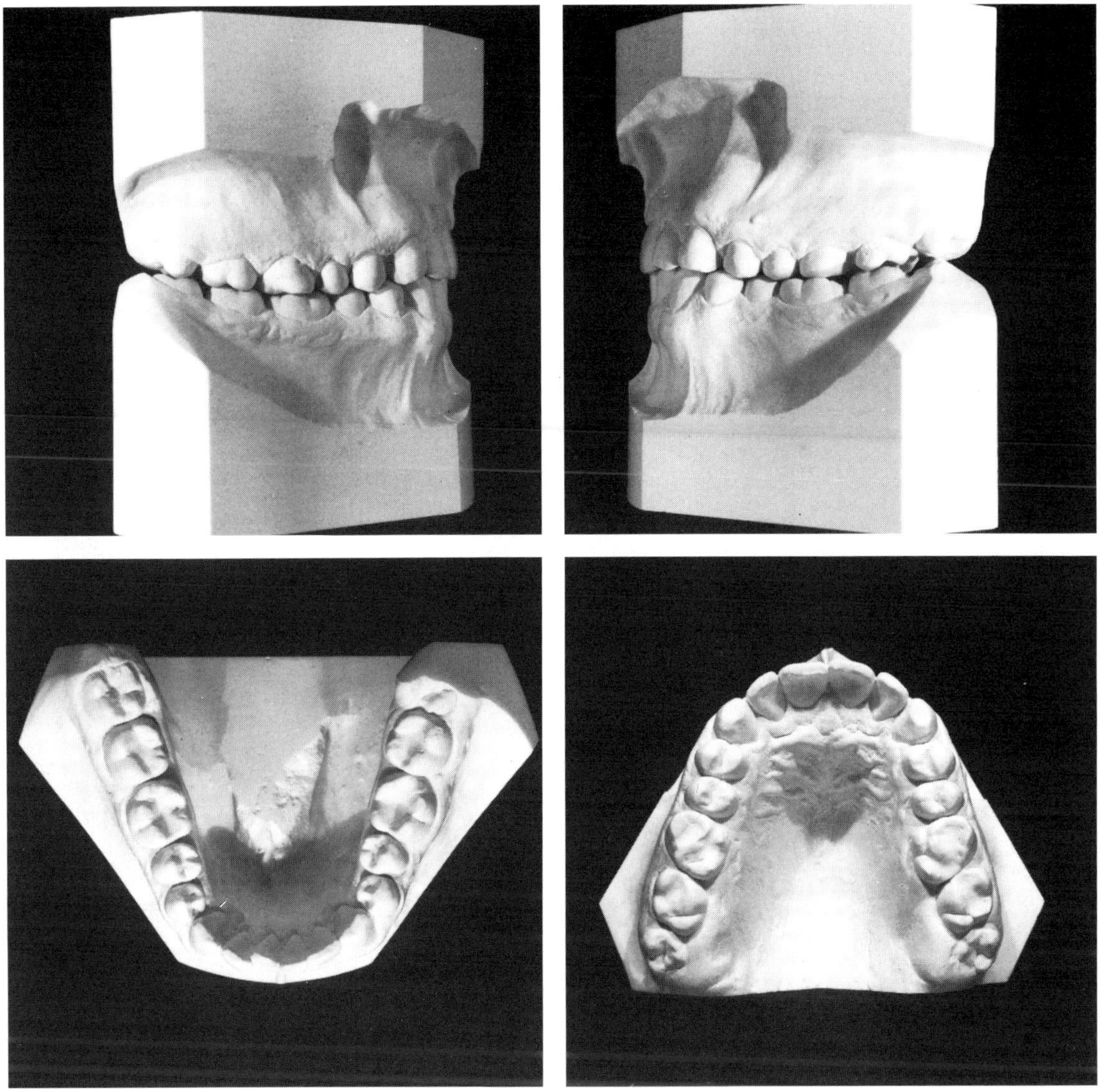

Figs 17-5 and 17-6 At the age of 21 y, 3 mo, the face appears longer due to the beard. The mandible has come further forward in relationship to the rest of the face and the mandibular dental arch occludes more mesially than it did five years previously. The occlusion on the right side is good; on the left the old pattern has returned in part, and the maxillary first permanent molar has gone again to palatal, which is not surprising when the triangular form and fragile contact with the second molar are considered. It is possible that the erupting third molar had a part to play. The most important observation is the lack of interdigitation, which is shown by the intraoral photographs and the dental casts. The interposition of the tongue between the lingual cusps is what is responsible.

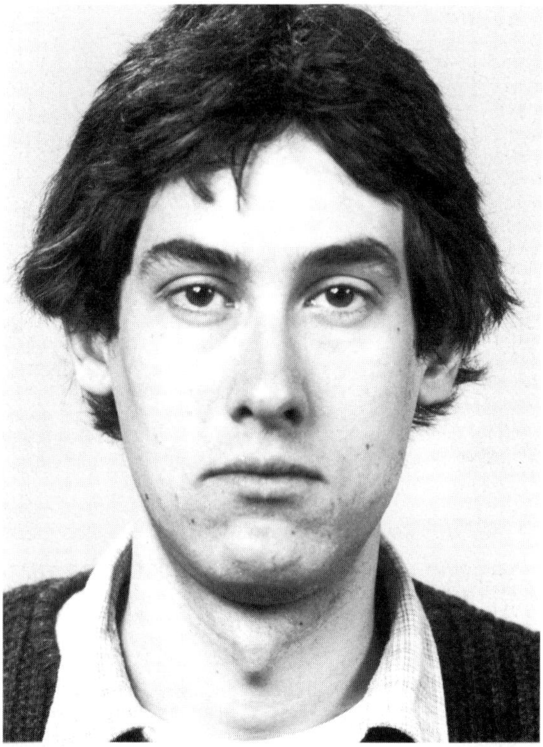

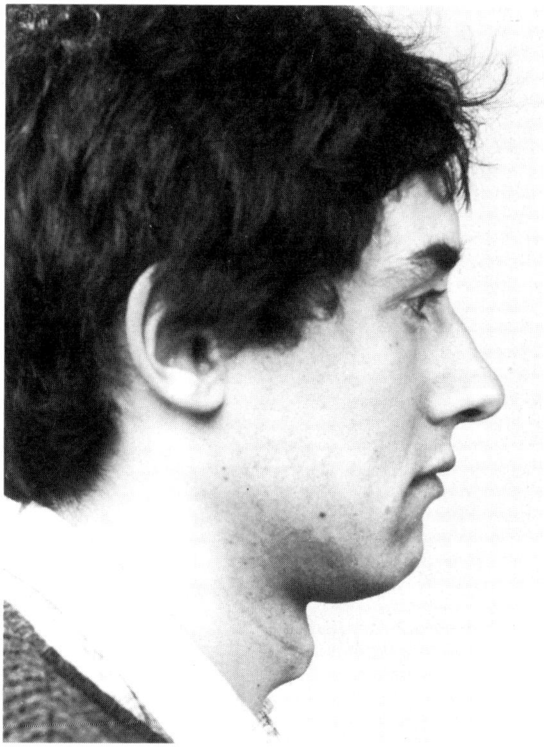

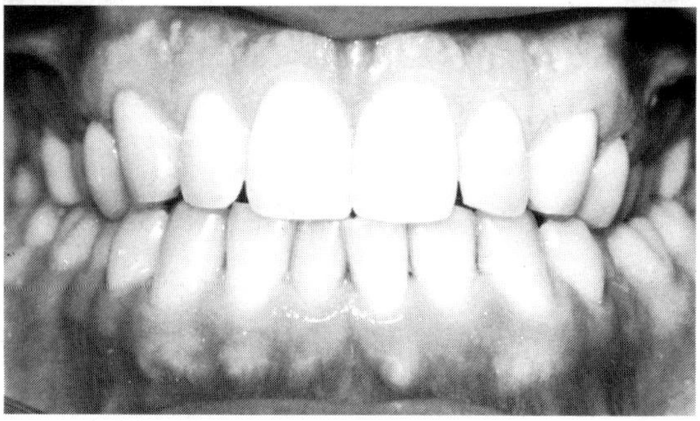

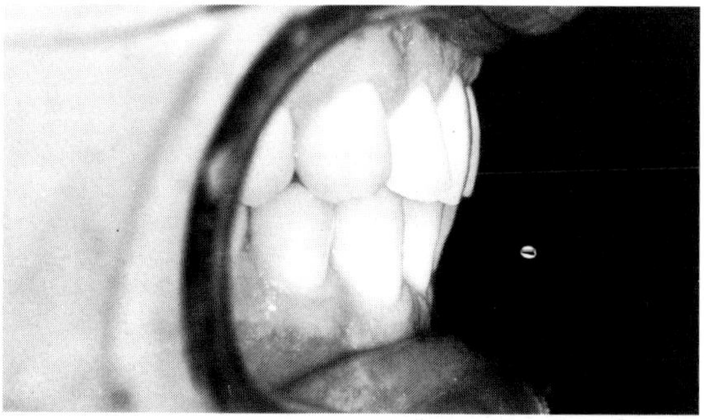

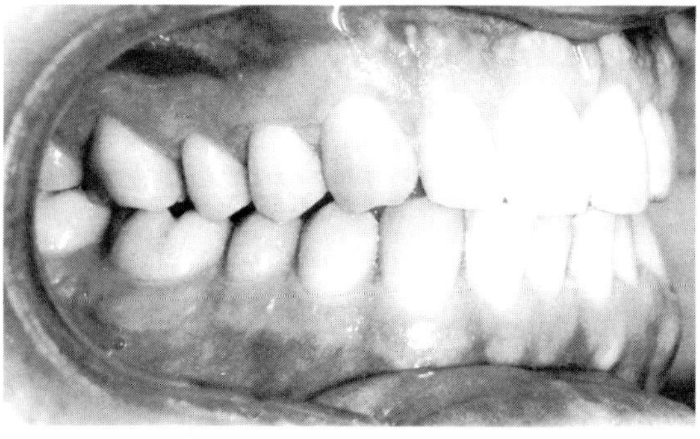

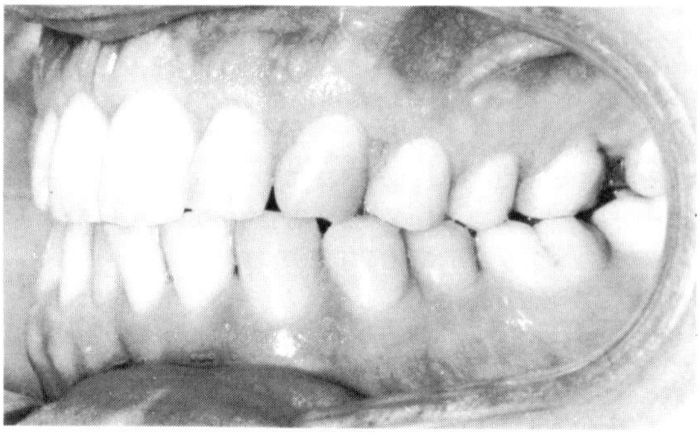

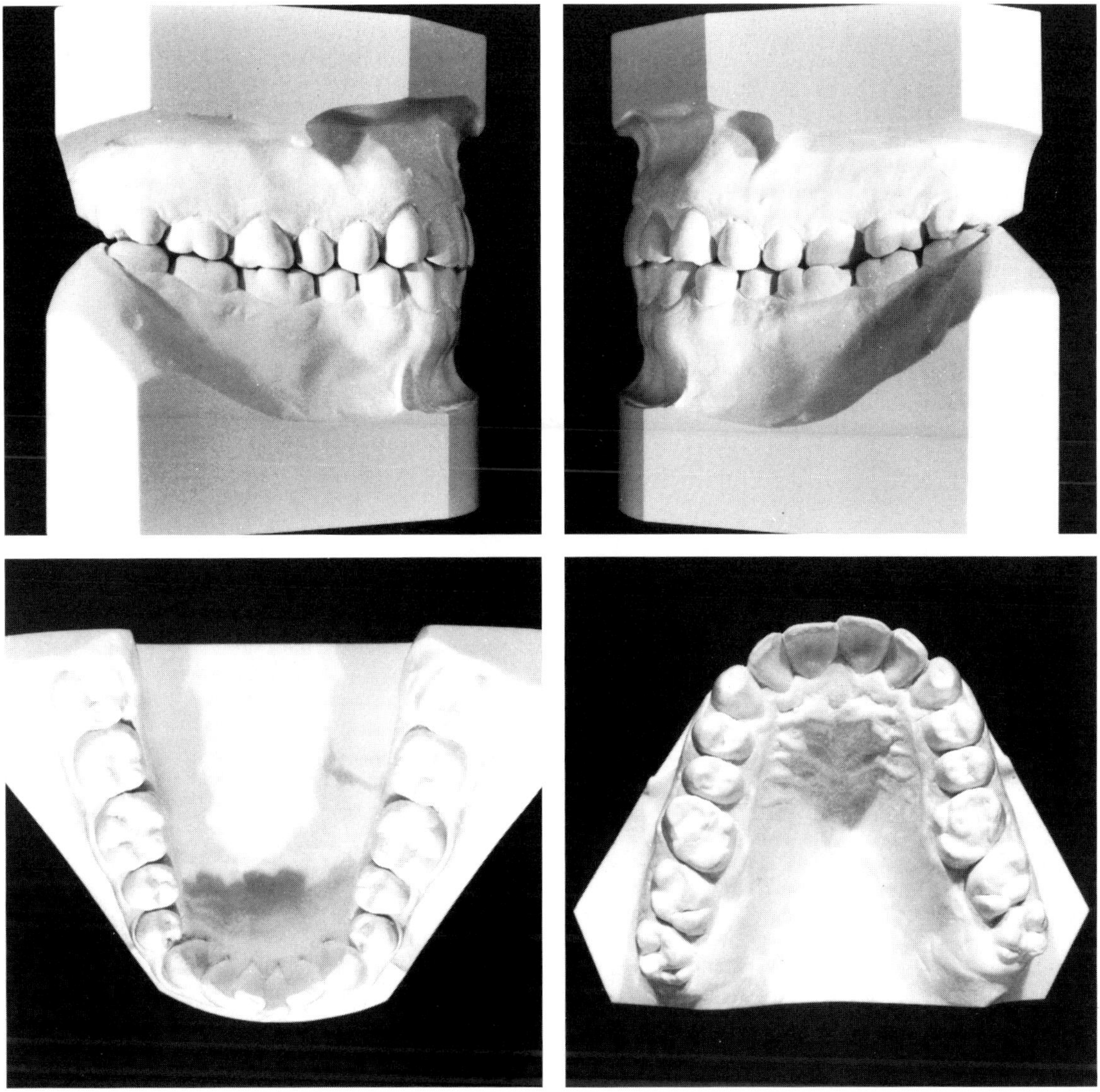

Figs 17-7 and 17-8 *At the age of 26 y, 3 mo, ten years after the conclusion of retention, the irregularities in the maxillary and mandibular anteriors have increased a little; they are not thought to be worthy of concern. The mandibular anteriors are hardly visible. The third molars have emerged fully, despite the fact that insufficient room for them is available in the maxilla to become well aligned in the arch. Because of the low cusp heights — as stated earlier — no definite interdigitation has developed. Moreover, the limited and unsatisfactory vertical contact between the molars on the left side, especially the first, can be blamed on the tongue interposition.*

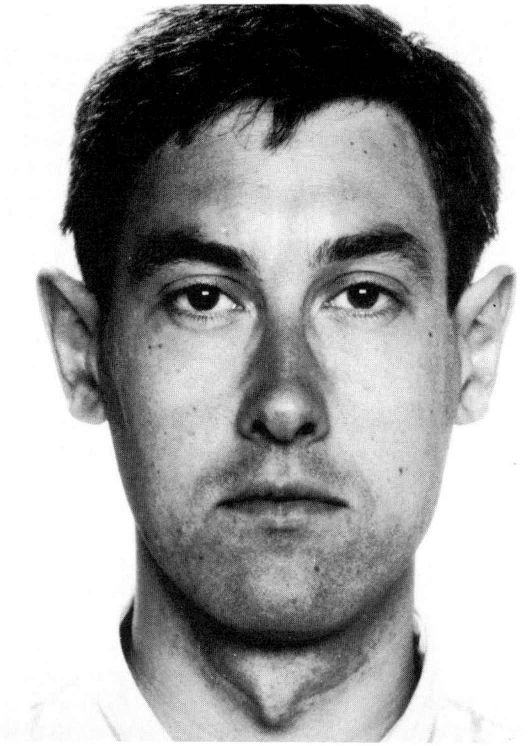
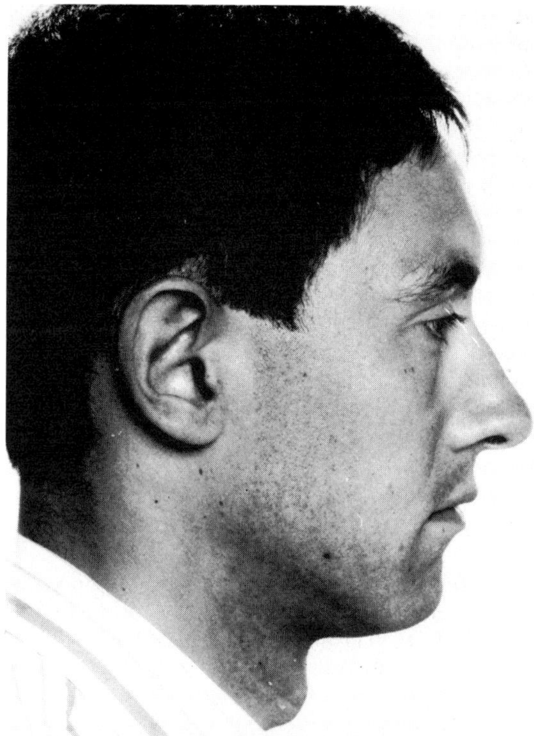
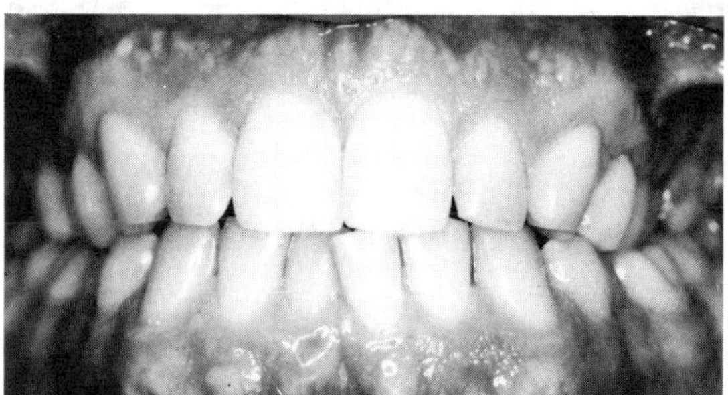
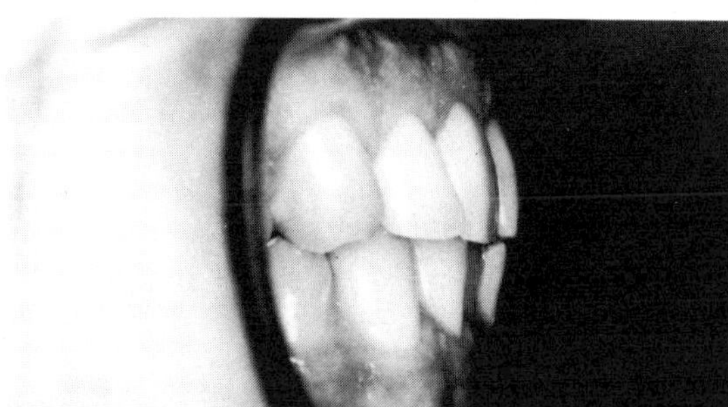
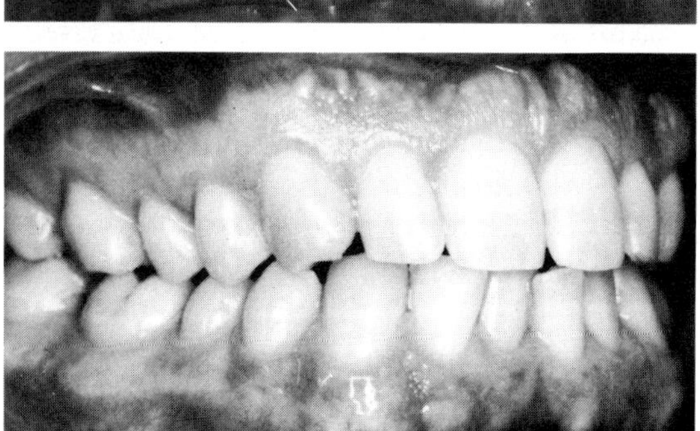
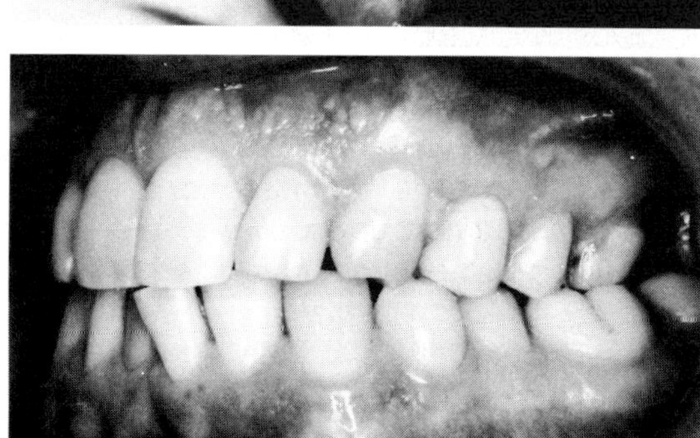

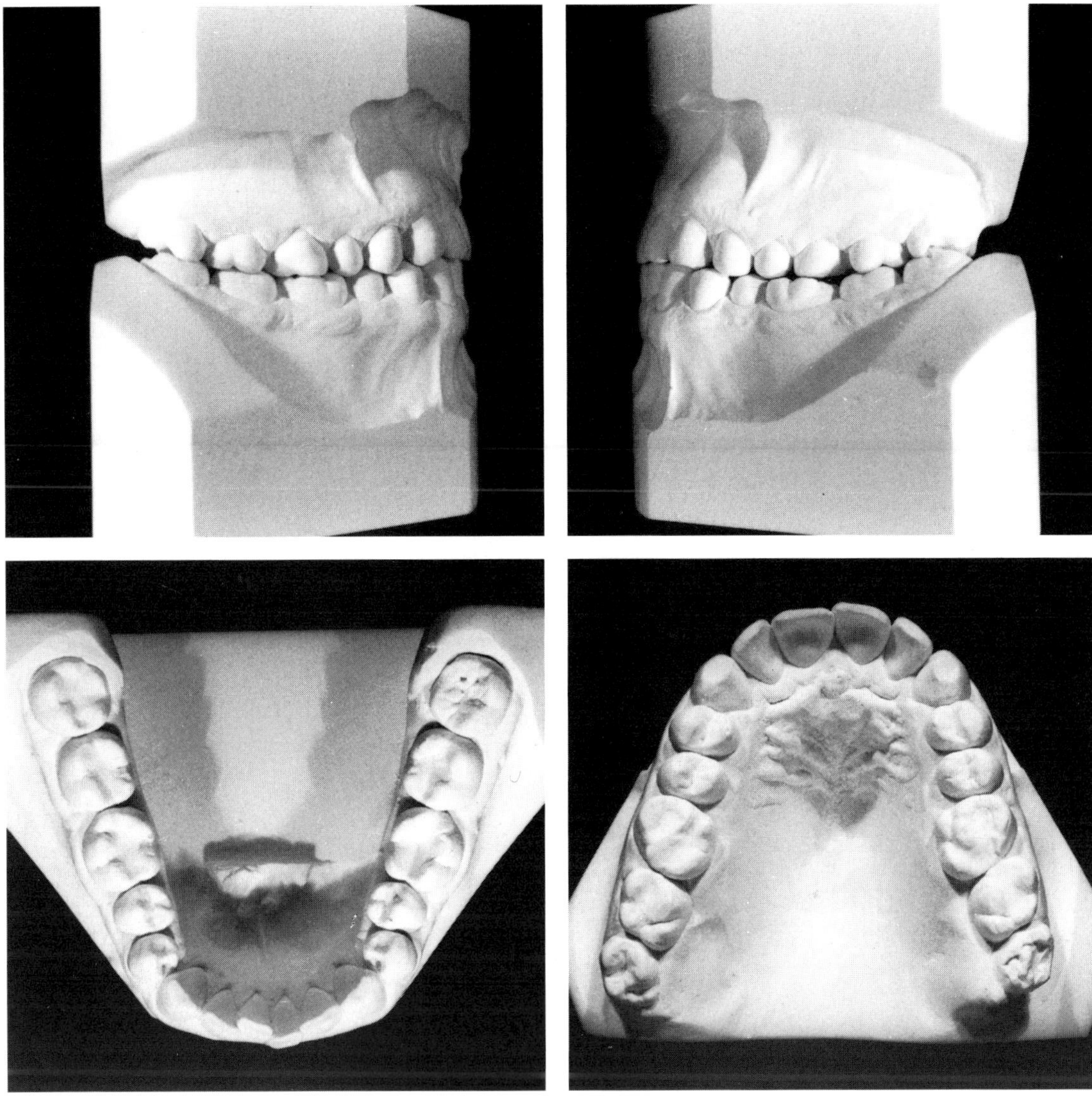

Figs 17-9 and 17-10 *At the age of 32 y, 5 mo, it appears that in the previous five years hardly anything has changed in the positions of the teeth. The interdigitation of the molars on the left has not improved. The mandibular right central incisor is located lingually, but parallel to the dental arch and not in supraposition. It does not disturb the patient. The minor labioposition of the maxillary left central incisor is not obvious.*

Figure 17-11a

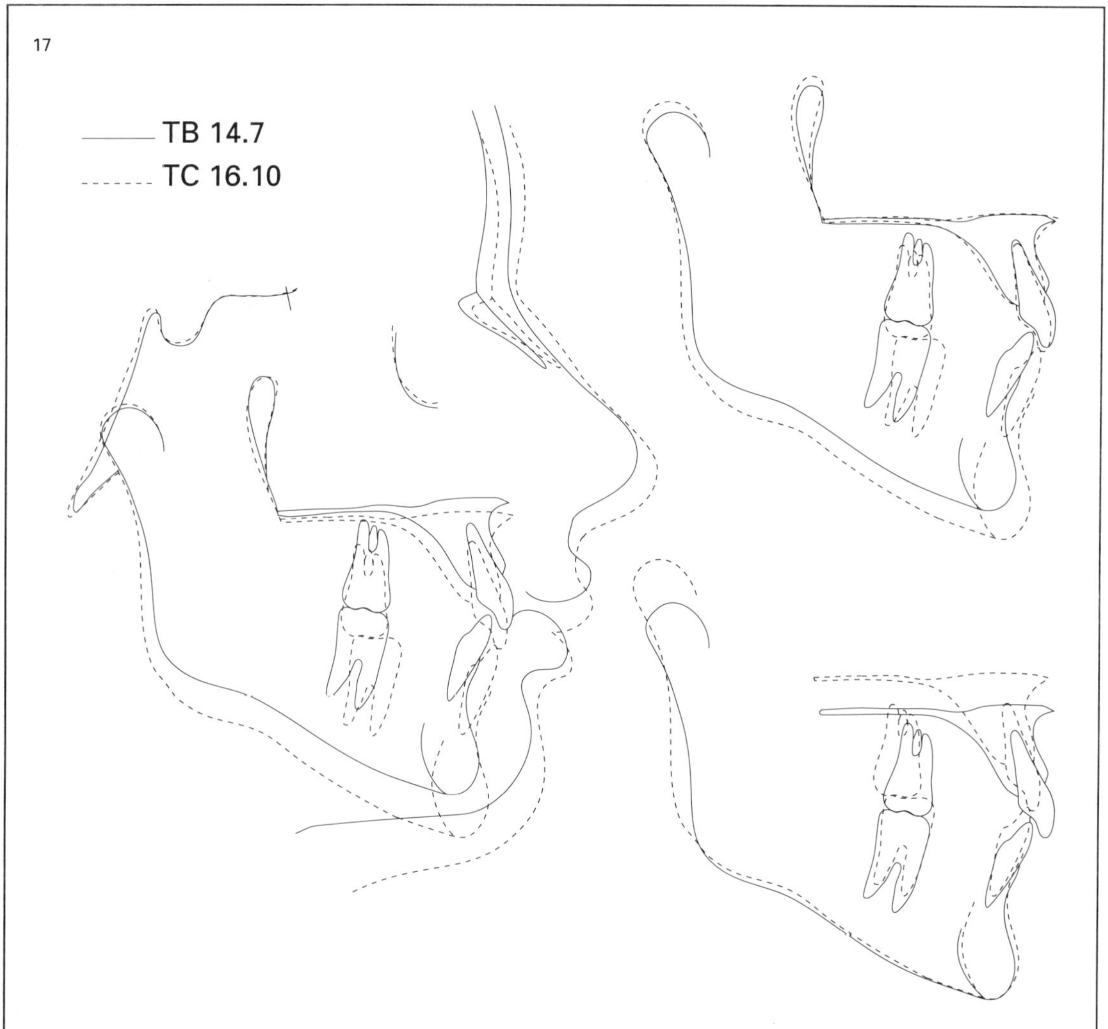

Fig 17-11 Superimpositions of tracings of cephalometric radiographs show that during treatment the ventral development of the maxilla was inhibited, the length of the mandible became much greater, and the face height increased. The lower face height increased significantly without the lower border of the mandible rotating to dorsal to any notable extent.
Following treatment, the facial growth continued vertically. The ventral positions of the jaws, teeth, and soft tissue contours barely changed at all.

Figure 17-11b

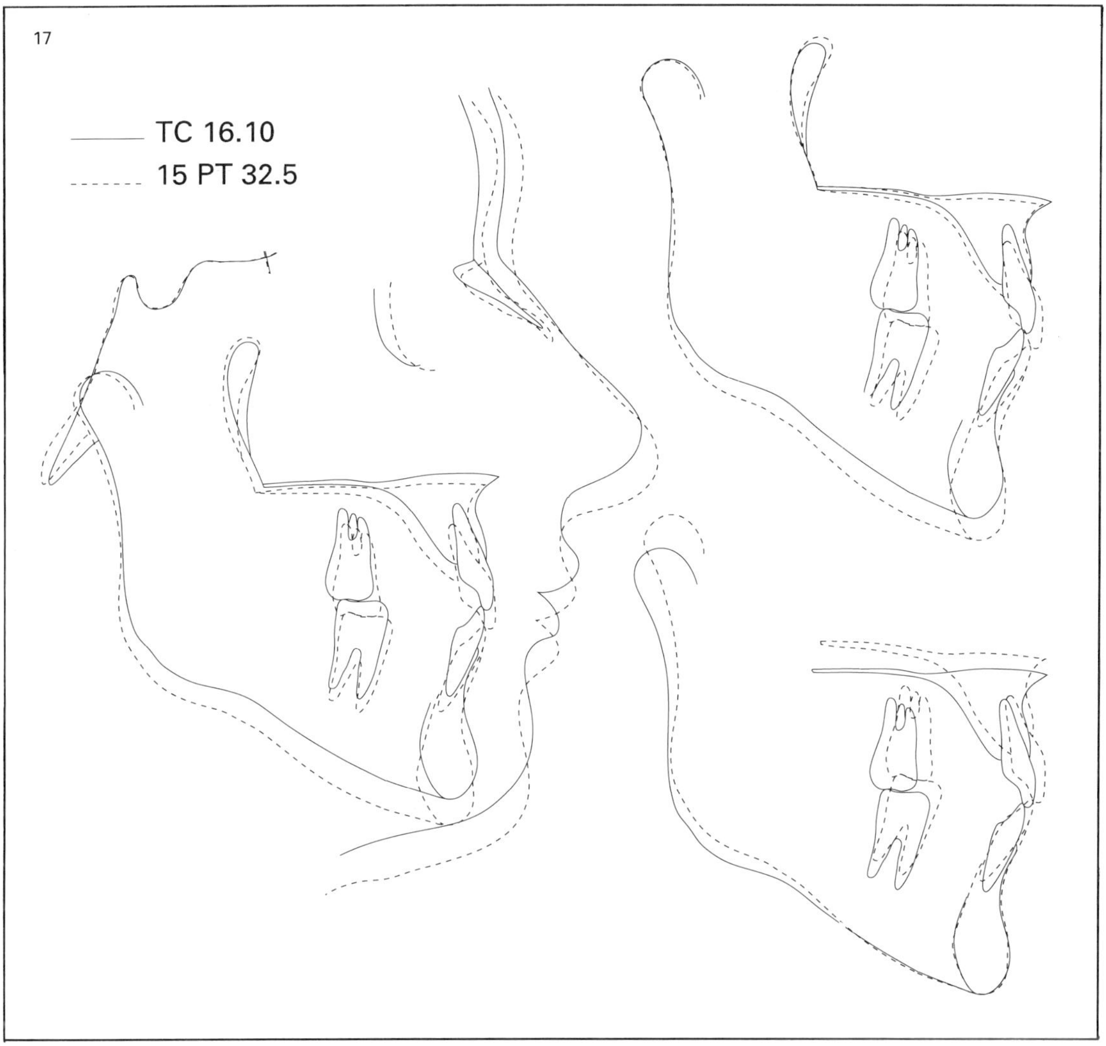

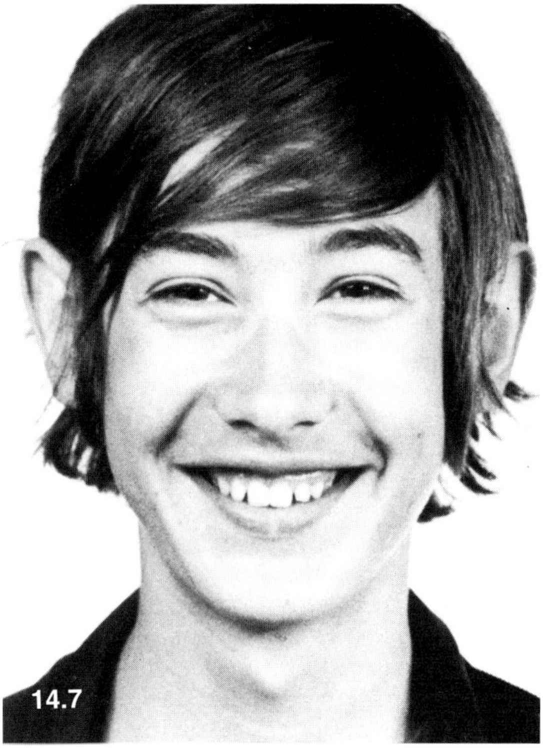
14.7

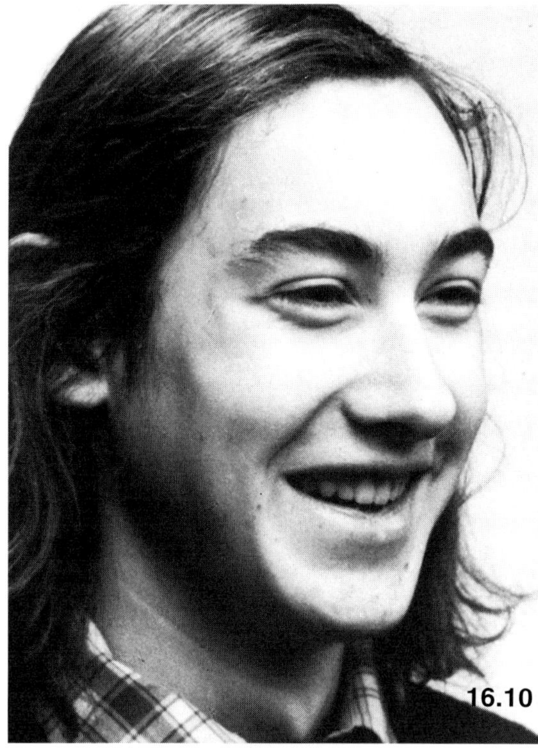
16.10

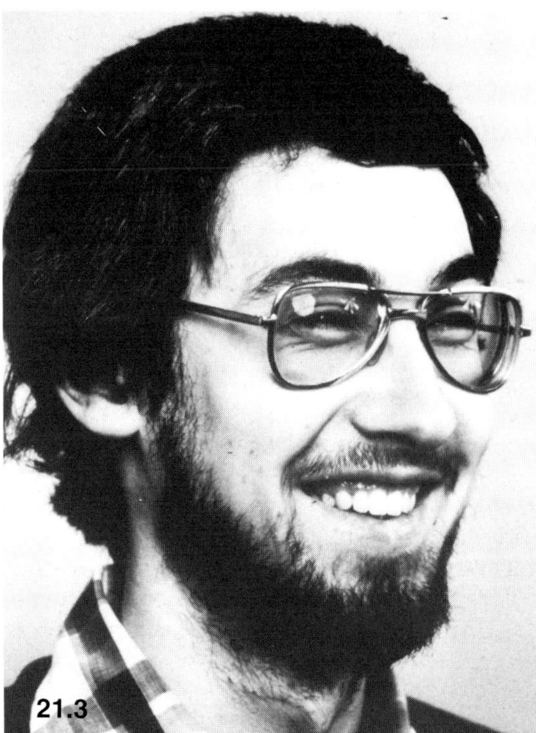
21.3

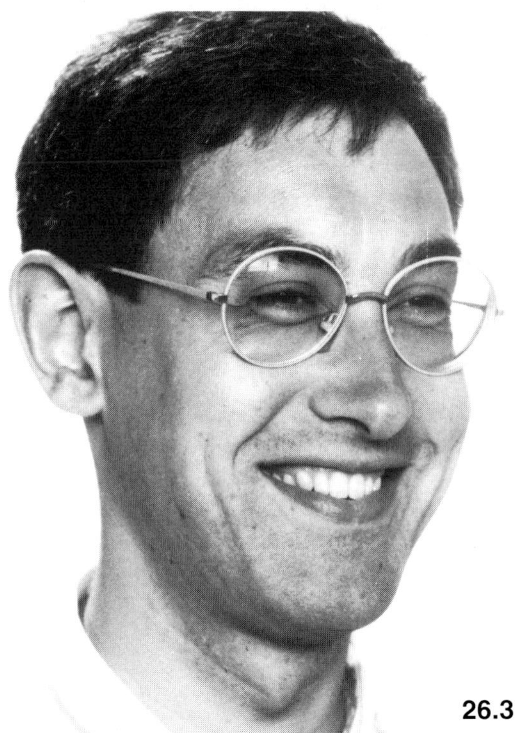
26.3

Fig 17-12 Note the changes that have taken place due to growth, treatment, and maturity.

dental arches that fit together well. In view of the limited cusp height, it was not clear if a solid interdigitation would develop. The maxillary left first permanent molar now stood in the line of the arch and occluded with its antagonist, which had rotated back a little (Figs 17.3 and 17.4).

In the next five years, the face developed further, particularly vertically, and the mandible attained a somewhat more ventral position with respect to the maxilla. At the age of 21 years, 3 months, the crown of the mandibular right third molar had fully emerged; those of the other three were partly through. The maxillary left first permanent molar had moved palatally and once more was in endo-occlusion. Tertiary crowding had developed in the mandibular anteriors while in the maxilla the lateral incisors had gone slightly to labial (Figs 17.5 and 17.6).

At the age of 26 years, 3 months, ten years after the conclusion of the retention period, several changes were in evidence; they were however not considered to be disturbing. The crowding in the mandibular anteriors had increased and the maxillary anteriors were somewhat malaligned (Figs 17.7 and 17.8). The overlapping in the front teeth of both jaws increased over the subsequent five years, but still remained acceptable (Figs 17.9 and 17.10). The tongue interposition between the molars on the left side persisted. The first permanent molars in that region barely are in contact; the second molars are in partial contact. Because of the shallow cusp heights no sharply defined interdigitation could be established either there or in those places where there is no tongue interposition. This explains why, despite the fact that the mandibular dental arch gradually had moved mesially in relationship to the maxillary arch as a result of the late growth of the mandible, the maxillary arch had not adapted in its breadth but had remained relatively narrow.

The superimposition of the cephalometric tracings shows that during treatment the ventral development of the maxilla had been inhibited, the mandible had become much longer, and the facial height had increased. Subsequent to treatment the face height became even greater (Fig. 17.11).

The photographs of the smiling face of this patient display the changes that resulted both from growth and from treatment (Fig 17.12). From this it is evident, just as from the superimpositions, that boys can exhibit considerable facial growth after the age of sixteen years.

Treatment was begun directly with an asymmetric headgear in this case for two reasons. The first reason was the age of the patient and the second is based on the concept that generally it is best to correct asymmetric occlusions as promptly as possible since in later stages of treatment it is more difficult and consumes more time. That applies also to transverse anomalies of the occlusion, except where — as was the case here — they originate from tongue interposition. As has already been mentioned, moving the maxillary first permanent molar to buccal made no sense since it was to be expected that due to the triangular crown form and the tongue interposition it would return palatally eventually. Moreover, the facial-orthopedic effect of headgears is greater if the thickness of the periodontal membrane of the molars to which the headgear is fitted is not increased by previous orthodontic movement. During the treatment it appeared that the maxillary left first permanent molar was only little displaced by the palatally directed forces generated by the asymmetric headgear. This tooth was subsequently easily moved into the arch with a spring mounted on the removable plate that was being used as a retainer.

Tongue interposition can frequently be found posteriorly but unless there is a distinct open bite it generally is overlooked. It is difficult to diagnose intraorally since often the effect is restricted to the lingual cusps. Tongue interposition usually is associated with an abnormal transverse occlusion (Fig. 17.13). In Dutch adolescents, 10% have an open bite in the posterior region and 18% have no solid interdigitation[12] In the adult population, 10% do not have maximal occlusion between the posterior teeth.[8] Tongue interposition can cease spontaneously during or after adolescence, but it is not possible to predict. In the majority of cases, tongue interposition probably will remain as a lifelong condition without posing any problem for the person concerned. It has never been shown that myofunctional therapy (tongue exercises) can result in permanent abolition of tongue interposition. The proposition that expansion of the maxillary arch can provide more room for the tongue and that this can eliminate tongue interposition appears not to be true in practice. Note also that caution should be exercised in the application of bulky acrylic appliances such as activators, since these certainly encroach on the intraoral space, and for that reason may not be able to be kept in place as required. Furthermore, a reduction in size of dental arches such as can occur when teeth are extracted can provoke an extension of the tongue interposition.

The course of orthodontic therapy and the stability of the result depends very much on the interdigitation. With a posterior open bite, it cannot be expected that changes in the position of involved teeth will be permanent. Such tooth movements have no justification. In addition, in cases with shallow cusp heights, a less stable result should be expected than where there are steep deep cusps interdigitating well. Both these aspects came into consideration in this case.

In retrospect, the question can be asked if stripping of the mandibular anteriors could have prevented the development of tertiary crowding. The TSD with relatively too much tooth material in the mandibular anteriors was an extra argument in favor of the procedure. However, at the end of treatment, a small vertical overbite that compensated for the TSD was present. The bite was stable and did not become deeper as time passed. The argument still remains that by stripping the mandibular anteriors, more stable interproximal support would be obtained (see Fig 12.15, page 192).

Tertiary crowding in the mandibular anteriors is still sometimes attributed to third molars, which in erupting and after emergence are thought to exert a mesial force on the dental arch. This has really never been proven, nor even that there is less tertiary crowding when third molars are absent. With the patient we have described it is also not clear whether or not the tertiary crowding would have been less if the third

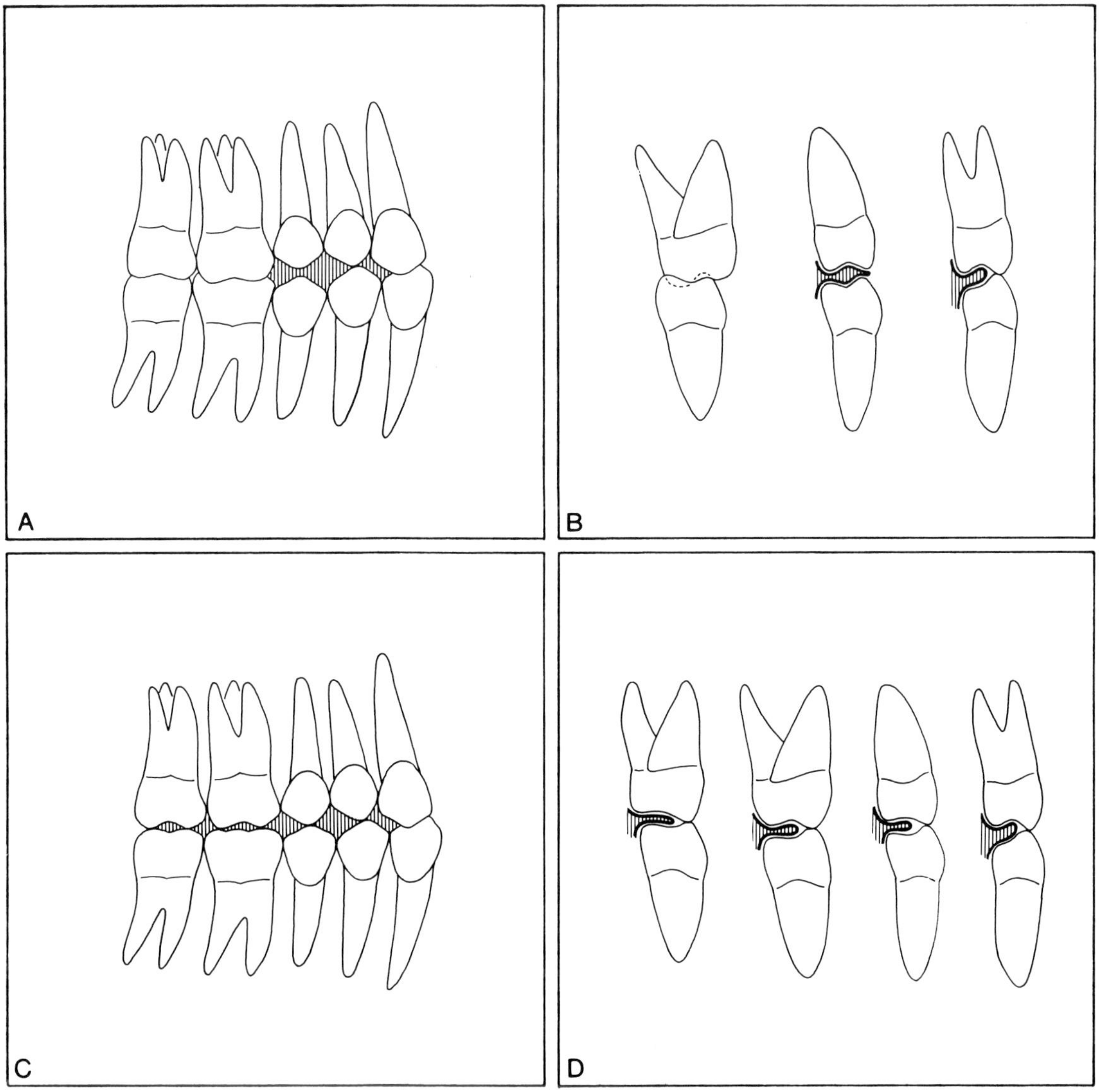

Fig 17-13 Simplified illustration of open bites in the posterior regions.

A,B Local open bite in the right posterior region, in which contact between the second premolars is totally lacking and is incomplete between the first ones. In contradistinction to the premolars, the first molars interdigitate quite well.

C,D Complete open bite over the whole length of the posterior region on the right. There is no, or inadequate, contact between the mandibular and maxillary teeth. No good occlusion nor interdigitation has developed transversely. Whenever the tongue takes a position between the buccal cusps, there will be no occlusal contact in that area.[30]

molars had been removed sooner. It is probable that the late growth of the mandible and its amount, the maturation of the facial musculature, and the increase in the pressure that the lower lip exerted were more important contributing factors.
In conclusion, this case was included because it is a clear example of how tongue interposition and lack of positive interdigitation can lead to the degeneration of a treatment result. Above all it shows the limited benefit gained by the treatment performed on this rather minor anomaly. Only the correction of the disto-occlusion on the left has been permanent; the other improvements have proven not to last. It can be suggested that the patient would not have been much worse off in the long term had no treatment been given.

Chapter 18

Class II/1, lower lip behind maxillary incisors
Cervical headgear, mandibular lip bumper, brackets 12, 11, 21, and 22
Female 10 years, 8 months to 27 years, 8 months

A girl of 10 years, 8 months with a broad, round face, a ventrally developed midface, and a dorsally placed chin exhibited a serious class II/1 anomaly with ¾ PW disto-occlusion. The lower lip at rest was located behind the maxillary central incisors and against their incisal edges. She could breathe easily through her nose. The overjet was 10 mm and the mandibular incisors were in contact with the palatal mucosa. There was slight crowding in both dental arches (Figs 18.1 and 18.2).

Taking into consideration the crowding in the maxillary arch, it was decided to correct the sagittal jaw relationship with a cervical headgear. If later on the patient could not hold her lower lip in front of the maxillary incisors, then a lip bumper would be applied in the mandible. A removable plate might be fitted later to the maxillary arch, followed by brackets on the incisors with an archwire designed to provide their controlled retraction.

At the age of 10 years, 10 months, the cervical headgear was fitted. After 8 months, a lip bumper was indeed provided in the mandible. A plate in the maxilla was not found necessary since the premolars and canines had spontaneously migrated distally and the depth of bite had decreased. Brackets were placed on the maxillary incisors and those teeth were retracted with an archwire of .019" × .026" following a .0175" twistflex arch. The retraction was performed with control of axial inclination and combined with some intrusion. At the age of 12 years, 7 months, after treatment of one year and nine months, all apparatus was removed and the maxillary canines were slightly ground incisally to correct their shape and location. Retention was considered unnecessary in view of the solid interdigitation and the normal relationship between the lower lip and the maxillary incisors. The facial improvement was striking even though the mouth still regularly was kept open. The maxillary incisors were a little too steeply positioned and made contact with the mandibular incisors. The crowding in the mandibular incisors had barely changed but the deep bite was eliminated. The alignment of the maxillary canines and one or two other teeth left something to be desired (Figs 18.3 and 18.4).

Two years later, it appeared that some of the shortcomings resulting from the appliances used had corrected spontaneously. Moreover the occlusion of the posterior teeth had been improved by ventral growth of the mandible (Figs 18.5 and 18.6). The records assembled 10 and 15 years after treatment display some minor

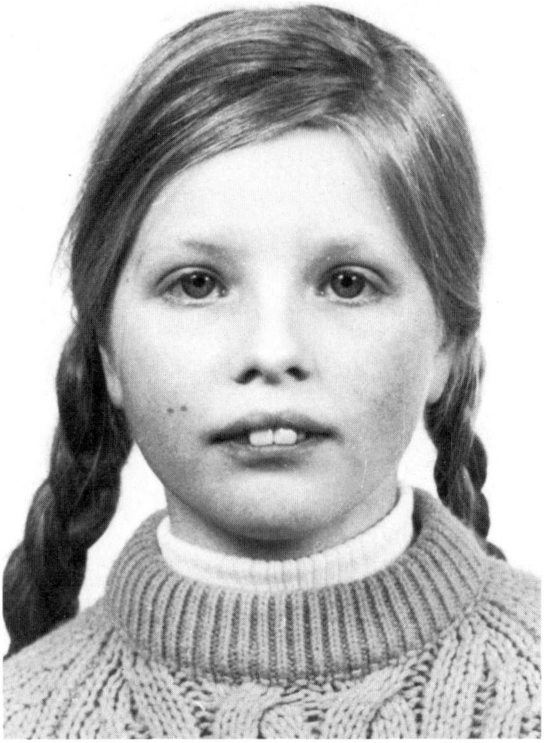

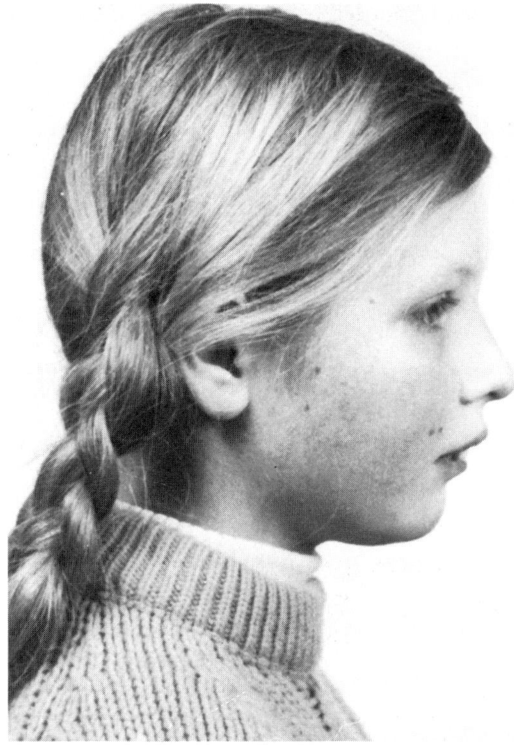

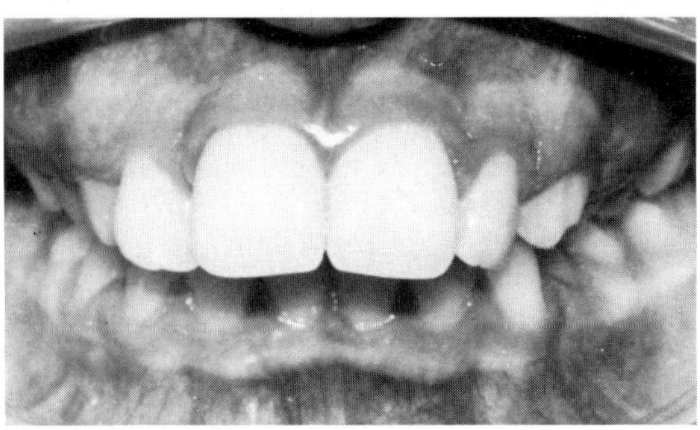

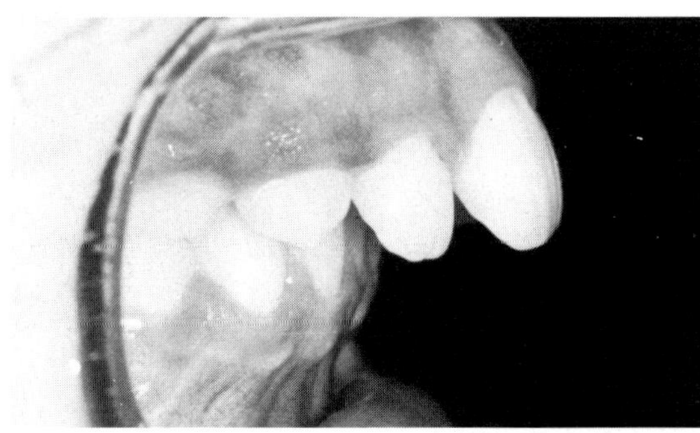

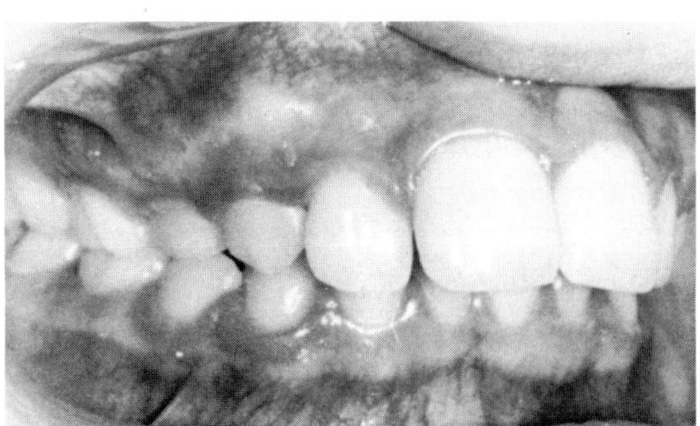

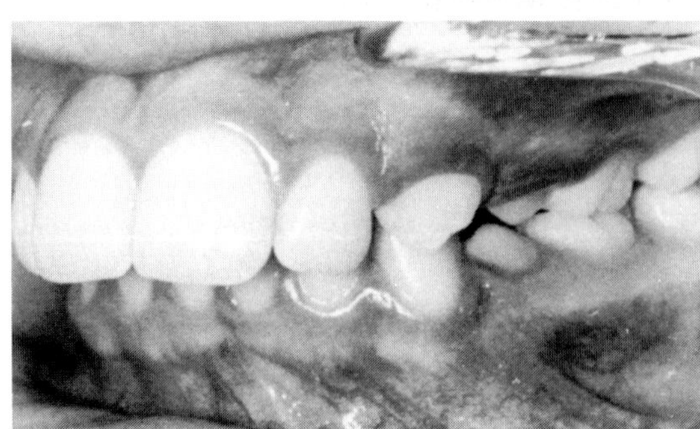

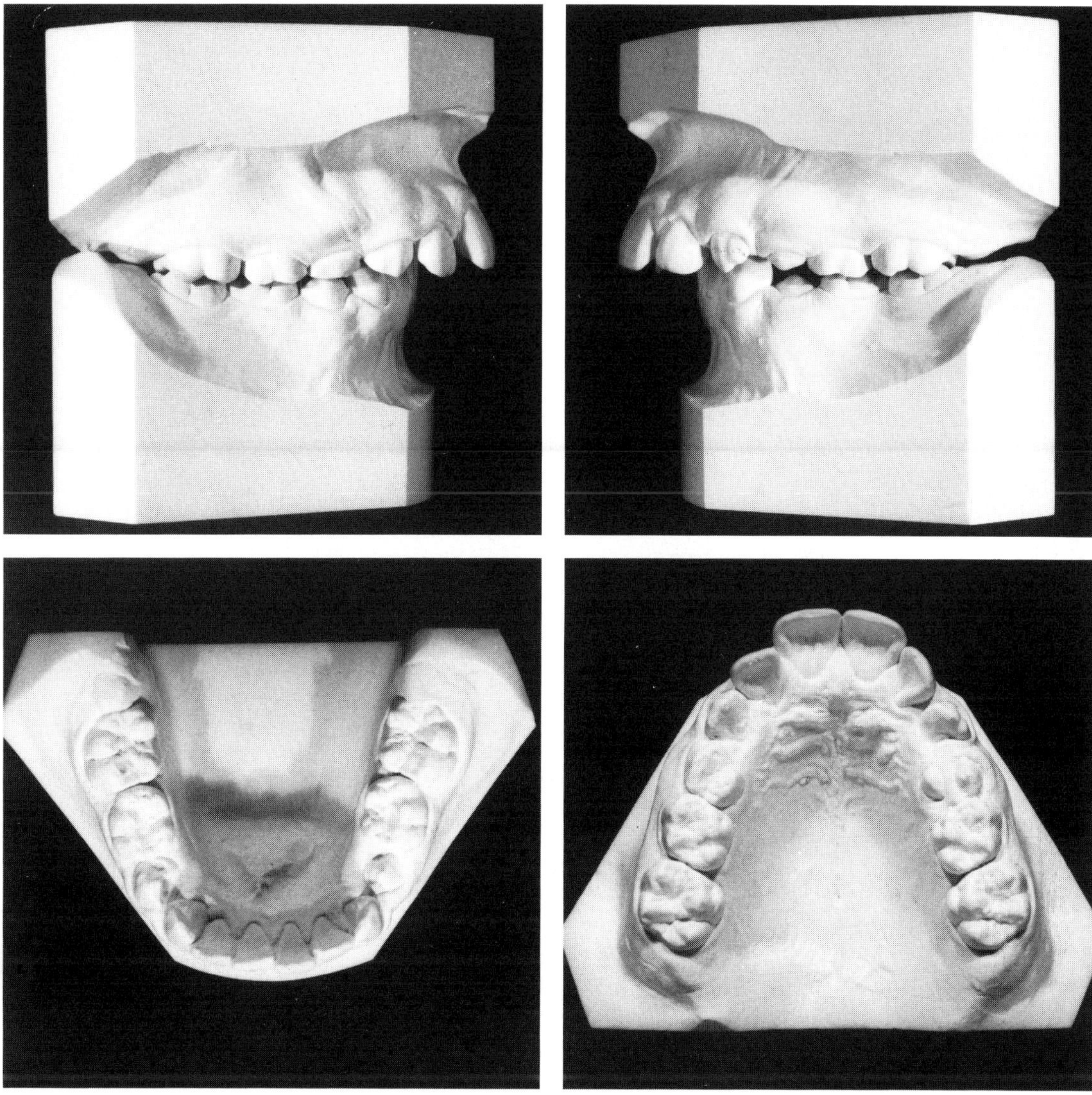

Fig 18-1 and 18-2 A girl of 10 y, 8 mo with a serious class II/1 anomaly of ¾ PW disto-occlusion and inadequate lip seal. The lower lip lies behind the maxillary incisors and is curled over. There is slight crowding in the mandibular anteriors. The second deciduous molars are broad. The maxillary dental arch is pointed, the central incisors are wide and the left canine has emerged rotated. The second deciduous molars are still present as is the maxillary right first deciduous molar. Only the cusps of the maxillary left first premolar have emerged. The gingiva remaining between the cusps indicates that the deciduous molar was lost prematurely. Normally a premolar emerges within the outline of the crown of its predecessor and the overlying mucosa does not need to be perforated. The presence of the second deciduous molars while the second permanent molars have not yet emerged is helpful for treatment.

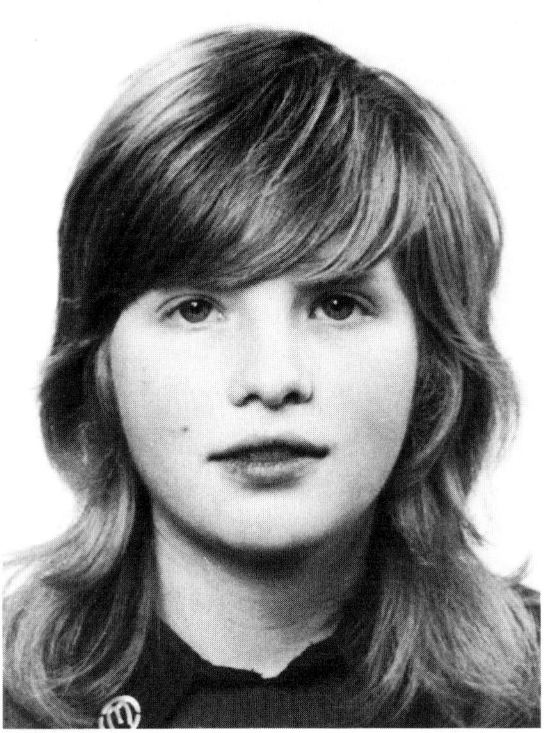

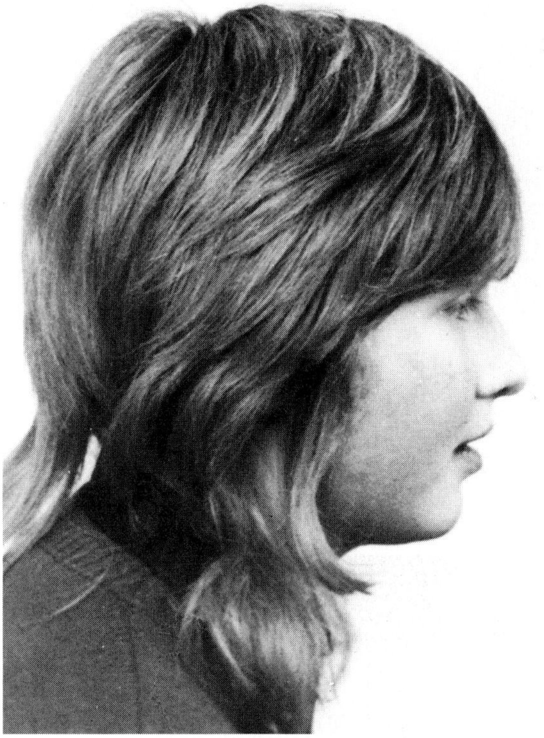

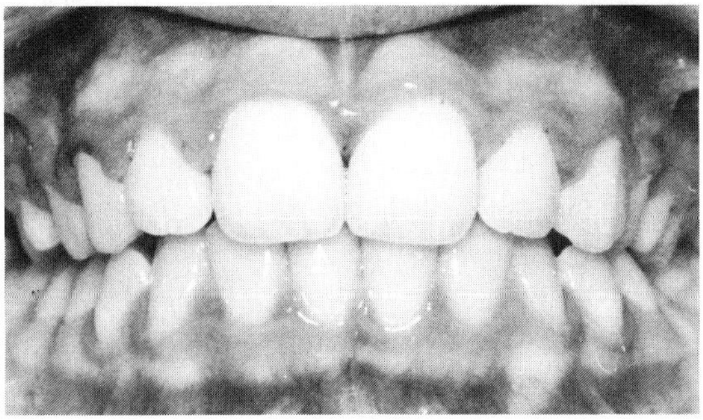

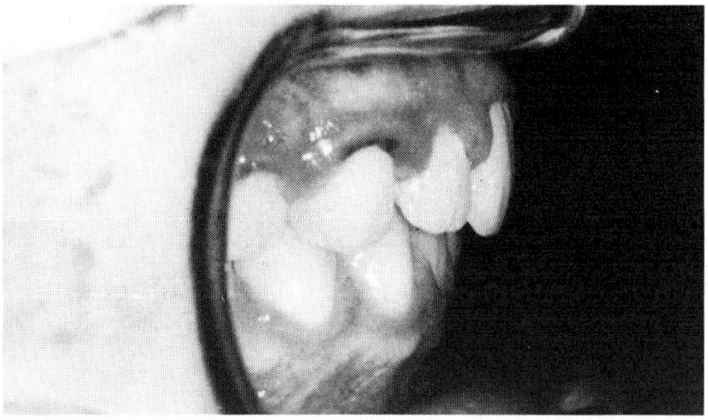

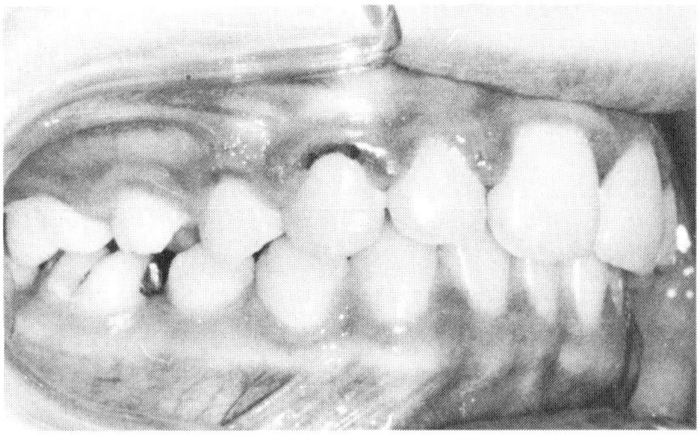

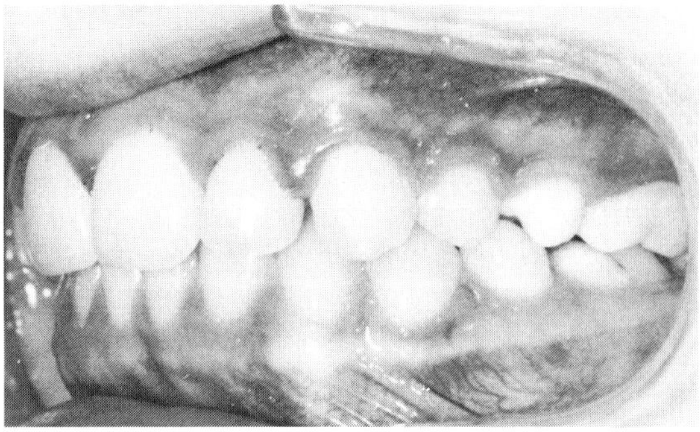

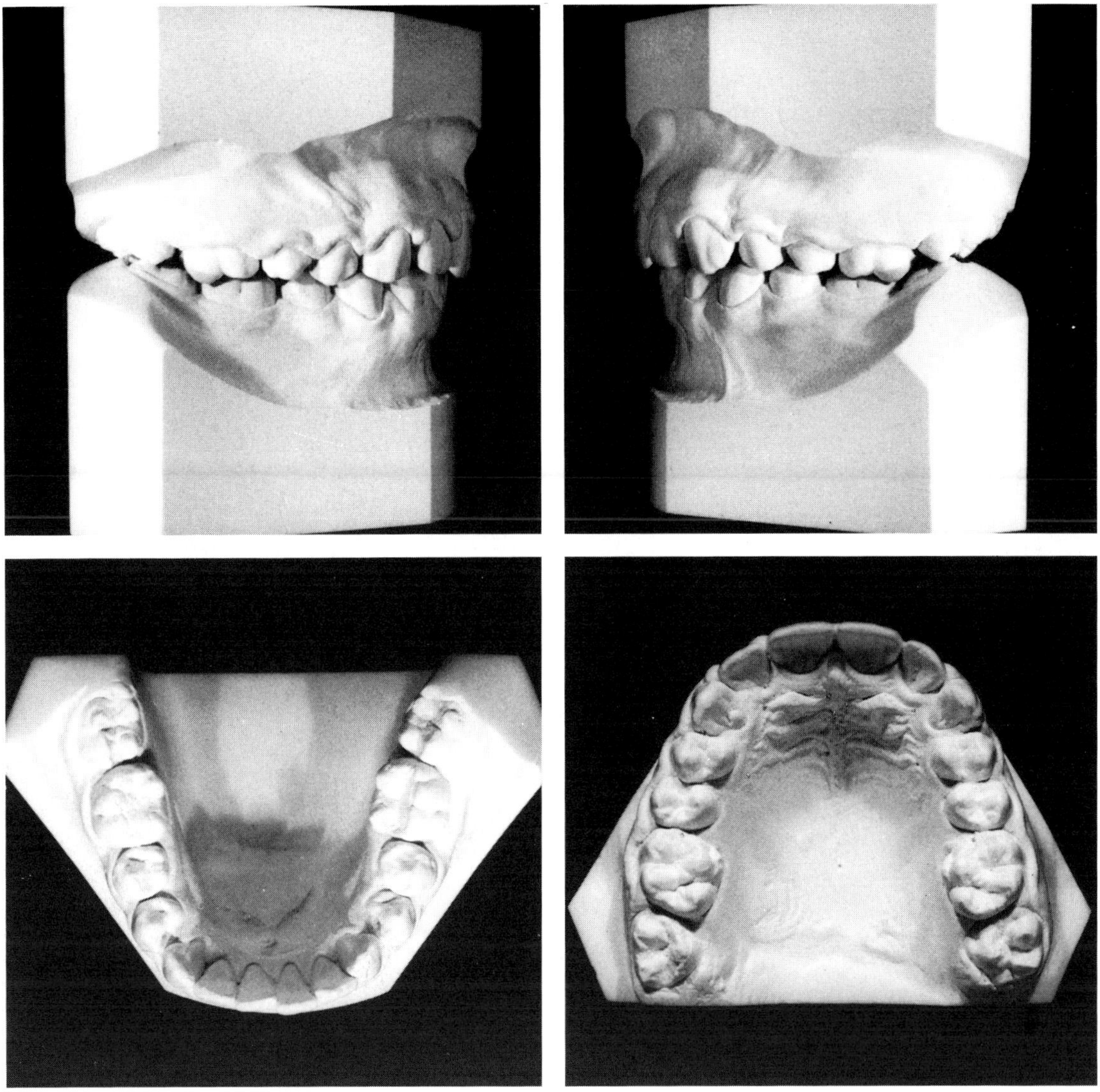

Figs 18-3 and 18-4 At the age of 12 y, 6 mo, the appearance of the patient's face and dentition is quite different. A serious anomaly has been corrected in a short time with simple means. The shortcomings of the appliances are mostly to be seen on the dental casts. The mandibular left first permanent molar has been tilted to lingual by the lip bumper. Such an effect is easily brought about, especially when the mandibular molars are tipped distally. An advantage of this is that the overbite is reduced. The alignment of the mandibular anteriors is not improved. The left maxillary canine is less rotated now than it was shortly after emergence. A limited mesiopalatal rotation of maxillary canines often is acceptable although rotation mesiolabially is not. The same applies to canines that are steeply positioned; it is often judicious not to attempt correction of the situation, the more so because complex appliances are required for uprighting movements and complications are inevitable.

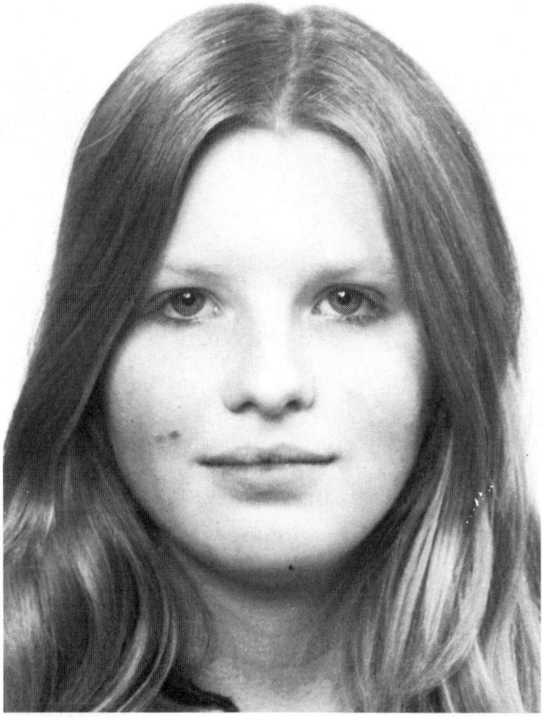

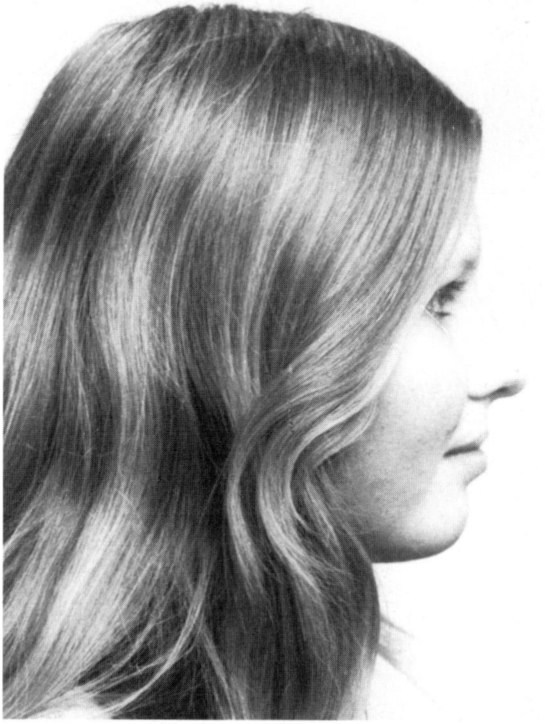

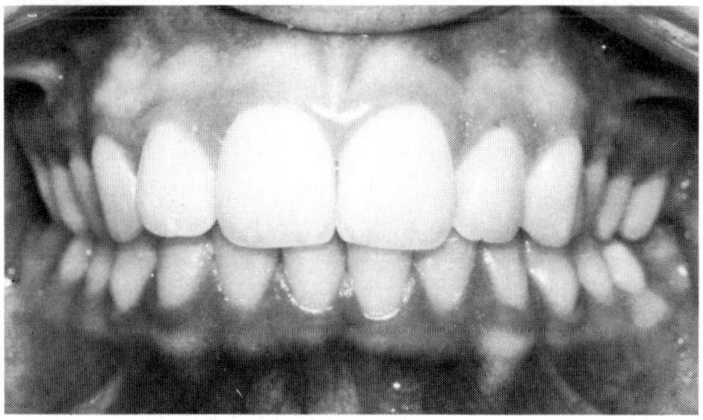

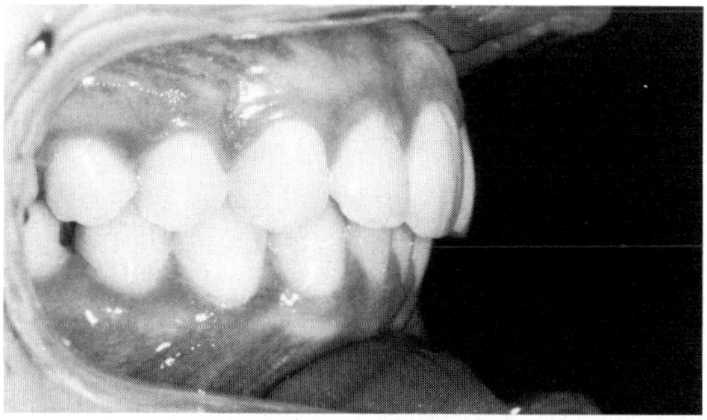

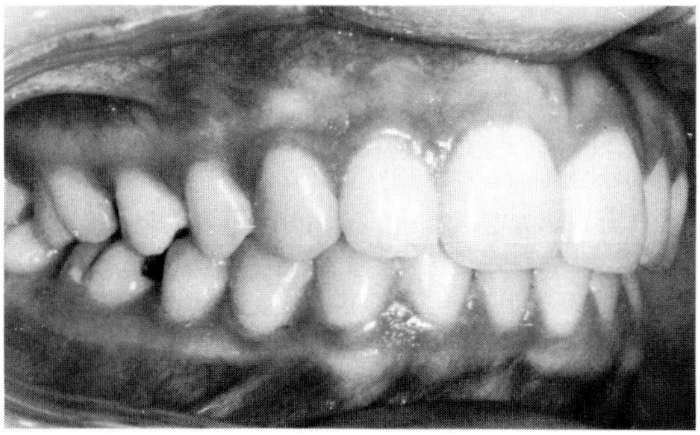

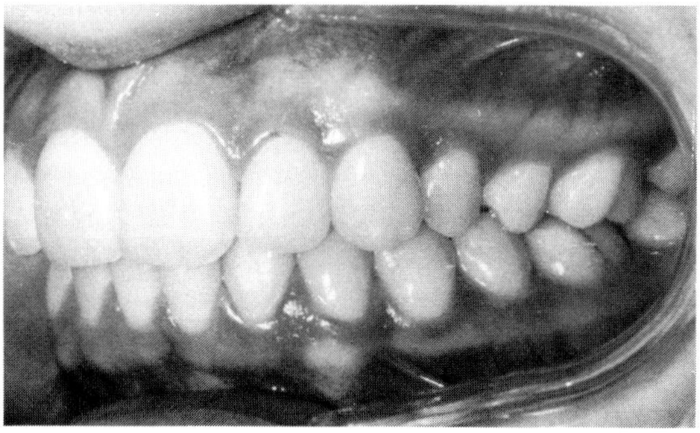

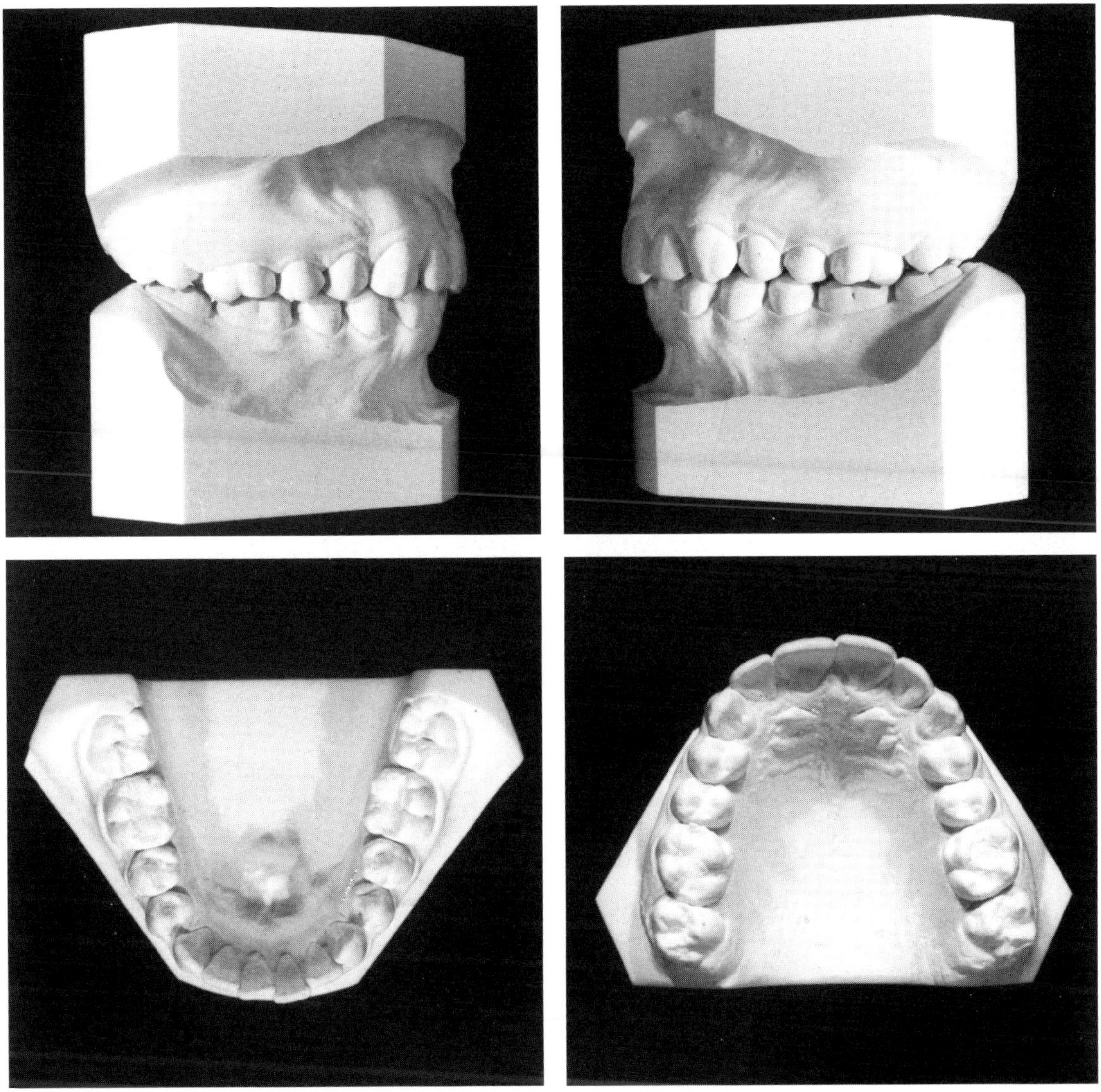

Figs 18-5 and 18-6 *At the age of 14 y, 7 mo, two years after treatment, the iatrogenic deficiencies have corrected themselves in part. The mandibular left first molar has uprighted, is once more in the line of the dental arch, and is in good occlusion. The occlusion overall has improved; premolars and molars have developed better interdigitation and the maxillary and mandibular incisors have tipped slightly to labial. The crowding in the mandibular anteriors has not increased. The mandibular left second molar has come into the arch properly.*

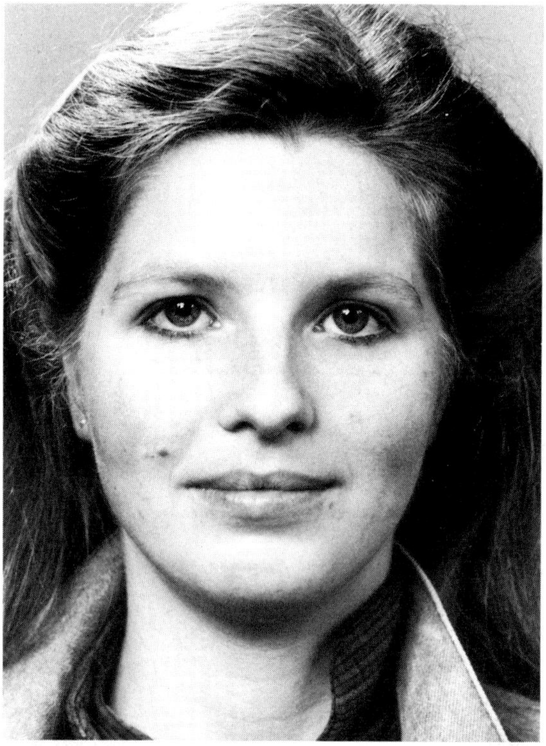

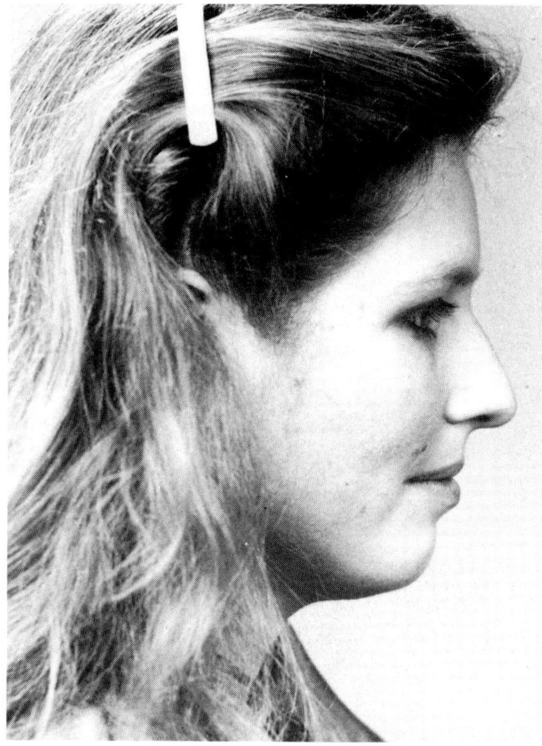

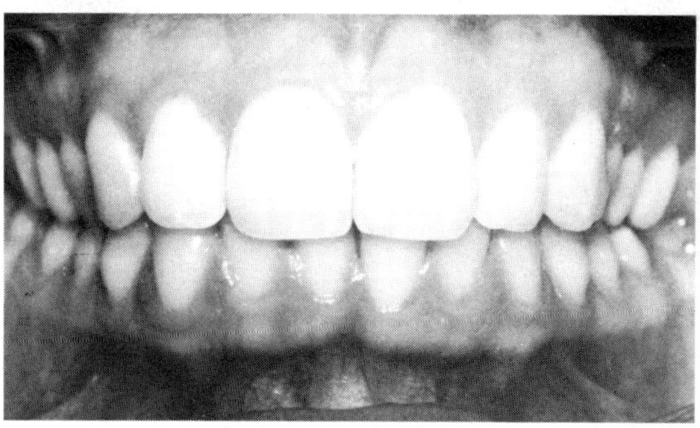

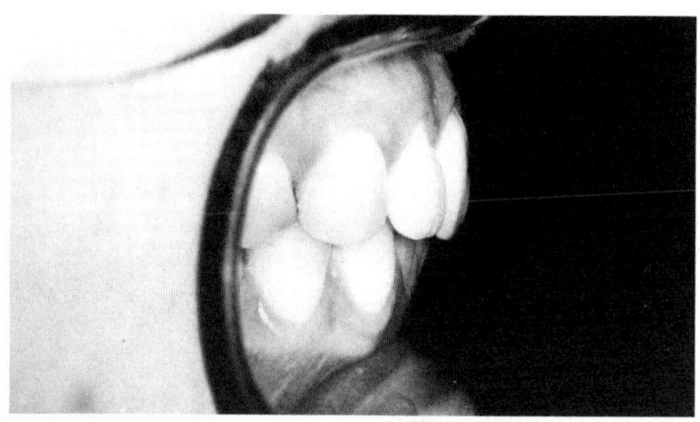

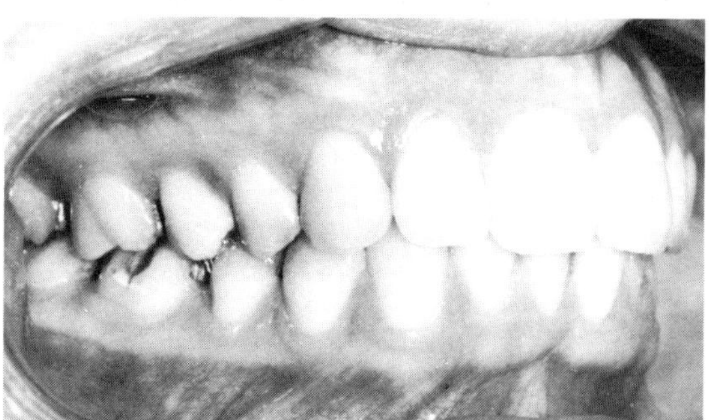

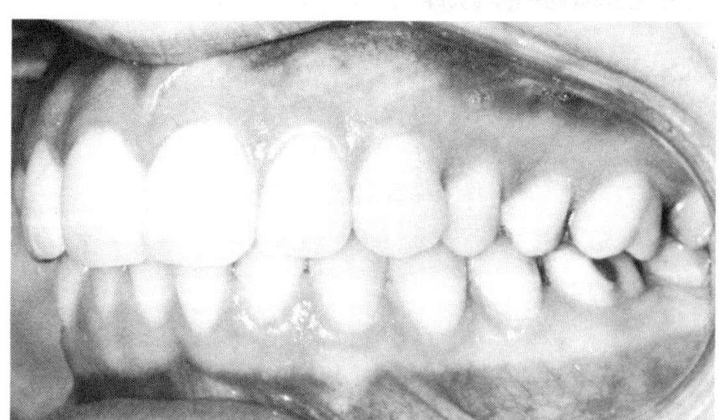

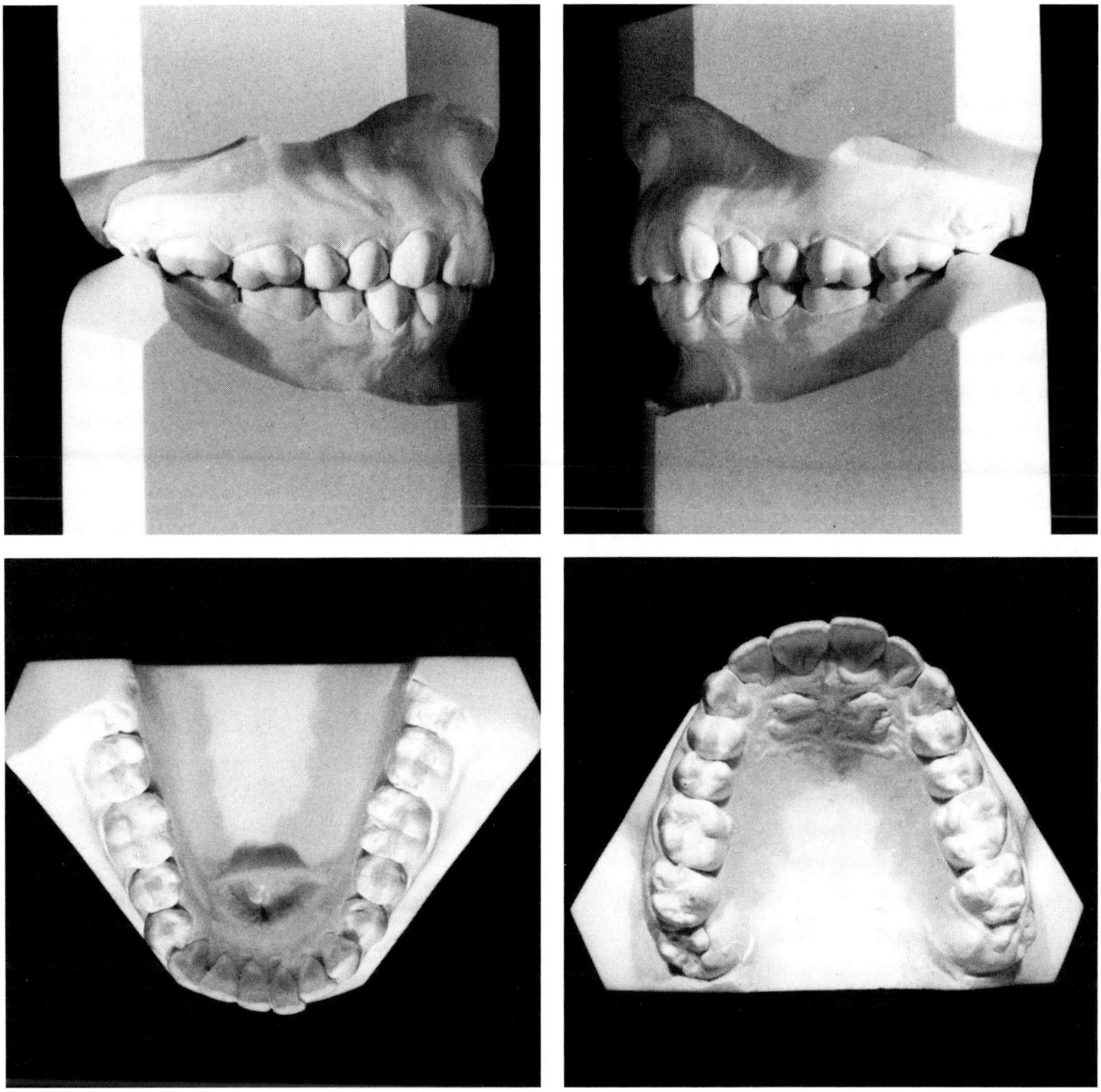

Figs 18-7 and 18-8 At the age of 22 y, 6 mo, ten years after treatment, a harmonious face and fine dentition are seen. The dental casts differ only minimally from those provided five years previously. The room available for the partly emerged third molars is insufficient. Their removal was advised.

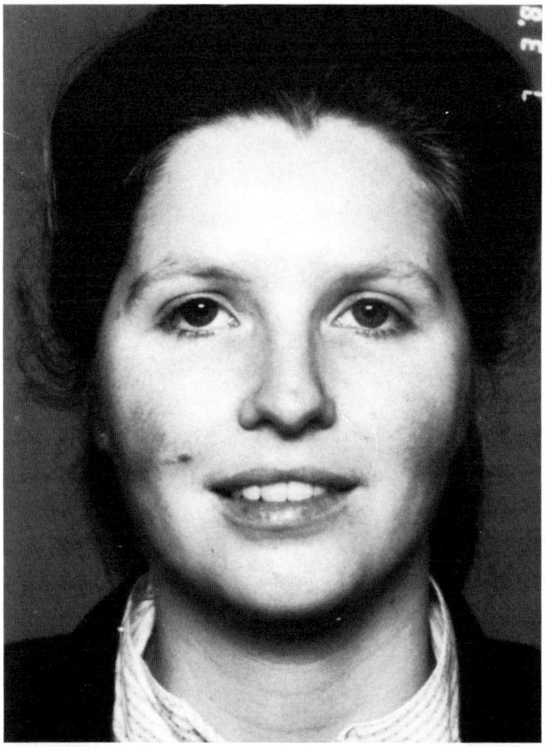

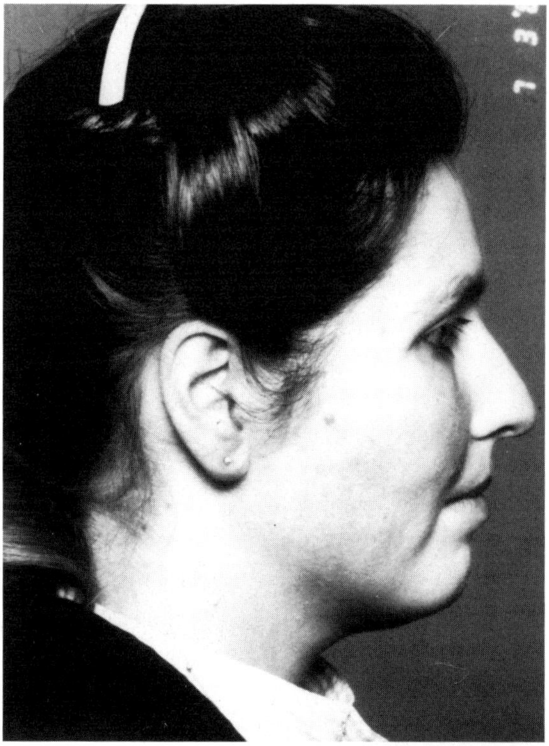

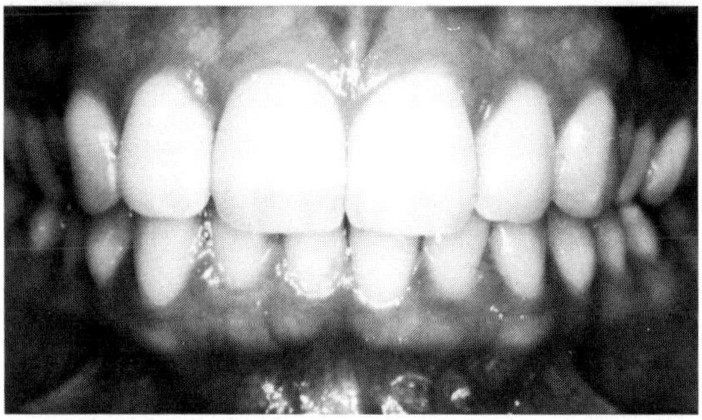

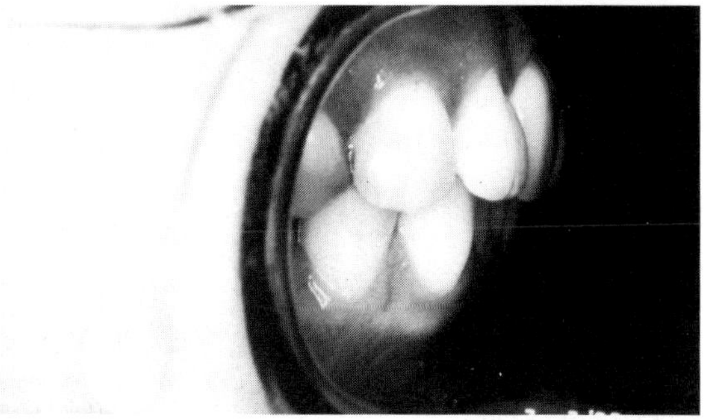

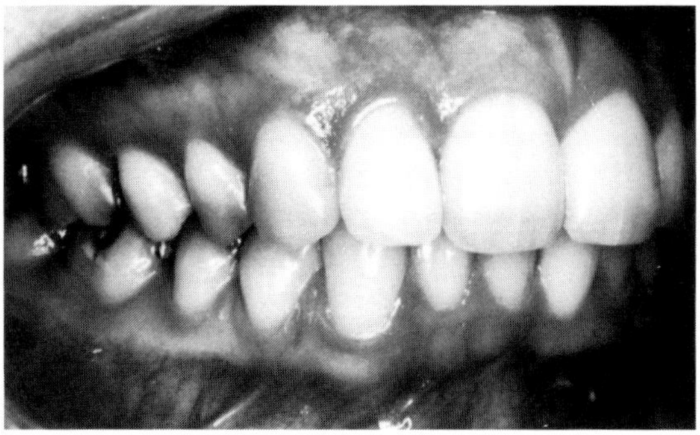

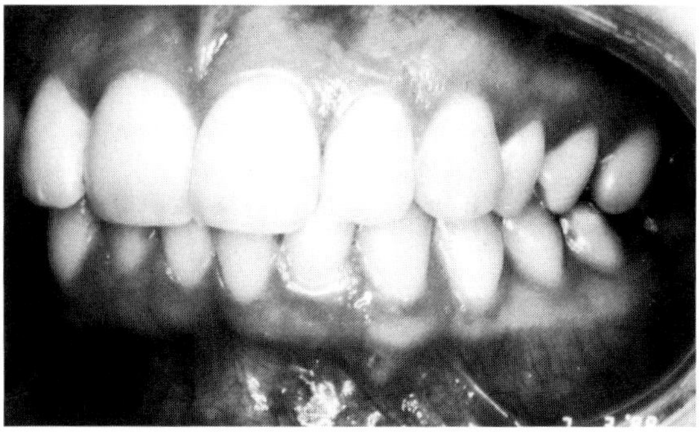

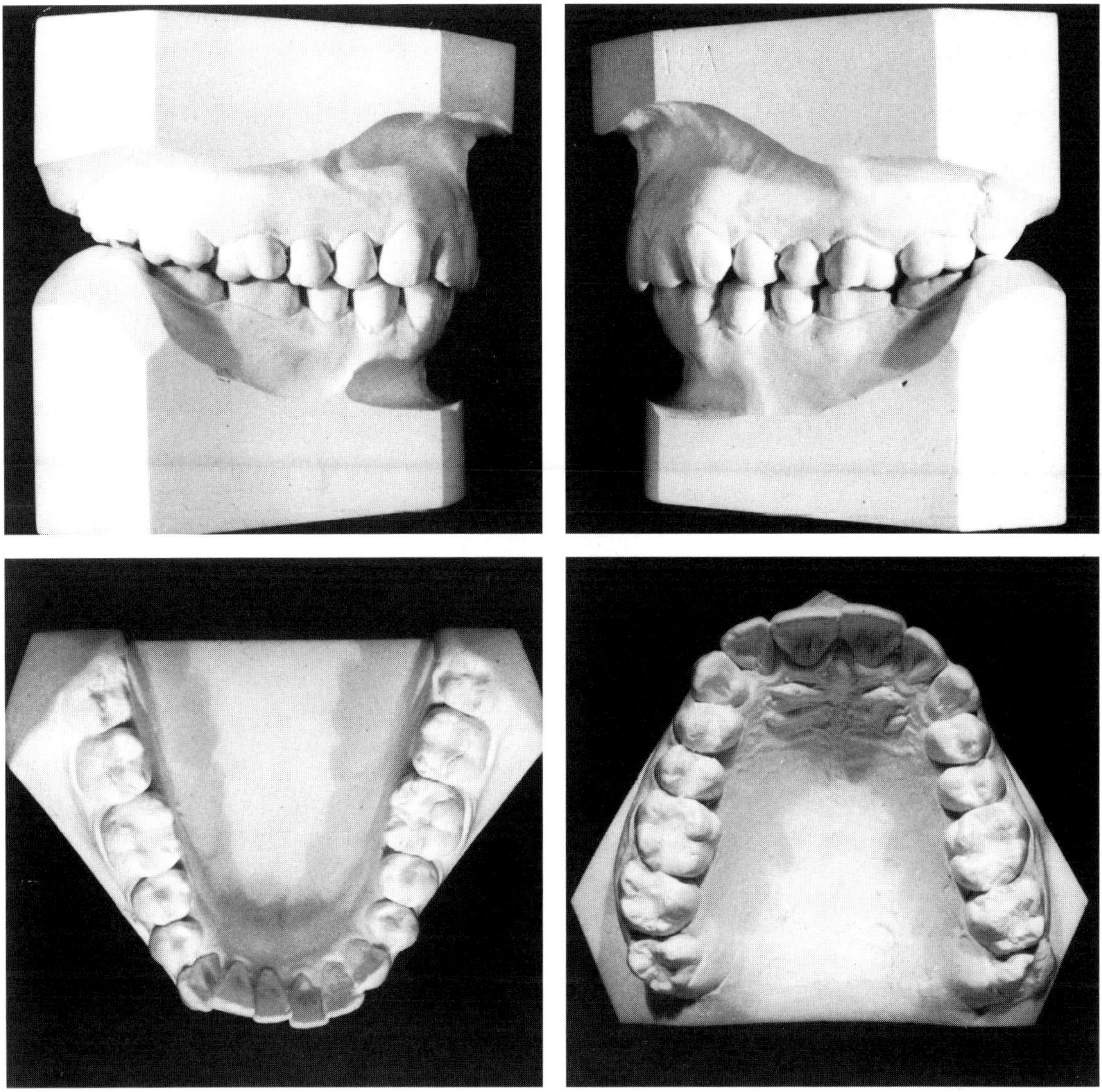

Figs 18-9 and 18-10 *At the age of 27 y, 8 mo, the third molars are still present. Perhaps the development of tertiary crowding in the mandibular anteriors and the minor changes evident in the maxillary anteriors can be attributed to this. For general dental reasons the third molars should have been removed either before emergence or shortly afterwards. Otherwise a good interdigitation exists and the dentition functions satisfactorily.*

Figure 18-11a

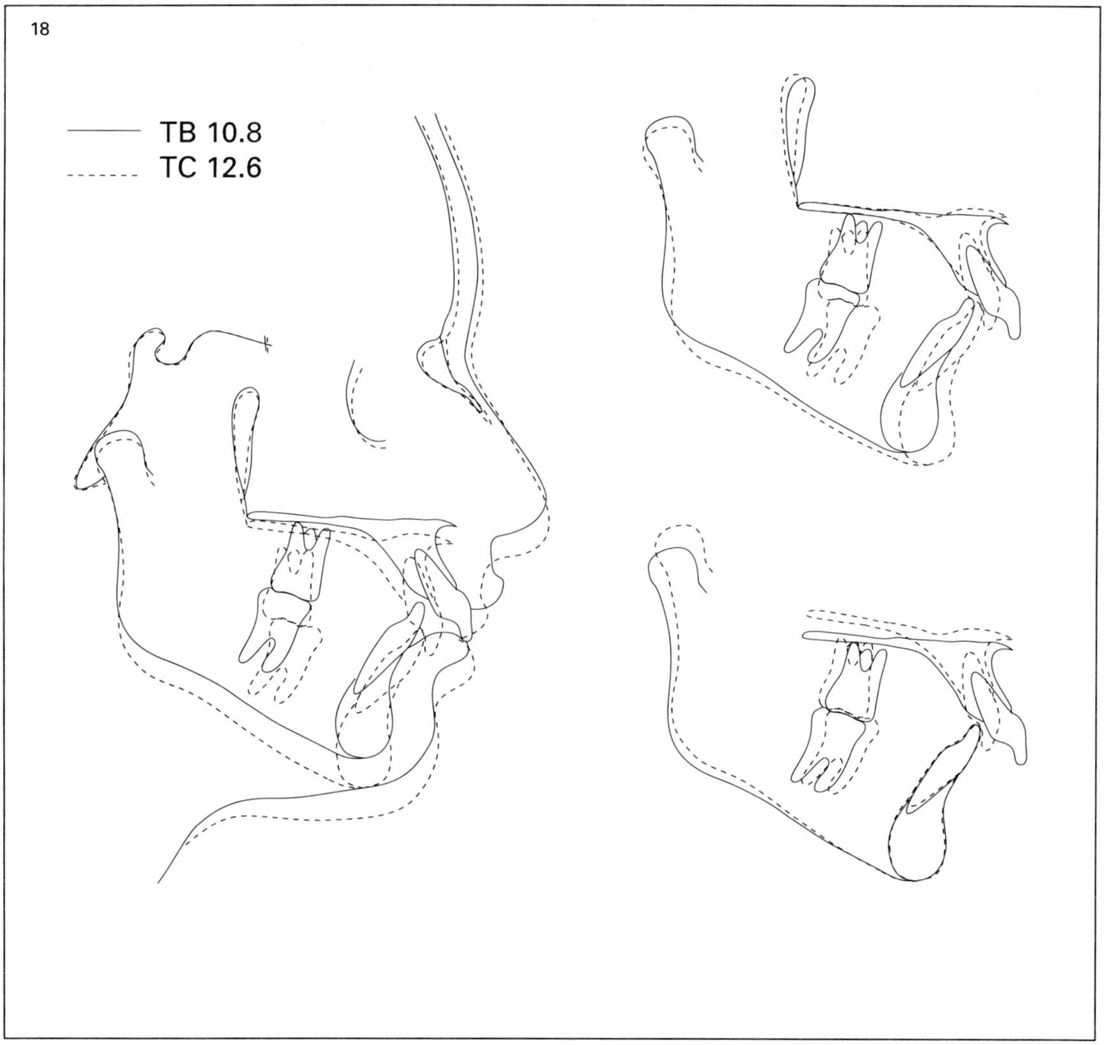

Fig 18-11 Superimposition of the cephalometric tracings shows that the mandible grew little during treatment and that growth was mostly vertical. The improvements devolve principally from the inhibition of the ventral development of the maxilla, the extrusion of the maxillary molars and the retraction of the maxillary incisors.
In the years subsequent to treatment the face continued to grow, also ventrally, and the labio-inclination of the maxillary and mandibular incisors increased.

Figure 18-11b

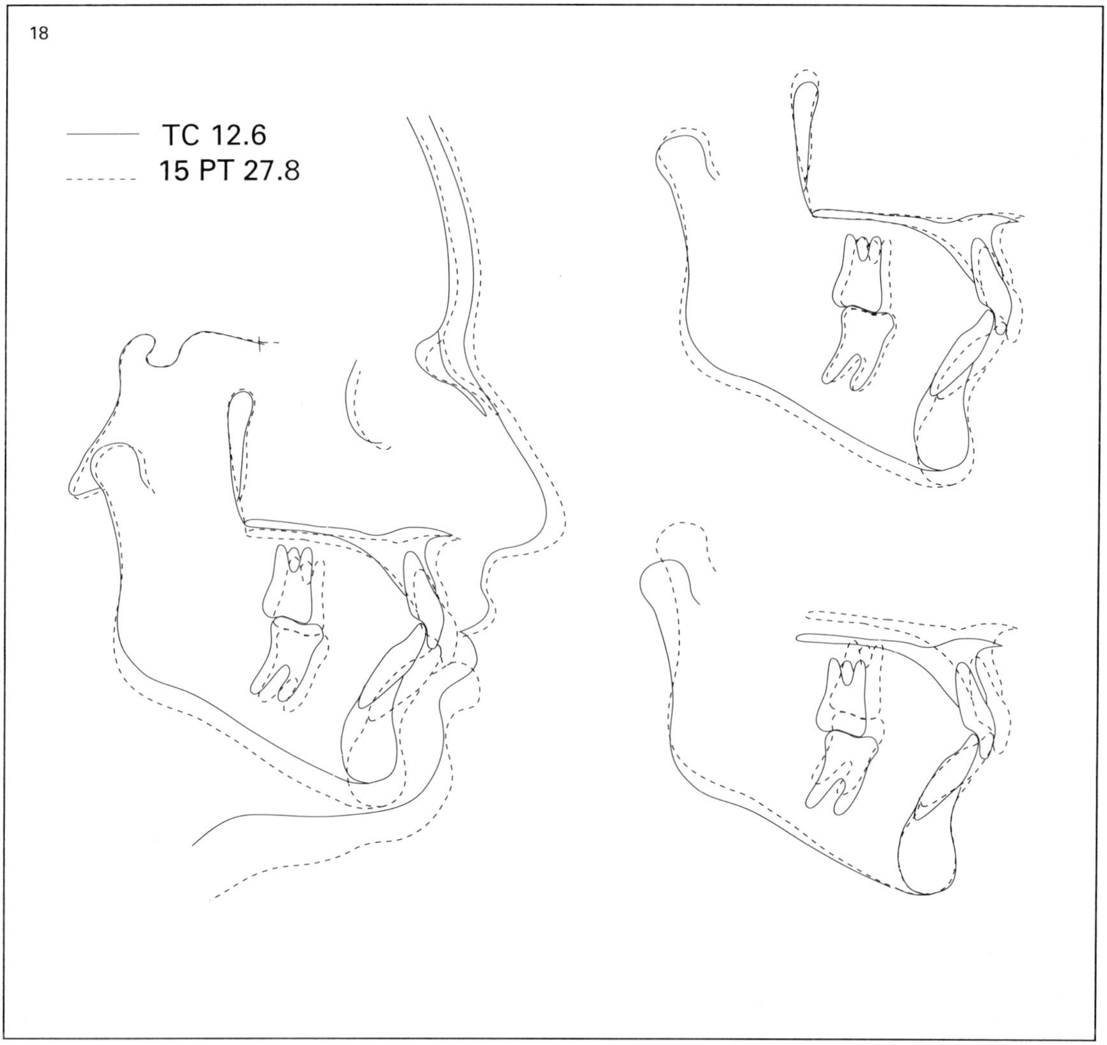

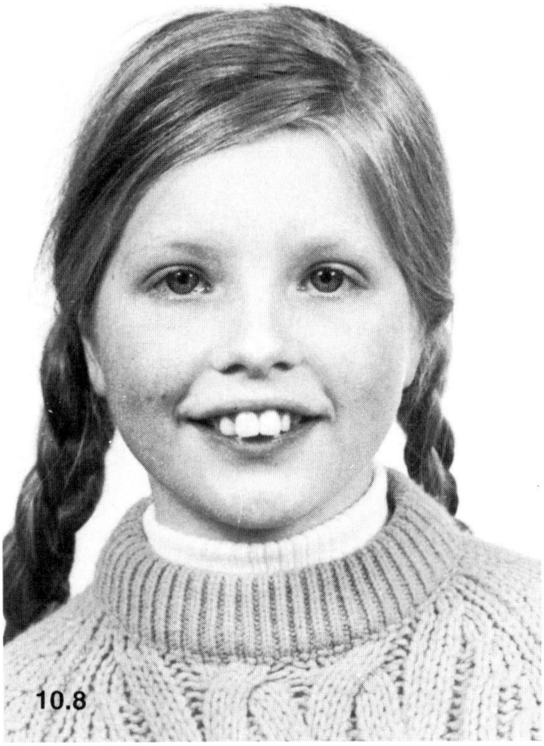
10.8

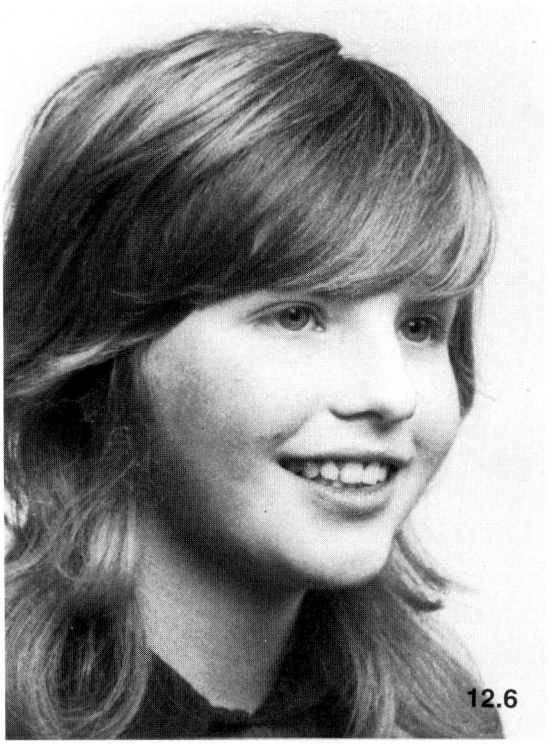
12.6

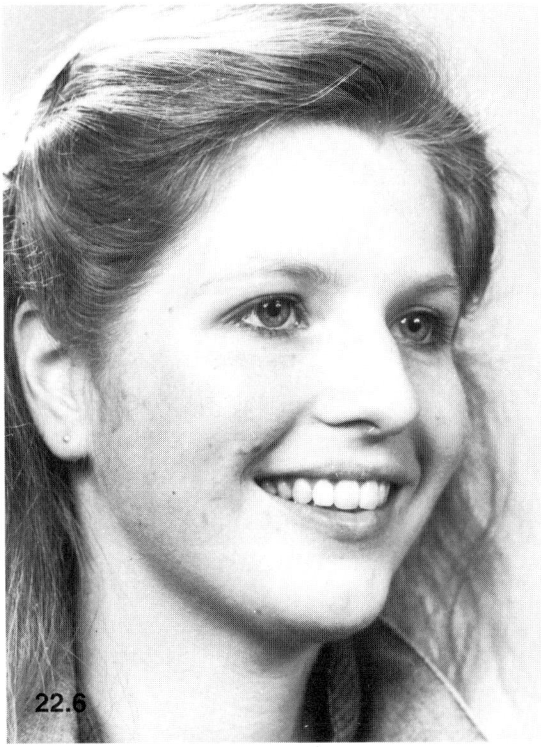
22.6

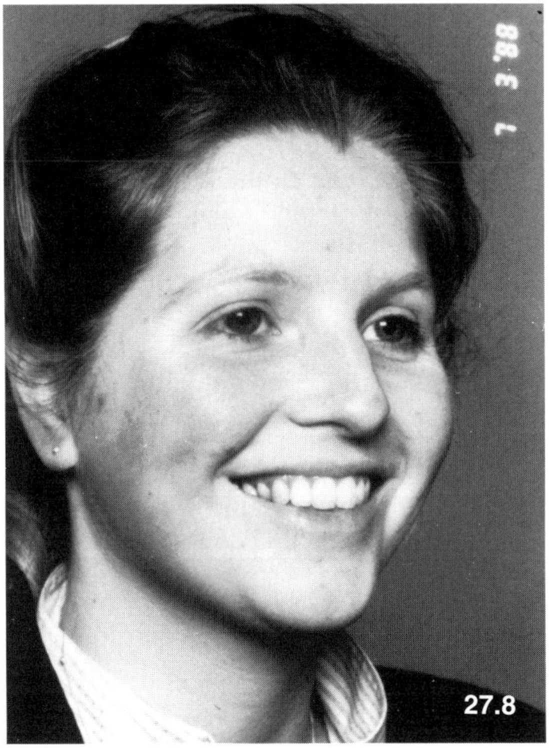
27.8

Fig 18-12 Note the marked changes that arose both in face and dentition during treatment and afterward.

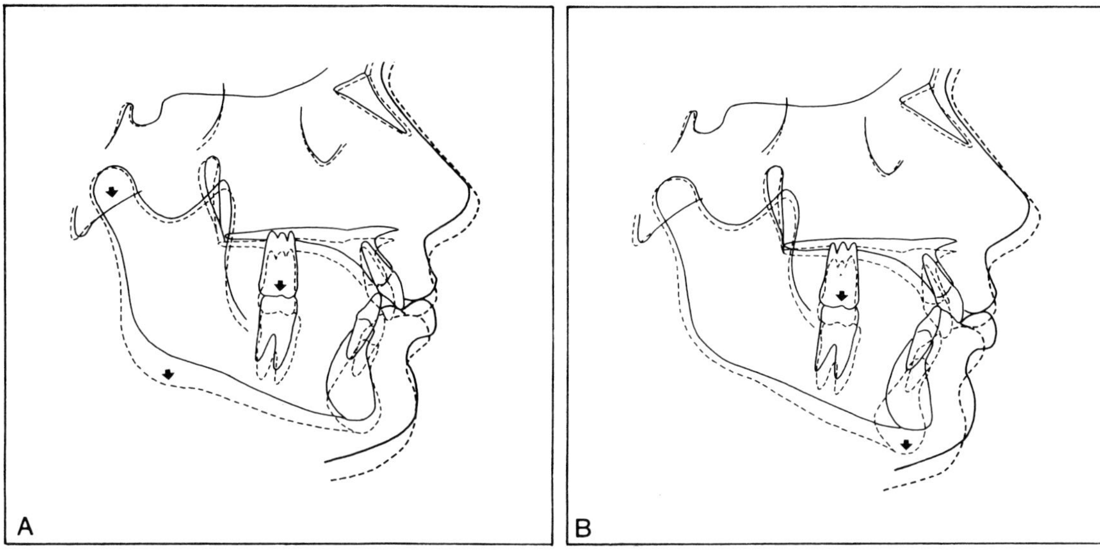

Fig 18-13 Diagrammatic representation of effects of the extrusion of first permanent molars in cervical headgear treatment.
A Extrusion of the maxillary molars stimulates the vertical growth of the condyles so that the ramus height increases more than it otherwise would have done.
B Extrusion of the maxillary molars leads to a backward rotation of the mandible, an increase in the slope of the inferior border of the mandible, a substantial addition to the lower face height and further recession of the chin. This pattern is characteristic of class II/1 anomalies, with an anterior open bite resulting from tongue interposition.[31]

changes (Figs 18.7 to 18.10). The result is satisfying, in both the short and the long term (Fig 18.12).

The superimposition of the cephalometric tracings shows that during treatment only limited mandibular growth took place, and that the improvement was due principally to inhibition of the ventral development of the maxilla and to the retraction of the maxillary incisors. Extrusion of the maxillary molars has contributed substantially to the reduction of the overbite (Fig. 18.11).

This case demonstrates that notable improvement in the end result can be seen after the conclusion of treatment. Molars and premolars that are moved to abnormal positions by means of the appliances can subsequently assume normal positions under the influence of the occlusion and the tongue and cheek musculature. Above all, with a solid interdigitation, the breadth of the maxillary dental arch is regulated by that of the mandibular dental arch when the latter moves mesially. In those circumstances, the mandibular teeth do indeed move into occlusion slightly more buccally.[27] If a solid interdigitation is absent in a particular zone, then the coordination between the antagonists will be lacking too, so opposing teeth will take up their positions independently of one another as demonstrated in the previous chapter.

If a cervical headgear is used, an extruding force is applied to the anchor molars with the advantage that this keeps the molars in occlusion. That is not the case when a parietal headgear is used. It has been suggested that the extrusive effect of a cervical headgear would lead to an increase in the height of the lower face that otherwise would not have occurred and especially not when a parietal headgear is used. Investigation of patients with a class II/1 anomaly and solid interdigitation who were treated with a cervical headgear did indeed show more increase of the lower face height than in a control group that received no treatment. The average picture corresponded with that in Figure 18.11. In the subsequent five years the treated group showed development that was directed ventrally for the most part, with only slight vertical development. Over the whole period of the investigation neither the lower face height nor the slope of the inferior border of the mandible showed a significant difference between the two groups.[16] These findings link with the research of Baumrind and his co-workers which indicated that in cervical headgear therapy the mandibular ramus grew more in length than when nothing or another form of therapy was used.[1] The extrusion of the maxillary molars probably stimulates the growth of the condyles, which following treatment is compensated for by growth directed more ventrally. However, class II/1 anomalies with an anterior open bite caused by tongue interposition do react somewhat differently to cervical headgear therapy. The lower border of the mandible slopes more steeply and the lower face height shows an increase that is not compensated for subsequently (Fig 18.13).

A number of remarks about lip bumpers have already been made in Chapter 11. In connection with this case, the following could be added. Lip bumpers that lie low in the vestibule exert not only a distal-driving but also a distally tipping force on the anchor molars. Such placement of the lip bumper is sometimes attempted to overcome excessive activity of the mentalis muscle (mentalis habit). Tipping the molars distally has the effect of opening the bite, especially when lip bumpers are fitted in both jaws. The effect is increased when elastics are placed vertically between hooks at the canine regions of each lip bumper. Not only is the bite opened anteriorly through the tipping distally of the first molars, but significantly more space is created in both arches.

Another effect of the lip bumper is that the mandibular left anchor molar has been tipped to lingual. Apparently there was inadequate checking of the breadth of the appliance in the molar region. It is not quite clear why this had no effect on the right side. In any case, the situation corrected itself eventually.

It is not advisable to fit brackets to canines unless adequate training in the use of full fixed appliances has been obtained. It seems a simple matter to provide brackets on the canines alongside the incisors. The wish to do so depends mostly on the need for the canine root to be tipped distally at its apex because it otherwise is too steeply oriented or even placed with the apex to mesial. Uprighting canines with a continuous archwire is likely to lead to elongation of the incisors, which is usually not desired. Steeply positioned canines are seldom ugly, certainly not when they are lightly ground as necessary (see Fig 19.5, page 317), something that also is indicated if they are too long relative to the incisors. Rotations of canines can be corrected by bonding a button onto the buccal surface and wearing an elastic between it and a suitable hook on a removable plate. Then the acrylic against the palatal of the canine should be ground to encourage the tooth to rotate. It should be noted that corrected rotations of canines have a great tendency to relapse. Fortunately it is possible to camouflage much by judicious grinding and altering contours with composite resins.

Chapter 19

Class II/1, scissorbite 14, 24, and 25

Cervical headgear, later with Kahn spur, maxillary removable plate, brackets 12, 11, 21 and 22, mandibular lingual arch with auxiliary springs Male 11 years, 7 months to 24 years, 8 months

A boy aged 11 years, 7 months, had a class II/1 anomaly with ½ PW disto-occlusion. Except for the disto-relation, his face was harmonious in form. Despite having a clear nasal airway he held his mouth open. Consequently his lower lip lay against the incisal edges of the maxillary anteriors, which were positioned too far to labial. He had sucked his thumb until the age of eight years. There was adequate space in the mandibular and the maxillary dental arches (ALD +1 and +2 mm, respectively) and the overjet was 6 mm. The mandibular incisors contacted the palatal mucosa. The mandibular dental arch was narrow; in the maxilla both first premolars and the left second premolar were in scissorbite (Figs 19.1 and 19.2).

It was decided to correct the disto-relation with a cervical headgear and to use a removable maxillary plate and a mandibular lingual arch to eliminate the scissorbite. A partial fixed appliance on the maxillary incisors would be used later as required if their correction were needed.

The cervical headgear was fitted at the age of 11 years, 9 months. Two months later the lingual arch and the plate were provided. The lingual arch was furnished with auxiliary springs to move the mandibular left first and second premolars and the right first premolar to buccal. The maxillary plate was provided with an anterior biteplane and springs that ran to buccal across the embrasures mesial to the first permanent molars, placing pressure on the buccal surfaces of the right first premolar and both the premolars on the left. On the left the spring was bent backward parallel to itself from the level of the mesial of the first premolar. Only the recursive portion of the horizontal loop was in contact with both the premolars. In this manner, it was possible to obtain a flexible spring that applied a gentle force to the premolars. Of course, the margin of the plate was trimmed away palatally where necessary to permit the teeth to move palatally. The biteplane was of such a thickness that the transverse movement of the premolars was not impeded by their antagonists.

After correction of the scissorbite, the biteplane was reduced in thickness to permit the cone-funnel mechanism to operate. Divided labial arches were added emerging distally to the canines and were used to retract the maxillary incisors and close the diastemata.

One year after the commencement of treatment, the disto-occlusion was largely eliminated and the remaining corrections had almost been achieved. The maxillary

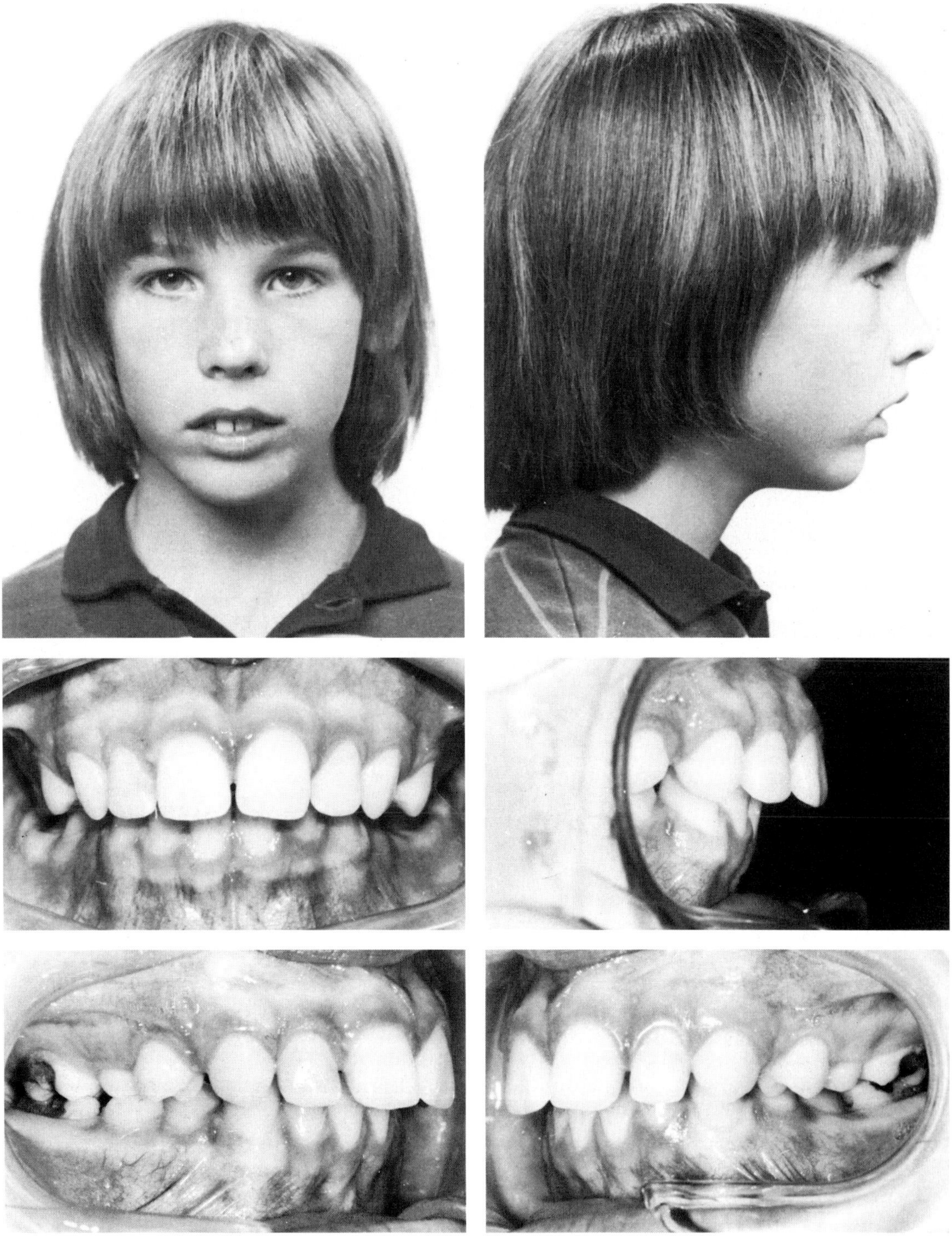

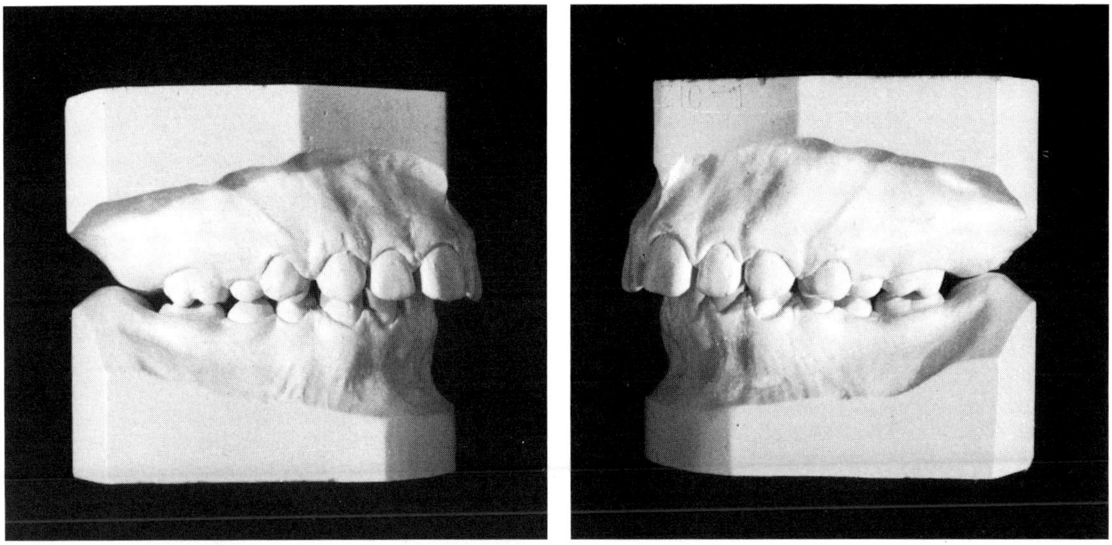

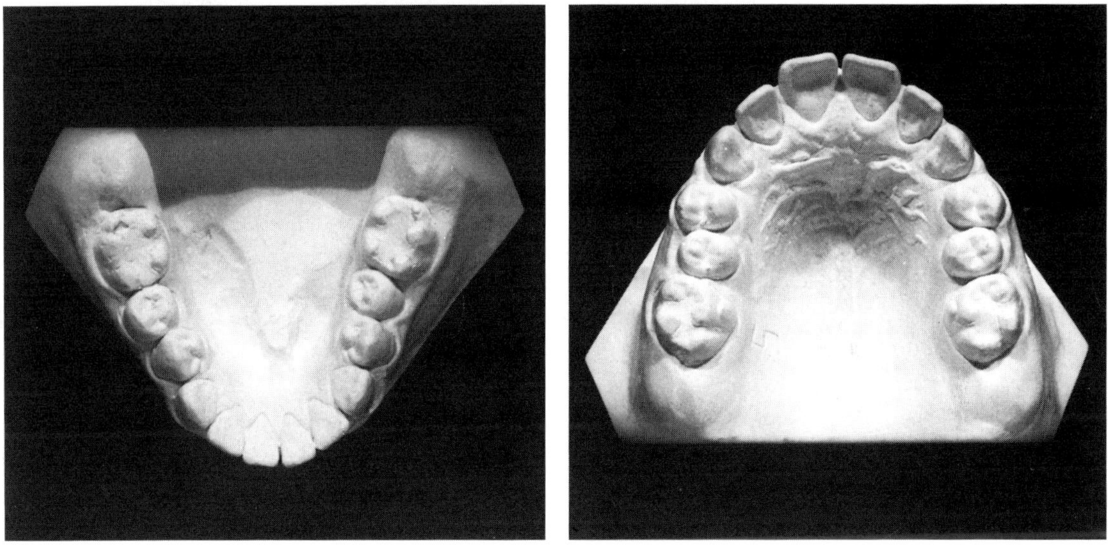

Figs 19-1 and 19-2 *A boy aged 11 y, 7 mo with a disto-relation. The lower lip lies against the incisal edge of the maxillary incisors. The upper lip is short, the lower lip curled over. There are no other functional aberrations. The disto-occlusion is of ½ PW. The maxillary anteriors are mildly labioverted, with spacing between them all. All maxillary premolars, except the second on the right, are in scissorbite and are tipped to buccal; their antagonists are tipped lingually. The second permanent molars have not yet emerged. The room available for them seems adequate as can be estimated in the maxilla from the distances from the distal surfaces of the first molars to the dorsal margins of the maxillary tuberosities.*

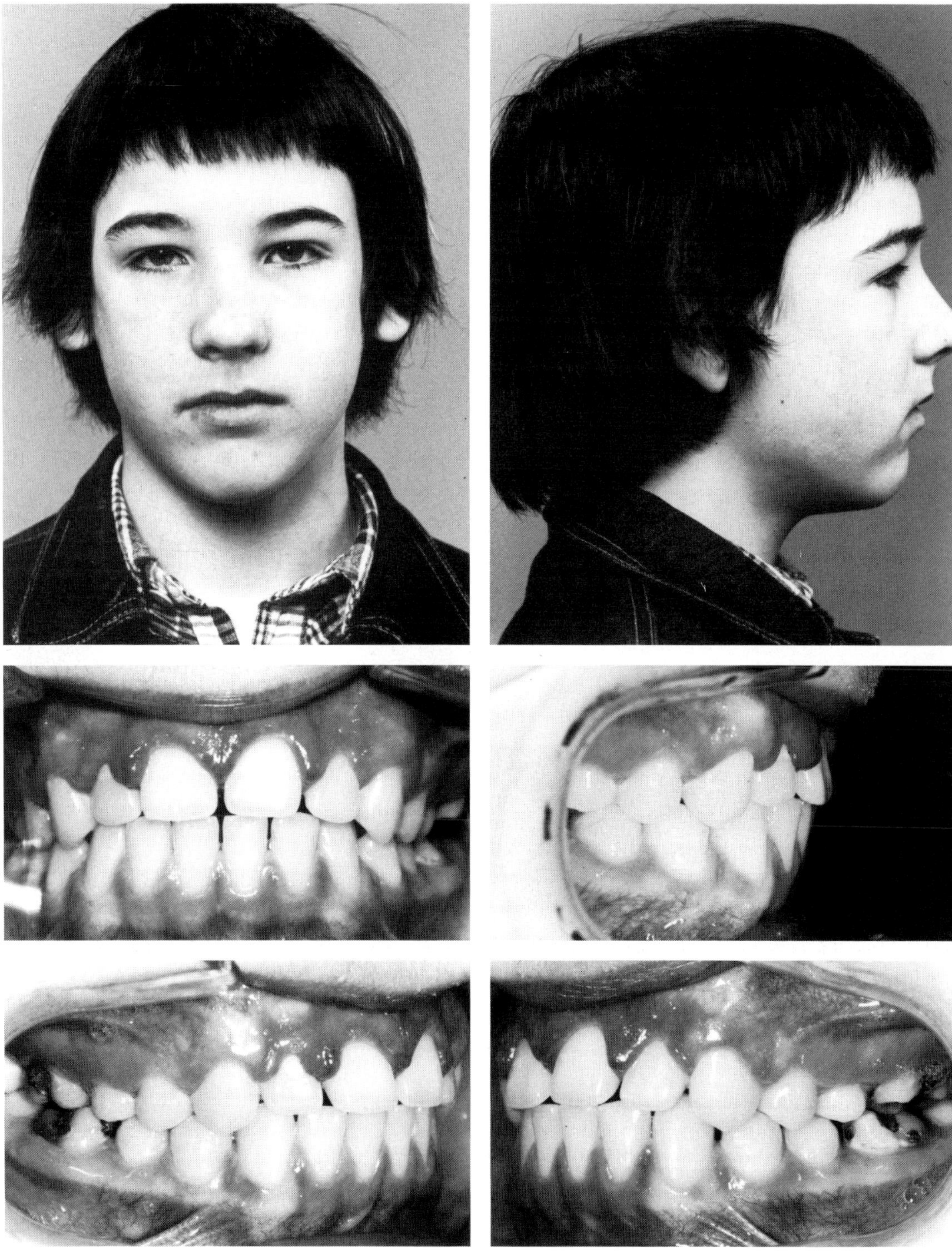

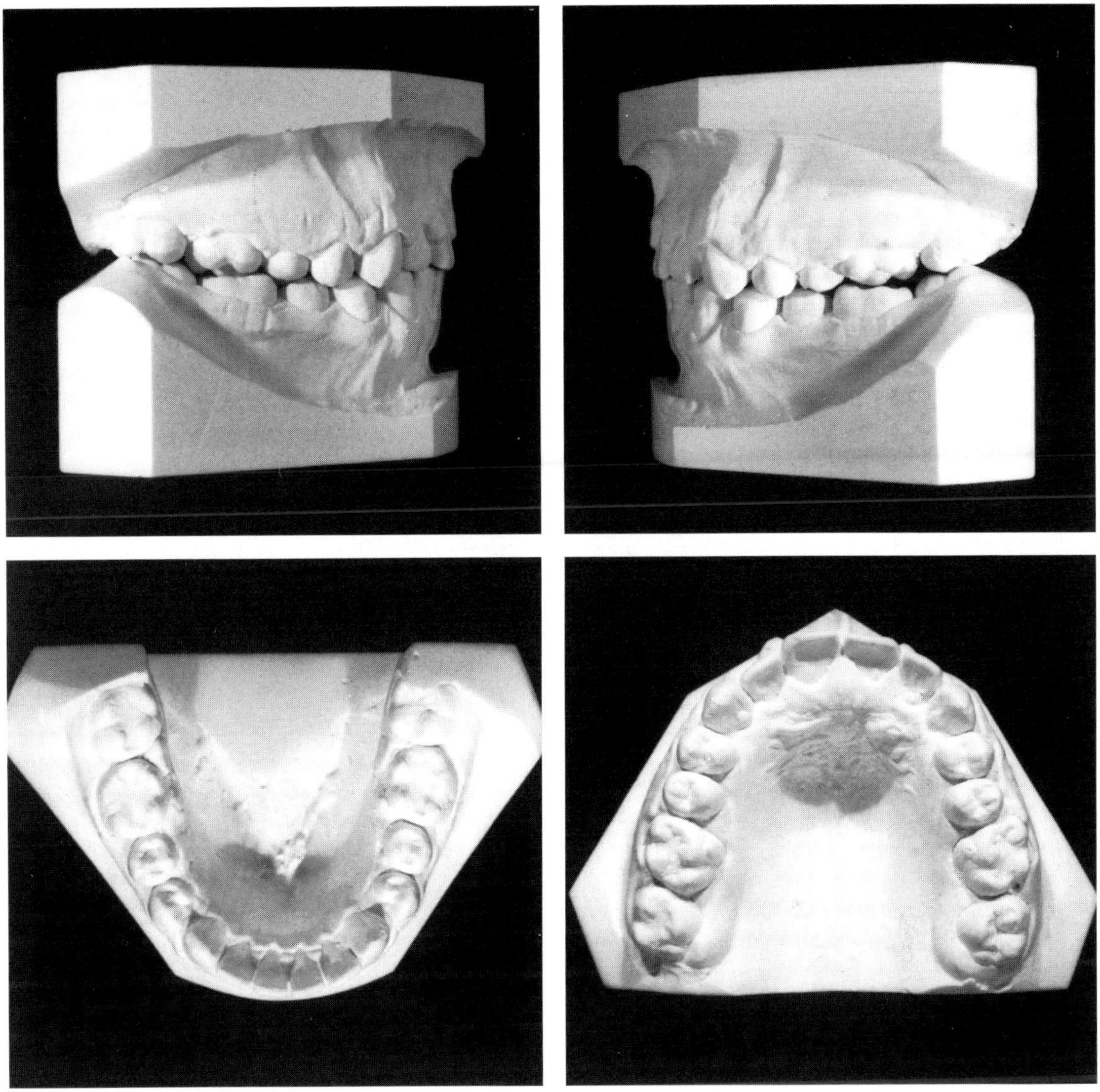

Figs 19-3 and 19-4 *At the age of 14 y, 10 mo, the treatment that had lasted 3½ years was concluded. The scissorbites had been eliminated, principally by increasing the breadth of the mandibular dental arch in the premolar regions. The maxillary incisors have been intruded and are positioned more to cranial than the canines. The first permanent molars do not occlude fully. In addition, the maxillary left first permanent molar is in buccoposition while the mandibular left first molar is in endoposition, something that is attributable to the use of the cervical headgear with a Kahn spur.*

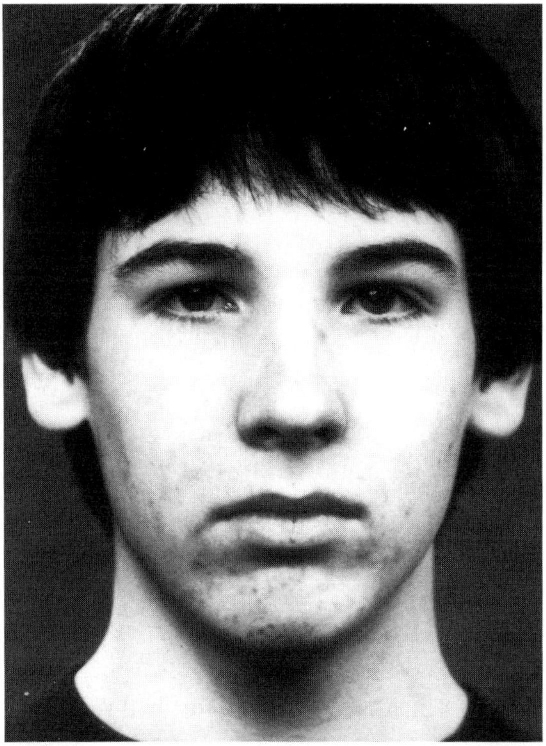
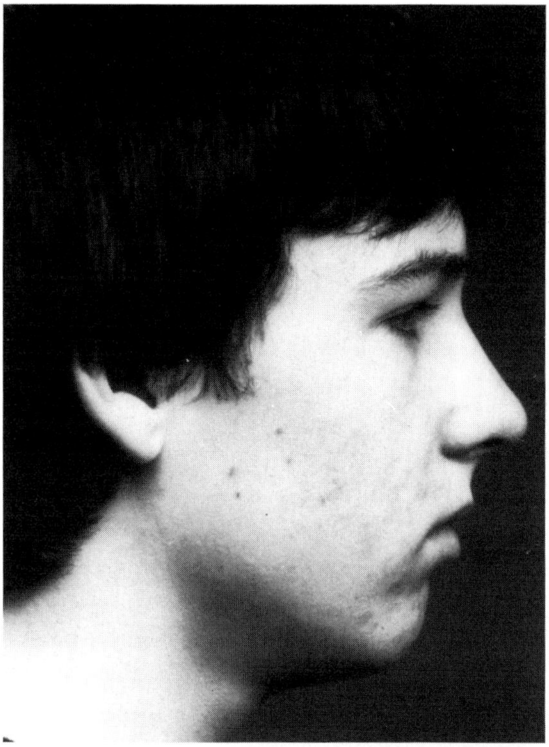
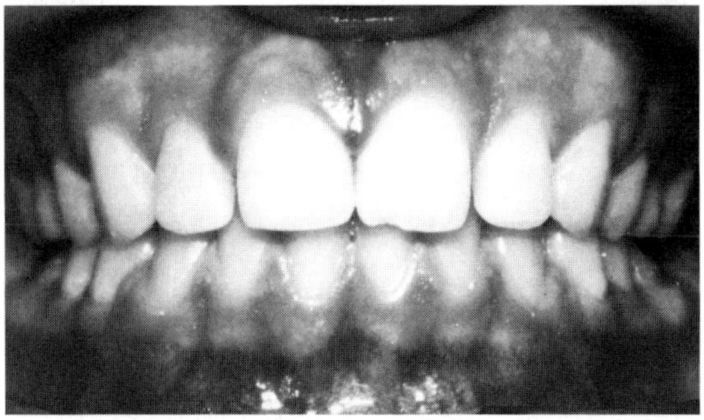
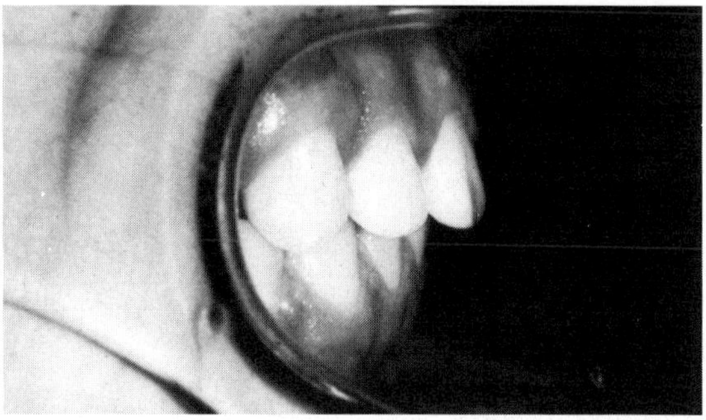
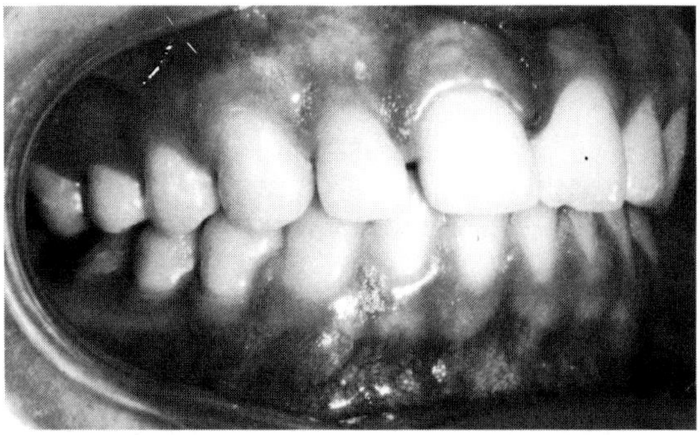
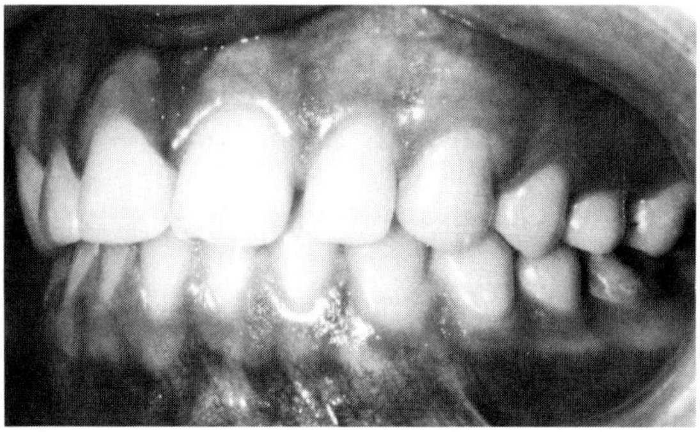

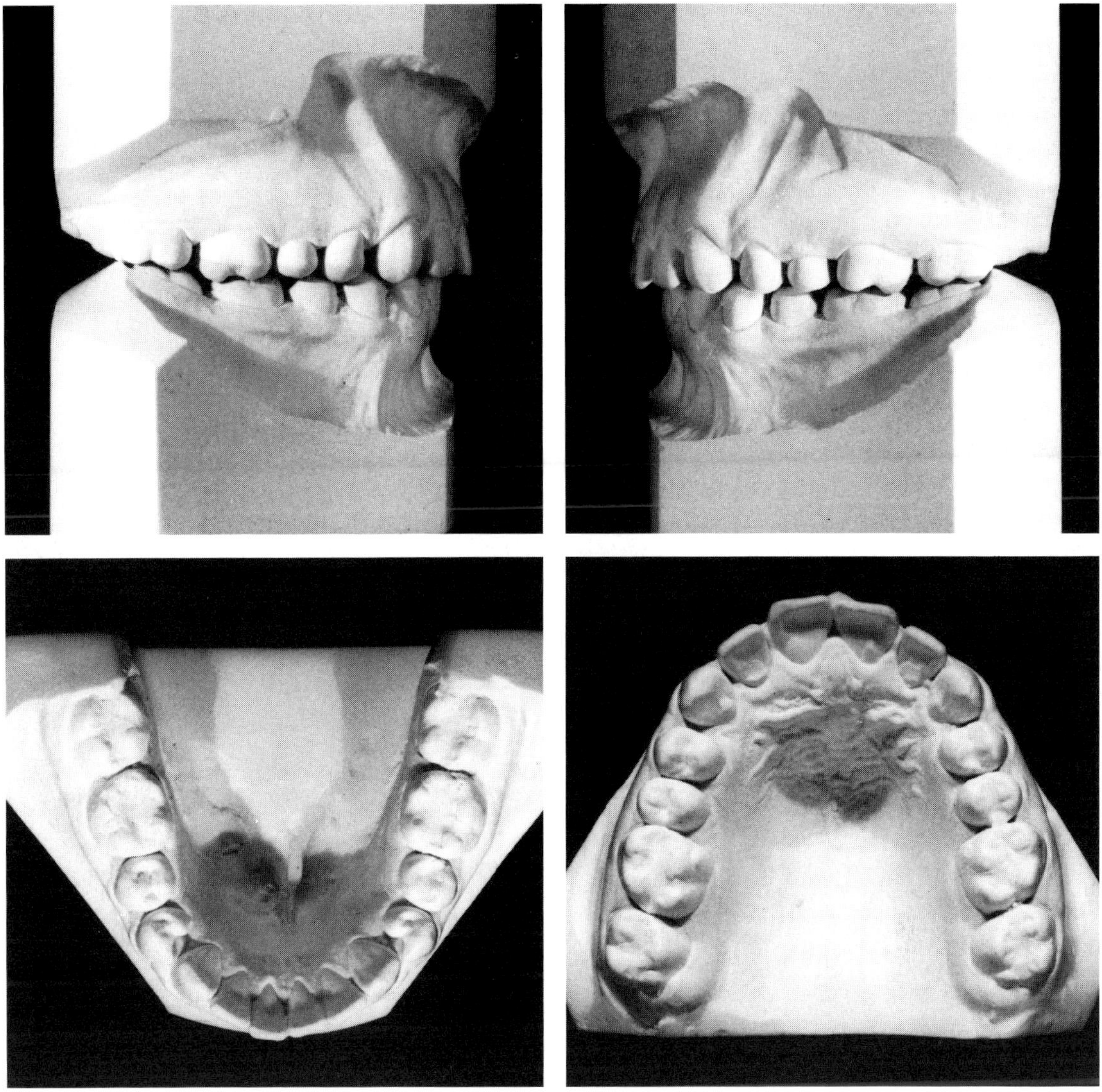

Figs 19-5 and 19-6 At the age of 16 y, 1 mo, two years after treatment was terminated, lip closure is normal. The upper lip is short. That being so, generally the maxillary incisors have to be intruded to achieve a good relationship between those teeth and stomion. The vertical angulation of the maxillary canines is not at all disturbing, particulary not after selective grinding of their cusps. The solid interdigitation consolidated the corrected scissorbites. The first permanent molars have improved in their occlusion, which resulted in the maxillary first molars improving their positions in the alveolar process. That applies also to the mandibular left first molar. Indeed sufficient room proved to be available in the maxilla for the second molars for their good emergence. There is now the question as to whether or not the same will apply to the third molars.

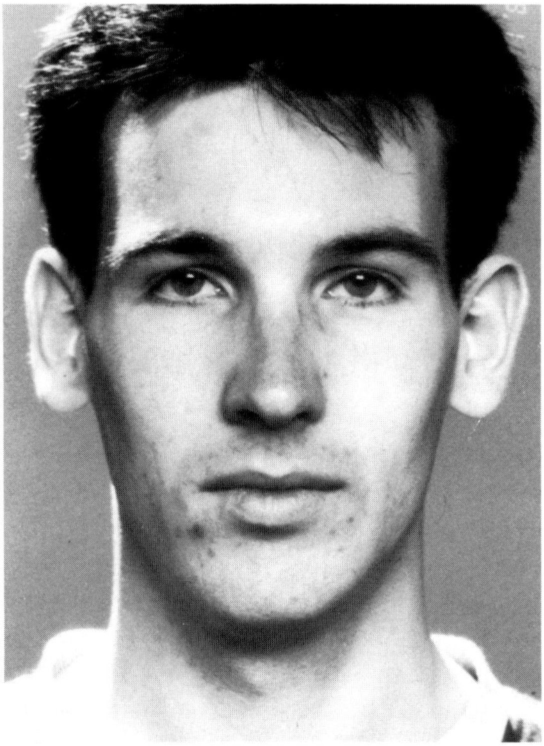
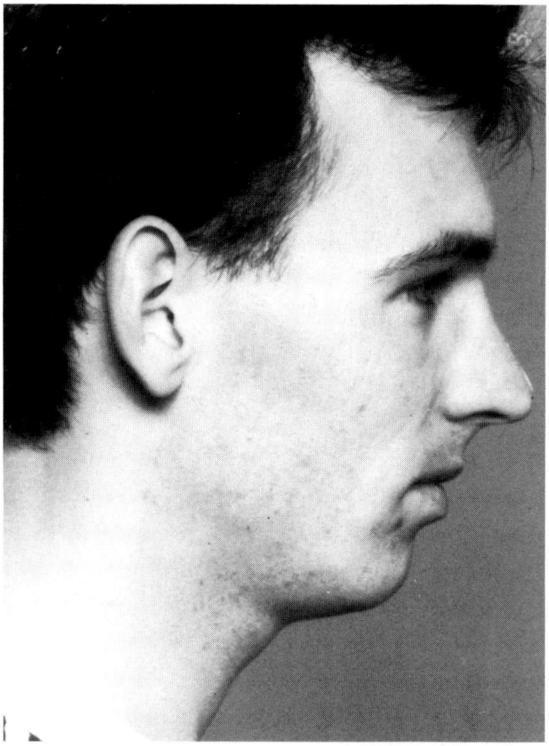
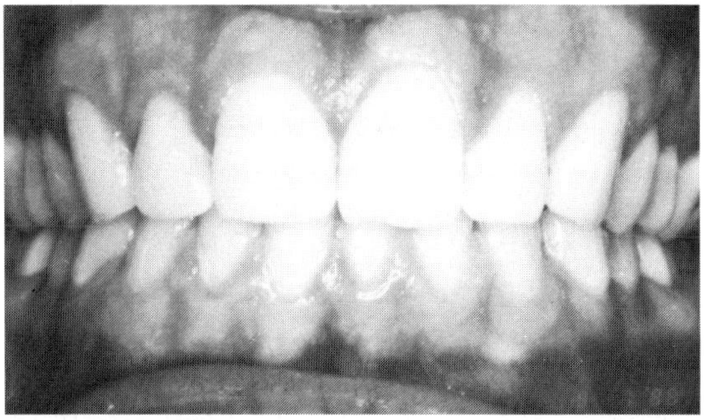
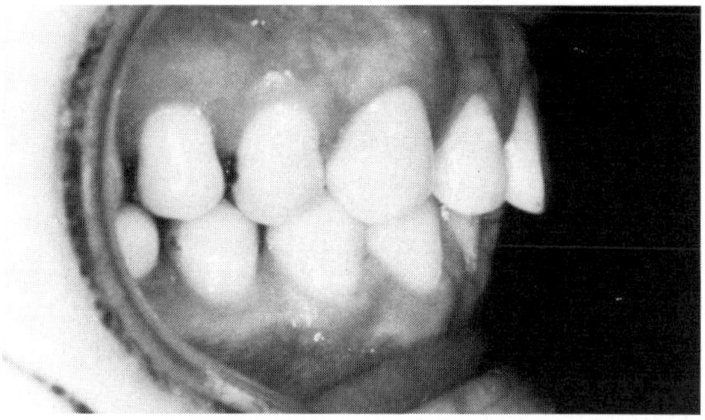
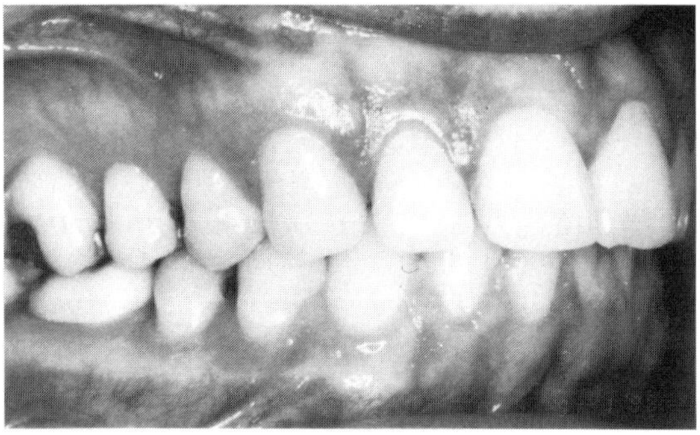
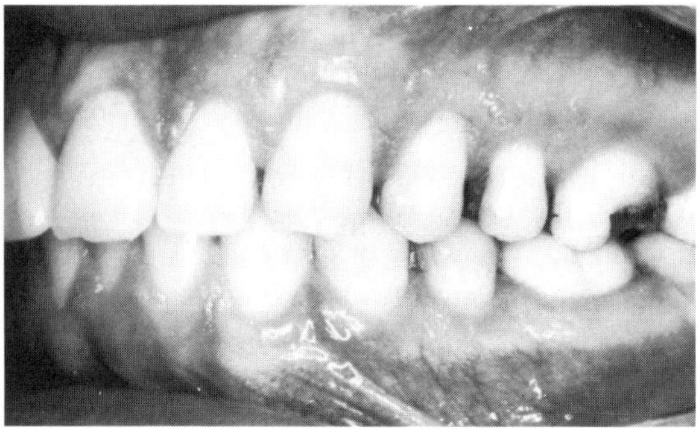

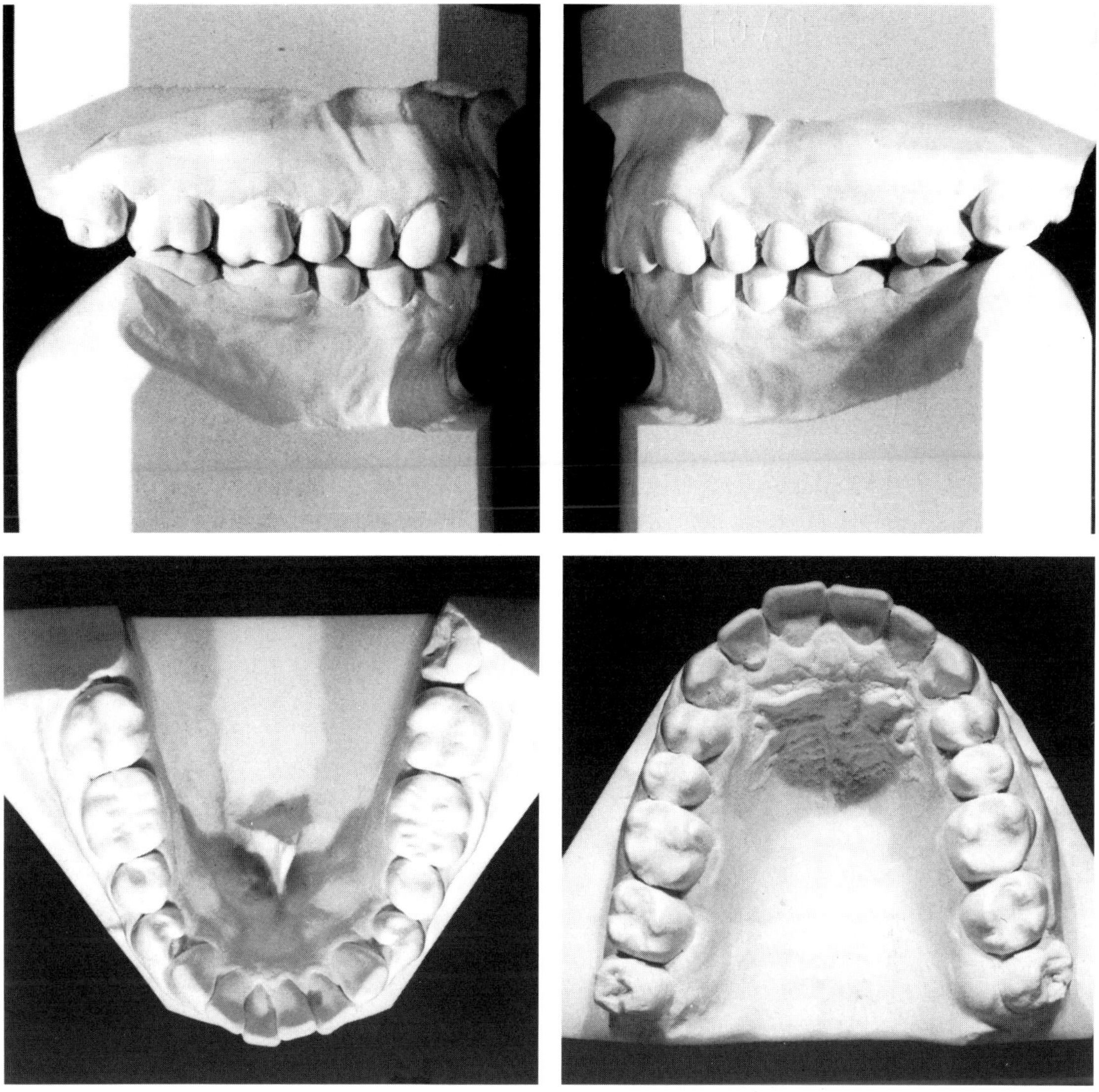

Figs 19-7 and 19-8 At the age of 24 y, 8 mo, ten years after treatment, there is a harmonious, though somewhat retrognathic, face. The mandibular incisors are in tertiary crowding. Their irregularity is however of no concern to the patient, possibly due to the fact that the incisal edges are level. The third molars do not have enough room. The removal of all four has been advised. The dental casts show clearly that the maxillary canines are perpendicular to the occlusal plane or even tilted slightly distally. In the bottom row of intraoral photographs, which were taken obliquely from the front, the canines seem to be inclined mesially more in accord with ideal occlusion. It is from this point of view that a dentition usually is seen. It is almost never seen from a truly lateral standpoint. Only in such a case will a perpendicular alignment of the maxillary canine be evident (intraoral photograph, middle right).

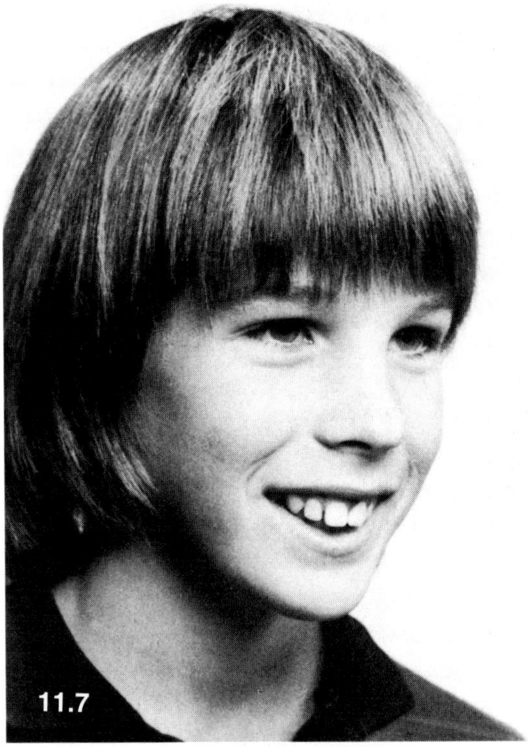

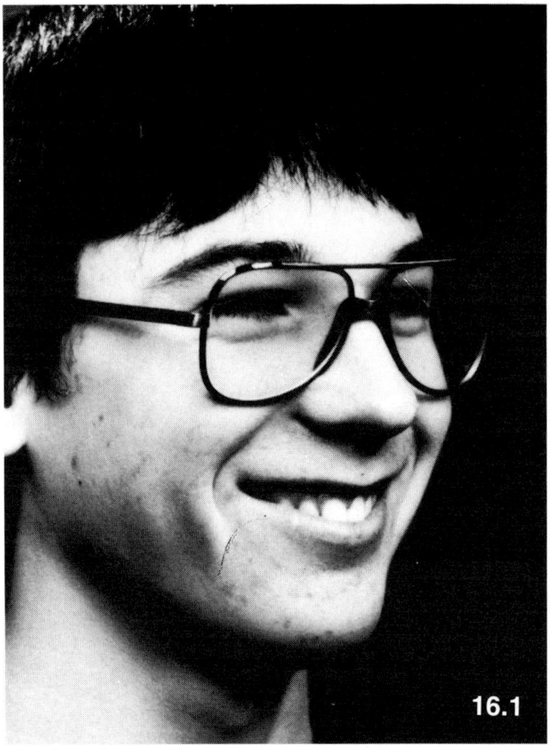

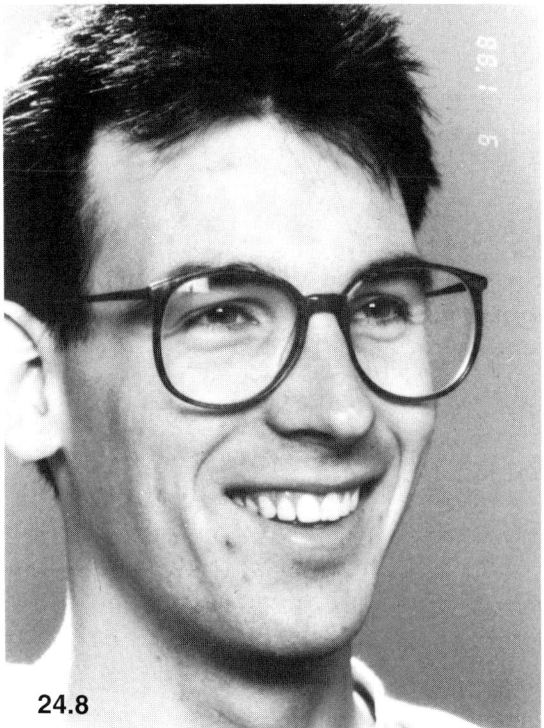

Fig 19-9 Note the changes in face and dentition.

incisors were in good alignment but were tipped back too much and had developed supraposition. At the age of 13 years 0 months, brackets were placed on the incisors to torque and intrude them,and consecutively a twistflex .0175" archwire and then a solid one of .019" x .026" were used for their correction. To support the torquing and intrusive action of the appliance, the headgear was replaced by one with a Kahn spur, which applied an upward force to the archwire between the brackets on the central incisors.

By the age of 14 years, 0 months, an acceptable result had been obtained and all appliances were removed, although there still were central diastemata in both dental arches and the maxillary left first molar was in buccoposition while the mandibular one was in linguoposition (Figs 19.3 and 19.4). Two years later, these diastemata had closed and the maxillary central incisors had moved forward a little. However, now slight spacing existed distal to the central incisors in the maxillary arch. In addition, the position of both maxillary and mandibular left first molars had improved and a good occlusion had developed between them (Figs 19.5 and 19.6).

At the age of 24 years, 8 months, ten years after treatment, the diastemata were practically closed. Tertiary crowding had developed in the mandibular dental arch but it was not considered objectionable (Figs 19.7 and 19.8). The treatment could be judged successful (Fig 19.9).

Scissorbites can be corrected in several ways. When opposing teeth need to be moved reciprocally it is possible, in cases with sufficient room in the dental arches, to achieve much in a short time with elastics through the bite. If mandibular first molars need to be uprighted or torqued, then the use of a lingual arch is the method of choice (see Chapter 13). In this case, it was not required so that elastics through the bite might have been used instead of the lingual arch.

In the treatment previously described, a cervical headgear with a Kahn spur was used to apply a vertical force to the maxillary incisors. Such a spur is made by soldering a short horizontal length of 0.045" wire to the center of the headgear, running dorsally and just long enough to rest securely under the maxillary archwire (see Figs 14.18C and D, page 236).

In the description that now follows of the mechanics involved, account has to be taken of the fact that there are other effects generated besides those moments described. This is due to the distal force derived from the neckstrap not being directed precisely through the center of resistance of the anchor molars. These moments can reinforce or diminish the effects produced by other forces. Reminders about this will not be repeated.

A cervical headgear has an outer arch with legs that project further dorsally than the ends of the inner arch. After the neckstrap is hooked to the outer arch, forces are generated that extrude and tip the maxillary molars. If the force runs cranial to the center of resistance, then the apices of the roots of the molars will tip distally. This can be seen from the way in which the headgear moves a little upward between the lips when the neckstrap is hooked on. This component of force can be used to intrude and torque the maxillary incisors through the medium of the Kahn spur. If the spur is resting passively against the incisal surface of the archwire in front, hooking on the neckstrap will not give rise to more tipping of the molar roots, but to an intrusive force on the anteriors. If when the headgear is inserted in the molar tubes it is

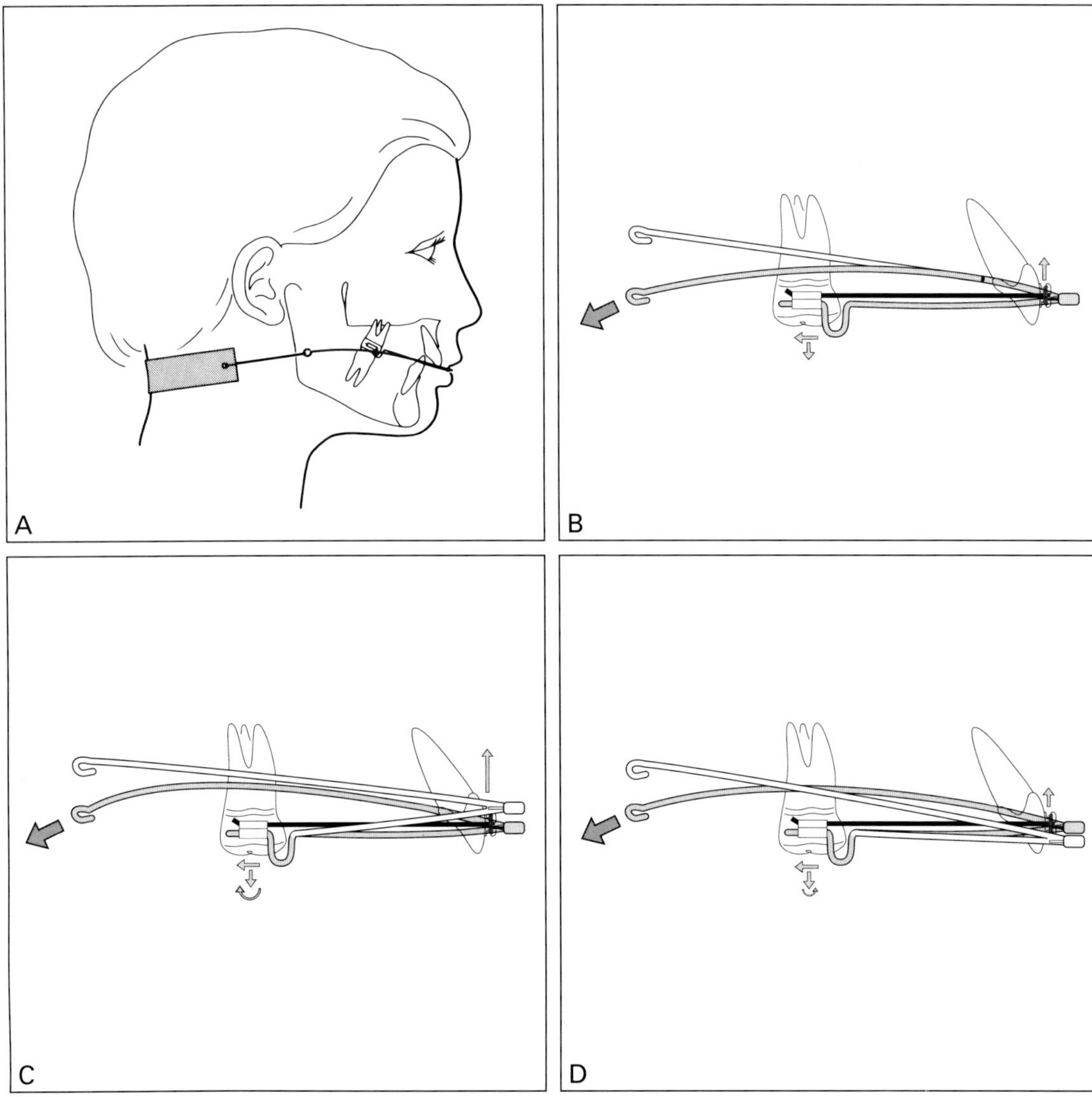
A
B
C
D

Fig 19-10 Mechanics involved in the application of cervical headgears with a Kahn spur in combination with fixed appliances for intrusion of the maxillary anteriors.

A The cervical headgear needs long outer arms which project further dorsally than the level of the maxillary first permanent molars to which it is connected. The force vector generated by the neckstrap should run above the trifurcation of the molar roots. When the neckstrap is activated, the outer arms are bent downward and the front of the headgear rises in the incisor region. There is a counterclockwise couple and a disto-occlusal force generated at the first molars. The result will be that the root apices of the molars will as a rule move more distally than the crowns do.

B With a cervical headgear fitted with a Kahn spur, which lies passively against the incisal side of an edgewise arch, activating the neckstrap does not produce a couple at the first molars apart from that provided by the edgewise arch itself, as long as the form of the inner arch of the headgear does not change. The spur pressing on the edgewise arch by activating the neckstrap produces a tilting action, which intrudes the incisors and extrudes the molars.

C If the headgear, which is adjusted so that the spur lies passively cervical to the archwire, is inserted with the spur now incisal to the archwire but without activating the neckstrap, the inner arch of the headgear will actively be intruding the incisors and be placing a clockwise couple on the molars. These forces will be added to the forces generated by the edgewise arch. If the neckstrap now is activated there is a danger that the additional forces will cause the molar root apices to move mesially while the crowns tip distally yet with little movement occurring in the incisors. Moreover an excessive force is being applied to the incisors that increases the risk of root resorption.

D Such problems can be avoided if the spur lies several millimeters incisal to the archwire when the headgear is passive. Then when the neckstrap is hooked on, the maxillary first molar roots will be loaded to distal and the clockwise couple due to the archwire will be countered. In activating the neckstrap, the height of the outer arms needs to be adjusted until only a gentle force (not more than 75 to 100 grams) is applied in a vertical direction to the anterior part of the edgewise arch by the spur.

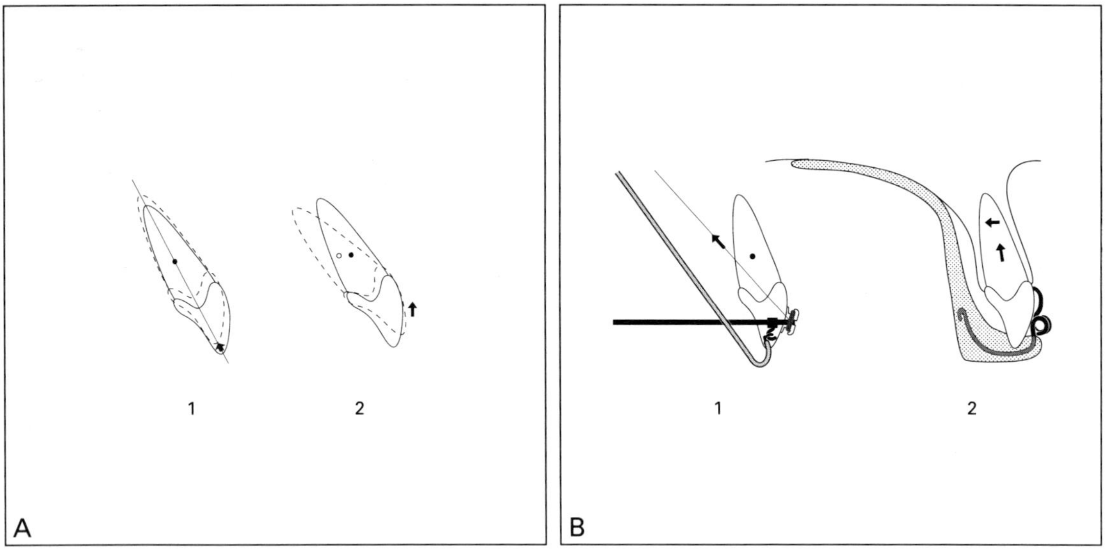

Fig 19-11 Effects of direction and point of application of intrusive forces on the movement of maxillary incisors.

A1. When the force acts in the direction of the root axis and passes through the center of resistance, intrusion occurs without labiolingual tipping.

2. If a vertical force runs at some distance ventral to the center of resistance and is applied at the labial surface of the tooth, then there will be not only an intrusive force but a tipping force. This will cause the crowns to move to labial. Since that movement is usually not wanted, it is prevented by tying the archwire back to the anchor molars. If in addition care is taken to prevent the molars moving mesially (headgear distal traction), the root apices of the incisors will be displaced to palatal, as illustrated.

B1. If a parietal headgear is attached with hooks to an edgewise arch, the direction of the force that will be transferred through the brackets to the teeth will be determined by the location on the archwire where the headgear hooks are fixed. Depending on the inclination of the incisors, the force will pass dorsal or ventral to the center of resistance. If the inclination of the teeth is normal, but especially if the maxillary incisors are steeply inclined, the force will run dorsally and cause the crowns to tip palatally. Intrusion will therefore be accompanied by palatal movement of the crowns unless the edgewise arch has compensating torque bent into it

2. If a parietal headgear is used that is attached to an appliance anteriorly, the direction of the force will probably run dorsally to the center of resistance and the intrusion will be accompanied by labial movement of the root apices unless a second moment is added to counteracts this. With the Bass plate, torquing springs are used to this end (see Fig 9-15, page 144).

necessary to bend it downward in the process of getting the spur to lie incisally to the archwire, then there will already be an intrusive force on the anteriors even before the neckstrap is hooked on. When the neckstrap is active, its effect is amplified and therefore much too great. Moreover there would then be an extruding and tipping force on the molar crowns. The unfavorable effect of this reaction is comparable to and amplifies that of the edgewise arch that is engaged in the brackets and for that reason should be avoided. It has already been pointed out that if the molars begin to tip distally, then the edgewise arch in front no longer has the desired effect (see Fig 14.16, page 232). Therefore the neutralizing of that reaction should be aimed for. That is possible by bending the inner arch of the headgear so that the spur when passive lies a few millimetres under the edgewise arch, and by bending the outer legs of the headgear upward. When the neckstrap is hooked on, the molar roots will not be tipped mesially but to distal. The height of the outer legs needs to be adjusted subsequently so that the intrusive force at the spur is the desired 75 to 100 g (Fig 19.10).

A further advantage of the Kahn spur is that the force is applied labial to the tooth crowns (since the edgewise arch is located there) and perpendicular to the occlusal plane. Because of this, a palatally directed force is applied to the incisor root apices even when the edgewise arch has no active torque built into it (Fig 19.11). Nonetheless, slight torque should be built into the arch since otherwise it would act as a brake on the palatal movement of the apices.

The intrusion of the maxillary anteriors needs to be done with care. Forces greater than 30 to 50 g per tooth (depending on the size of the attached root surface) need to be avoided, paying consideration to the fact that the bone surface area being subjected to that intrusive force is rather small. If a Kahn spur is used, then the intrusive force derived from it and the edgewise arch need to be very limited because large intrusive forces can cause significant root resorption.

From the foregoing material it does appear that the system of forces involved in this application is complicated. Additional factors become involved, such as the breadth of the arches, the rotation of anchor molars, differences between left and right sides, influences of tongue and lips, and the forces generated in swallowing and chewing. The manner in which patients use their headgear (for example in inserting and removing it) also will have an effect. Rough handling can negate any "fine-tuning" to the appliance. It cannot be too often reiterated that at each visit all aspects of the therapy should be closely examined to check on the need for adjustments. The avoidance of any large forces is also necessary. If anything should go awry, then there is a hope that any mishap between two visits would be small in its effect and better able to be corrected than if large forces had been at work.

To conclude, attention is paid again to the steepness in the position of maxillary canines. As mentioned in Chapter 12, it is technically difficult to move the apices of these teeth to distal without producing undesirable consequences. Steeply positioned maxillary canines do not cause problems in the excursions of the mandible, and if necessary can be ground for enhanced performance. Any esthetic problem with steeply inclined maxillary canines can be discounted, as is illustrated by Figure 19.7. The position of the canines can indeed be disturbing if they are positioned outside the dental arch or are rotated mesiolabially. Correction of such a situation is sensible. That can often be done orthodontically without brackets.

Moreover it is possible to camouflage an abnormal position by reshaping with grinding and addition of composite. That applies not only to abnormal positioning, but also to many other esthetic imperfections.[25]

Chapter 20

Class II/1, ventral forced bite over 12
Extraction 53, tongue blade, cervical headgear, brackets 12, 11, 21, and 22
Female 8 years, 2 months to 28 years, 5 months

A girl aged 8 years and 2 months with a harmonious face and adequate lip seal displayed a class II/1 anomaly, which was masked to some extent by a forced bite to ventral caused by the maxillary right lateral incisor. The patient could not close into occlusion in centric relation due to the interference of that lateral incisor. Beside the ventral forced bite, there were no functional abnormalities. She had sucked her thumb till she was 6 years old. The mandibular arch had diastemata in the anterior region and the maxillary arch had insufficient room to accommodate the right lateral incisor, which had emerged palatally. The interdigitation of the posterior teeth was solid (Figs. 20.1 and 20.2).

It was decided to correct the ventral forced bite as soon as possible. To provide space for the labial movement of the maxillary right lateral incisor, the adjacent deciduous canine was extracted. The class II/1 anomaly would be corrected at a later stage. For that purpose a cervical headgear would be used, eventually combined with a maxillary removable plate and in the last phase with brackets on the four maxillary incisors. The patient was instructed to use a wooden tongue blade at least three times a day for five minutes each time to wedge the lateral incisor to labial (Fig 20.3). As soon as she could close her mandibular teeth behind the lateral, she should clench her teeth together in that position as much as possible. After two weeks, the reversed overbite had been corrected and the teeth adapted to their new habitual occlusion (Figs 20.4 and 20.5).

The treatment of the class II/1 anomaly was delayed until shortly before the end of the second transitional period because with mild disto-occlusions the headgear therapy can best be initiated while the maxillary second deciduous molars are still present and the second permanent molars not yet emerged. In this case, the headgear was placed at the age of 10 years and 2 months (Figs. 20.6 and 20.7). The aim was to use the cervical headgear to correct the disto-occlusion, to prevent the first permanent molars from migrating mesially, and to increase the dental arch perimeter to provide enough space for the maxillary permanent canines (Fig 20.18). There was no need to use a maxillary removable plate. At the age of 13 years 0 months, brackets were placed on the maxillary central incisors and those teeth were intruded (see Chapter 14). Two months later, they had reached the level of the lateral incisors, whereupon they too were provided with brackets to intrude them simultaneously with the central incissors. The edgewise arch was bent inward to

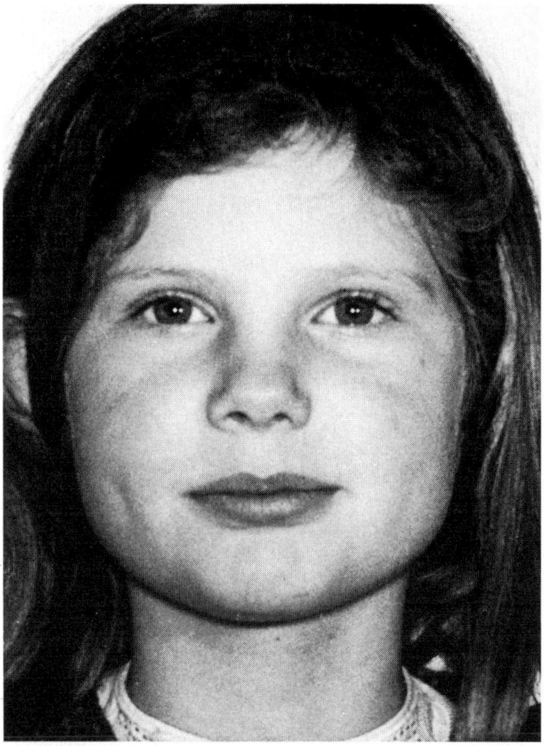

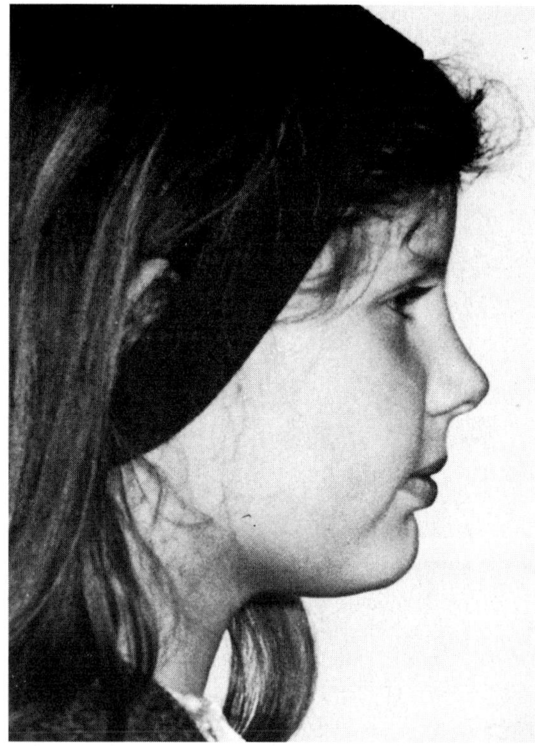

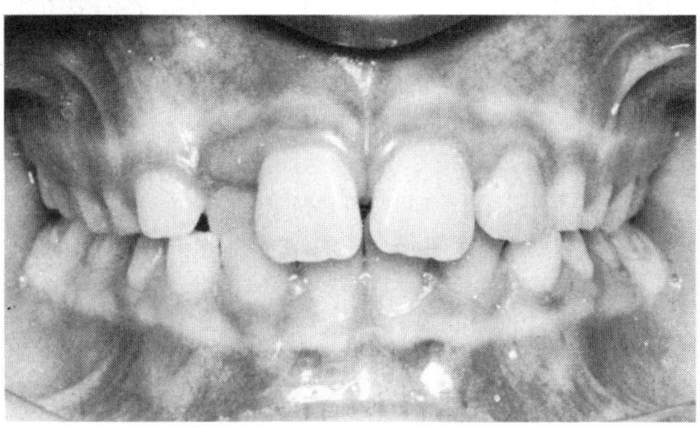

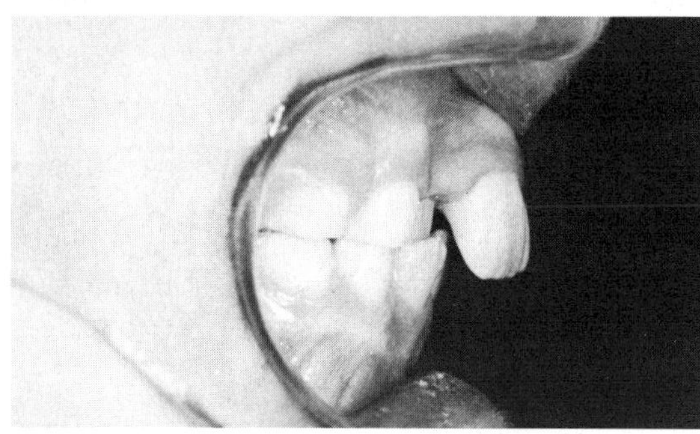

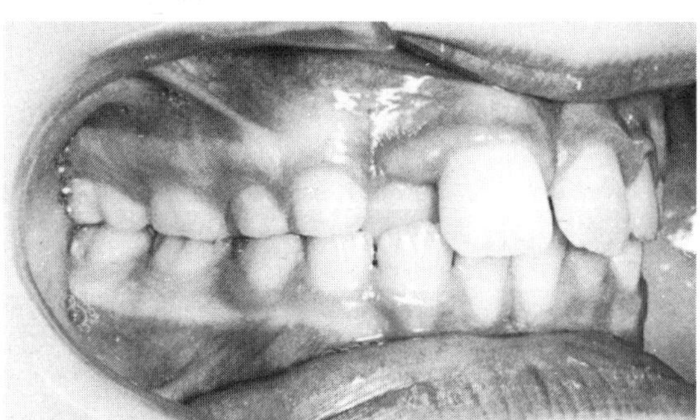

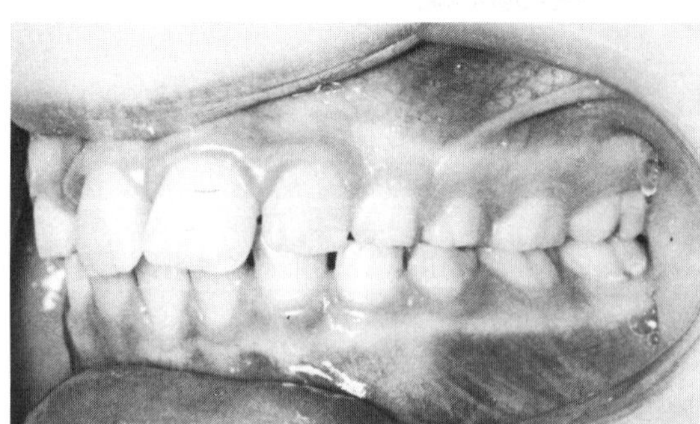

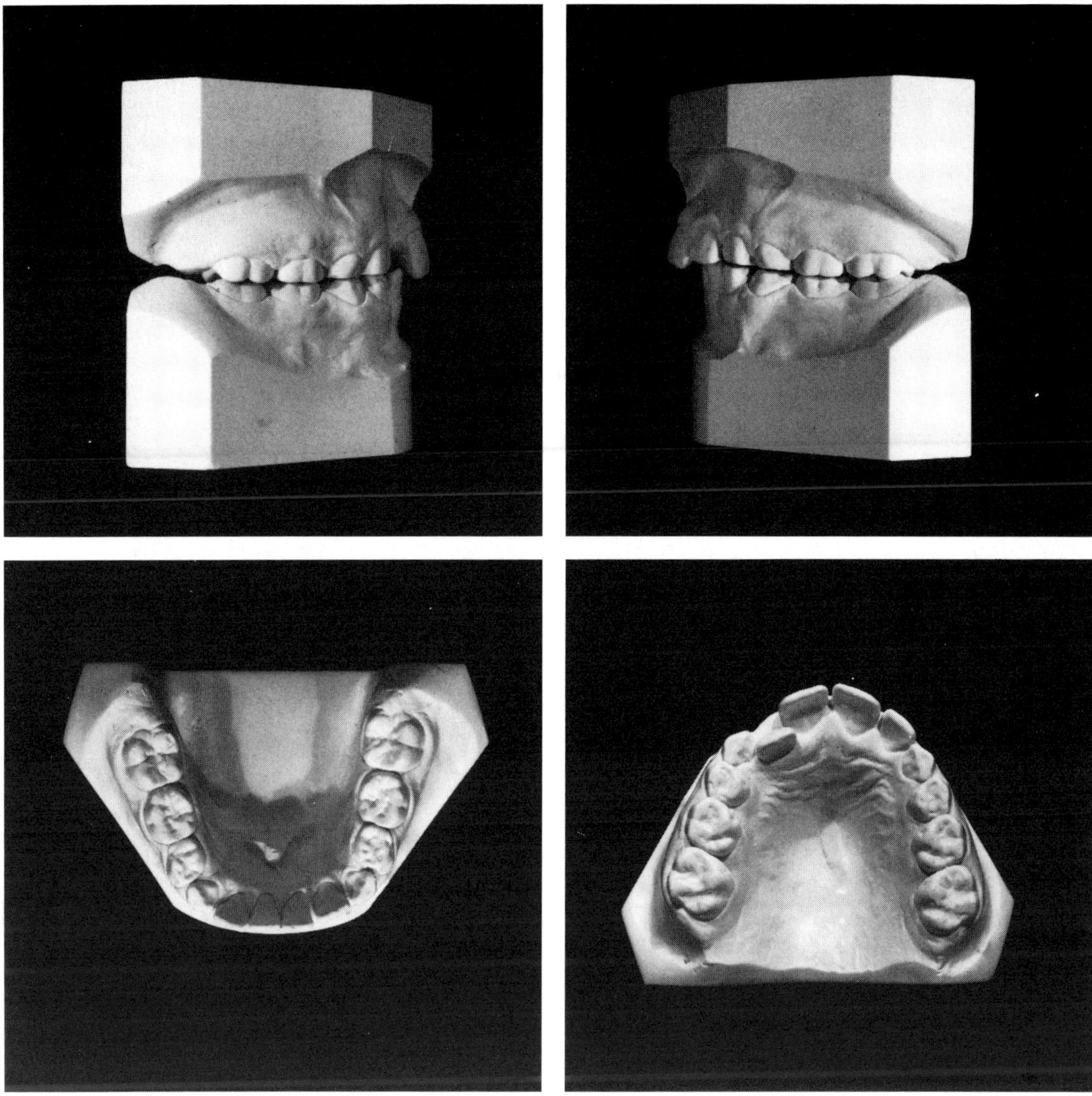

Figs 20-1 and 20-2 *A girl aged 8 y, and 2 mo with a harmonious face, prominent cheek bones, a small nose, and well-positioned lips that are closed at rest. She has a class II/1 anomaly that is disguised by the presence of a ventral forced bite. She cannot close her teeth behind the maxillary right lateral incisor, which has emerged palatally. The maxillary teeth on the right are located more mesially than those on the left. The habitual occlusion (in forced bite) is 4mm ventral to the central relation. With maximal retroposition of the mandible, the incisal edges of the opposing right lateral incisors meet edge-to-edge. The dentition overall has adapted to the forced bite. The posterior teeth are in solid interdigitation and have normal inclinations.*

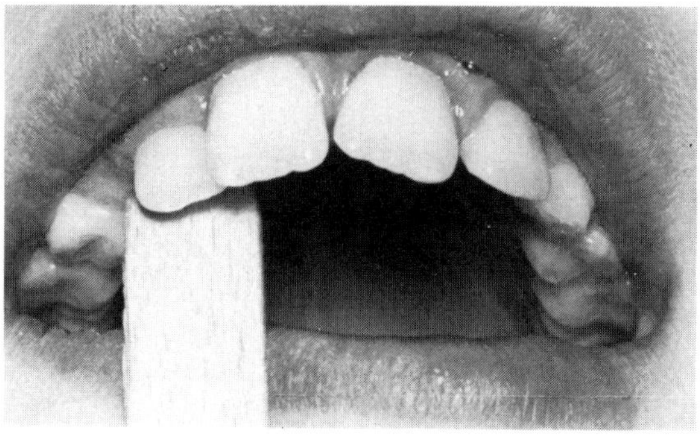

Fig 20-3 The reversed overbite of the maxillary right lateral incisor is being corrected with a wooden tongue blade, which has been made narrower to avoid it putting pressure on the adjoining teeth. The patient must put intermittent pressure to labial on the tooth concerned, using the mandibular incisors as a fulcrum. The blade should be held at a steep angle to enhance the labial acting force and reduce the force that would cause intrusion. The correction of the reversed overbite is only sensible if subsequently sufficient vertical overbite is present to maintain the improvement. When insufficient room is available for the tooth to be displaced labially, that room must be provided. In this case, the room was obtained by extracting the deciduous canine.

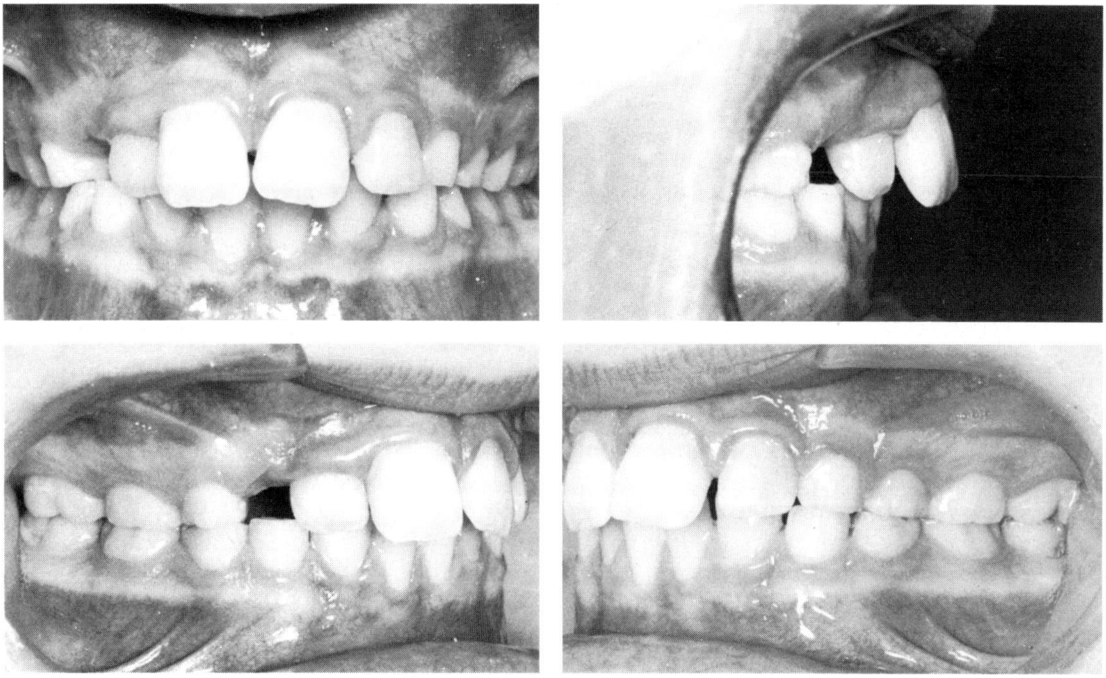

Fig 20-4

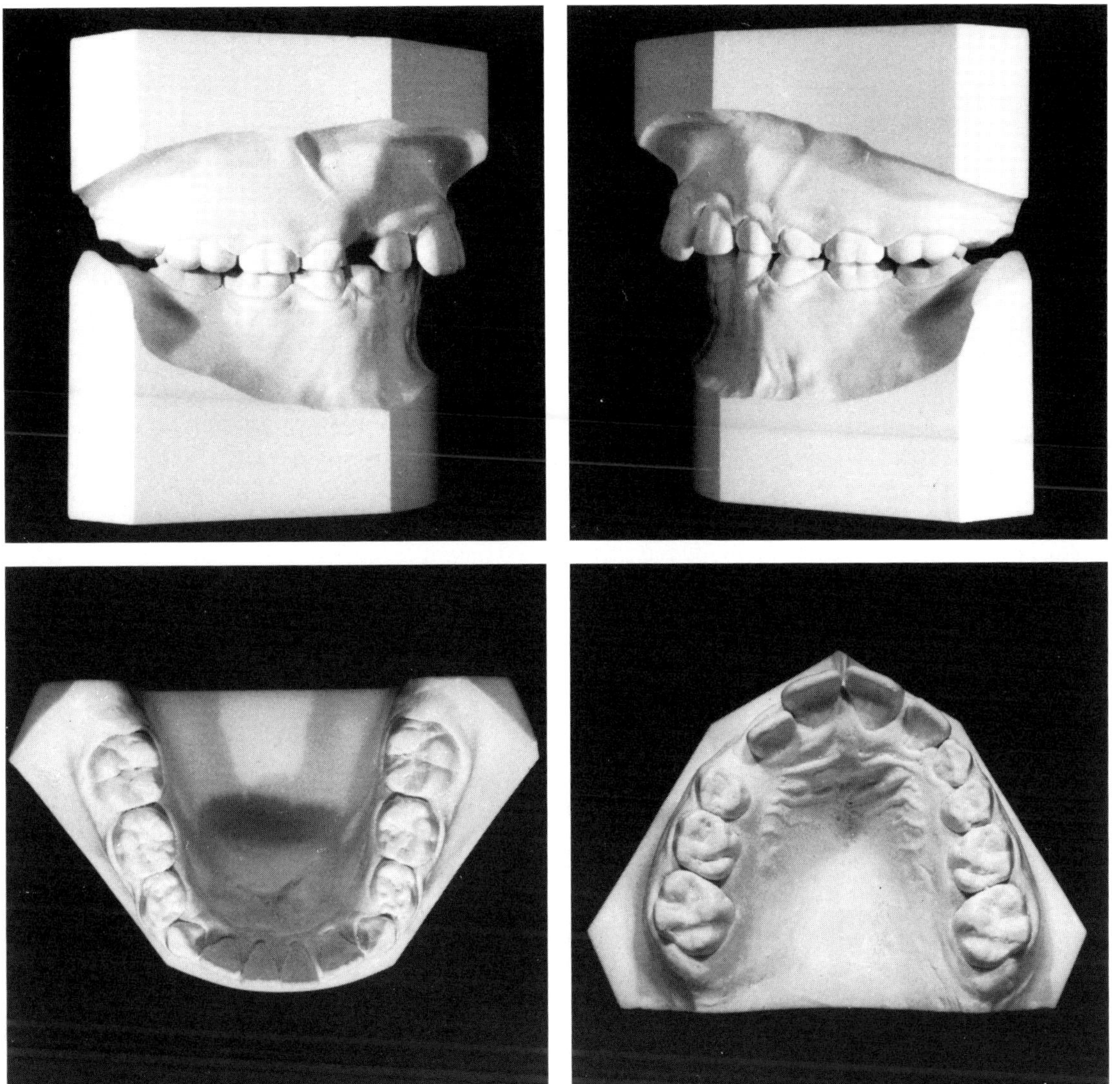

Figs 20-4 and 20-5 At the age of 8 y, 9 mo, six months after correction of the reversed overbite of the maxillary right lateral incisor, the habitual occlusion has adapted itself to correspond with the central relation. The overjet is now greater than it was when the forced bite was present. The more dorsal position of the mandibular dental arch is associated with an increase in the disto-occlusion. Due to the altered interdigitation, the inclination of the posterior teeth has changed. A result of the unilateral extraction of the deciduous canine on the right has been an increase in asymmetry in the maxillary arch. Now insufficient space is available for the maxillary permanent canine, which will emerge labial to the arch if nothing is done about it.

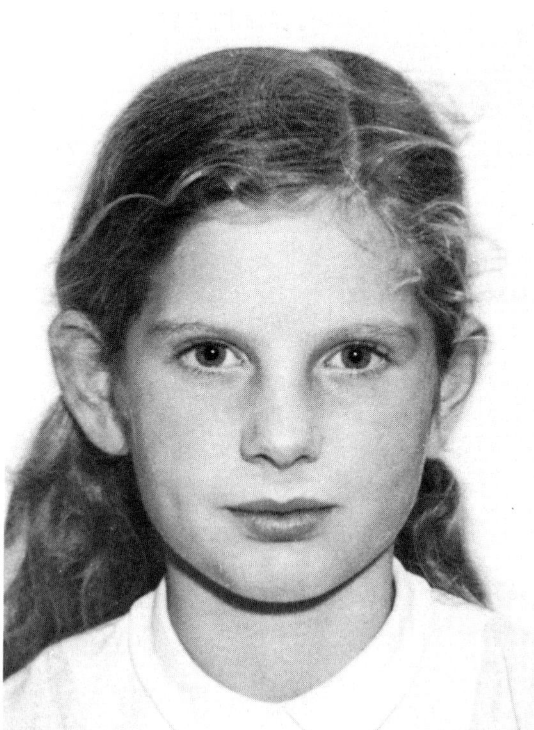
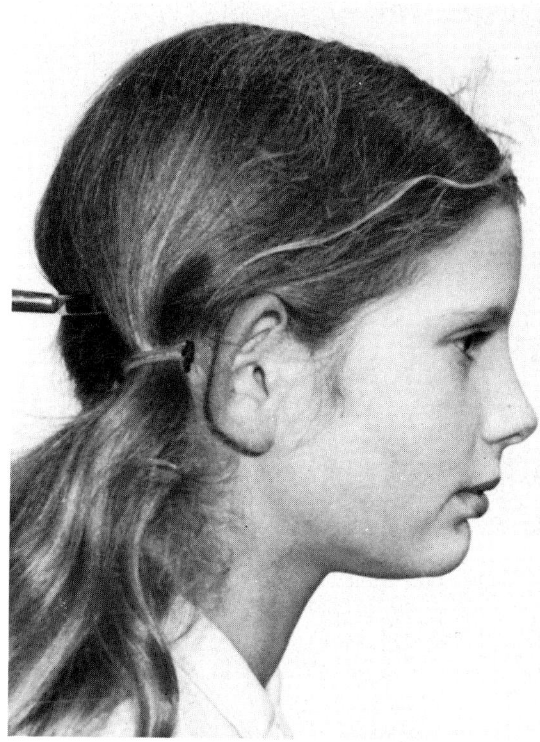
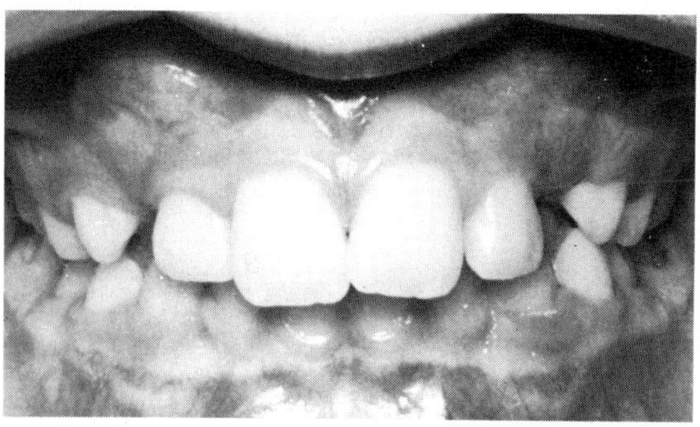
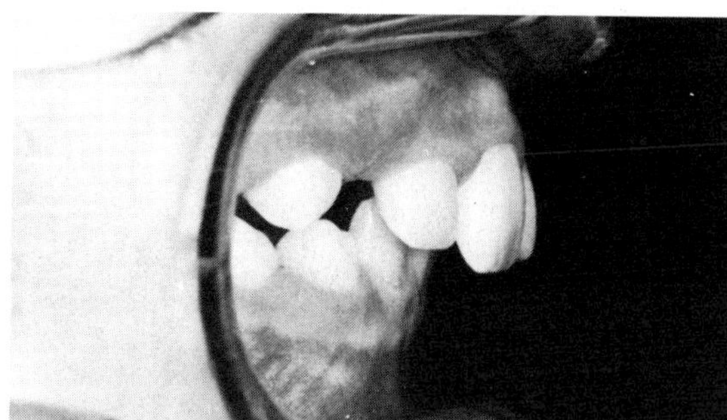
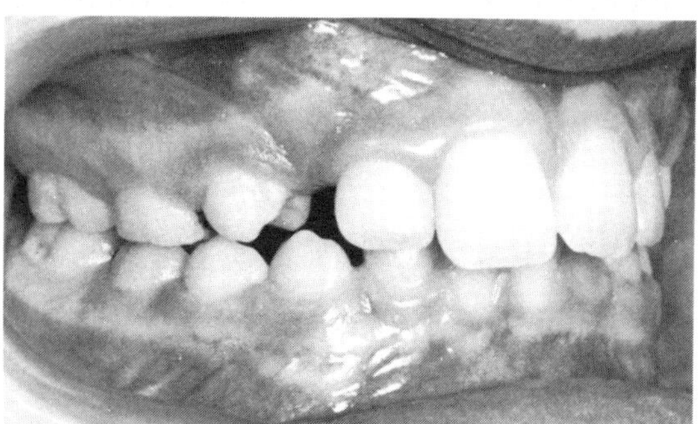
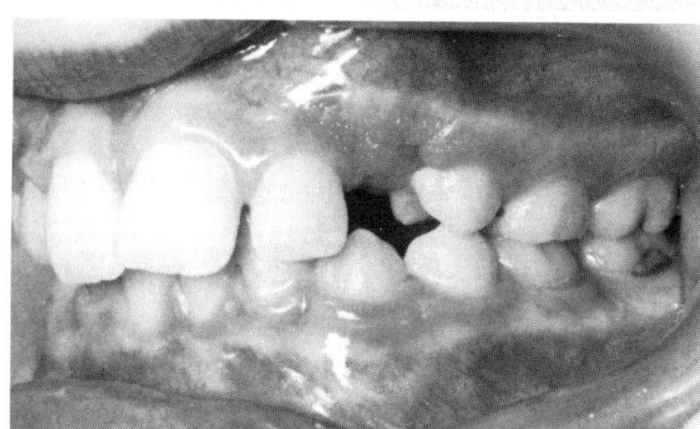

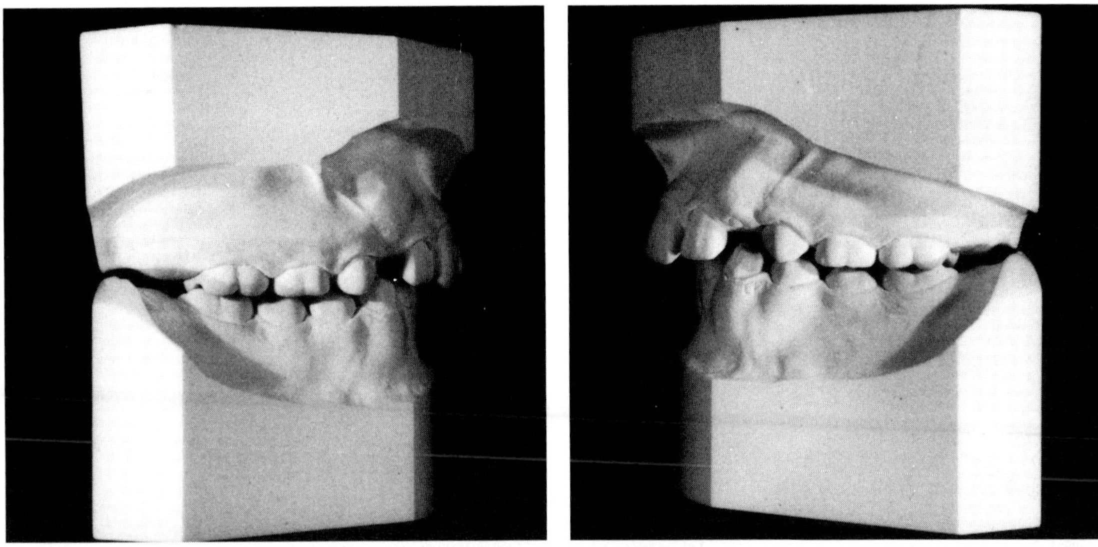

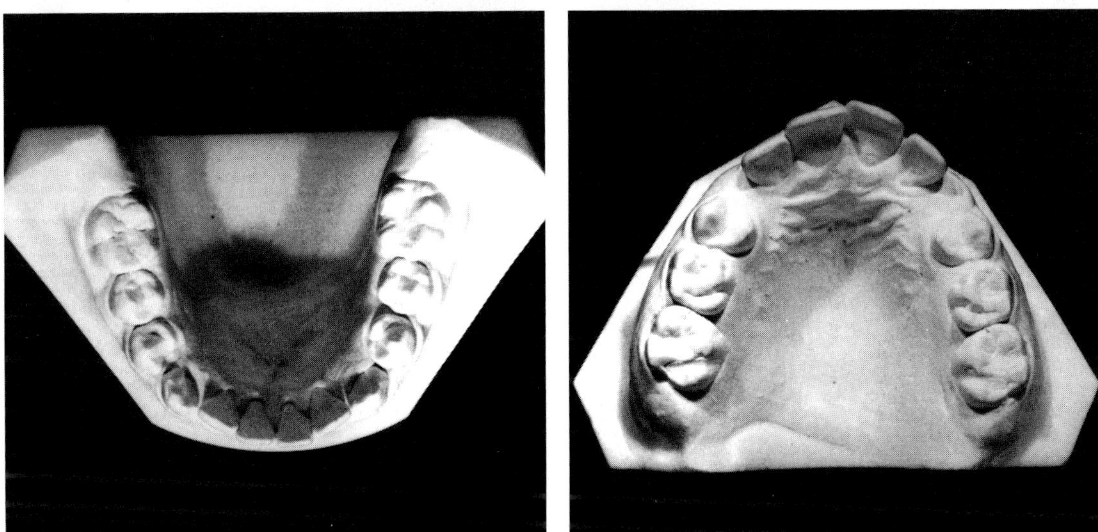

Figs 20-6 and 20-7 *At the age of 10 y, 2 mo, the time to initiate headgear therapy had arrived. The second transitional phase was complete in the mandible where a good arch existed. In the maxilla the second deciduous molars were still present and the second permanent molars had not yet emerged. By placing a cervical headgear at this stage it would be possible to prevent the mesial migration of the permanent first molars that otherwise would consume the extra space that becomes available at exfoliation of the second deciduous molars. The maxillary incisors have not moved further into supraposition because the lower lip has opposed it.*

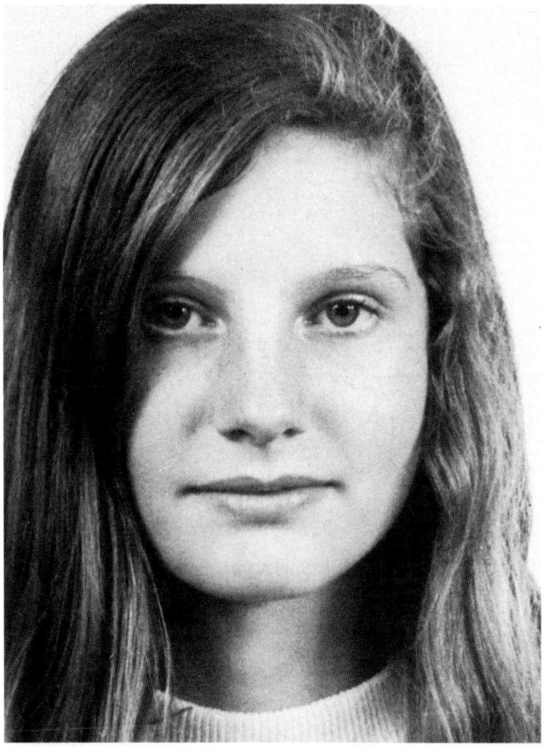
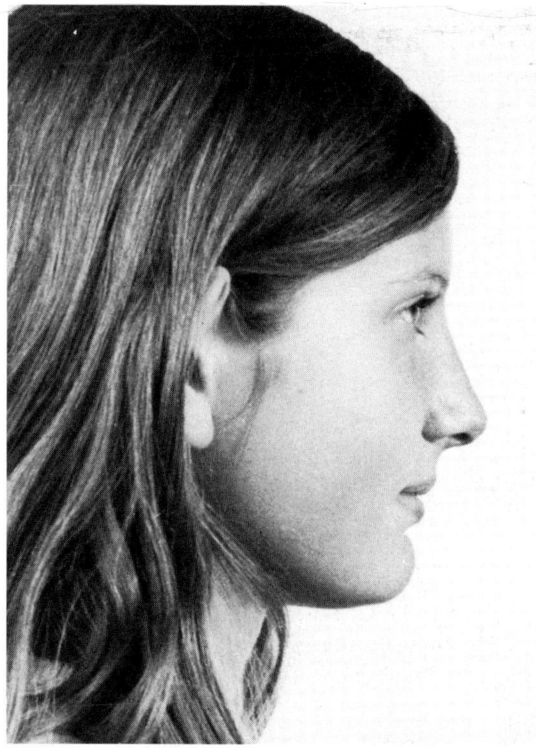
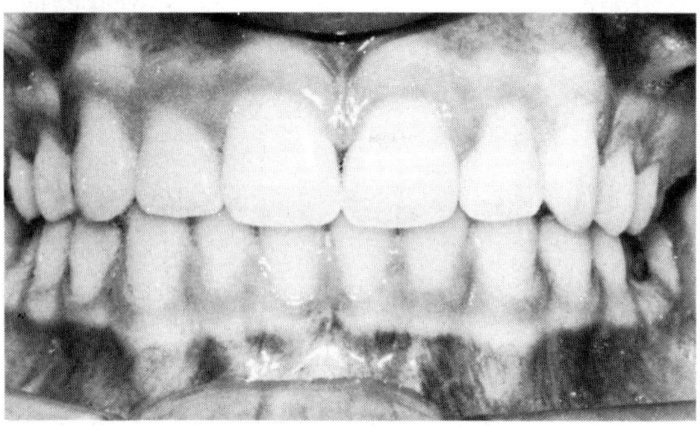
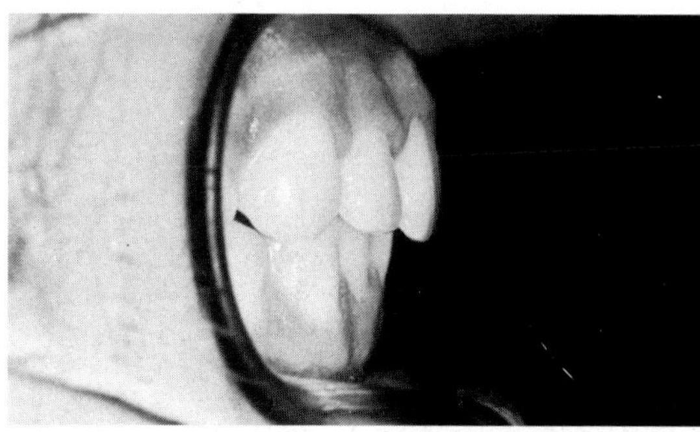
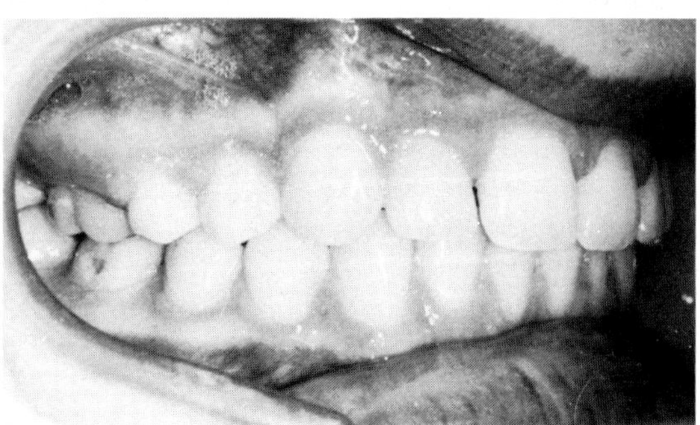
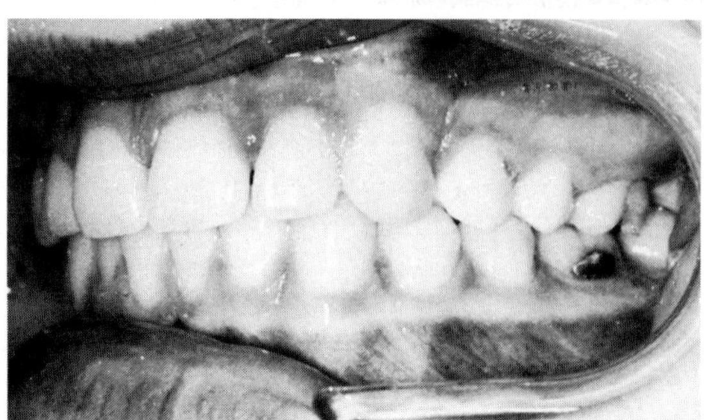

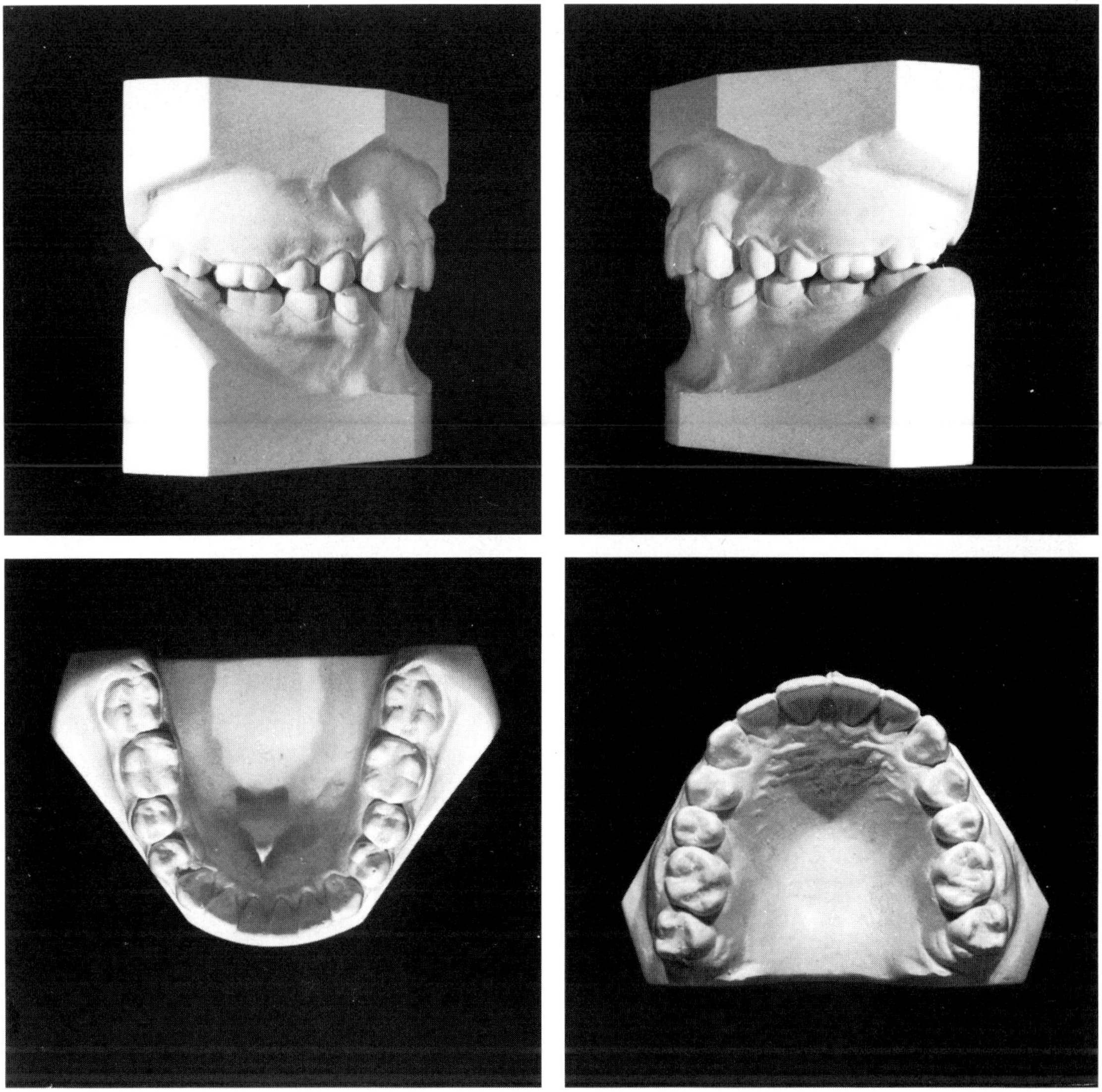

Figs 20-8 and 20-9 At the age of 13 y, 7 mo, after treatment for two years and four months, the patient has an excellent dentition that fits well into her harmonious face. The premolars and canines exhibit a good occlusion and solid interdigitation. Relapse of the disto-occlusion need not be feared. Whether or not the incisors will become irregular in the course of time is not possible to foretell. Certainly some changes in alignment are to be expected.

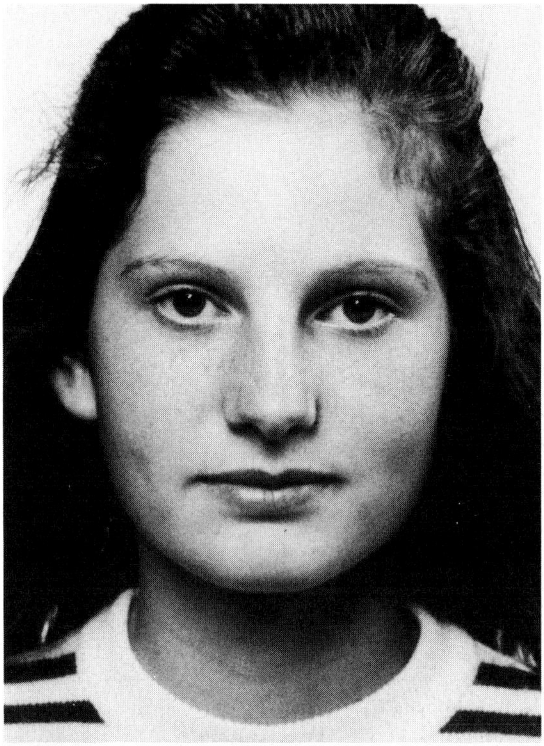
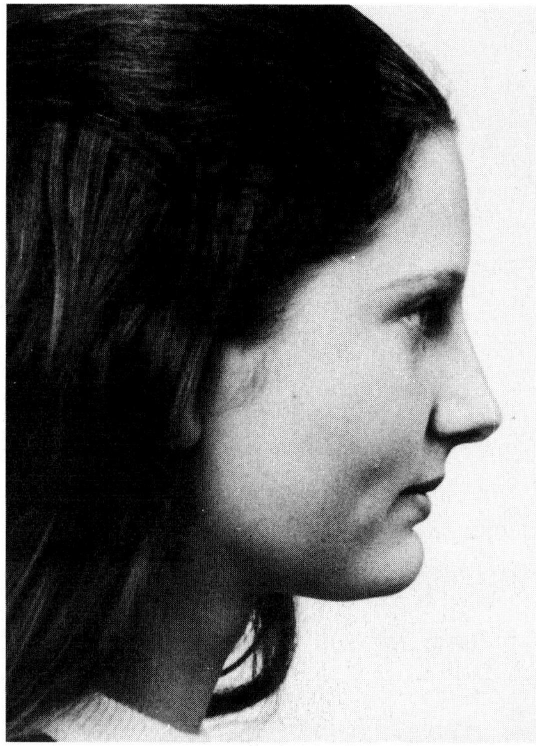
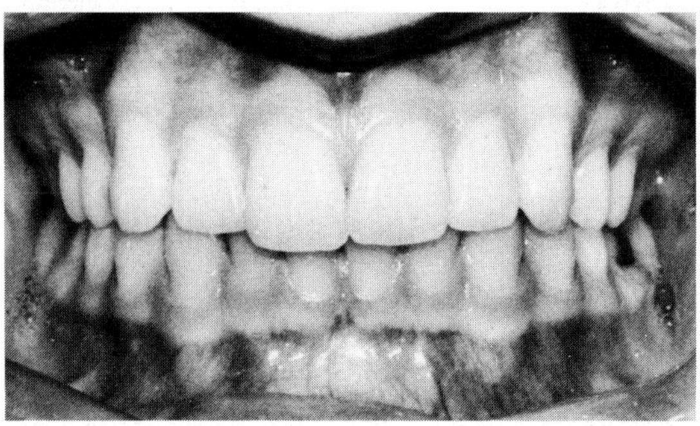
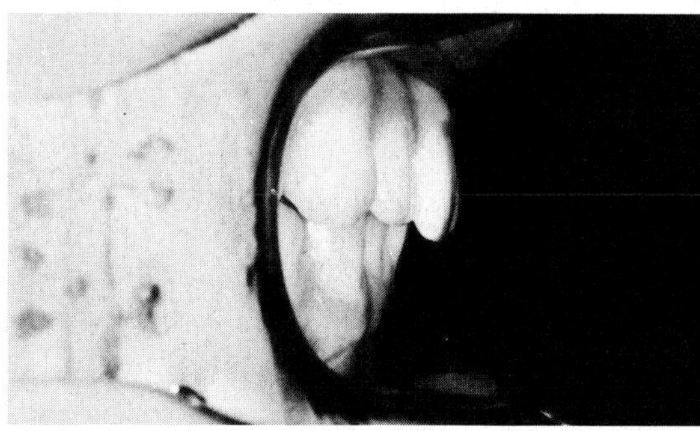
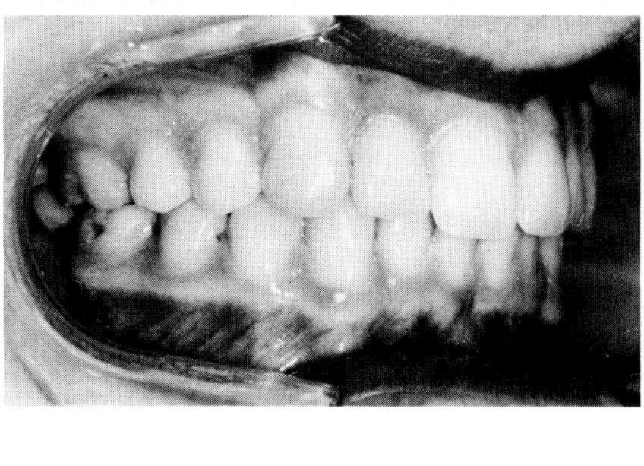
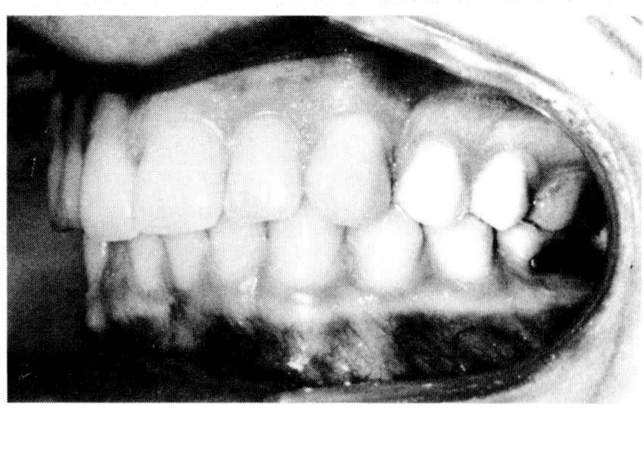

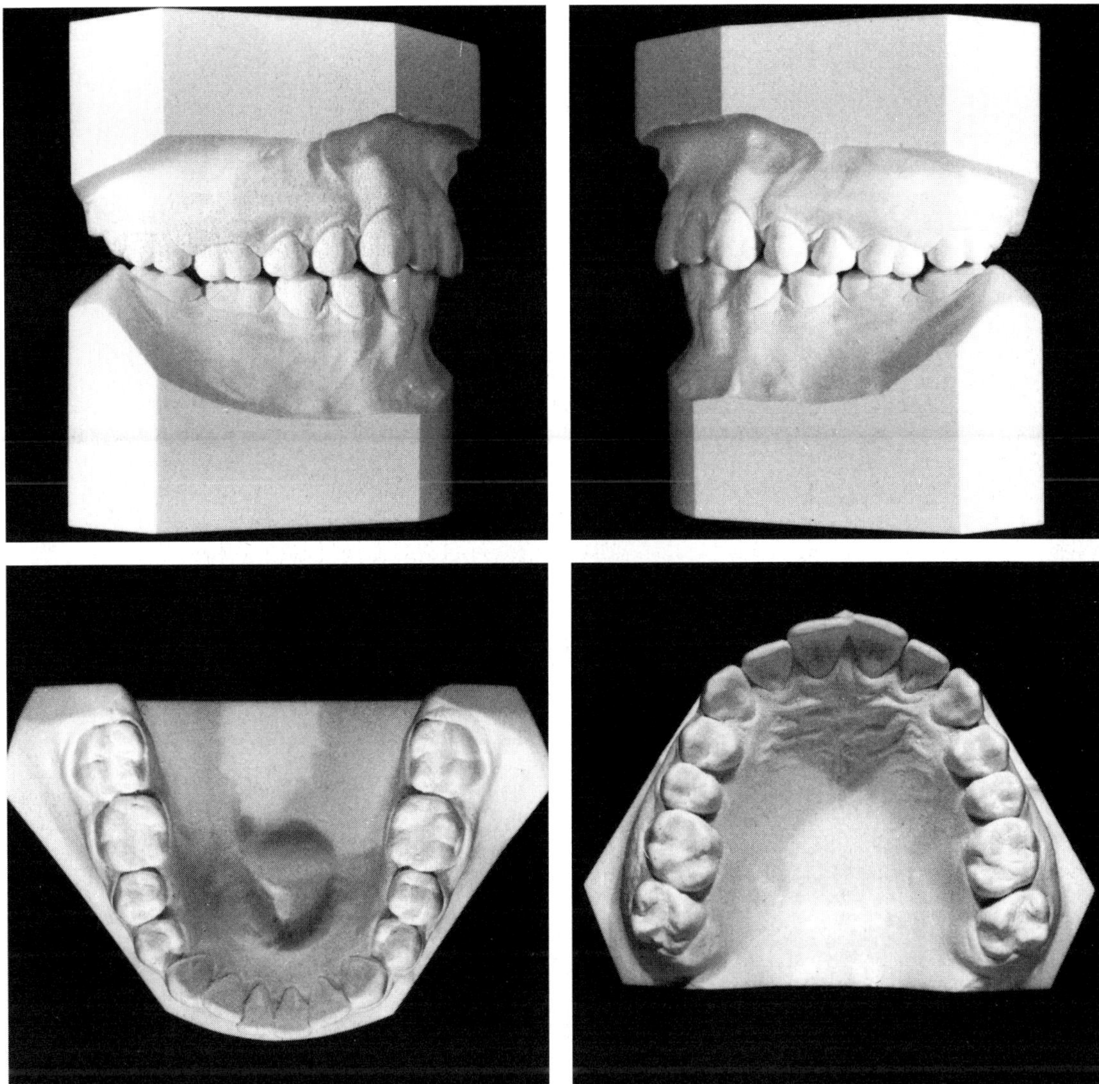

Figs 20-10 and 20-11 *At the age of 15 y, 6 mo, two years following treatment, the vertical overbite has increased. The maxillary right central incisor has extruded slightly. Apart from that, little has changed.*

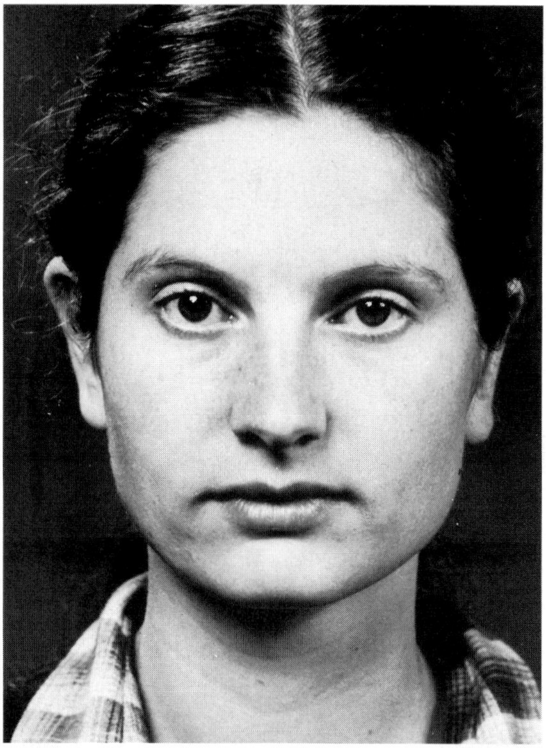
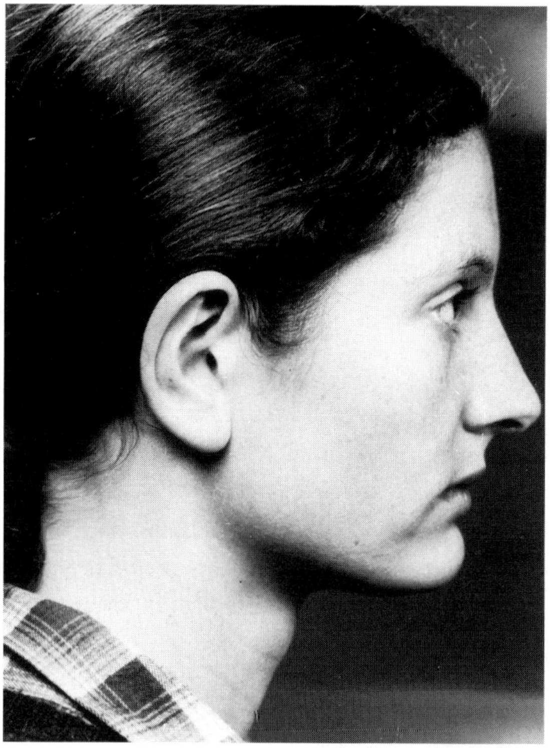
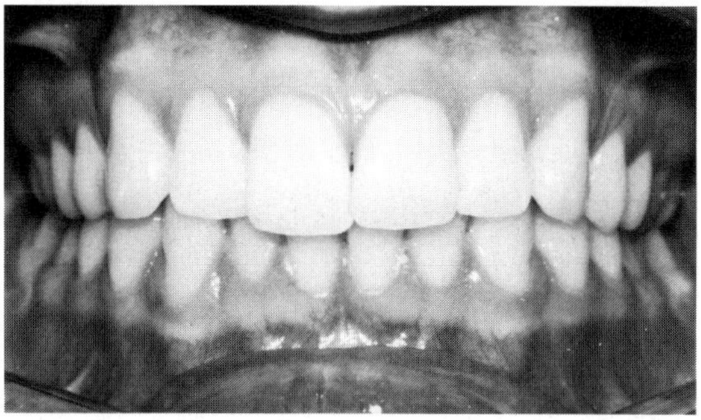
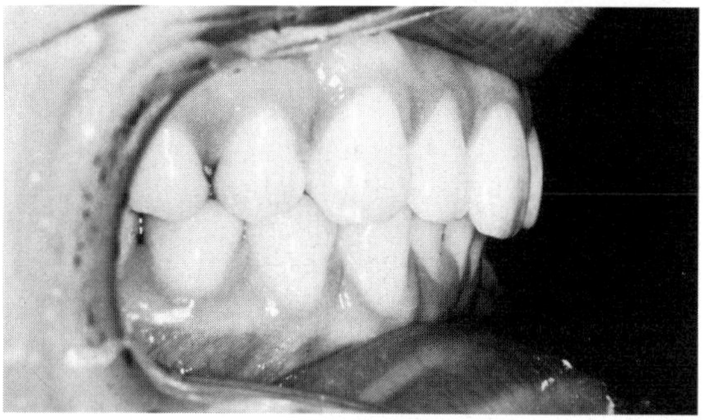
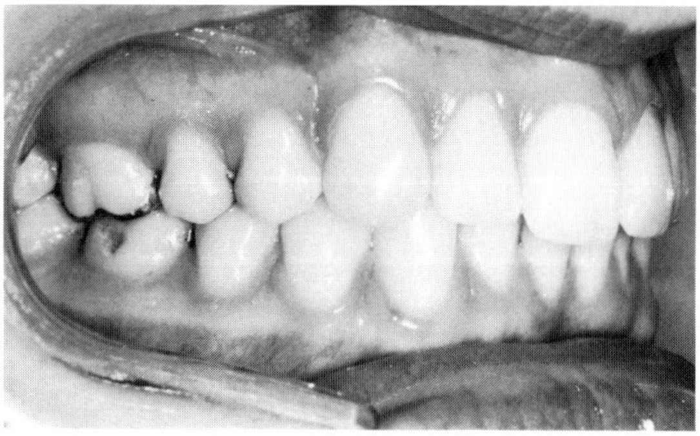
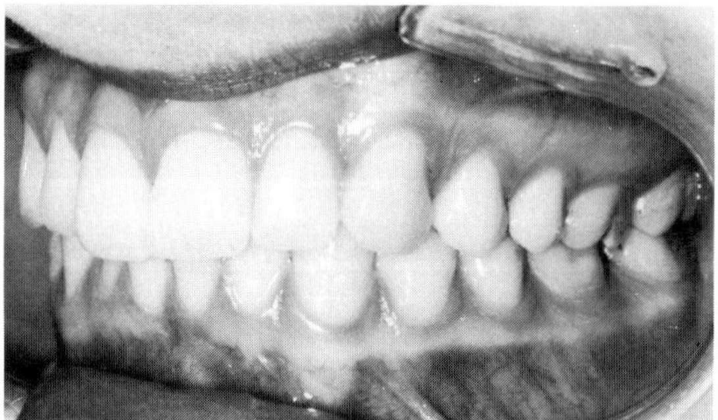

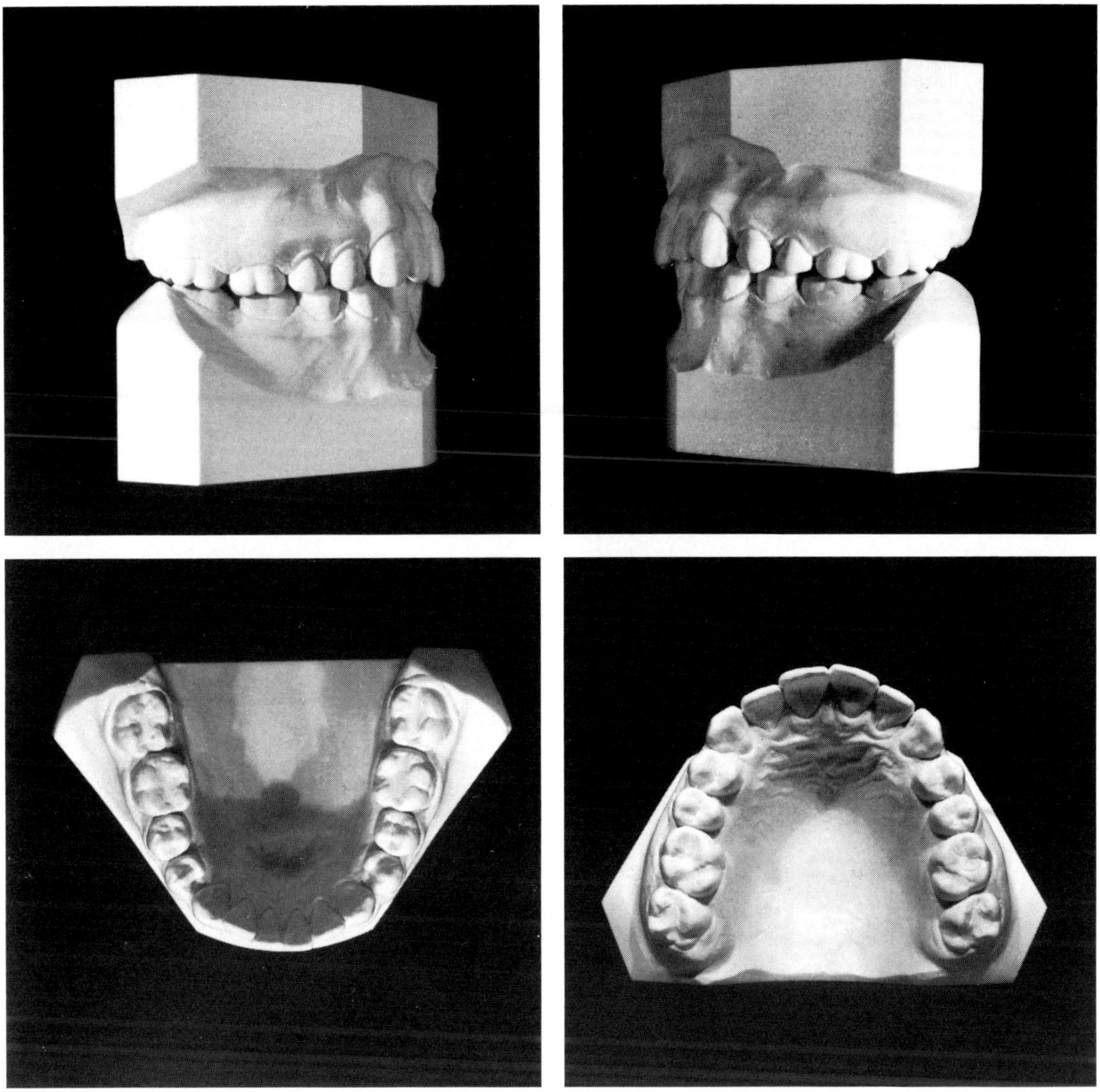

Figs 20-12 and 20-13 *At the age of 23 y, 4 mo, ten years after treatment, the picture has scarcely changed. Mild tertiary crowding has appeared in the mandibular incisors. The mandibular right lateral incisor has moved to lingual; the left lateral has also, although less so.*

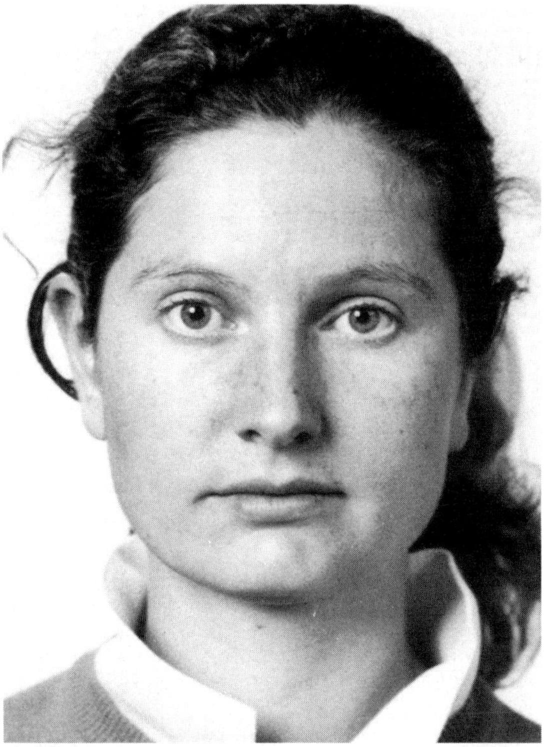

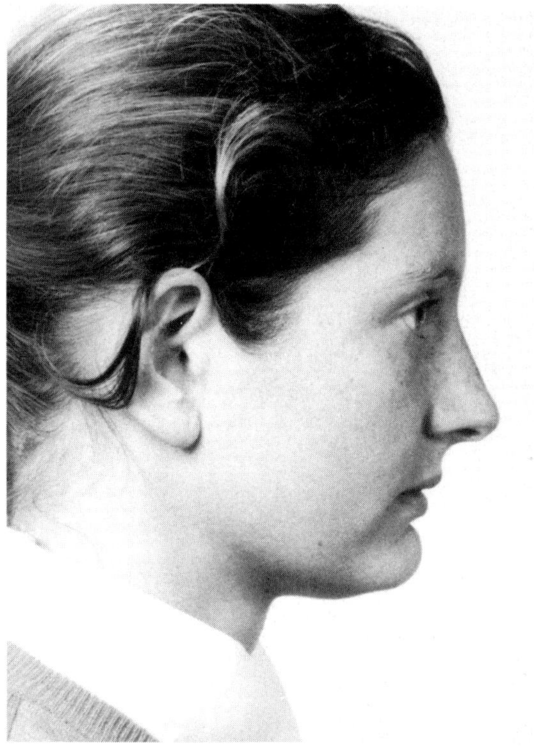

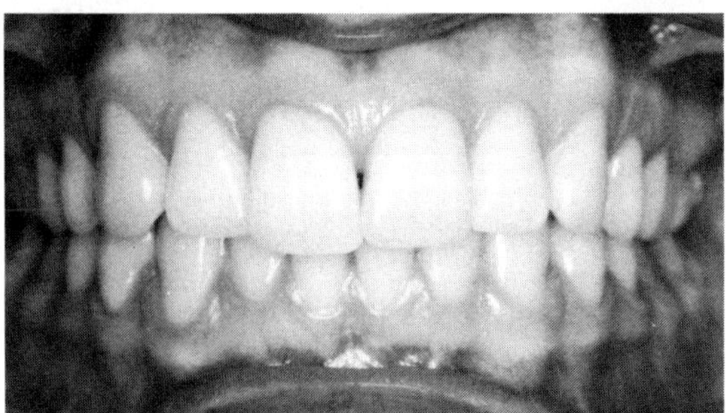

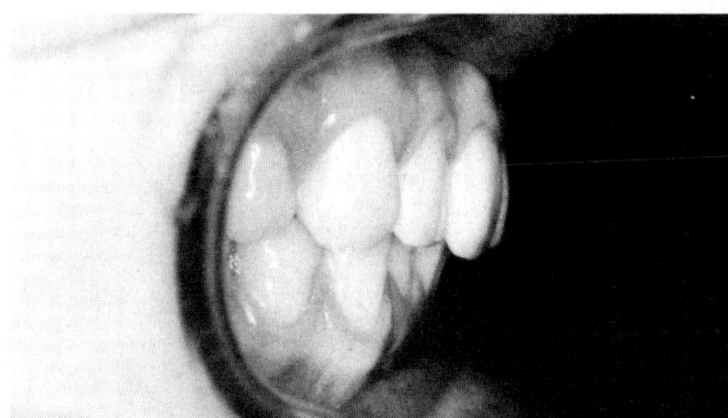

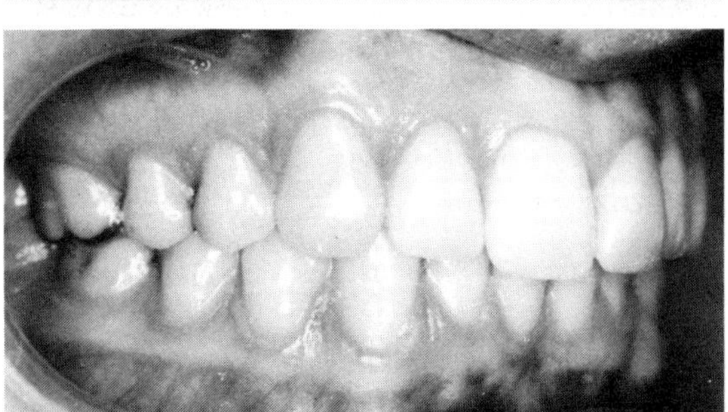

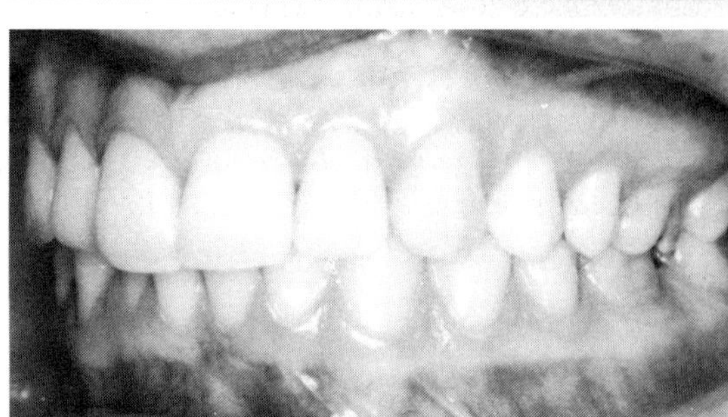

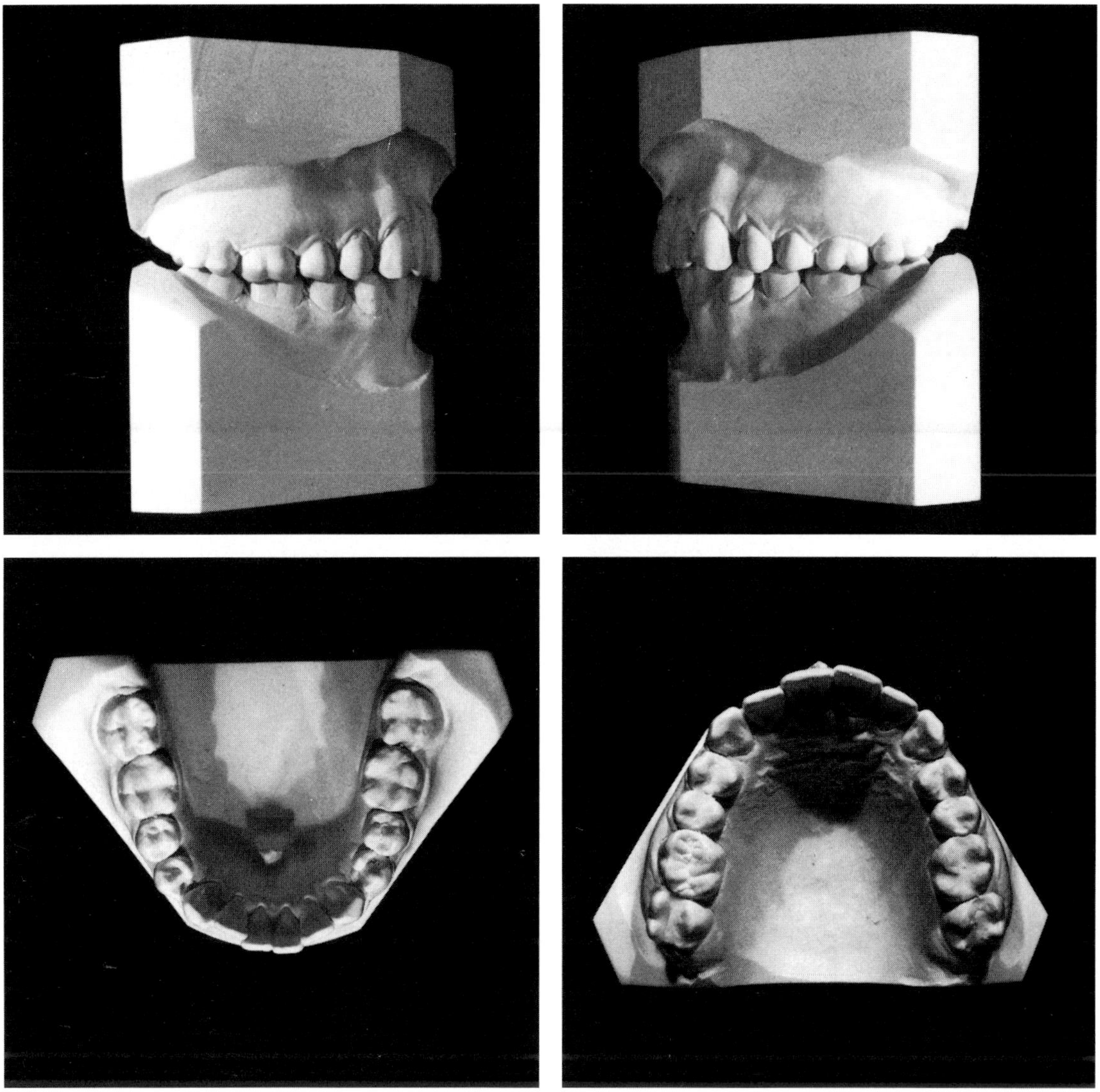

Figs 20-14 and 20-15 *At the age of 28 y, 5 mo, fifteen years after treatment, the tertiary crowding in the mandibular incisors has increased somewhat. Both lateral incisors in the mandible have moved a little more lingually. The maxillary incisors have become mildly irregular, although it is not obtrusive.*

Figure 20-16a

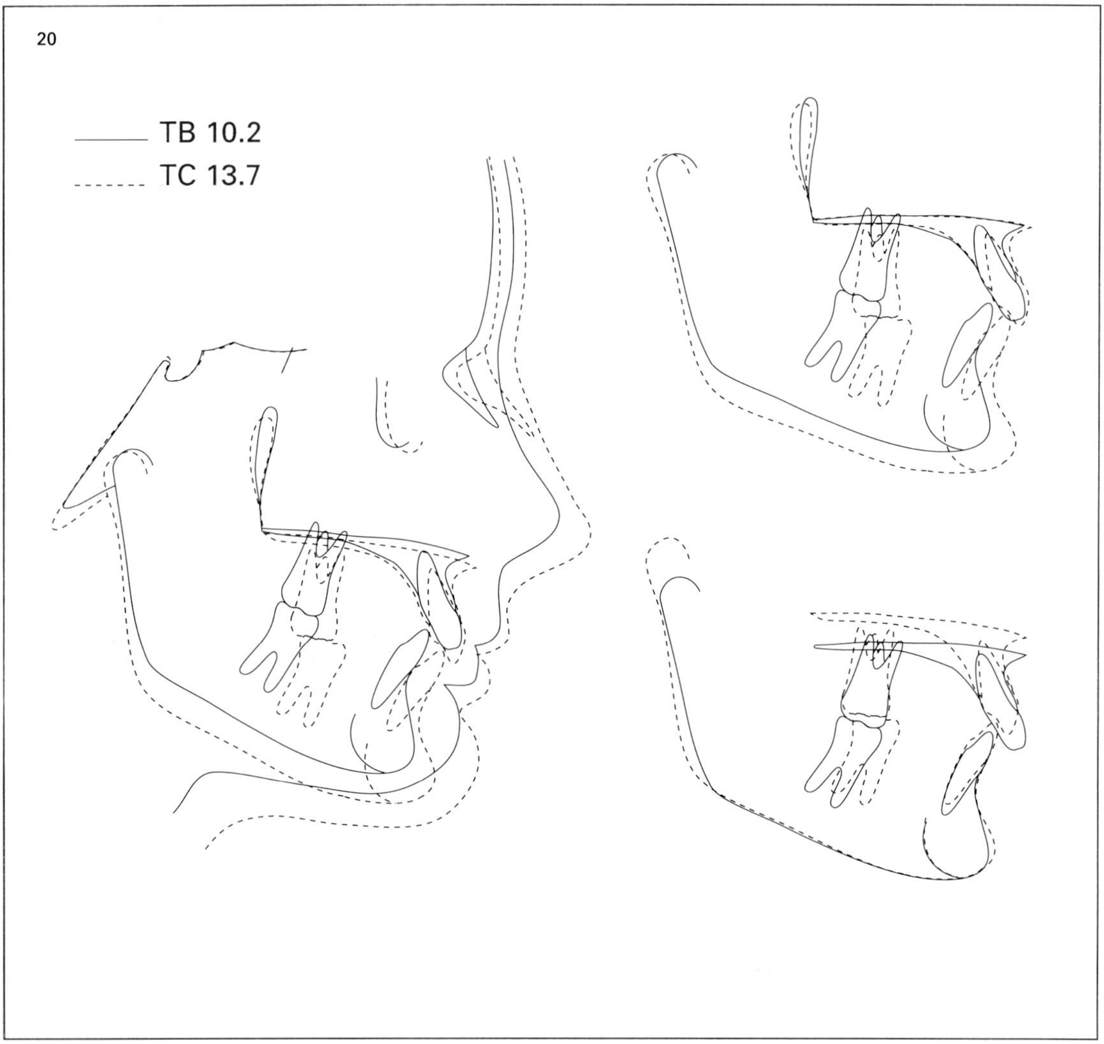

Fig 20-16 Superimpositions of tracings of cephalometric radiographs show that during treatment the mandible grew significantly ventrally and vertically, while the ventral development of the maxillary complex was restrained. Subsequent to treatment, growth was essentially ventrally directed.

Figure 20-16b

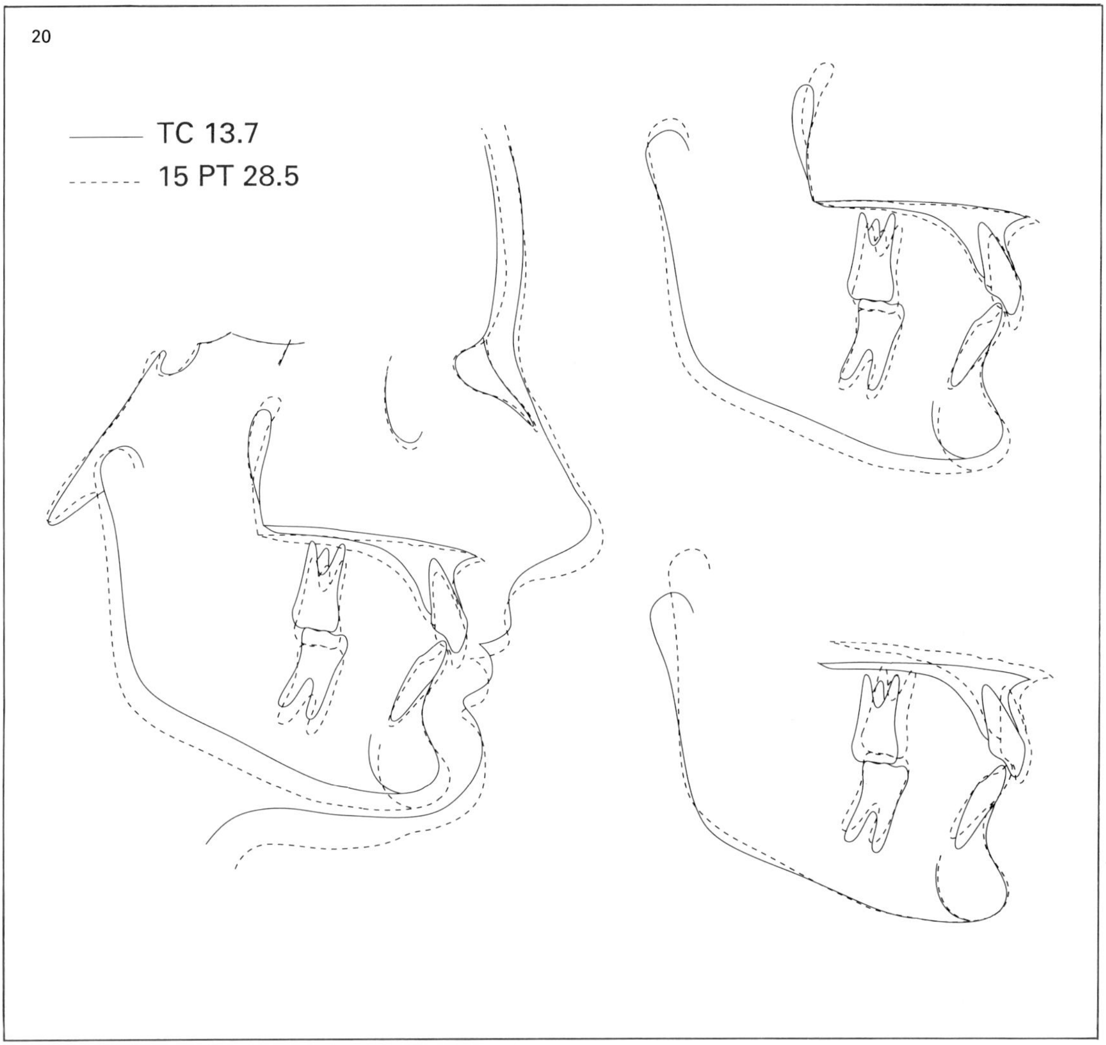

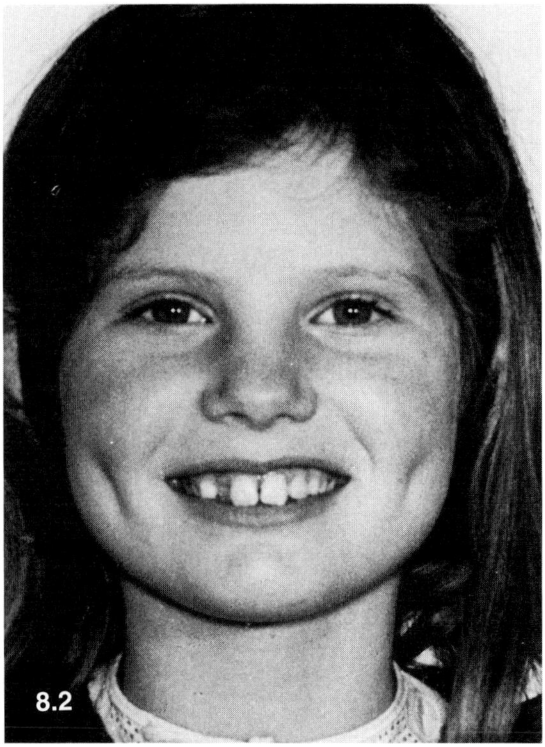

8.2

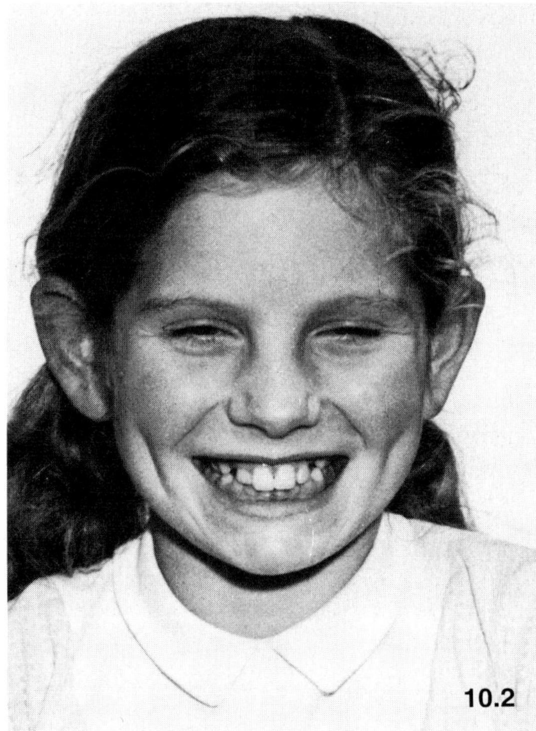

10.2

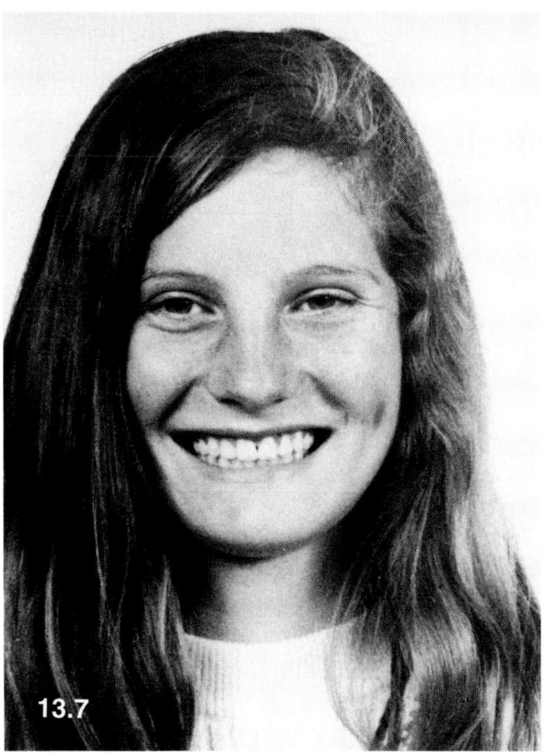

13.7

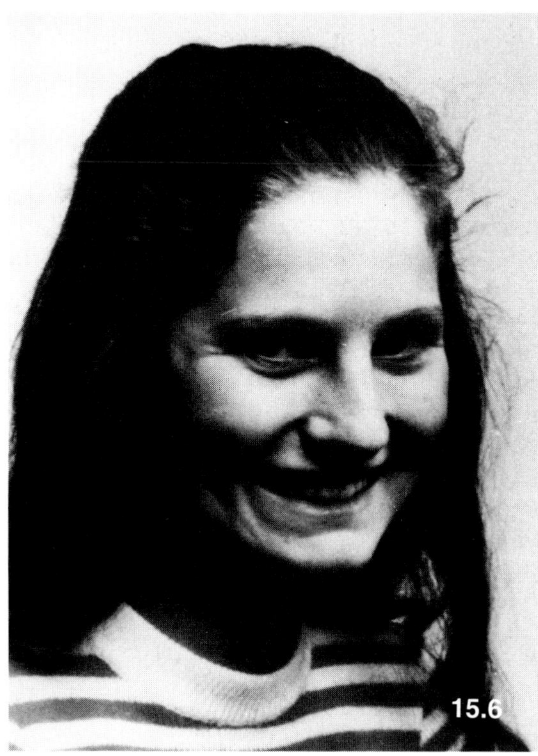

15.6

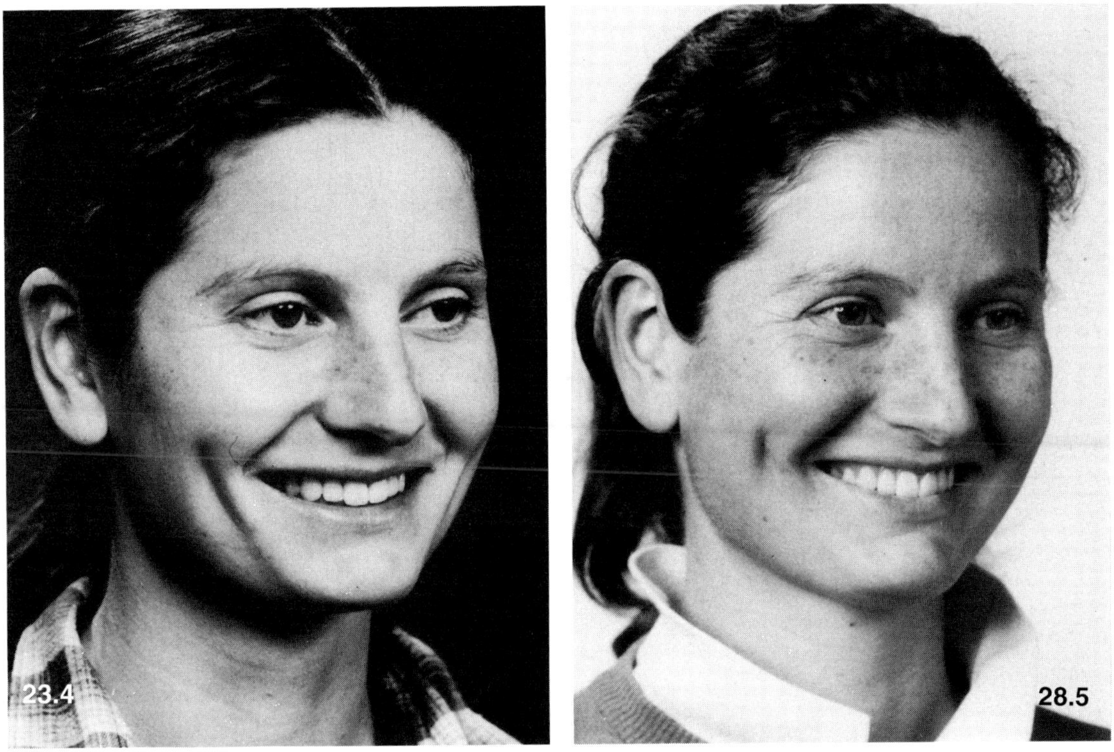

Fig 20-17 Note the changes that occurred in 20 years with growth and treatment.

contact the canines and used to displace those teeth a little to palatal. When the patient was 13 years 6 months, a satisfactory result had been achieved and all appliances were removed (Figs 20.8 and 20.9).

Two years later little had changed; just the maxillary right central incisor had over-erupted slightly (Figs 20.10 and 20.11). Ten years after treatment ,the mandibular incisors showed mild tertiary crowding; the mandibular right lateral incisor had moved lingually and the left one had too, but less so (Figs 20.12 and 20.13). Another five years later, the tertiary crowding has increased, with the right lateral incisor as well as the left one being in linguoposition (Figs 20.14 and 20.15). With the mandibular tertiary crowding, the maxillary incisors have also become mildly irregular. Nevertheless, the treatment is still found to be satisfactory after fifteen years. The superimposition of the tracings shows the effects of growth and treatment (Fig 20.16). The photographs of her smiling face show the changes over many years (Fig 20.17).

If a maxillary lateral incisor is in reversed overbite, it is necessary to investigate whether or not there is a ventral forced bite. This generally concerns a class II/1

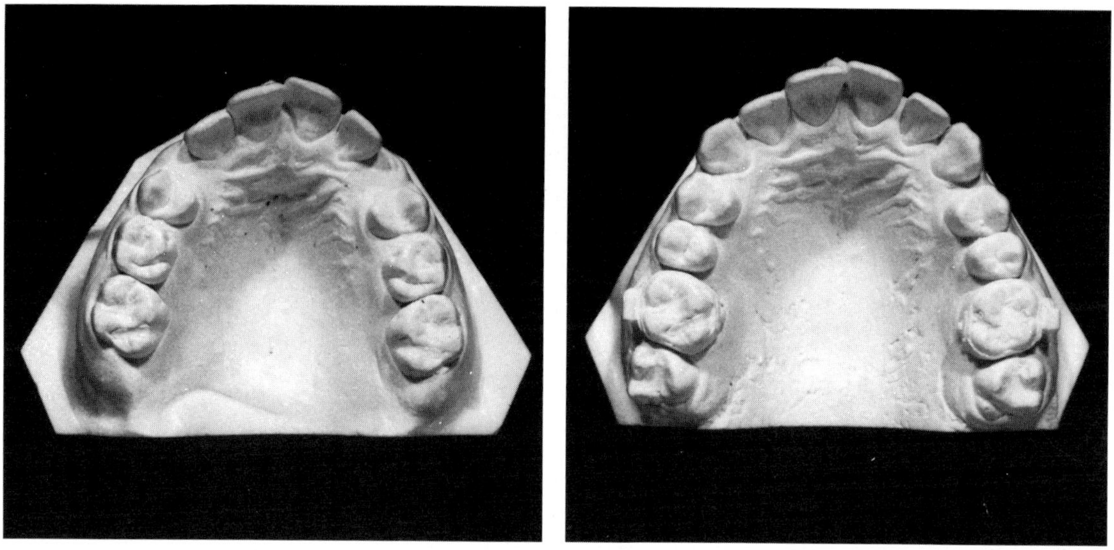

Fig 20-18 Thanks to the cervical headgear, the dental arch perimeter has been increased significantly over 1½ years. The maxillary dental arch has become broader as the result of the cheeks being held away and the rail mechanism working (see Fig 7-9, page 108). By preventing mesial migration of the first permanent molars, the space in the premolar region has been retained. Moreover, the first permanent molars have been moved a little to distal and distally rotated.

anomaly, which due to the forced bite may give the appearance of being a neutro-occlusion (Fig 20.19). Such forced bites can be combined with a lateral forced bite — then a midline deviation and occasionally a unilateral crossbite are usually seen.

Biting on a tongue blade or similar thin spatula is a reasonably effective and certainly the least expensive method of correcting the reversed overbite of a single tooth, particularly when the antagonist may be displaced in the opposite direction. That method can also be applied to the reversed overbite of two adjacent maxillary incisors. It then depends rather more than in the correction of a single tooth on the understanding of the patient of the purpose of the tongue blade biting and the enthusiasm that is brought to it. This is particularly so in the critical phase when it is just possible to close the mandibular teeth behind the maxillary ones. The chance of success is increased if buttons are placed on the teeth that require reciprocal movement so that the patient can fit crossbite elastics as soon as it is possible to close the mandibular teeth behind the maxillary ones. It has to be emphasised that improvement can only be achieved if there is enough space and if the vertical overbite after correction is sufficient to prevent a relapse. Moreover, it is essential to ensure that the unerupted canine is clear of the lateral incisor alongside it.

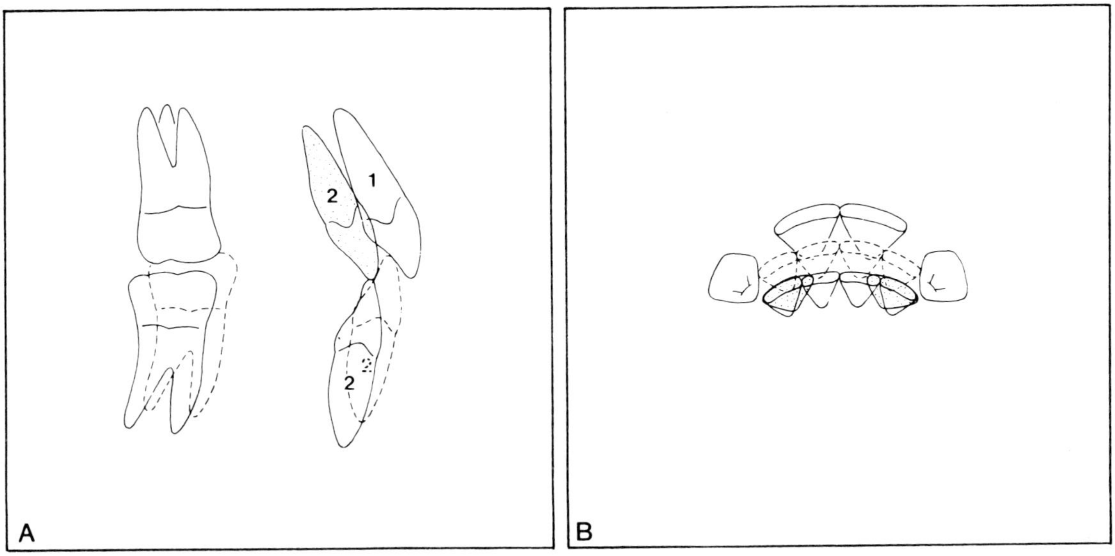

Fig 20-19 Diagrammatic illustration of a ventral forced bite in association with a class II/1 anomaly, resulting in a neutro-occlusion.

A In normal closing movements of the mandible, the incisal edges of the lateral incisors strike each other. Maximal occlusion occurs more to ventral, with the mandibular lateral incisor between the maxillary lateral and central incisors. The molars take up a neutro-occlusion.

B Occlusal view of the maxilla with the four mandibular incisors drawn in with continuous lines to depict initial contact with normal closure. Maximal occlusion is shown with broken lines. The maxillary lateral incisors are hatched to relate them to A.

The picture illustrated here can be seen in class II/1 anomalies with marked crowding in the maxilla, when the eruption and emergence of the maxillary permanent central incisor is associated with premature loss of the deciduous lateral incisors. In the maxilla, the distance between the deciduous canines becomes a little greater and the permanent maxillary lateral incisors emerge palatally. If subsequently contact develops between them and the mandibular arch, then the lateral incisors can go even further to palatal and the mandibular incisors slide over these teeth to ventral. The occlusion of the other teeth then is adapted to that situation.[30]

Most orthodontic treatment can only be concluded when the premolars and canines are in good occlusion. That applies particularly to the correction of disto-occlusions. If treatment was begun at an early age, then it may be many years before the previously mentioned point is reached. It is not possible to accelerate the eruption of premolars and canines. It is clearly desirable to delay the provision of appliances for as long as appropriate, to avoid unnecessarily long treatment times. If an early start is wished for, then if it is at all possible the treatment should be split into phases with rest periods without appliances.
Among other situations, such a case would be a serious class II/1 anomaly with the lower lip behind the maxillary incisors, where there is a great risk that the protruding maxillary incisors will be fractured. In this case there was deliberate delay until the second transitional phase was almost complete. After correction of the reversed overbite, there was no reason for beginning treatment early. One of the objectives of this strategy is to avoid treatment fatigue.
A last point requiring emphasis is that after extraction of deciduous canines it is usually necessary to ensure that sufficient room is made available for the permanent canines. In class II/1 cases, this can be achieved in the maxilla with the use of a cervical headgear, simultaneously with such other treatment aims as might be dealt with by that appliance.

Chapter 21

Class I with class II/2 tendency, reversed overbite with ventral forced bite over 11 and 21

Tongue blade, cervical headgear later with Kahn spur, maxillary removable plate, brackets on 12, 11, 21 and 22, maxillary removable retainer

Male 8 years, 5 months to 29 years, 0 months

A boy aged 8 years, 5 months exhibited a class I anomaly with a ventral forced bite, with no other functional abnormalities. He could bring his mandible sufficiently far back for the incisal edges of the right central incisors to meet. In that situation, there was a slight disto-occlusion. The maxillary second deciduous molars were badly carious, with the result that the mesiodistal size of those teeth was reduced (Figs 21.1 and 21.2).

It was decided to correct the reversed overbite as quickly as possible, also with the object of preventing the lateral incisors making faulty contacts as they emerged further. In view of the considerable overbite and the desired reciprocal displacement of the involved teeth, the use of a tongue blade was an obvious solution (see Fig 20.3, page 330). After two weeks, both the reversed overbite and the ventral forced bite had been eliminated and the mandibular dental arch occluded a few millimeters further to distal (Figs 21.3 and 21.4). The further eruption of the lateral incisors needed no guidance and there were no other reasons for active intervention. It would be sufficient to maintain observation of his dental development and facial growth. It would not be until the second transitional period that orthodontic treatment might be initiated.

During the five-year period of observation, the situation in the maxillary and mandibular anteriors did not improve as much as expected. Although adequate space was available in the dental arches and the occlusion did not present impediments, spontaneous corrections barely came about. Gradually the spacing vanished and an increasing degree of crowding developed. The carious deciduous molars were neither restored nor extracted (Figs 21.5 and 21.6).

At age 12 years, 10 months, the lingually tipped mandibular left second deciduous molar and the persistent maxillary right deciduous canine were removed (Figs 21.7 and 21.8). Ten months later, a cervical headgear was fitted and eight months later a maxillary removable plate was inserted. The latter was replaced by brackets on the maxillary incisors four months later, incorporating a .0175" twistflex arch-wire. To intrude the maxillary incisors and apply torque to them, a .019" × .026" archwire was subsequently fitted and a Kahn spur was added to the cervical headgear. After active

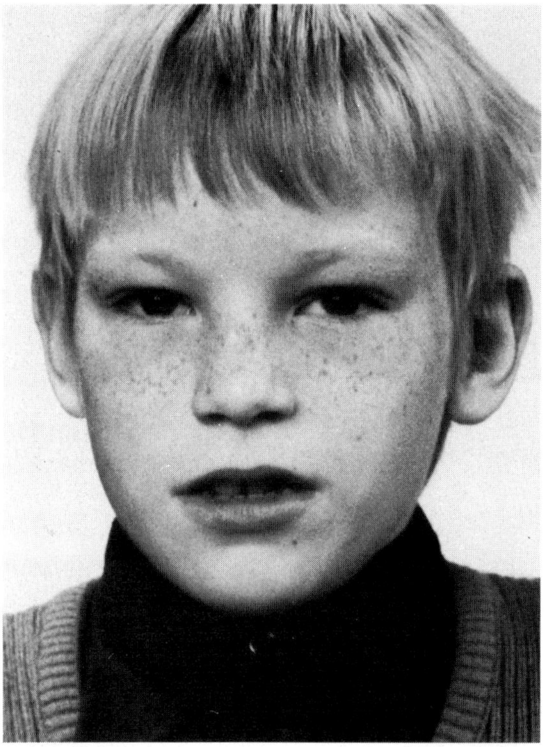

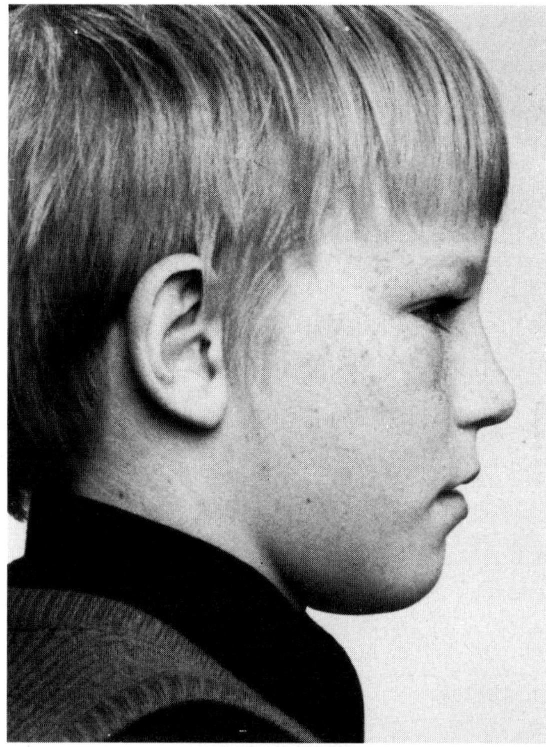

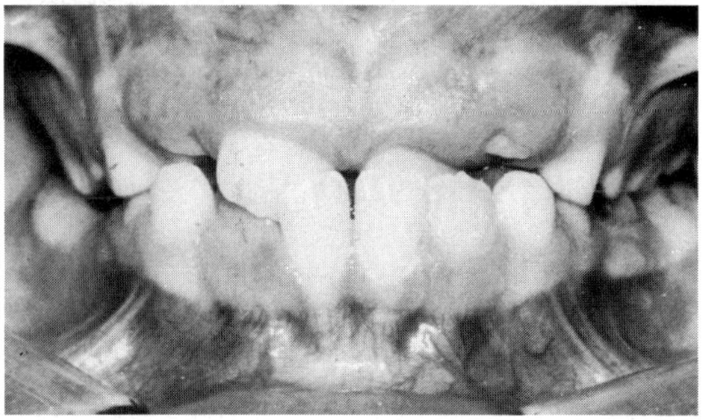

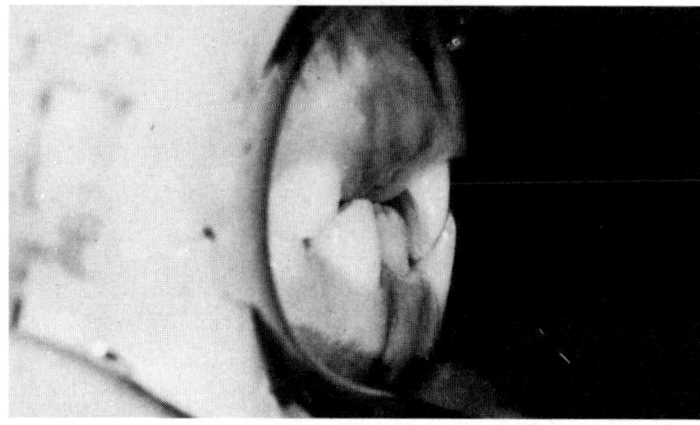

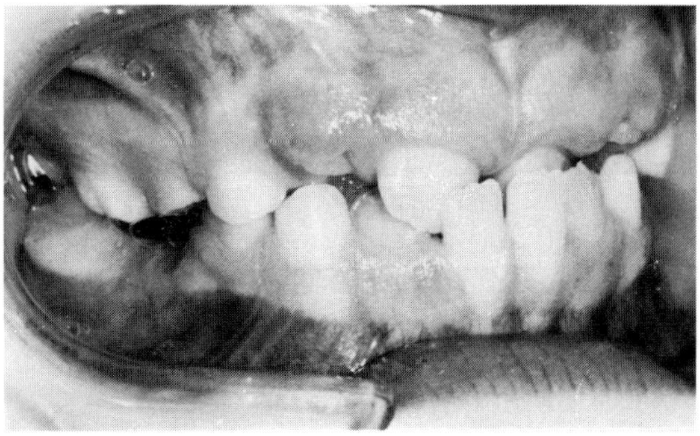

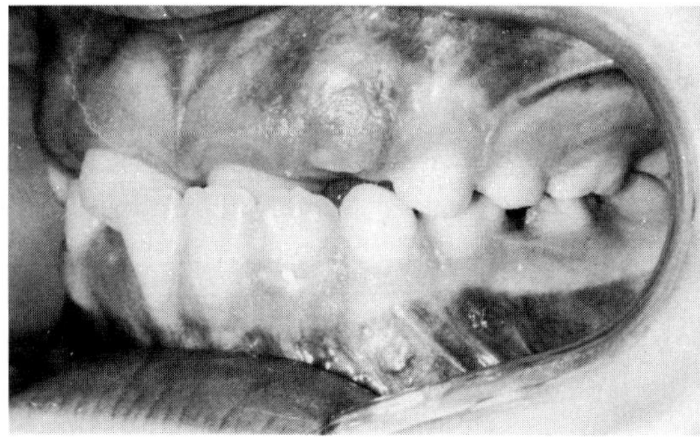

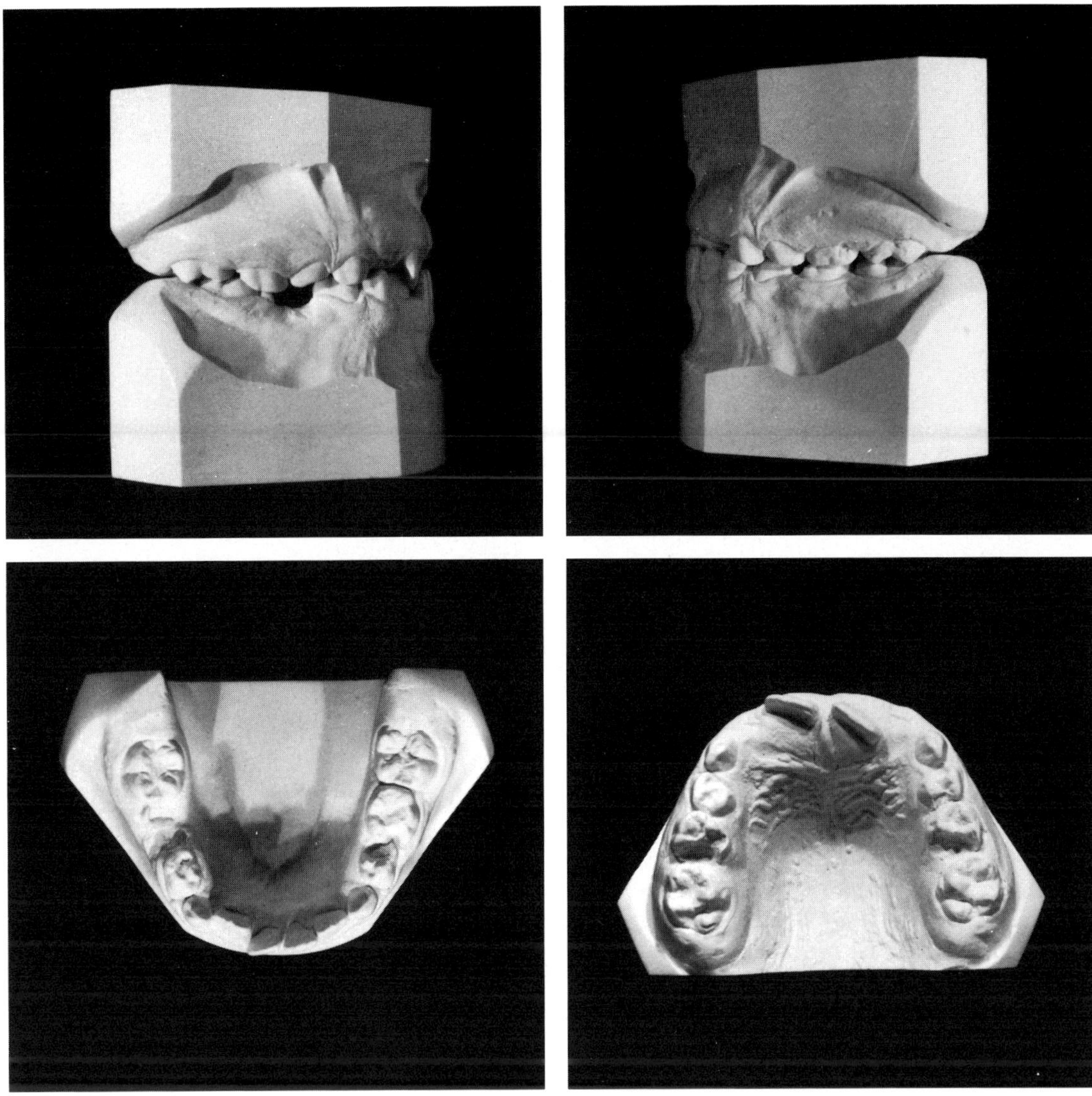

Figs 21-1 and 21-2 *A boy of 8 y, 5 mo with a reversed anterior overbite associated with a ventral forced bite, so that a slight disto-relation has been masked. He can bite in a sufficiently retruded position so that the right central incisors meet edge-to-edge. The dental arch perimeters both have been reduced by caries of the deciduous molars. The central incisors in the mandible are tipped a little to labial and those in the maxilla are mildly tipped palatally. In reversed overbite, the incisors make contact with the right maxillary central incisor lingual to the mandibular central incisor but labial to the lateral incisor. In the maxilla, the lateral incisors have only recently emerged and have not yet established contact with the opposing teeth.*

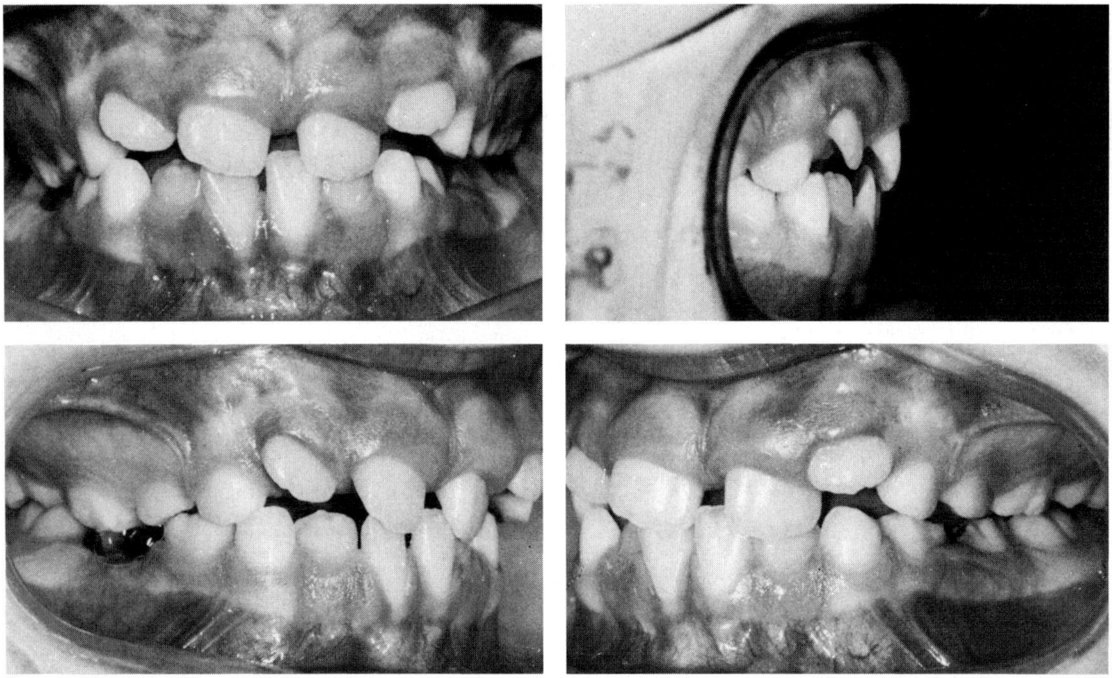

Figure 21-3

treatment for one year and ten months, the appliances were removed and a maxillary removable retainer was provided. This retainer was worn continuously for three months and for the next three months only at night. At the age of 16 year, 0 months, a satisfactory result had been obtained (Figs 21.9 and 21.10). In the two years following the end of retention, some crowding of the mandibular anteriors became evident and subsequently increased only a little. The inclination of the maxillary incisors barely changed, which can be attributed to the normal vertical position of stomion (Figs 21.11, 21.12, and 21.16). At the age of 25 years, nine years after the end of retention, a satisfying situation exists (Figs 21.13 and 21.14). The facial changes are shown in Figure 21.15.

A reversed overbite of the incisors that is associated with a ventral forced bite should preferably be corrected during the first transitional period. A cooperative patient can usually procure the desired tooth movements with the use of a tongue blade (wooden spatula) and subsequently the development of the dentition can proceed normally. Some time later consideration should be given to the need for further orthodontic treatment, and, if it is necessary, then when it should best be performed. This case is an exception concerning the limited tendency for spontaneous reduction of the irregularity of the maxillary and mandibular incisors following correction of the reversed overbite. Normally the influence of the tongue and lips is sufficient to bring about re-alignment of incisors as long as there is adequate room for such

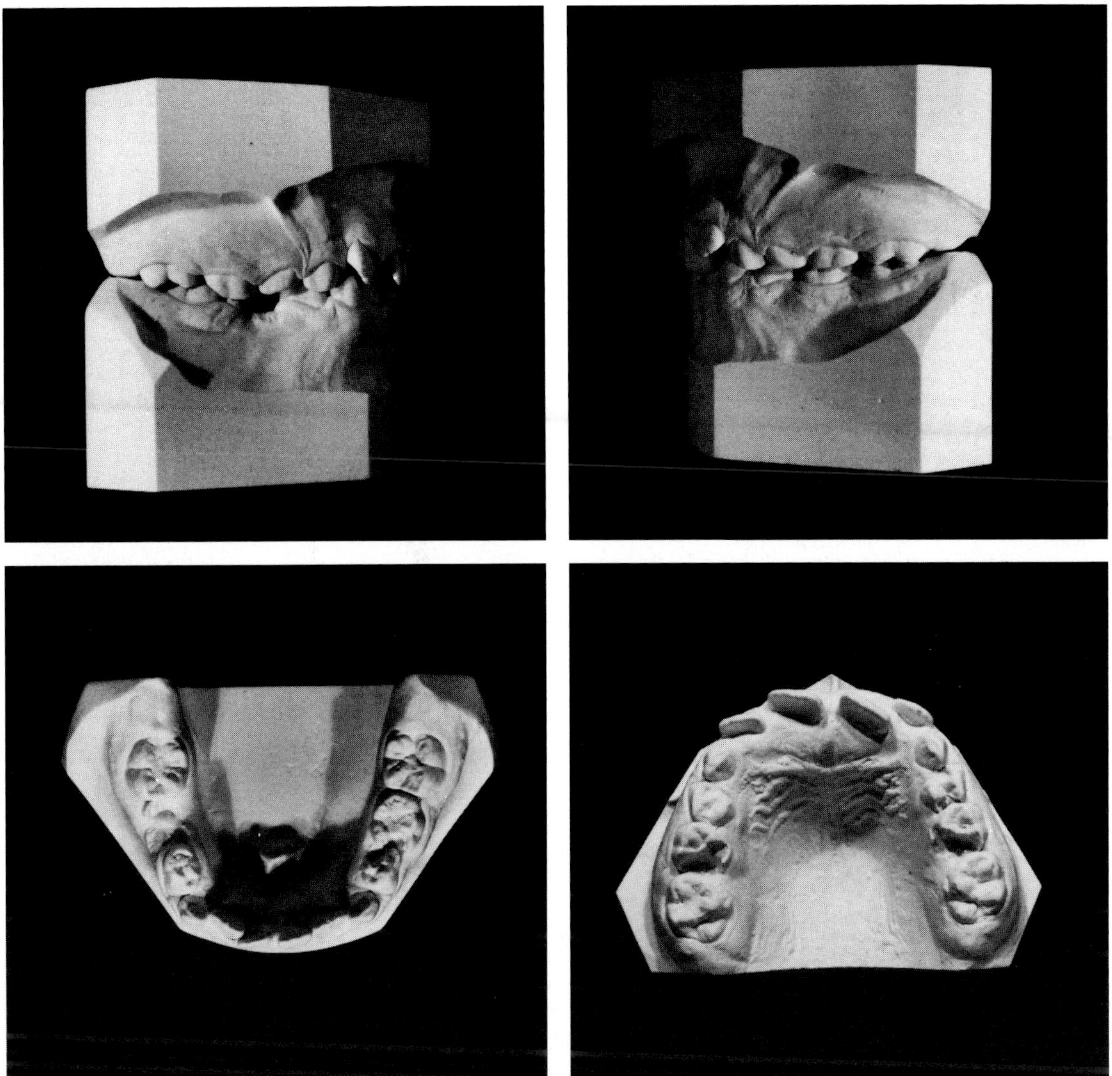

Figs 21-3 and 21-4 *At the age of 8 y, 6 mo, use of a tongue blade for only two weeks has secured correction of the reversed anterior overbite. In the mandible, the two central incisors and the left lateral incisor have moved lingually. In the maxilla, both central incisors have moved labially and as they erupt both lateral incissors will assume contact labially to the mandibular incisors.*

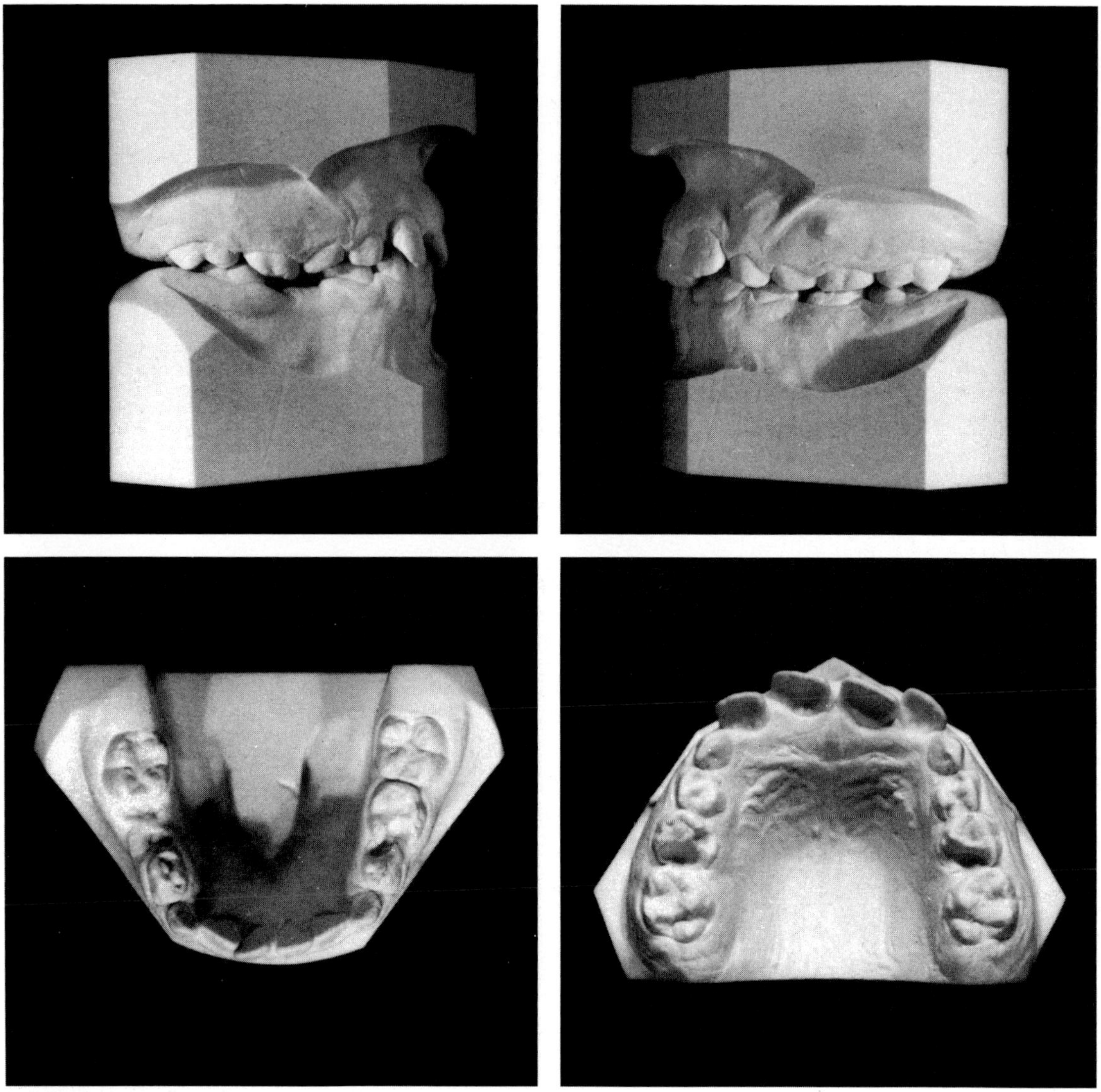

Figure 21-5 At the age of 9 yr, 3 m, the neutro-occlusion has changed little. By overerupting the maxillary right second deciduous molar with its large disto-occlusal cavity has prevented too much mesial drifting of the mandibular right first permanent molar. The position of the mandibular right central incisor has not improved in the last nine months despite the space available and the absence of impediment from the occlusion. It can be seen that subsequent to the correction of the reversed anterior overbite minimal spontaneous corrections have followed. Only the irregularities of the maxillary incisors are slightly reduced.

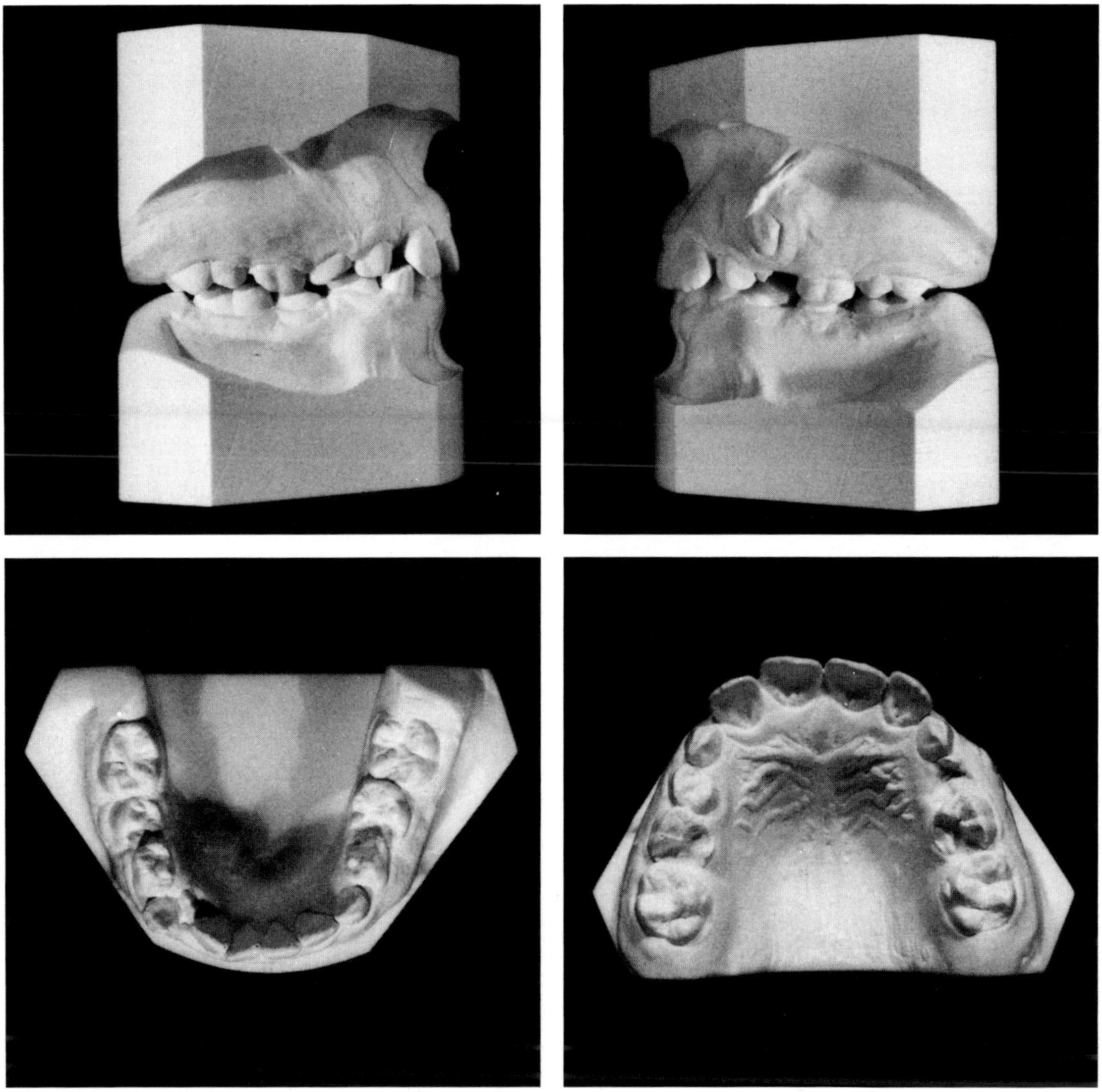

Figure 21-6 *At the age of 11 y, 3 mo, the extra room in the region of the right mandibular central incisor has vanished and the overall crowding of the mandibular anteriors has increased slightly. The permanent canine on the right has emerged lingually. Sufficient room is available in the dental arch on the right for the mandibular second premolar. The left maxillary first premolar has emerged too far to buccal, probably in association with the persistent root fragment of its precursor. The maxillary incisors are now aligned regularly and the rotations of the central incisors are no longer apparent.*

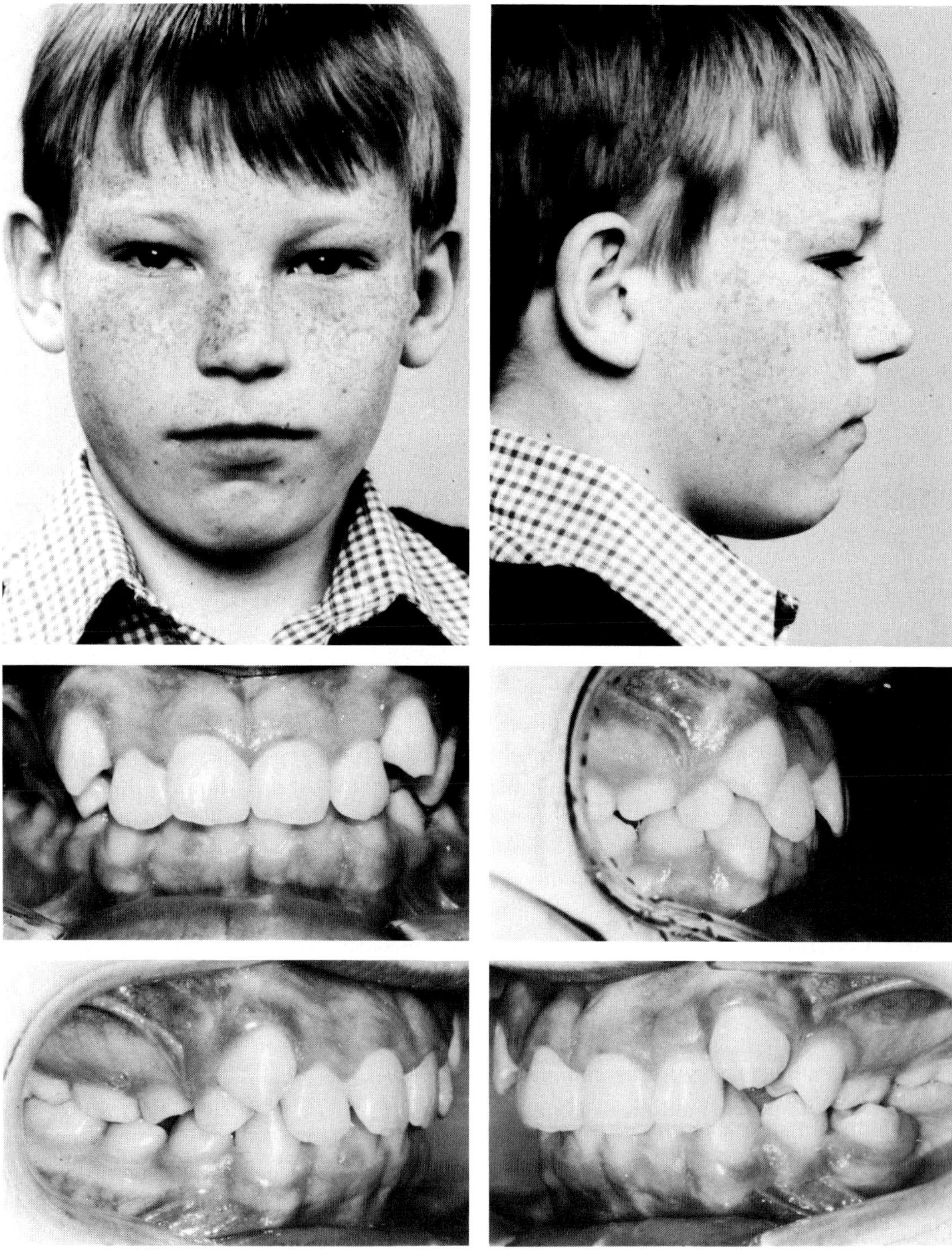

Tongue blade, cervical headgear later with Kahn spur, maxillary removable plate, brackets on 12, 11, 21 and 22, maxillary removable retainer

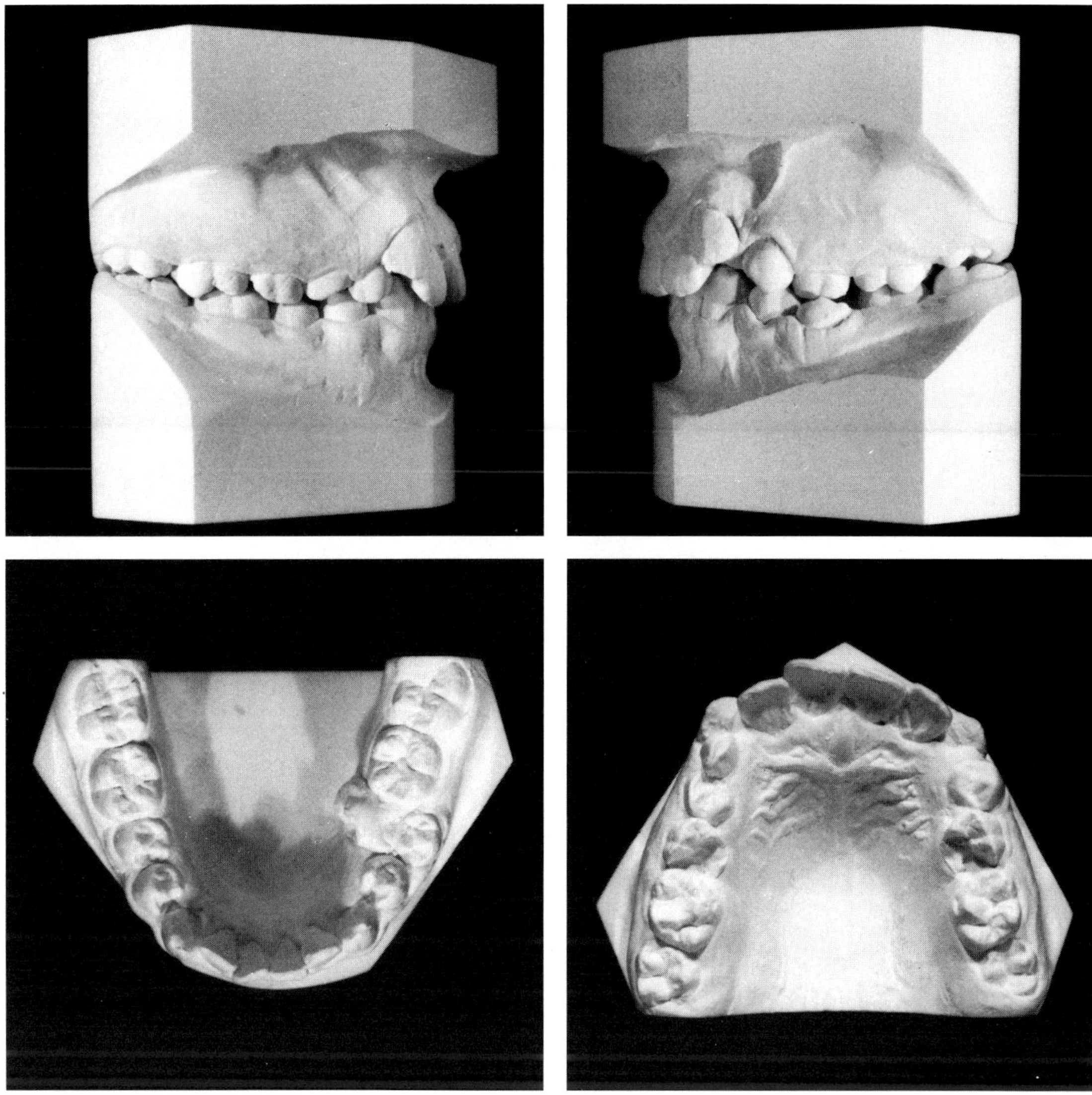

Figs 21-7 and 21-8 *At the age of 12 y, 10 mo, the maxillary canines have emerged ectostomatically. On the left there is not enough room, in contrast to the right where the deciduous canine has remained. The carious maxillary second deciduous molars are still present, as is the mandibular second deciduous molar on the left; the latter has been forced to lingual by the eruption of the premolar. The maxillary incisors are steeply positioned, the bite is deep and the maxillary right lateral incisor has overerupted. On the right, there is neutro-occlusion, left a disto-occlusion of ½ PW, while nonetheless the midlines of both dental arches match quite well. The difference in occlusion corresponds with the crowding in the second quadrant and with the mesial migration and rotation of the maxillary left first permanent molar.*

Class I with class II/2 tendency, reversed overbite with ventral forced bite over 11 and 21

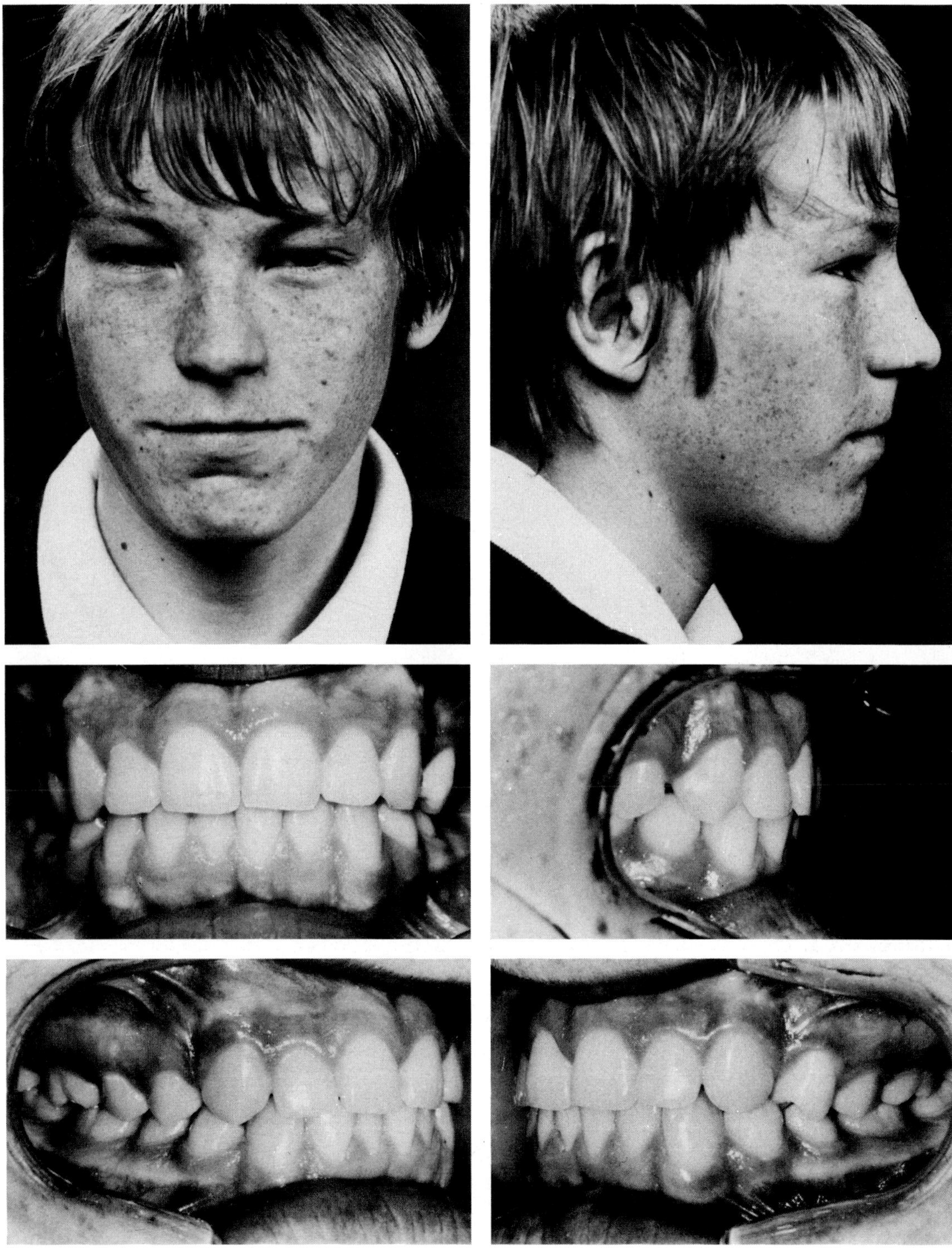

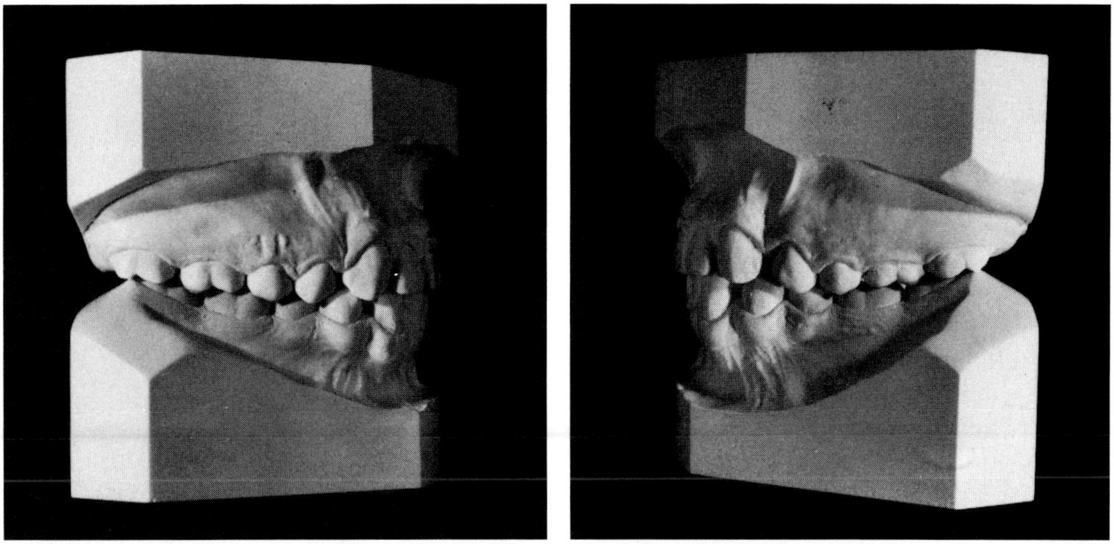

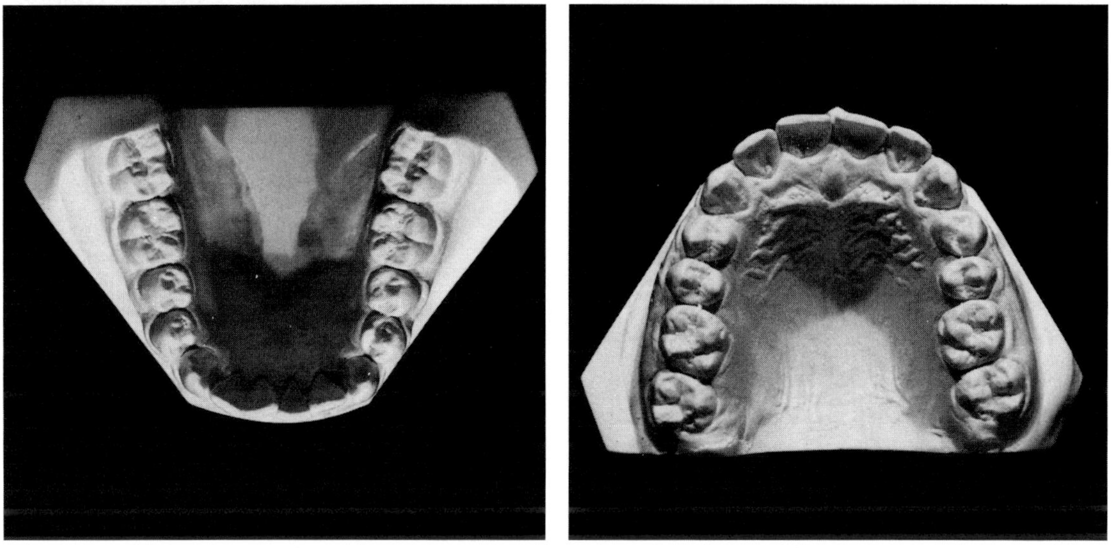

Figs 21-9 and 21-10 *At the age of 16 y, 0 mo, after a treatment time of one year and ten months with a retention period of six months, a good result has been obtained with solid interdigitation of the posterior teeth. In the mandibular arch, spontaneous improvements have occurred that could be attributed to the intrusion and protrusion of the maxillary incisors. Only the mandibular right central incisor has rotated a little more. The clinical crown of the maxillary first premolar that originally emerged buccally is longer than that on the right side.*

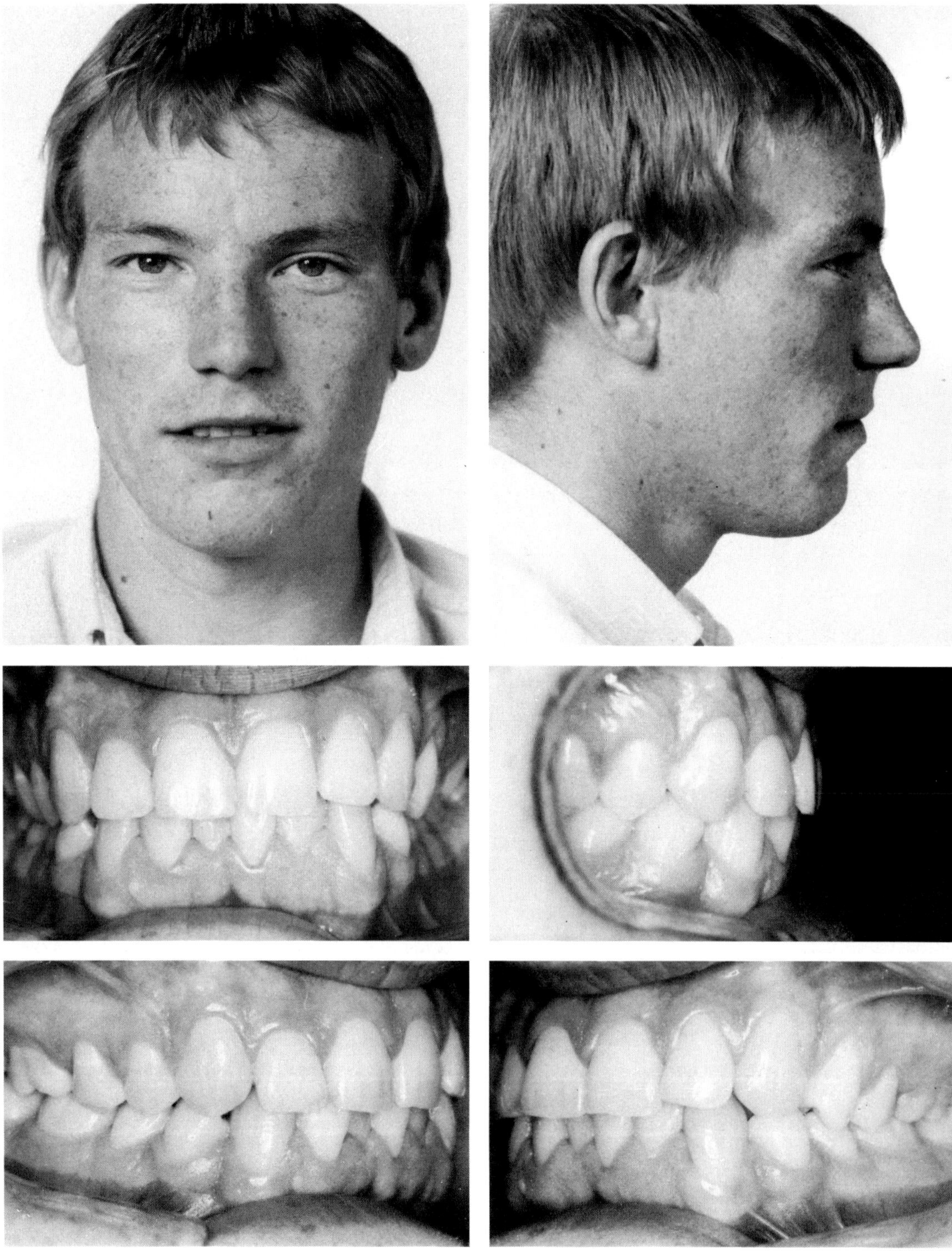

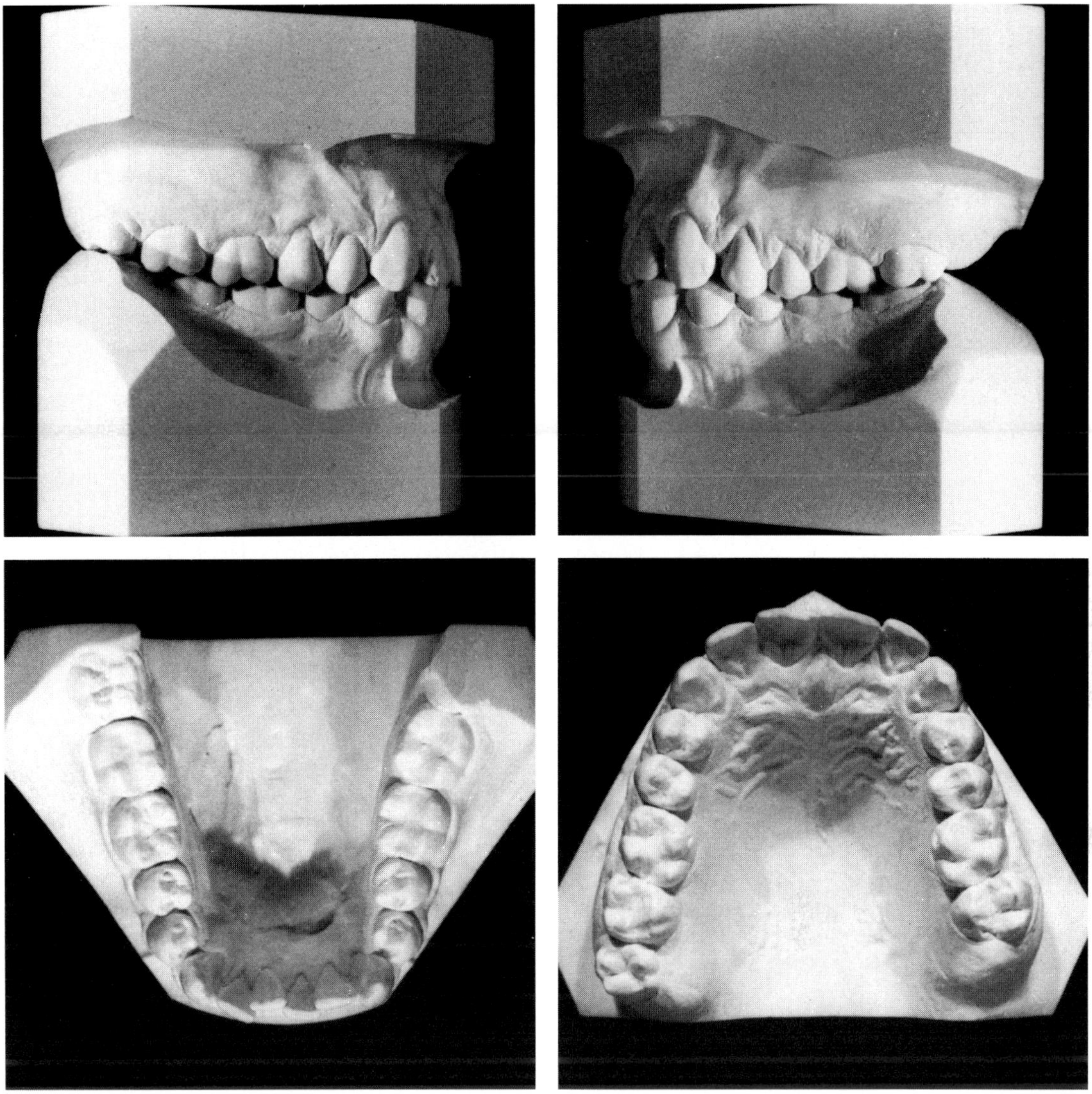

Figs 21-11 and 21-12 At the age of 21 y, 1 mo, the mandibular lateral incisors are more lingually placed than they were five years previously. The tertiary crowding present at the age of 18 has become more evident and is unrelated to the treatment but probably is due to the late growth of the mandible and not to the third molars for which insufficient room exists. In the maxilla, where the third molar on the right has emerged, little has changed.

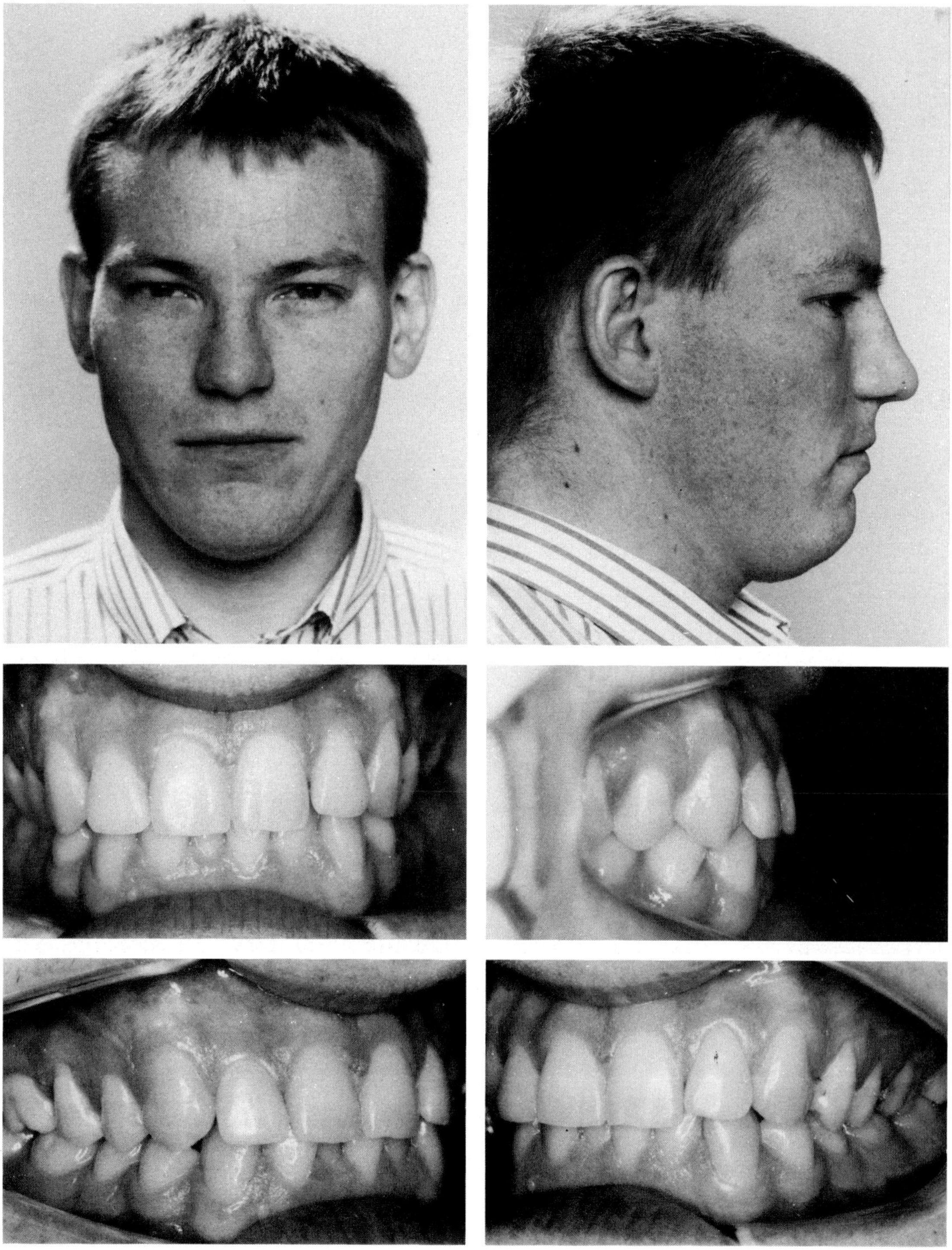

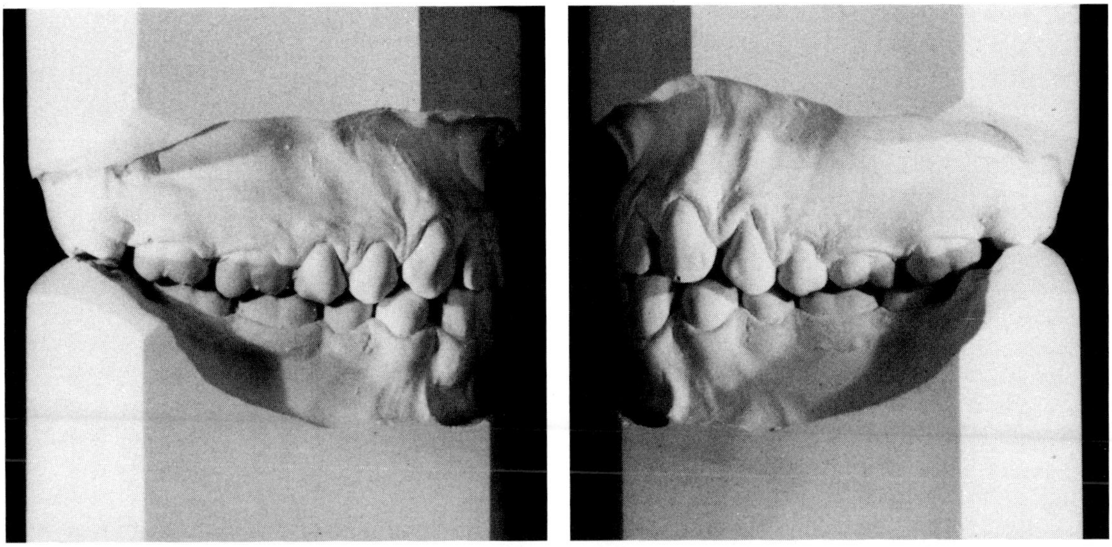

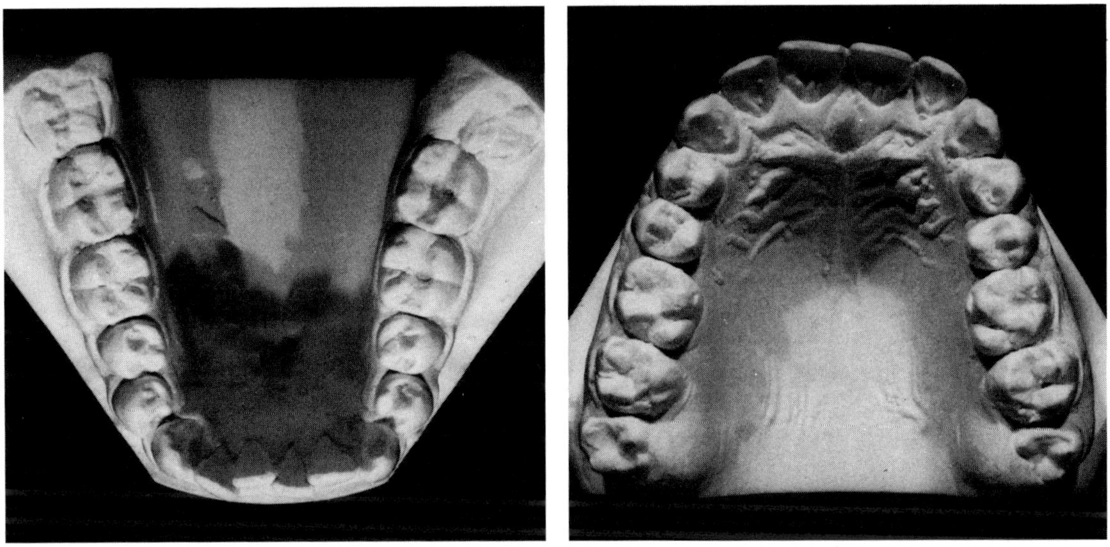

Figs 21-13 and 21-14 *Aged 25 yr. 1 m., nine years after termination of retention, the result is satisfactory; the mandibular incisor crowding is not considered objectionable. Insufficient room is available for third molars on the left and both should be removed.*

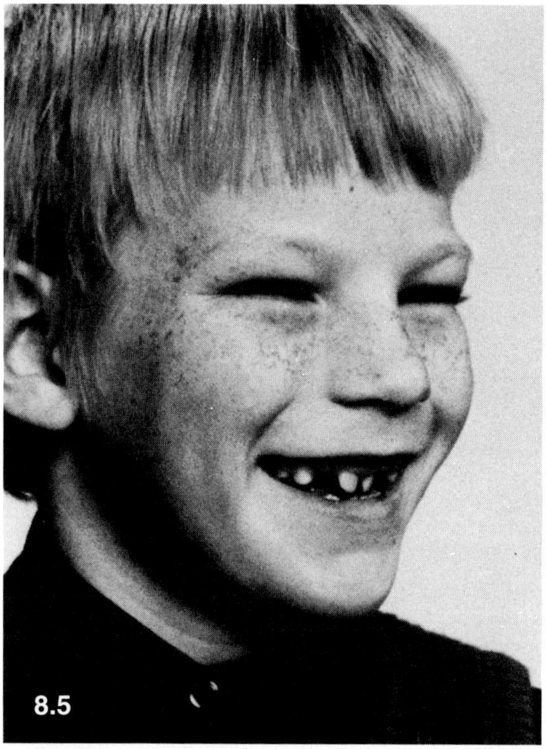
8.5

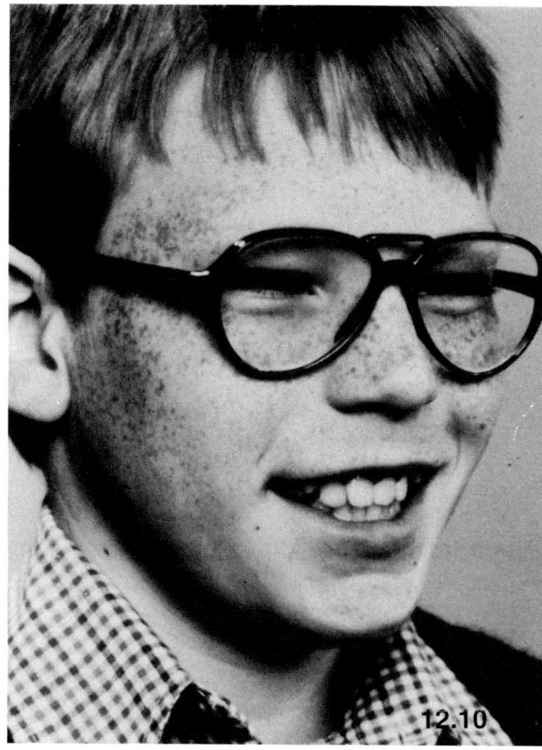
12.10

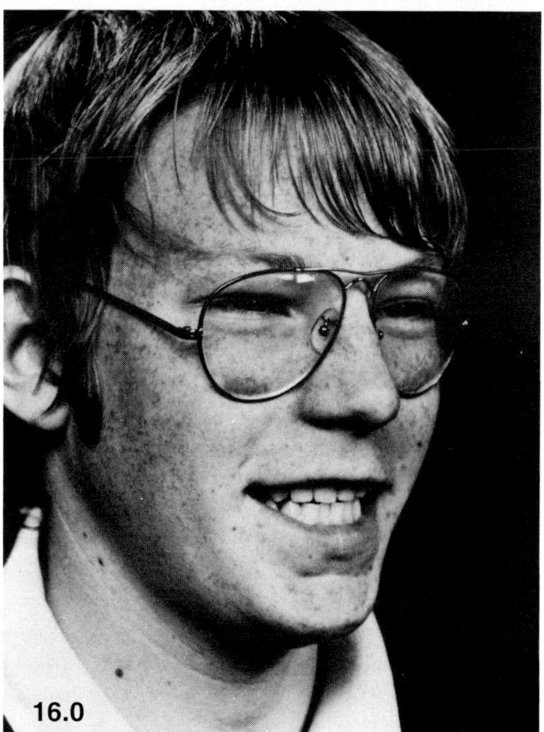
16.0

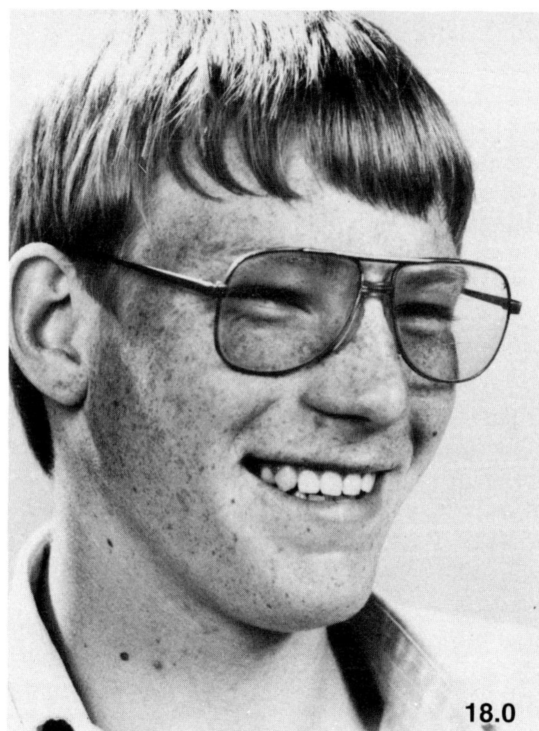
18.0

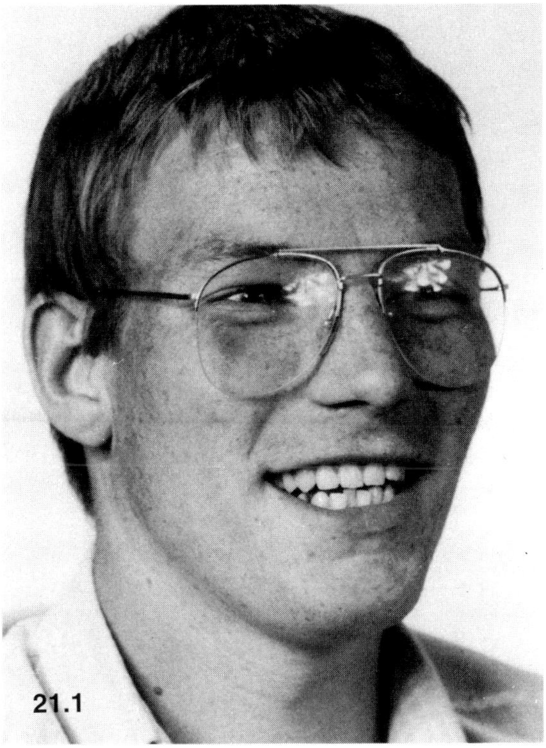

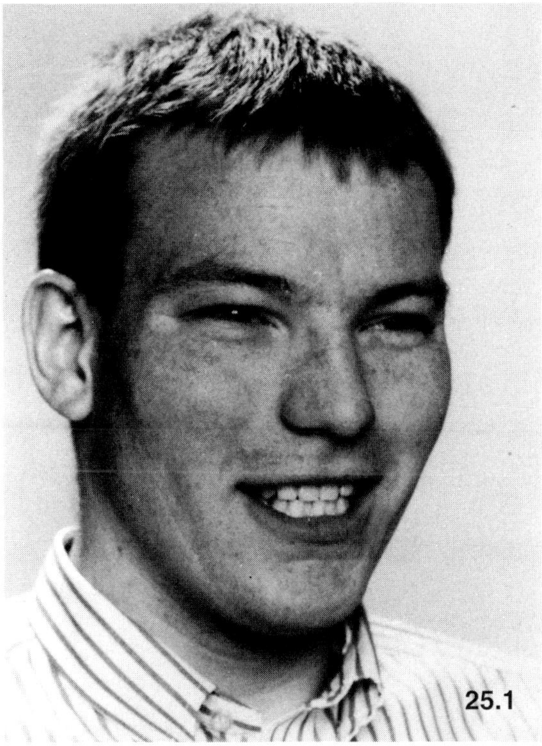

Fig 21-15 Note the changes that follow growth and treatment.

movement and neither the occlusion nor thumb- or finger-sucking inhibit it. Should these changes not occur, consideration should be given to a relatively early start to active treatment although that usually leads to prolonged treatment time. Such a decision should only be made in exceptional circumstances, in particular in cases with marked rotation of maxillary central incisors. Such a case is described in the next chapter.

An essential element in treatment such as that outlined in this chapter is the intrusion of the maxillary incisors. A cervical headgear with a Kahn spur serves well in this regard (see Fig 19.10, page 322). Patients whose treatment is stopped with the maxillary incisors still in supraposition can develop a deep bite and an arrangement of the maxillary incisors as seen in class II/2 anomalies (coverbites). The may finally end up with a situation that is less satisfactory than it would have been had no treatment been done (see Chapter 35). Therefore it is essential that in all orthodontic treatment the level of stomion is kept under surveillance (see Fig 21.16).

In general, it is unwise not to treat deciduous molars that have periapical inflammation. They should preferably be restored or otherwise extracted. Nevertheless, untreated carious deciduous molars can have their place in restricting the loss of

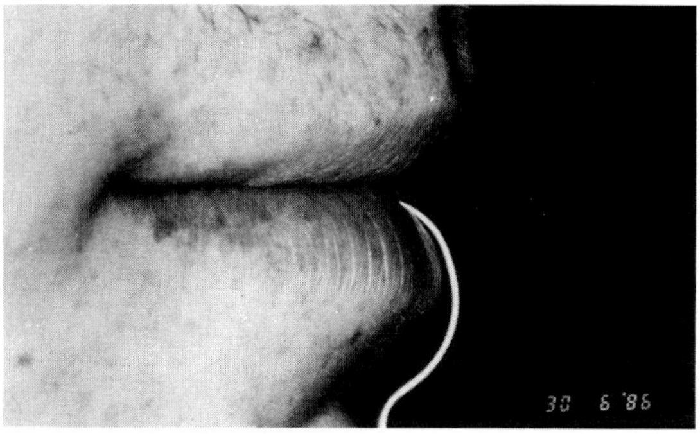

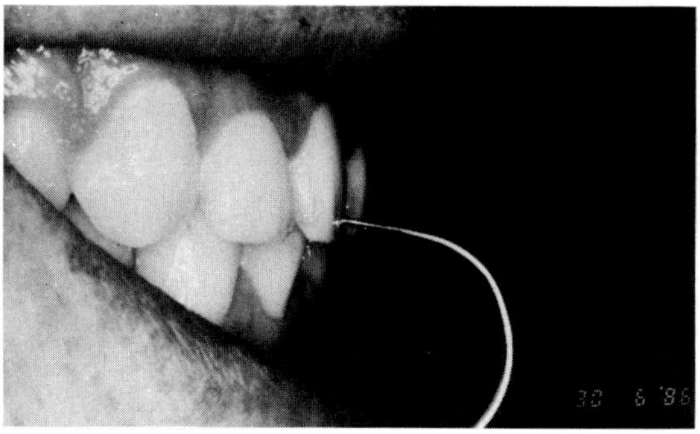

Figures 21-16 At the age of 21 y, 1 mo, stomion is located 2 mm above the incisal edges of the maxillary central incisors, something that is essential for a stable inclination of the maxillary incisors. If these teeth had not been intruded by the treatment then stomion would have been higher, with a considerable chance that the maxillary incisors would have been tipped palatally and, as a consequence, forced the mandibular incisors to lingual.

space even though crown material has been lost. That does not only apply to the dental arch in which they lie, but also the opposing arch, in which drifting can be prevented by overeruption of pertinent teeth. This applies especially in the case of the maxillary second deciduous molar which can impede mesial migration of the mandibular first permanent molar if the adjacent deciduous second molar has been lost early and the maxillary tooth has over-erupted. In the patient described here, such circumstances arose on the right side.

Finally it is again emphasized that where a reversed overbite is associated with a forced bite to ventral, the earliest possible correction should be sought so that dental development subsequently will progress normally. Following that intervention it is important to delay any further treatment, should it be necessary, until it will be most effective and efficient. Indeed treatment usually can be concluded only after the second transitional period is complete. If treatment is begun too early, then its duration must be unnecessarily long.

Chapter 22

Class II/1, agenesis 35, rotations 11 and 21
Cervical headgear, brackets 12, 11, 21, and 22
Female: 8 years, 11 months to 29 years, 5 months

A girl 8 years 11 months of age, with a slightly receding chin, exhibited a class II/1 anomaly (¾ PW disto-occlusion). There was marked mesiopalatal rotation of the maxillary central incisors. She could breathe easily through her nose and kept her mouth closed. The mandibular left second premolar was congenitally absent. Mild crowding existed in the anterior of both dental arches (Figs 22.1 and 22.2).
It was decided to engage in treatment immediately and to correct the rotations of the maxillary central incisors before they erupted fully. The disto-occlusion would be corrected with a cervical headgear. Whether or not to retain the mandibular left second deciduous molar would depend on the degree of root resorption. A decision in this regard would be postponed for the time being.
At the age of 9 years, 0 months, bands with double molar tubes were fitted to the maxillary first permanent molars and brackets were placed on the four maxillary incisors. A 0.015″ twistflex arch was installed. In conjunction with this, the maxillary deciduous canines were extracted. This provided room to overcorrect the maxillary incisors. It was unlikely that the permanent canines would be displaced palatally by the lateral incisors, since palpation showed that the canines lay buccally. After two months a .0175" twistflex arch was placed. During subsequent visits, the arch was activated. A cervical headgear was fitted to correct the disto-occlusion. Overcorrection of the rotations was obtained with the use of a .019" × .026" archwire and later use of wedges placed at the distal sides of the brackets between the brackets and the archwire (see Fig.14.14D, page 228). Then offsets were placed in the archwire itself. After seven months, the desired overcorrection had been achieved and this was maintained for a further ten months (Fig. 22.3).
The partial fixed appliance was removed at the age of 10 years, 7 months, and the treatment continued just with the headgear to correct the remaining disto-occlusion and obtain more space to accommodate the canines (Fig 22.4). It was hoped that the maxillary central incisors would not rotate back too much, but they did indeed relapse somewhat. So, at the age of 11 years, 9 months, the central incisors had some slight mesiopalatal rotation once more. In the meantime, the disto-occlusion had been eliminated and there was sufficient room for the maxillary permanent canines to take up a good position spontaneously (Fig 22.5). The mandibular left second deciduous molar was in good function, was not ankylosed, and the roots showed hardly any resorption since the beginning of treatment. It was decided to

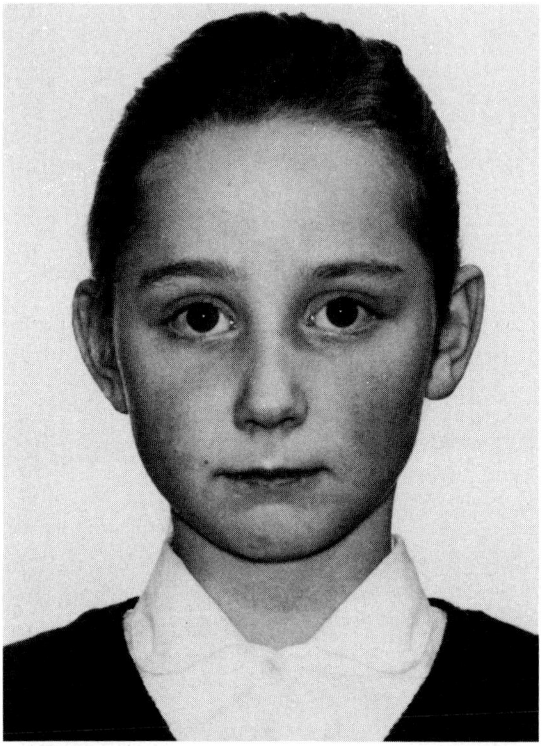

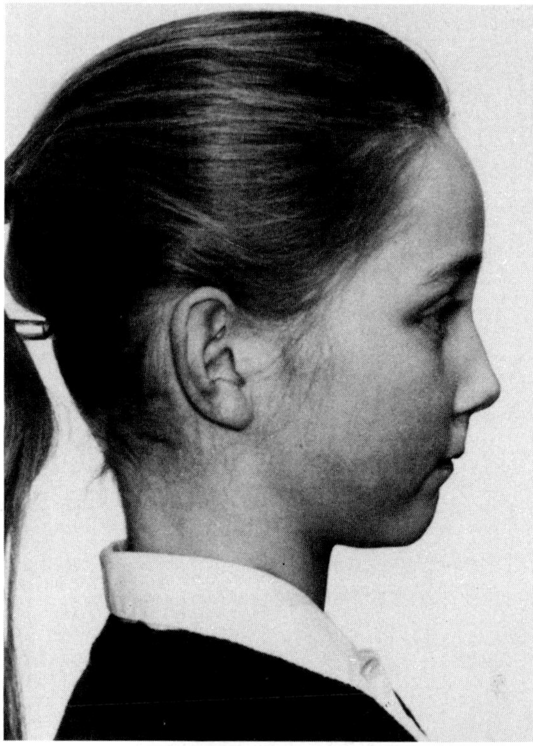

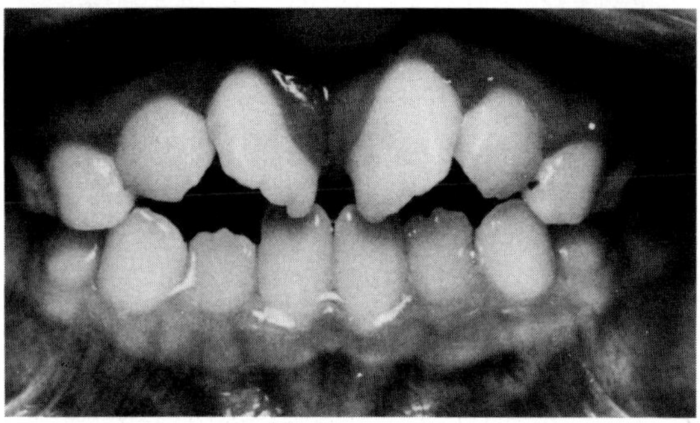

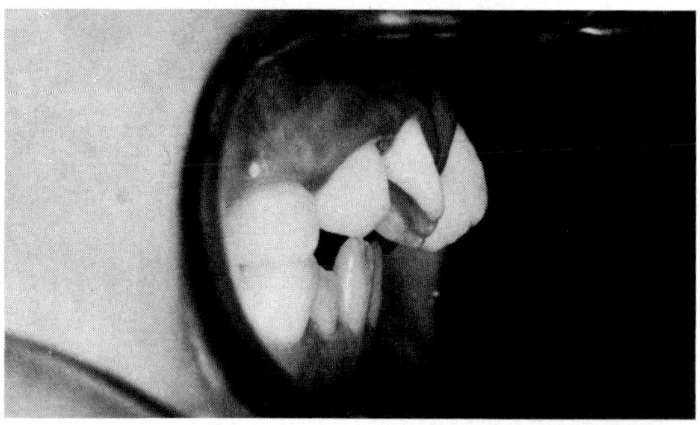

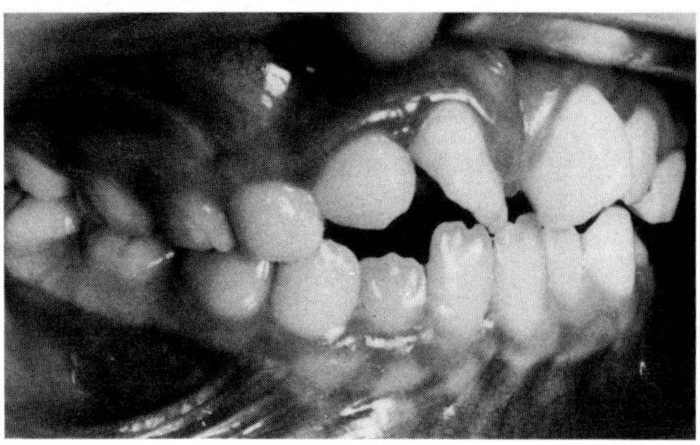

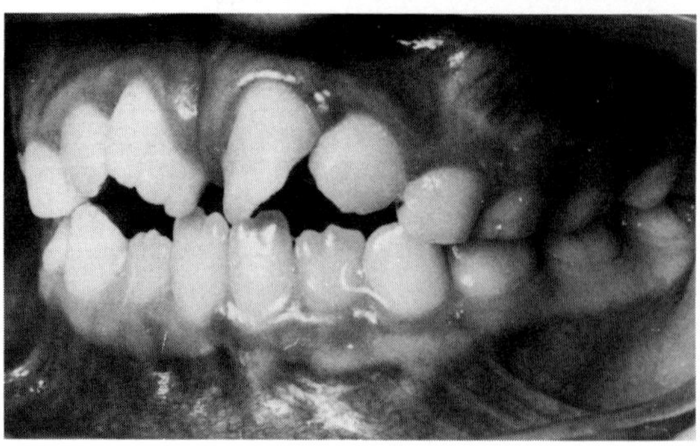

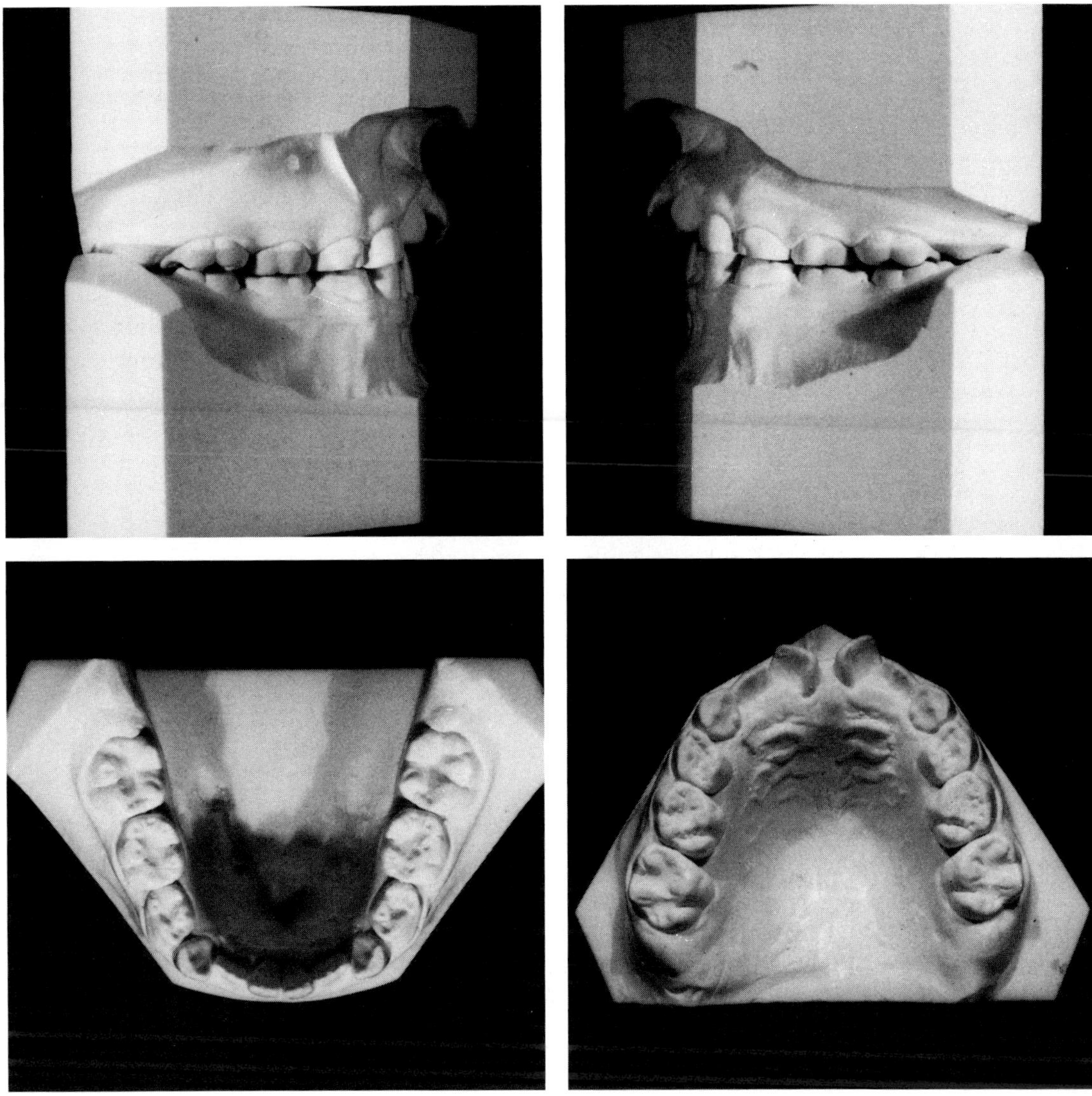

Figs 22-1 and 22-2 *A girl aged 8 y, 11 mo with a class II/1 anomaly and markedly rotated maxillary central incisors. She can breathe well through her nose and has competent lip seal. The chin lies somewhat caudally with respect to the rest of the face. Only the mandibular central incisors are fully erupted; the rest are still half-covered by the gingiva. Both dental arches are well-formed and show little abnormality except for the mesiopalatal rotation of the maxillary central incisors. There is solid interdigitation of the posterior teeth.*

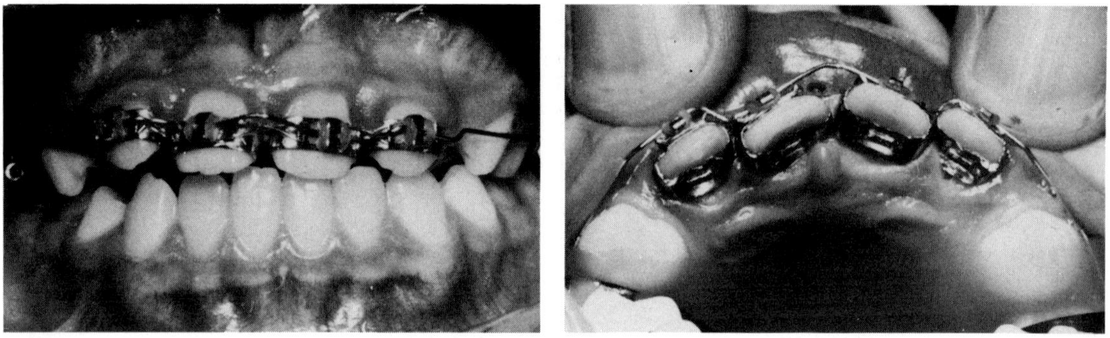

Fig 22-3 At the age of 10 y, 7 mo the maxillary incisors have been over-corrected and already in retention for ten months.

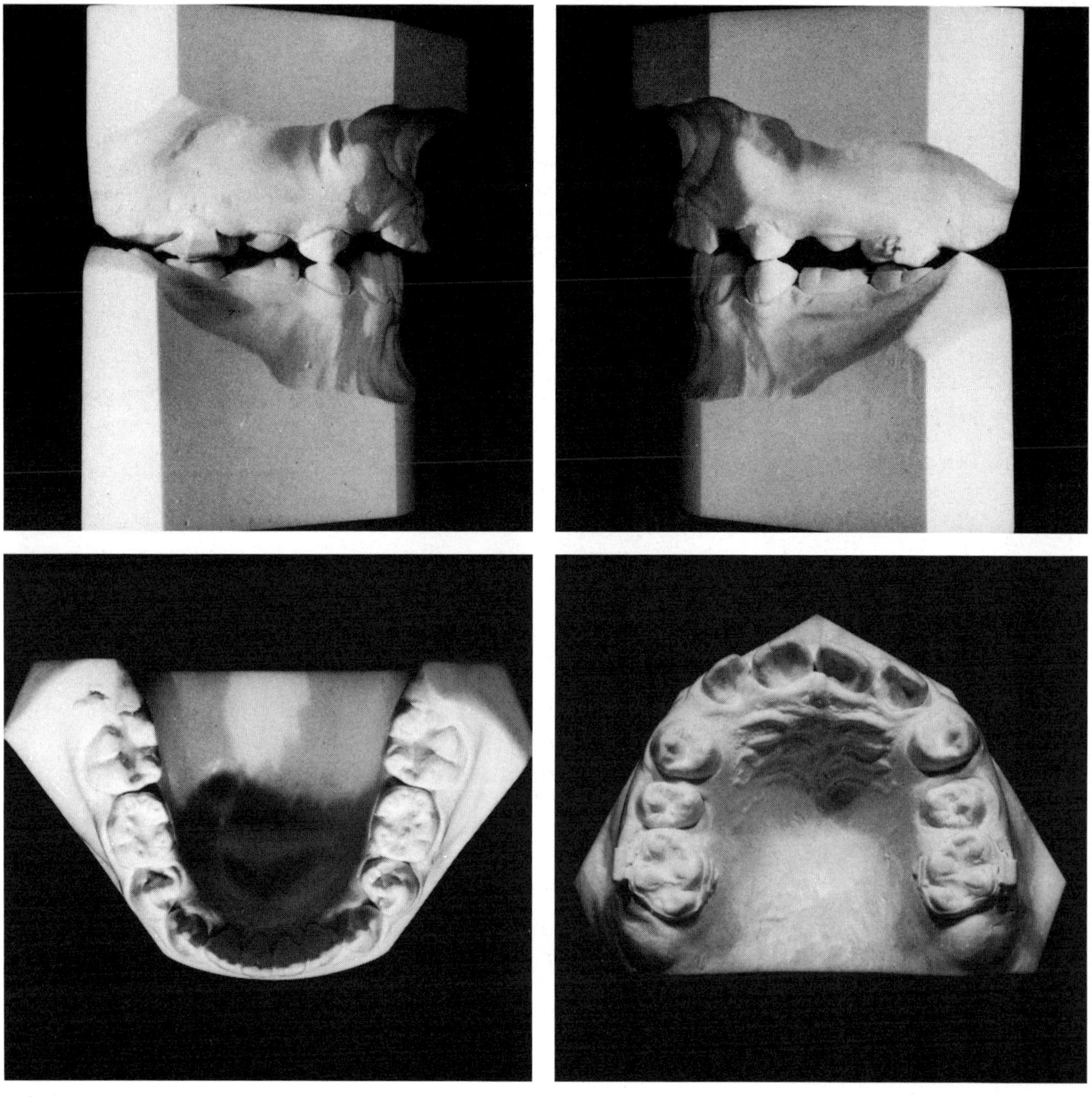

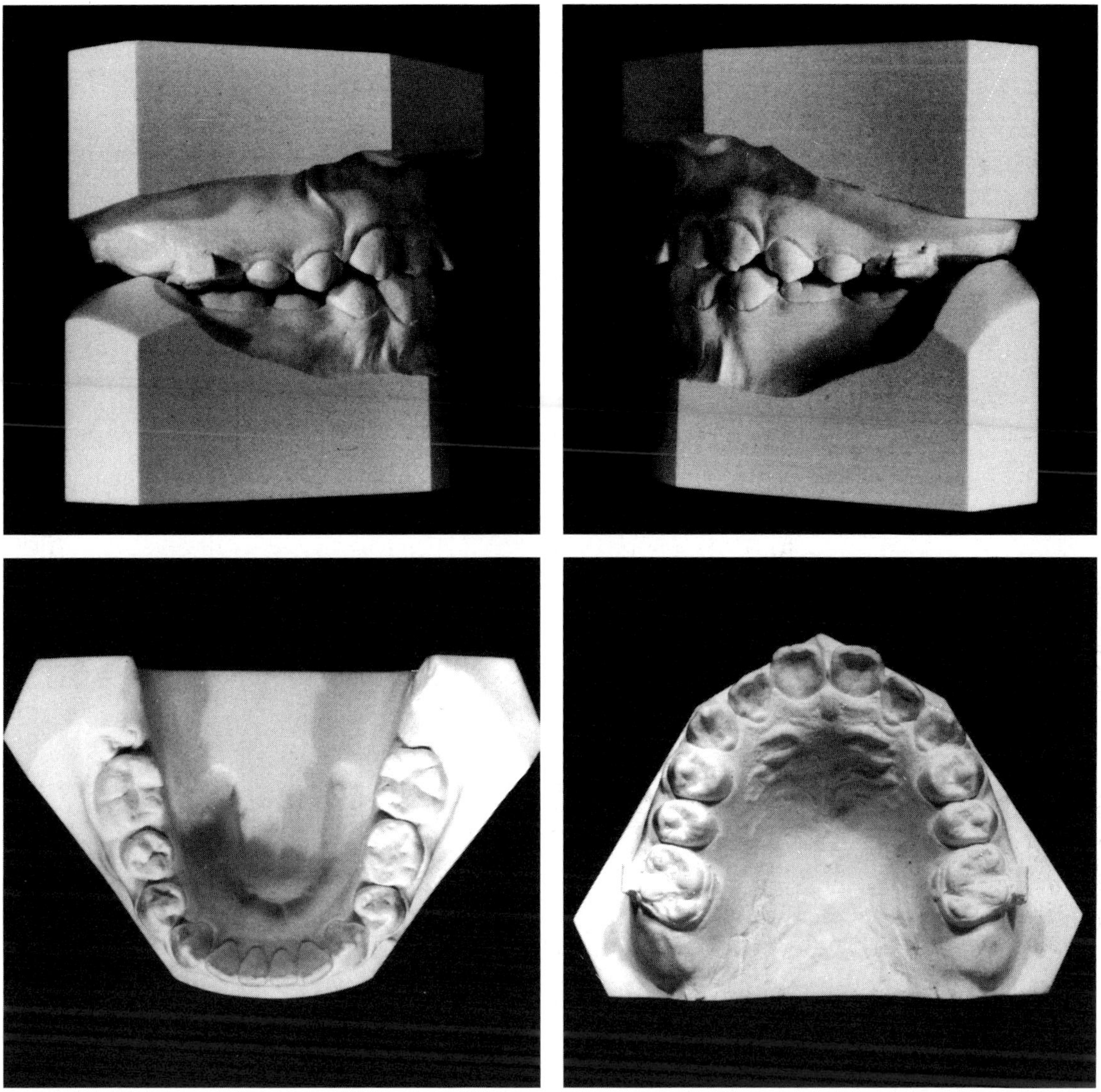

Fig 22-5 At the age of 11 y, 9 mo there is neutro-occlusion and sufficient space has been gained to accommodate the maxillary permanent canines. The maxillary central incisors have only rotated back a small amount, and now are in acceptable alignment although a little too far inclined to labial.

Fig 22-4 The dental casts at age 10 y, 7 mo, after removal of the bands and brackets, show that there is inadequate room for the maxillary canines, which are located buccally in the alveolar process at the level of the reflection of the mucosa.

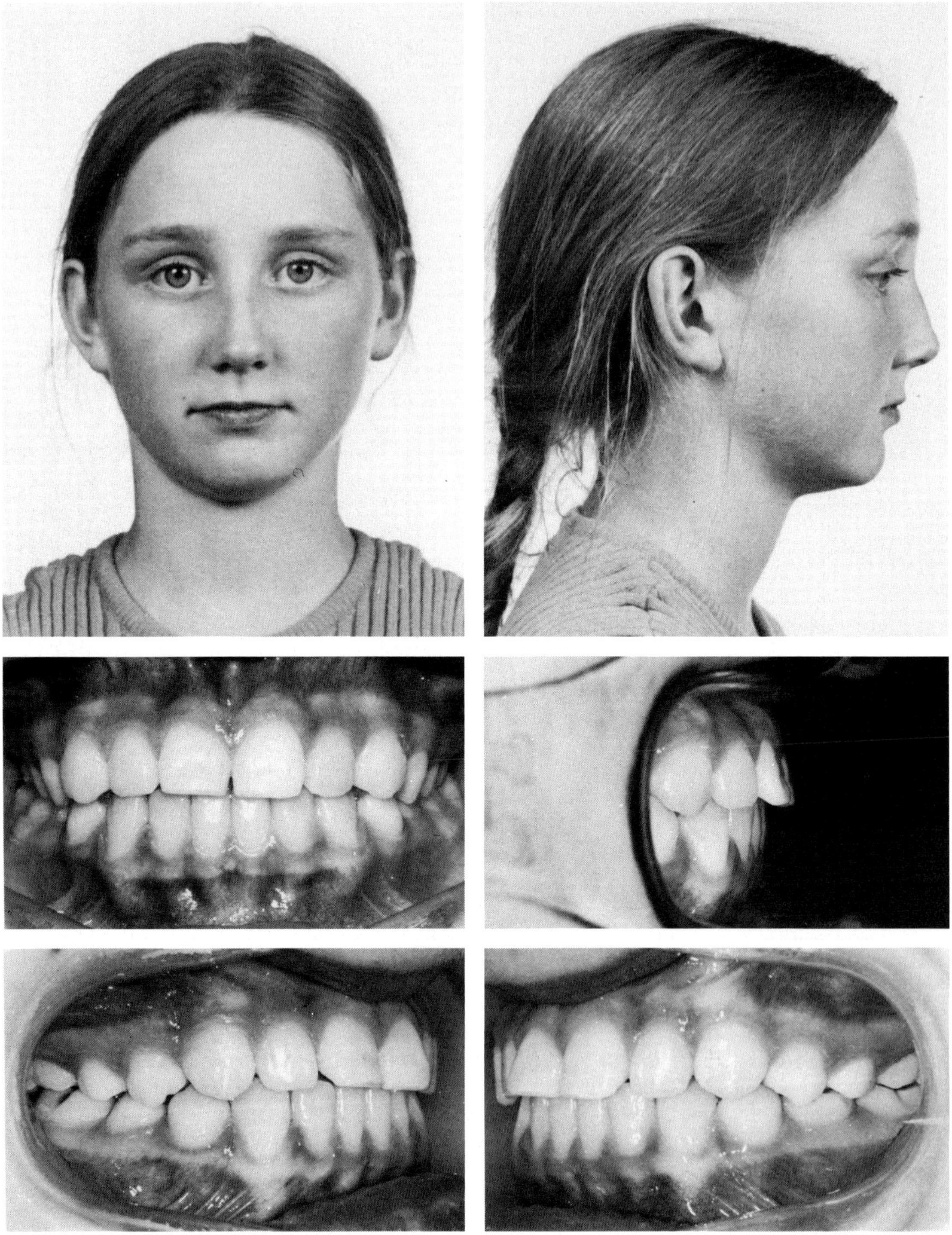

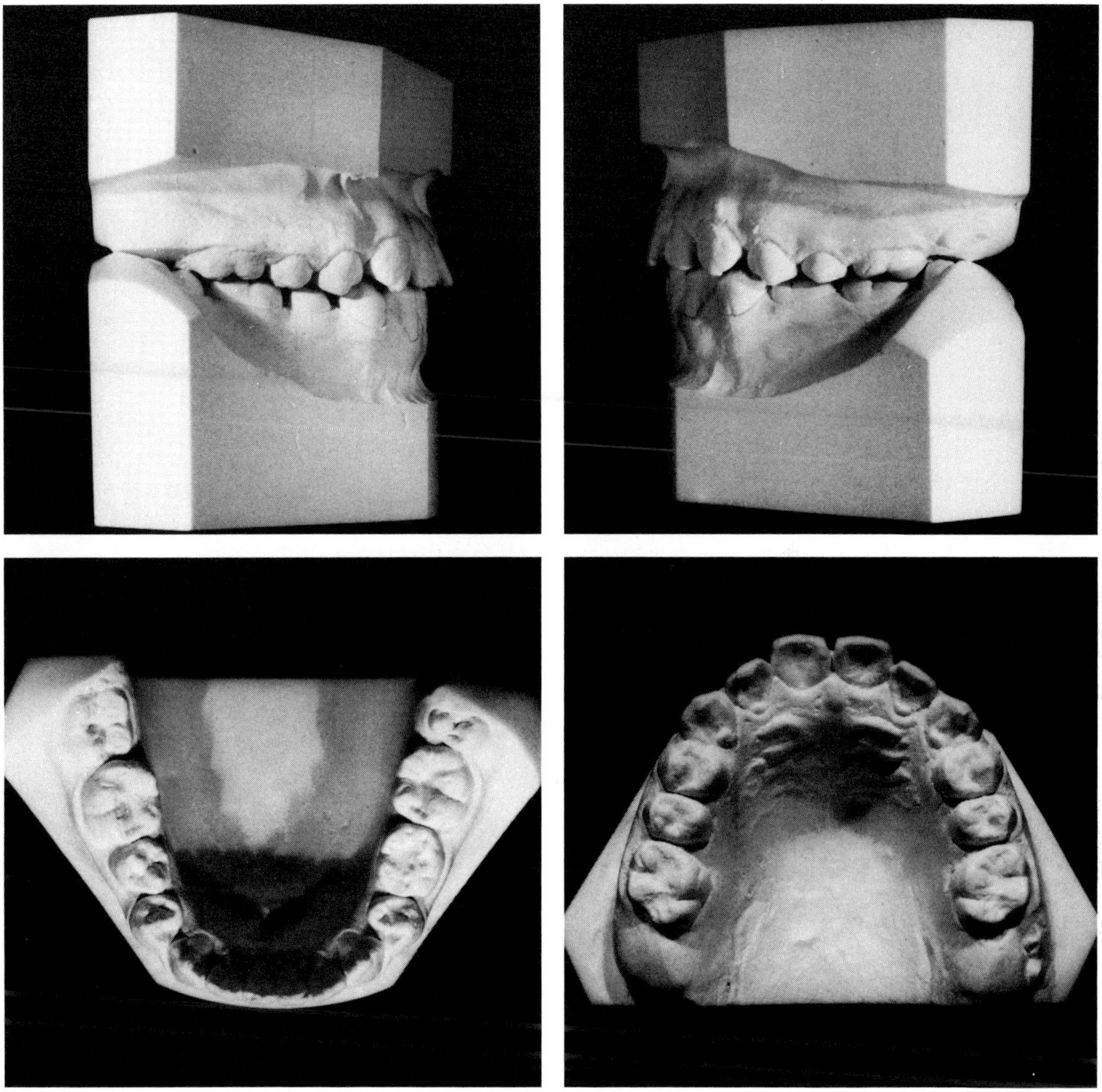

Figs 22-6 and 2-7 Aged 12 y, 8 mo the patient shows a good result with solid interdigitation achieved. The maxillary canines are mildly mesiopalatally rotated, but that is not found objectionable. The mandibular left second deciduous molar is functioning well; it does however prevent the first permanent molars on that side moving into neutro-occlusion. The abnormal crown forms of the maxillary central incisors have been improved somewhat by grinding.

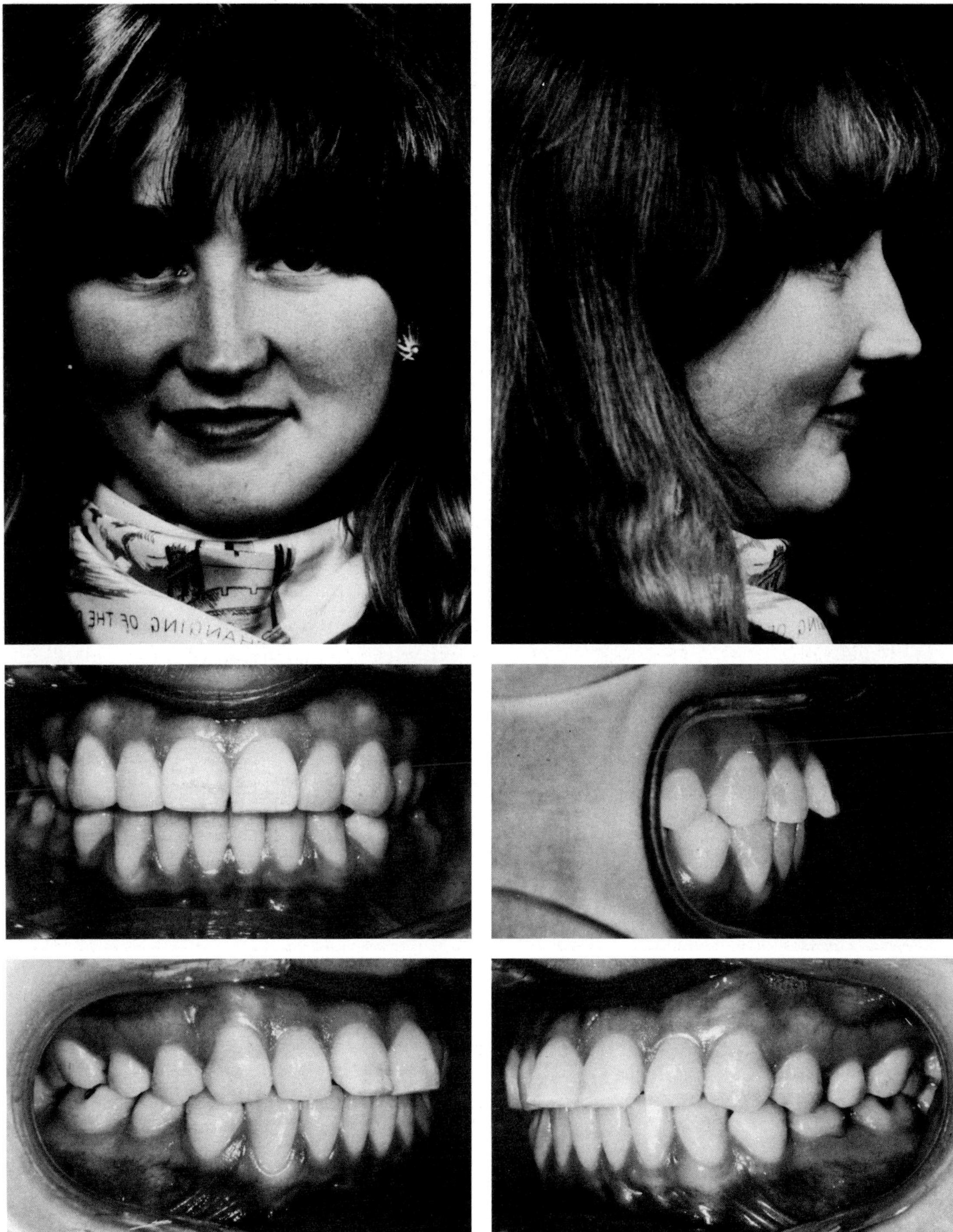

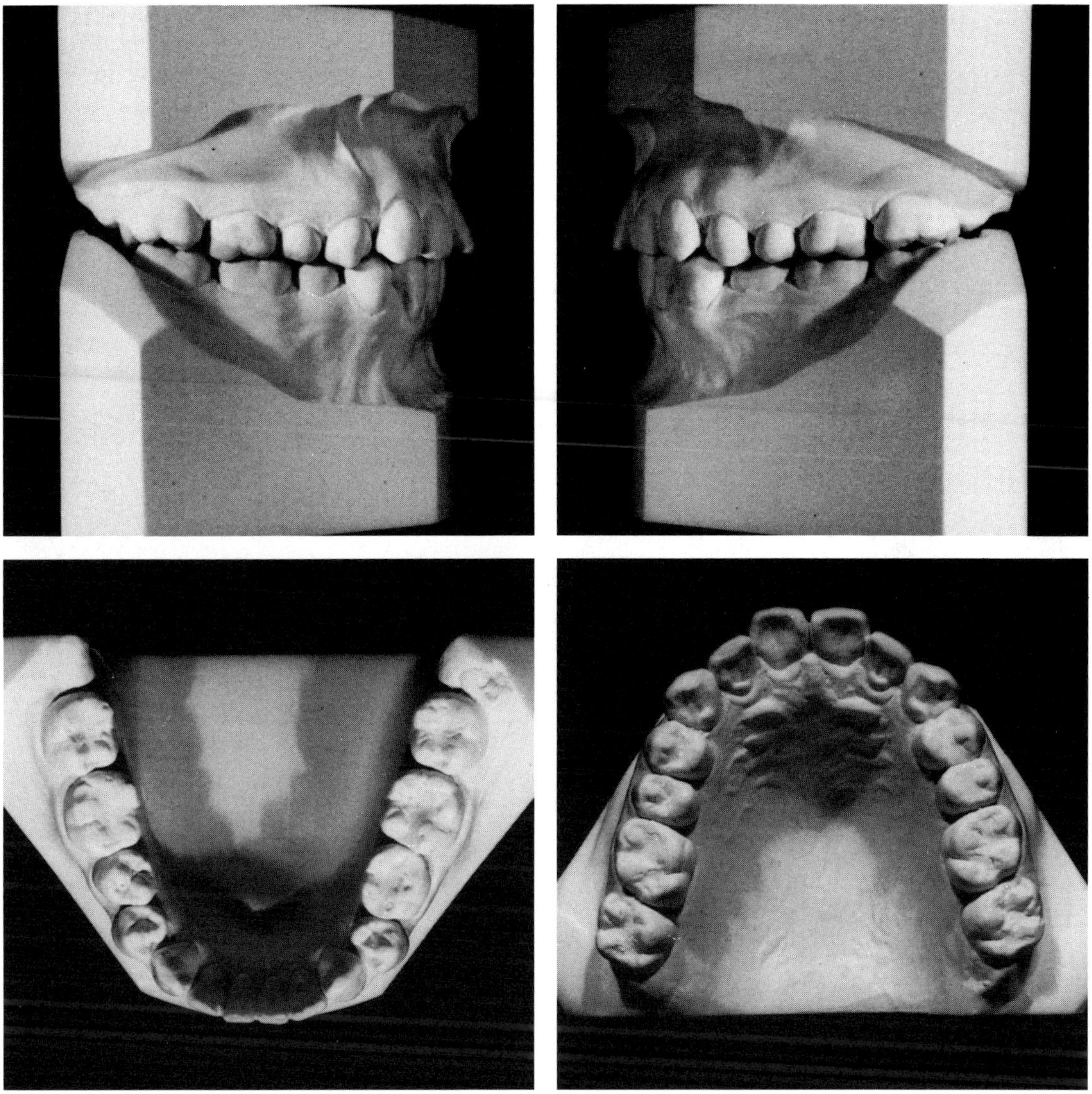

Figs 22-8 and 22-9 *At the age of 22 y, 10 mo, ten years after treatment, there is an esthetically acceptable, well-functioning dentition in a harmonious face. The small irregularities in tooth alignment are not objected to. That applies not only to the minor crowding and rotation of the mandibular premolars but also to the mesiopalatally rotated maxillary canines and the slightly labially inclined maxillary central incisors.*

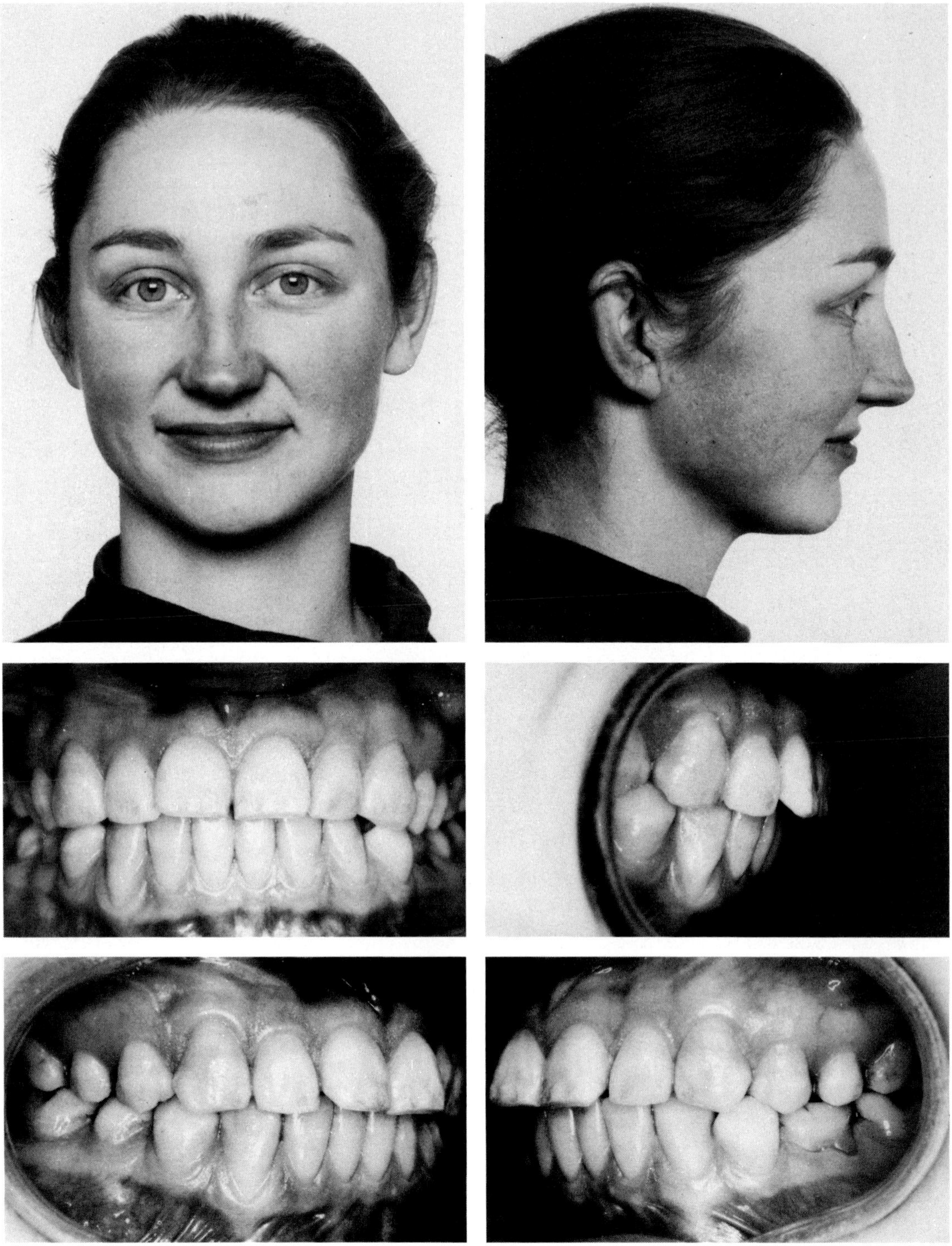

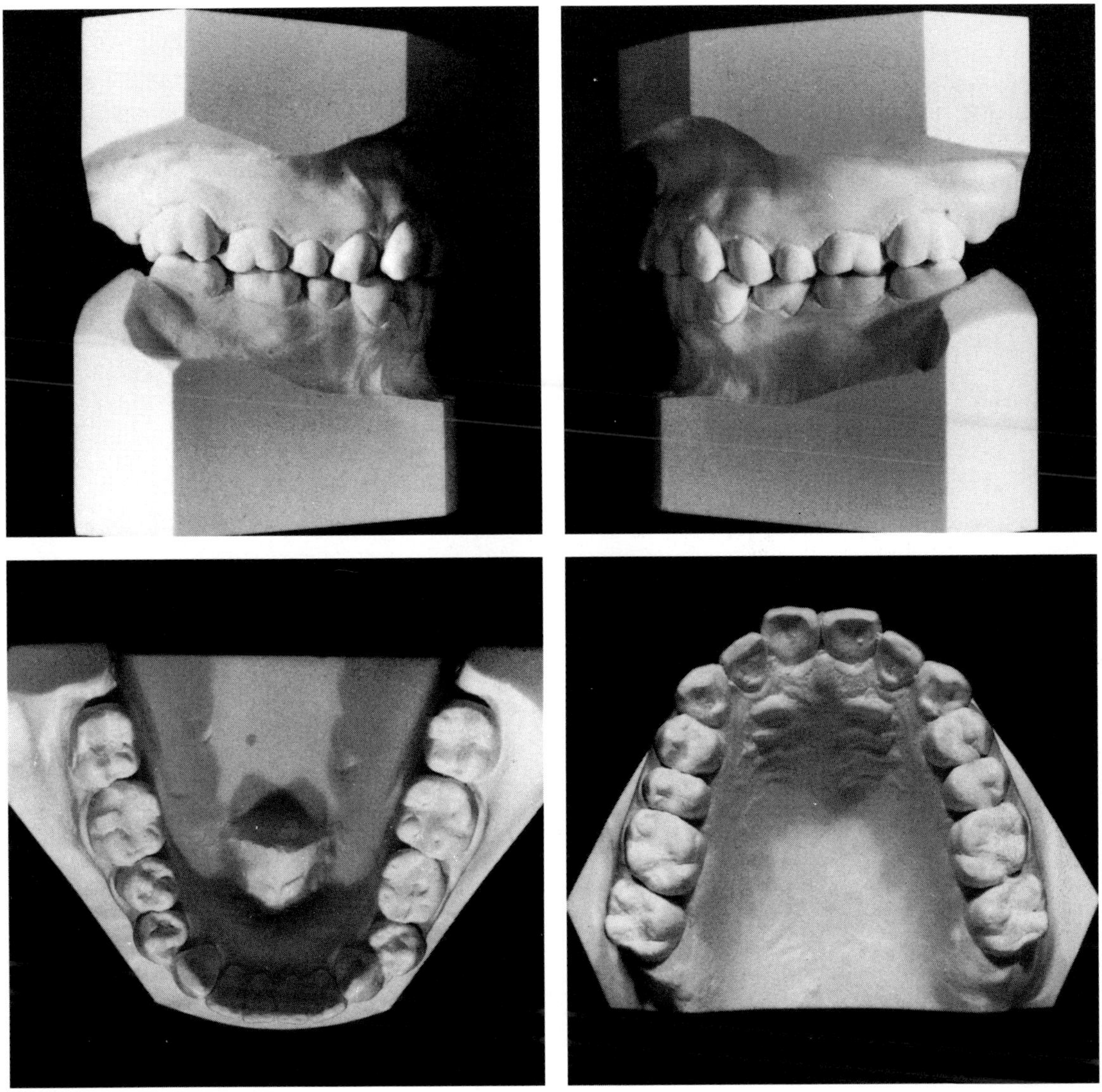

Figs 22-10 and 22-11 Now at the age of 29 y, 5 mo, sixteen years after treatment, there is little change in the picture. The mandibular left second deciduous molar is still in good function. There has been some gingival recession distobuccally, exposing the root a little.

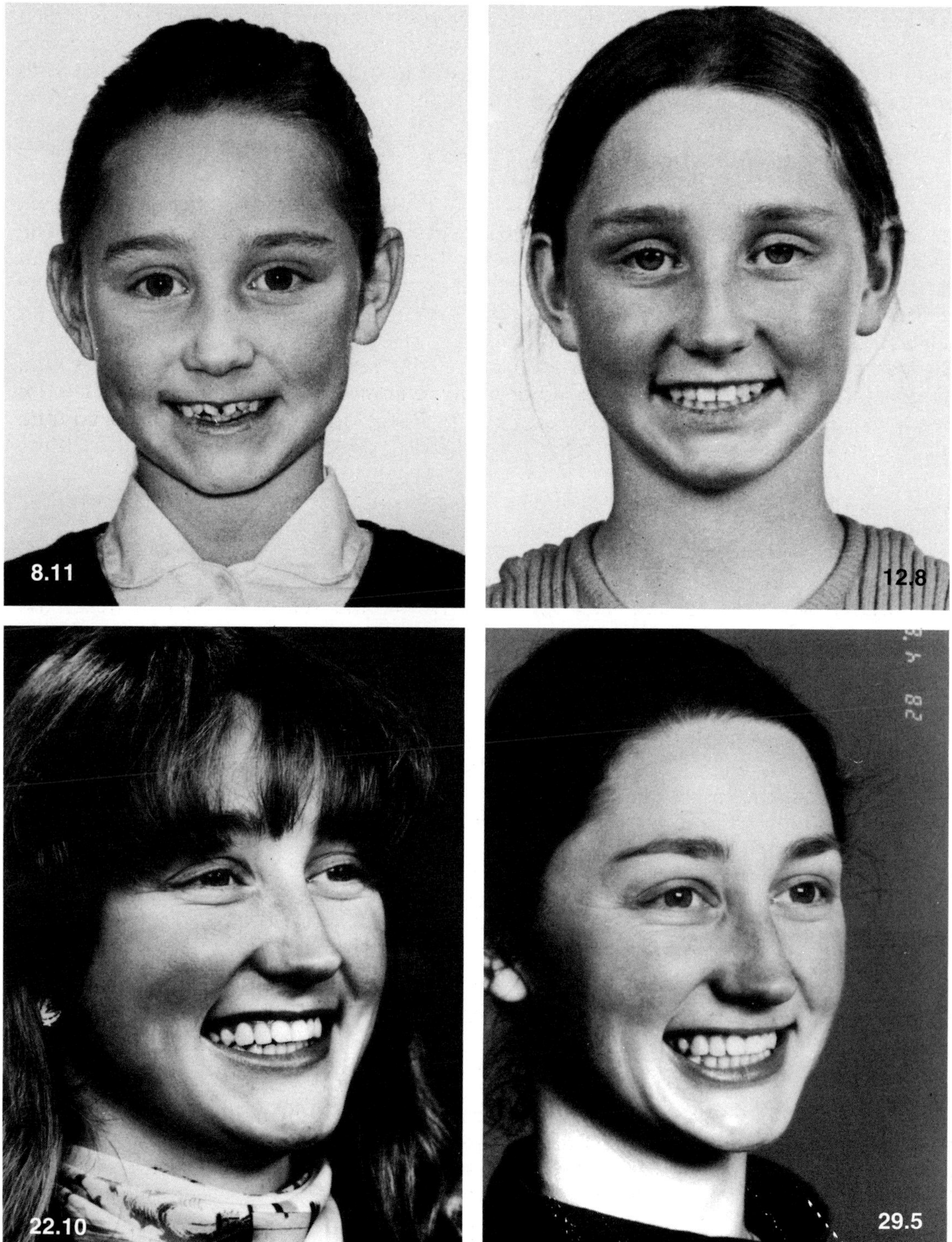

Fig 22-12 Note the retention of improvement at different ages.

retain that deciduous tooth. If it should be lost in the future, then something such as a bridge could be provided in its place. The relapsed rotations of the maxillary incisors were not corrected with a fixed appliance — at the request of the patient — but with elastics attached to the headgear (Fig 22.14). After five months, they were again in good alignment and it was proposed that the headgear and elastics be worn less. At the age of 12 years 8 months, a good result had been obtained and treatment was terminated (Figs 22.6 and 22.7).

Ten years later, the distal incisal angles of the maxillary incisors appeared to have moved labially somewhat; they were nonetheless in acceptable alignment. The second permanent molars had emerged well. Since it appeared as if there would not be enough space for the third molars to emerge properly, it was advised that the mandibular left third molar, which was the only one that was present, be removed (Figs 22.8 and 22.9).

Six years later, at the age of nearly 30 years, the picture had barely changed. The gingiva of the retained deciduous molar showed some recession and the roots were partly exposed buccally (Figs 22.10 and 22.11). Radiologically the roots showed little resorption compared with their condition 21 years previously, while marginal bone loss also was limited (Fig 22.13).

The photographs of the smiling patient show not only the improvements secured by treatment, but also the maturation and growth that took place (Fig 22.12).

Rotations of maxillary permanent incisors are usually considered to be ugly, particularly when there also are spaces between the teeth. In such a case, the prognosis for a permanent correction is unfavorable since the possibility available for spontaneous correction for whatever reason has not been utilized. Where there is crowding, the possibility of spontaneous correction does not exist, but if space becomes available when deciduous canines are extracted (provided that for other reasons it is not contraindicated), then the teeth may indeed take up better positions. Spontaneous corrections generally will be maintained, and they usually take place in the first six months following the extraction of deciduous or permanent teeth.

It is principally in situations with an excess of space that active movement and over-rotation at an early age have advantages. The clinical crowns are still short and the roots are not yet fully formed. With prolonged retention, the roots and periodontal structures may proceed with their development in the new positions. A disadvantage however is that length of the treatment must be increased because it cannot be finished until the premolars and canines have developed a good occlusion.

In addition to correction at an early age and use of prolonged retention, section of the supra-alveolar periodontal fibers reduces the chance of relapse. Those fibers run between the teeth and between the teeth and their encircling soft tissues and, in comparison with the fibers that run from tooth to alveolar bone, show very little adaptation to orthodontic tooth movements. After tooth movement, and in particular after rotation, these fibers are placed under tension from which they tend to return to their original lengths. This leads to relapse. The sectioning of these supra-alveolar fibers after tooth movement eliminates this stress so that the tissue structure adapts to the new situation.[5, 6, 9] The technique of supra-alveolar section is illustrated in Figure 22.15.

Supra-alveolar fiber sectioning should be contemplated particularly in cases such as

A B C

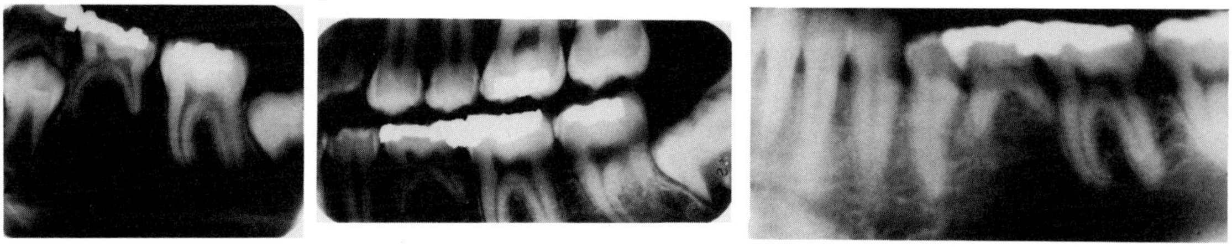

Fig 22-13 Radiographs of the mandibular left second deciduous molar at different ages.

A Periapical radiograph at the age of 8 y, 11 mo The roots of the mandibular left second deciduous molar show limited resorption. There is an amalgam restoration mesio-occlusally.

B Bitewing radiograph at the age of 17 y, 9 mo, five years after treatment. The roots have diminished little. The amalgam restoration now embraces the distal.

C Part of an orthopantomogram at the age of 29 y, 5 mo The roots of the mandibular left second deciduous molar appear to have resorbed little further. It also shows that the marginal bone loss is minimal.

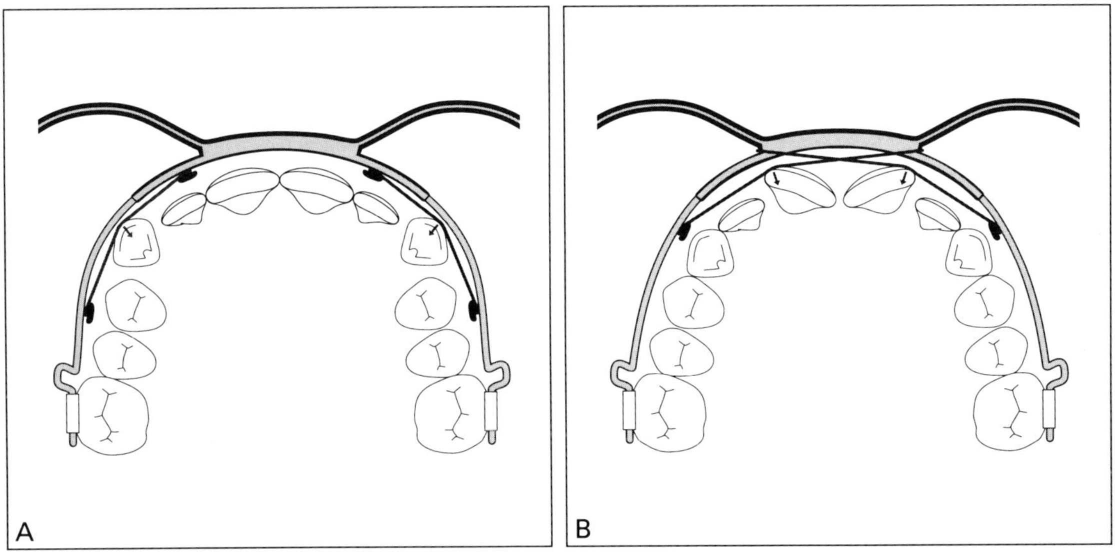

Fig 22-14 Combination of elastics with a headgear to apply labial forces on maxillary teeth in class II/1 anomalies that are being treated with a headgear and where teeth are not moving spontaneously into better positions.

A Canines that have erupted labially can be moved palatally with elastics hooked onto the inner arch of the headgear where strategically placed hooks have been affixed. The elastics should only contact the teeth that need to be moved. If that cannot be assured, the tooth in question can temporarily be built up with composite.

B In a comparable way, the maxillary incisors can be retracted and rotated. In this this case, the elastics can be stretched from the junction of the inner and outer headgear bows to appropriate hooks on the inner arch as illustrated.

It only makes sense to attempt to move teeth with elastics and the headgear, if there is sufficient space and the occlusion does not inhibit the movements wished for. Moreover, the tension in the neckstrap has to be sufficient to prevent the force of the elastics moving the headgear forward in the molar tubes. When the neckstrap is undone to remove the headgear, the patient should be careful to hold the headgear back in the tubes by pressing on the headgear in front at the solder-joint to prevent accidental injury to the mucosa if the elastics cause the inner arch to jump out of the tubes unexpectedly. Of course the headgear must be worn the proper number of hours (approximately 14 per day) to secure the desired result.

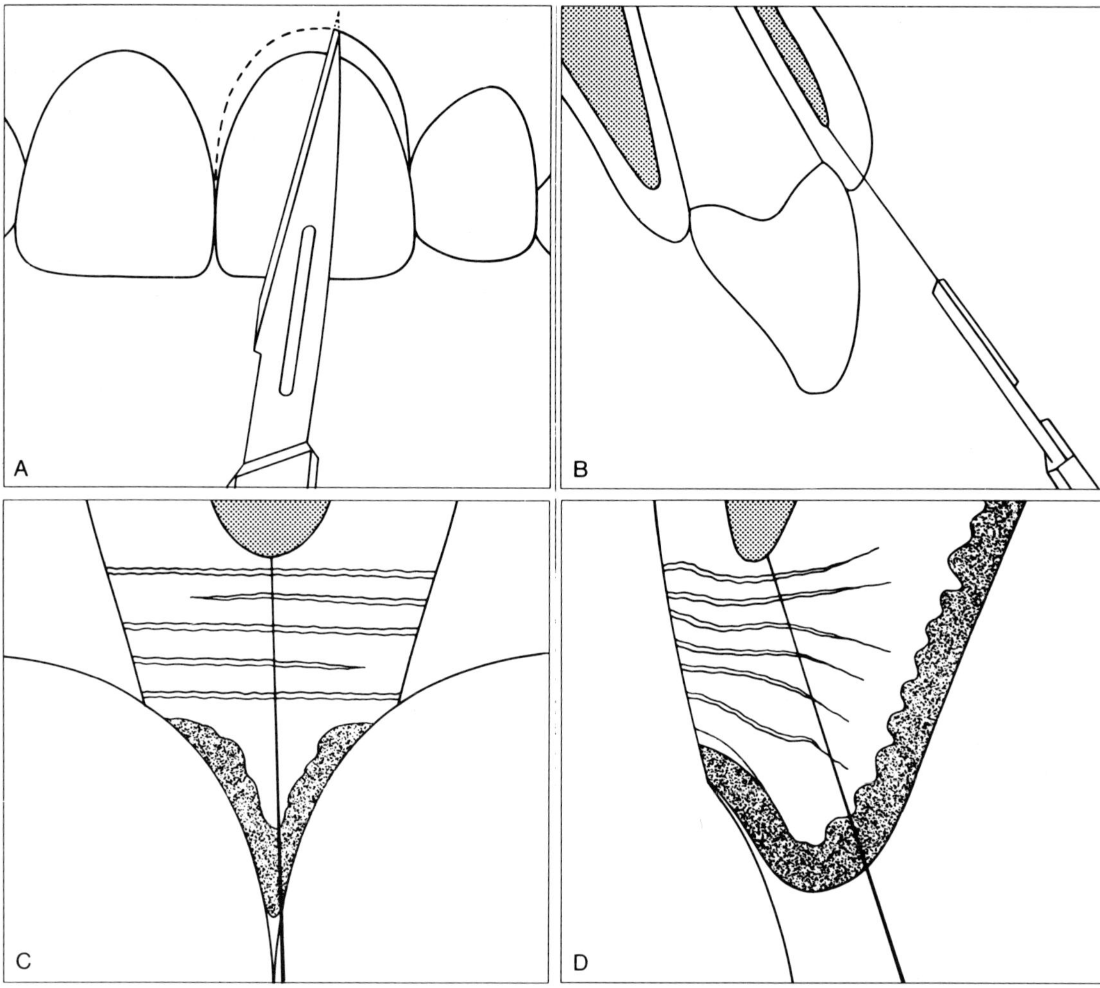

Fig 22-15 *The sectioning of supra-alveolar fibers to overcome relapse of rotations.*
A, B The incision is made down to the bony margin of the alveolus.
C, D The interdental fibers, and those that terminate in the gingiva, are cut through.[33]

this, where the teeth are rotated distolabially. These rotations show a greater tendency to relapse than those that are mesiolabial.[17]

It is accepted that pericision of these fibers in a well-cared for mouth will have no unfavorable effects on the periodontal tissues.[24] The effect of sectioning of interdental soft tissues on preventing closed diastemata from reopening is limited.[18]

If limited relapse does occur, it is not necessarily unacceptable for the patient. Quite often it is thought to be a personal trait, especially since most relapse is only partial but has the same characteristics as the original deviation. Nor does everyone wish to have a "film star smile," but values their teeth having a more individual appearance. Where a patient finds a relapse to be unacceptable, then the choice must be to re-treat and install a form of permanent retention, or to mask the imperfection by means of grinding and/or recontouring the teeth with composite resin.[25] The latter method is relatively inexpensive while taking little time, and is not susceptible to relapse. Furthermore, the uncertainties and disadvantages of permanent retention are avoided.

Moving maxillary incisors with fixed appliances before the emergence of the adjacent permanent canines can be risky. The roots of the lateral incisors usually lie close to the canine crowns. If the unerupted canines are not located buccally, moving the lateral incisors can result in the canines being impacted. Therefore, it is essential to locate the canines by palpation before considering the use of fixed appliances on the incisors. Also, in such cases consideration should be given to extraction of the deciduous canines, not just to provide space for the incisor movements but also to reduce the chance of impaction of the permanent canines.[10]

When a premolar is congenitally absent, the question arises as to how long the corresponding deciduous tooth can remain functional. When it concerns only one tooth and there is no other reason to perform orthodontic treatment on the dental arch involved, then preservation of the deciduous molar is the appropriate objective. If the roots are not resorbed and the crown is well-restored and caries-free, such a tooth can last until an advanced age. Critical matters are whether or not ankylosis sets in before the completion of facial growth, or loss of periodontal attachment exposes the bifurcation of the roots which lies closer to the cemento-enamel junction in deciduous molars than in permanent ones.

Chapter 23

Class II/1, agenesis 15, 25, 35, and 45

Cervical headgear, brackets 12, 11, 21, and 22, maxillary removable retainer
Female: 12 years, 4 months to 28 years, 4 months

A girl of 12 years, 4 months, attended because she and her parents were dissatisfied with the irregularity of her maxillary incisors. She had a class II/1 anomaly with a disto-occlusion of ½ PW and a harmonious face with normal function. All second premolars were congenitally absent. The second deciduous molars were restored with amalgam. Their roots were good and exhibited barely any signs of resorption. The mandibular and maxillary anteriors were slightly crowded (ALD –2 mm and –3 mm, respectively). The maxillary left central incisor was tipped labially and was excluded from the dental arch. This exclusion also applied, although to a lesser extent, to the maxillary canines (Figs 23.1 and 23.2).

It was decided to preserve the second deciduous molars and to correct the disto-occlusion with a cervical headgear; this would also provide room for the maxillary left central incisor and the canines. Second, the four maxillary incisors would be moved to their correct places with a partial fixed appliance.

At the age of 12 years, 6 months, a cervical headgear was provided. Six months later, brackets were placed on the four maxillary incisors and a .0175" twistflex archwire was fitted. After four weeks the twistflex was replaced with a .019" × .026" arch. In another month the desired result had been obtained and the appliance was removed (Figs 23.3 and 23.4). A removable plate was worn for six months for retention, day and night for the first three months and only while sleeping for the remaining three months.

Eleven years later, at the age of 24 years 9 months, the maxillary central incisors have become a little prominent and the crowding in the mandibular anteriors, especially on the left, has increased. Consequently the midline of the mandibular dental arch has moved further to the left with respect to that of the maxillary arch. The patient was satisfied with the appearance of her teeth and had not noticed that the mandibular left second deciduous molar no longer was in occlusion (Figs. 23.5 and 23.6).

At the age of 28 years, 4 months, it was also apparent that the mandibular right second deciduous molar had ankylosed and no longer made occlusal contact. The roots of the maxillary left second deciduous molar had become further exposed. There were no pockets, neither there nor associated with the other deciduous molars, the roots of which were still totally covered by the gingiva. The positions of the other teeth had not changed visibly (Figs 23.7 and 23.8). It might be expected that

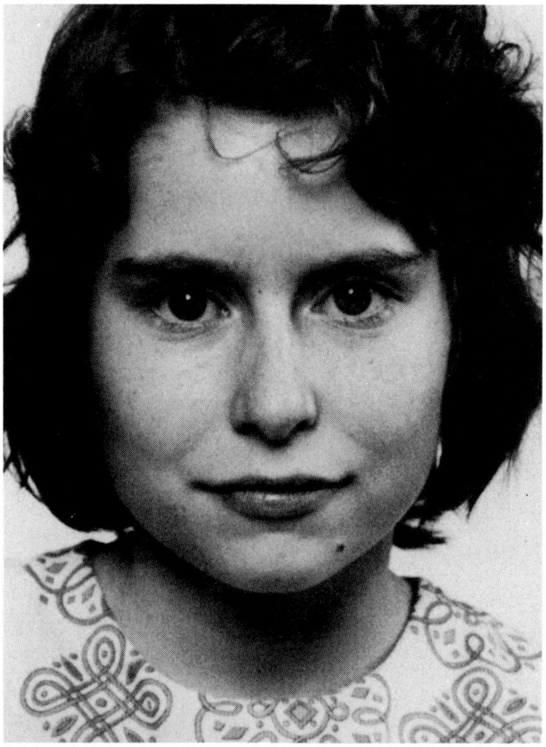
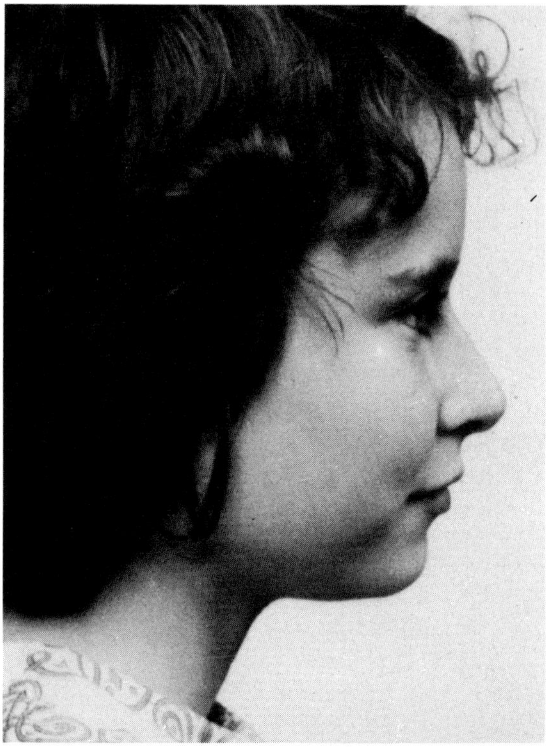
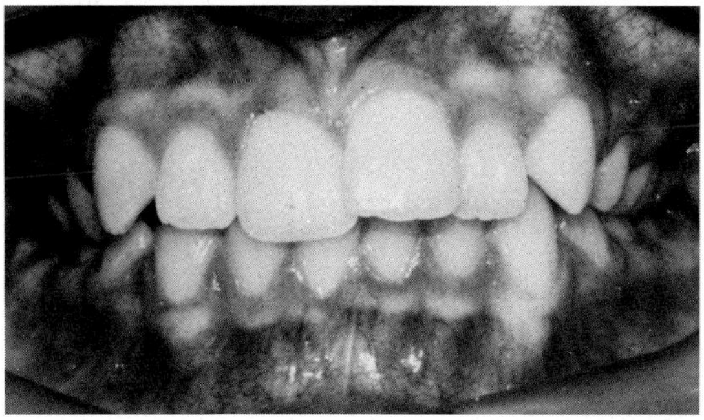
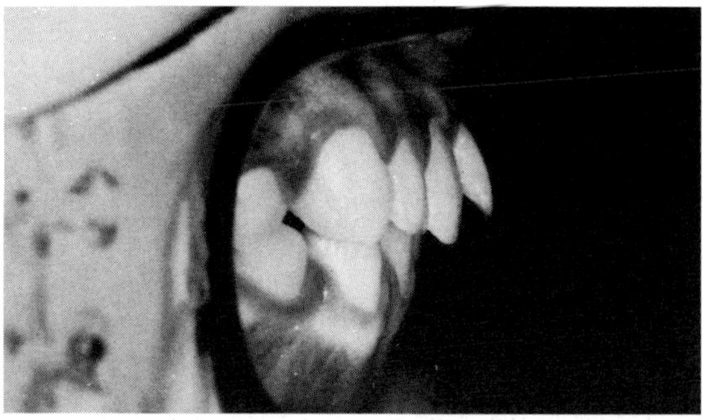
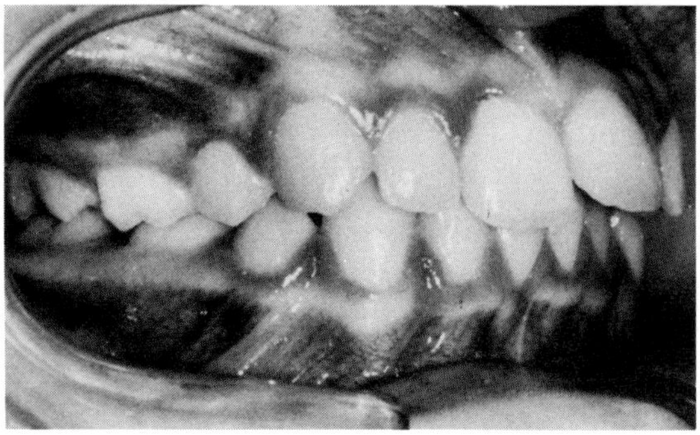
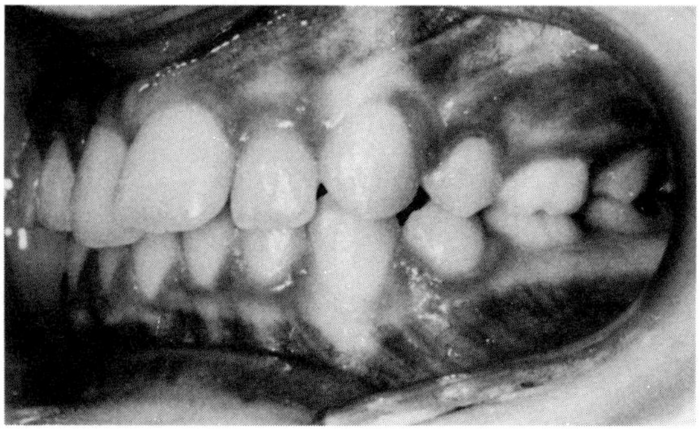

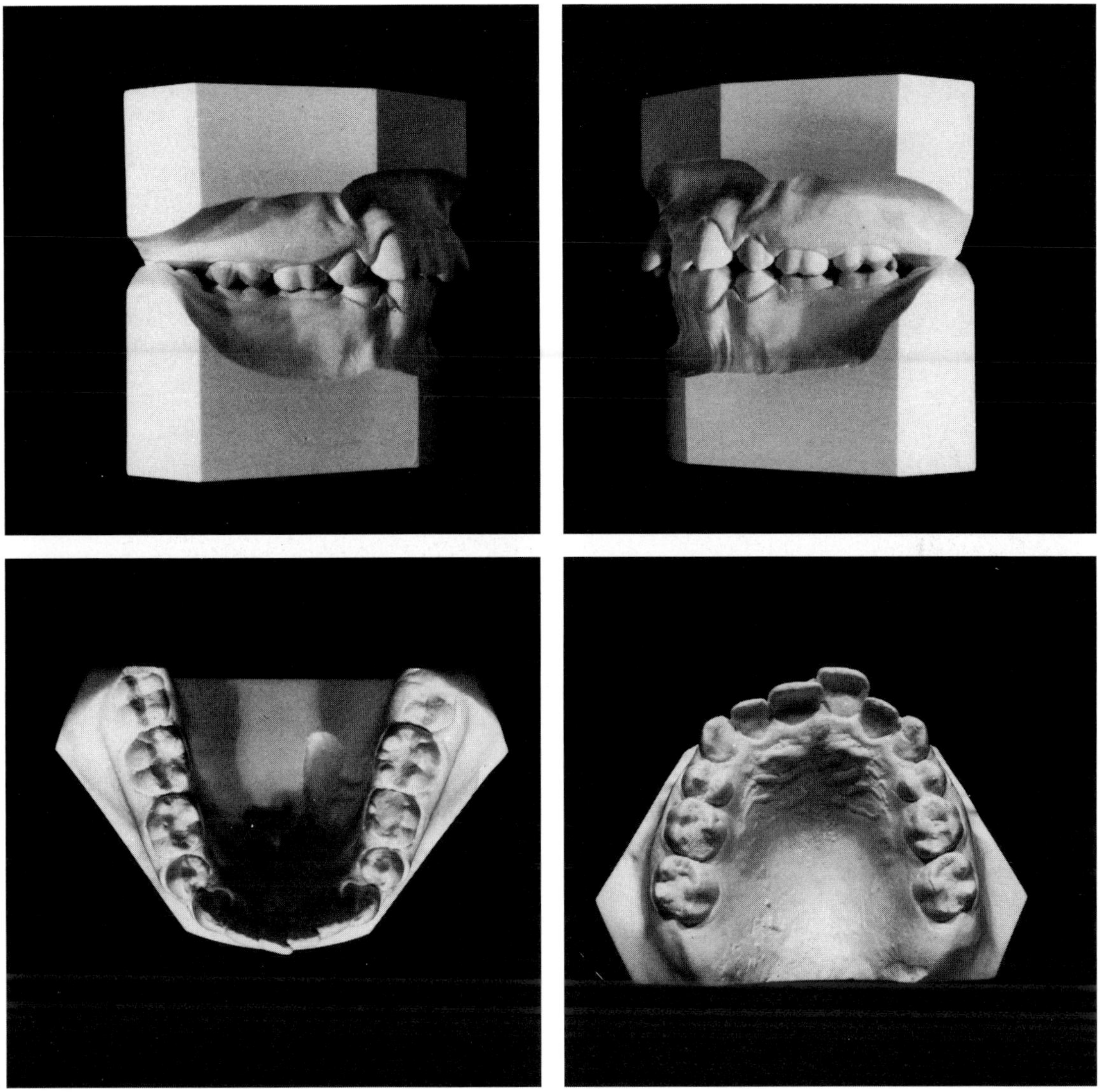

Figs 23-1 and 23-2 *A girl of 12 y, 4 mo with a class II/1 anomaly (disto-occlusion ½ PW), a good face, and normal function. All second premolars are congenitally absent. Both dental arches have mild crowding in the anterior region, which is evidenced in the maxilla by the left central incisor and both canines being outside the line of the arch. The patient and parents find this undesirable. The mid-line of the mandibular arch is displaced to the left of that of the maxilla. The posterior section of the apical area in the maxilla seems unlikely to provide sufficient space for proper emergence of the second permanent molars.*

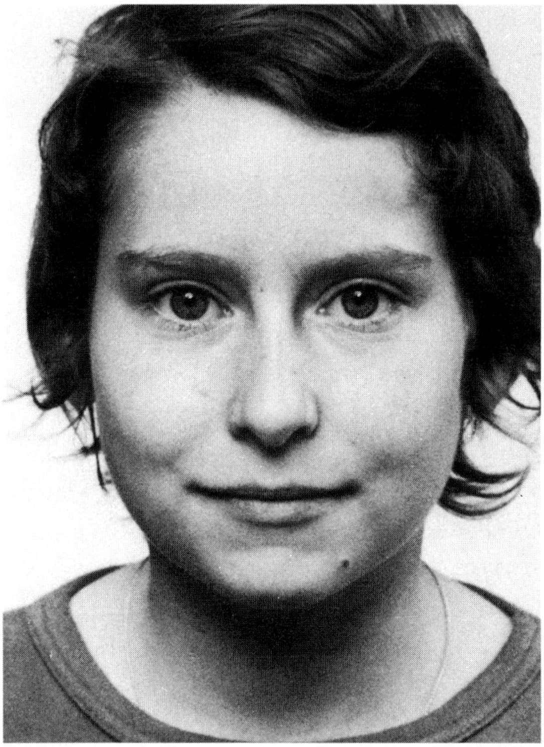

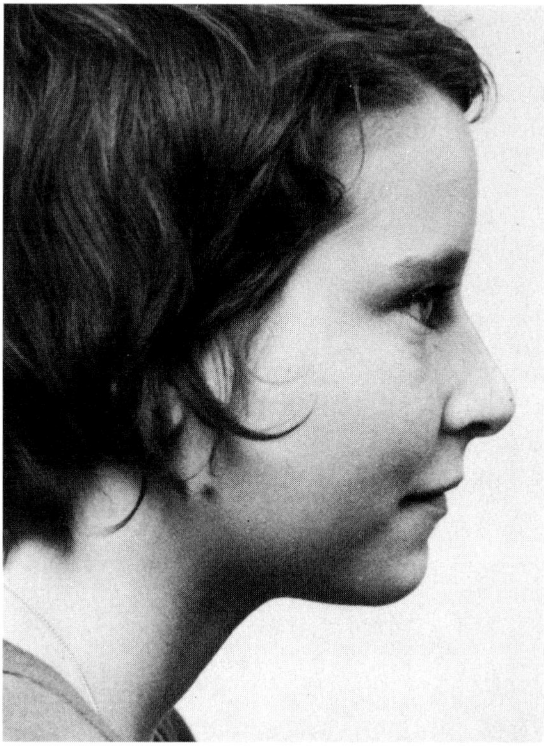

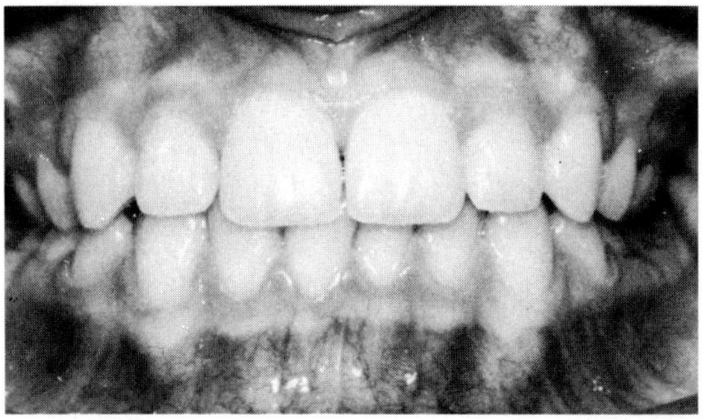

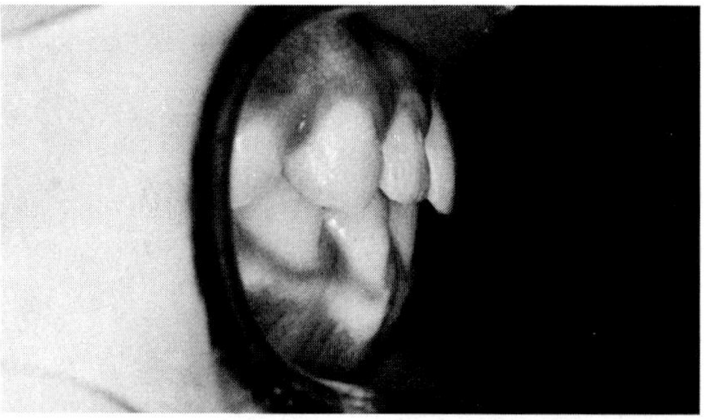

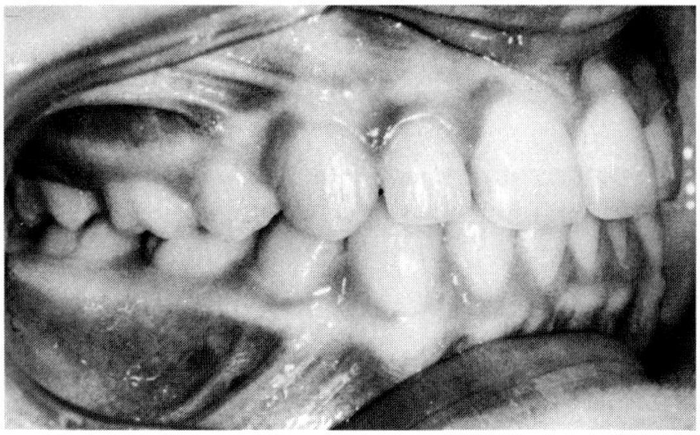

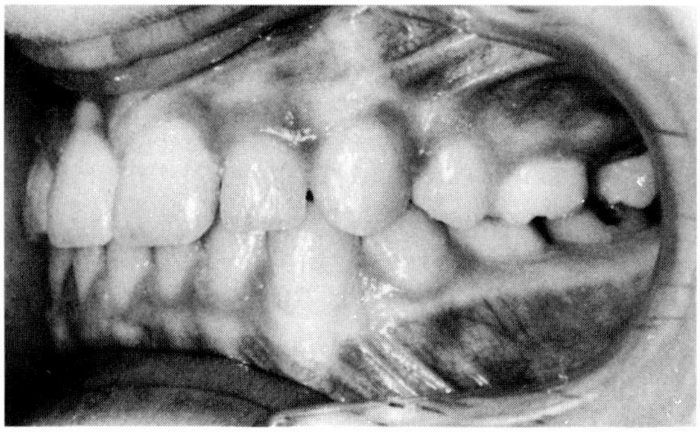

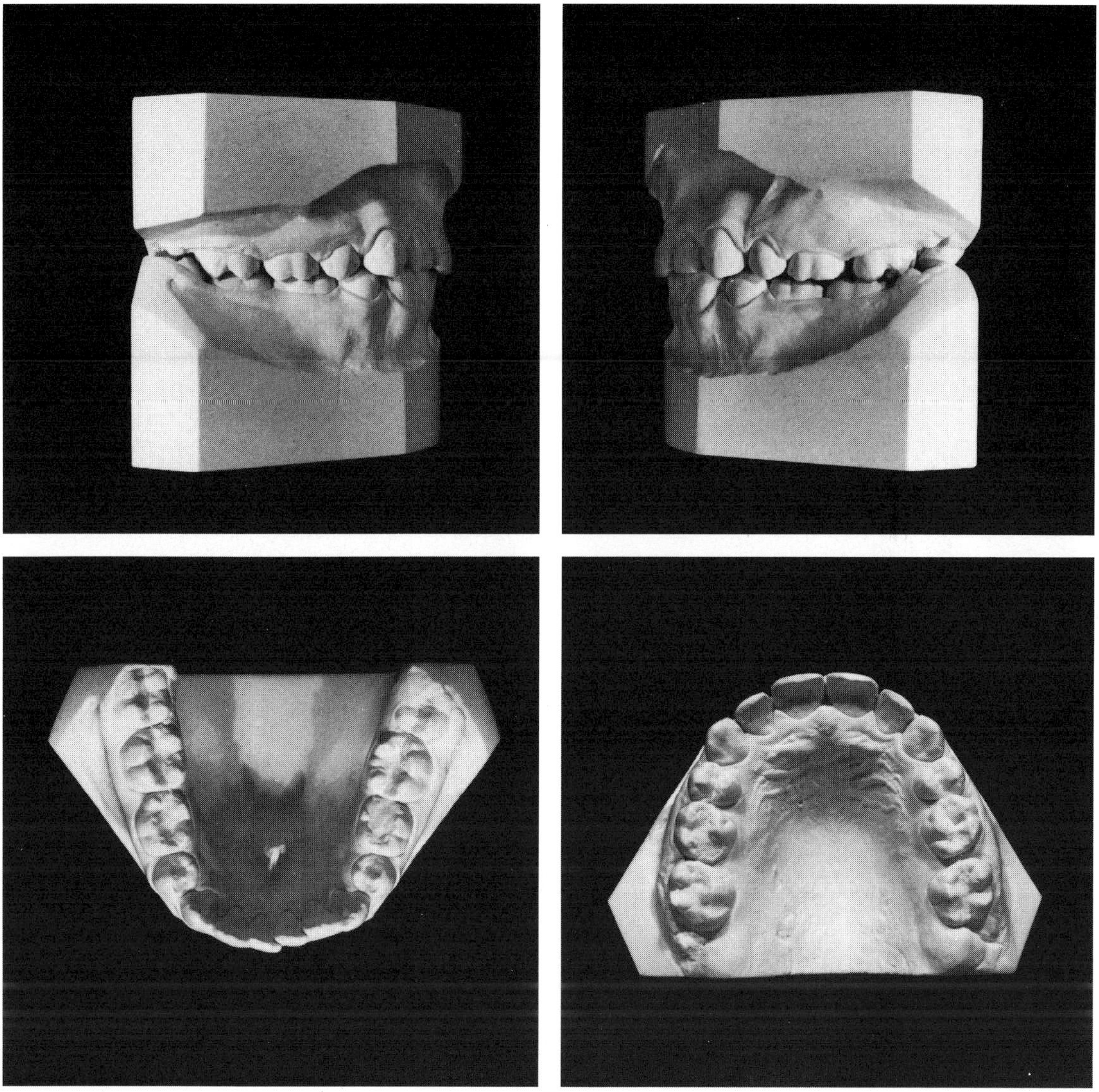

Figs 23-3 and 23-4 *At the age of 13 y, 2 mo, the desired result has been reached after eight months of active treatment. The maxillary anteriors are well-aligned, and the posterior teeth are in excellent occlusion. The crowns of the second deciduous molars are similar in form with those of the first permanent molars and occlude well. That is not the case if a deciduous molar has a premolar as antagonist (see Fig 22-7, page 373). At this stage, the second permanent molars have too little room in the maxilla to emerge properly. The situation in the mandibular arch has not changed noticeably.*

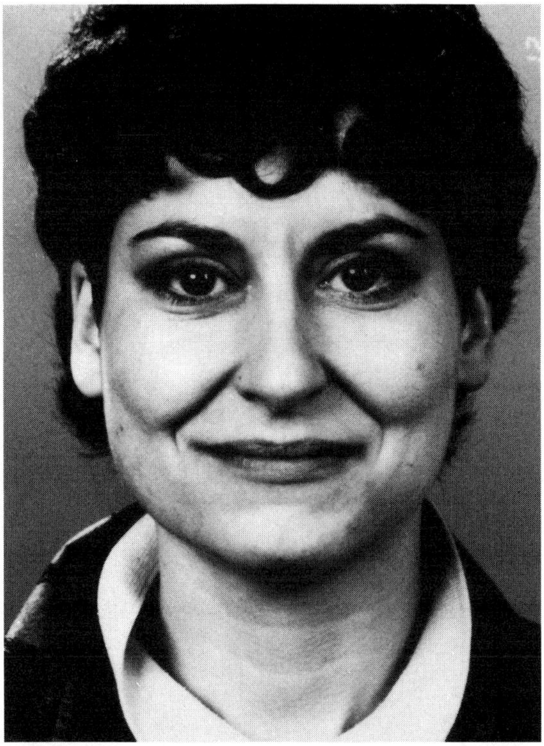

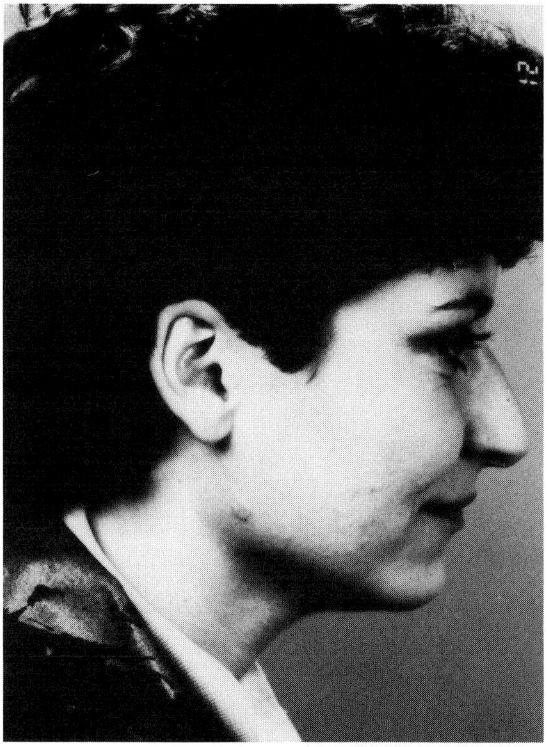

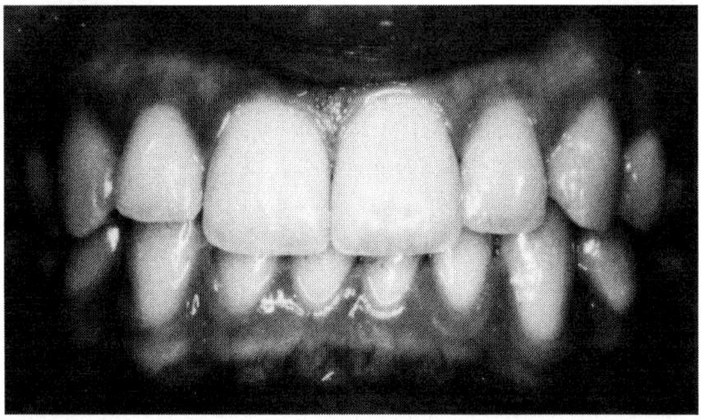

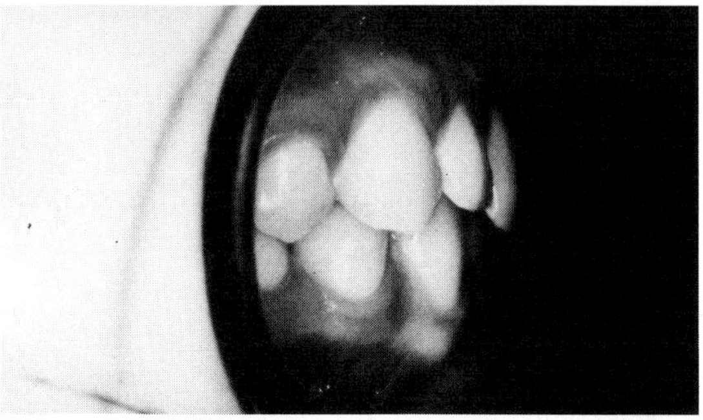

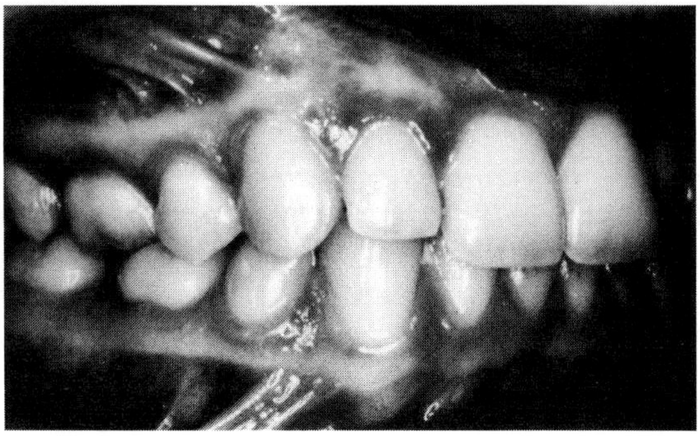

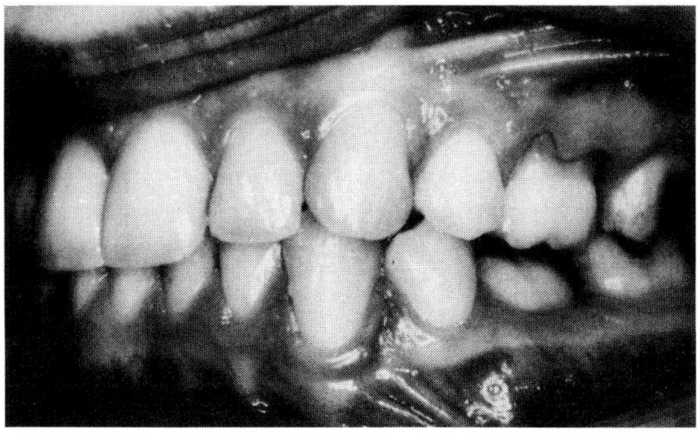

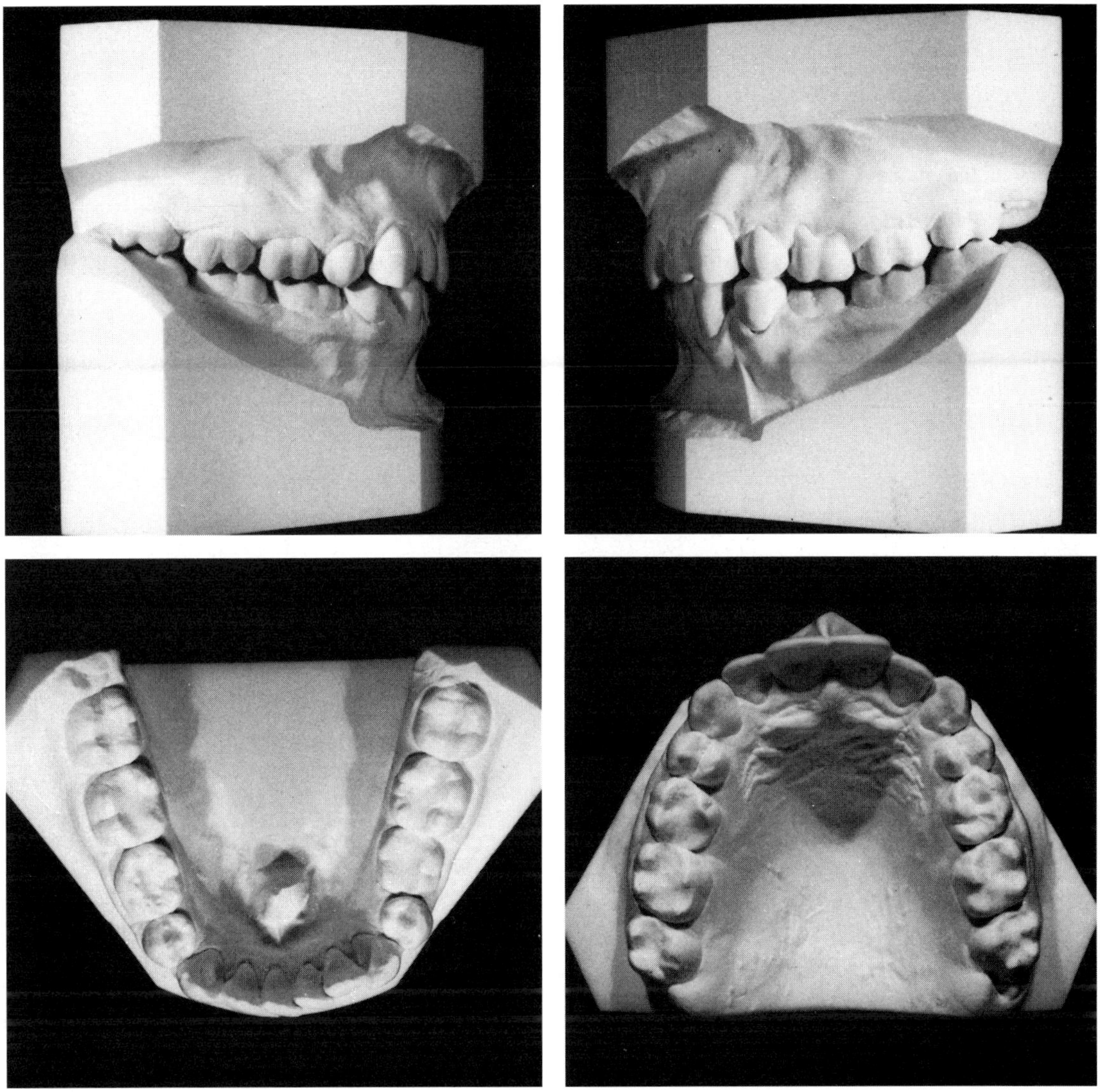

Figs 23-5 and 23-6 At the age of 24 y, 9 mo, eleven years after treatment, few changes can be noted that might be considered to be relapse. The patient is satisfied. The mild supraposition of the maxillary central incisors was not considered disturbing as also was true of the increased crowding of the mandibular anteriors. The infra-position of the ankylosed mandibular left second deciduous molar had not been observed by the patient, although the retraction of the gingiva of its antagonist had been seen. The maxillary right third molar had not formed, and on the left not enough room was available for the third molar to emerge. Removal of that third molar, and eventually both mandibular third molars, was advised.

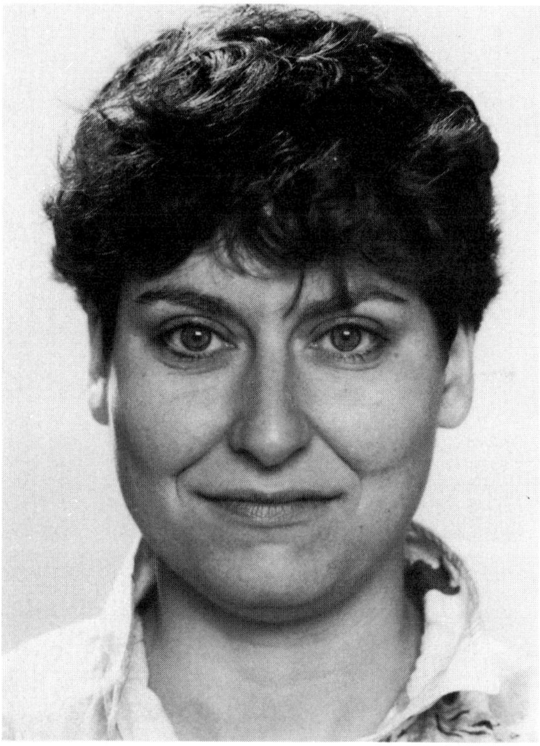
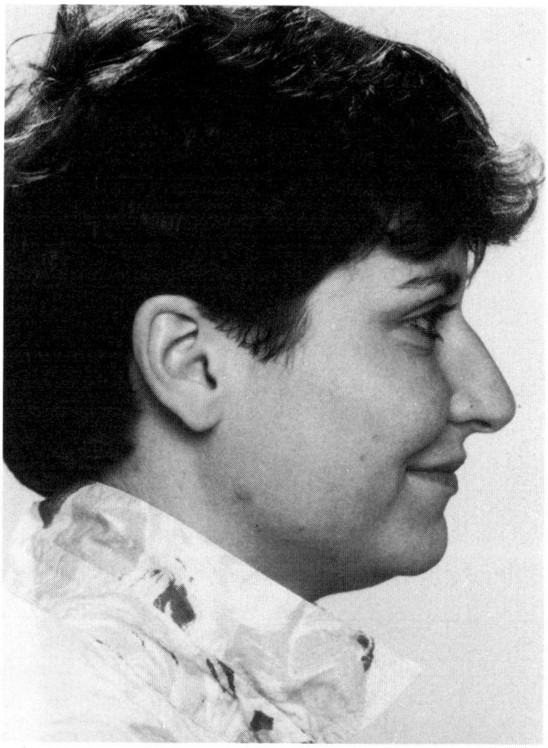
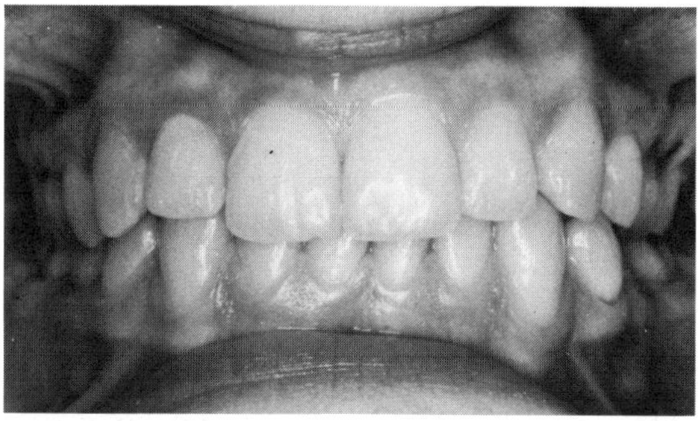
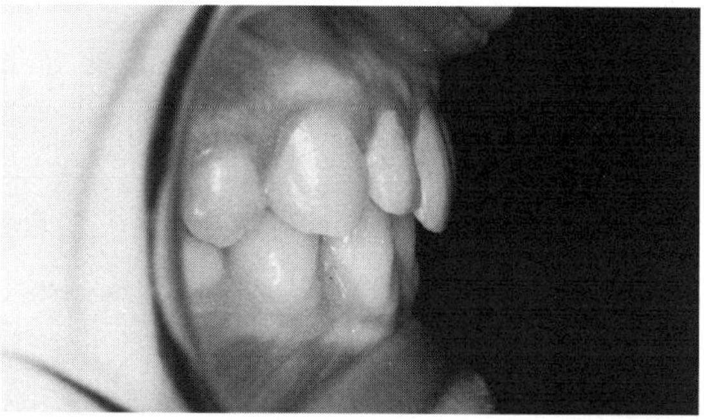
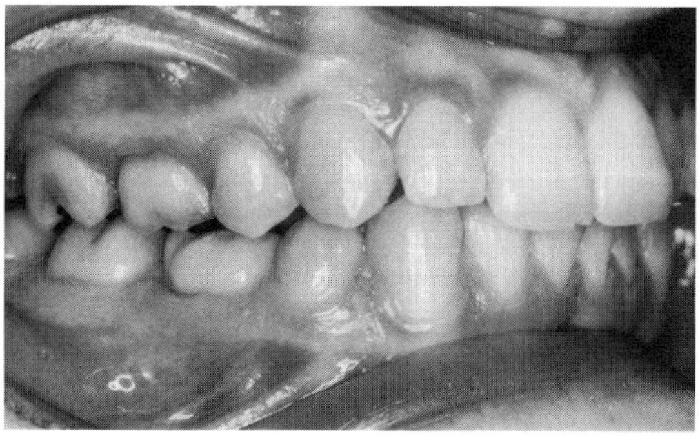
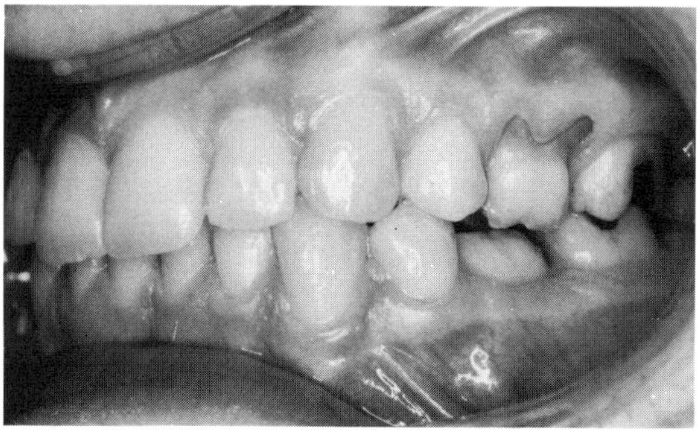

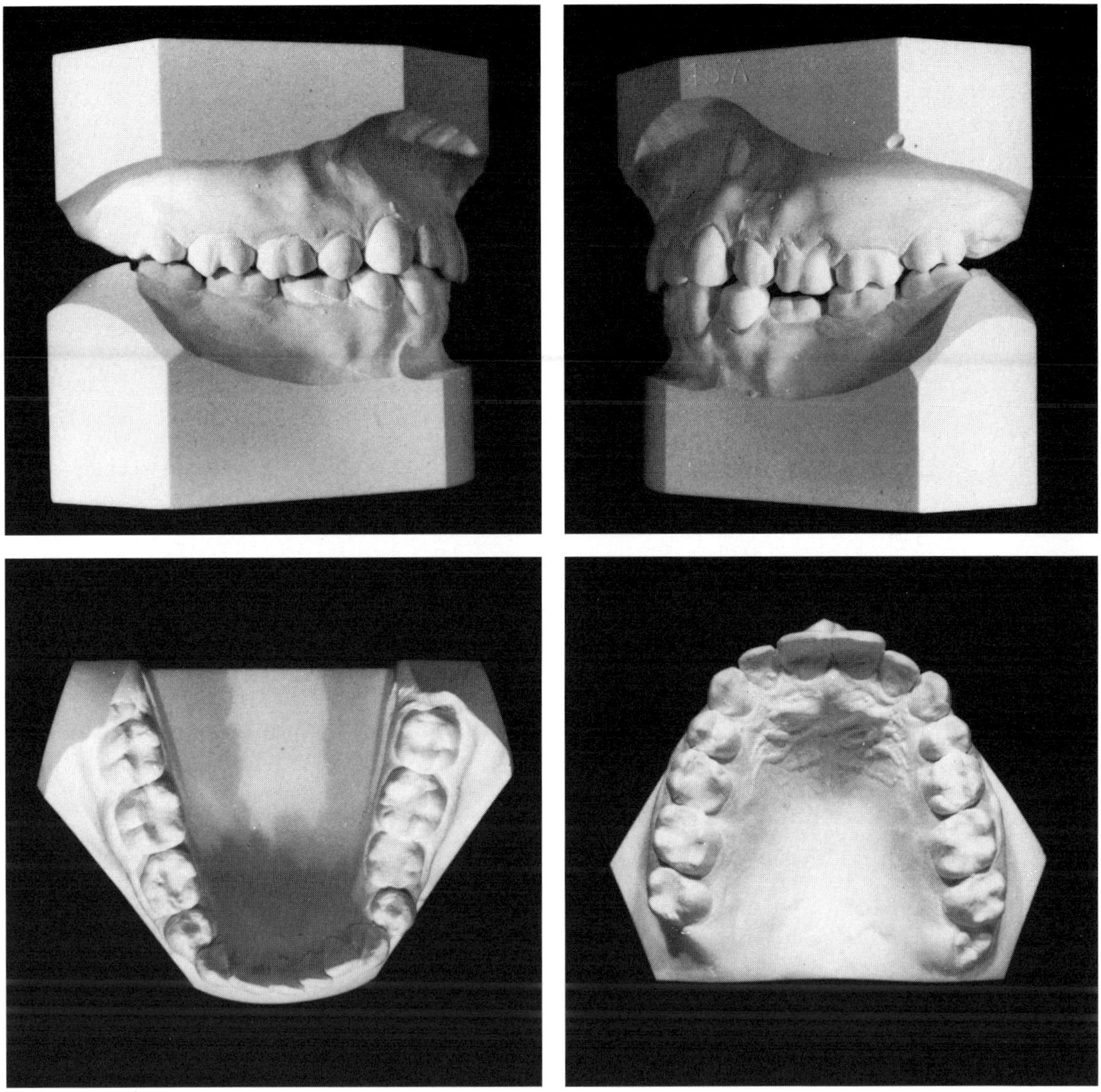

Figs 23-7 and 23-8 *At the age of 28 y, 5 mo, fifteen years after treatment, the second deciduous molars are still present. In the mandible, the right second deciduous molar has become ankylosed and is no longer in occlusion. The gingiva has receded further on the buccal of the roots of the maxillary left second deciduous molar. The roots of the other deciduous molars are still fully covered. The alignment of the teeth in general has not changed visibly; just the crown of the maxillary left third molar, which is still present, has emerged somewhat.*

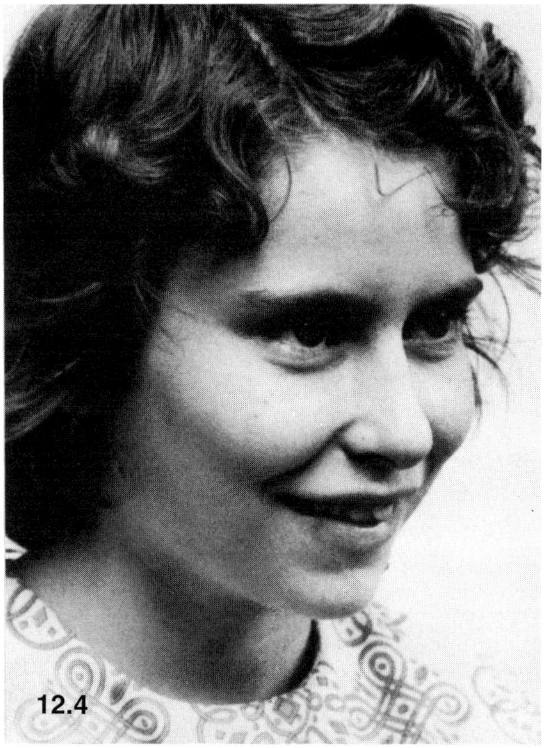

12.4

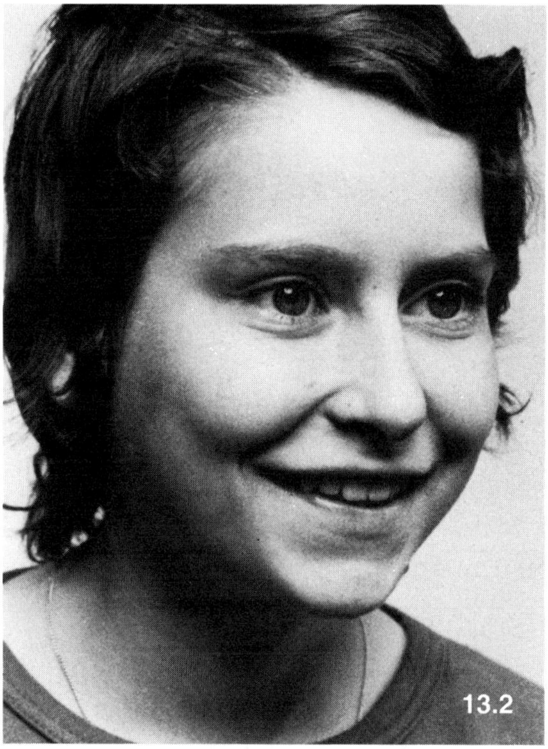

13.2

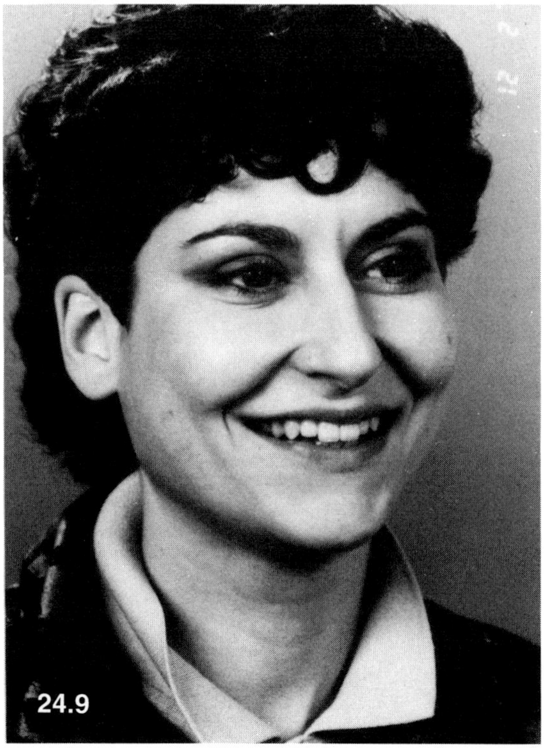

24.9

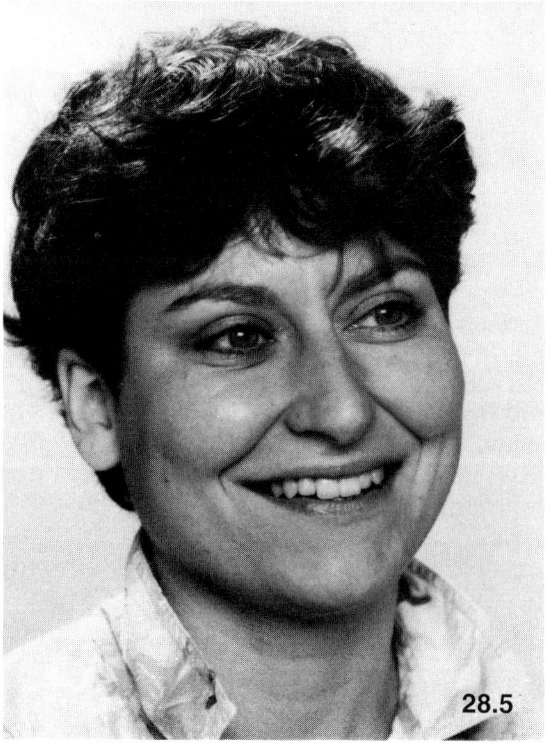

28.5

Fig 23-9 Note the changes that have taken place over sixteen years.

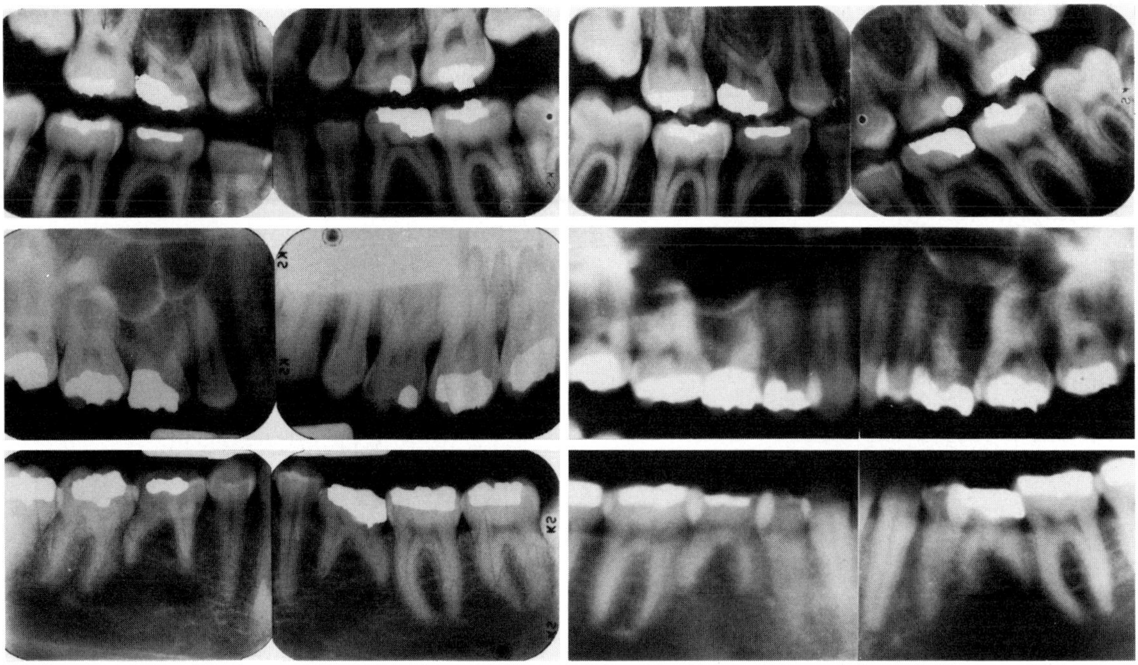

Fig 23-10 Radiographs at different ages show that the deciduous molars have lost little root substance in the sixteen y, and that marginal bone loss has remained minimal.
A 12 y, 4 mo.
B 13 y, 1 mo.
C 24 y, 9 mo.
D 28 y, 5 mo.

the deciduous teeth would continue to function for many years since their roots showed minimal resorption (Fig. 23.10).

The photographs of the smiling patient illustrate the long-term effect of a relatively simple and brief therapy (Fig 23.9). Above all, these photographs show better than could be seen in the "en face" and profile pictures that extraction of deciduous molars and the closure of the spaces would have led to a falling back of the dentition in relationship to the face. The consequence would have been a reduction in facial animation and expressivity.

In the book, *Problems and Procedures in Dentofacial Orthopedics*, a chapter is devoted to the congenital absence of premolars, and the various treatment possibilities are dealt with at length.[33] Therefore it is considered that remarks need only be made here that apply to the case under consideration.

In class I anomalies with crowding and labioversion combined with prominent lips, or with labioposition of the maxillary and mandibular anteriors, the treatment planning for cases of agenesis of premolars is relatively simple. If four second premolars are missing, extraction of all second deciduous molars and closure of the spaces are indicated unless an unacceptable unfavorable influence on the profile can be expected. If all four premolars are not absent, then a first or second premolar needs to be removed in the quadrants that are complete.

In class II/1 anomalies with no reasons to extract in the mandible, the absence of maxillary premolars can be used to advantage to move the teeth mesial to the space distally into the resulting diastema. Then the molars should attain a disto-occlusion of 1 PW. In unilateral agenesis, one premolar on the contralateral side can be extracted. The reverse applies to class III anomalies with agenesis in the mandible.

These considerations apply only if all the remaining teeth are sound and well-formed. If that is not the case (for example, a poor first permanent molar), then the removal of another tooth rather than the premolar should be considered.

As a rule, congenital absence of teeth is not associated with crowding and labio-version, nor with labioposition of incisors. In agenesis, the dimensions of the other teeth are often smaller than normal. In cases with otherwise no indication to extract permanent teeth, the presence of agenesis induces the question for how long the deciduous molars might be expected to function. The answer to that question depends on four relevant aspects: caries susceptibility, root resorption, retraction of the gingiva, and development of ankylosis.

Deciduous molars that become carious show more root resorption than those with sound crowns. Why root resorption occurs in some deciduous molars without a successor but not in others is not clear. There is great variation in that respect. The recession of gingiva can differ markedly not only between persons but in the same mouth. In deciduous molars, the furcation is closer to the crown than in permanent molars so that retraction of the gingiva more readily gives rise to problems. The development of ankylosis of deciduous molars is most critical when vertical development of the lower face has not been completed. They can then come to lie so far in infra-position that the periodontal structures of the neighboring teeth are damaged. Where ankylosis occurs in adulthood, the undesirable effects are less severe. An ankylotic deciduous molar that does not occlude can be kept, without problems, for many years.

If a deciduous molar is lost in later years, it can be replaced, if desired, by an adhesive bridge, any other appropriate prosthesis, or an implant.

In general, in cases of congenital absence of premolars it is not desirable to extract corresponding deciduous molars that have a good prognosis, unless orthodontic treatment with full fixed appliances is indicated for other reasons. If extractions are indeed performed and the spaces closed, as much as possible should be done to prevent dorsal movement of the mandibular and maxillary anterior teeth, if such movements would lead to a sunken mouth, resulting in a reduction of facial animation and expressivity. Otherwise a prematurely old face is likely to develop.

Chapter 24

Class II/1, high gum-line

Bass-plate with parietal headgear, cervical headgear, brackets 12, 11, 21, and 22
Female: 10 years, 0 months to 23 years, 4 months

A girl aged 10 years, 0 mohths displayed a class II/1 anomaly with a relatively retruded mandible. She held her mouth open, and at rest her lower lip lay behind the maxillary incisors, which were overerupted. She could breathe easily through her nose. A disto-occlusion of 1 PW was associated with an overjet of 9 mm and an overbite of 6 mm. The mandibular incisors contacted the palate, and when asked to close her teeth together and close her mouth, stomion was found to be slightly above the middle of the maxillary central incisor crowns. The upper lip was short and when smiling about 2 mm of the gum was visible. In the maxillary dental arch, in which the first permanent molars were rotated mesiopalatally, sufficient room was available for all teeth. There was a TSD of 2 mm in the anteriors with relatively broad mandibular incisors that were crowded (Figs 24.1 and 24.2).

It was decided to commence treatment as soon as possible to correct the disto-relation and intrude the maxillary incisors, and to finish treatment with the use of brackets on the maxillary incisors. At the age of 10 years, 1 month, a Bass-plate was placed in association with a parietal headgear which fitted onto the front of the plate (Fig 24.3; see Fig 9.15, page 144). Disadvantages of this technique are that an anterior open bite, page 144 is created, and the maxillary teeth that are held in the clasps are unable to move to buccal in response to the rail mechanism as the disto-occlusion is corrected. The latter may lead through the occlusion to undesired transverse movements of the antagonists (Figs 24.4 and 24.5). If the Bass-plate is then left out after enough intrusion has been attained, and the parietal headgear is replaced with a cervical one, then the forces of the tongue and cheeks combined with those of the occlusion are free to stimulate improvements in the positions of the teeth. The tendency of artificially displaced teeth to return to their original positions assists these improvements (Fig. 24.6). Moreover, a cervical headgear can be adapted to apply more force on one side than the other, as is required in asymmetry such as this (Figs 24.7 and 24.8).

The treatment comprised ten months of Bass-plate combined with parietal headgear, and ten months of cervical headgear during the last six months of which the headgear was made asymmetric. In addition, during the last three months of use of the cervical headgear, a partial fixed appliance was used on the maxillary incisors to retract and properly position these teeth. The treatment was concluded at the age of 12 years, 1 month. The result was satisfactory (Figs 24.9 and 24.10). The maxillary

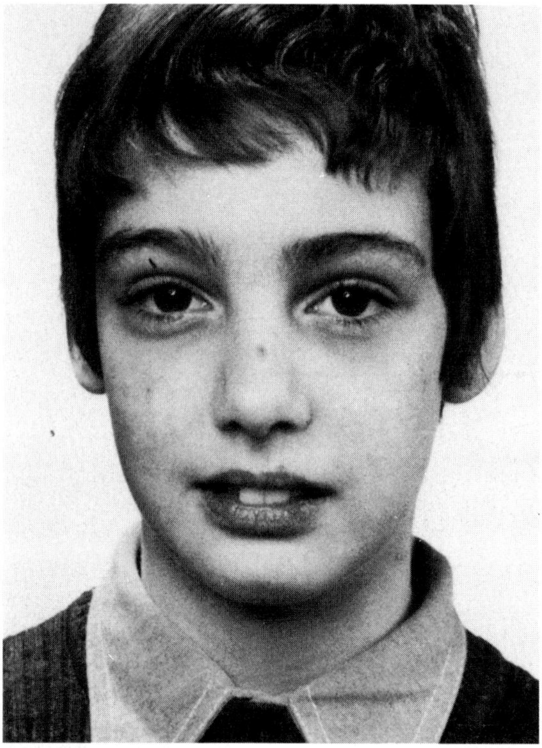
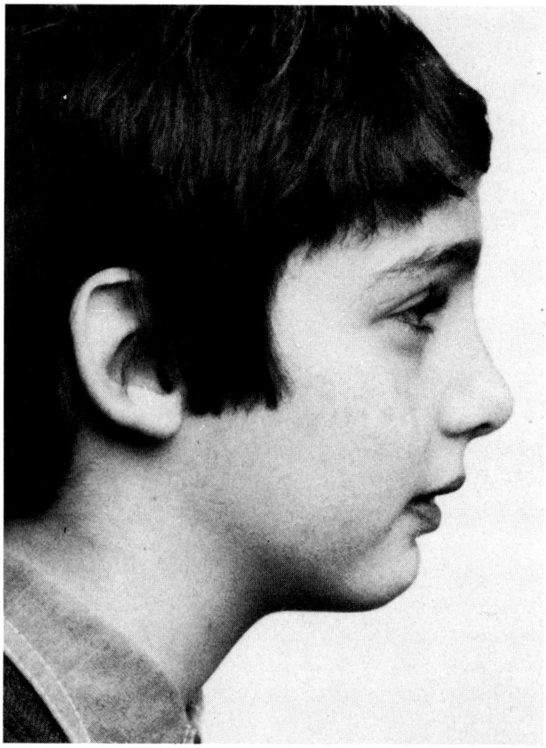
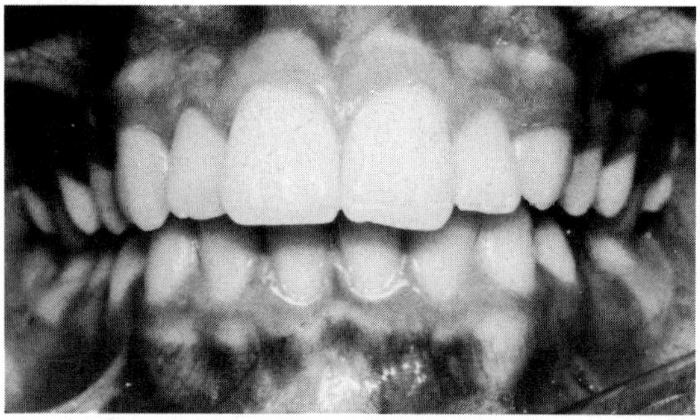
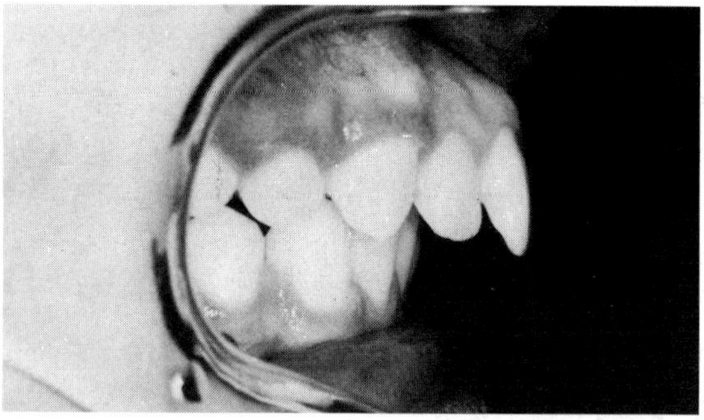
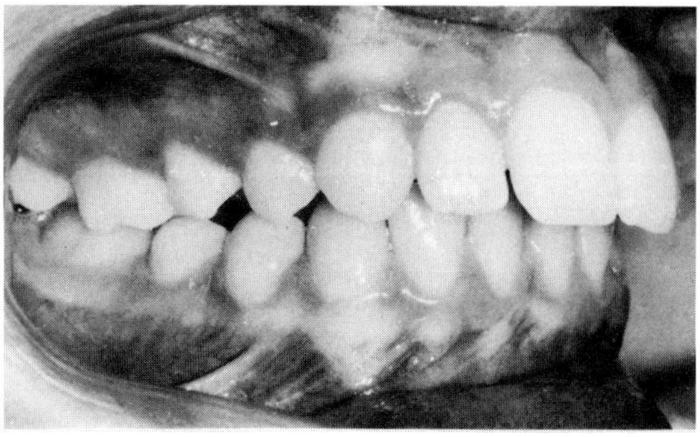
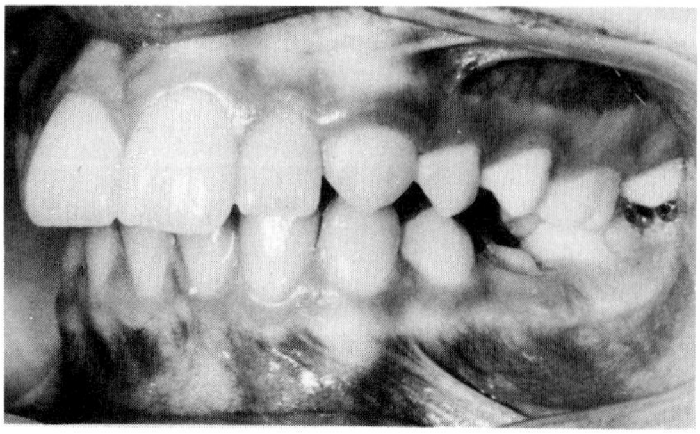

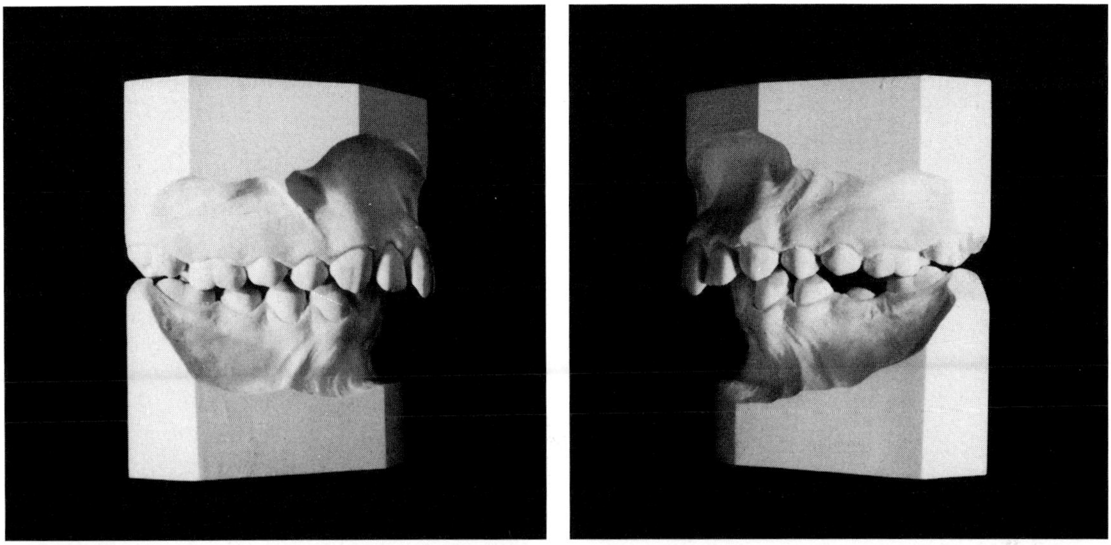

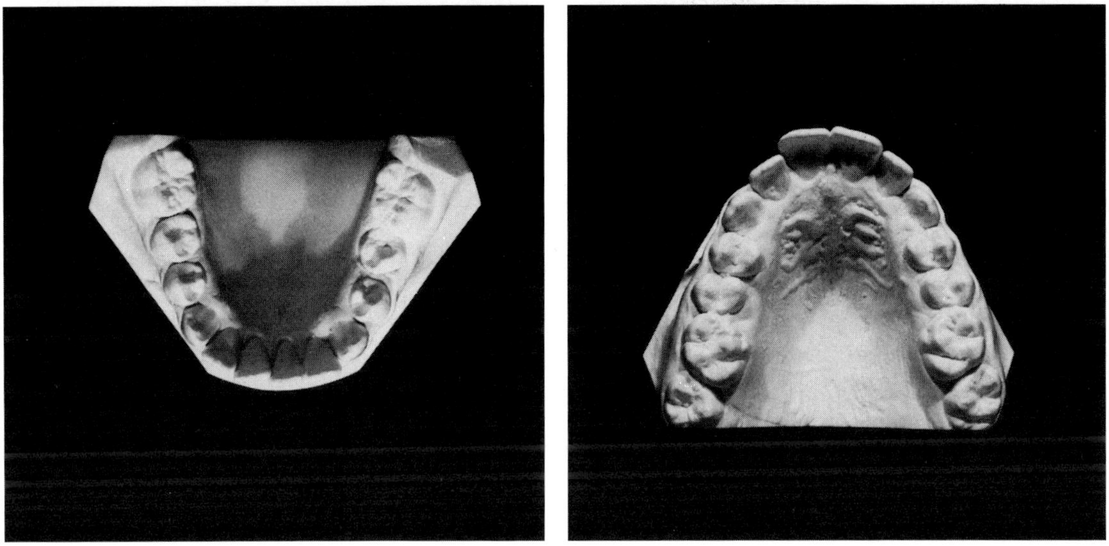

Figs 24-1 and 24-2 *A girl aged 10 y, 0 mo with a class II/1 anomaly, the lower lip behind the prominent and overerupted maxillary incisors, a clear nasal passage, and a 2 mm high gum-line when smiling. The premolars and permanent canines, as well as the maxillary second permanent molars, have already emerged. The maxillary first permanent molars are rotated mesiopalatally. A disto-occlusion of 1 PW is combined with a solid interdigitation, except between the premolars, which have only recently emerged. The mandibular arch shows an ALD of –2mm, while a TSD is present with a 2 mm relative excess of tooth material in the mandibular anteriors.*

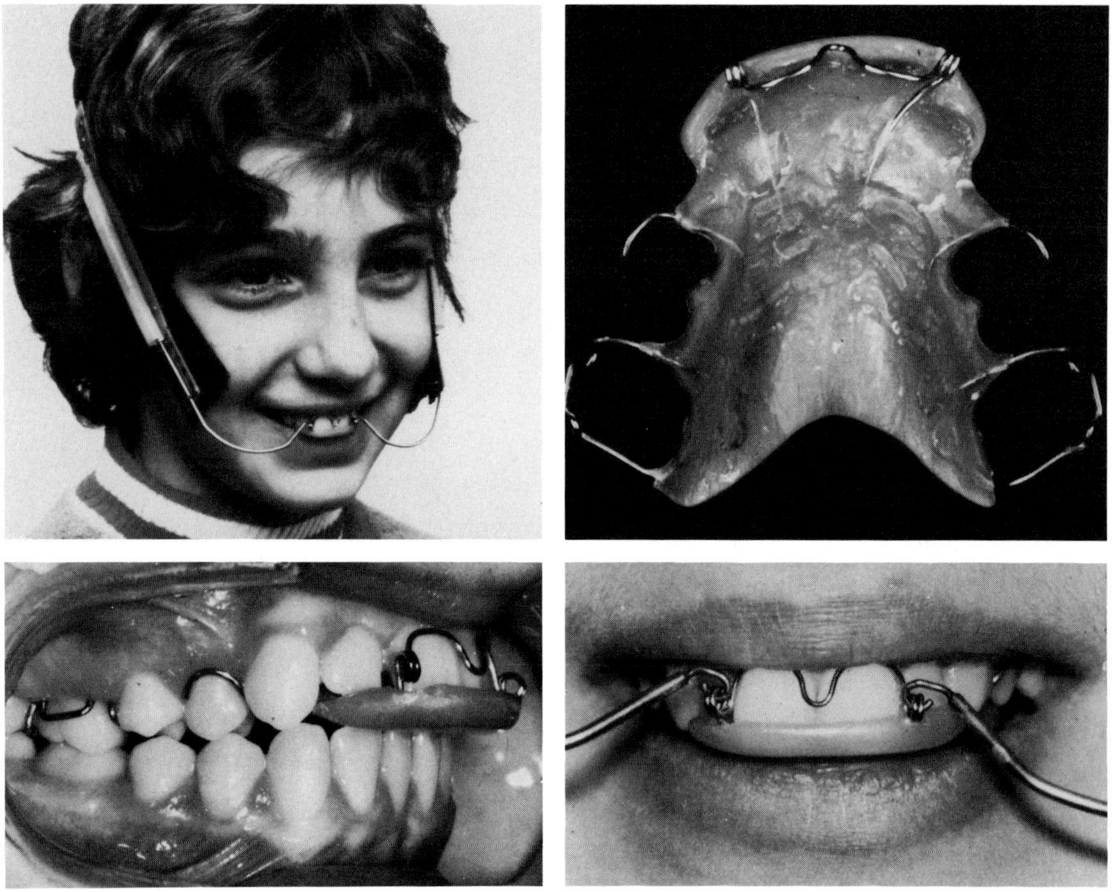

Fig 24-3 A Bass-plate with parietal headgear in use.

A The headgear is hooked onto the plate anteriorly, and due to the direction of the applied force, the maxilla is held back and the maxillary incisors are intruded.

B The plate is firmly retained by clasps on the posterior teeth and by the torquing springs on the incisors.

C The acrylic that caps the maxillary incisors should be sufficiently thick to ensure that the wire elements onto which the headgear is hooked will not be dislodged. A disadvantage of this construction is that the biteplane is rather high and an anterior open bite is promoted.

D The hooks from the headgear are fitted into the coils of the incisor torquing springs, which should be slightly active to prevent the incisors being tipped backwards. The plate has to be worn at all times, and the headgear at least 14 hours per day.

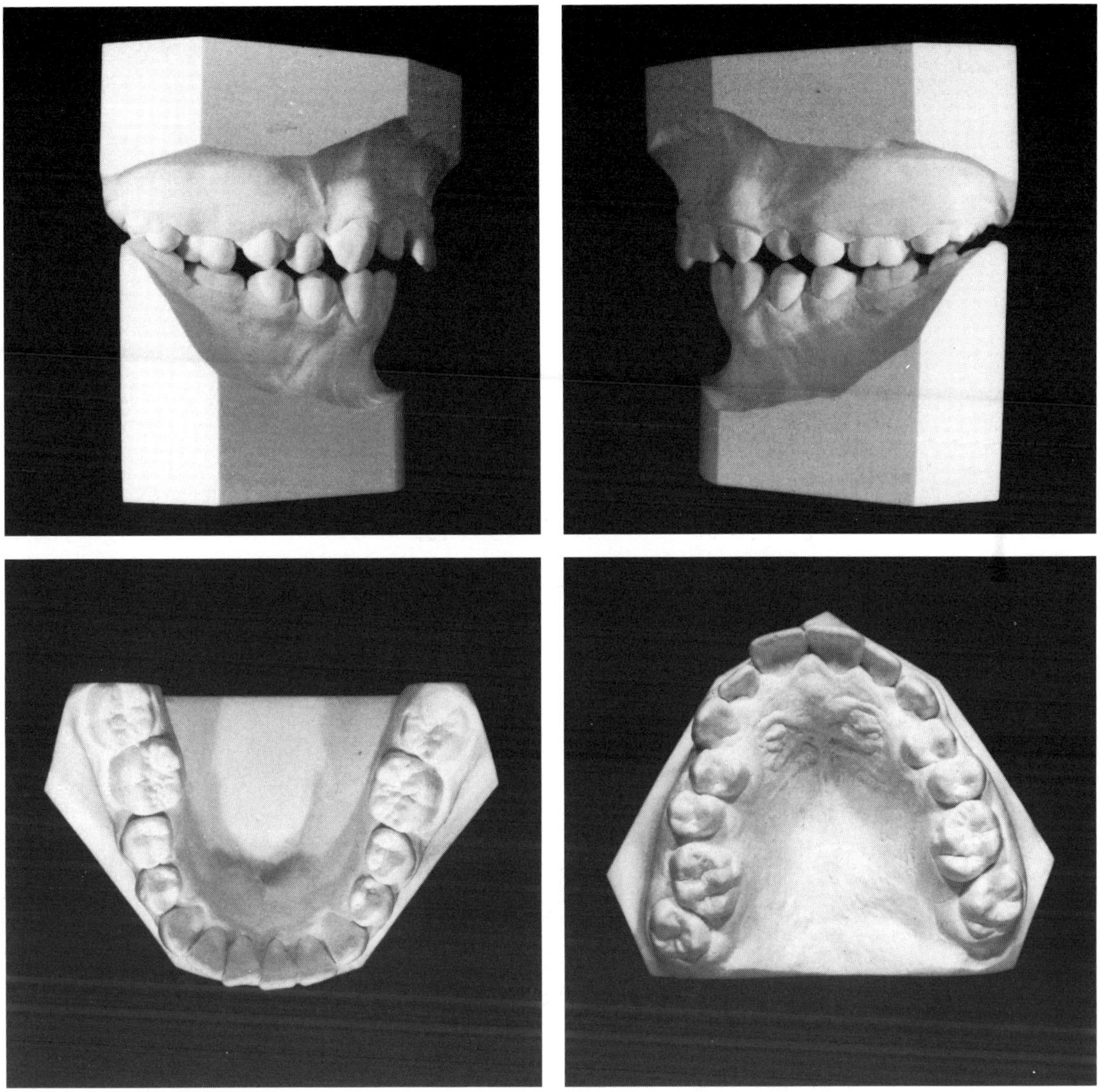

Fig 24-4 At the age of 10 y, 6 mo, after five months treatment with a Bass-plate and parietal headgear, the disto-occlusion has improved little on the left side. The curve of Spee in the mandibular dental arch has been leveled partially by the Bass-plate being worn continuously. The open bite has been produced mainly by intrusion of the maxillary incisors. The clasps on the first premolars and first molars impede any movement to buccal that these teeth normally would have undergone as the response to the rail mechanism. Instead, their antagonists have moved to lingual. To limit this effect, the clasps on the first permanent molars were removed after the appliance had been worn for eight months.

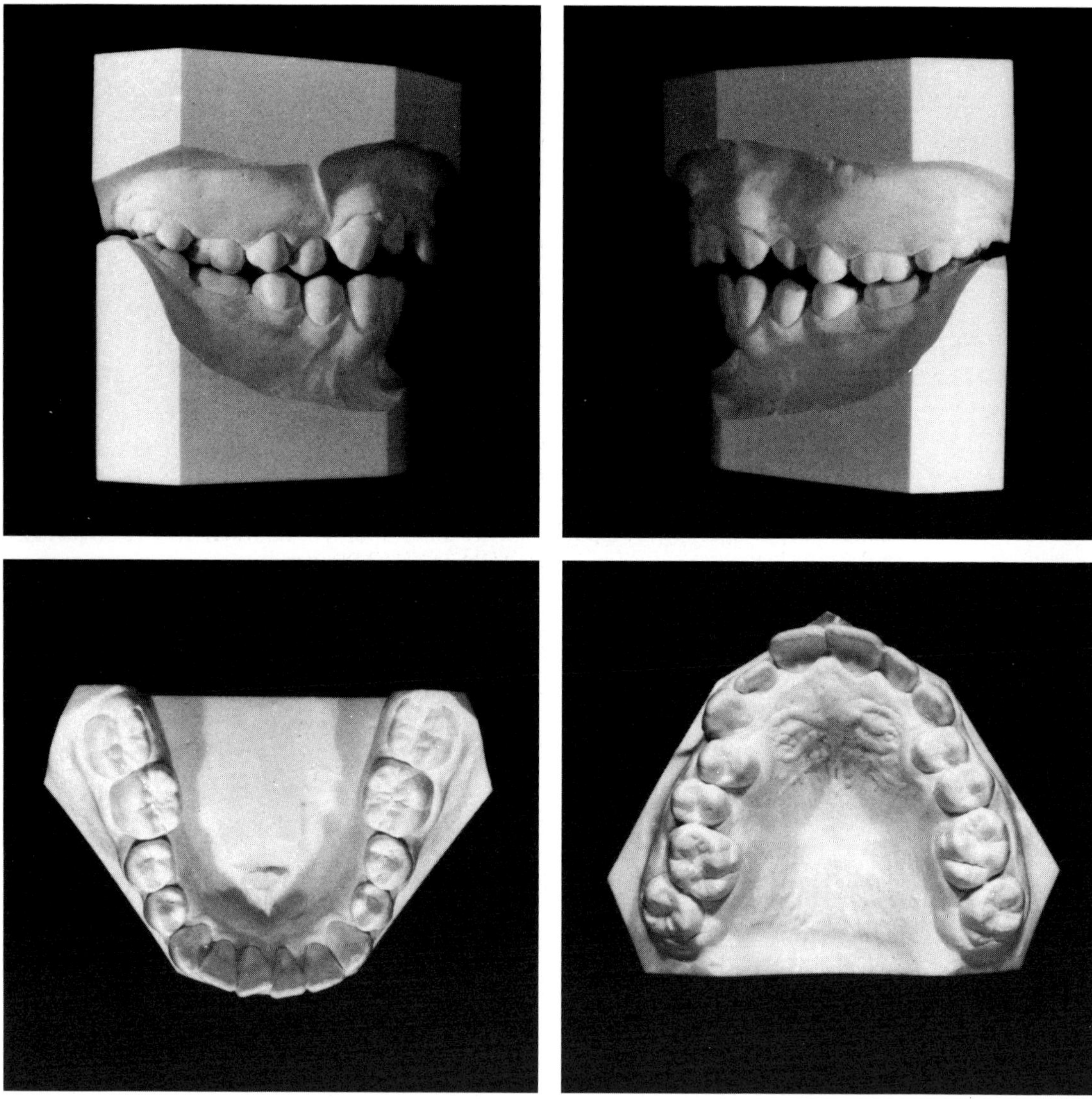

Fig 24-5 At the age of 10 y, 11 mo, the disto-occlusion and the overjet have further improved. The anterior open bite has certainly not become less since the thickness of the Bass-plate has not been changed. Due to the interdigitation of the posterior teeth and the fixation of the maxillary first premolars and first molars by the clasps embracing them, the rail mechanism has worked in reverse. The antagonists have adapted themselves transversely to the maxillary teeth by moving lingually. The premolars on the right are nearly in neutro-occlusion, but on the left they are still ½ PW in disto-occlusion. Correspondingly, the midline of the maxillary arch is 2 mm left of the mandibular midline. To give the posterior teeth the opportunity to assume better buccolingual positions, the Bass-plate was discarded and the parietal headgear was replaced with a cervical one.

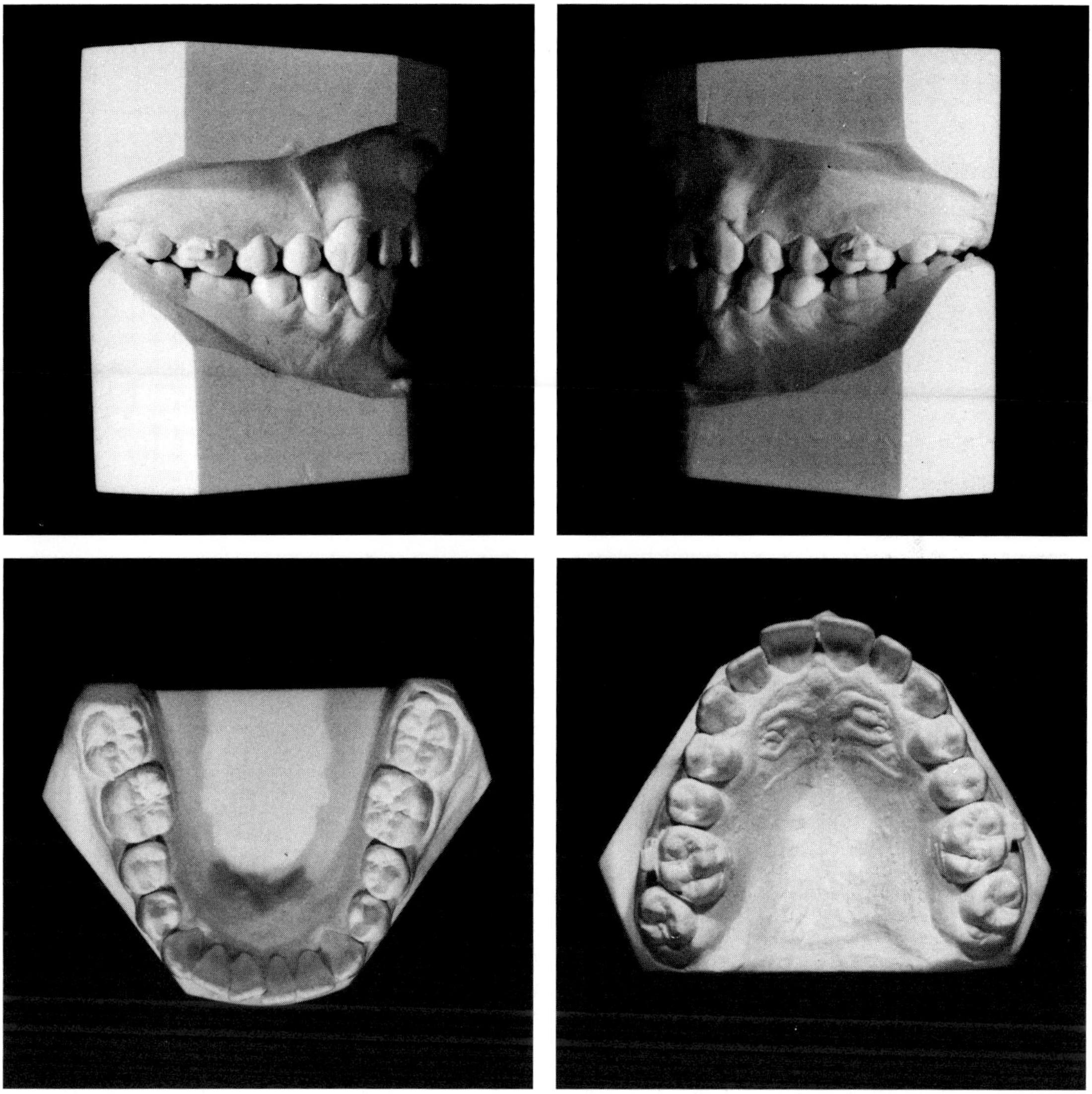

Fig 24-6 *At the age of 11 y, 3 mo the teeth had been free to assume better positions over four months. The first permanent molars have moved buccally both in the maxilla and the mandible. The same applies to the first premolars, which also have taken up better positions in the dental arches. To correct the existing asymmetry in the occlusion, the cervical headgear was modified to produce asymmetric forces.*

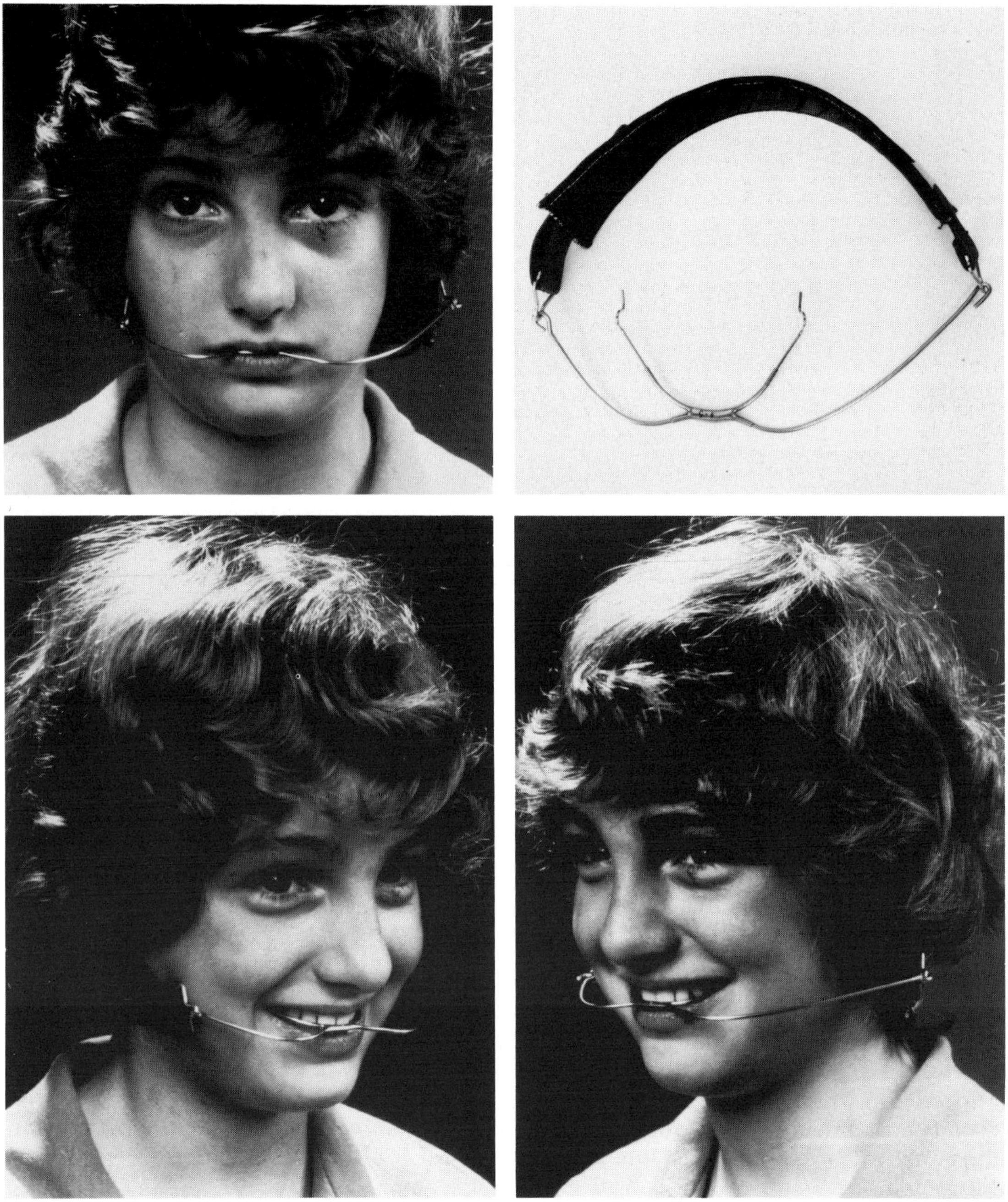

Fig 24-7 The asymmetric cervical headgear in use with a shortened right outer bow and the left bow bent outward.

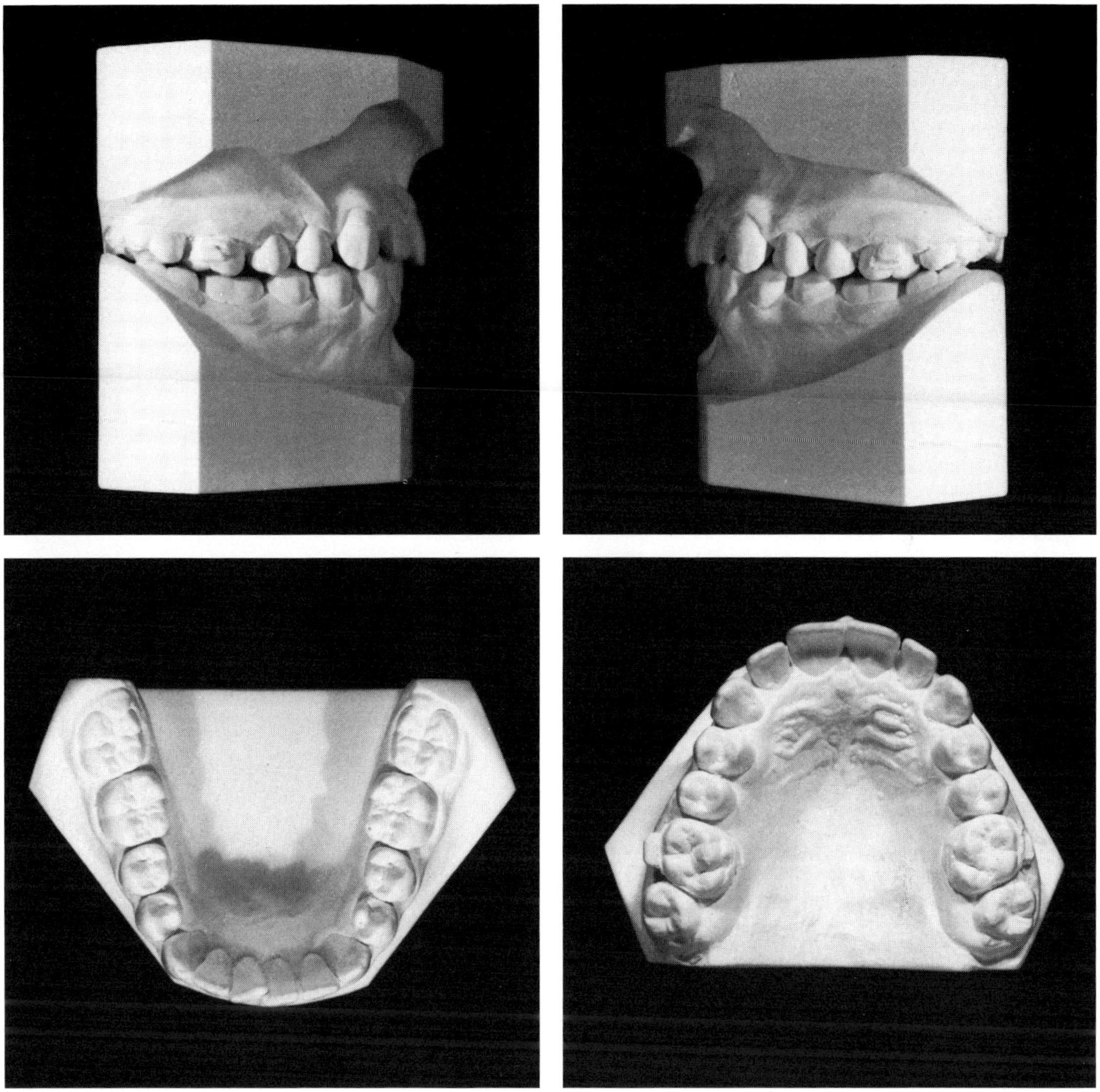

Fig 24-8 At the age of 11 y, 9 mo, after six months of use of asymmetric headgear, there is now neutro-occlusion on the left side too. As the result of the interdigitation and the influence exerted by the tongue and cheek musculature, the positions of the first premolars and first molars in both jaws have been improved. To retract the maxillary incisors and place them in optimal positions, brackets were provided on those teeth and an archwire was fitted. After three months, all appliances were removed and no retention was provided subsequently.

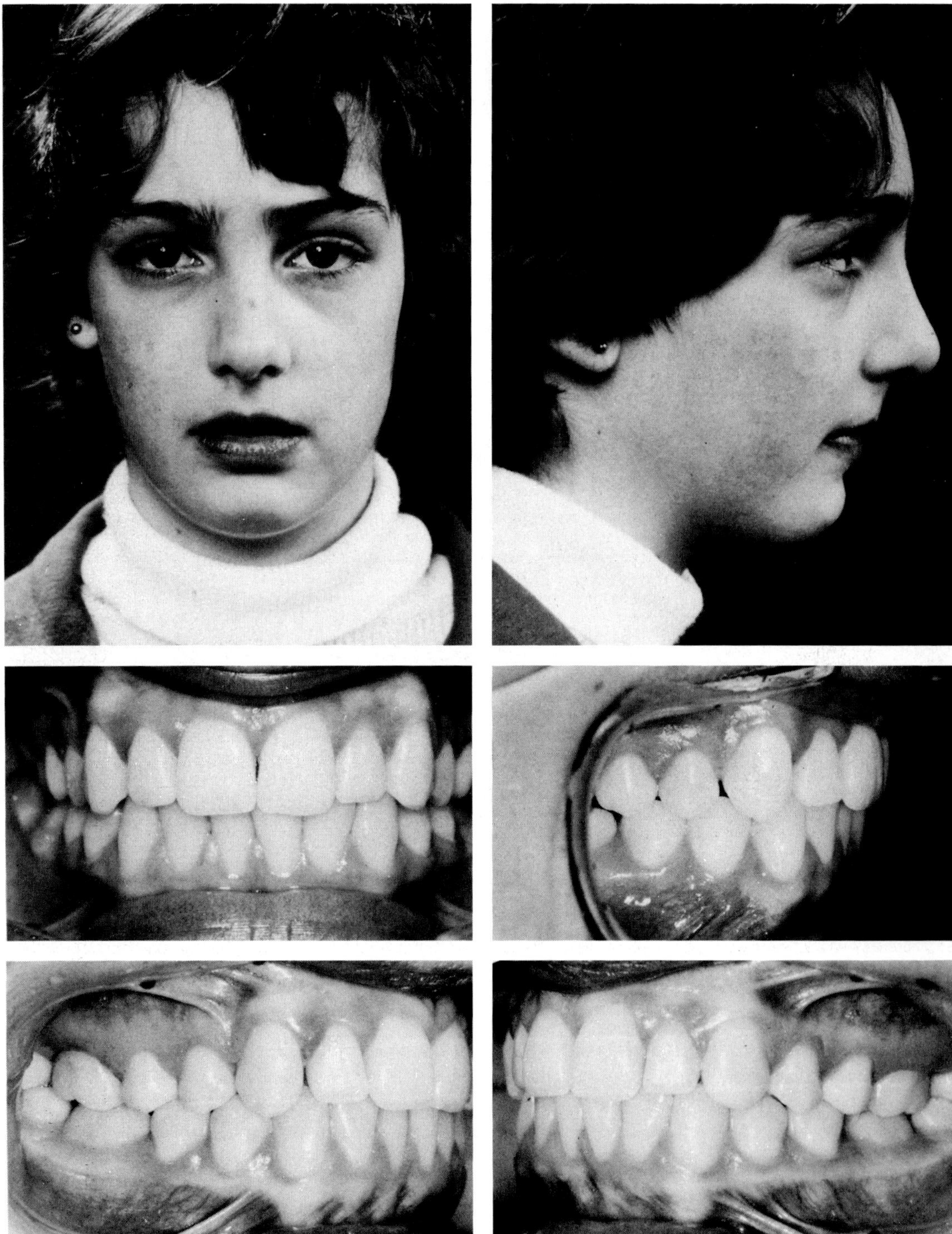

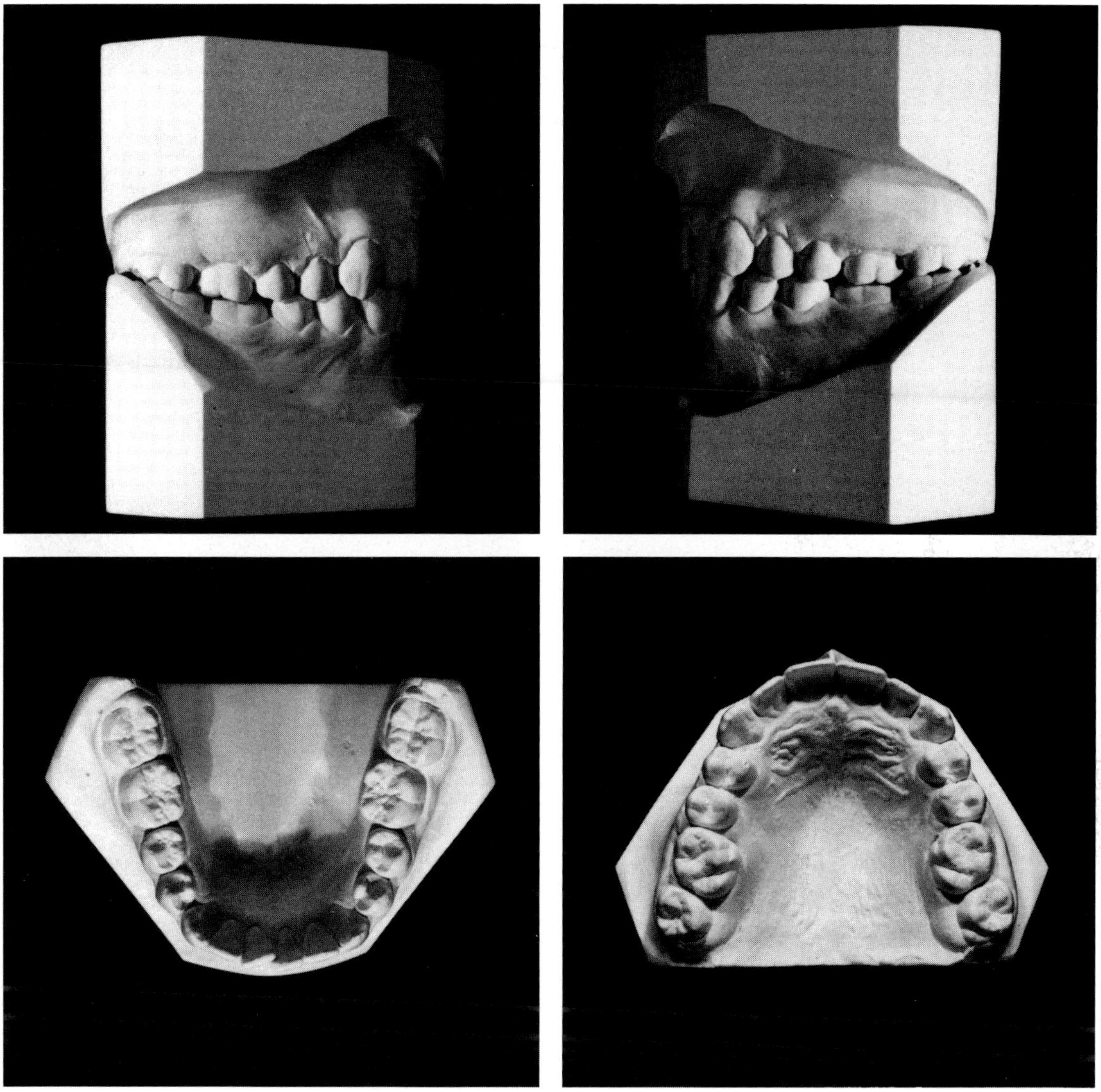

Figs 24-9 and 24-10 At the age of 12 y, 1 mo, after two years of treatment, a satisfactory result has been achieved with adequate lip seal and solid posterior interdigitation, while the lower lip does not overlap the maxillary incisors excessively. Stomion is about 1 mm above the incisal edges of the maxillary incisors. The rotation of the maxillary first permanent molars has been corrected. They and their antagonists are in a slight linguo-position, as was the case originally. The mandibular incisor crowding has increased somewhat and the right central incisor has rotated.

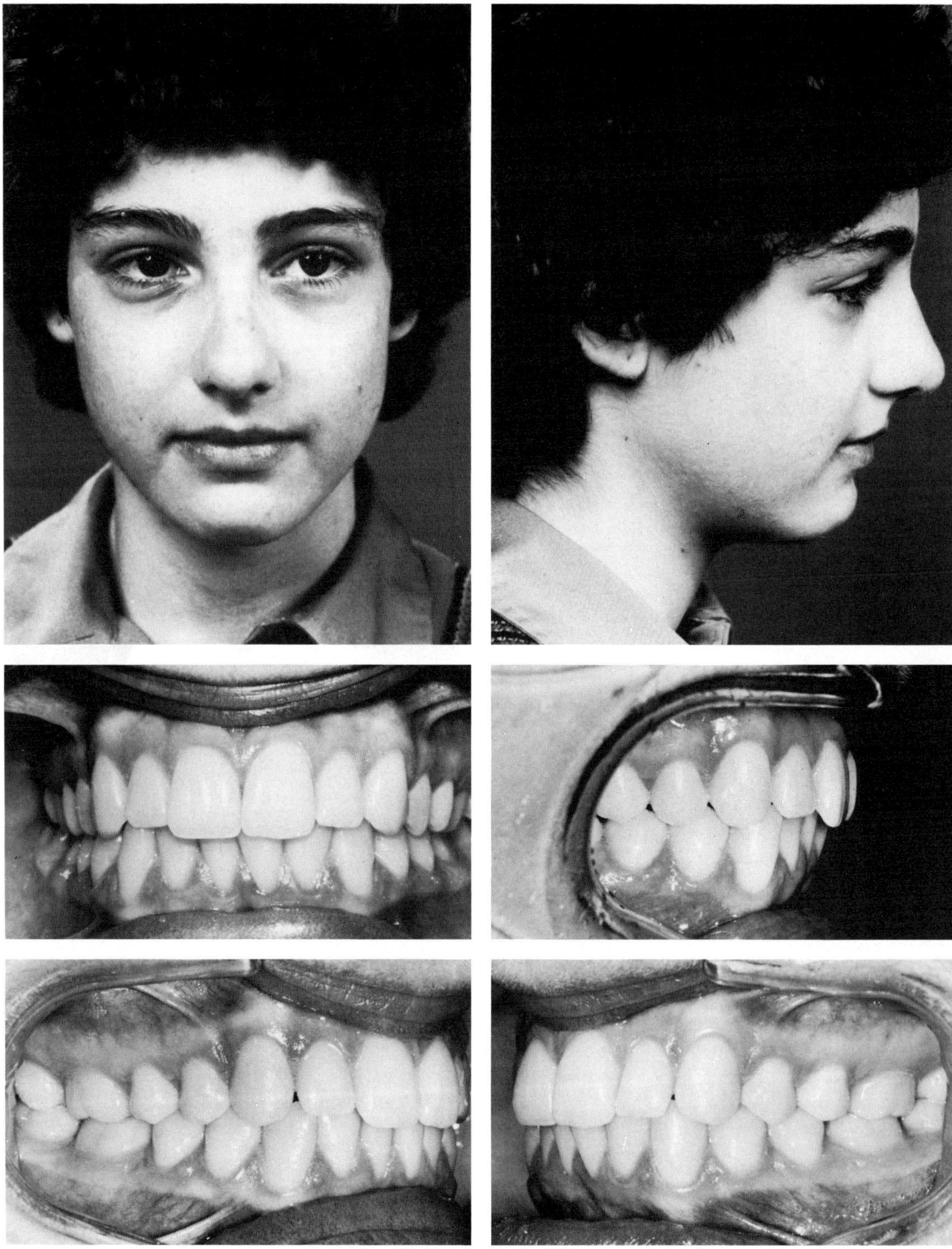

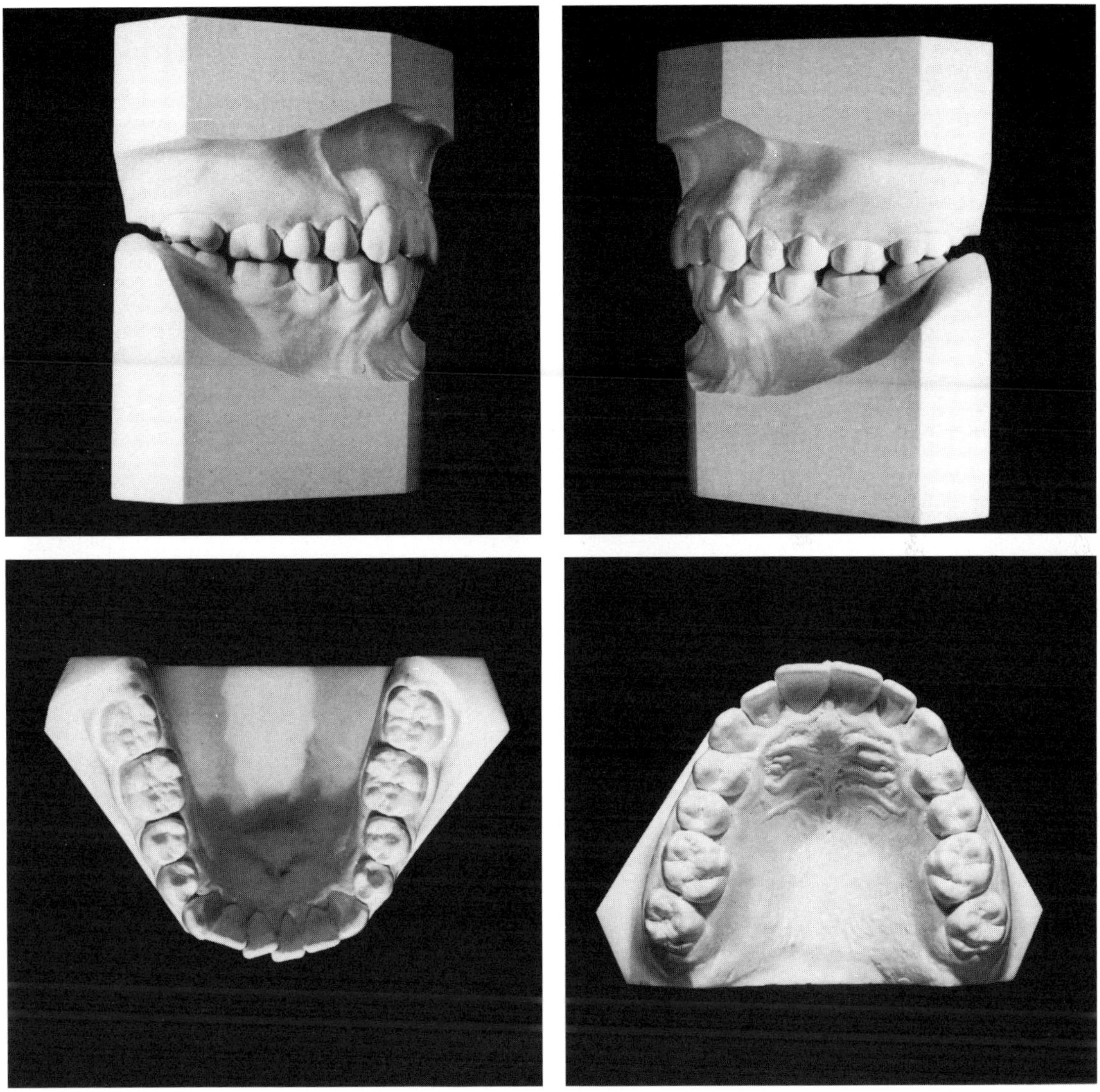

Figs 24-11 and 24-12 *At the age of 14 y, 3 mo, two years after treatment, the maxillary incisors have become slightly more in supraposition. The one on the right has returned partly toward its original position and the distal side has rotated to labial. In the maxilla, the posterior section of the apical area is small; it will increase in size only a little so that insufficient space will become available for the third molars.*

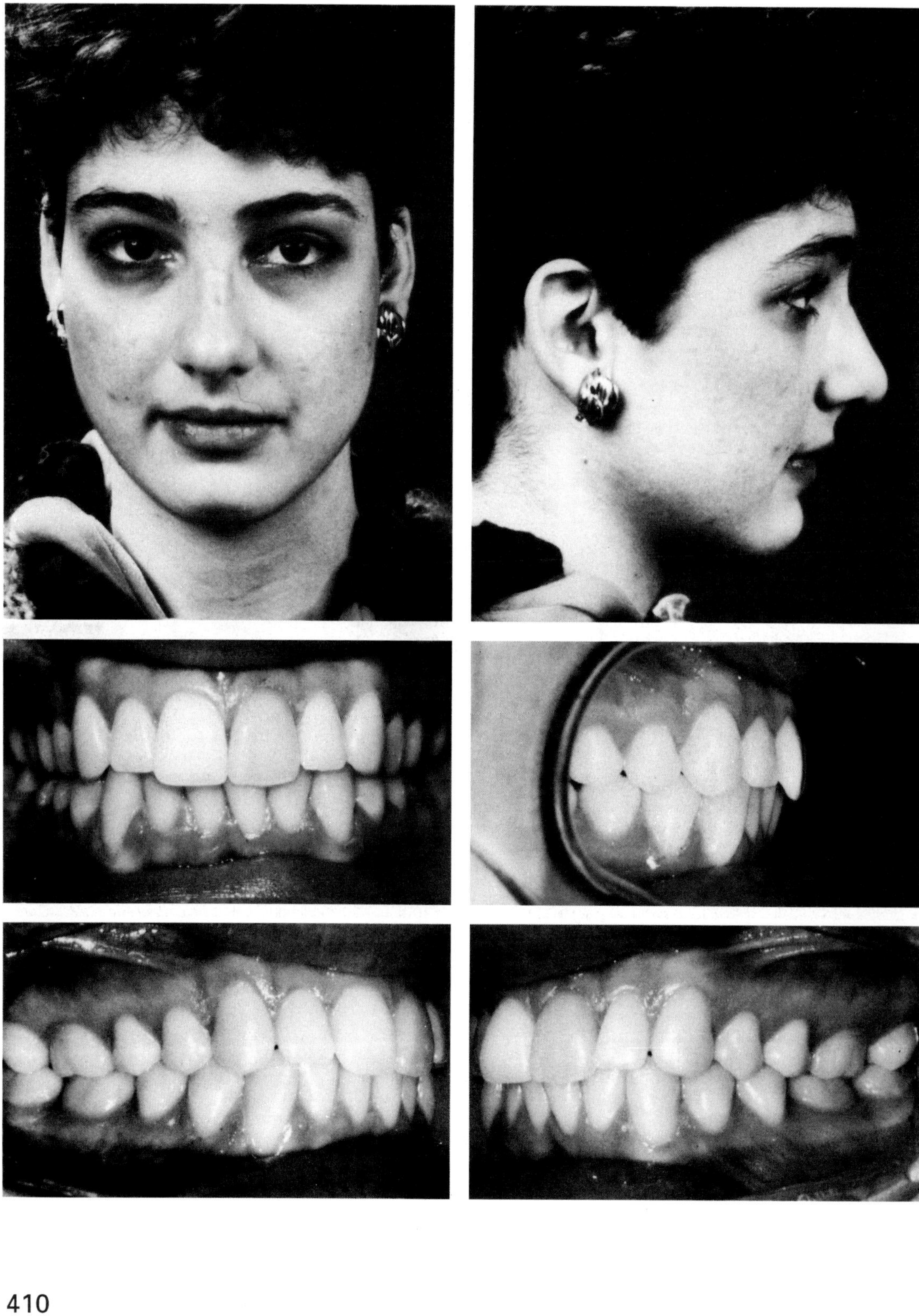

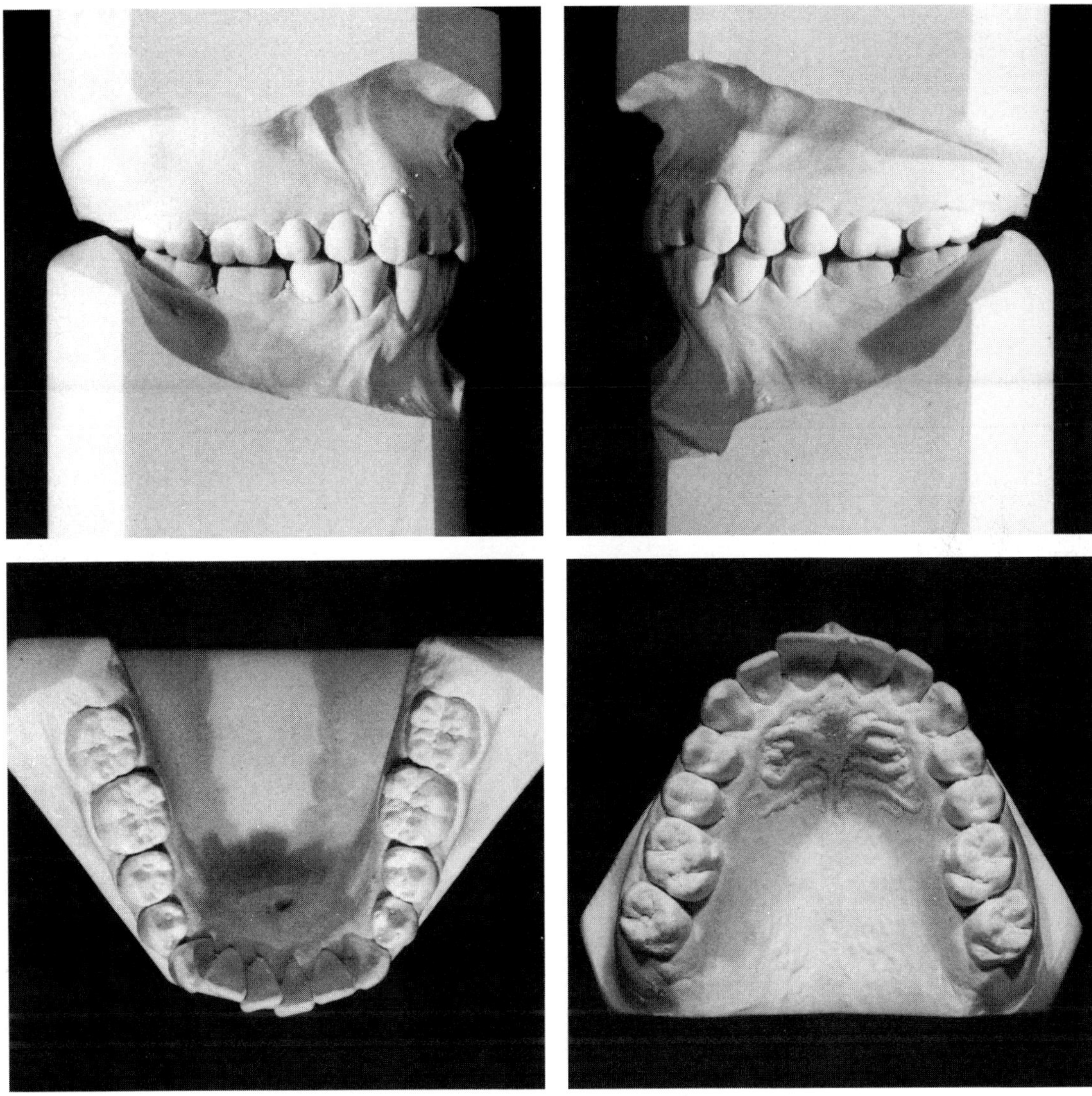

Figs 24-13 and 24-14 *At the age of 17 y, 2 mo, five years after treatment, the irregularity of the anteriors has increased somewhat. The maxillary left central incisor has become non vital as the result of some trauma, after which it was treated endodontically and became discolored. The maxillary right central incisor has moved more to labial at the distal. The mandibular incisor crowding has also increased but is not considered objectionable. The lip closure is adequate even though the upper lip is short.*

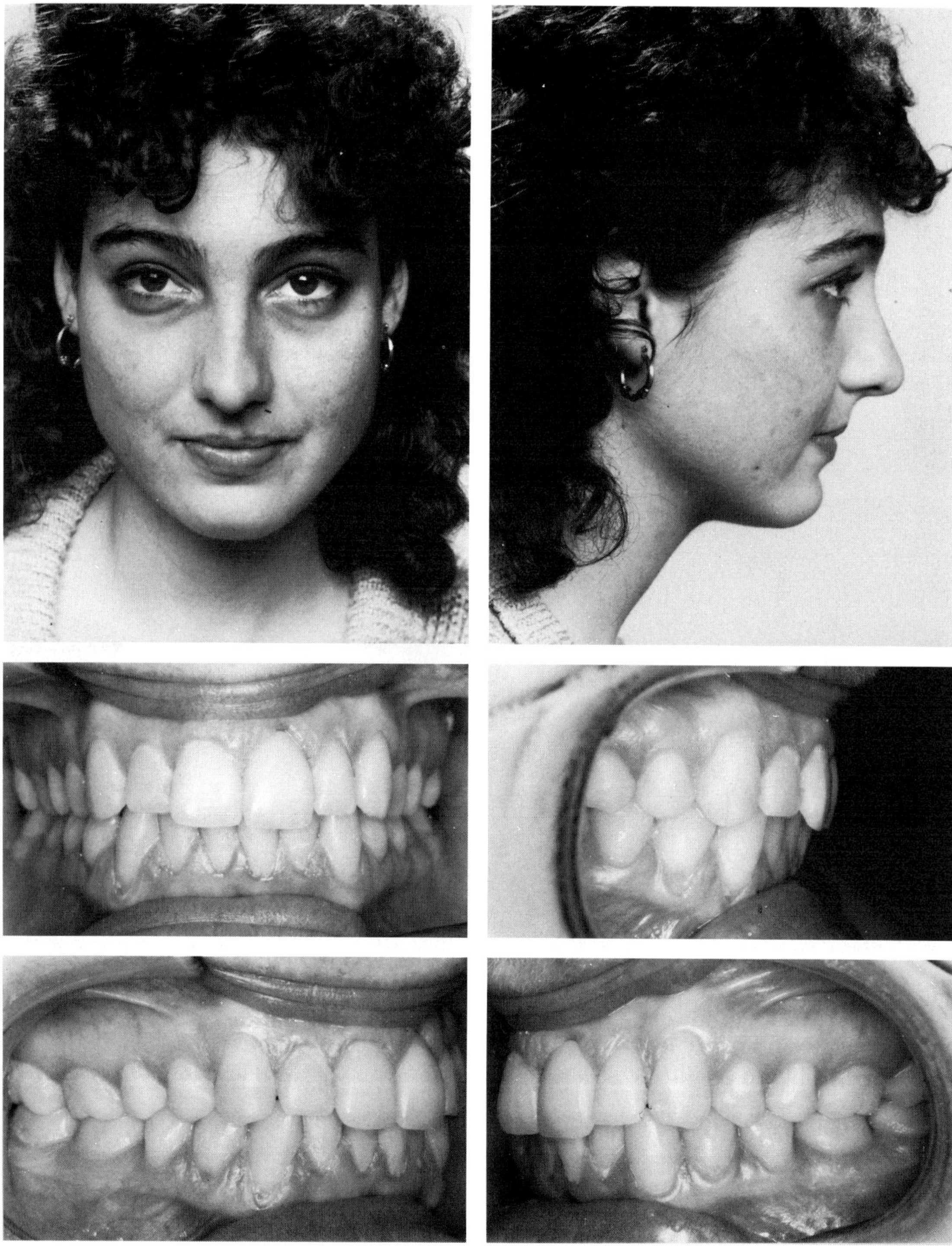

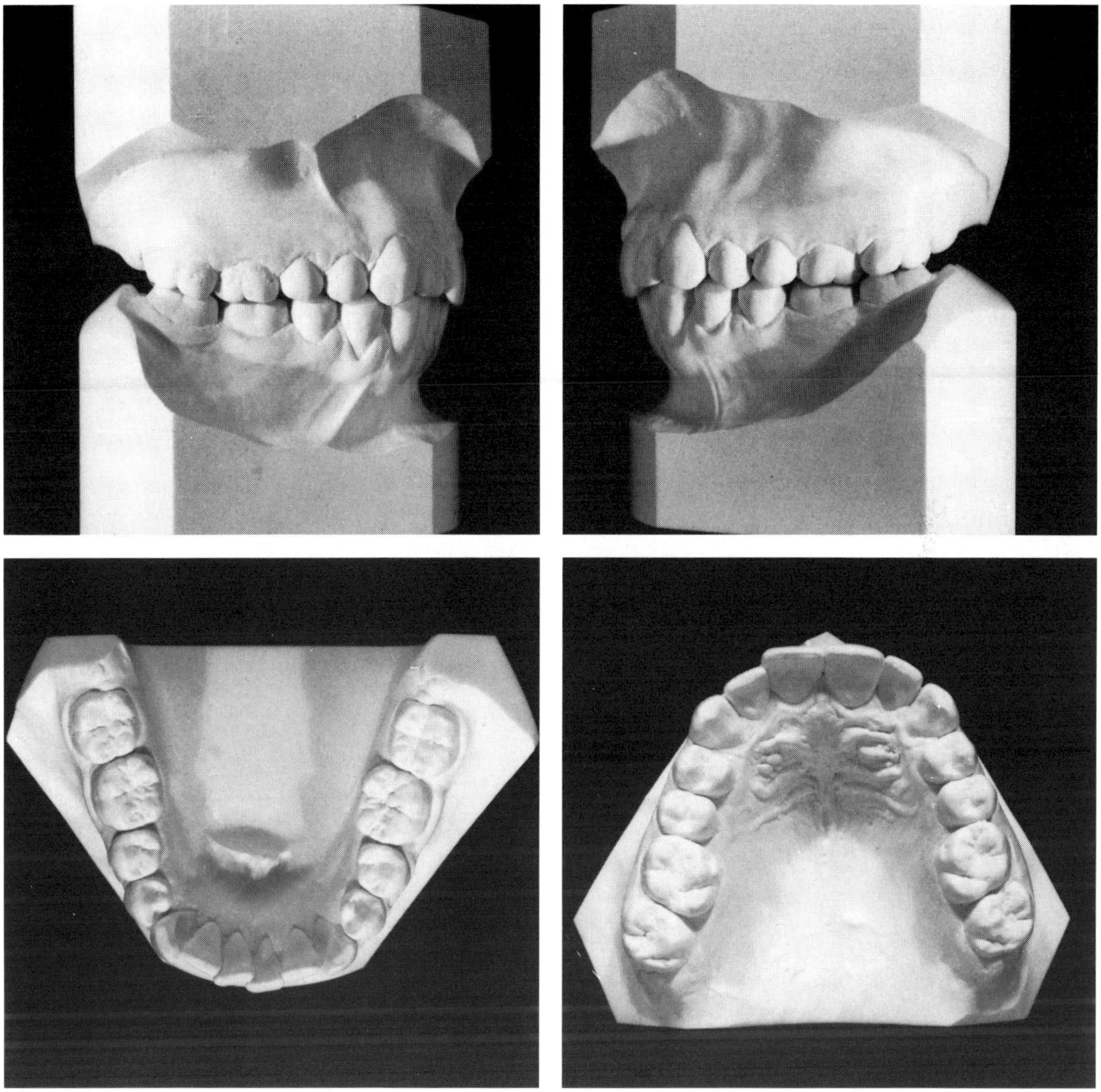

Figs 24-15 and 24-16 *At the age of 23 y, 4 mo, eleven years after treatment, little change can be noticed. The crown of the maxillary left central incisor was fractured in a fall and restored by means of a metal core and porcelain jacket crown. The third molars in both jaws were removed in the meantime. The patient is satisfied with the result.*

Figure 24-17a

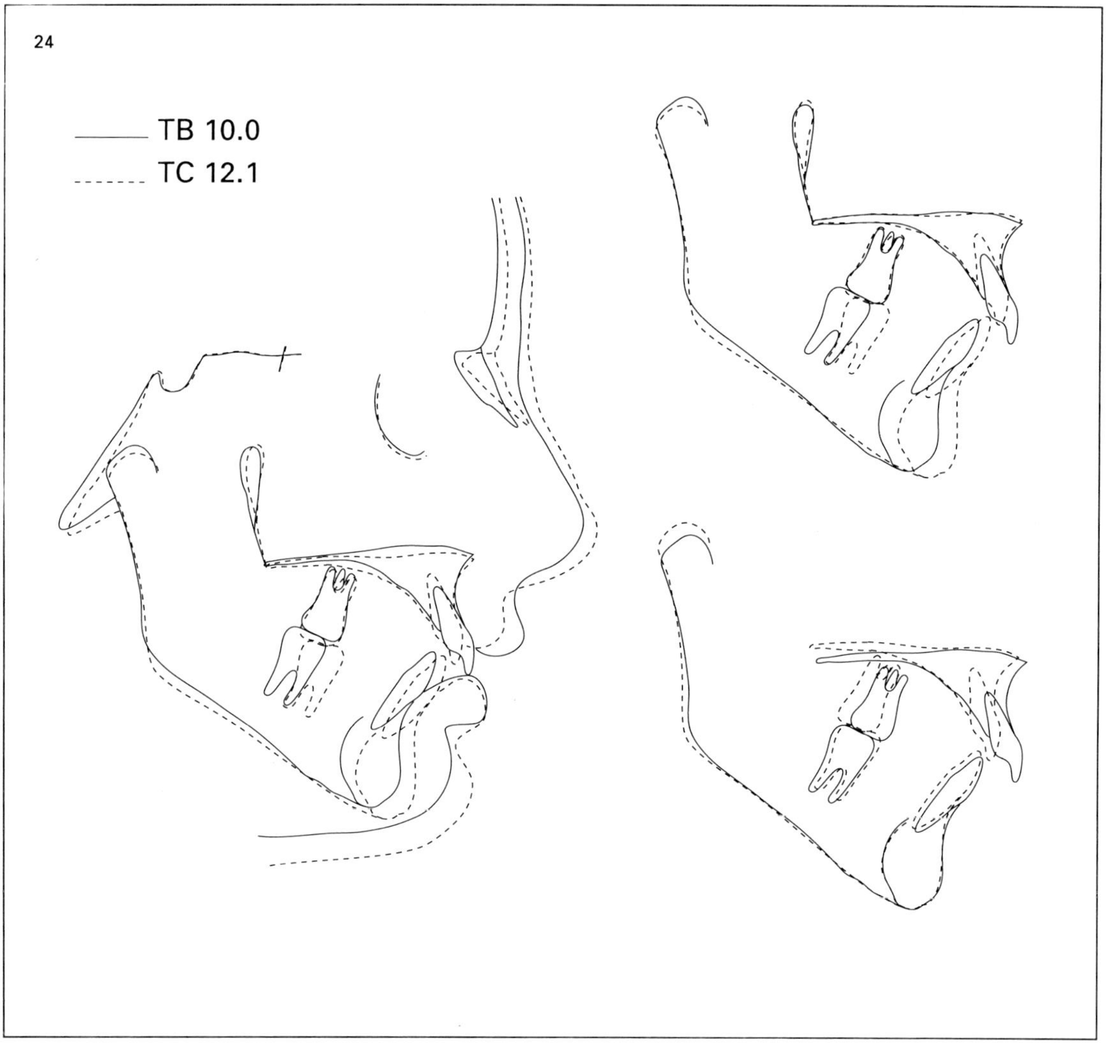

Fig 24-17 Tracings of the cephalometric radiographs show the changes that occurred during growth and treatment. The ventral development of the maxilla was inhibited and the maxillary incisors intruded significantly. The mandible exhibited good ventral development; the height of the face, in particular that of the lower third, increased very little. The marked growth that is shown here in the eleven years since treatment, took place mostly between the ages of 12 and 14 years. In this period, the height of the face and the length of the mandible increased greatly.

Figure 24-17b

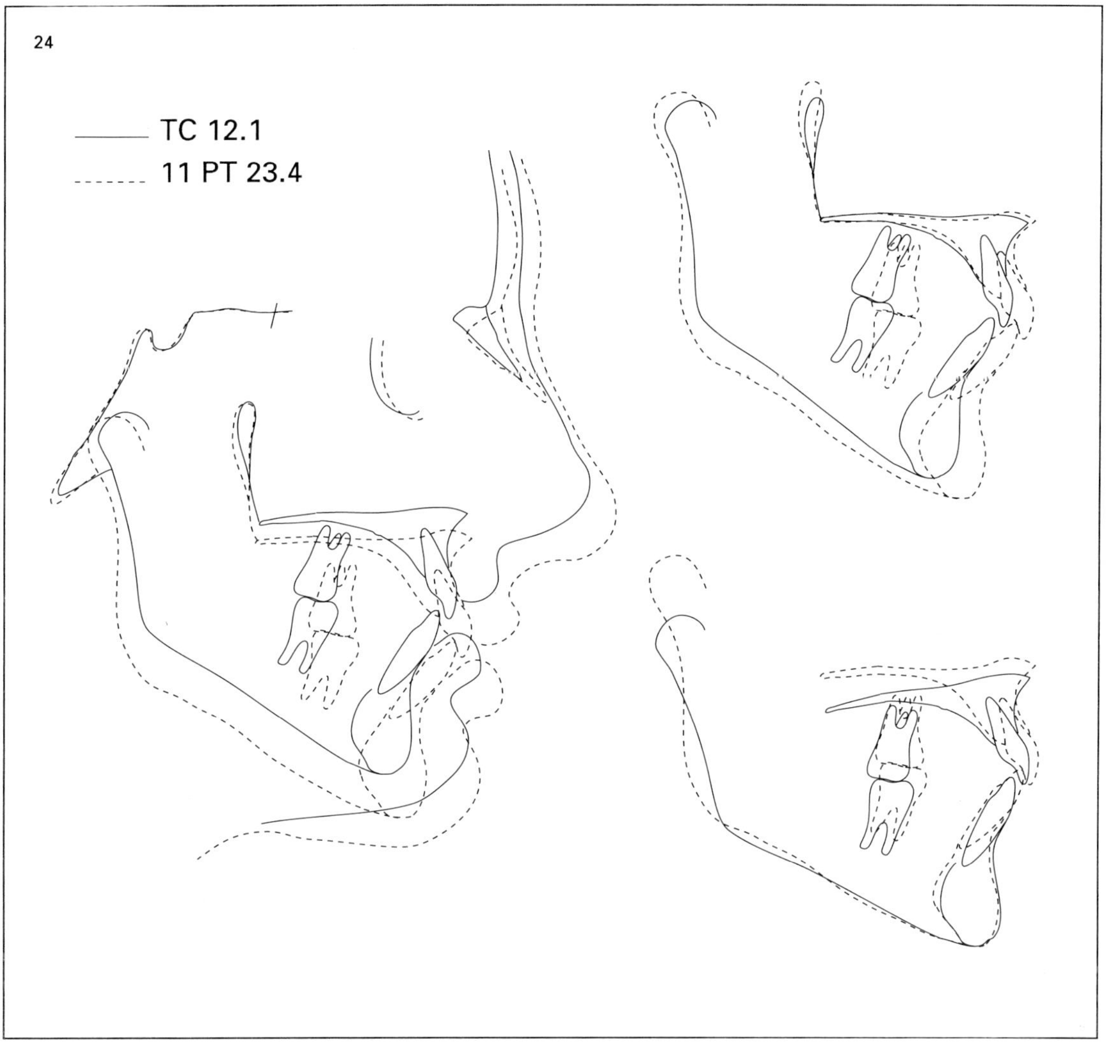

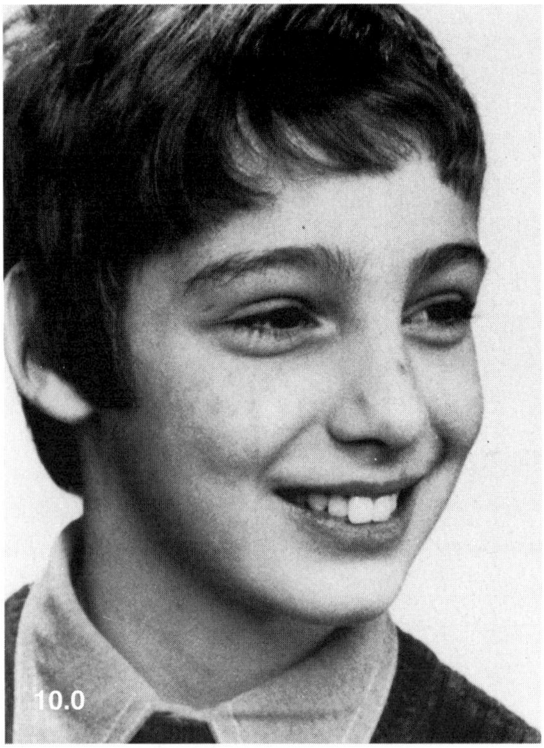
10.0

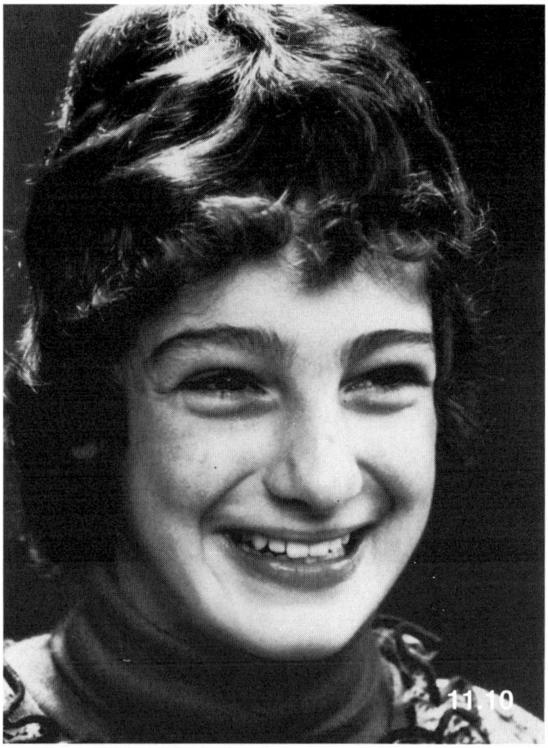
11.10

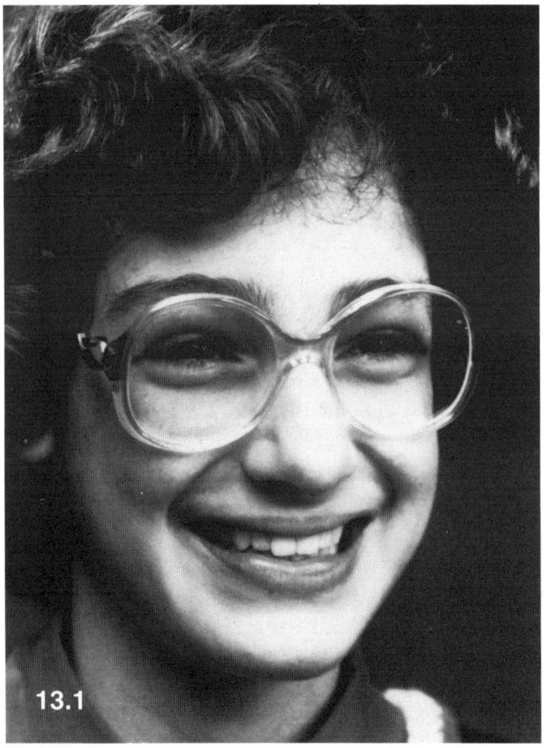
13.1

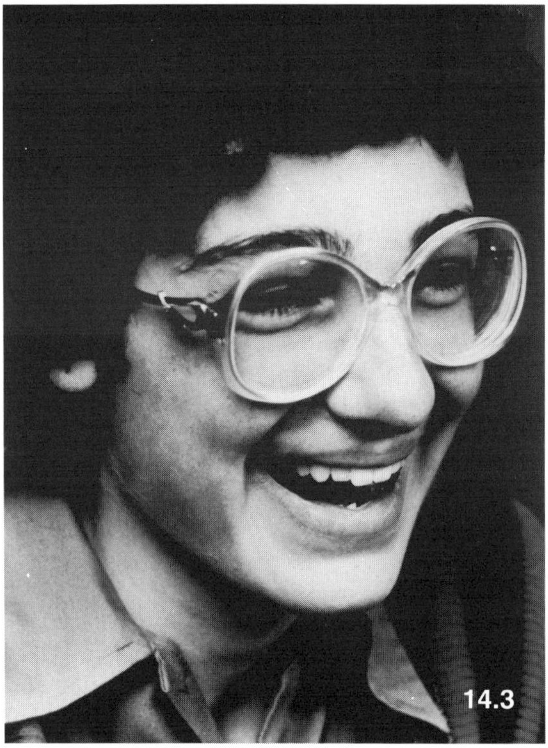
14.3

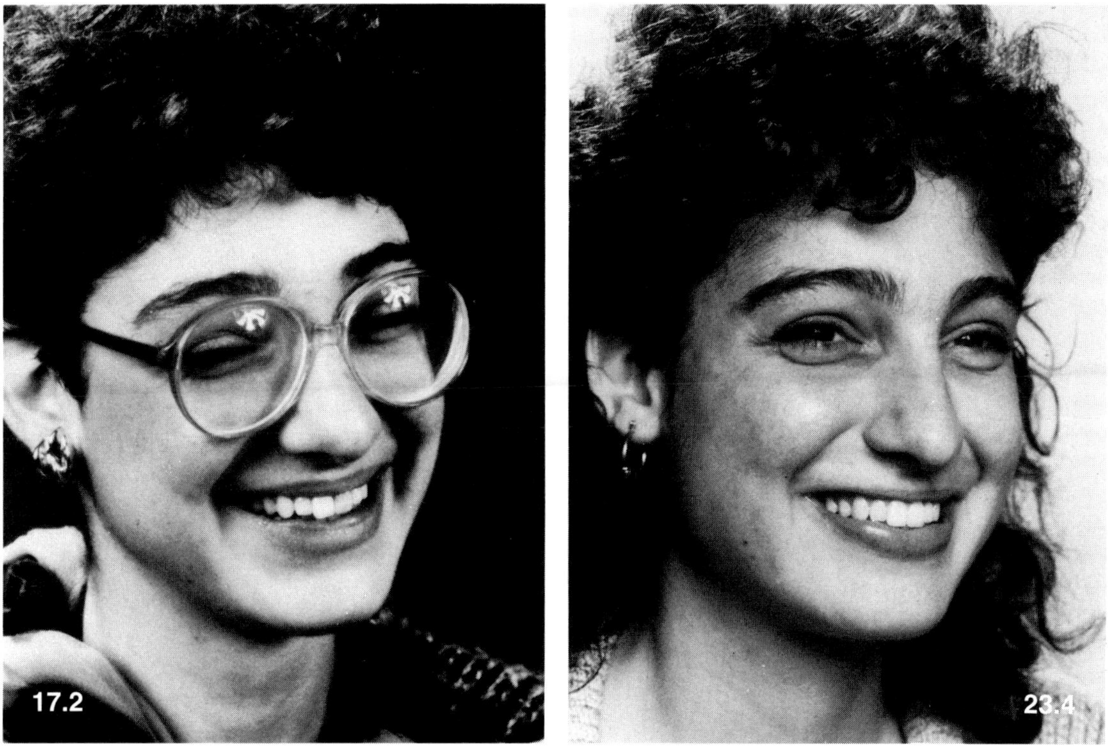

Fig 24.18 Note the improvements, in particular the elimination of the "high gum-line" when smiling.

complex had been restrained in its ventral development, the maxillary incisors intruded, and the mandible grew considerably, especially ventrally (Fig 24.17). Retention was not provided since a good interdigitation was achieved and the incisors were aligned well originally. Moreover, stomion now was at the correct height. In the years that followed, the distal side of the maxillary right central incisor moved again a little labially, and tertiary crowding developed in the mandibular incisors. The latter was not considered a problem (Figs. 24.11 to 24.16).
Superimposition of the tracings of the cephalometric radiographs show the effect of growth and treatment, particularly the incisor intrusion in the maxilla (Fig 24.17). The photographs of the smiling face illustrate the improvement in appearance and the lowering of the "high gum-line" (Fig 24.18), while in Figure 24.19, the position of stomion directly after treatment and eleven years later can be seen. The correct position of stomion is not only of importance in reducing the exposure of gum when smiling, but also as mentioned previously, to avoid the later development of an overlapping deep bite (coverbite), typical for class II/2 anomalies. This unfavorable development after treatment can occur when there is a combination of a short upper

A B C D

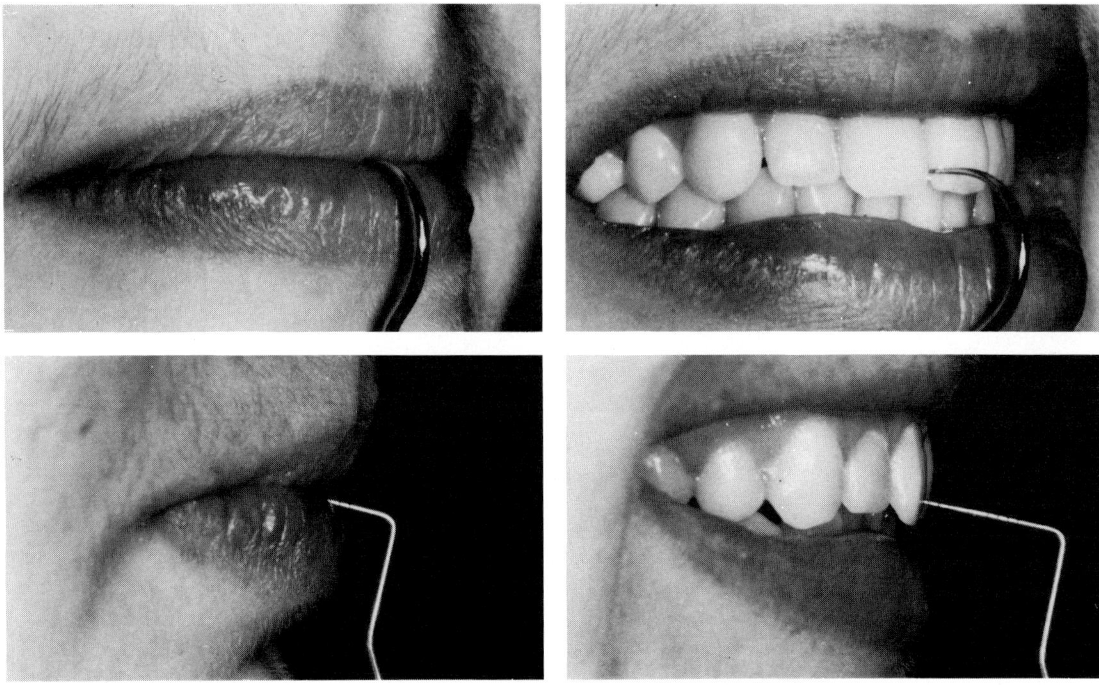

Fig 24-19 The maxillary incisors were so far intruded that a good position for stomion was obtained (A,B: after treatment; age 12 y, 1 mo) which remained subsequently (C,D: eleven years after treatment, age 23 y, 4 mo).

lip, competent lip seal, and excessive coverage of the maxillary incisors by the lower lip (see Chapter 35).

This treatment has been presented with the purpose of emphasizing that when prominent overerupted maxillary incisors are retracted, they must also be intruded. It is also to show the influence of interdigitation when spontaneous corrections are obstructed by appliances. The clasps of the Bass-plate impeded buccal movement of the first molars and first premolars, with the result that the adjustments due to the rail mechanism occurred not in the maxillary arch but in the mandible. The opposing mandibular teeth moved lingually while under normal conditions only the maxillary teeth change their positions. Once the obstructing appliances were eliminated, the maxillary teeth moved buccally together with their antagonists.
The use of a Bass-plate has several disadvantages. It brings about a sudden bite-opening, which is inconvenient for the patient. Furthermore, the occlusal contact between opposing teeth is eliminated for some time. In addition, transverse tooth movement is blocked as previously described. Nonetheless, the Bass-plate in combination with a parietal headgear is a worthwhile addition to the orthodontic armamentarium because it can secure intrusion of the maxillary incisors.

Chapter 25

Class II/1, open bite
Parietal headgear (full-time), brackets 12, 11, 21, and 22, positioner
Female 13 years, 2 months to 29 years, 1 month

A girl aged 13 years, 2 months attended with an increased lower-third facial height combined with a class II/1 anomaly and an anterior open bite. She had recently stopped sucking her thumb and although she kept her mouth open she could breathe freely through her nose. Her upper lip was short and passive; the slightly everted lower lip lay against the incisal edges of the maxillary incisors. The tip of her tongue rested on the mandibular incisors; those teeth also were everted and had spaces between them. There was a disto-occlusion on the right of ¾ PW, a little more on the left. An overjet of 8 mm and an overbite of 0 mm existed. A surplus of space was available in the dental arches (ALD of +3 mm in both) (Figs 25.1 and 25.2).

In view of the large lower face height and the anterior open bite, it was decided to apply a parietal headgear. Because the patient wished to avoid prolonged treatment and because all the permanent teeth had emerged except the third molars, and also because it was not expected that she would grow much more, it was proposed that the headgear should be worn at all times except during meals. At the beginning of treatment, a partial fixed appliance would be fitted to the maxillary arch to counter the possibility that the continuous wearing of the headgear would cause too much space to be created in that arch, and would tip the first permanent molars too far distally.

Two weeks after the first consultation, the maxillary first permanent molars were banded and a parietal headgear was fitted. Six weeks later, brackets were placed on the maxillary incisors and a .0175" twistflex arch tied into them. That archwire was replaced with a .019" × .026" archwire at the next visit. After eight months, treatment was concluded. The disto-occlusion had been over-corrected and the height of the lower face had increased little. In the central relationship, the incisal edges of the maxillary and mandibular incisors were in contact, the mandibular ones slightly ventral to the maxillary ones. Because of the action of the parietal headgear, the maxillary first permanent molars were in infra-position and infra-occlusion (Figs 25.3 and 25.4).

To obtain a better alignment of the teeth and to provide retention of the sagittal corrections, a positioner was used. For two months, the positioner was worn four hours during the day as well as during the entire night. For the following two months, it was worn only during sleep. After that, the maxillary incisors were less steeply inclined, the reversed sagittal overbite had gone, and the occlusion was

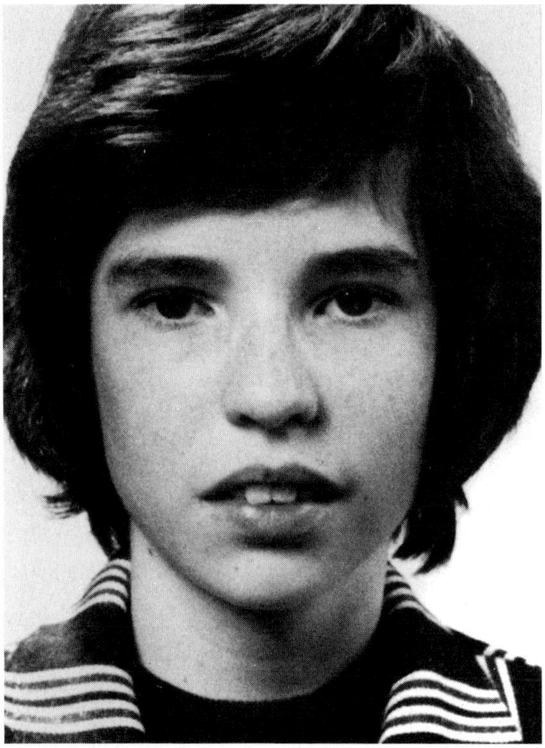
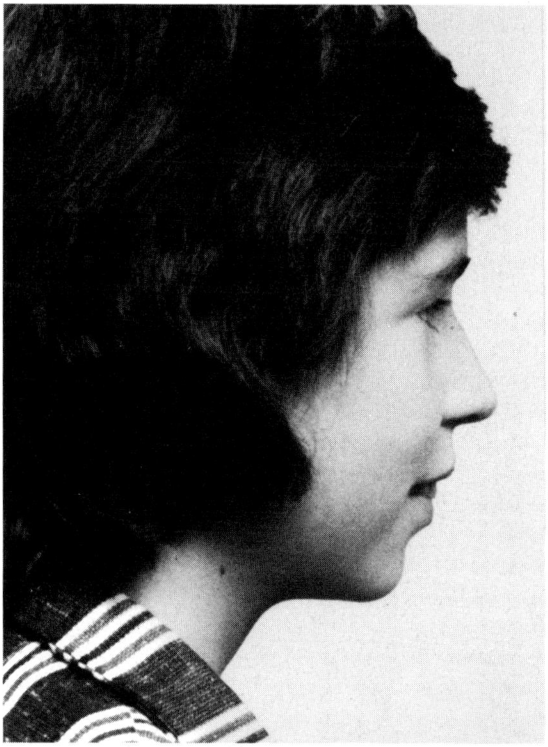
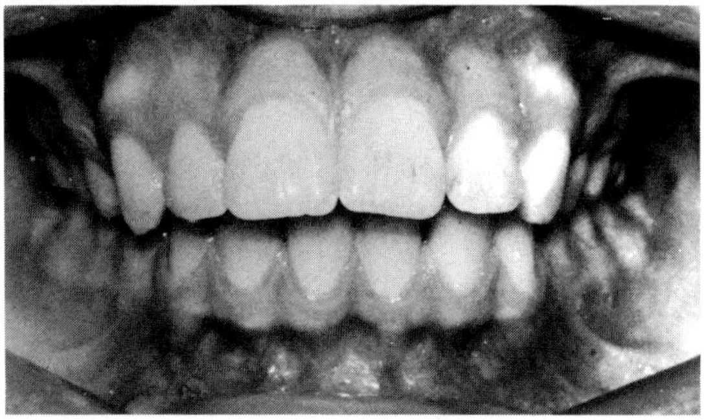
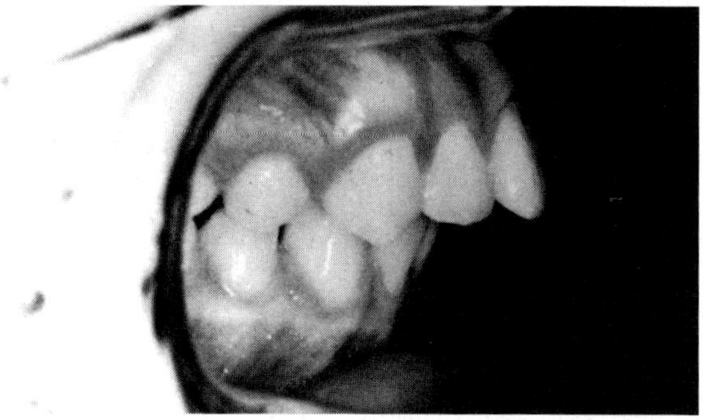
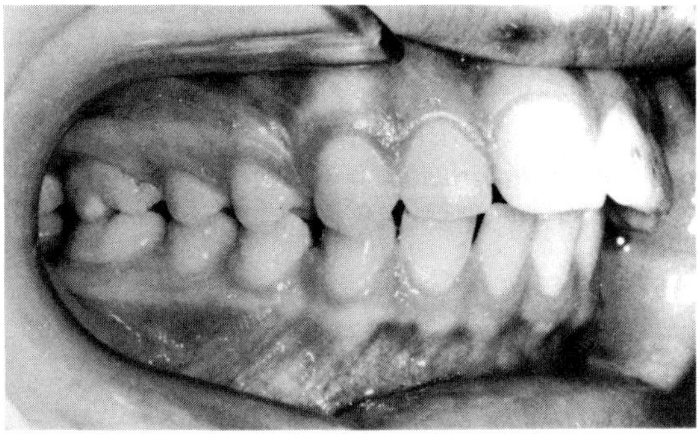
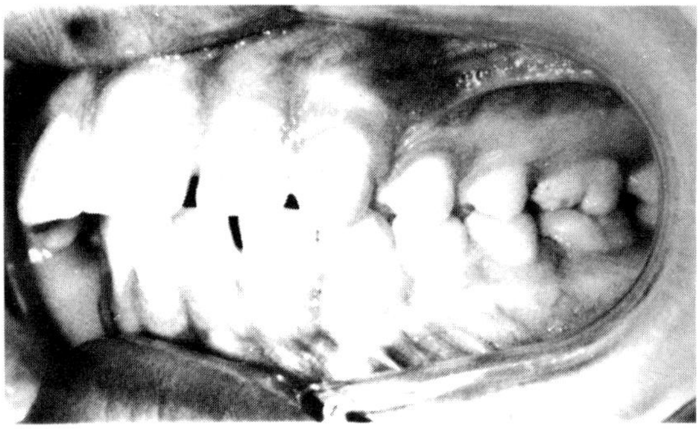

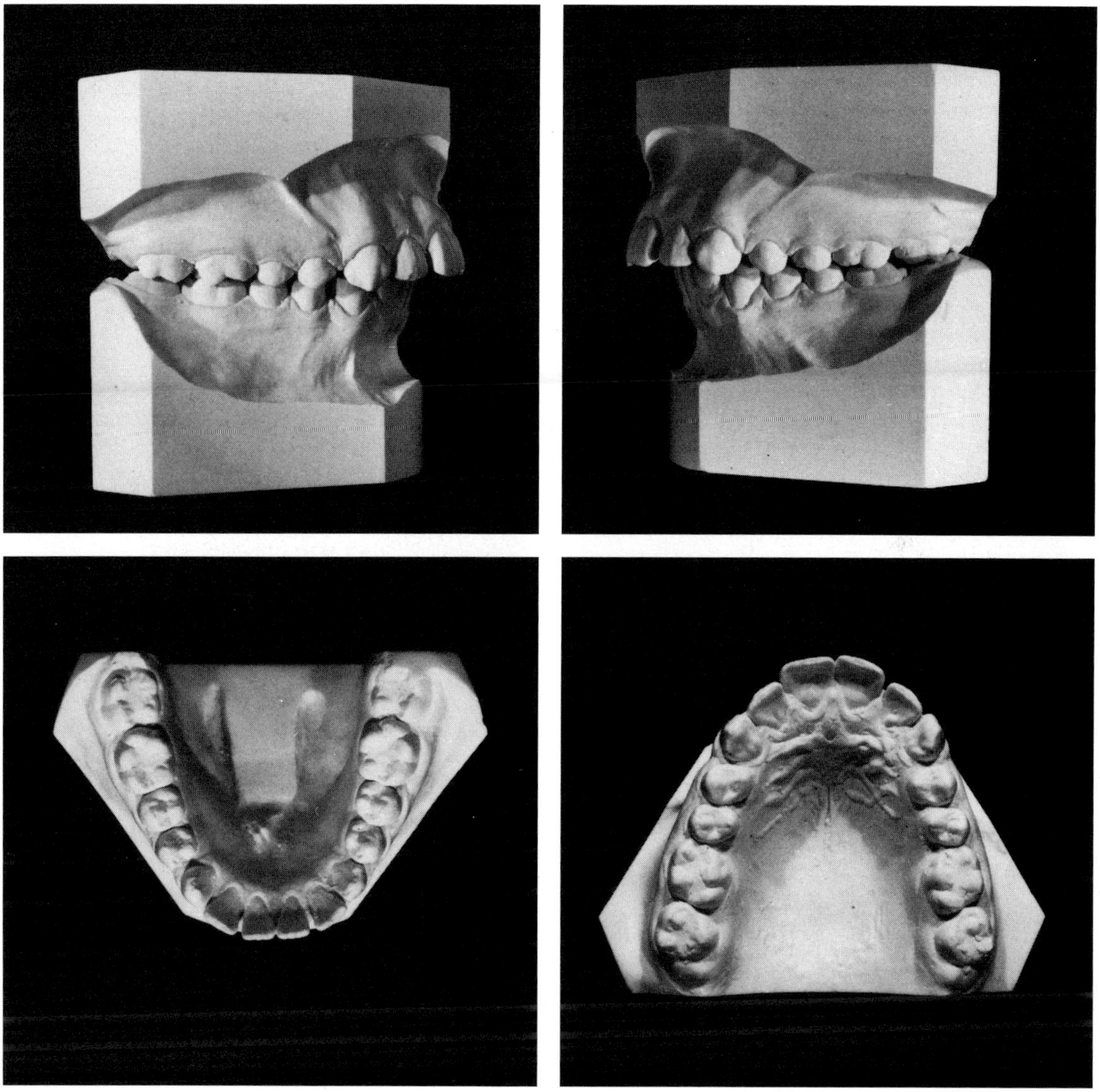

Figs 25-1 and 25-2 *A girl of 13 y, 2 mo with a class II/1 anomaly, a disto-occlusion of ¾ PW on the right and almost 1 PW on the left, an anterior open bite (she had sucked her thumb until recently) and a relatively receding mandible. Both dental arches are well-formed, exhibiting a solid interdigitation of the posterior teeth and eversion of the incisors with slight anterior diastemata. The incisors in both jaws do not overlap vertically; their incisal edges are at the same heights.*

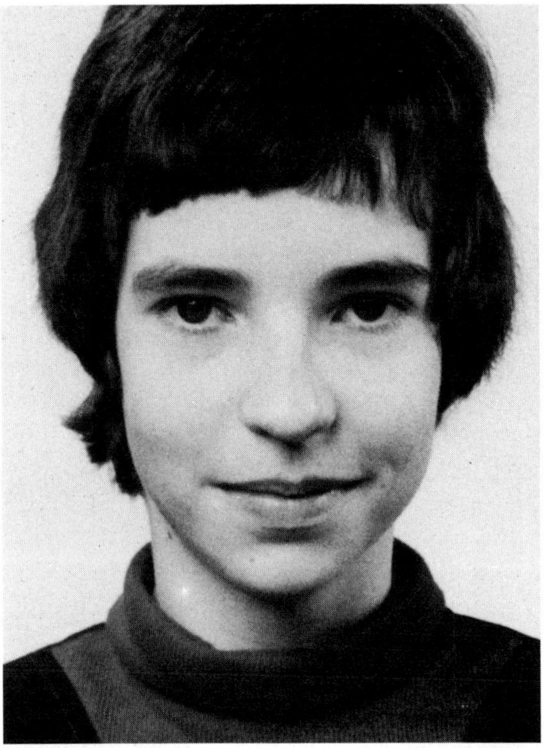
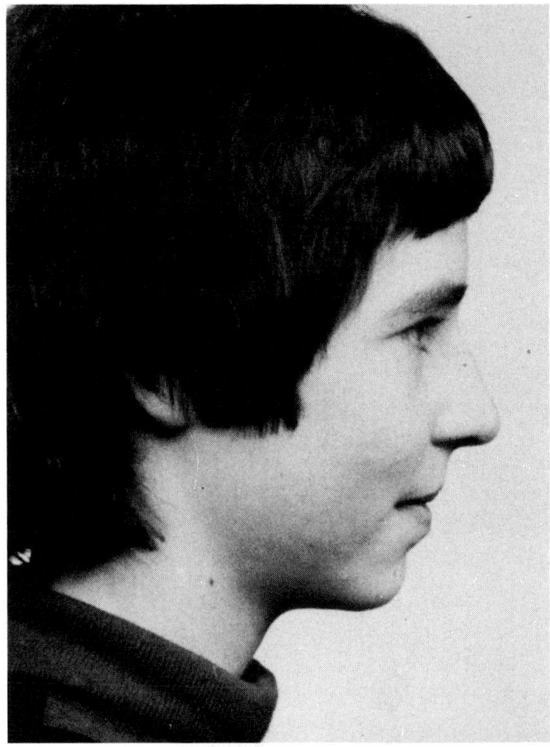
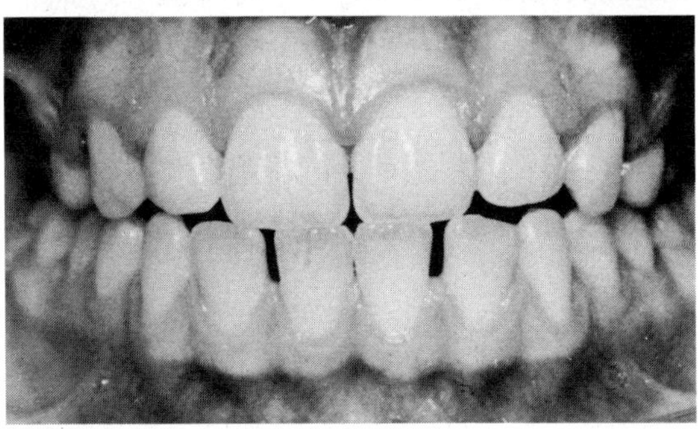
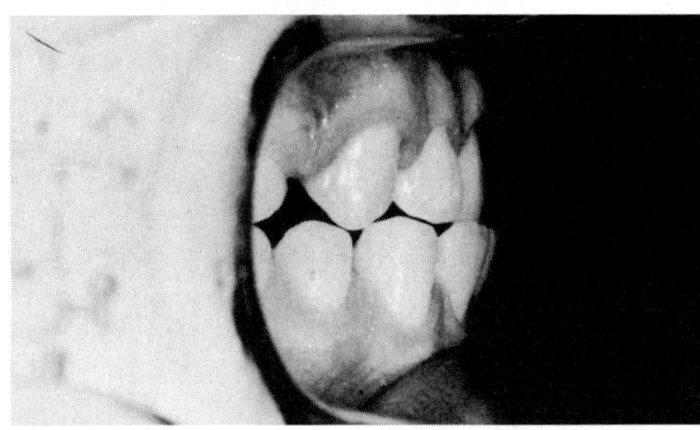
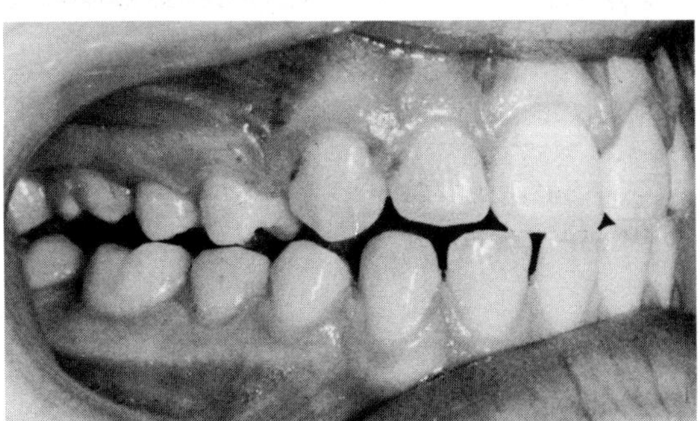
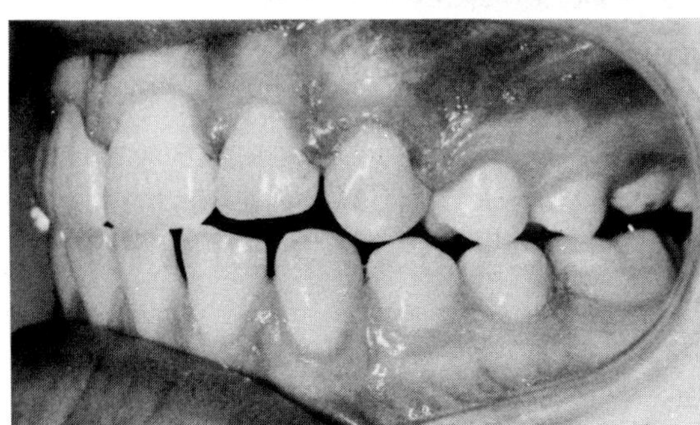

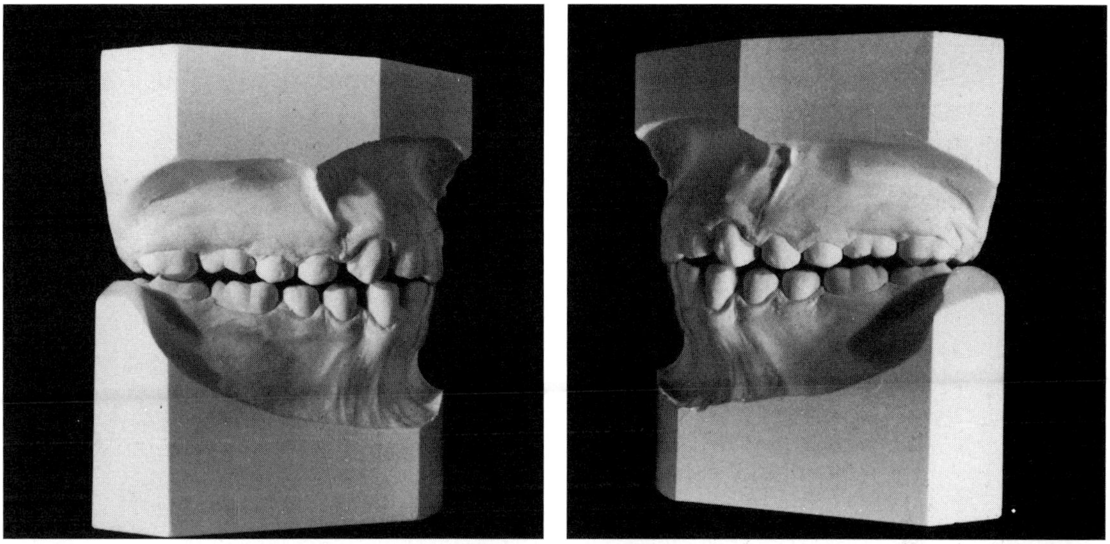

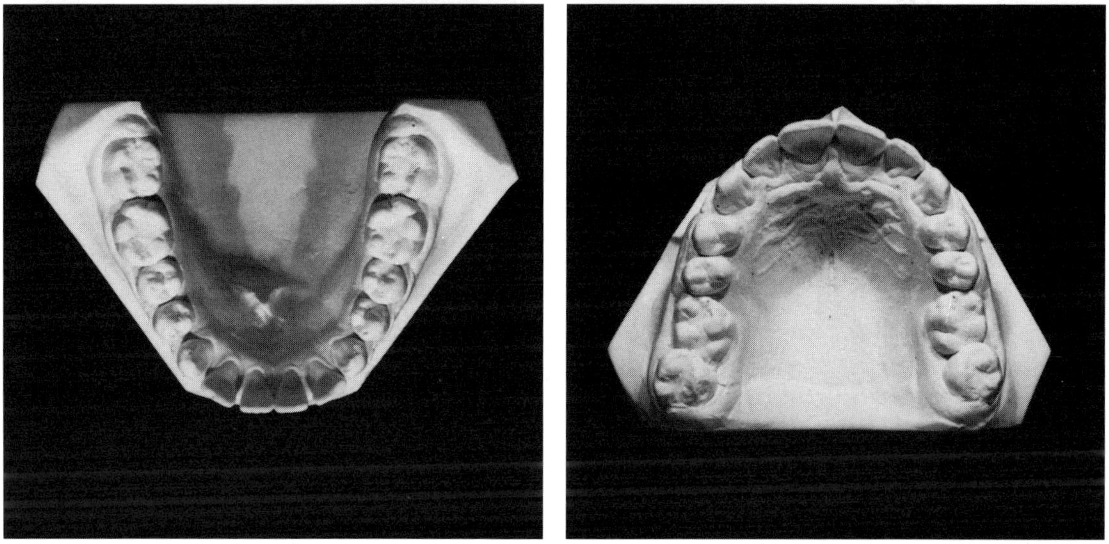

Figs 25-3 and 25-4 *At the age of 13 y, 10 mo, after eight months of treatment, the disto-occlusion had been overcorrected. The incisal edges of the incisors are located directly opposite each other in central relation (in the intraoral photograph taken from the side the patient is holding her jaw too far to ventral). The maxillary first permanent molars are in infra-position and infra-occlusion and are too far palatally. The dental arches show no abnormalities except for the diastemata between the mandibular incisors. Because of the overcorrection of the disto-occlusion, the arches do not fit together well. In addition, the maxillary incisors are a little too steeply inclined.*

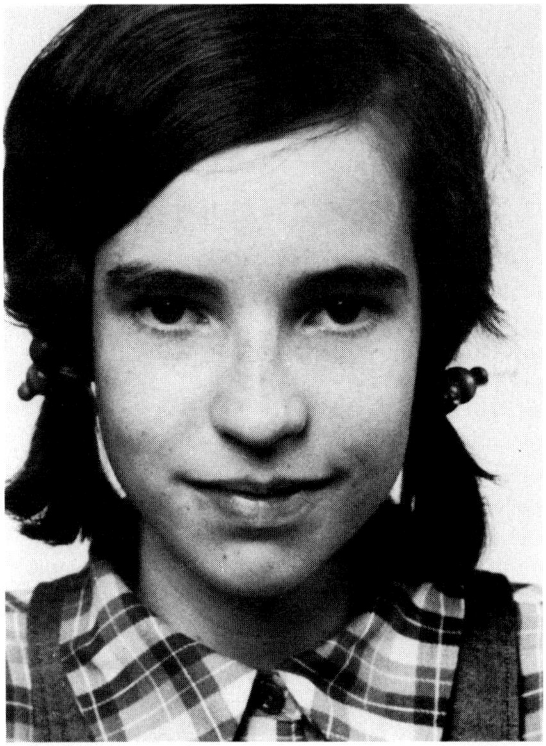

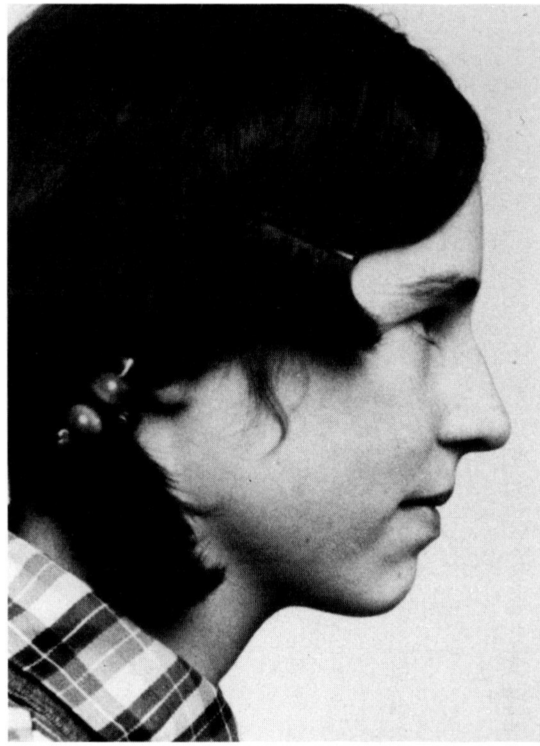

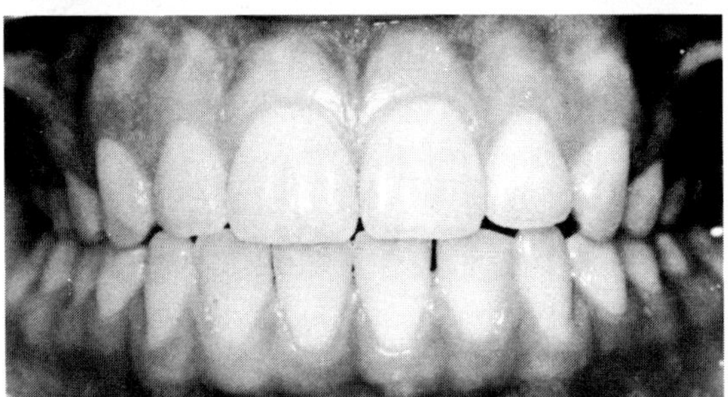

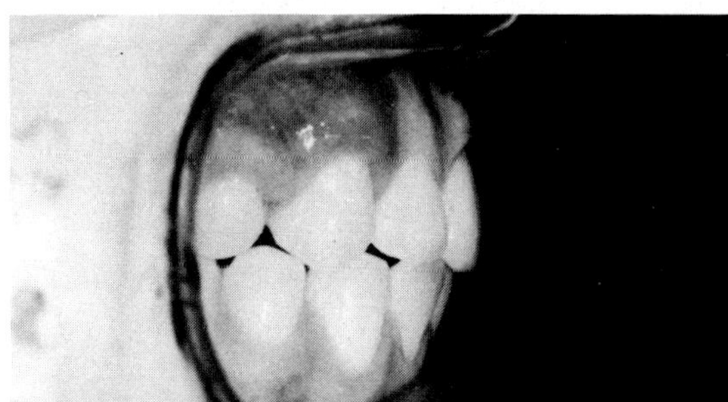

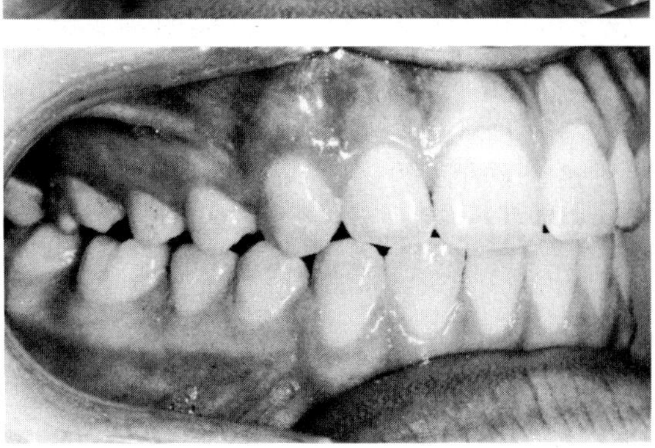

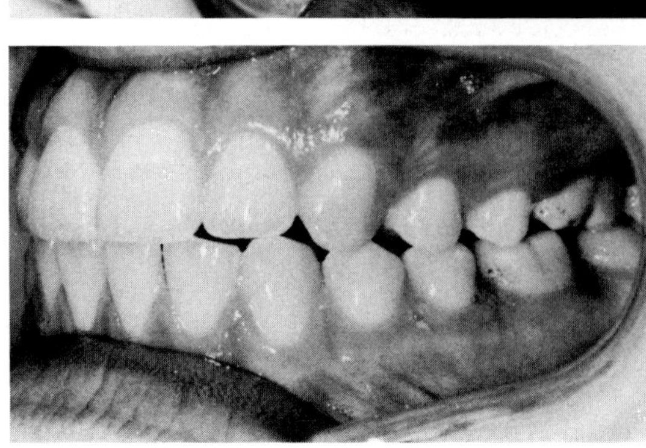

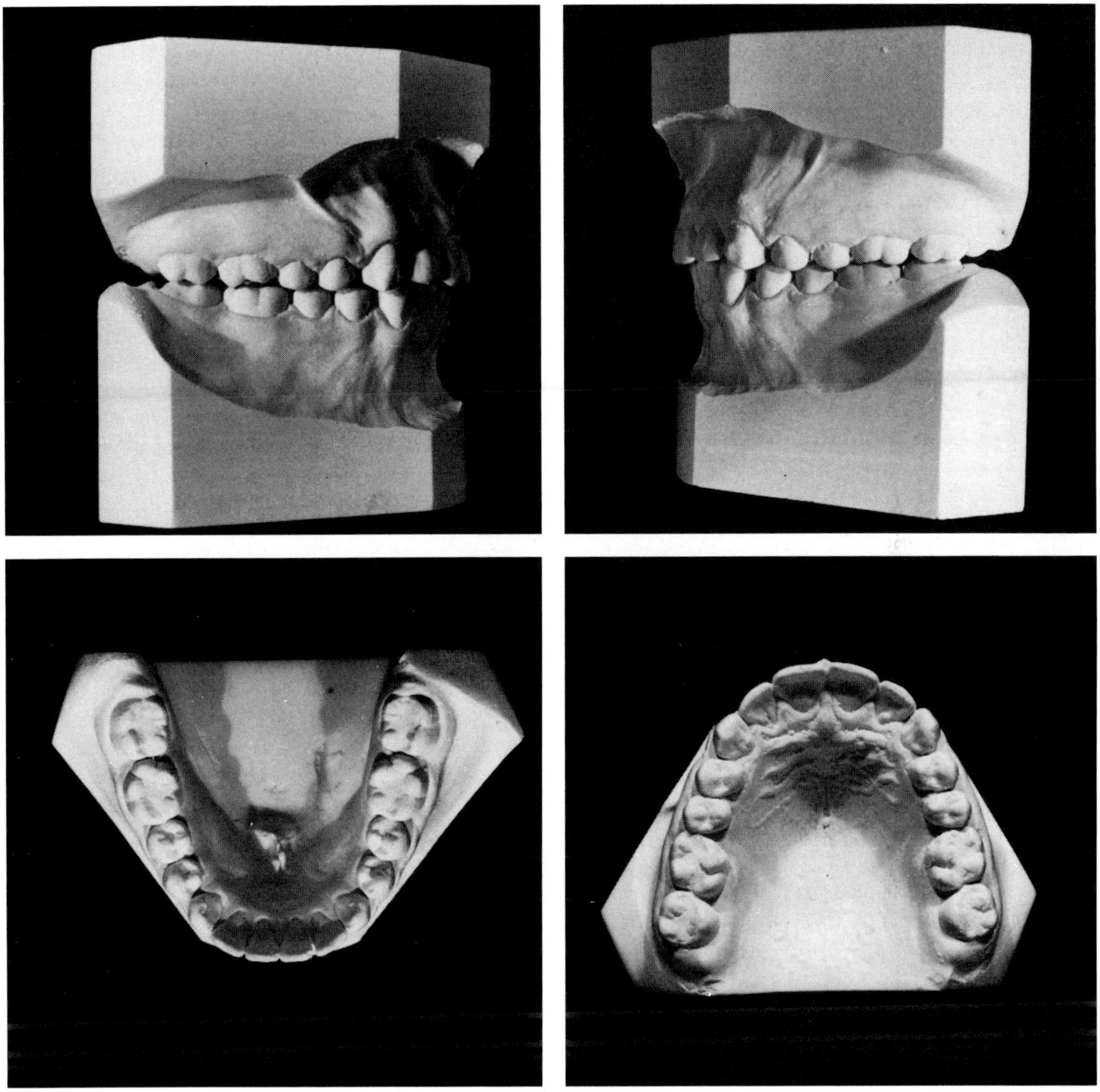

Figs 25-5 and 25-6 *At the age of 14 y, 4 mo, the occlusion has been improved after wearing a positioner for six months. The first permanent molars are in their correct positions and make vertical contact. The maxillary incisors are less steep and there is a slight overjet and overbite.*

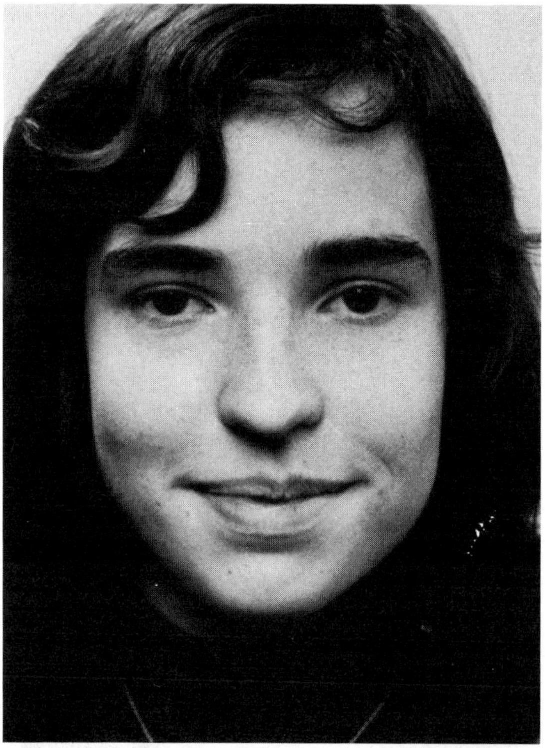

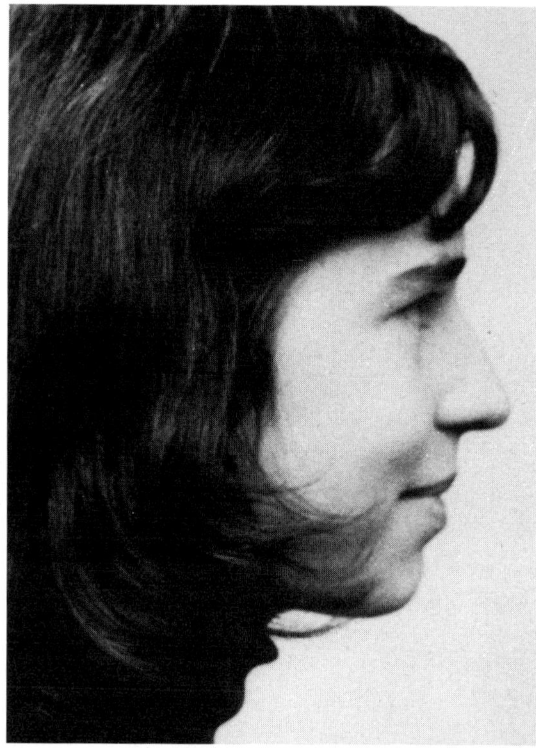

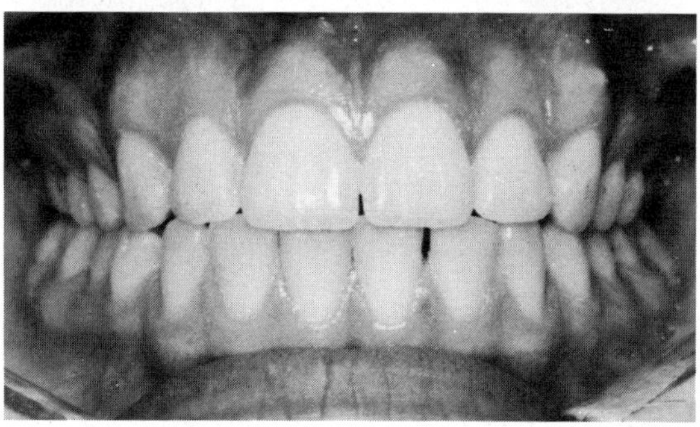

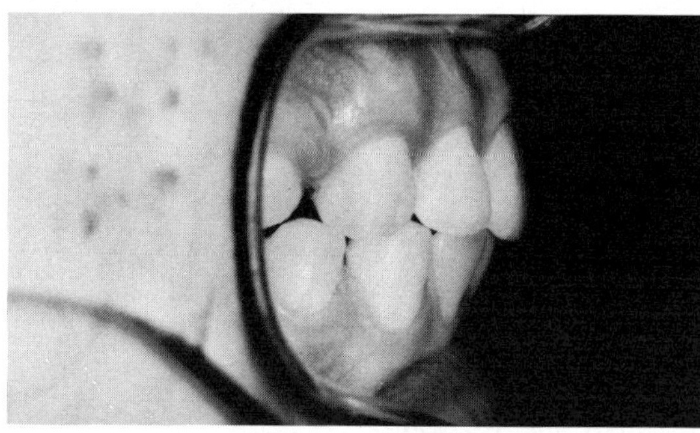

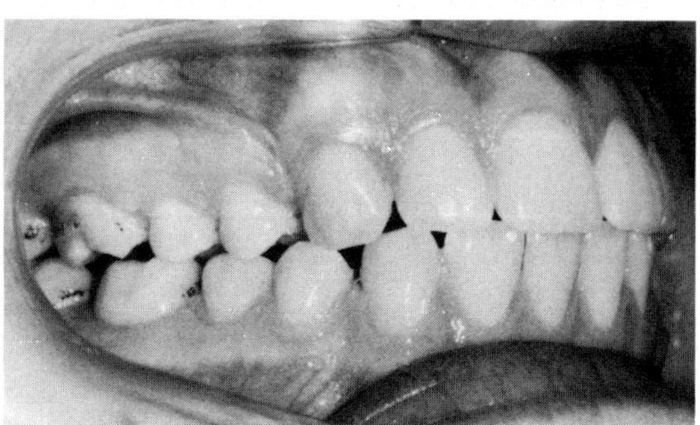

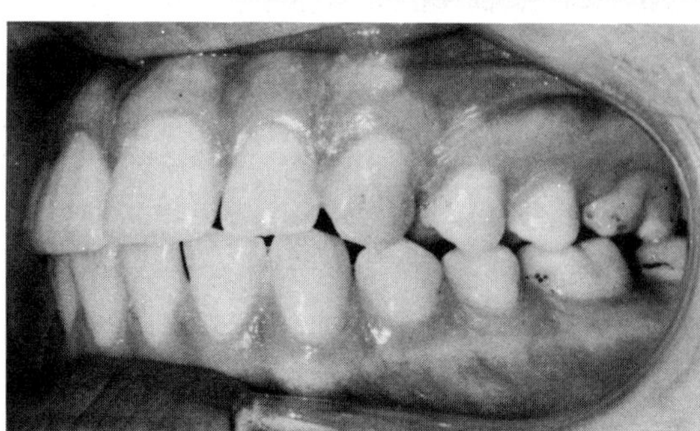

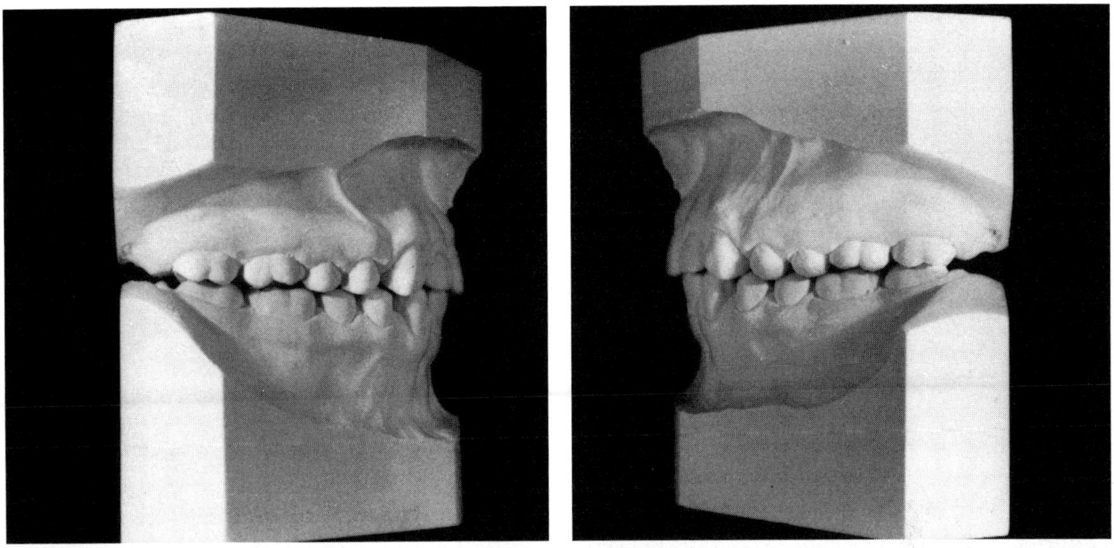

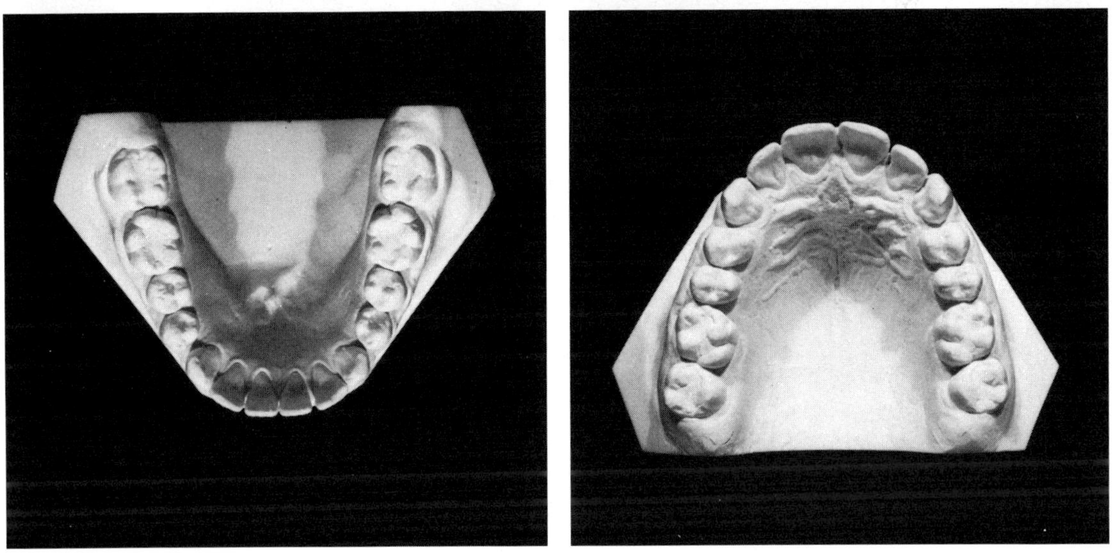

Figs 25-7 and 25-8 *At the age of 16 y, 6 mo, the occlusion has settled in further with a very minor disto-occlusion of the molars on the right. This corresponds with the slight displacement of the midlines of the dental arches relative to one another.*

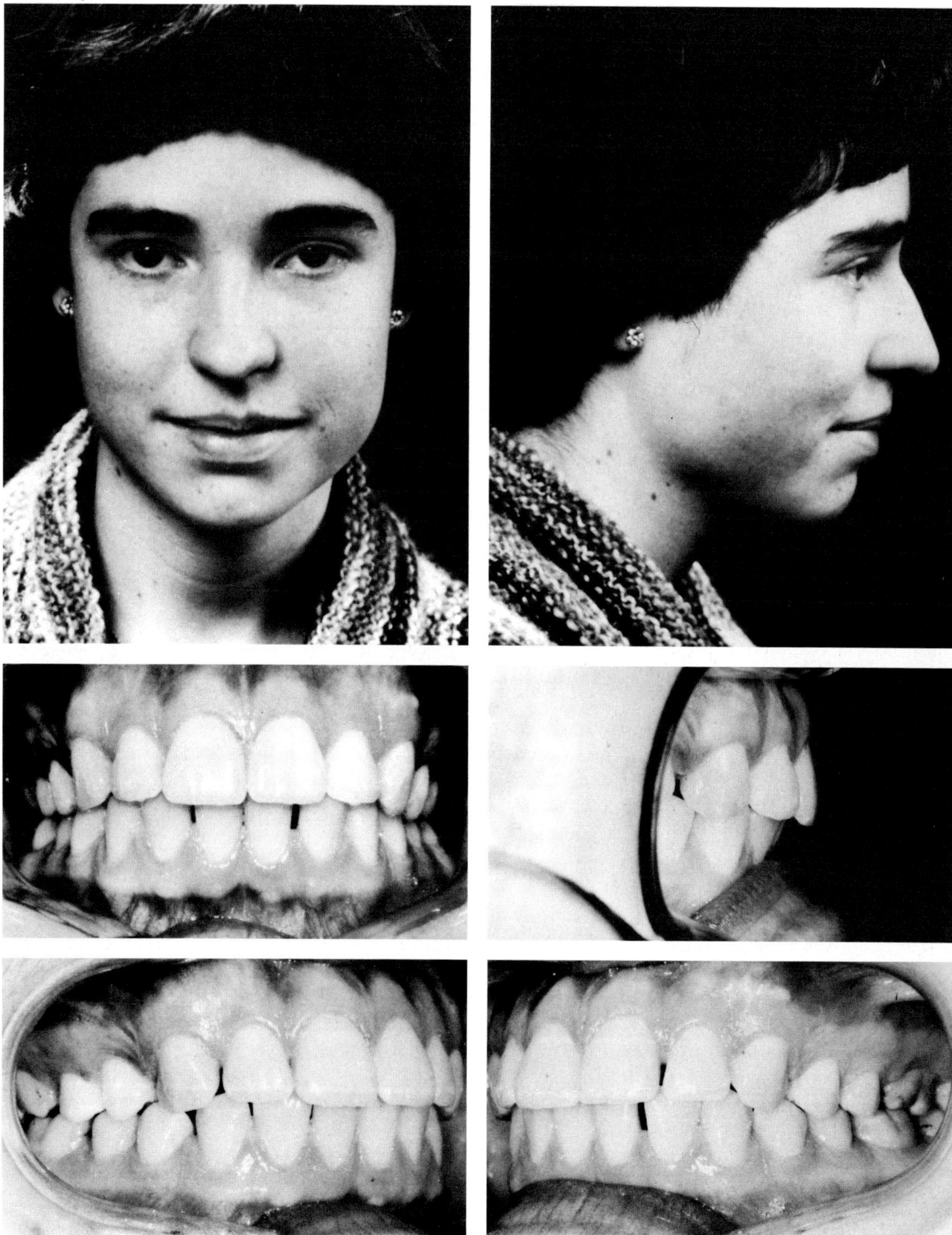

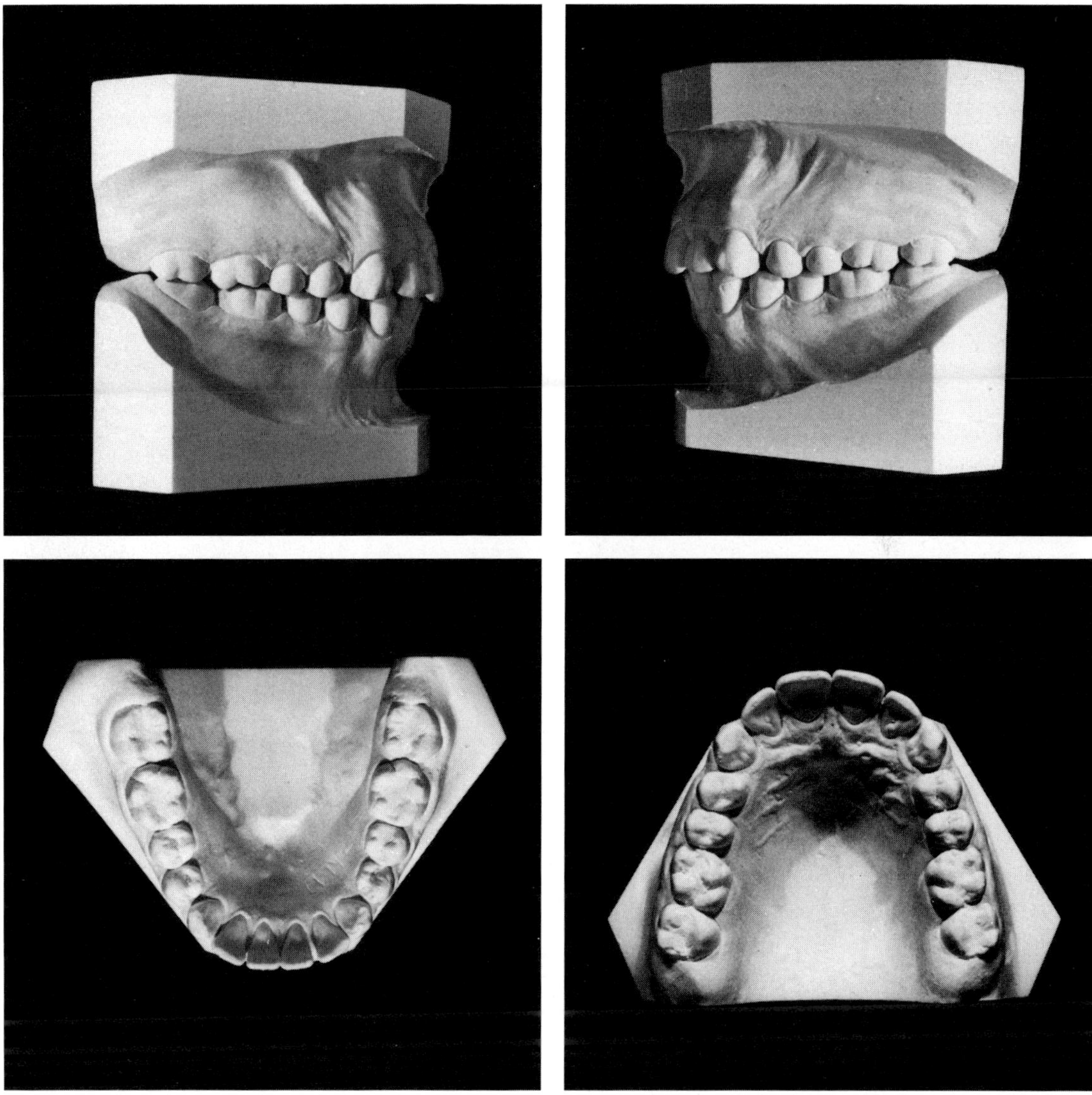

Figs 25-9 and 25-10 *At the age of 19 y, 6 mo, five years after treatment, an esthetically and functionally excellent dentition with solid interdigitation exists and fits well in a harmonious face.*

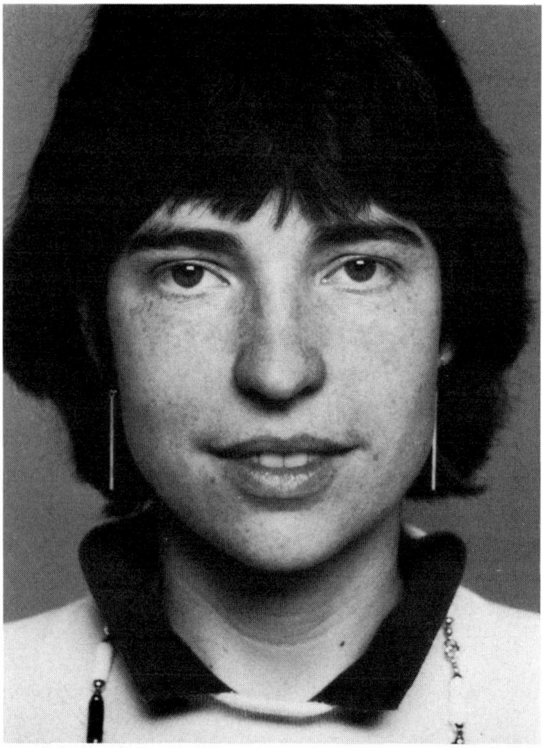
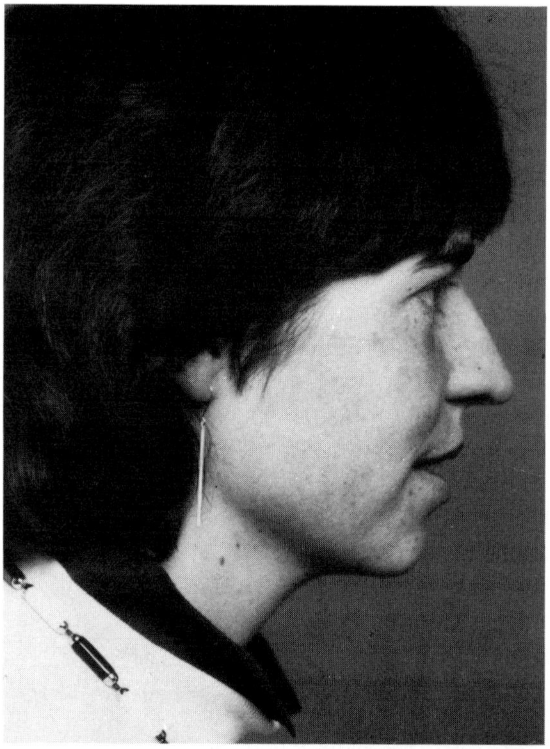
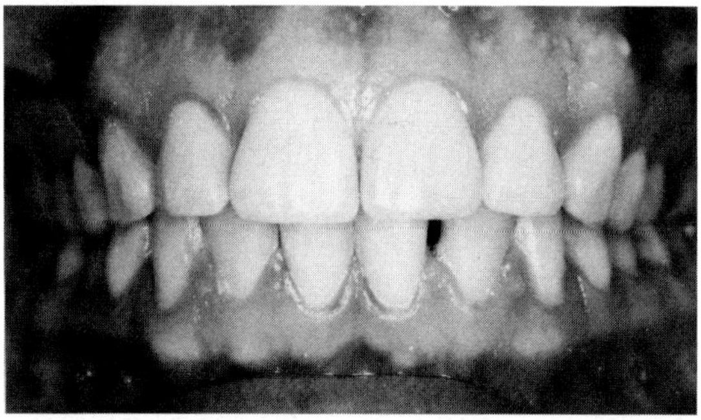
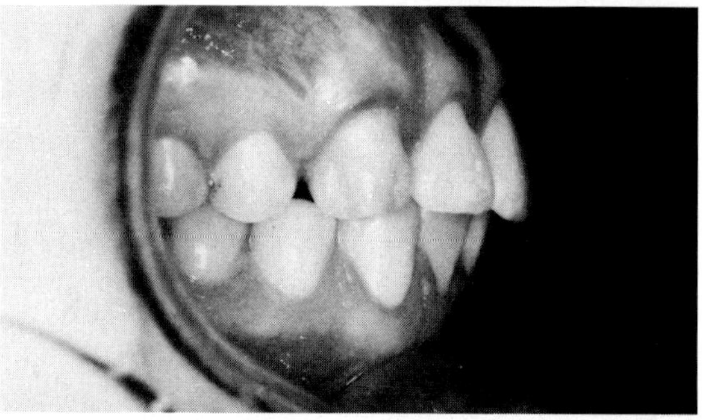
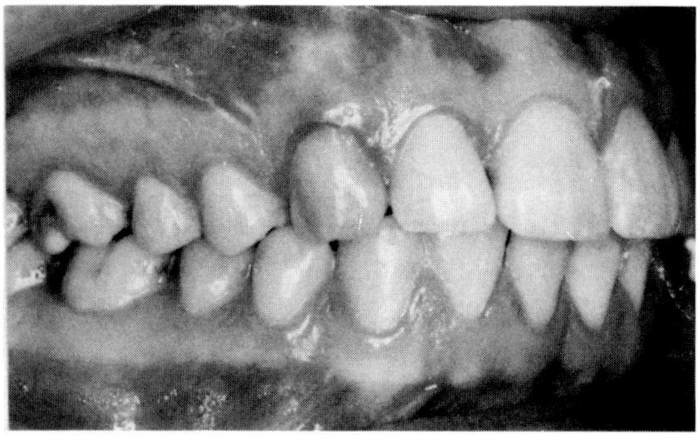
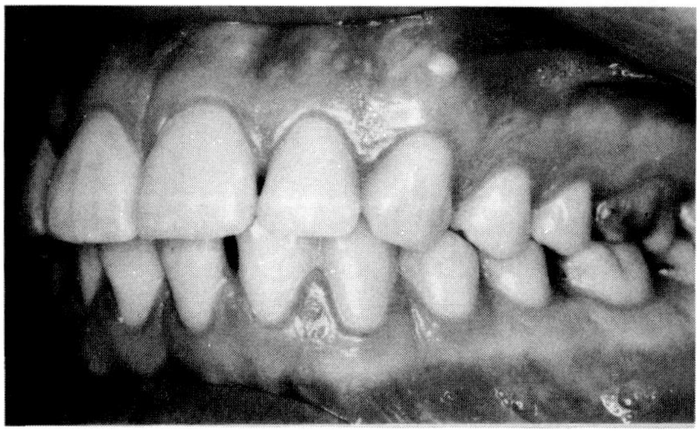

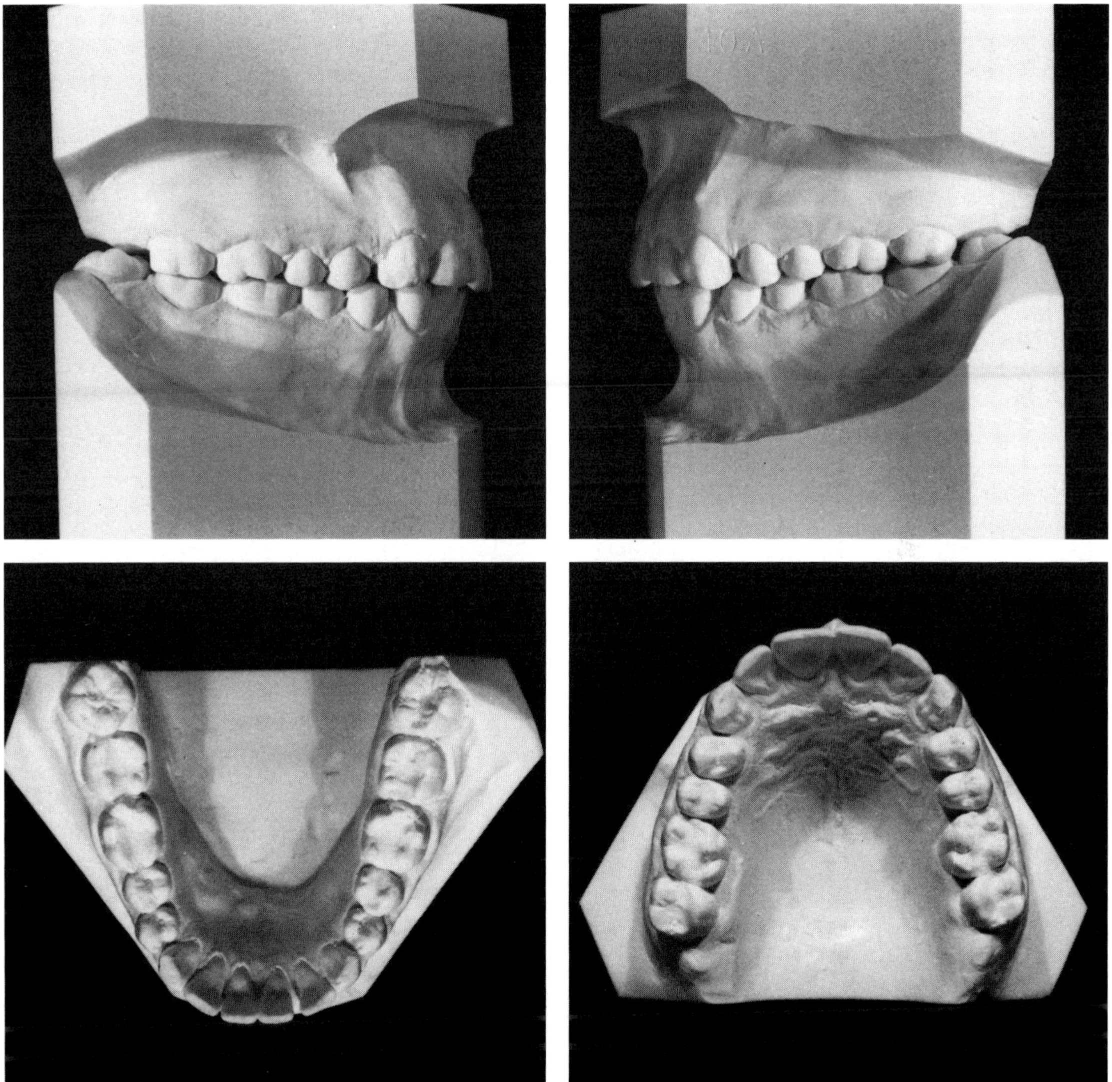

Figs 25-11 and 25-12 *At the age of 29 y, 1 mo the only teeth that are positioned abnormally are the mandibular third molars, which have emerged in the interim. It was advised that they be extracted, especially since the maxillary third molars had already been removed on emerging. The diastema between the two mandibular left incisors was not considered objectionable.*

Figure 25-13a

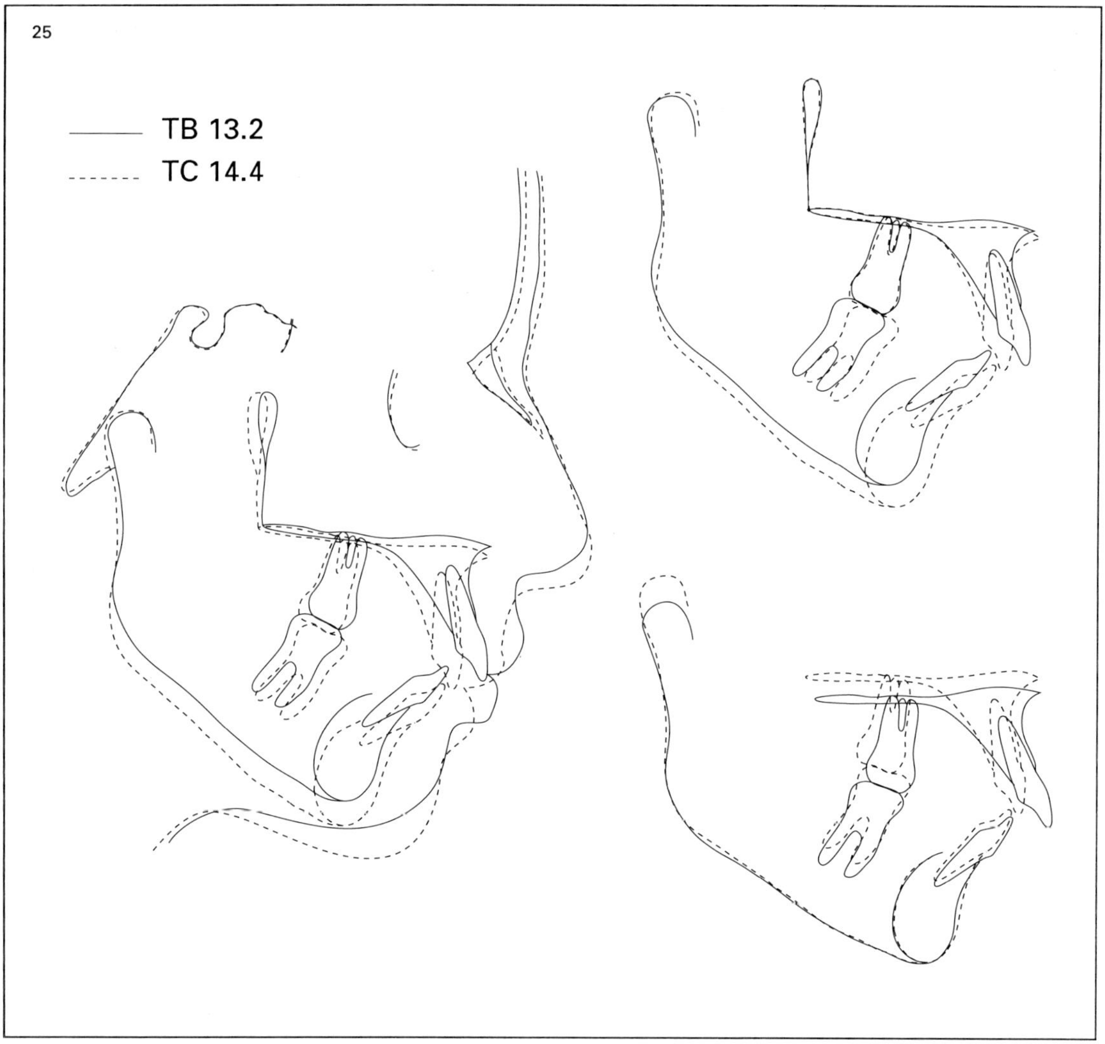

Fig 25-13 The tracings of lateral cephalometric radiographs show that no ventral development occurred in the maxilla during treatment, while the maxillary incisors were significantly retruded. The lower-face height increased only slightly and the slope of the lower border of the mandible had not steepened. The maxillary first permanent molars have moved very little occlusally. The direction of growth of the mandible was normal, and not excessively to caudal. This tendency in development had continued after the end of treatment.

Figure 25-13b

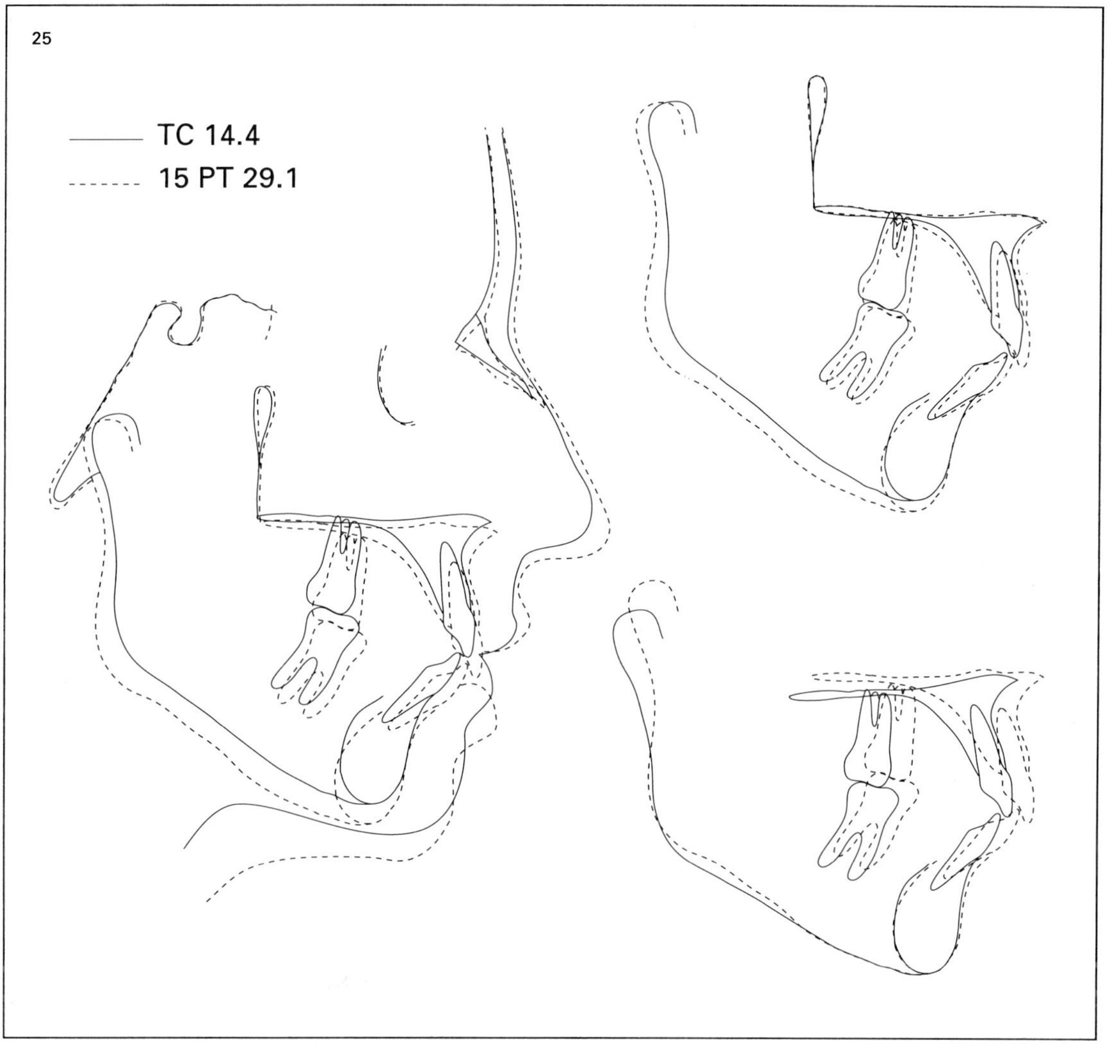

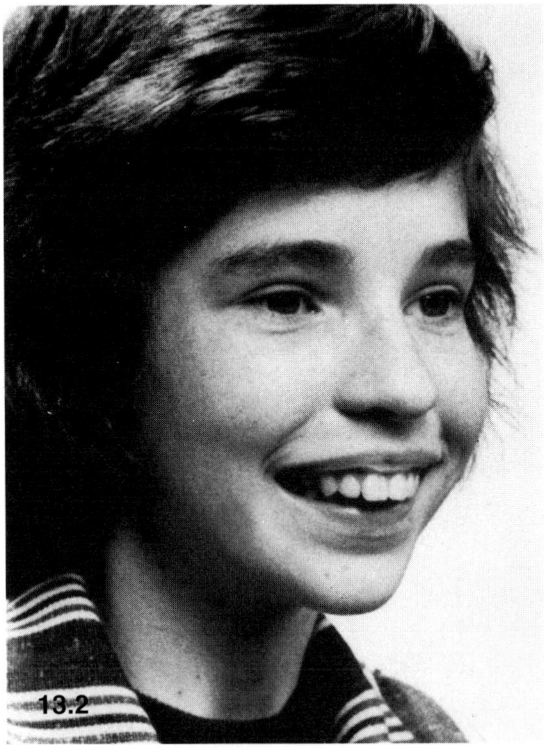
13.2

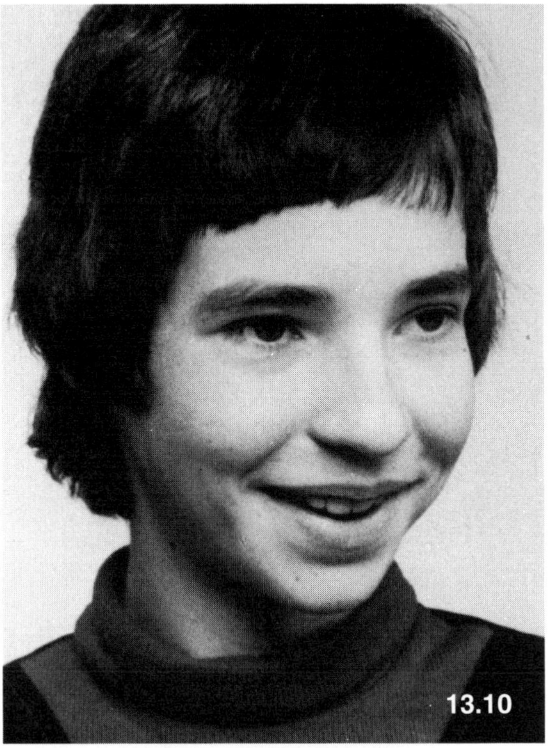
13.10

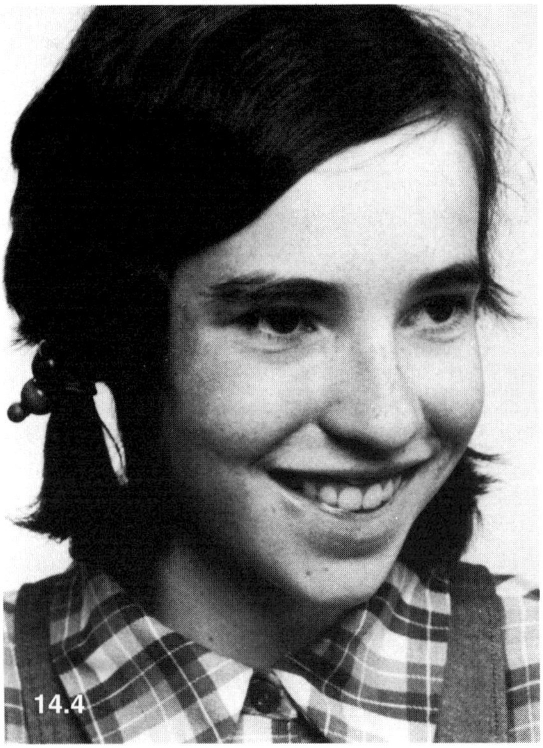
14.4

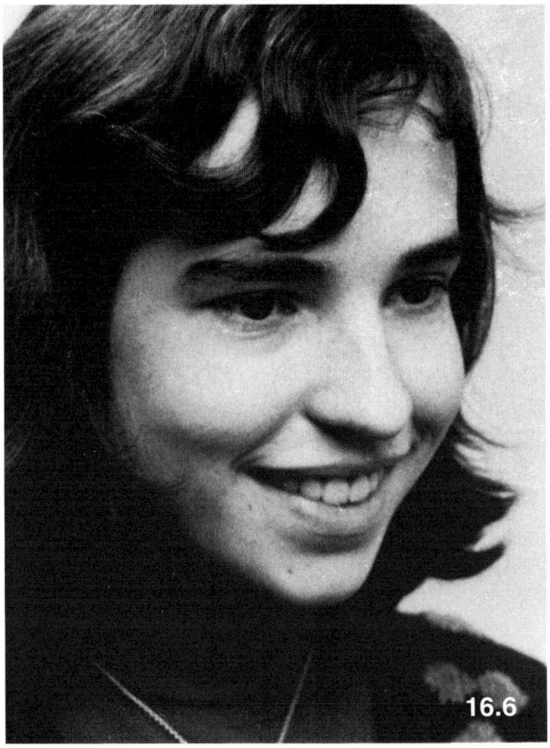
16.6

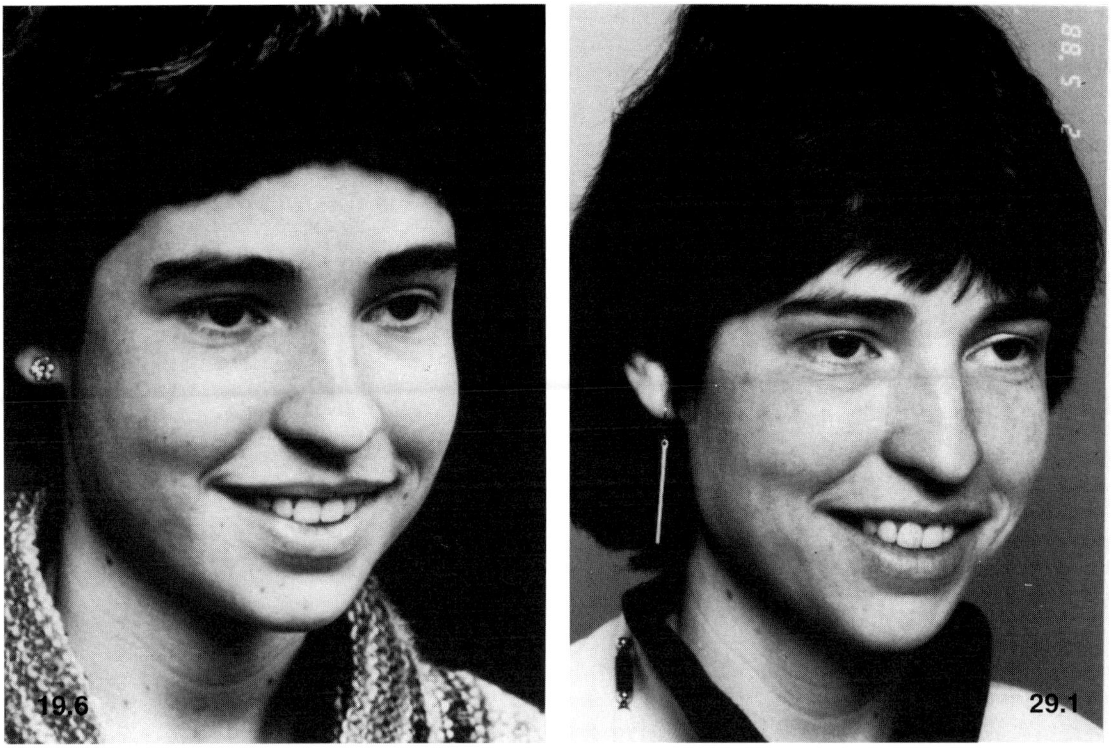

Fig 25-14 Note the changes that have become evident during and after treatment.

substantially improved (Figs 25.5 and 25.6). Two years later, a neutro-occlusion with solid interdigitation had been established and the incisor contact had again improved (Figs 25.7 and 25.8). Five years after treatment, there was a harmonious face and an almost ideal occlusion was present (Figs 25.9 and 25.10). Ten years later at almost 30 years of age, the same situation existed (Figs 25.11 and 25.12).
The superimpositions of the tracings of the cephalometric radiographs show that during treatment the maxilla did not develop ventrally, the maxillary first permanent molars did not move occlusally, and the maxillary incisors had been retruded. The improvement had been provided largely by the relatively marked growth of the mandible in a short time, which occurred in a favorable direction. In the two years following treatment, the face still developed significantly, while the lower face only added very little to its height (Fig 25.13). The photographs of the smiling face show the changes that can be attributed to growth, treatment, and maturity (Fig. 25.14).

It was not clear to what degree the anterior open bite depended on the tongue posture, or alternatively the thumb-sucking that was indulged in until shortly before treatment began. The relatively large lower face height and the eversion of the mandibular incisors with diastemata justified the supposition that the interposition of the tongue was not the consequence of the distortion due to the thumb-sucking, but was an independent phenomenon in its own right that was unlikely to diminish. On the basis of this supposition, the parietal headgear was chosen in preference to a cervical headgear, which would have encouraged an increase in the lower-face height due its tendency to extrude the anchor molars. Considering the reaction to the treatment and the facts that the open bite did not relapse and the height of the face did not increase much following treatment, it seems that the original supposition was unwarranted. It is more likely that the tongue interposition was a secondary change in function to adapt to the open bite caused by the thumb-sucking.

In hindsight, it would appear that the patient could have been treated as effectively or even better with a cervical headgear, which would not have disturbed the occlusion of the first permanent molars. Cases in which the anterior tongue interposition is primary, and above all in which there is impeded nasal breathing and an open mouth, react differently to treatment and growth than did this case. Also, even if a parietal headgear is used, a marked increase in lower-face height can stil occur after treatment. Moreover, following treatment, maxillary incisors that have been retracted return labially if the lips are not held closed (see Chapter 26).

The continuous wearing of extraoral and functional appliances has the advantage that results are obtained more quickly, possibly due in part to more dental than skeletal changes being achieved. Against this is the fact that part of the result obtained subsequently will be lost. Probably the point at which relapse takes place — the boundaries of the biologically acceptable equilibrium — is not transgressed if a facial orthopedic appliance is only worn 14 hours a day. In the ten hours remaining each day a return within the boundaries of biologic acceptable equilibrium is assumed to take place, which cannot occur while the appliance is being worn continuously. When the continuous wearing of the appliance is terminated, a considerable return toward the original position will occur, rather than no or only a minor return following the termination of the use of an intermittently worn facial orthopedic appliance. Observation of patients who have worn their headgear more or less continuously supports this idea. Even where a solid interdigitation had developed, partial relapse of disto-occlusion was seen. That held also for patients whose disto-occlusion had been corrected with class II elastics. If in such cases the disto-occlusion had not been overcorrected to the extent that a slight reversed overbite had been reached, a partial relapse of the disto-occlusion would be seen subsequently.

From the previous considerations it would appear that it does not make much sense to wear a headgear more or less continuously, since in the end the disto-occlusion must be overcorrected to such a degree that the dental arches no longer match well. Little is gained except a relatively short time under active treatment, an aspect that had merit in this case due to her age and the advanced developmental stage she had reached. However, it would have been better if her treatment could have begun at an earlier age and thus made it possible not to wear the facial-orthopedic appliance continuously.

Chapter 26

Class II/1, anterior open bite
Parietal headgear, maxillary removable plate
Male 11 years, 7 months to 21 years 7 months

A boy aged 11 years, 7 months exhibited a class II/1 anomaly and anterior open bite. He had a long, narrow face, a small nose, an increased lower-face height with a retruded chin, and a steeply inclined lower mandibular border. When relaxed, his mouth was open and his tongue lay between the maxillary and mandibular incisors. He had sucked his thumb until he was nine years old. His short upper lip was almost functionless, while the lower lip was everted and had no contact with the maxillary incisors. Despite a clear nasal airway, he breathed through his mouth most of the time (Figs 26.1 and 26.2).

Taking into account the excessive lower-face height and the inadequate lip seal, it was decided to correct the disto-occlusion with a parietal headgear. At a later stage a removable plate would be used in the maxilla to move the premolars and canines distally and to retract the maxillary incisors.

At the age of 12 years, 8 months, the headgear was fitted, and within a short time an obvious improvement was secured. Eight months later, the maxillary second deciduous molars were superseded by the premolars. There and elsewhere in the dental arch was spacing. At that juncture a plate was provided (see Figure 7.12, page 112). It was used first to move distally the premolars and subsequently the canines; finally, the incisors were retracted and the anterior spaces closed. At the age of 13 years, 1 month, after a treatment time of one year and five months, a satisfactory result had been obtained and all appliances were removed. No retention was used. A good occlusion and solid interdigitation of the posterior teeth were realized, and the maxillary anterior teeth were almost in contact with the mandibular ones. The perioral musculature had changed little; the mouth still remained open, the upper lip was scarcely used and mouth-breathing persisted (Figs 26.3 and 26.4).

Four months after the conclusion of treatment, the maxillary incisors had moved a little to labial and the anterior diastemata had returned. He was advised to do lip exercises with a wooden spatula, and to try to keep his mouth closed as much as possible. Moreover, it was recommended that he applied sticking plaster at night to hold his mouth closed. By the next check-up eight months later, the maxillary anteriors were found to have moved more to labial. The patient said that he was afraid of suffocating if plaster was put over his mouth and he could not get around to doing lip exercises.

Approximately 2½ years later the patient was seen again. The neutro-occlusion with

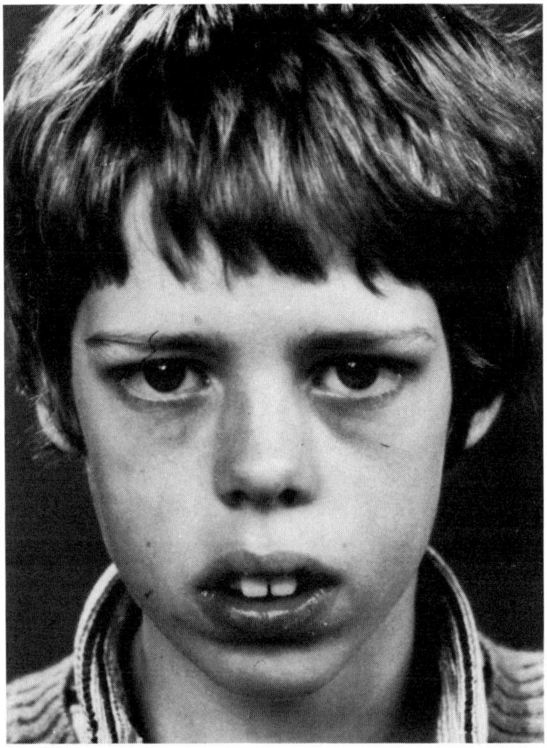
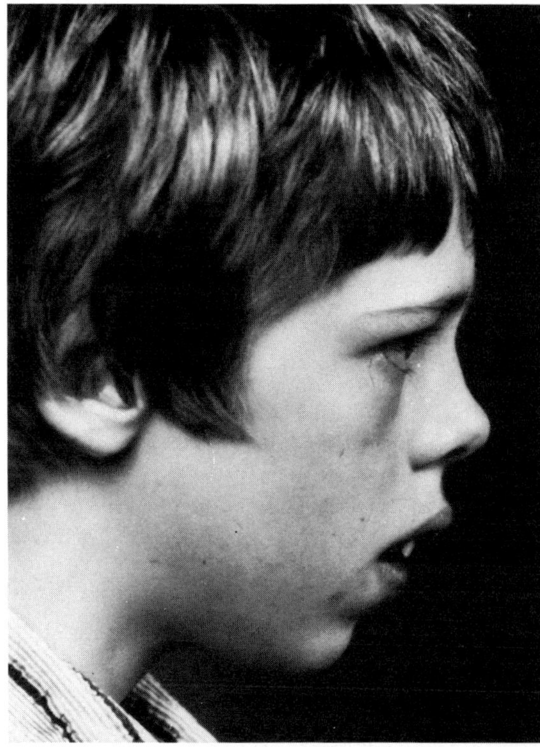
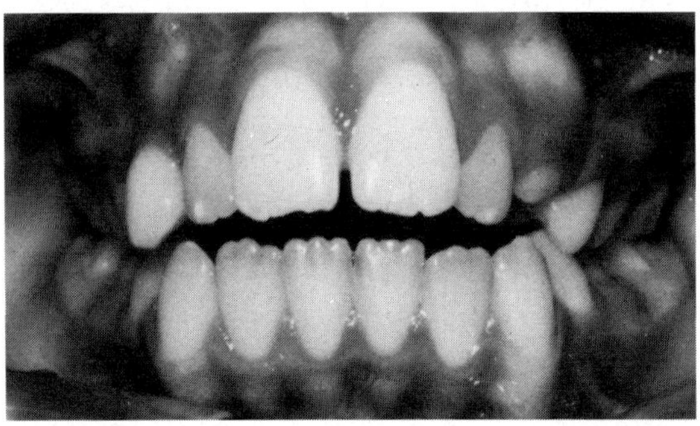
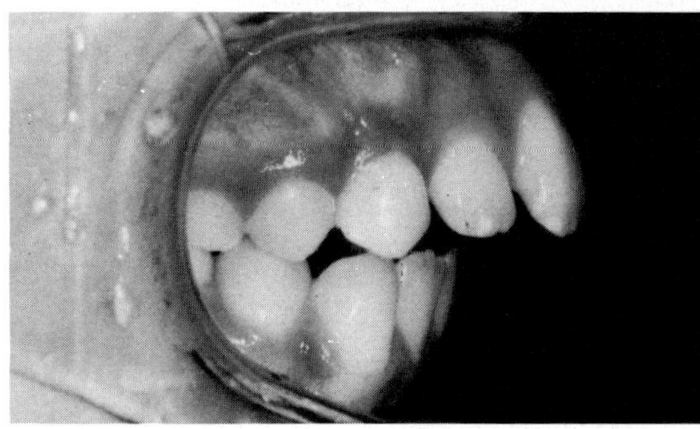
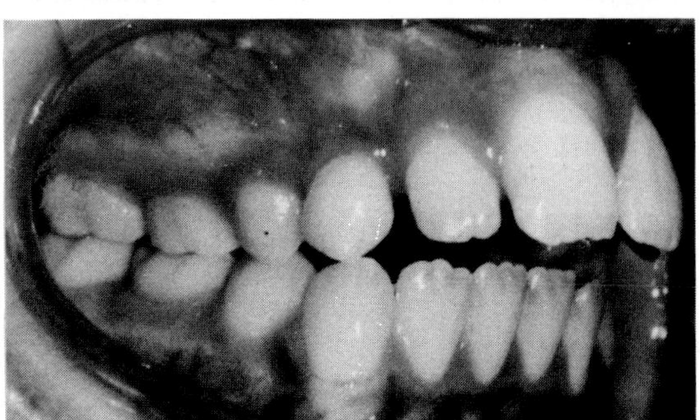
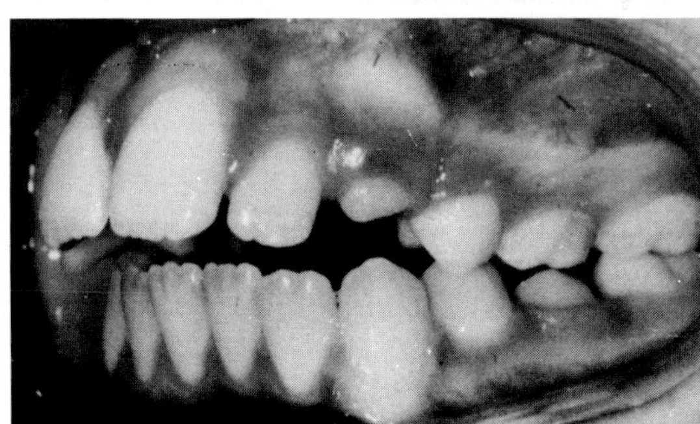

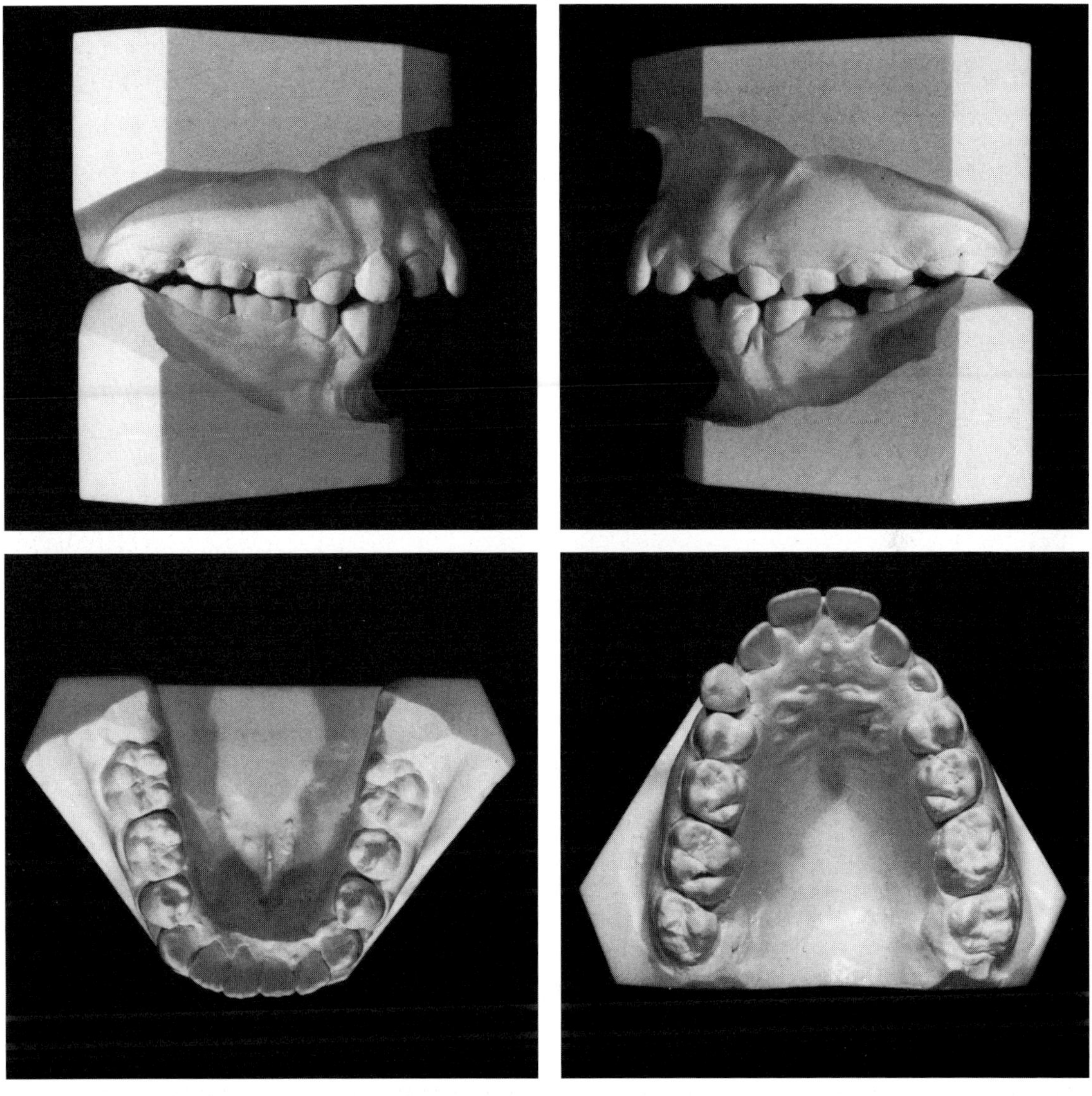

Figs 26-1 and 26-2 A boy aged 11 y, 7 mo with a long, narrow face, an excessive lower-face height, and a receding and underdeveloped chin. He made little use of his oral musculature; his mouth was always kept open. A disto-occlusion of about 1 PW (left a little more than on the right), is combined with a pronounced eversion of the maxillary anteriors, an overjet of 11 mm and an overbite of –2 mm. The mandibular dental arch is normal, the maxillary arch is narrow but matches the mandibular arch buccolingually. Diastemata are present between the maxillary incisors. The maxillary right deciduous canine is loose, and the maxillary permanent canine on the left has already emerged.

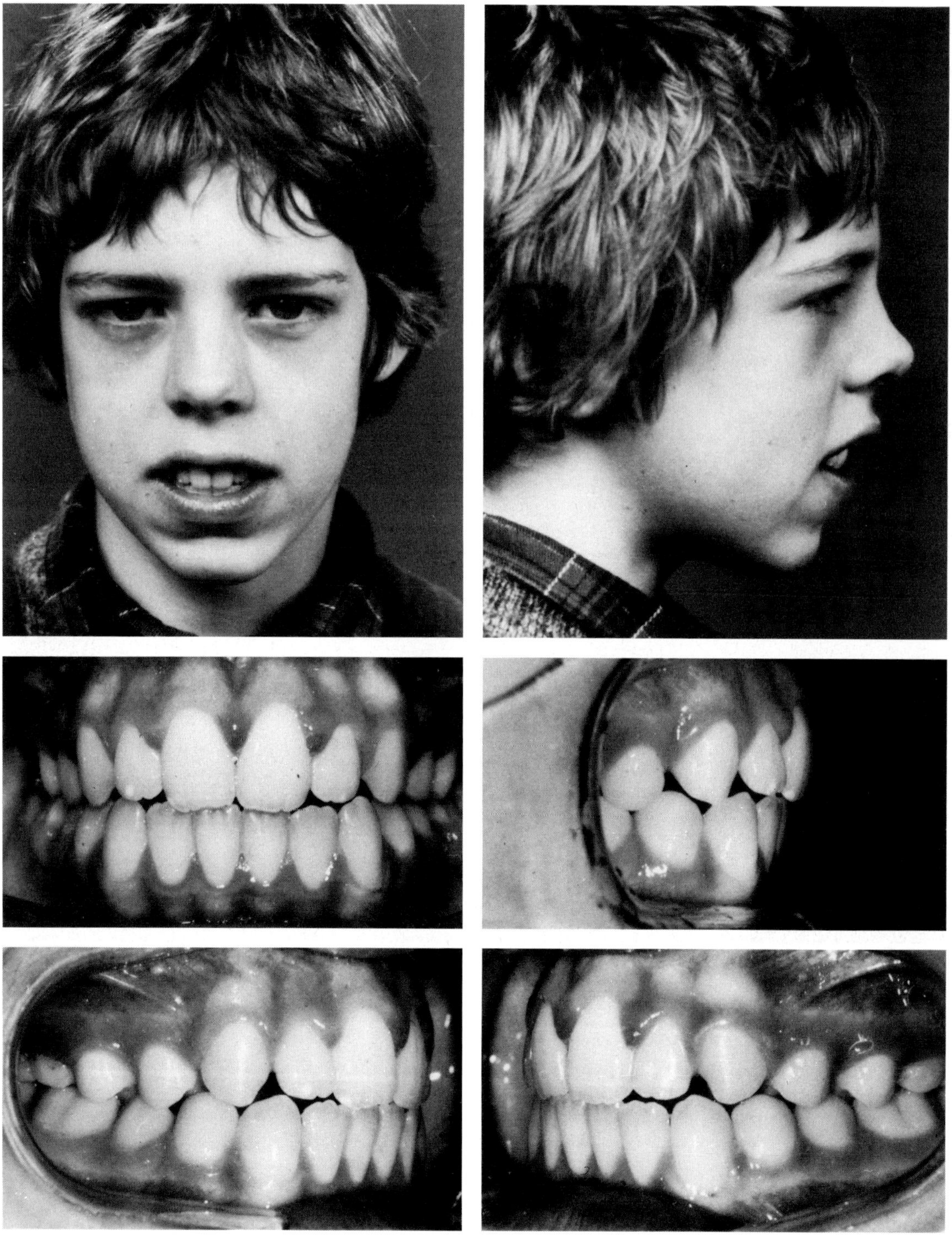

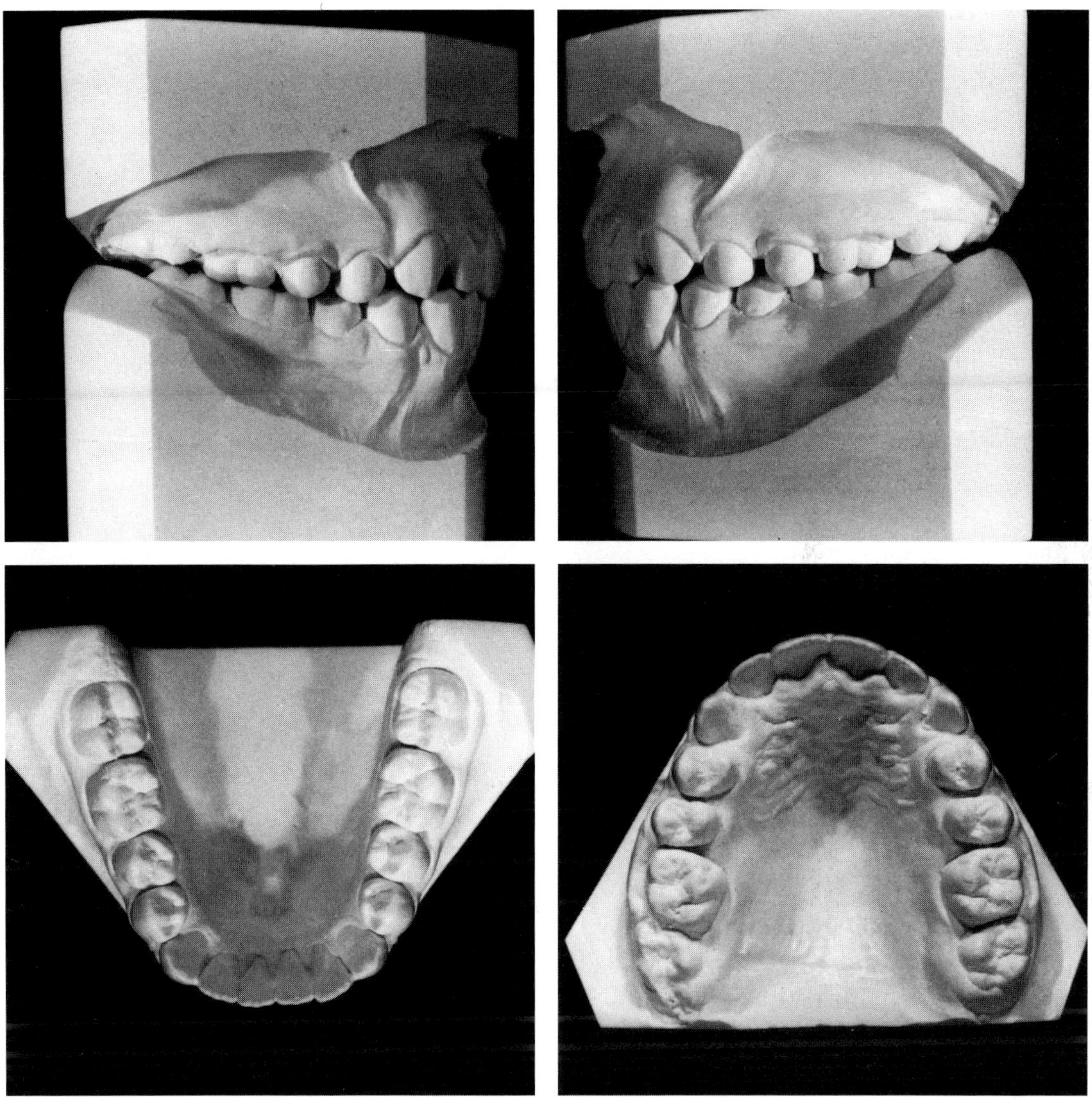

Figs 26-3 and 26-4 At the age of 13 y, 1 mo, the disto-occlusion has been corrected without any obvious improvement in facial appearance. The open mouth, atonic and immobile upper lip, and the everted lower lip with a much exposed vermilion border continue to form a largely unattractive picture. The dental arches display few shortcomings and occlude well.

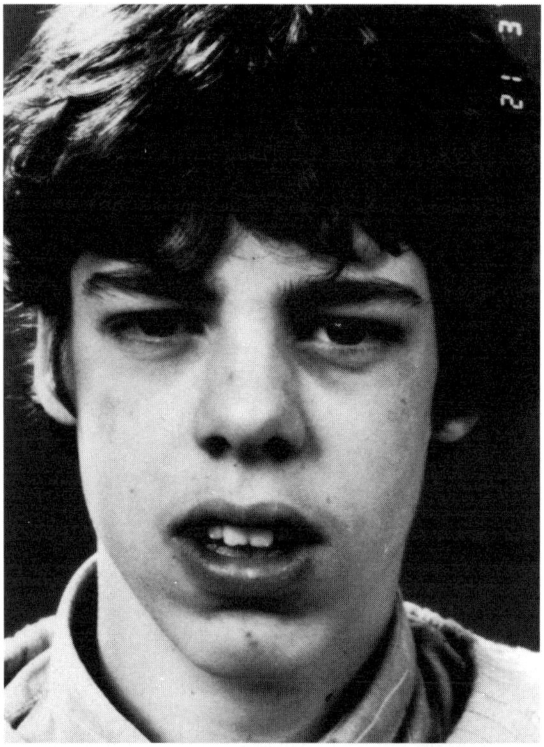
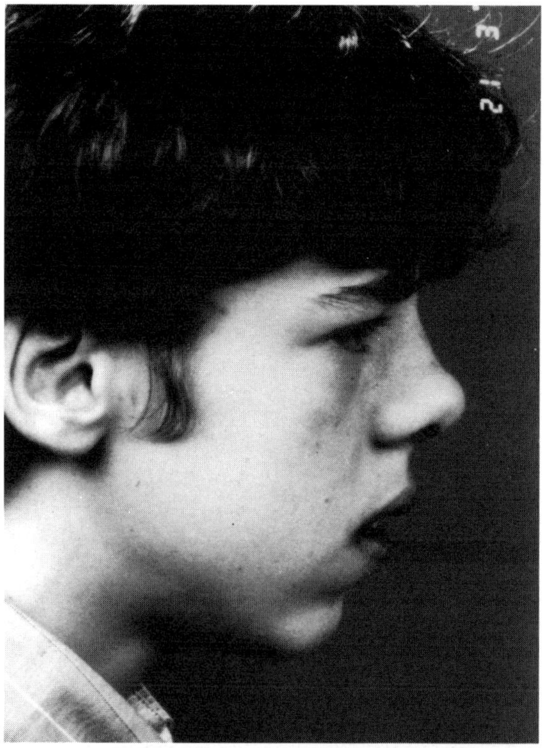
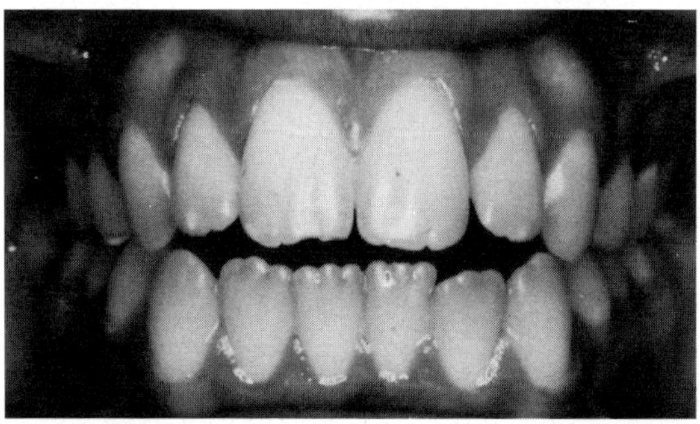
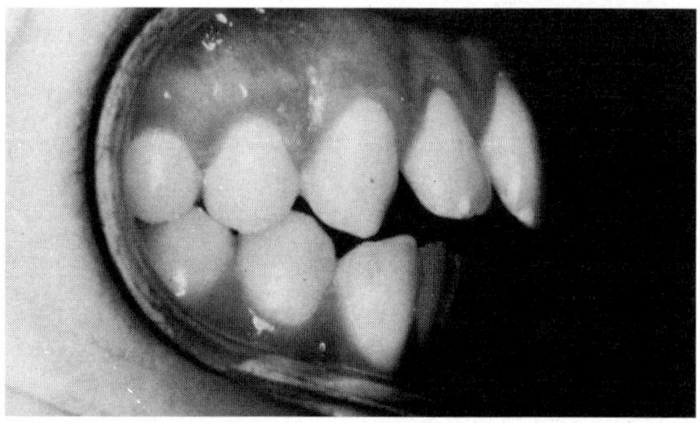
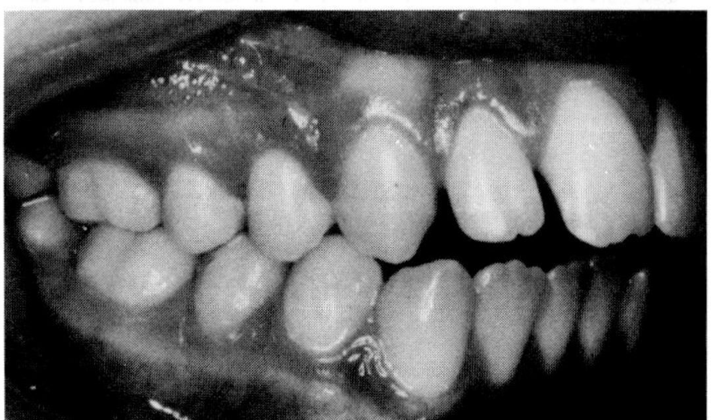
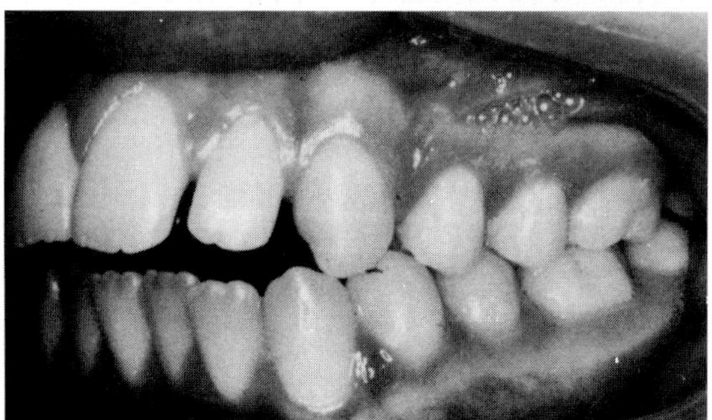

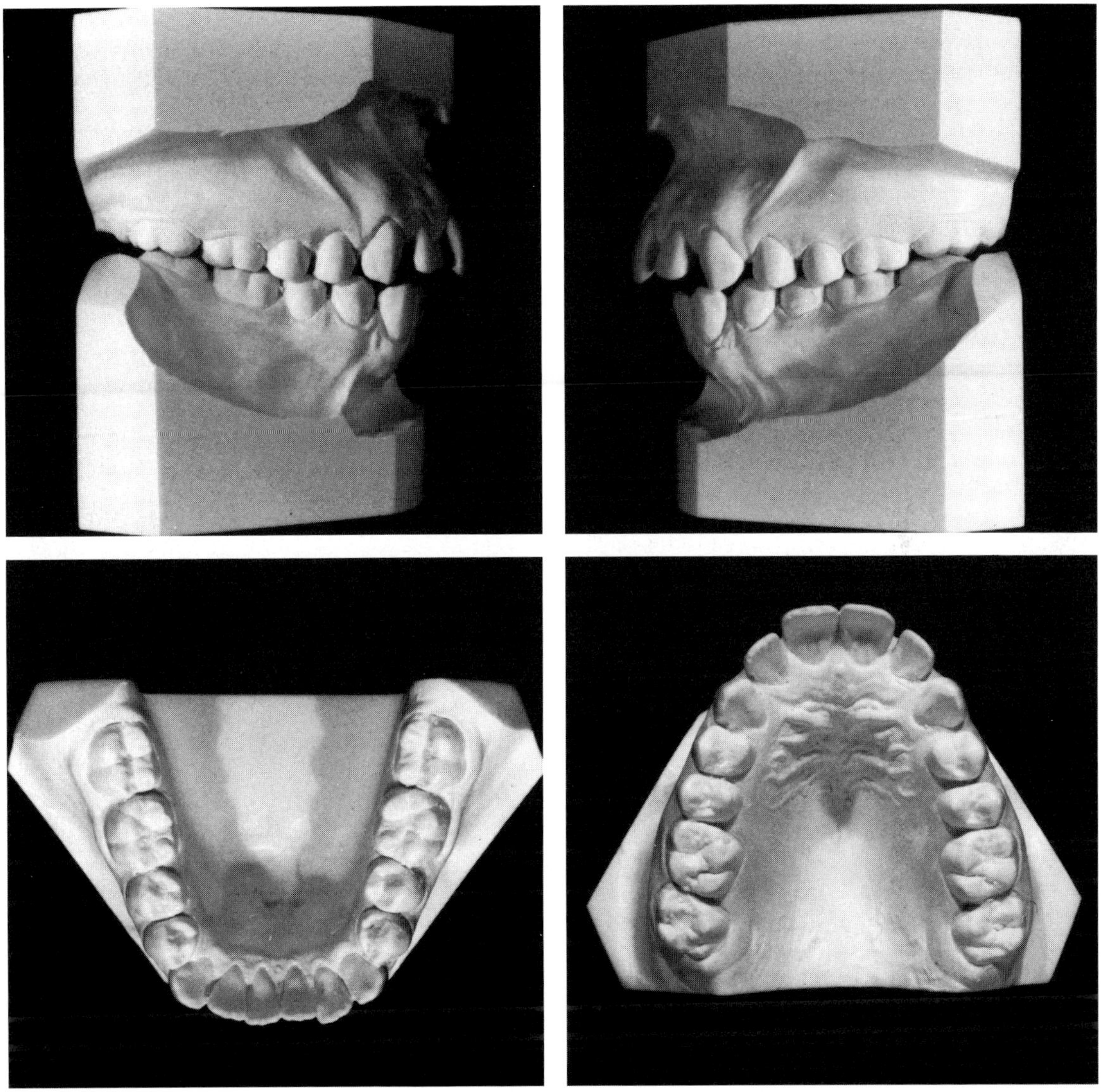

Figs 26-5 and 26-6 At the age of 16 y, 5 mo, three years and four months after the end of treatment, the improvements in the posterior occlusion seem stable, which can be attributed to the solid interdigitation of the premolars and molars. The anterior open bite has relapsed. The eversion of the maxillary incisors has largely returned, and with it the diastemata on both sides of the lateral incisors. The face has matured, but functional conditions have changed little.

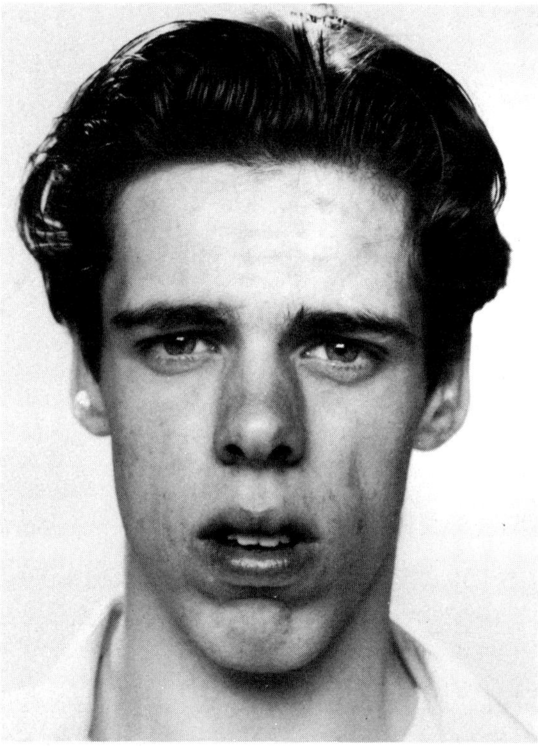
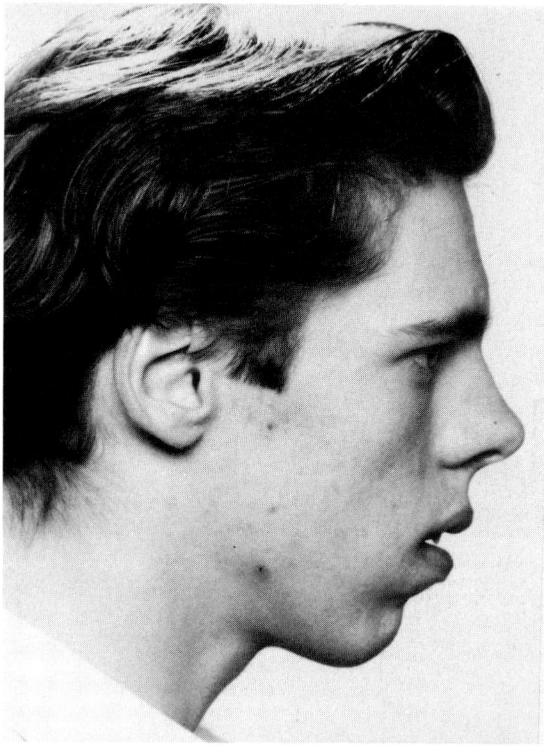
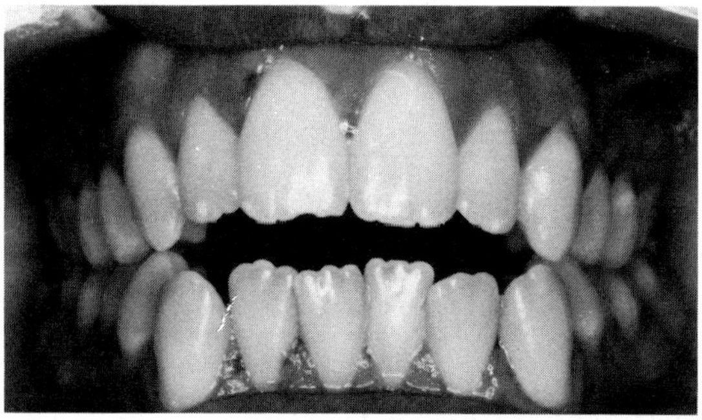
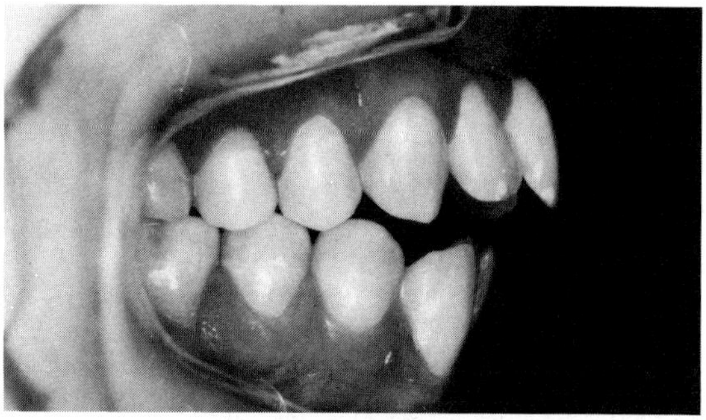
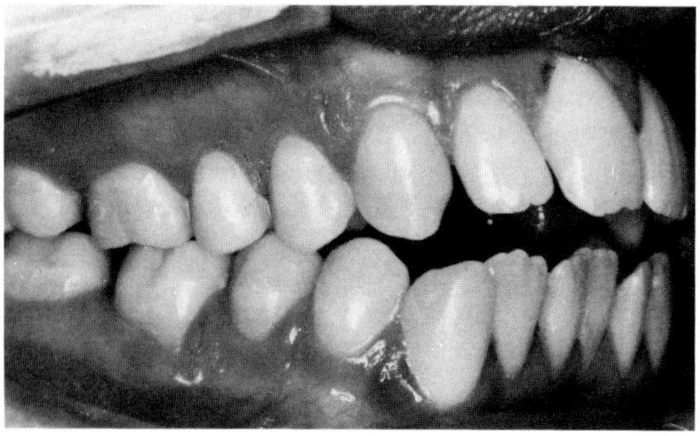
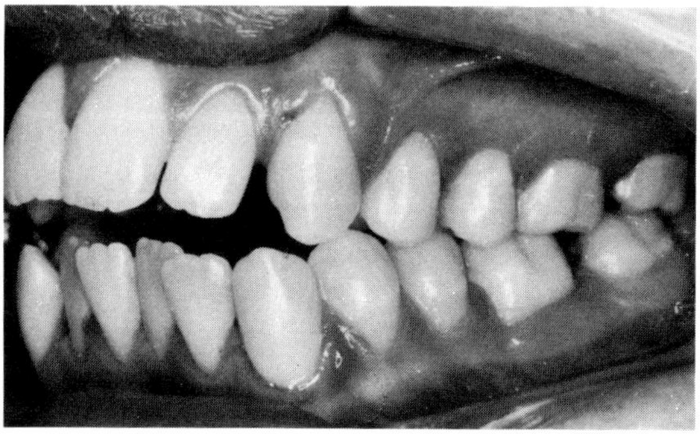

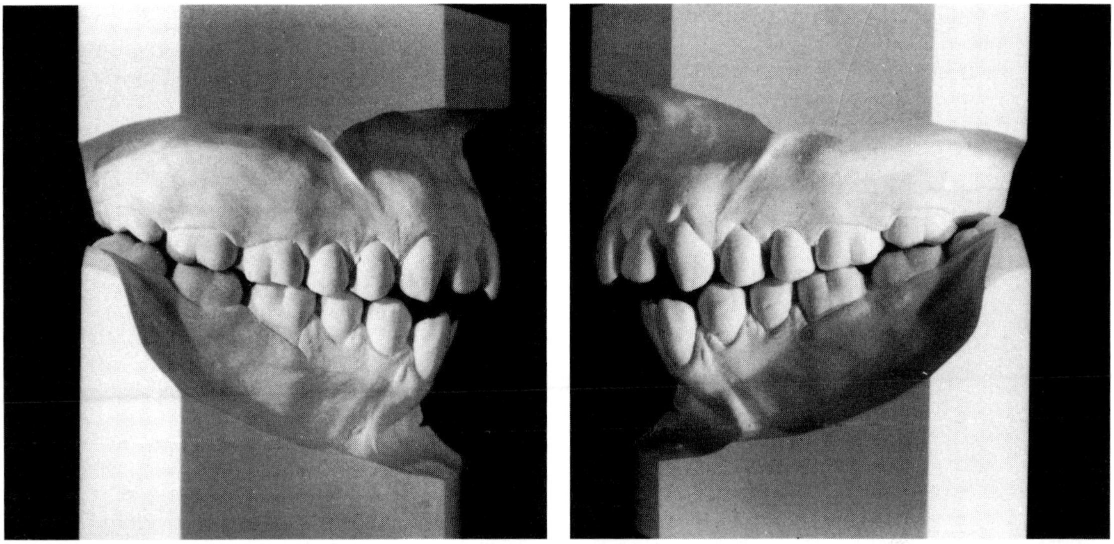

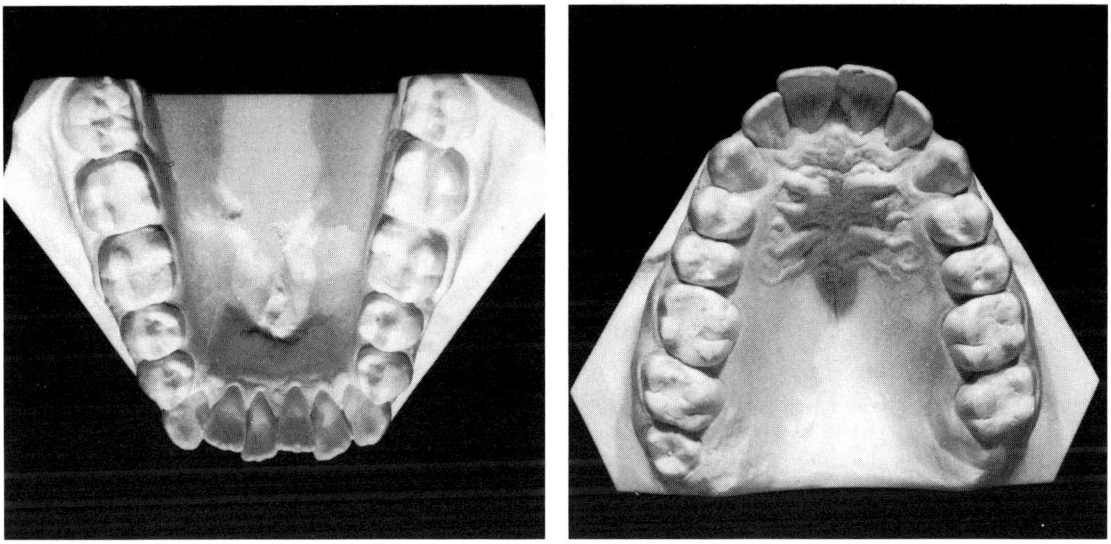

Figs 26-7 and 26-8 *At the age of 21 y, 7 mo, 8½ after treatment, the face has become larger and the lips have begun to cover the teeth better. The tongue interposition and the associated open bite are still present, just as is the mouth-breathing. The occlusion has barely changed, but the crowding in the mandibular anteriors has increased.*

Figure 26-9a

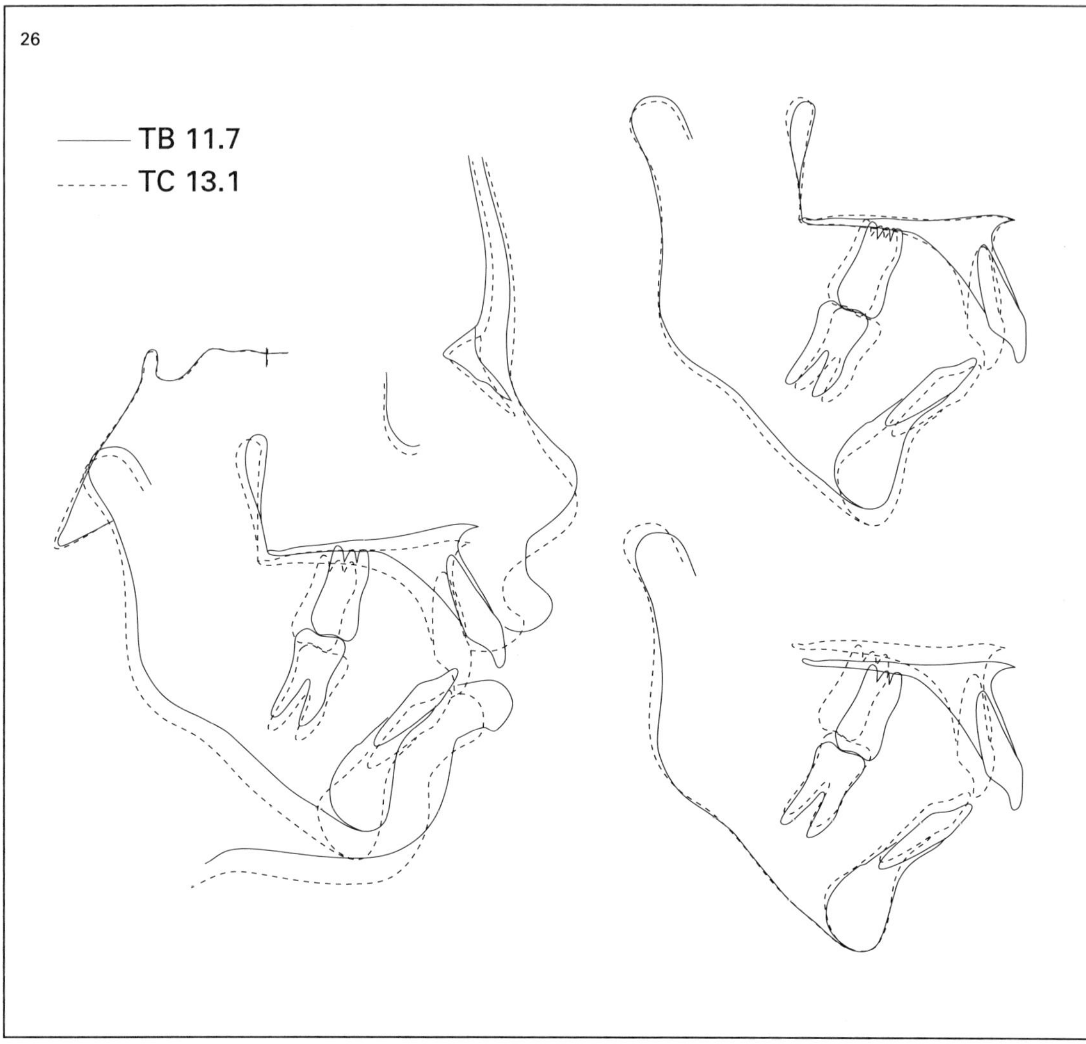

Fig 26-9 Superimpositions of the tracings from cephalometric radiographs show that during treatment the maxilla was restrained in its ventral development and the maxillary anteriors have been retracted and elongated. The mid-face has become slightly longer, but the maxillary first permanent molars have not erupted further. The mandible has moved more ventrally, while the ramus height increased minimally.

Figure 26-9b

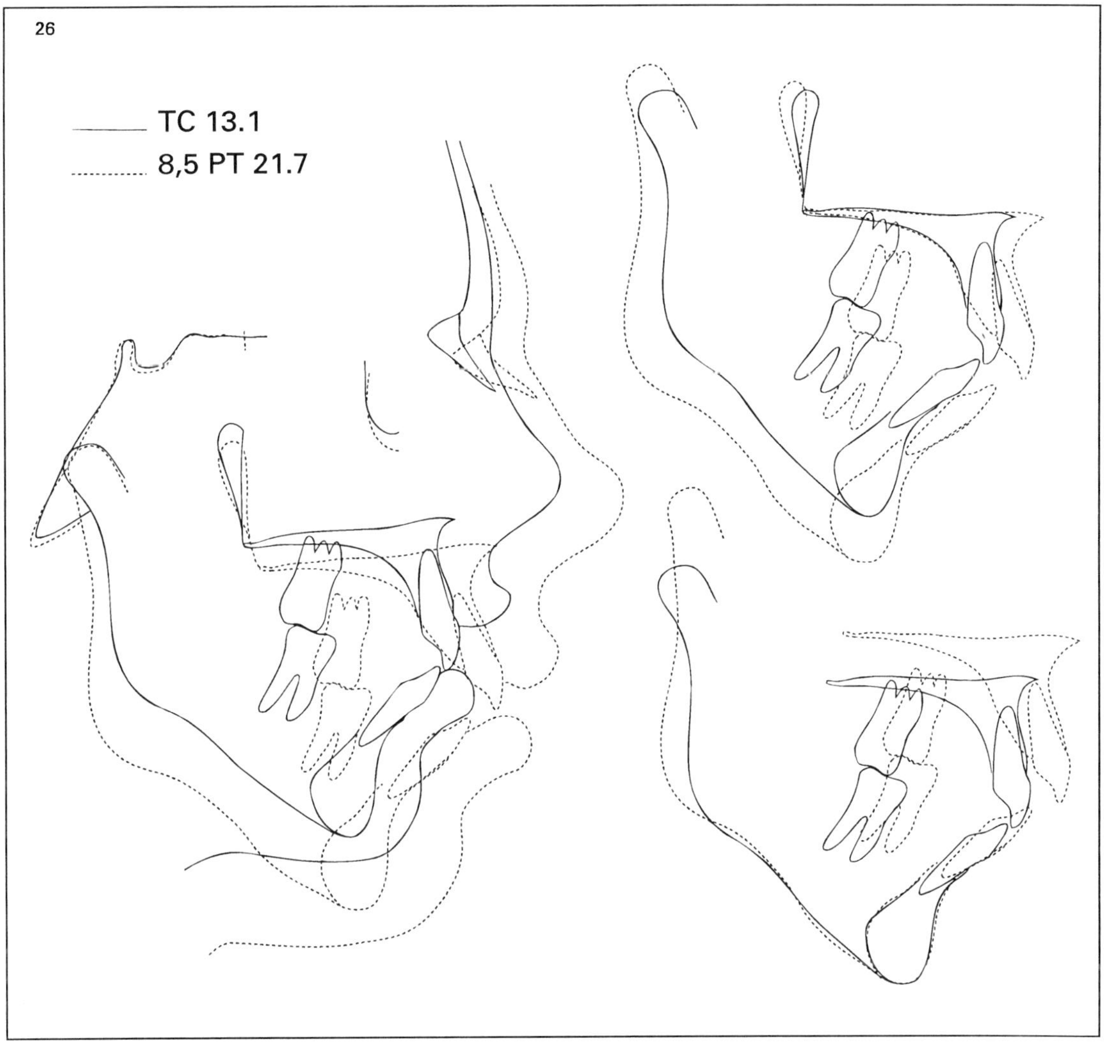

In the 8½ years following treatment, the face experienced an extreme vertical growth. The lengths of the mid-face and the ramus increased markedly. The maxillary incisors moved labially, but elongated only slightly. On the other hand, the first molars in both jaws, and also the mandibular anteriors overerupted considerably. The increase in height had occurred more in the anterior part of the face than posteriorly as evidenced in the increase in steepness of the lower border of the mandible. The excessive vertical development of the face took place mainly in the first 3½ years after treatment.

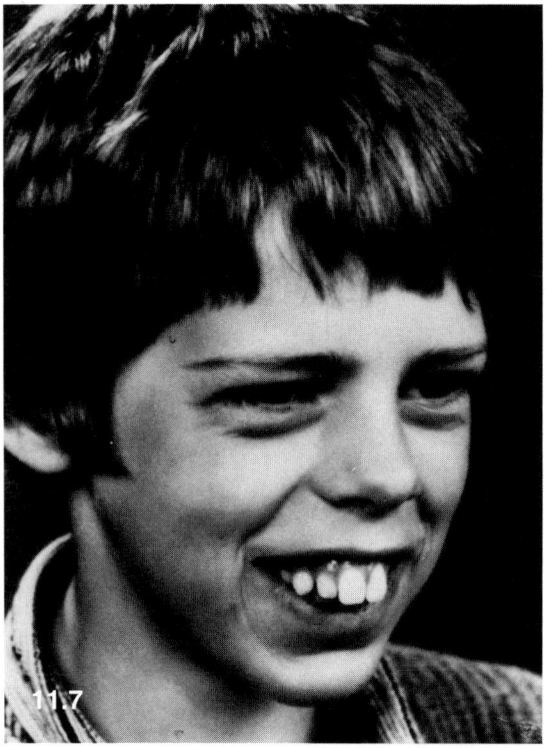
11.7

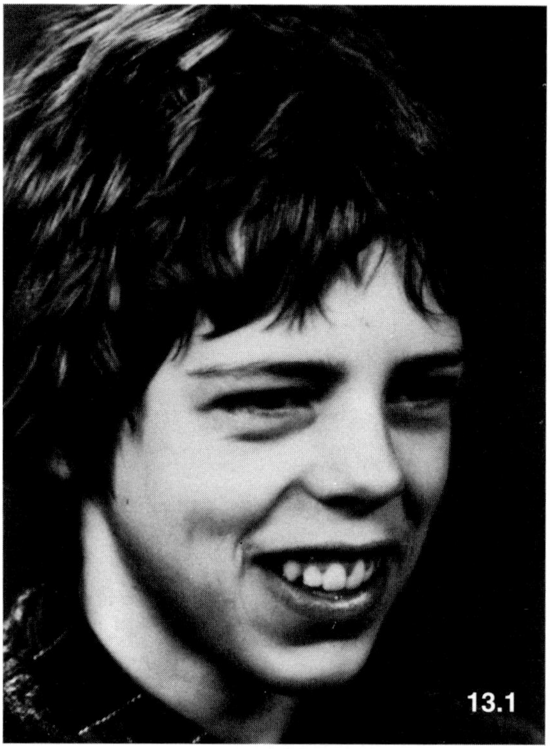
13.1

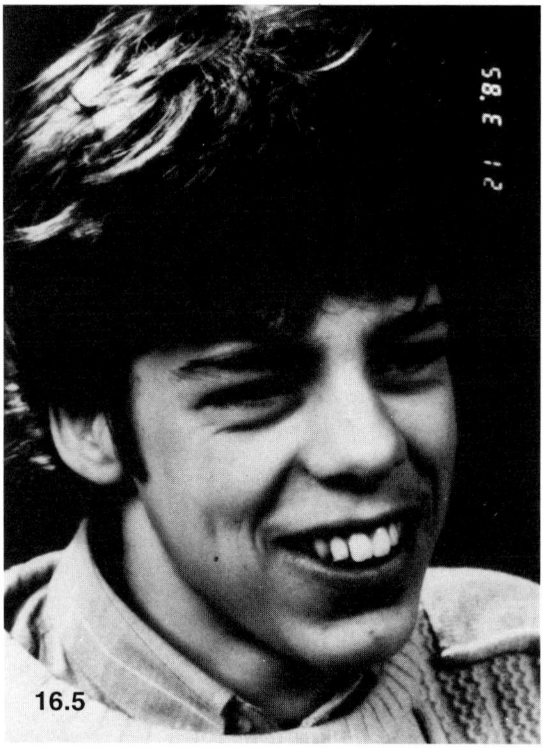
16.5

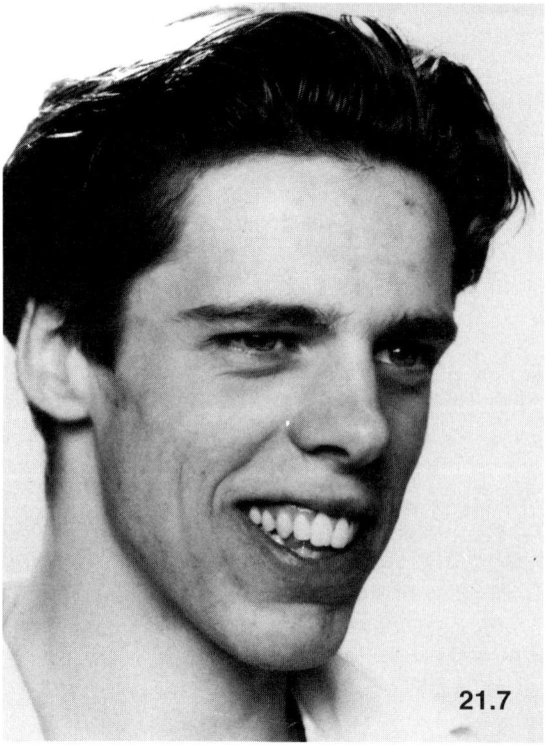
21.7

Fig 26-10 Note the changes associated with growth and treatment. The increased face height is accentuated in the last photo by the different hairstyle.

solid posterior interdigitation had remained stable. The overjet amounted to 6 mm and the overbite was –2 mm. His face had matured but little had changed from a functional point of view. Lip seal was still inadequate and tongue interposition persisted anteriorly (Figs 26.5 and 26.6). The height of the lower third of the face seemed to have increased, which was confirmed with superimposition of tracings of cephalometric radiographs (Fig 26.9).
Five years later, the situation had only slightly changed. His mouth remained open when relaxed, but his lips had grown longer and functioned better (Figs 26.7 and 26.8).
The photographs of the smiling patient demonstrate less clearly the excessive vertical development of the face than the superimpositions of the tracings (Fig 26.10).

The parietal headgear had worked well for this patient in correction of the disto-occlusion and had prevented extrusion of the maxillary molars to which the headgear was applied. The height of the lower face had not increased noticeably and the skeletal correction can be attributed principally to a ventral development of the mandible while the development of the maxilla had been inhibited in both ventral and vertical directions.
If a cervical headgear had been used in this case, the maxillary molars would probably have been extruded, and the height of the mid-face would have increased and the mandibular ramus would have grown more vertically. The result then would have been rather less satisfactory. However, it is questionable as to whether or not the picture 3½ years later would have been any different from the present one. Perhaps the marked vertical development that became evident following treatment might instead have occurred during treatment and the subsequent development might have been more ventrally directed.
When patients have a tongue interposition, an anterior open bite, inadequate lip seal, an increased lower-face height, and a steeply inclined lower border of the mandible, they often also seem to display an excessive vertical growth in the years after being treated with other forms of facial-orthopedic appliances. That also can happen incidentally, when in a disto-occlusion two maxillary premolars are extracted and the incisors are retracted. It is not possible to give a good explanation of this phenomenon. Perhaps a decrease in the intraoral space for any reason, including the wearing of a plate, promotes compensation vertically, or perhaps before treatment was begun, the situation was already an expression of the domination of intraoral functional components over extraoral ones. During treatment, the vertical effects could still be restrained by the appliances being used but subsequently be free to play an influential role. With these suggestions in mind, it may have been better to provide brackets on the maxillary incisors and retract them with an archwire through the molar tubes, to avoid the temporary reduction of intraoral space that the use of a plate involves.

In retrospect, it was unwise not to provide retention. In the absence of adequate lip closure, account needs to be taken of a partial relapse of the incisors. One can prevent relapse by the wearing of a removable retainer at night until adequate lip seal is achieved or the face is fully grown. A disadvantage of such a plate would be, as previously indicated, that it reduces the intraoral space. Therefore it might be better to hold the incisors and canines in their corrected positions with a thin twistflex wire bonded to those teeth palatally with composite. If the maxillary anteriors are unified in this way they can only move labially or cervically "en bloc" and diastemata will not develop between them. More stability is obtained by incorporating the first premolars in this approach. The twistflex would in that case have to run on the palatal surfaces of the premolars, or in the occlusal fossae. Then grooves would need to be ground in them since the mandibular antagonists would otherwise bite onto the twistflex. The inclusion of premolars in the retention does provide the additional possibility of controlling vertical relapse.

Anterior open bites that are caused by tongue interposition and are associated with inadequate lip seal can exhibit not only a tendency to excessive vertical facial growth but to relapse of the incisors. Such limitations should be taken into consideration from the start.

If the problem lies in an unacceptable alignment of the teeth, then after correction a permanent form of retention is required. If the request for treatment is based primarily on dissatisfaction with the facial configuration, then it is wise to put aside any thought of facial-orthopedic intervention; treatment should be delayed until the completion of growth and then a combination of orthodontic and surgical treatment will solve the problem.

It should be remarked in conclusion that on the basis of the records available at the age of 21 years 7 months, the pros and cons of combined orthodontic and surgical therapy were fully discussed with this patient. He was not inclined to undergo surgery, since his facial appearance did not upset him and the eversion of his maxillary incisors and the associated crowding of the mandibular incisors were not strong enough reasons to justify intervention. He was encouraged in his decision by the assurance that in the process of growing older his teeth would become less conspicuous.

Chapter 27

Class II/1, anterior open bite

Extraction 17 and 27, cervical headgear, maxillary removable plate
Female: 14 years, 2 months to 35 years, 8 months

A girl aged 14 years, 2 months, whose growth was almost complete, attended with a mild class II/1 anomaly and an anterior open bite. Her mid-face was ventrally placed in relationship to the face as a whole and a slight double protrusion was evident. At the age of six years, her adenoids had been removed and subsequently she had ceased thumb-sucking. She had no difficulty breathing through her nose. Notwithstanding the eversion of the maxillary incisors and the overjet of 6 mm she had an adequate lip seal and kept her mouth closed. During speech and swallowing, but also when at rest, the tip of the tongue lay between the maxillary and mandibular incisors. The arch forms were essentially normal and any abnormalities in alignment were limited. The maxillary incisors were everted and barely overlapped the mandibular incisors vertically. She had a high caries activity. All the permanent molars had large restorations and the maxillary second permanent molars were partly decalcified buccally. The third molars were present but the room available for their proper emergence was inadequate (Figs 27.1 and 27.2).

In view of the poor quality of the second permanent molars, and the presence of well-formed third molars for which insufficient room was available, it was decided that the maxillary second permanent molars should be extracted and that a cervical headgear would then be used with a maxillary removable plate to correct the abnormality. A contributory factor in deciding on extraction of the second molars was that only little further growth could be expected so that correction of the disto-occlusion had to rely almost entirely on tooth movements.

At the age of 14 years, 4 months, after removal of the maxillary second molars had been performed, a cervical headgear was fitted. Six months later a plate with divided labial arches was provided in the maxilla and the incisors were retracted and the diastemata closed. After one year and five months, the desired result had been reached, and the plate was used for another six months for retention purposes.

At the age of 16 years, 4 months, the prominence of the mid-face had been reduced and a good occlusion with incisor contact was established. The crowding in the mandibular anteriors had increased somewhat (Figs 27.3 and 27.4). Eight months later, the maxillary left third molar had emerged and the maxillary incisors had moved labially a little. Furthermore, a central diastema had returned but did not worry the patient. The angulation of the maxillary third molars did improve in the subsequent years (Fig 27.10), and the rotation of the mandibular second molars corrected itself after the mandibular third molars had been removed.

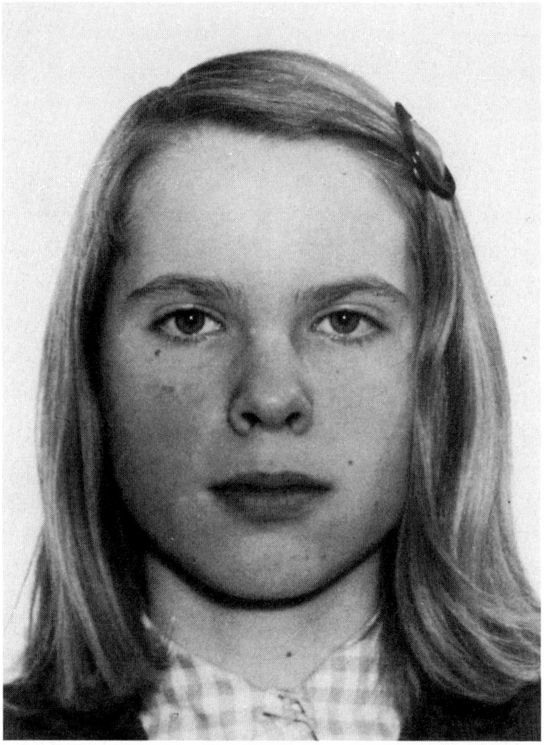

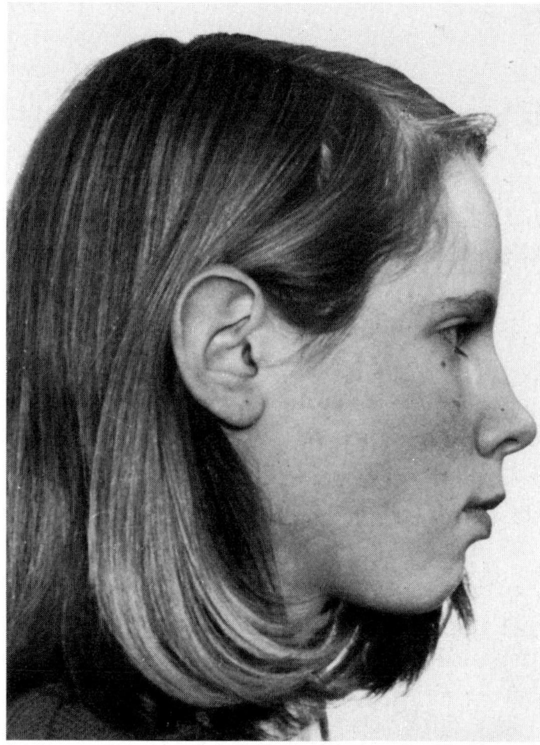

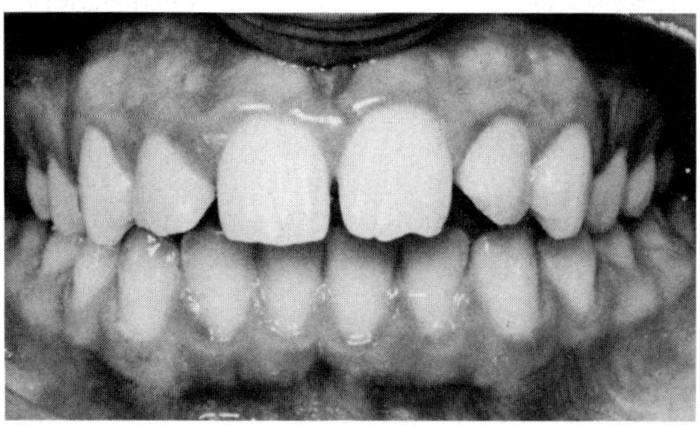

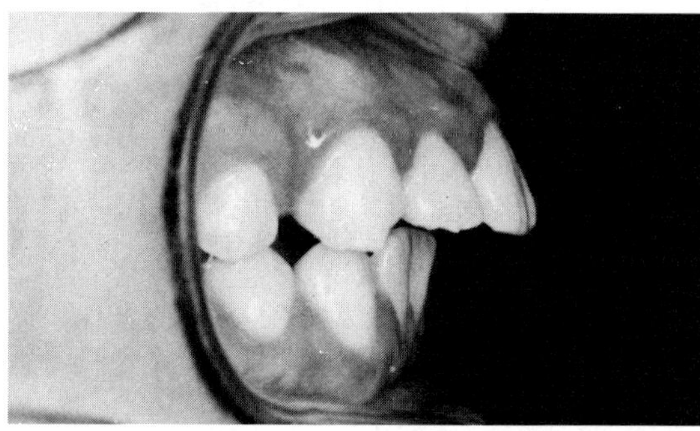

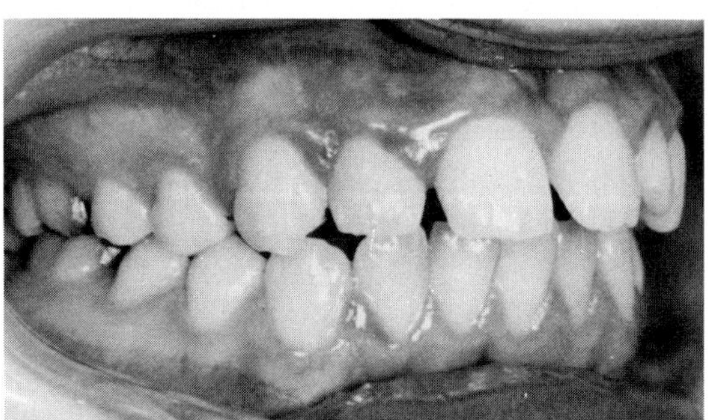

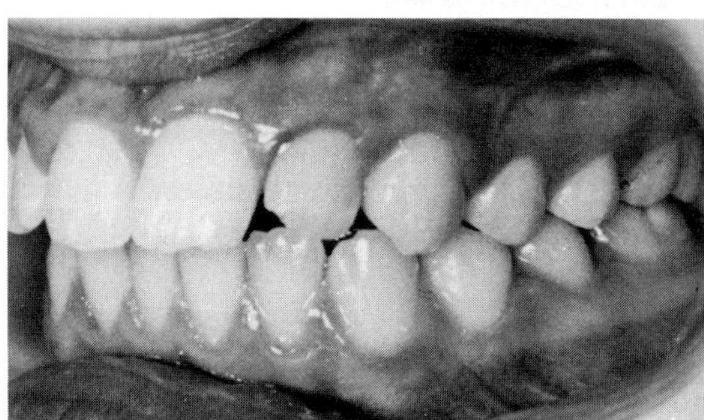

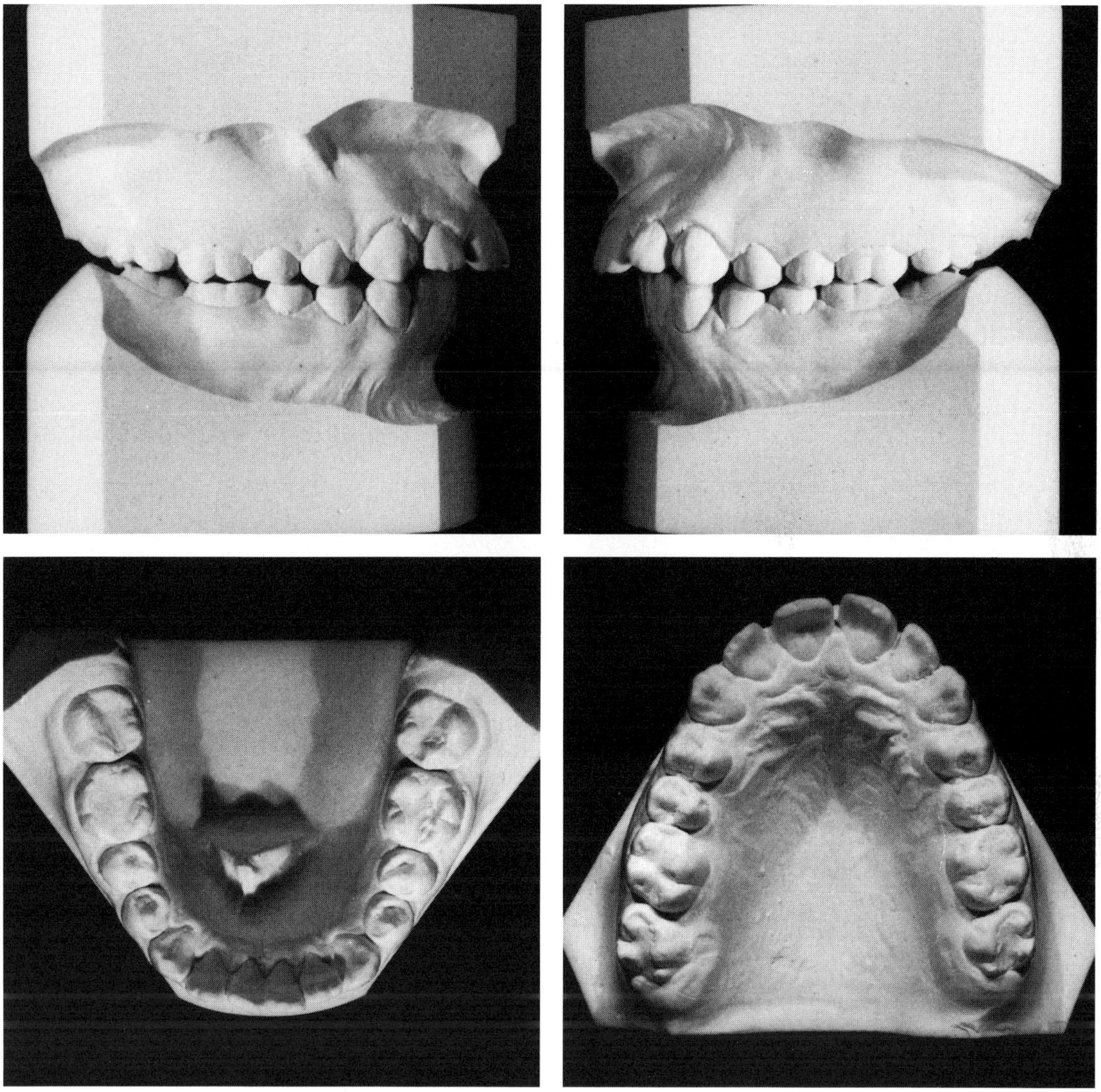

Figs 27-1 and 27-2 A girl aged 14 y, 2 mo with a class II/1 anomaly (¼ PW) and an anterior open bite. In relationship to the rest of her face, the mid-face is a little too far to ventral. She has adequate lip seal but during swallowing and at rest she holds her tongue on the incisal edges of the mandibular anteriors. The everted maxillary incisors show diastemata. In the maxilla, the distance between the distal surface of the second permanent molar and the dorsal limit of the tuberosity is short on both sides, and that space will not increase sufficiently to permit the third molars to emerge properly. The posterior section of the apical area of the mandible also is too small, which is expressed by the rotation of the second permanent molars (see Fig 27.10). In addition, the mandibular incisors show some crowding.

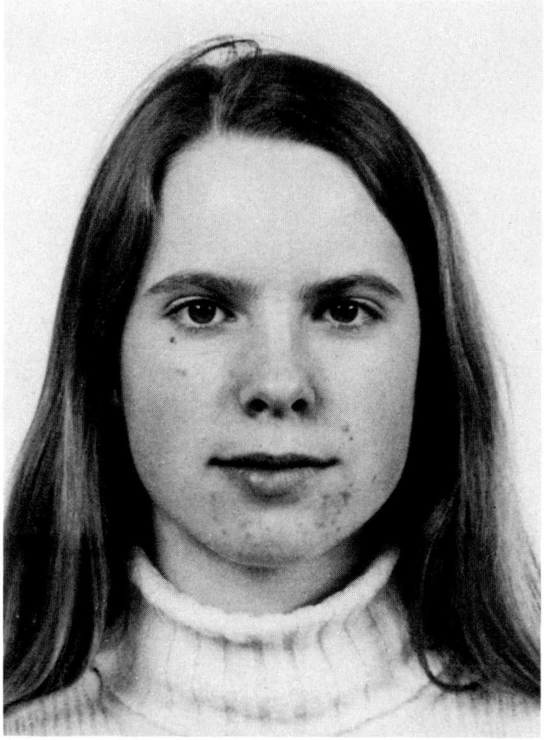

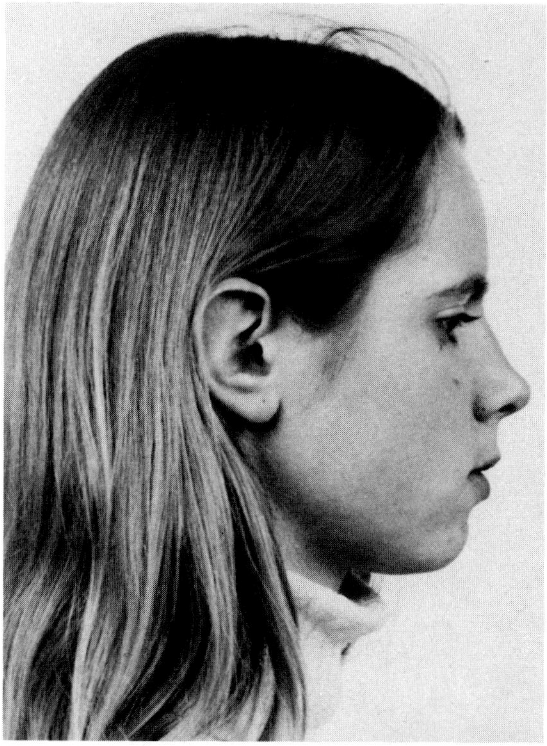

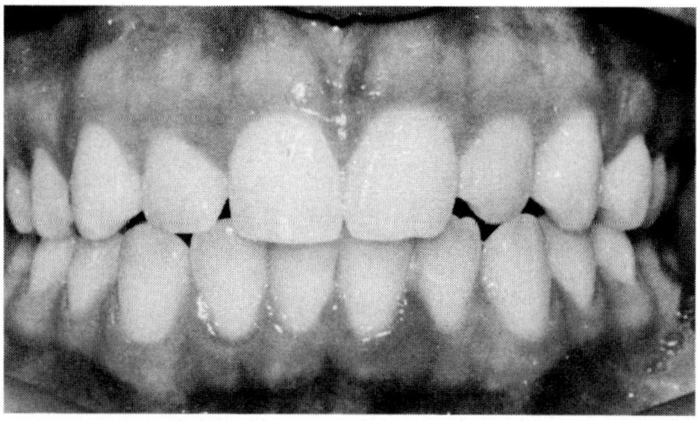

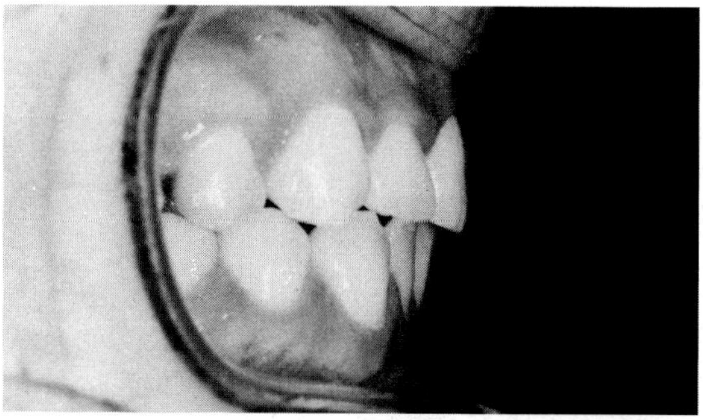

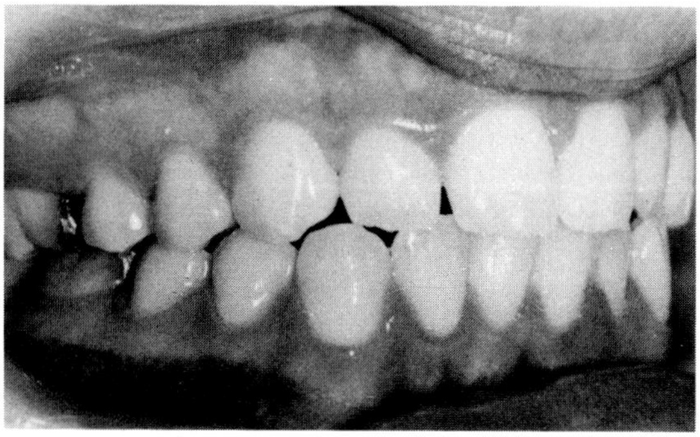

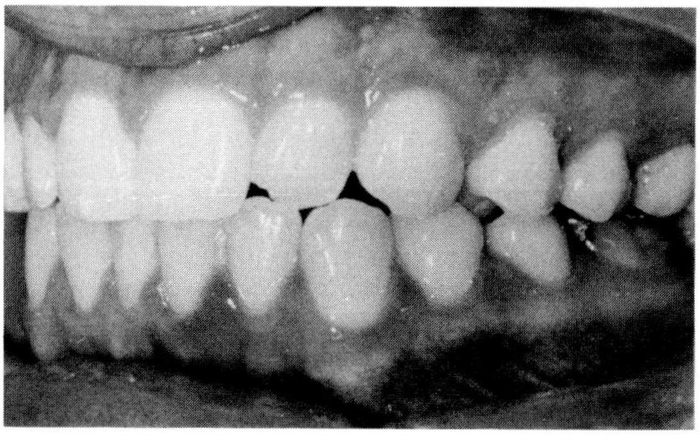

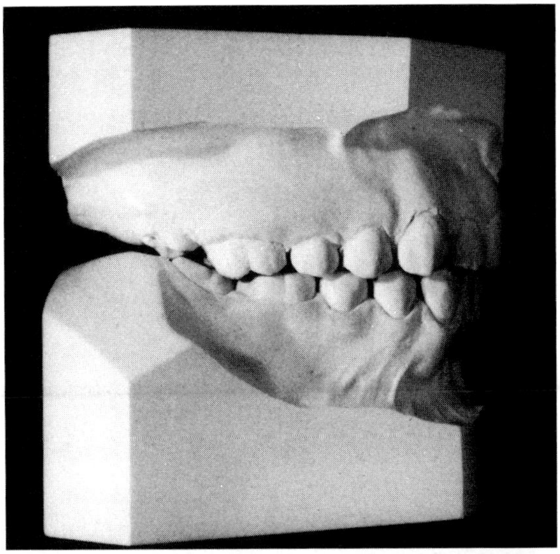

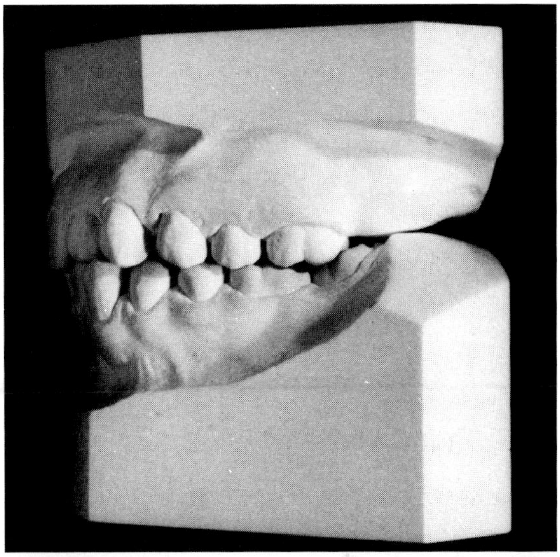

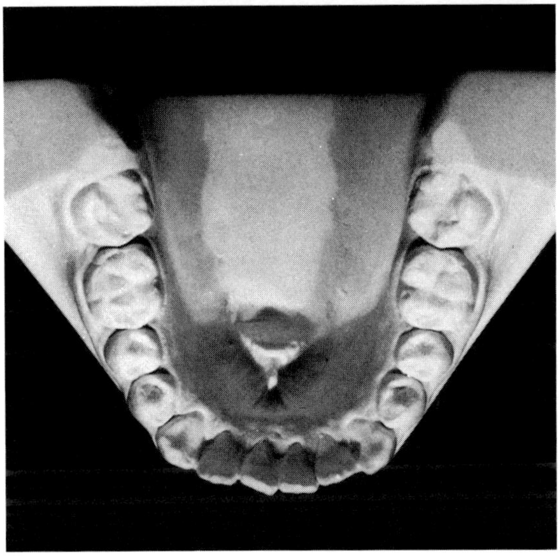

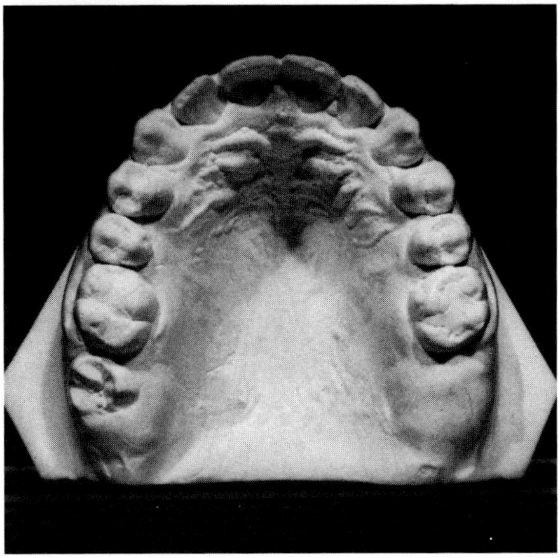

Figs 27-3 and 27-4 *At the age of 16 y, 4 mo, the mid-face is relatively less ventrally placed, and a good posterior occlusion has been realized. The mandibular and maxillary incisors make contact. The overbite is however somewhat meager. In the mandible, the incisor crowding has increased and the two second permanent molars remain rotated still. More than enough room is available for the maxillary third molars, the right one having emerged already.*

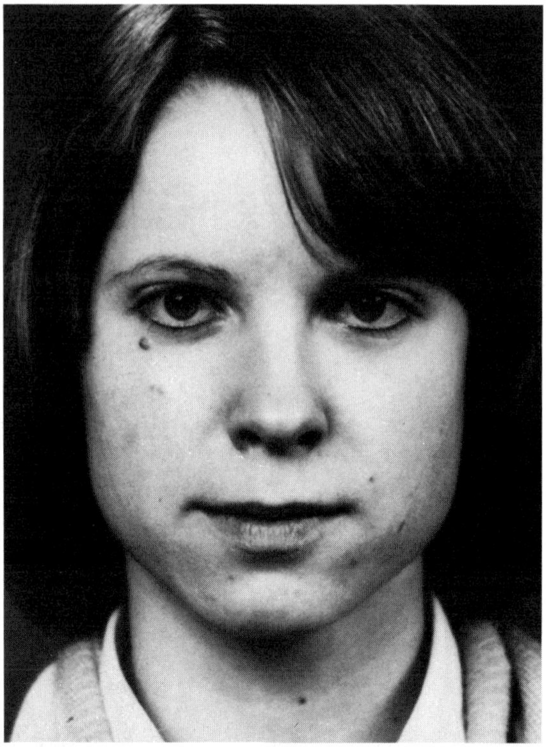

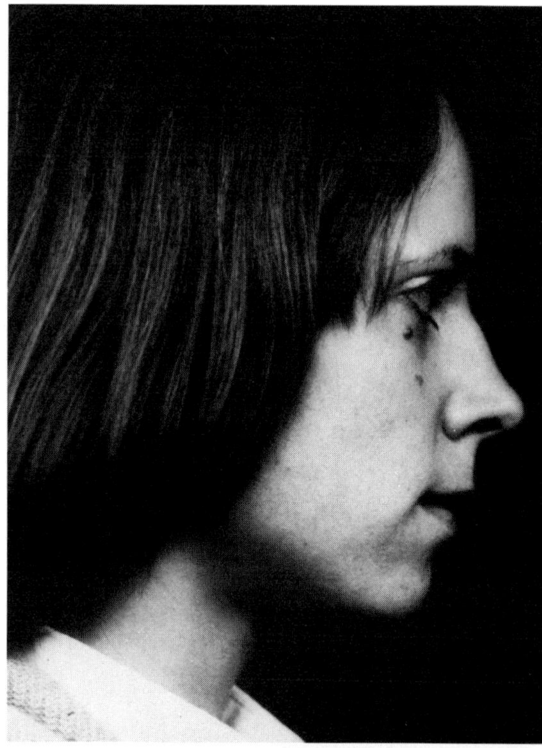

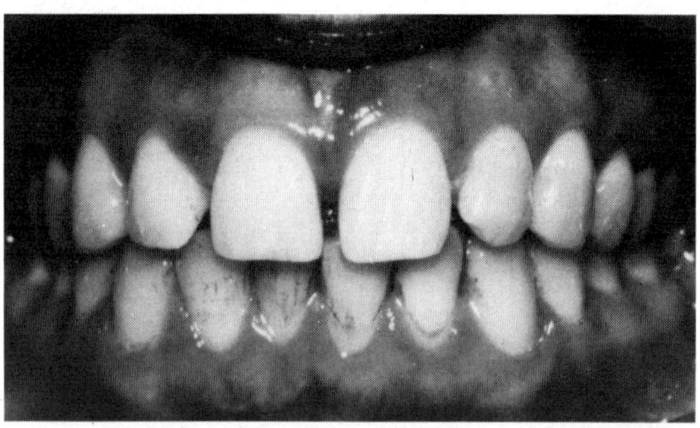

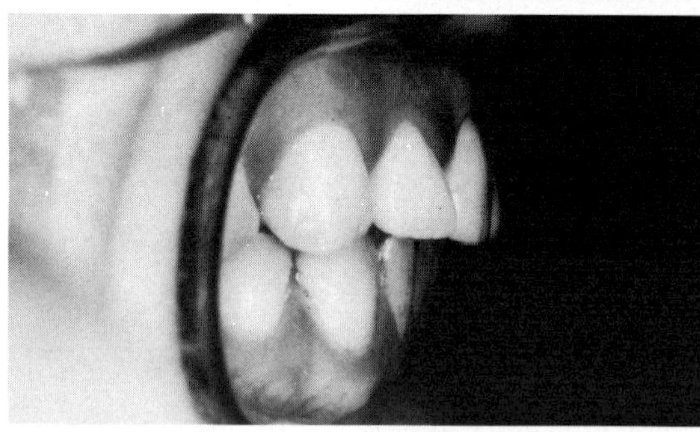

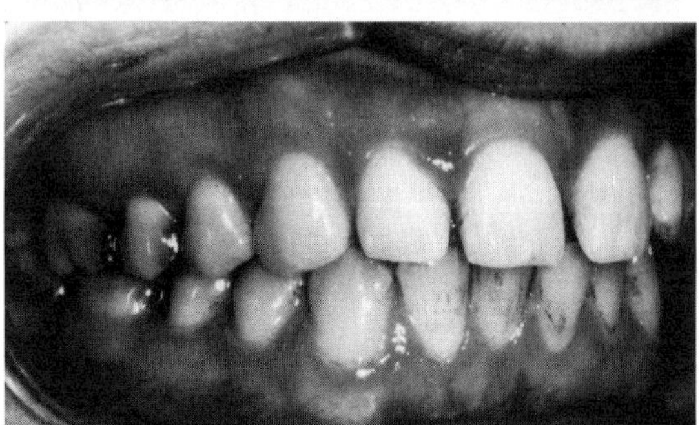

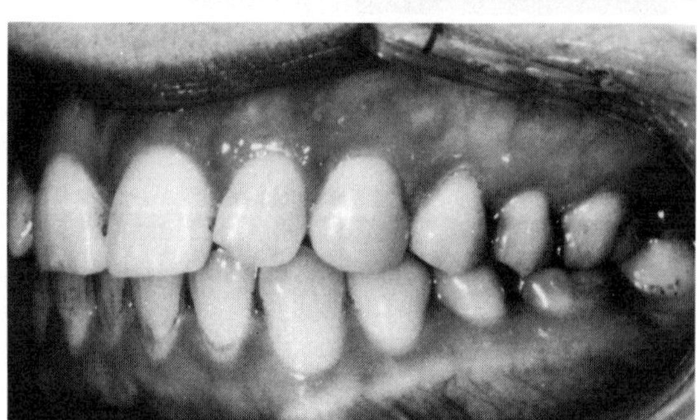

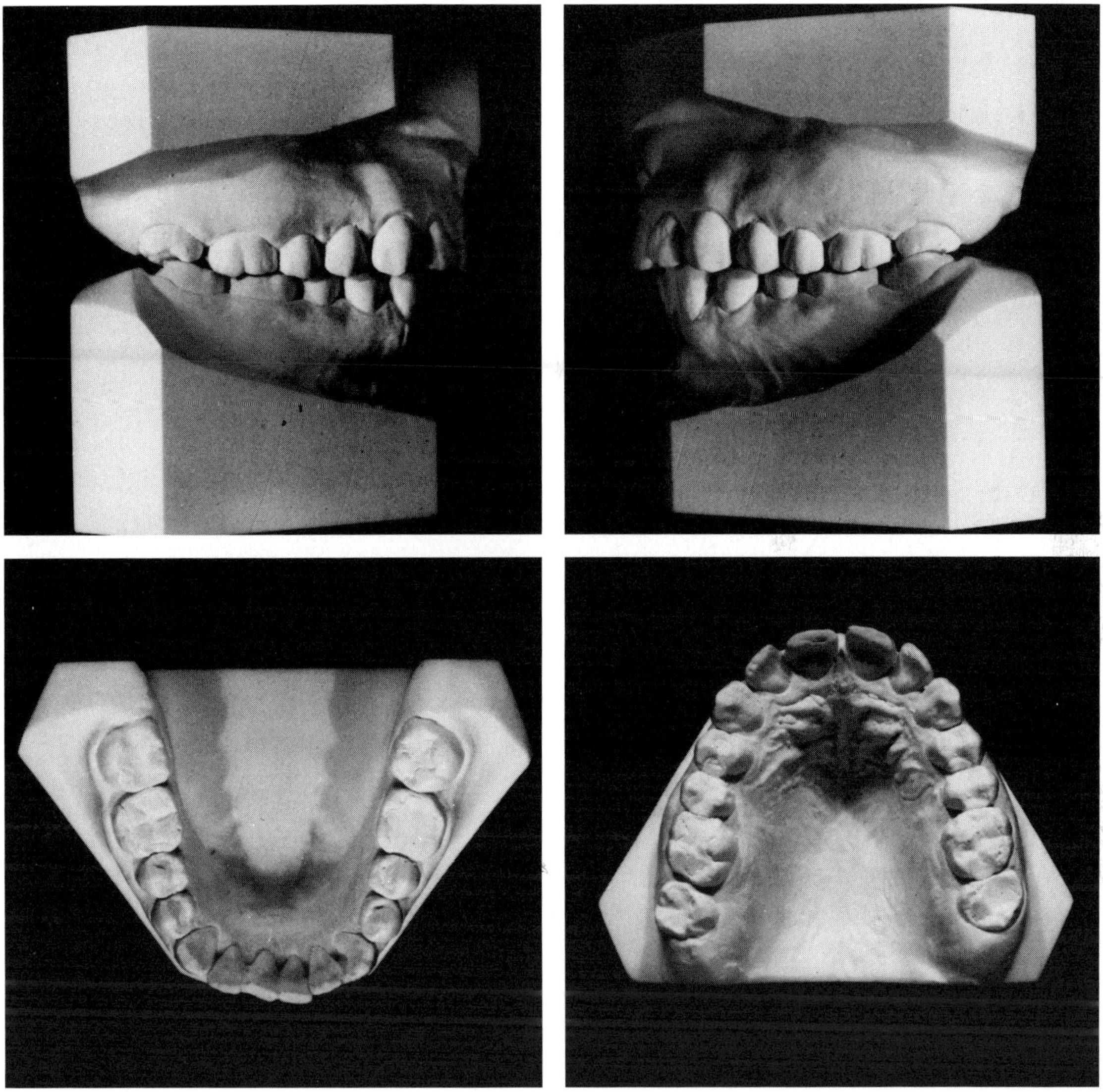

Figs 27-5 and 27-6 *At the age of 26 y, 5 mo, ten years after treatment, tongue interposition is still present. That applies also to the open bite now combined with an increased overjet. There is once again a central diastema, which at this age is not considered a problem. After the third molars in the mandible had been removed the mandibular second permanent molars took up better positions, no doubt under the influence of their occlusion with the maxillary third molars.*

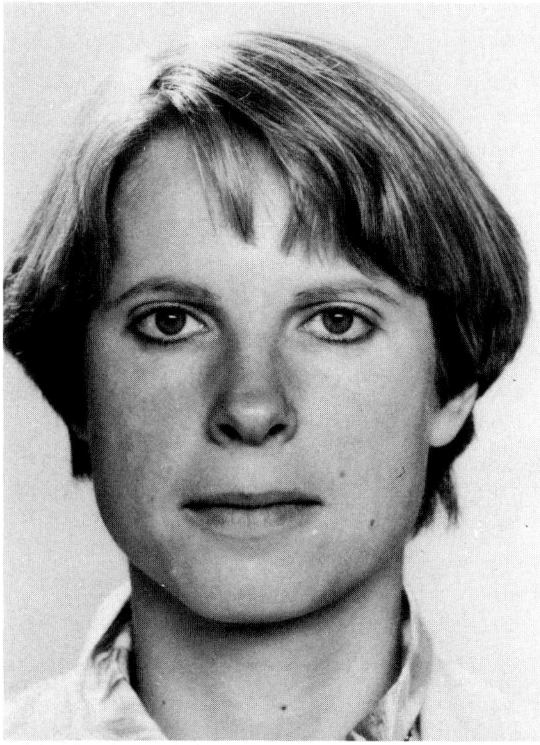

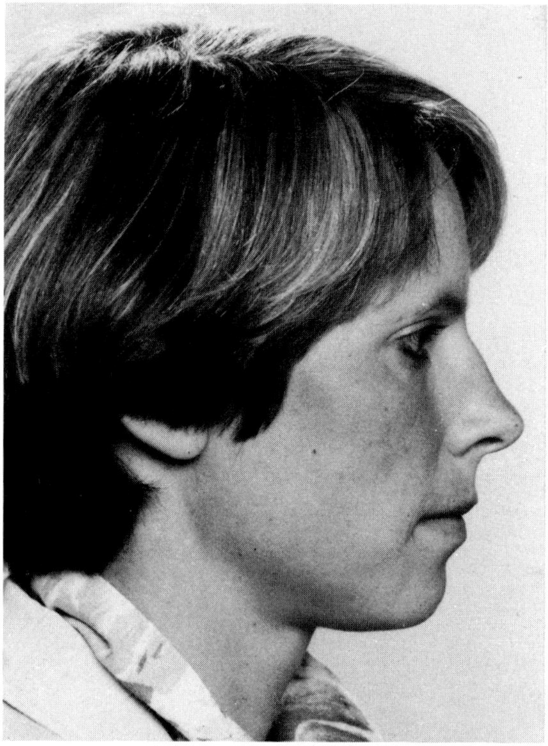

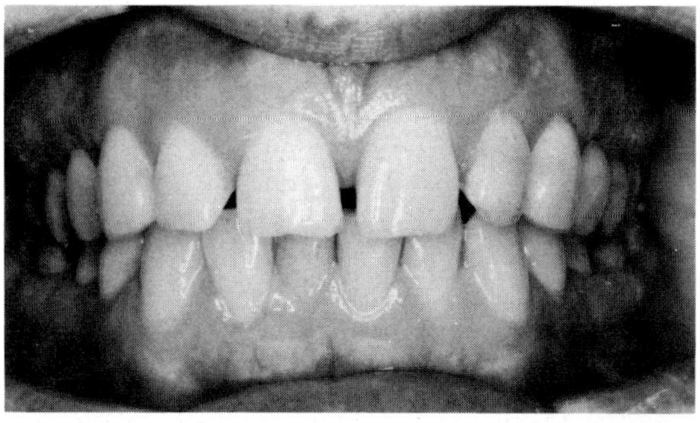

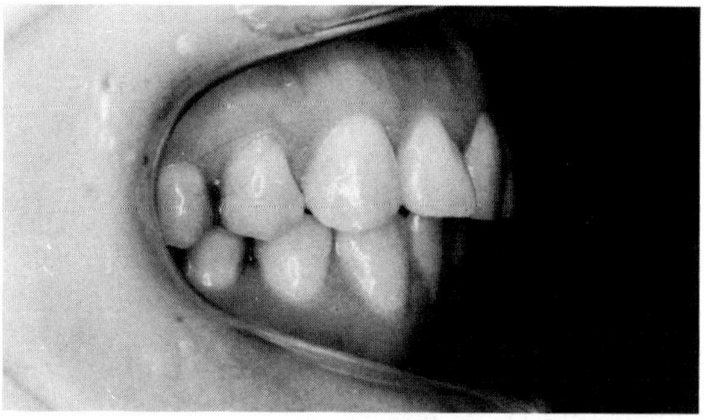

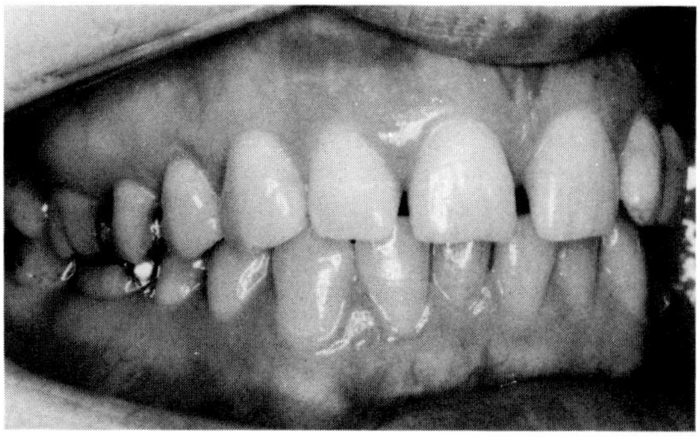

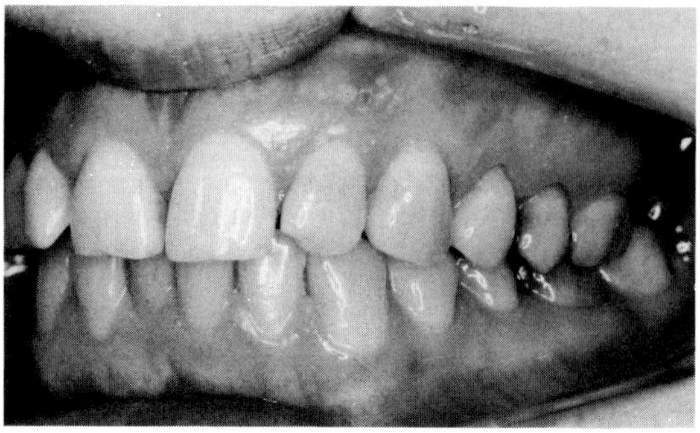

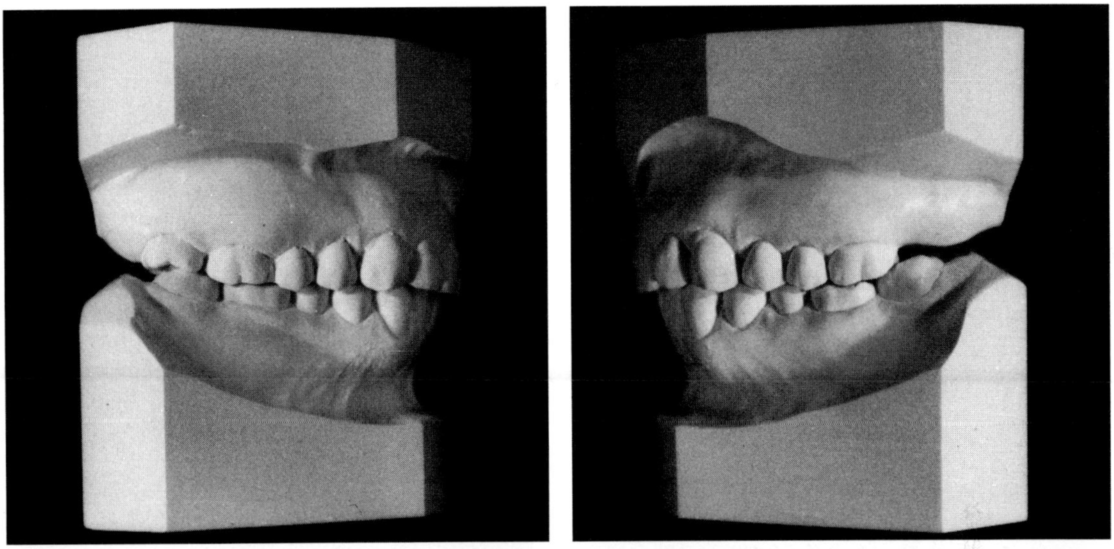

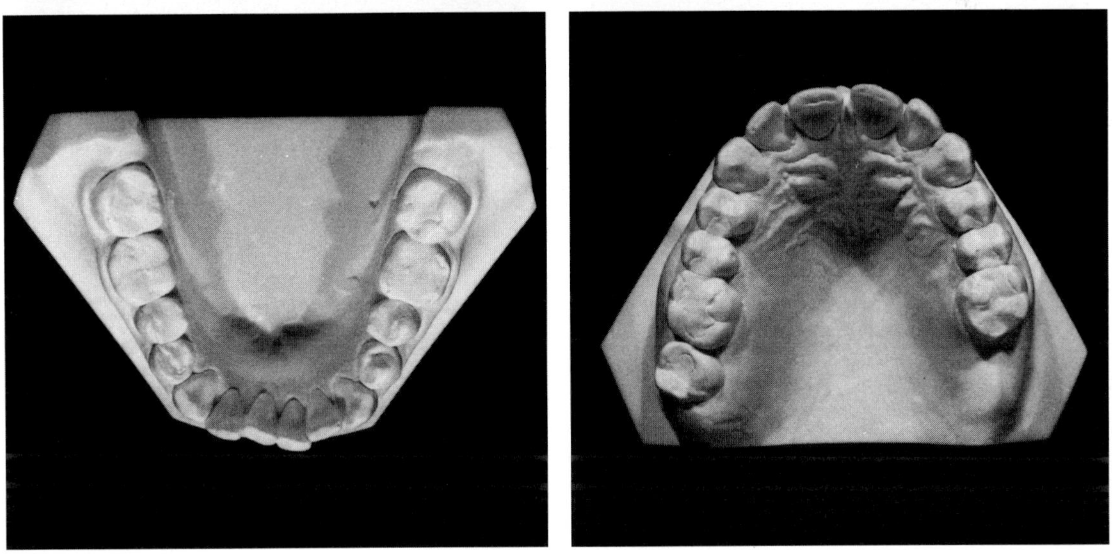

Figs 27-7 and 27-8 *At the age of 35 y, 8 mo, nineteen years after treatment, a harmonious face matching a well set-up dentition is to be seen. The anterior open bite is still evident, although it has become smaller. Unfortunately, the maxillary left third molar had been extracted in the interim. After it was proposed to eliminate the central diastema by building up the incisor crowns with composite, the patient declined to go ahead because she "would rather remain herself."*

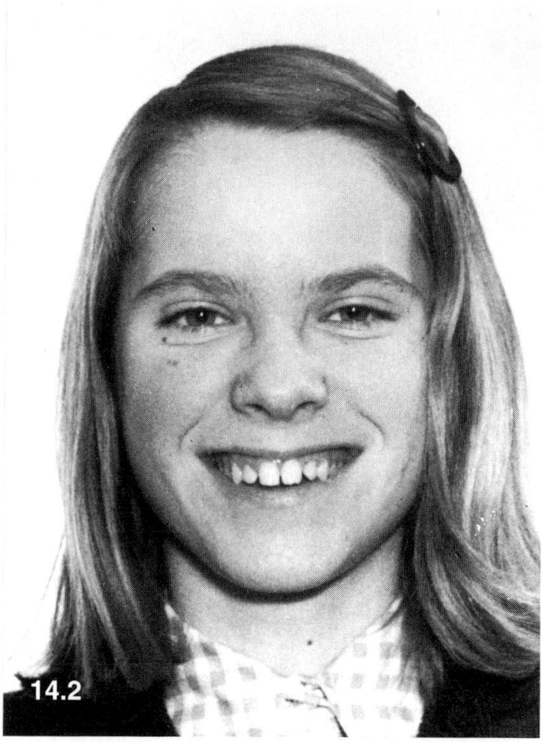
14.2

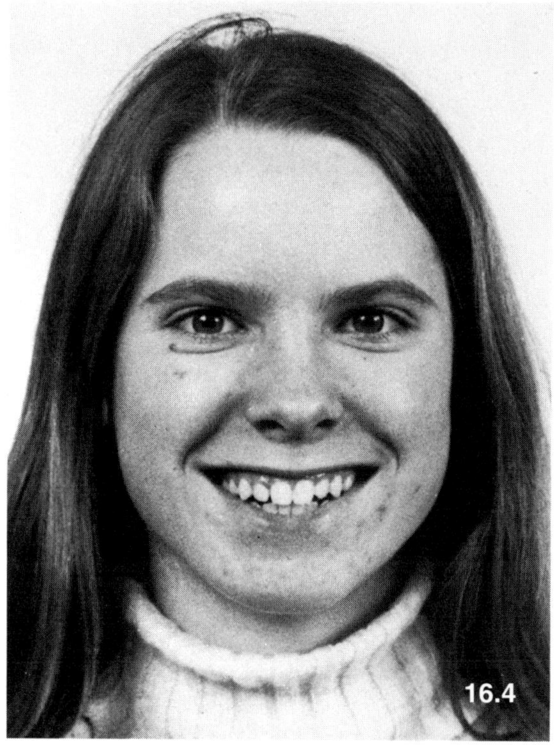
16.4

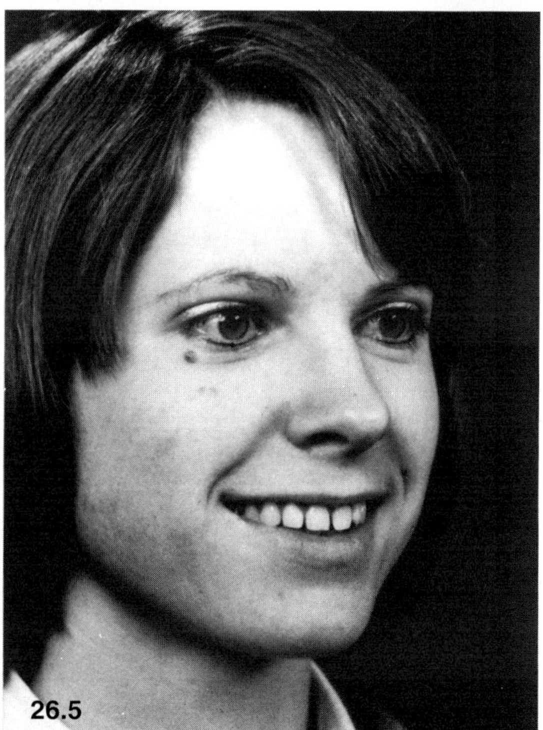
26.5

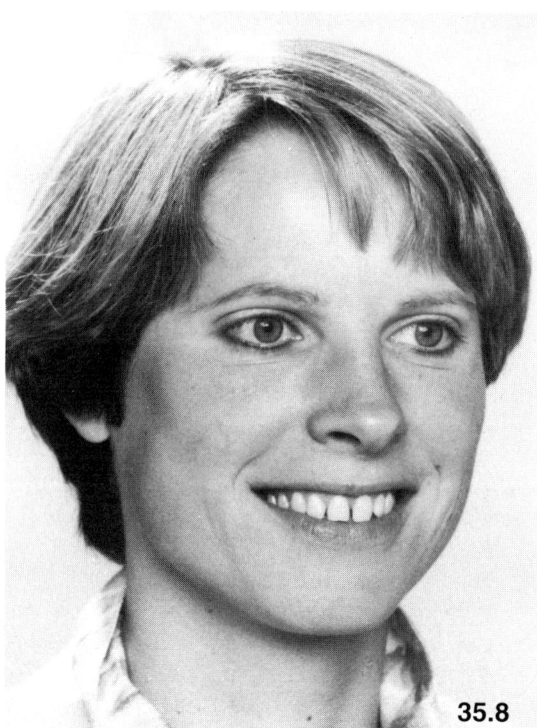
35.8

Fig 27-9 Note the changes that might be attributed to treatment and maturity. There is little change in facial character because growth had more or less finished by the time treatment began.

Ten years after treatment, the tongue interposition persisted, as did the anterior open bite, the eversion of the maxillary incisors, and the central diastema. The situation in the mandibular incisors had not changed. There was solid interdigitation of the posterior teeth, with the maxillary third molars well positioned in good occlusion with the mandibular second molars (Figs 27.5 and 27.6). At the age of 35 years, 8 months, 19 years after treatment, the open bite is still present although it is slightly less. The central diastema could still be seen, but at this age, it was accepted without complaint. However, when the possibility of correcting it (with the development in the interim of composite resins and acid etching of the enamel) by building out the contours of the incisor crowns was explained to her, the patient showed interest and an appointment was made to carry it out. However, the patient later cancelled the appointment, saying that she preferred after all to keep her own characteristic appearance (Figs 27.7 and 27.8).
From comparisons of the photographs of the smiling face it can be concluded that growth had indeed been more or less complete when the treatment had been initiated (Fig 27.9).

Interposition of the tongue leads to a different distribution of forces than in situations in which the tongue lies within the dental arches. If other functional conditions are normal then the influence of tongue position on the location of the maxillary incisor teeth is less than when inadequate lip closure accompanies it, as was demonstrated in the previous chapter. In that case it was seen how following treatment the maxillary incisors relapsed markedly to labial, while in the present case the relapse was limited. Unfortunately, the latter relapse was associated with the occurrence of a central diastema that was larger after treatment than it was originally. At the outset, this diastema was not thought to be objectionable. If this had become of concern it would have been necessary after re-treatment, to hold it closed by bonding a piece of thin twistflex wire palatally to the incisors.
As has already been pointed out, anterior open bites are quite common in the Dutch population. From a country-wide epidemiologic study in the 1980s, it came to light that 40% of 2,273 persons between 15 and 70 years of age had no contact between the mandibular incisors and either their antagonists or the palate.[8] Of the 525 adolescents in the study (between 15 and 20 years of age), 59% had no vertical contact between incisor teeth in maxilla and mandible. In 39% there was indeed vertical contact, and in 2% the mandibular incisors impinged on the palatal mucosa behind the maxillary anteriors.[12] From these data, it became evident that not only do anterior open bites often occur, at least in the Netherlands, but also that as age increases the prevalence decrease only slightly. As a generality it can be said: for two thirds of the population applies, once an open bite, always an open bite.
Taking into consideration the great prevalence of anterior open bites, the question is, should this condition be considered abnormal, or just a variation of the norm? An additional aspect is that open bites are seldom even noticed by the patients, so mostly not found to be something to be disturbed about. Moreover, an open bite has

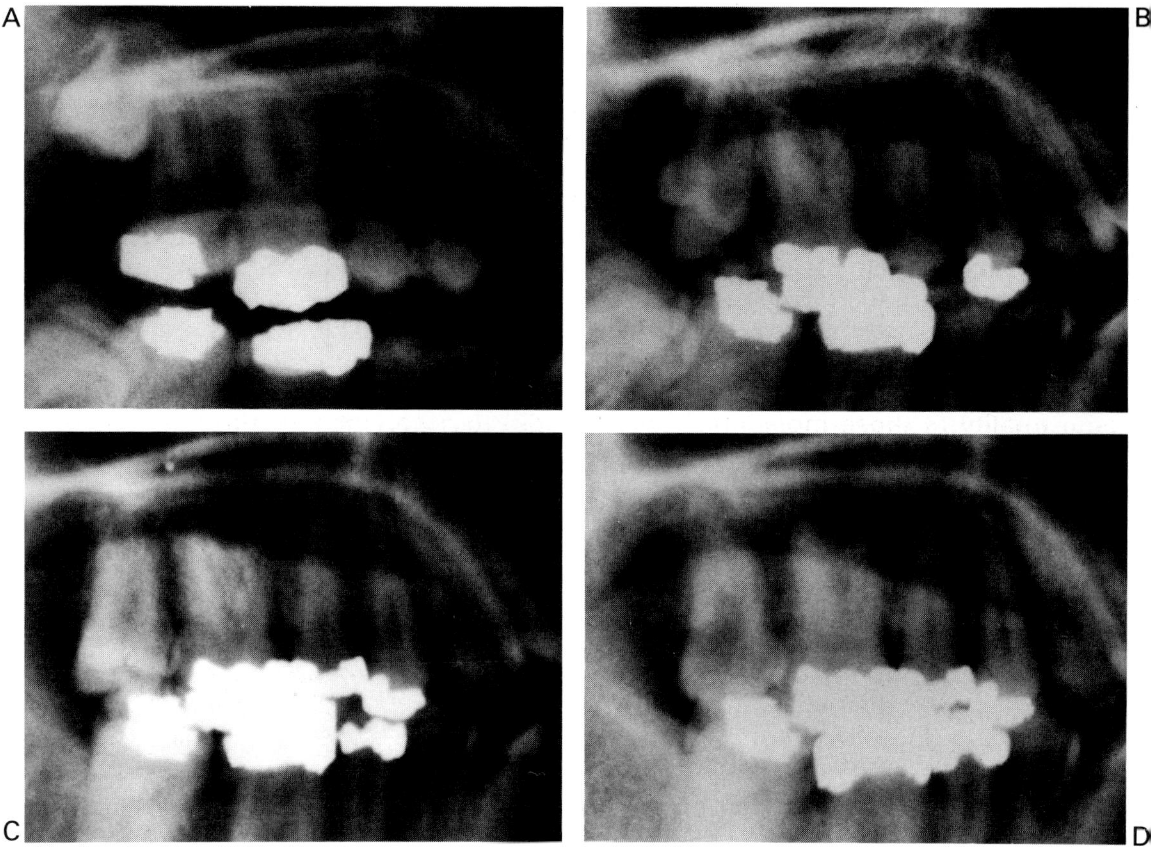

Fig 27-10 Parts of lateral cephalometric radiographs that illustrate the effect of removing the maxillary second permanent molars and mandibular third molars. On the radiographs, the left and right sides are superimposed, which makes interpretation a little difficult.

A At the age of 14 y, 2 mo, the maxillary third molars are distally angulated and located close by the apices of the second molars. In the mandible, the third molars are impacted and overlap the second molars. It was at this stage that the maxillary second molars were extracted.

B Two years four months later (16 y, 6 mo), the maxillary first permanent molars have been moved a little to distal at the conclusion of treatment.
The right maxillary third molar has emerged already, but the left one has erupted less far. They have drifted mesially from their original locations, reducing their angulation to distal. The mandibular third molars were removed shortly after this radiograph was taken.

C Two y later (18 y, 7 mo), the maxillary third molars occlude well with the mandibular second molars, which have improved in position and angulation.

D Another three years later (21 y, 7 mo) the roots of the molars have been evenly distributed within the available space. The third molars in the maxilla are now angulated to mesial.

no detrimental effects on function. To treat an open bite that is not associated with esthetically objectionable aspects is therefore usually unwise and should be avoided especially having regard to the great likelihood of root resorption taking place.
If an open bite is treated because the patient finds the abnormal alignment of the teeth to be unacceptable, then an estimate should be made of the degree of relapse to be expected. If the chance is great, and no relapse would be acceptable, then permanent retention will have to be used. This can be achieved by fixing a thin twistflex archwire palatally to the relevant teeth with composite. Another possibility is to mask later deficiencies by recontouring the teeth with composite additions. However, lengthening the crowns with composite provides only a temporary solution, since the tongue will exert pressure between the teeth once more.
The extraction of second permanent molars in the maxilla in a class II/1 anomaly can simplify orthodontic treatment. Reasons to consider this course of action might be poor quality of those molars and lack of room to accommodate all three molars in that quadrant. However, before extractions are performed, evidence should be obtained that the third molars are indeed present, well-formed, and normally located. In connection with the estimation of the space available for the three molars, it should be realized that use of a headgear will lead to a lessening of the growth of the posterior apical area.[31] In addition, the buccal tubes projecting from the first permanent molars will make it difficult to keep the buccal surfaces of the second molars well-cleaned. Furthermore, it has been demonstrated that after extraction of second permanent molars in the maxilla, the third molars — as long as they are not abnormally placed — will almost always assume a good position in the dental arch.[7] The time at which this procedure is done is not important as long as it is delayed until it is certain that the third molar crowns are well-formed.
Unilateral extraction of a second permanent molar in the maxilla should be considered in a class II/1 subdivision. The extraction of the second permanent molar on the side of the greater disto-occlusion makes it easier to correct the asymmetry. With a cervical headgear, whether or not supported by a maxillary plate, the first permanent molar and the premolars on that side can be moved to distal.
It seldom is the case that there is insufficient space for the third molars in the maxilla yet adequate space in the mandible. Whenever at an early age it is clear that it will not be possible for the third molars to come into the arch in the mandible, then a germectomy might be considered. The third molar germs can be removed with a relatively simple operation, with use of a sucker, as long as they are as yet uncalcified. This must be done at about the age of eight or nine years, so psychological concerns may provide a contraindication to such a procedure.
To conclude, it might be observed that the patient described here might not have looked much different in the long run if she had not had orthodontic treatment. Perhaps a late development of her face could have led to a reduction of the rather limited disto-occlusion, and maturity of her lip musculature might have caused her maxillary incisors to fall back a little. In the years during which she was treated, the information about tongue interposition previously given and in earlier cases was not yet available. At that time, it was considered that the tongue activity would be reduced as treatment proceeded. One can only entertain that hope if thumb-, finger-, or lip-sucking had been indulged in till about the time treatment was begun.

Chapter 28

Class II/1, anterior open bite
Parietal headgear, brackets 12, 11, 21, and 22, positioner
Female: 11 years, 1 month to 30 years, 6 months

A girl aged 11 years, 1 month exhibiting a disto-relation, had a class II/1 anomaly combined with an open bite extending from, and including, the canines on the left to the first premolars on the right. The involved teeth showed no vertical overlap and a gap of 3 to 4 mm existed between the opposing incisors. She sucked two fingers intensively with the lips closing around those fingers when they were in place. From this it was evident that she could breathe freely through her nose although generally she kept her mouth open. Her tongue, which appeared to be relatively large, was pressed between the anterior teeth during swallowing and lay between them when at rest. There was a suggestion of a lisp, though it could been due to the existence of the open bite rather than being a basic speech defect. A disto-occlusion of ½ PW existed on both sides with an overjet of 7 mm. Enamel hypoplasia could be seen on the maxillary incisors (Figs 28.1 and 28.2).

The decision was made to attempt to eliminate the finger-sucking and to correct the abnormal jaw relationship with the use of a parietal headgear. At a later stage it would be necessary to use a partial fixed appliance to retract and extrude the maxillary incisors.

At the age of 11 years, 3 months, the headgear was fitted. The finger-sucking had stopped by that time. Six months later, the maxillary anteriors were banded with the band material extended cervically to the gingival margins to protect the enamel. To begin with a .0175" twistflex archwire was used; three months later, this was replaced with a solid .019" × .026" archwire (Figs 28.3 and 28.4).

At the age of 12 years, 9 months, the appliances were discarded. A positioner was provided for minor corrections (Figs 28.5 and 28.6). This positioner was worn for two months for some hours during the day, and all night. After this, the positioner was worn at night only and with reducing frequency for seven months. The records obtained subsequently show a slight return of the open bite with an accompanying increase in the overjet (Figs 28.7 and 28.8).

Five years later at the age of 18 years 6 months, the picture was barely altered. There is tertiary crowding now in the mandibular anteriors and the posterior teeth occlude slightly more mesially, especially on the right. In addition, the midline deviation has more or less vanished as has the lisping (Figs 28.9 and 28.10). The records taken ten years later indicate that the situation at the time just described was already stable. It satisfied the needs of function and esthetics, particularly in the latter after composite

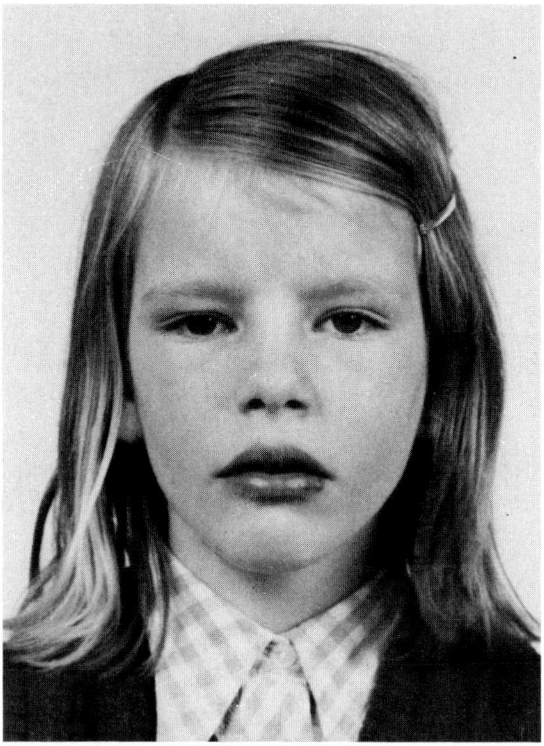
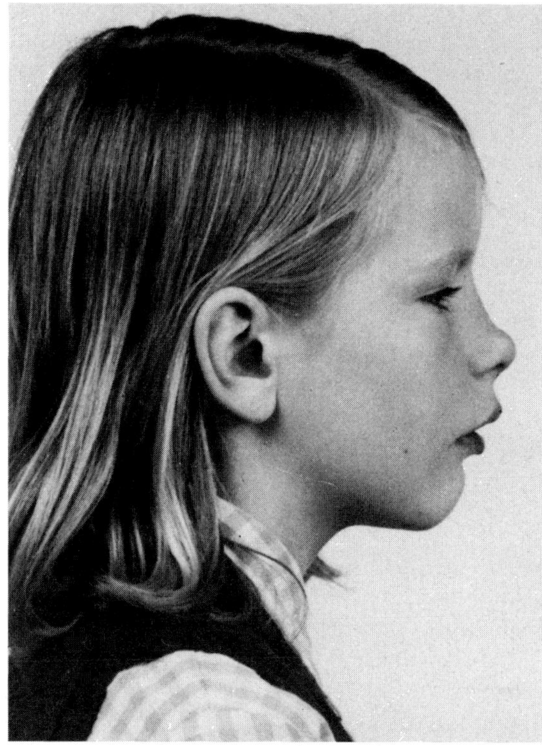
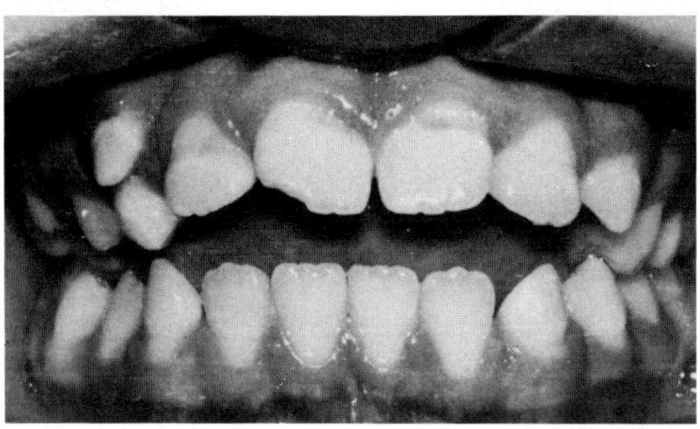
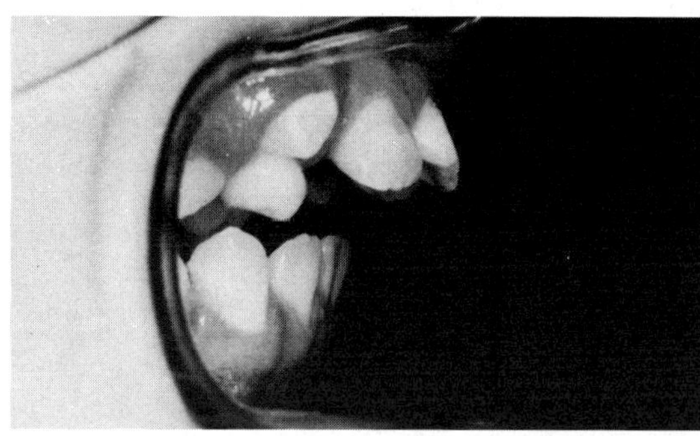
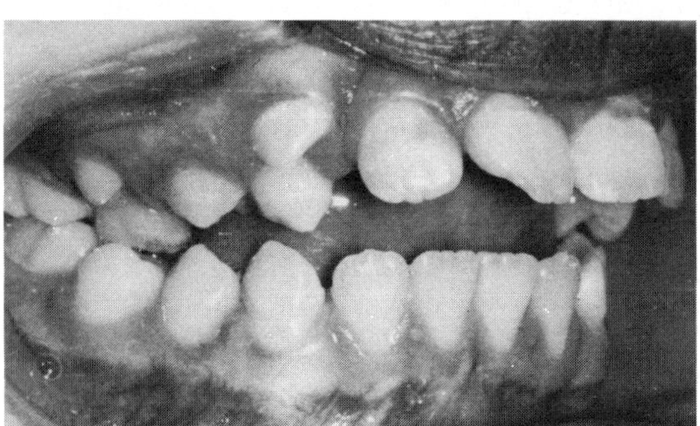
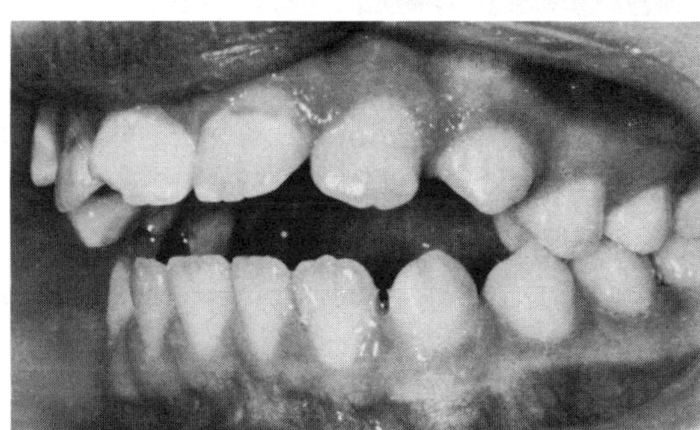

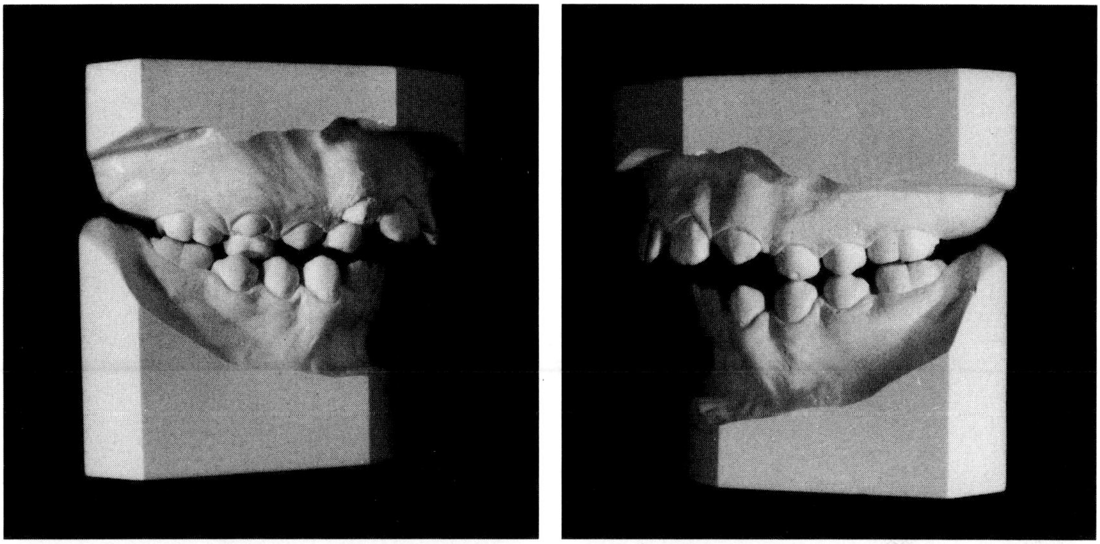

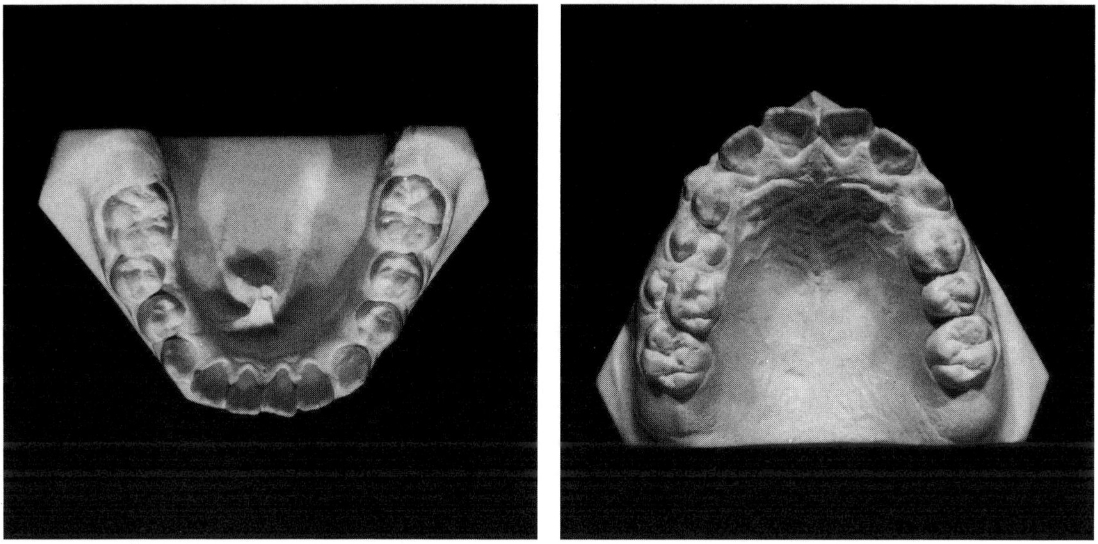

Figs 28-1 and 28-2 *A girl aged 11 y, 1 mo presented with a disto-relation, a class II/1 anomaly of ½ PW and an anterior open bite from, and including, the canines on the left to the first premolars on the right. She sucked vigorously on two fingers and if she was not doing that she held the anterior part of her tongue between the dental arches when at rest, but particularly during swallowing and speaking. The maxillary incisors show enamel hypoplasia and the distal incisal angle of the maxillary right central incisor has been fractured. The overjet is 7 mm and the middle of the mandibular dental arch is 2 mm to the right of that of the maxillary arch (the intraoral photograph of the left side was taken with the mandible posed too far ventrally).*

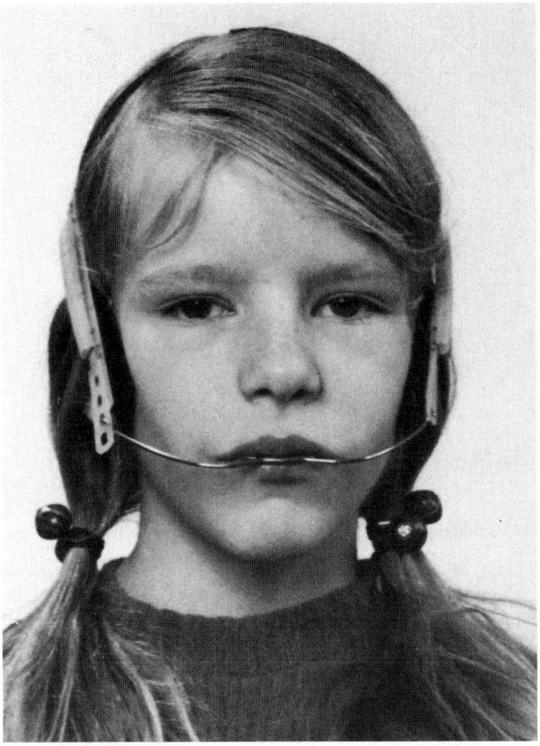

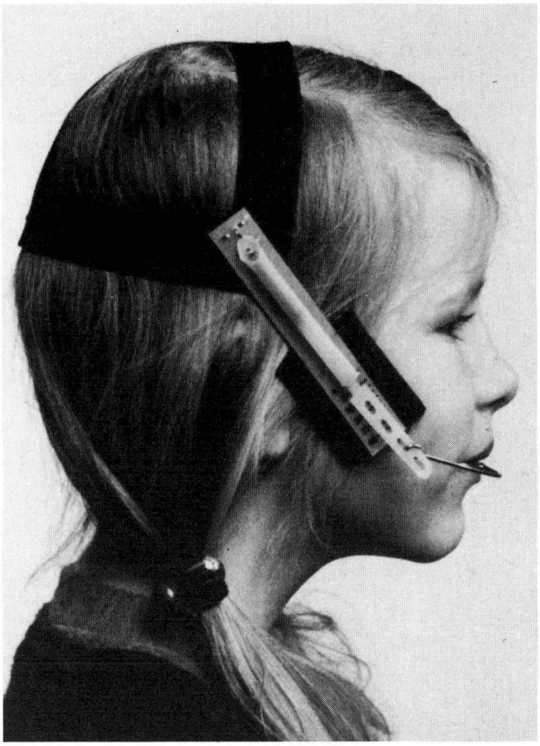

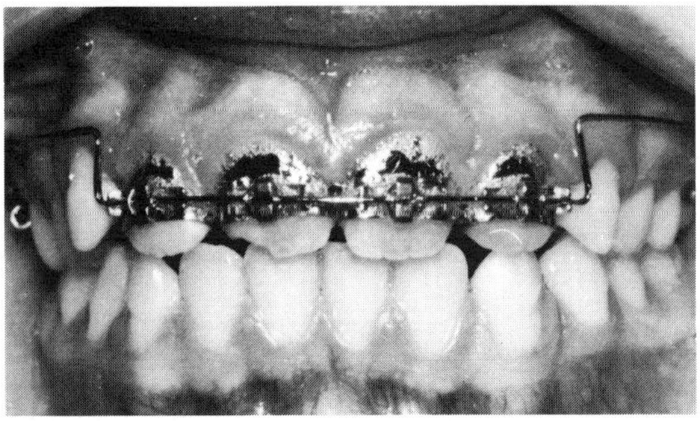

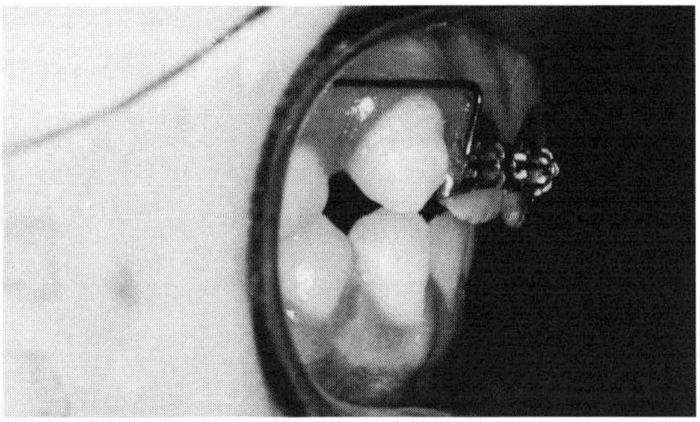

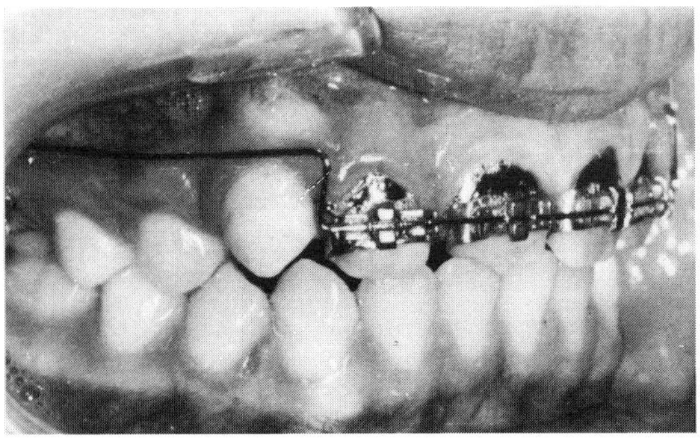

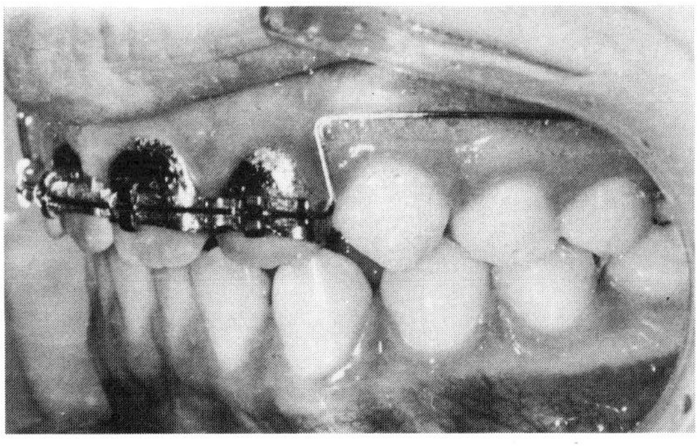

Fig 28-3 The situation at the age of 12 y, 2 mo, eleven months after the beginning of treatment. Bands with edgewise brackets have been placed on the maxillary incisors. Initially a .0175" twistflex archwire was used and thereafter a .019" × .026" rectangular arch to retract and intrude the maxillary incisors. The bands have been extended to the cervical margins labially to protect the hypoplastic enamel. A parietal headgear could be used via double molar tubes.

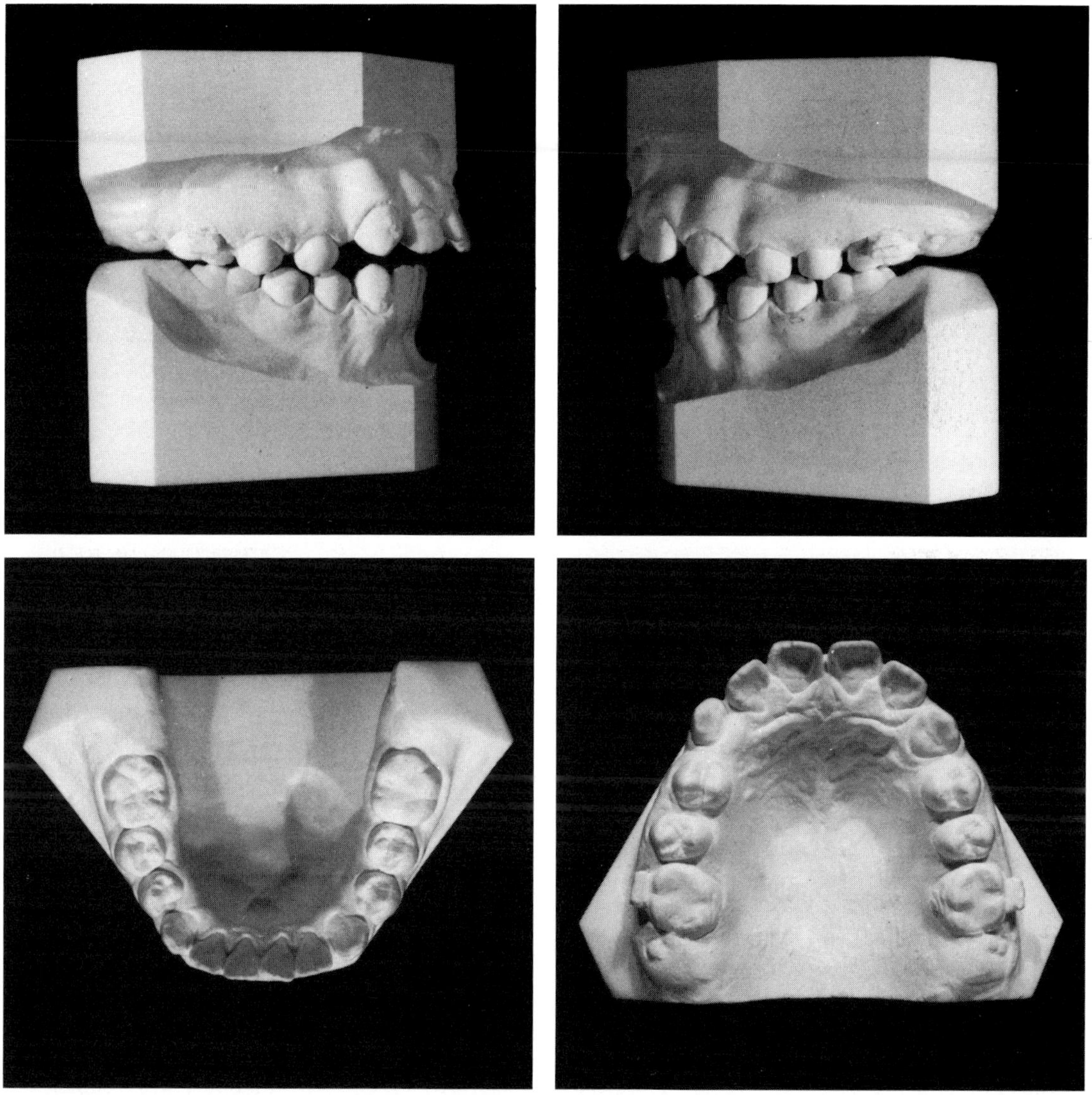

Fig 28-4 Dental casts of the situation prior to fitting the partial fixed appliance, at the age of 11 y, 9 mo. In the molar region a neutro-occlusion has been obtained but the anterior open bite has been only minimally reduced.

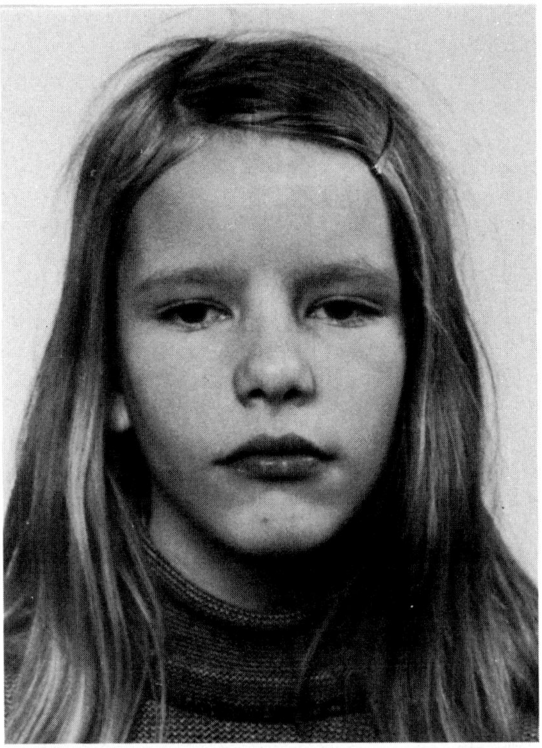
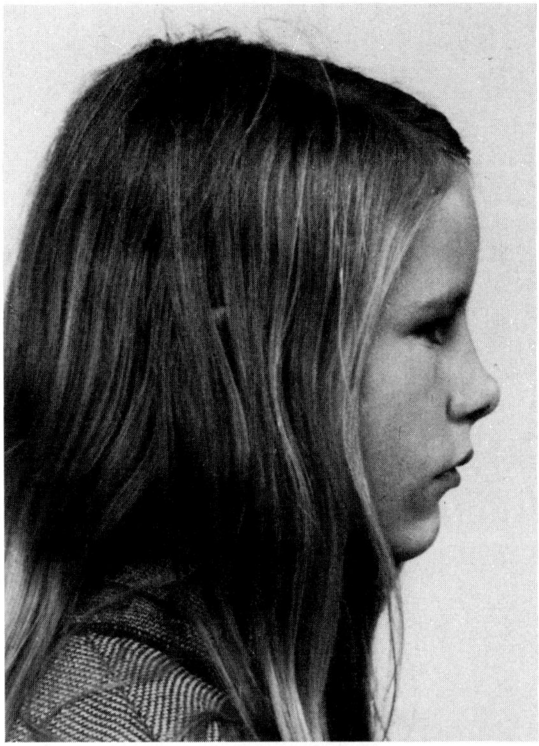
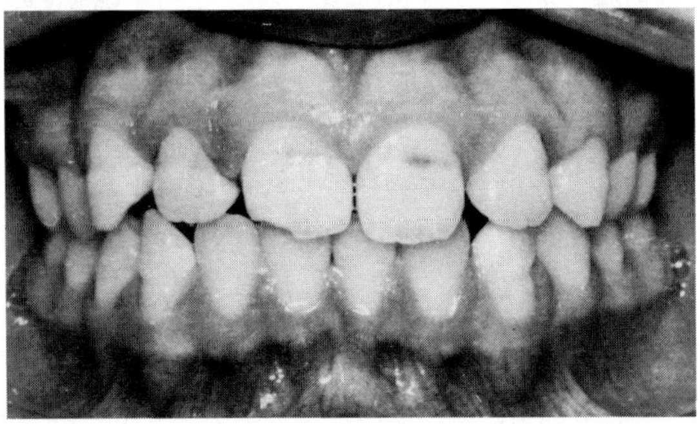
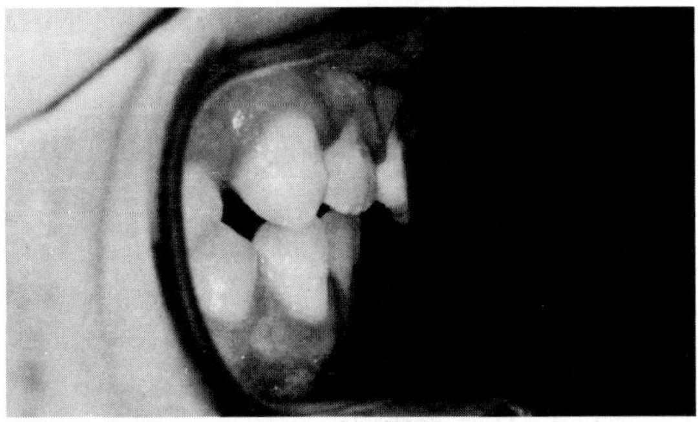
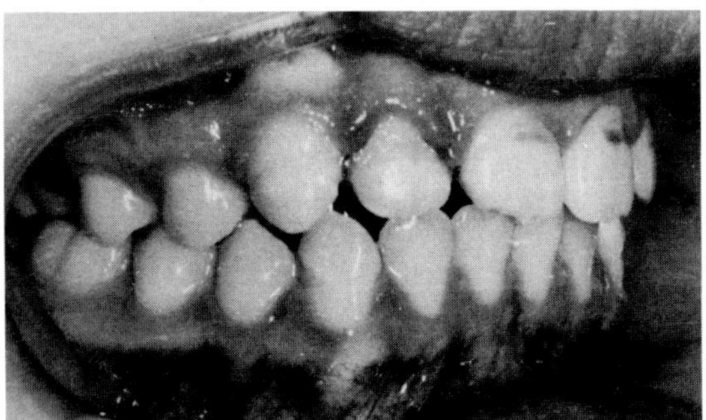
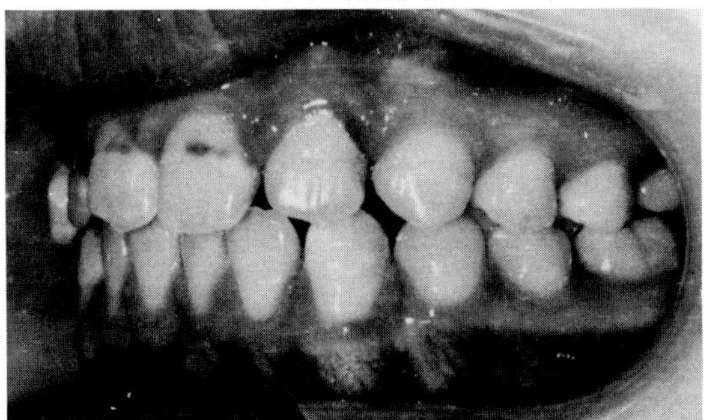

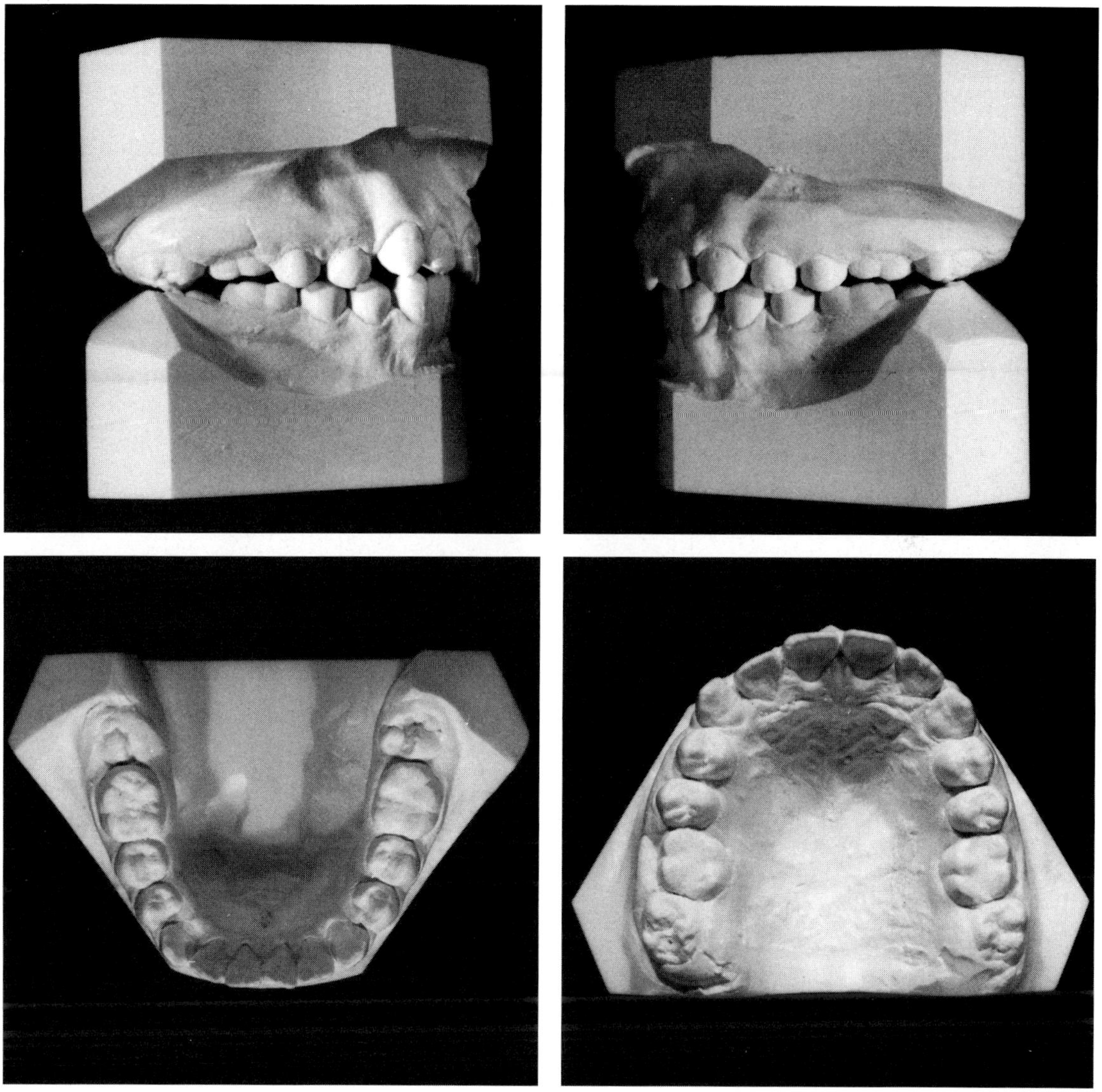

Figs 28-5 and 28-6 At the age of 12 y, 9 mo after an active treatment time of 1½ years the appliances have been removed and a positioner provided. The patient, who had stopped sucking her fingers before treatment commenced had by now learned to keep her mouth closed at rest. The profile is noticeably improved. The maxillary and mandibular incisors make contact, although the overbite is shallow. The parietal headgear has caused the maxillary first permanent molars to assume an infraposition. Moreover they are now too far palatally, something that in part can be attributed to the lack of occlusal contact. Because of the fact that the maxillary canines were not included in the appliance, the position of the canine on the right is not ideal. Nor has the midline discrepancy been corrected.

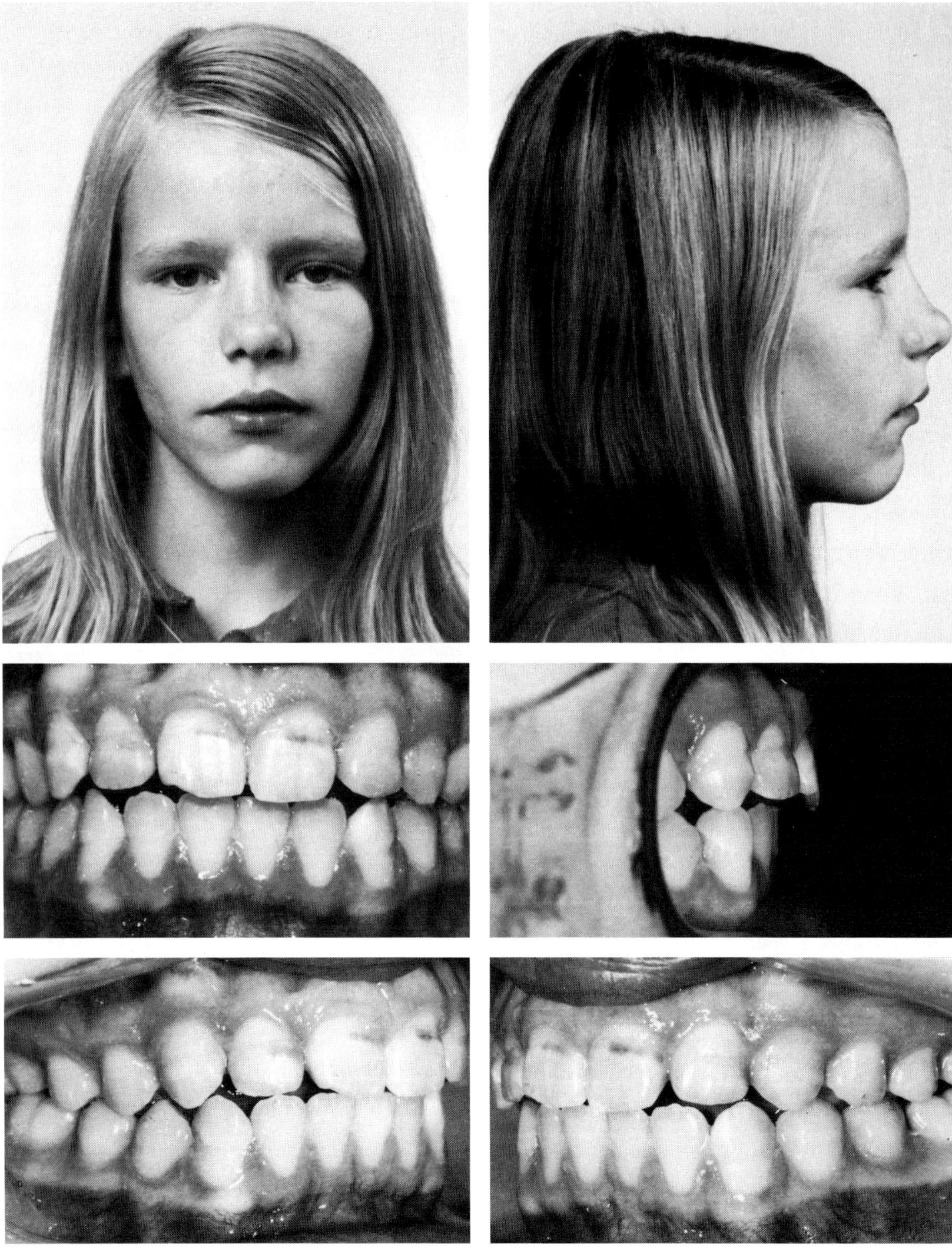

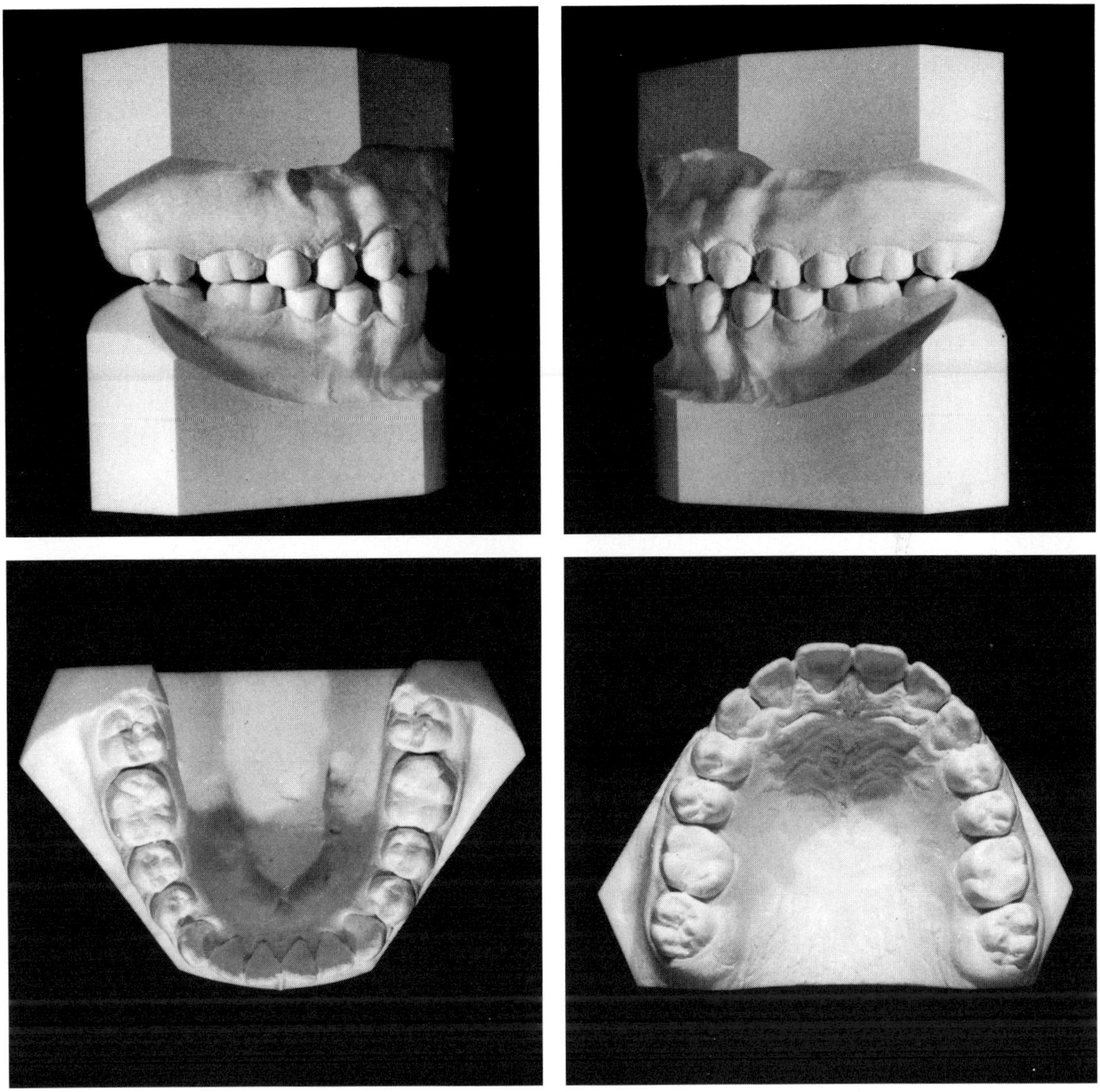

Figs 28-7 and 28-8 At the age of 13 y, 6 mo the use of the positioner has been stopped after a gradual reduction in wearing time. There is a slight open bite anteriorly again due to the maxillary incisors moving into mild infra-position and the overjet increasing. The use of the positioner has resulted in an improvement in the positions of the maxillary canines, with partial correction of the midline deviation. Furthermore, the position of the maxillary first molars has been changed. The latter depended primarily on the working of the cone-funnel mechanism once occlusal contact had been reestablished and probably would have occurred even if the positioner had not been used.

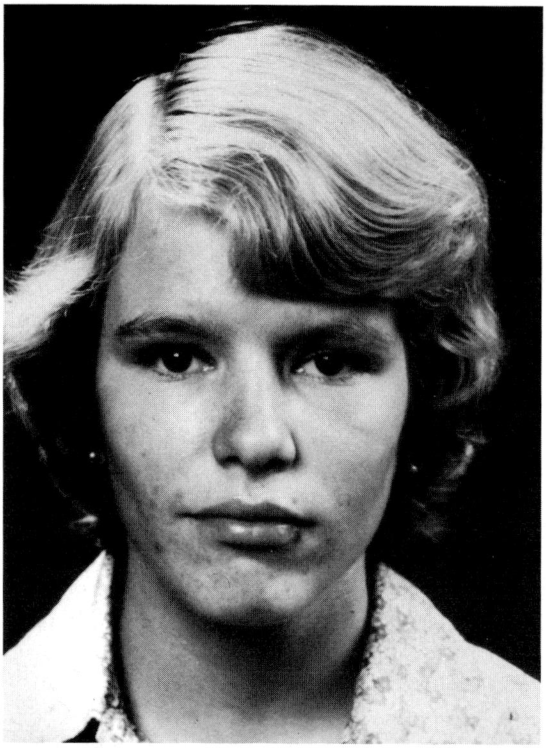
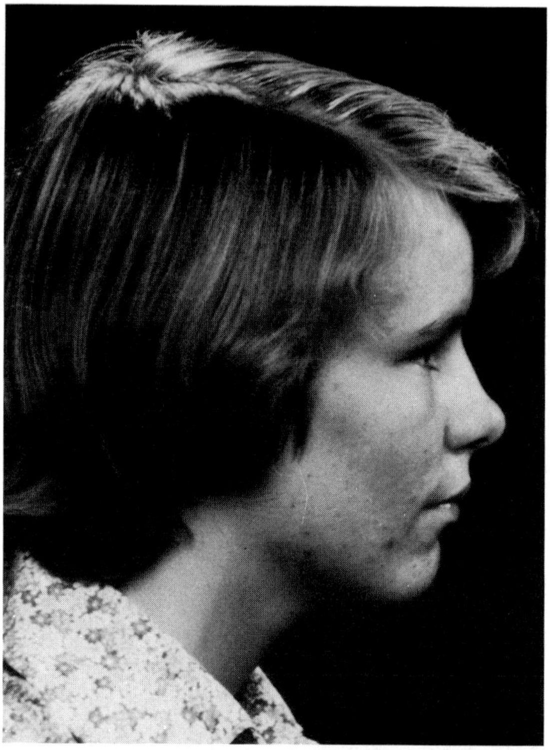
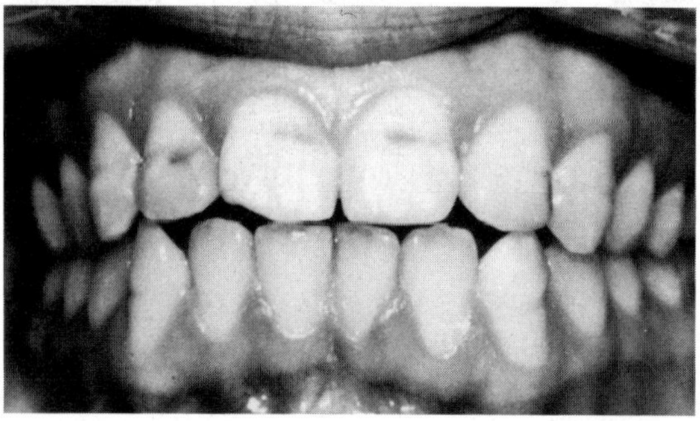
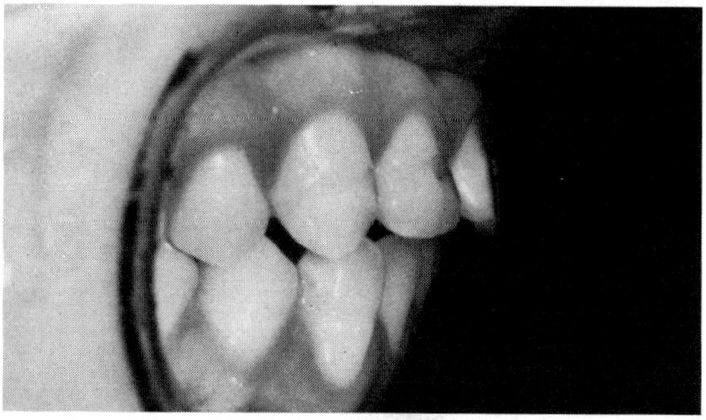
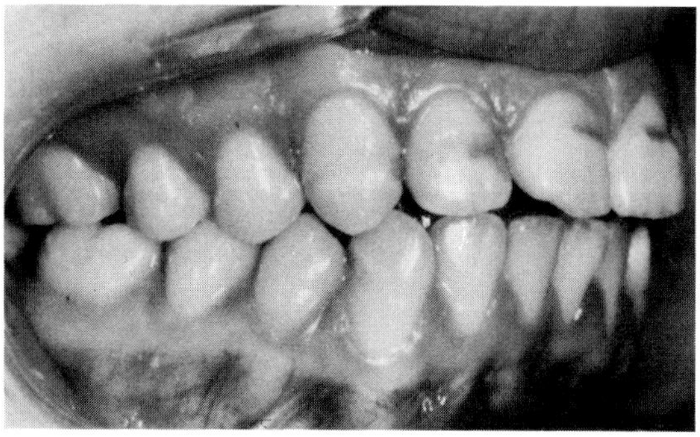
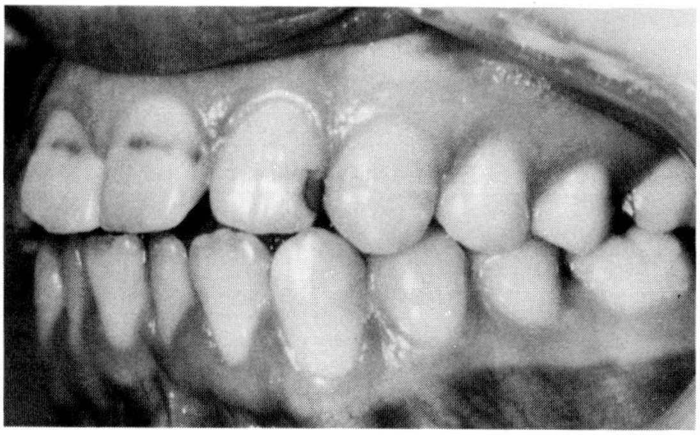

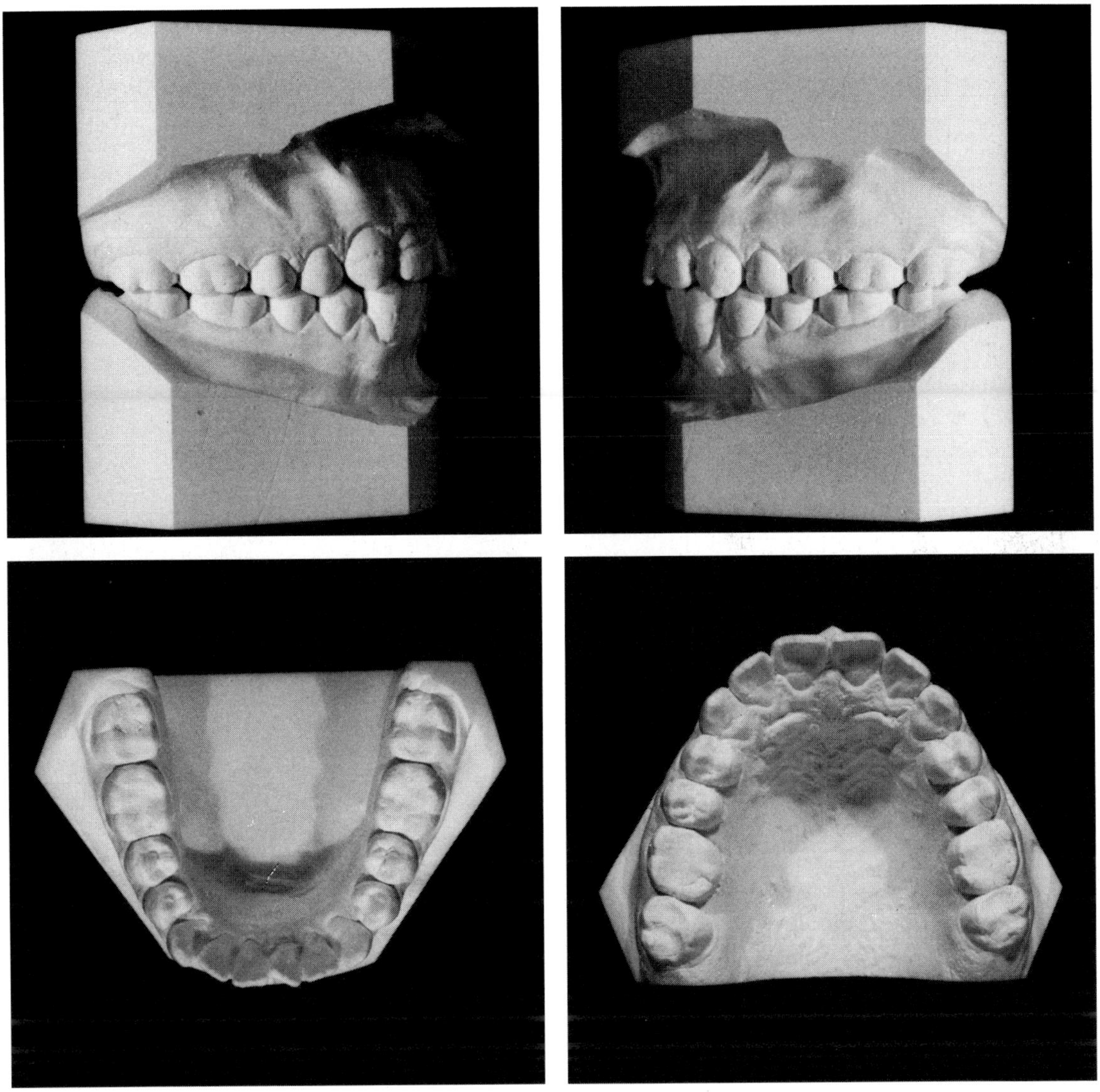

Figs 28-9 and 28-10 At the age of 18 y, 7 mo, five years after the use of the positioner had stopped, her face has matured. The mandibular dental arch has moved somewhat to mesial, especially on the right. There also exists a solid interdigitation of the posterior teeth and canines on the left. The mild crowding that originally was present in the mandibular anteriors has increased in the past five years; in particular, the mandibular left central incisor has rotated more. In addition the midline deviation has now more or less vanished.

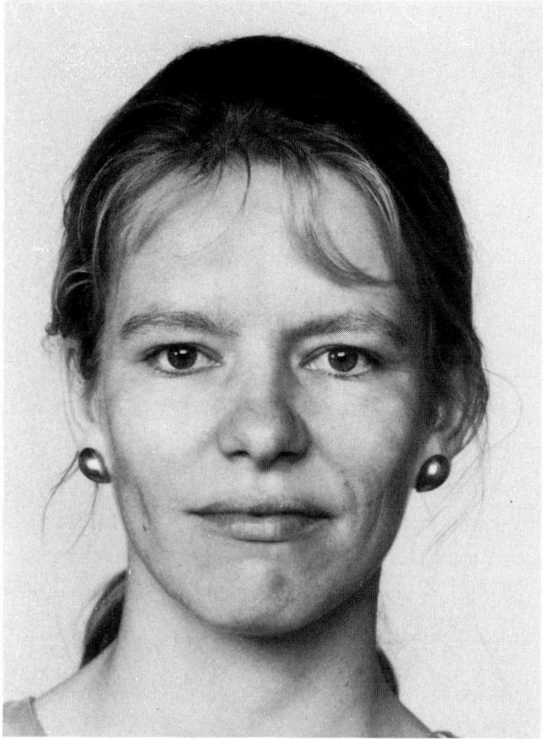

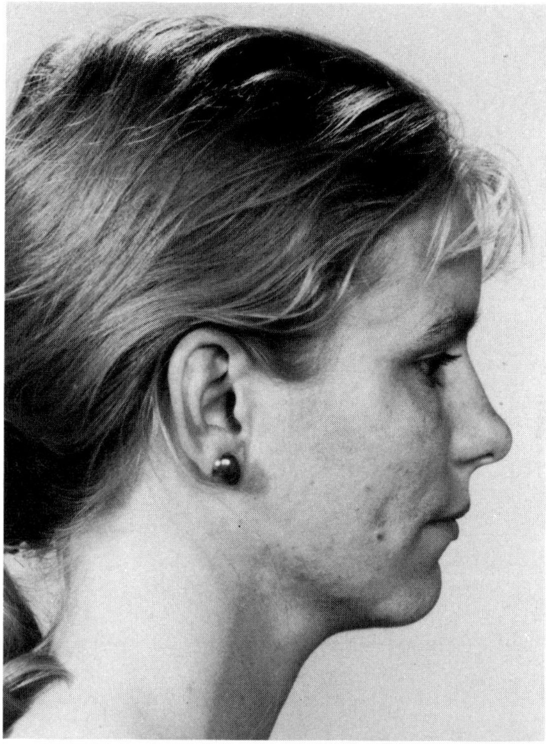

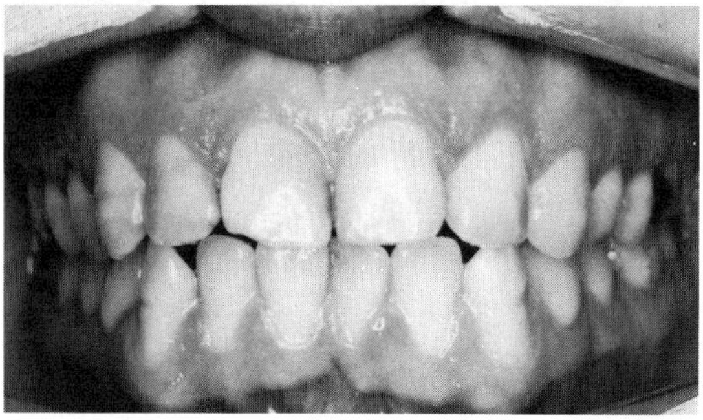

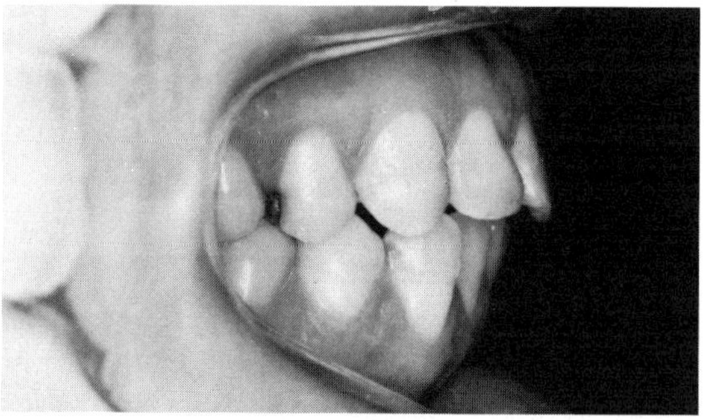

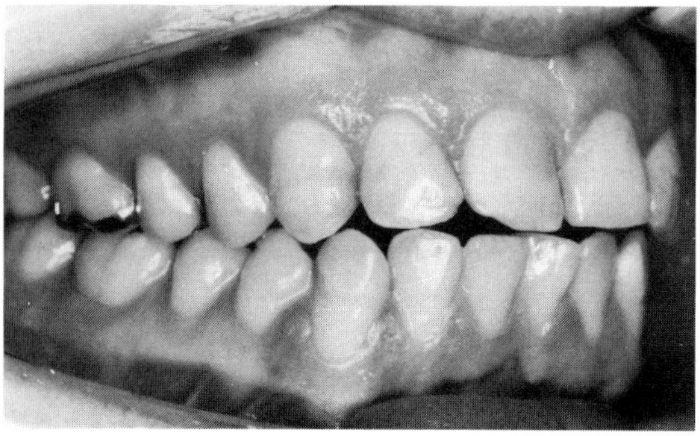

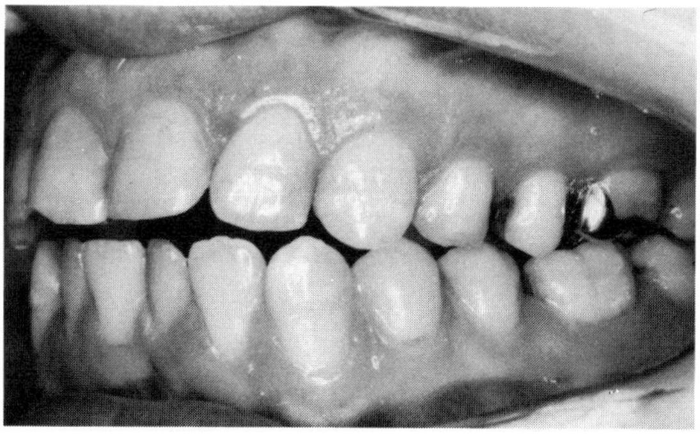

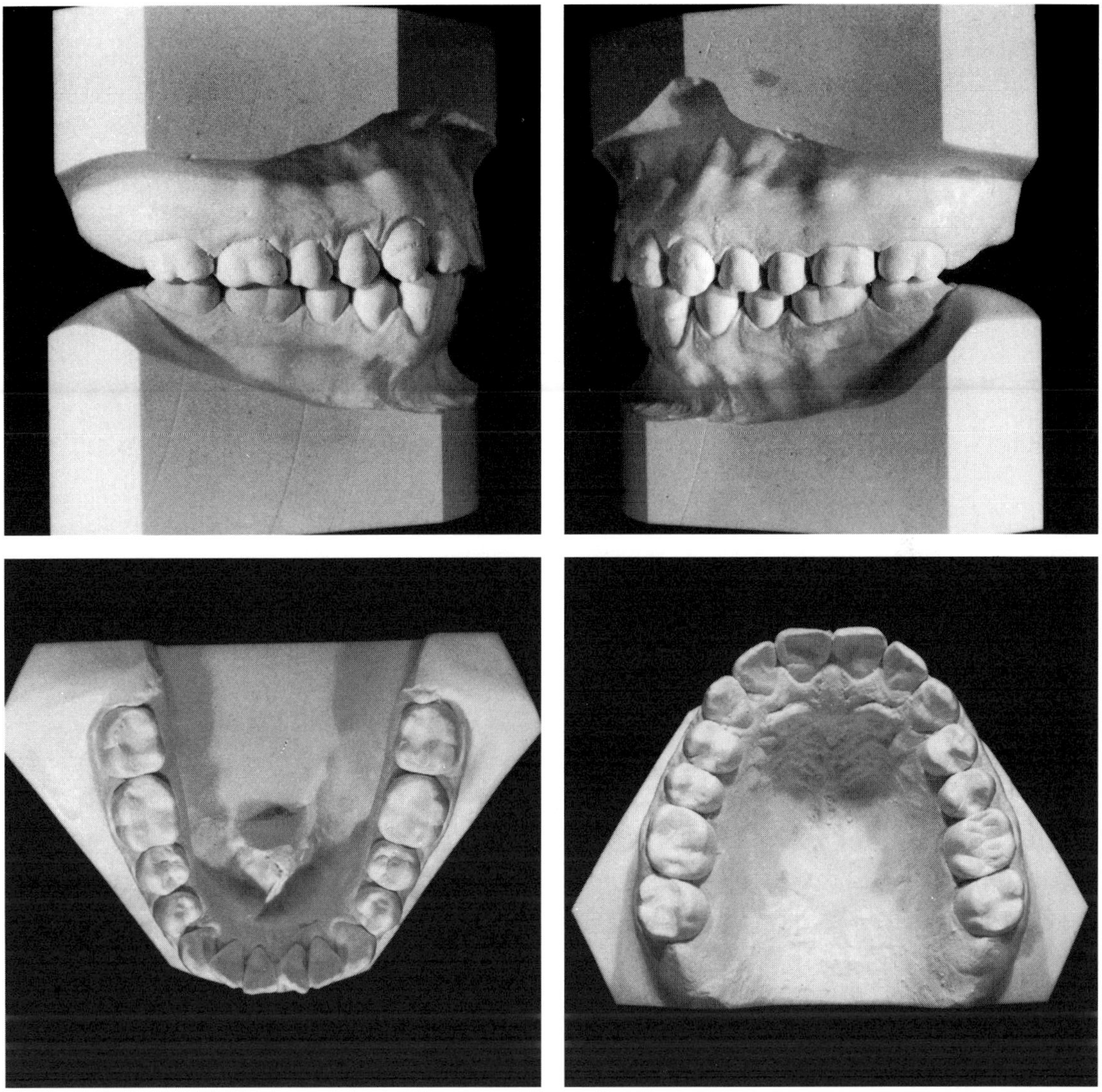

Figs 28-11 and 28-12 *At the age of 30 y, 6 mo, the situation is satisfactory. A harmonious face is combined with a presentable dentition; this has been complemented by the use of composite to restore the hypoplastic defects in the enamel of the maxillary incisors. The teeth function well and the anterior open bite presents no problems. (The intraoral photograph of the left side is not in habitual occlusion.)*

Figure 28-13a

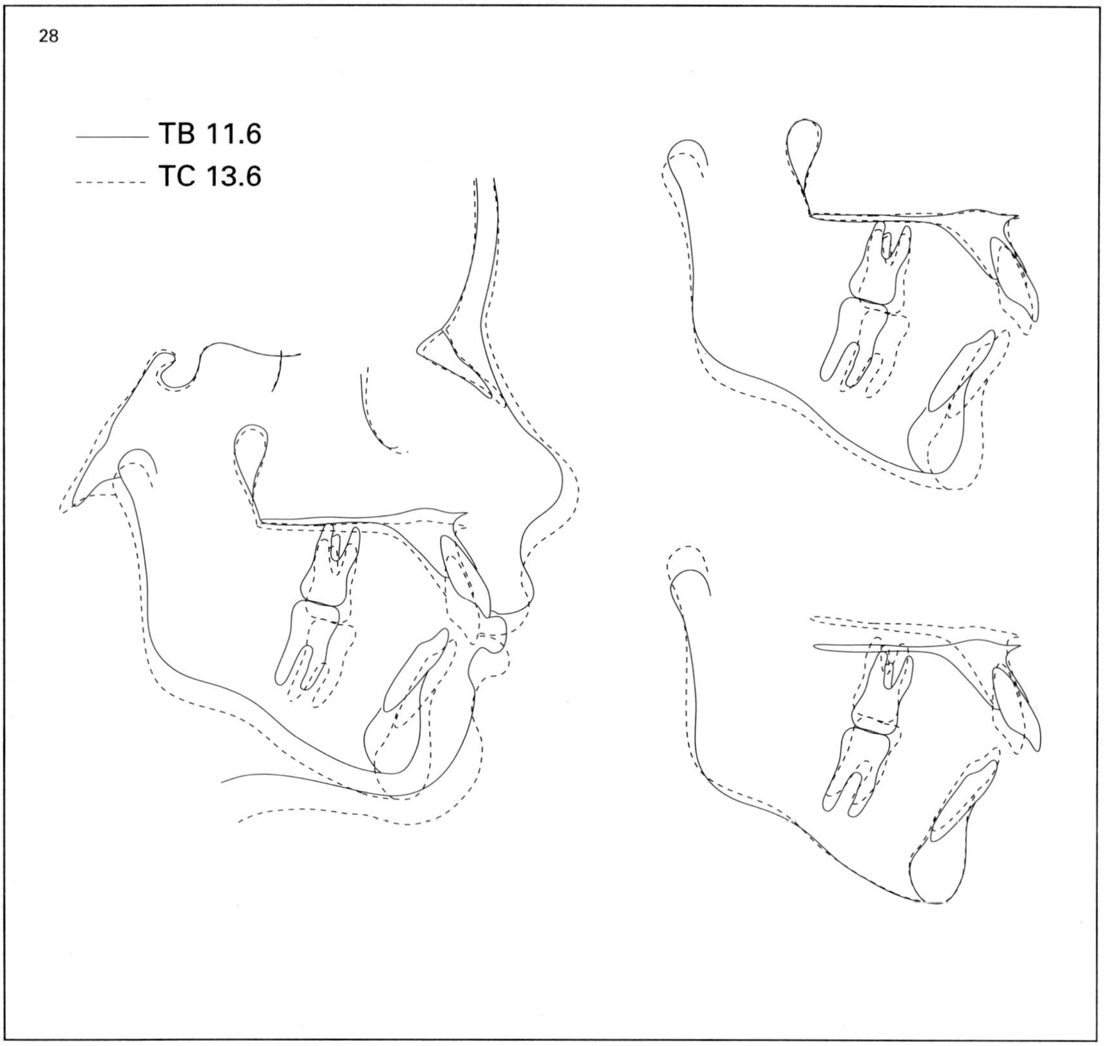

Fig 28-13 Superimposition of tracings of the cephalometric radiographs. During treatment, the ventral development of the maxilla was impeded while the mandible grew ventrally and caudally. The maxillary anteriors have been retracted and extruded. The lower-face height has only increased a little and the steepness of the lower border of the mandible has decreased. The growth that followed the treatment was normal; there is no indication at all of excessive vertical growth.

Figure 28-13b

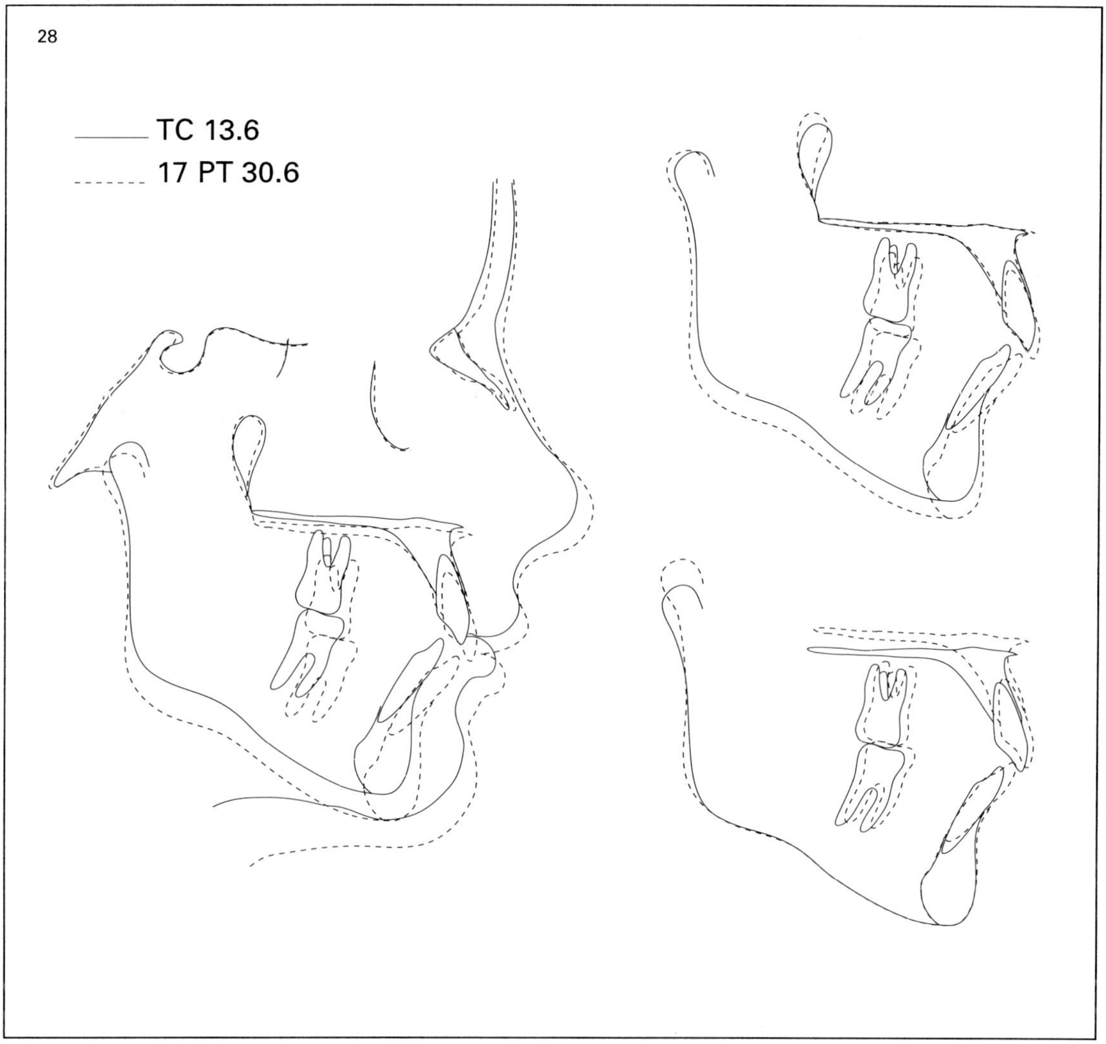

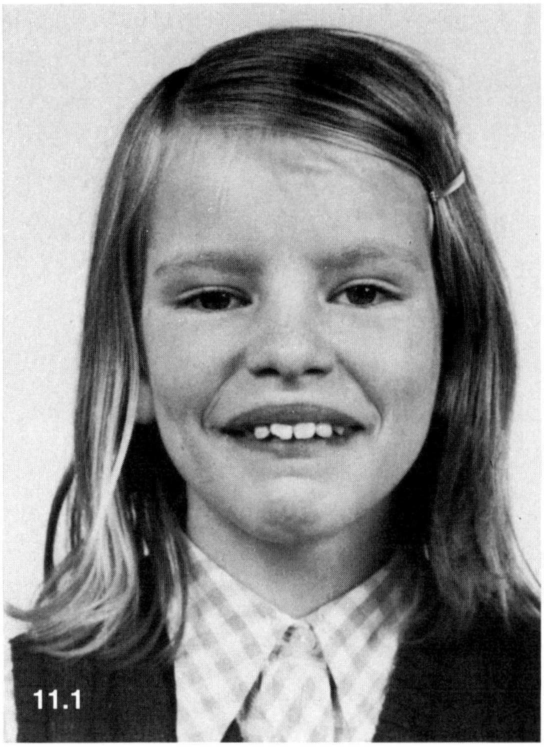
11.1

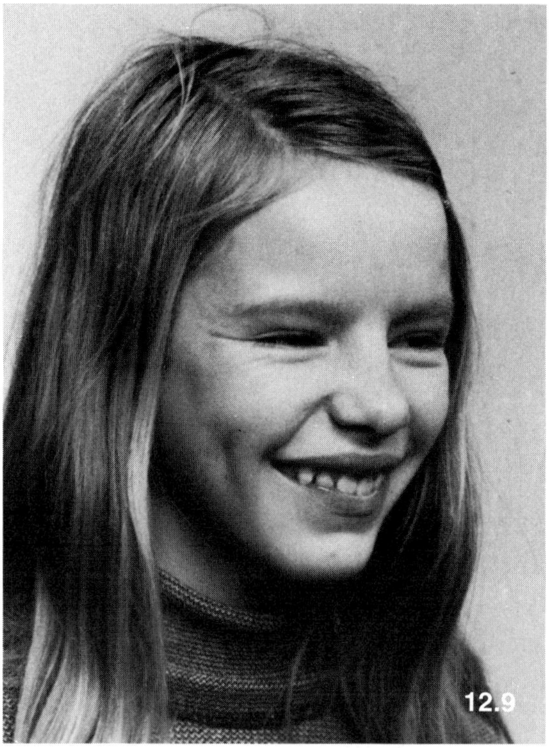
12.9

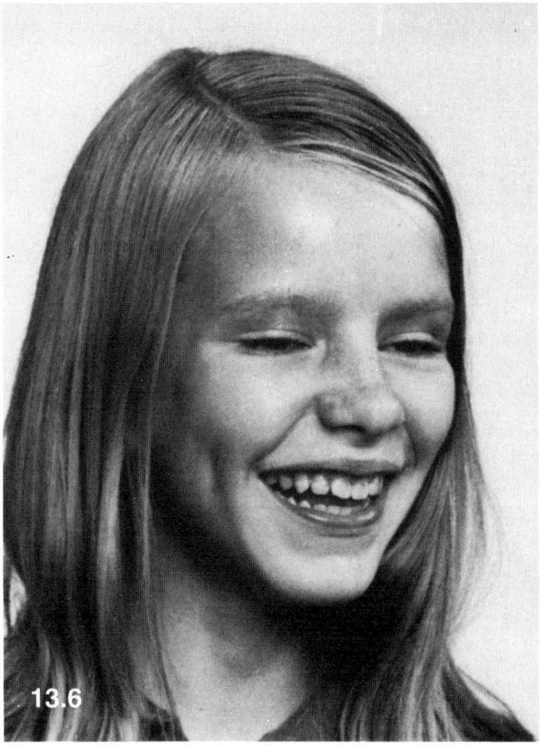
13.6

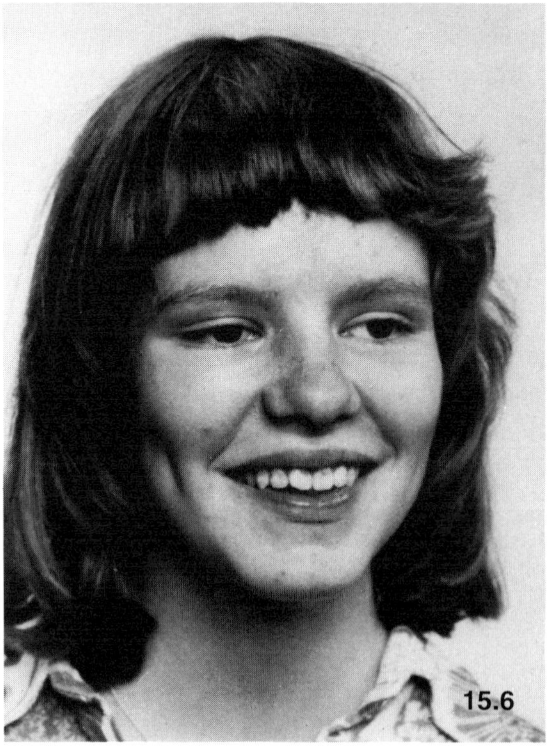
15.6

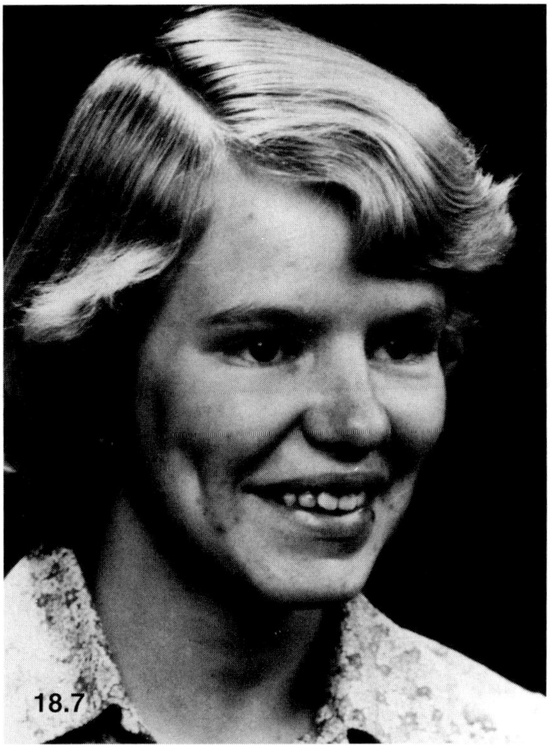

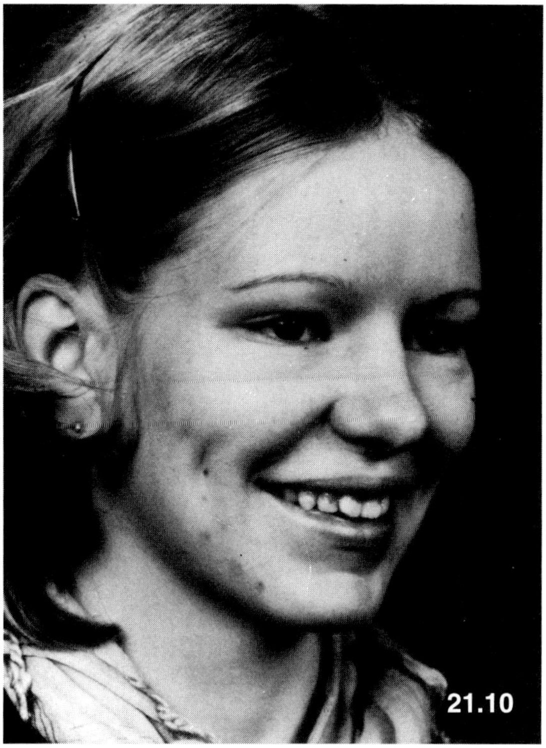

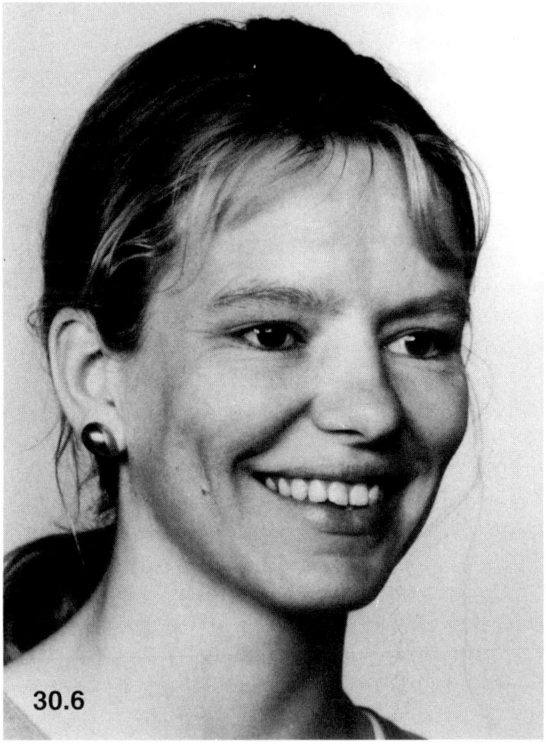

Fig 28-14 Note the changes that accompanied the treatment and growth. The effect of different hairstyles on her appearance is evident. Here is a harmonious face with dentition that functions well.

had been used to hide the hypoplastic defects in the enamel of the incisors (Figs 28.11 and 28.12).
Superimposition of the tracings from cephalometric radiographs, as well as examination of the photographs of the patient's smiling face, show that during treatment and the subsequent growth, the lower face height did not increase abnormally. Indeed, the steepness of the inclination of the lower border of the mandible had decreased (Figs 28.13 and 28.14).

As has already been pointed out, the prognosis for treatment of an anterior open bite is relatively favorable when the patient has been sucking thumb or fingers and given up the habit recently. This is especially true when the patient has been closing the lips around the thumb or fingers to secure a good seal, thus indicating that a clear nasal airway is available. If in addition the face, particularly the lower face, is not unduly high and the mandible is of normal form with a reasonably horizontal slope of the mandibular lower border, one can expect that orthodontic treatment will not lead to a deterioration of the facial configuration and external appearance. That is, excessive lengthening of the face and especially of the lower third of the face need not be feared. A slight relapse of the open bite after it has been closed is by no means unlikely. That depends on whether or not tongue interposition is still present after treatment has ceased. If the original tongue behavior was of a secondary character, being used to close off the open bite caused by the thumb-sucking, rather than creating the open bite by interposition, then a relapse is unlikely. If the sucking habit had been associated with tongue interposition of a neuromuscular origin (primary), then relapse, even partially, of the open bite can be anticipated. As described in the previous chapter, there is a return after intervention to the environment that existed originally.
It is only some time after concluding treatment that it can be determined if an open bite that was associated with thumb- or finger-sucking incorporated tongue interposition of neuromuscular origin. It is wise to begin with the assumption that this is the case, since that would require a treatment strategy that anticipates a partial relapse of the open bite and malalignment of the incisors. It is also important that normal lip closure be developed since if that is present it will substantially reduce any tendency of the maxillary incisors to move labially again.
A tongue that appears a little too large at the beginning of treatment is not in itself a bad sign. In a few years, the picture can change naturally. Maturation of the face involves different rates of growth in its components so that the skeleton may grow more than the tongue as occurred in this case.
This patient was given no permanent retention because adequate lip closure was evident during treatment and the alignment of the maxillary incisors prior to banding was not irregular. Moreover, as the retention provided by the positioner was gradually reduced, no significant changes occurred.
In retrospect, the question can be asked whether or not a cervical headgear could have been used instead of the parietal one. It can be supposed that the eventual result would have been little different; but during treatment, the first permanent molars would have remained in occlusion and not moved palatally. However, it was still valid to choose a parietal headgear in view of the size and extent of the open bite and the risk that the extrusion of the anchor molars that a cervical headgear can

produce — at least during treatment — might have resulted in an undesirable increase in the length of the face, in particular the lower face.
This case shows similarities with the one of Chapter 26 in that they both had a class II/1 anomaly and a large anterior open bite. They differed considerably, however, where functional conditions were concerned, in facial configuration, the form of the mandible, the steepness of the lower border of the mandible, and the course of the treatment and the development that followed.
It is difficult to differentiate between the two kinds of patients with an open bite. Besides the factors previously mentioned, there are less obvious differences: differences in head posture, facial animation, the use of facial musculature, lip posture, manner of speaking, smiling and swallowing, the position and movements of the tongue and lips together, all of which combine to make a picture whose elements must be taken into account when attempting to categorize these patients.
Not all patients with an open bite can be placed together into one group. In making the diagnosis, it is desirable to make the best possible estimate of whether or not the progress of treatment can be expected to be favorable. If the outlook is not favorable, then serious consideration should be given to refraining from intervening. Should it nevertheless appear that treatment is indicated, it must be decided if that treatment should best be limited to correcting disturbing malalignment of teeth and then providing permanent retention.
Finally, some remarks are in order regarding the possibilities and limitations of myofunctional therapy in providing the permanent elimination of tongue interposition.
It is repeatedly and emphatically proven that it is possible by means of speech therapy to obtain a permanent correction of tongue behavior during speech and for the learned pattern of behavior to become subconscious. However, there is a significant difference in this between speaking and swallowing. Speaking is a learned, controlled, conscious activity; swallowing is a subconscious automatic function that originates in reflexes. There are no data from which it can be concluded that the pattern of swallowing can be permanently influenced by myofunctional exercises, nor that by such means an orthodontic anomaly can be ameliorated. It can be maintained that the implementation of those forms of myofunctional therapy that have been developed to date with the purpose of correcting so-called aberrant patterns of swallowing is of no value. If nonetheless one thinks that such an attempt should be made, it would be wise to limit that activity to an attempt to improve the rest position of the tongue and lips and not to undertake that until after the age of 10 years is reached.[19, 22, 29]

Chapter 29

Class II/1, total open bite
Suture expansion, cervical headgear, maxillary plate
Male: 13 years, 1 month to 26 years, 2 months

A boy aged 13 years, 1 month exhibited a class II/1 anomaly and facial asymmetry with a more ventral development of the mid-face on the right than on the left side. He was able to breathe through his nose easily and still sucked his thumb regularly. His tongue was large and at rest lay between the occlusal surfaces of the posterior teeth, also covering the mandibular incisors. When swallowing, and during speech, the tongue was held between the dental arches both anteriorly and posteriorly. There was an open bite overall and the dental arches only came into contact fortuitously. Consequently, the maxillary and mandibular dental arches did not match, with the result that the too narrow maxillary arch did not meet the mandibular arch properly. Upon closure into central relationship, the midlines of the dental arches coincided but the only contact was between the buccal cusps of the first permanent molars. When asked to close the teeth together, occlusion was achieved through swinging the mandible to the right until the canines on that side came into contact. As a consequence, the midline of the mandibular dental arch was then displaced 3 mm to the right (Figs 29.1 and 29.2).

To secure a significant broadening of the maxilla in a short time, rapid maxillary expansion was chosen. Subsequently, the disto-occlusion would be corrected with a cervical headgear. Because the oral hygiene left something to be desired originally, and several cavities still needed restoration, it was not until the age of 13 years, 9 months that the expansion appliance was cemented in place. The thumb-sucking had in the meantime been abandoned. After four weeks, the expansion screw had almost reached its limit without achieving the increase in width required. Therefore the acrylic of the plate on one side was cut through in the mouth, the screw turned back, and the two halves of the plate re-united with rapid-curing self-polymerizing resin so that the expansion could be continued (Fig 29.11). By the age of 13 years, 11 months, the necessary width had been reached and a cervical headgear was fitted. Three months later, the expansion plate was removed. It was assumed that by then the reorganization of the bone in the region of the midpalatal suture had been completed and that if a plate was used with divided labial arches to retract the maxillary incisors, it would also provide adequate retention to maintain the expansion. The first permanent molars were rebanded with the object of continuing to wear the cervical headgear. Eight months later, a new plate was provided, embodying a "tongue barrier" on each side with the intention to alter the position of the tongue.

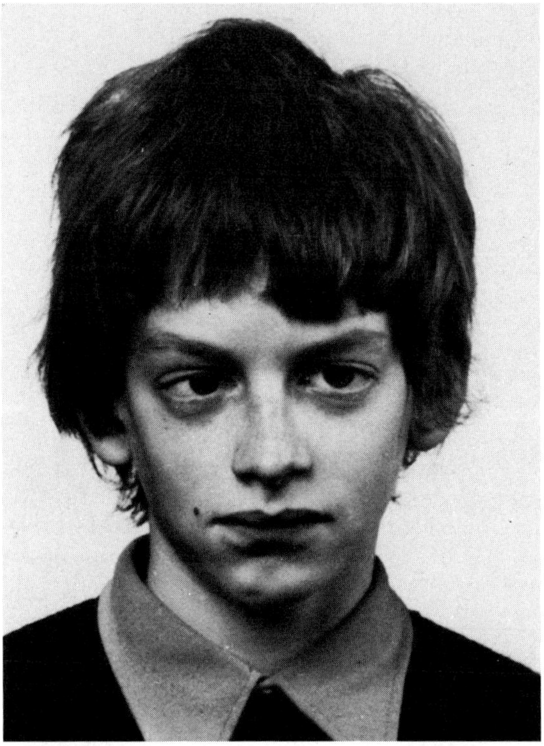

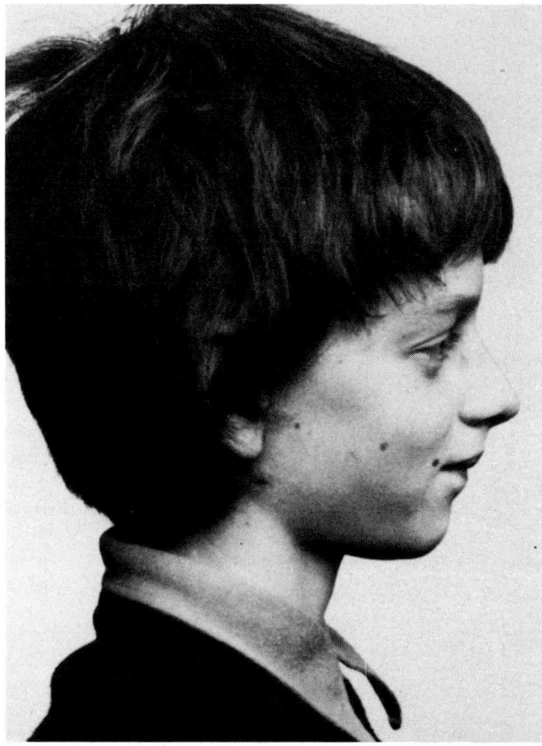

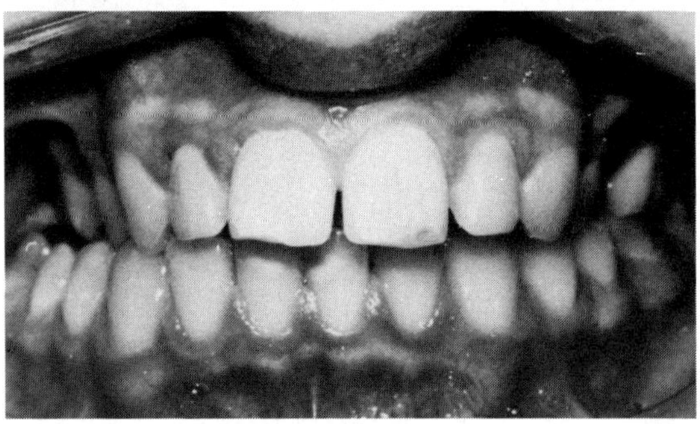

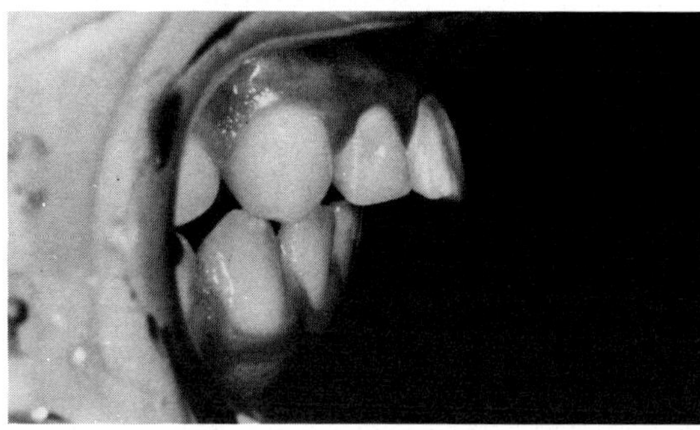

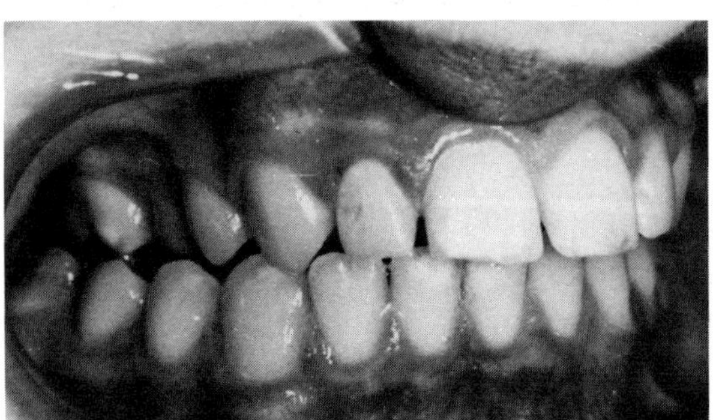

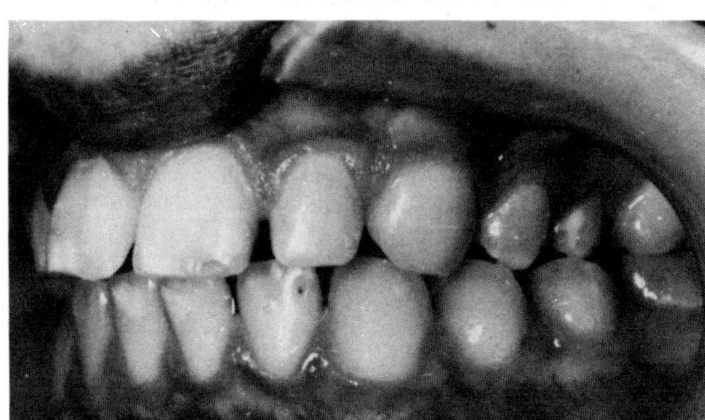

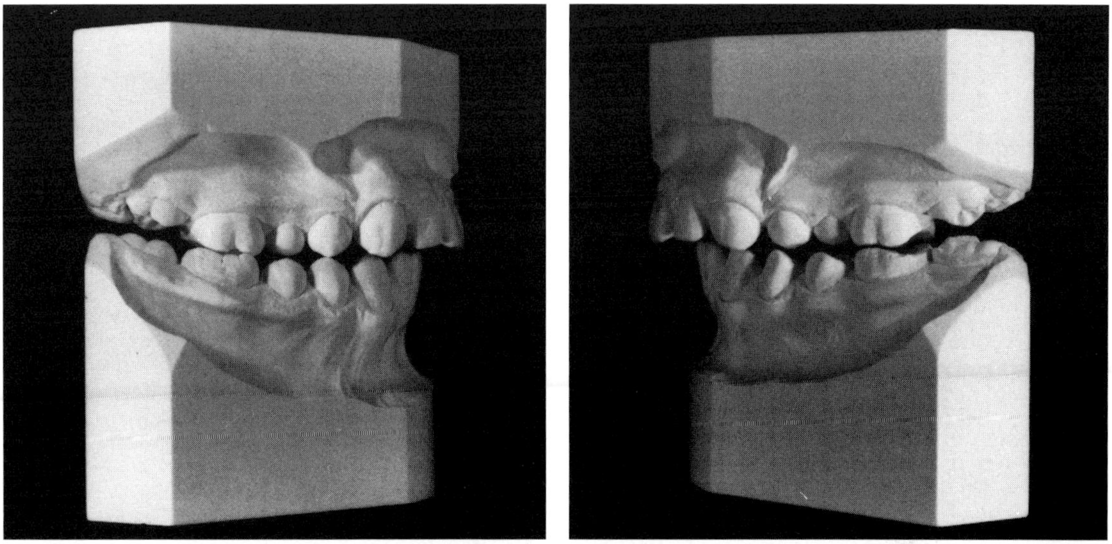

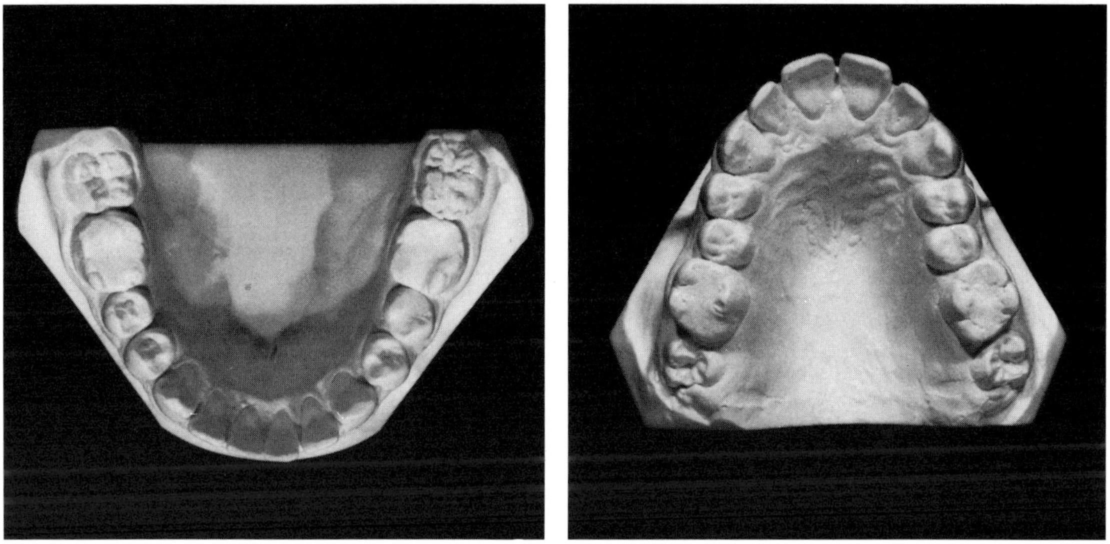

Figs 29-1 and 29-2 *A boy aged 13 y, 1.mo presented with facial asymmetry, a class II/1 anomaly (¾ PW disto), clear nasal airway and adequate lip closure. The intraoral photographs were taken after asking him to close his teeth together, which resulted in one contact on both sides between the first molars and on the right between the canines. In this process, the mandibular arch midline came to be 3 mm further to the right than when in central relation. Because the tongue lay between the teeth at rest and when swallowing, there had been no mutual adaptation between the maxillary and mandibular dental arches. The dental casts have been photographed in central relation; in so doing ,they make contact artificially in just a few places. The mandibular dental arch displays hardly any abnormality. The maxillary arch is too narrow and shows labioversion of the incisors. The overjet is 8 mm while the maxillary and mandibular incisors barely overlap vertically.*

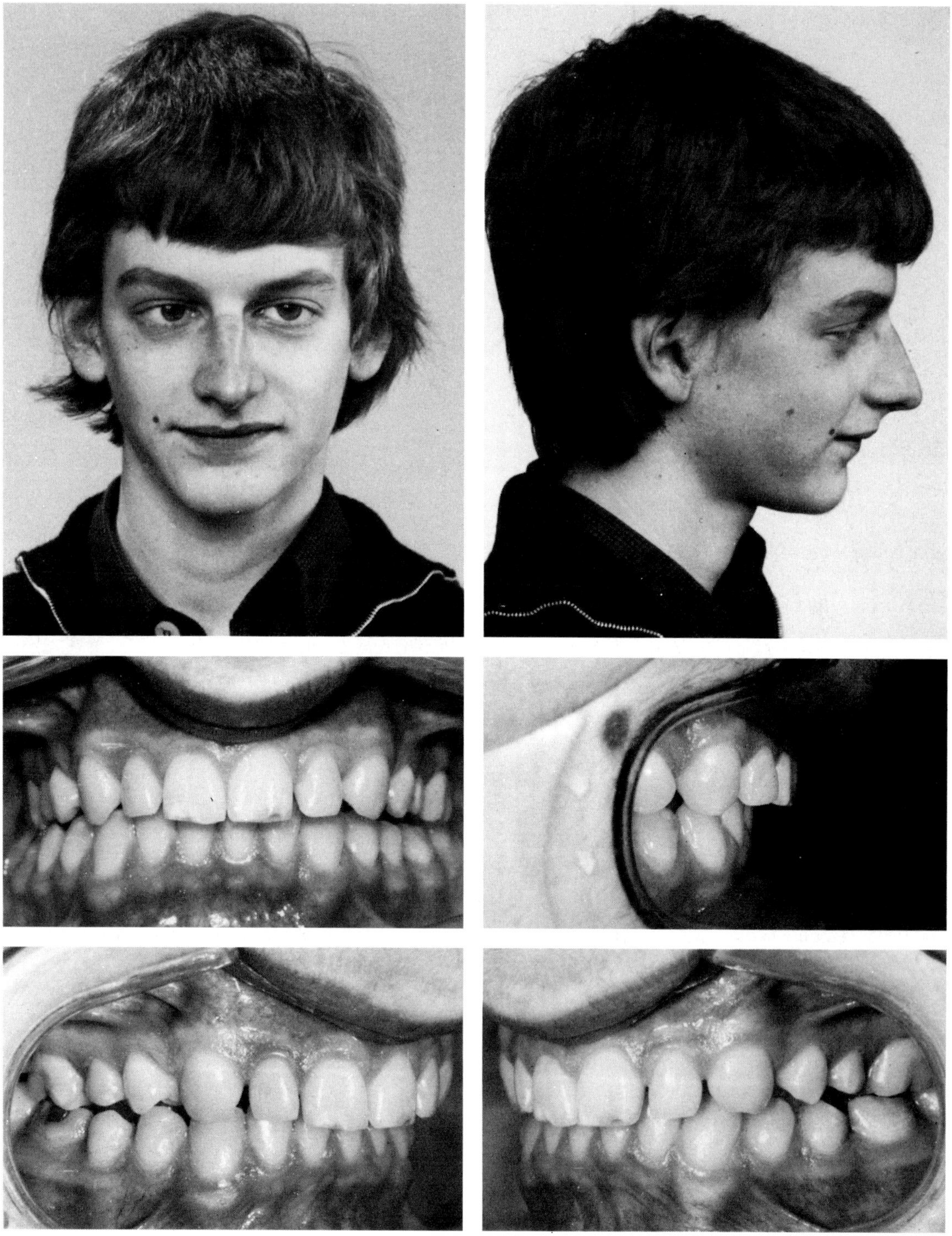

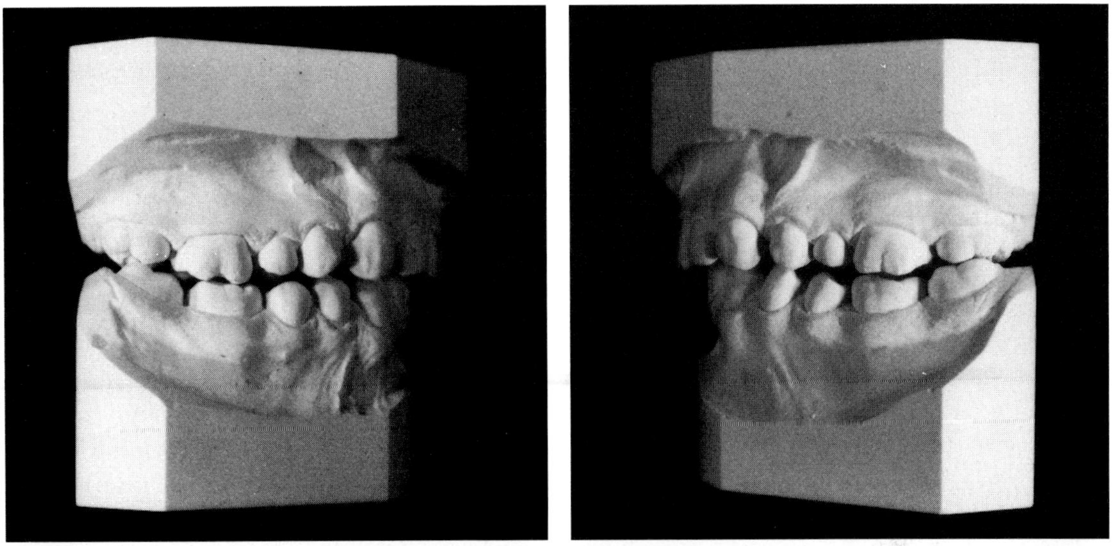

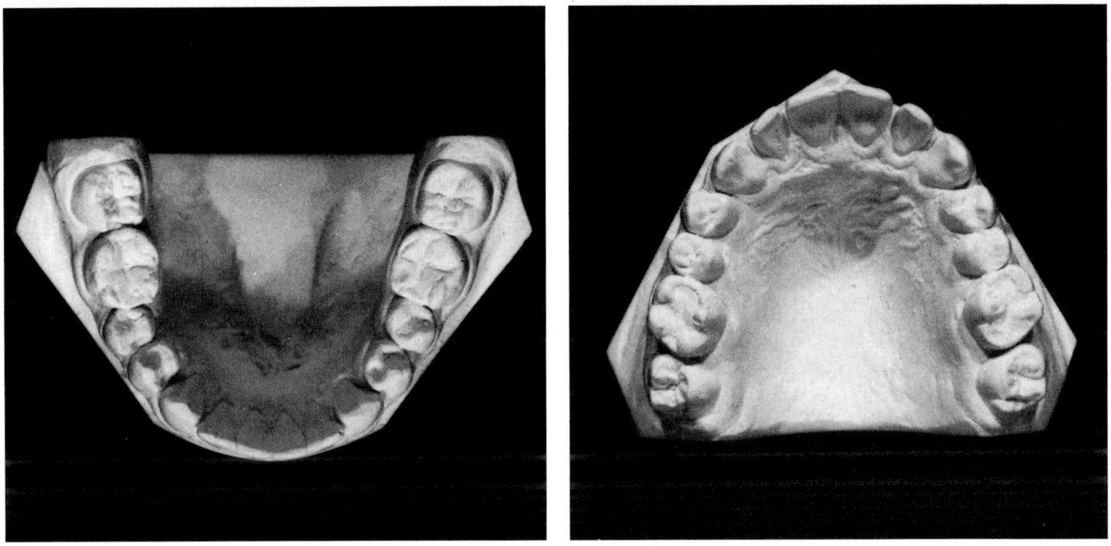

Figs 29-3 and 29-4 *At the age of 16 y, 3 mo, after treatment for 2½ years, the mandible has taken up a more ventral position. The maxillary dental arch now matches the mandibular arch reasonably well in width but the occlusion does not show satisfactory interdigitation. The teeth only meet in a few places when the patient is asked to close his teeth together. The plaster models have been photographed in artificial relationship. Both dental arches are of normal shape but have no mutual coordination in their occlusion. The overbite has increased a little.*

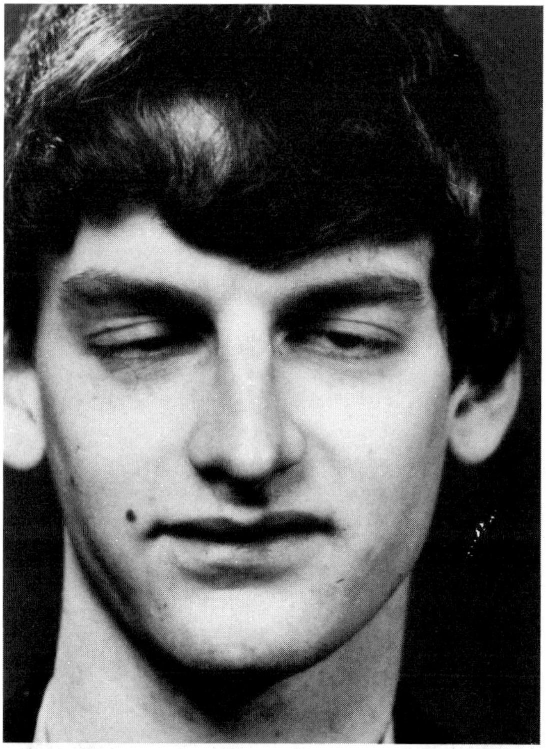
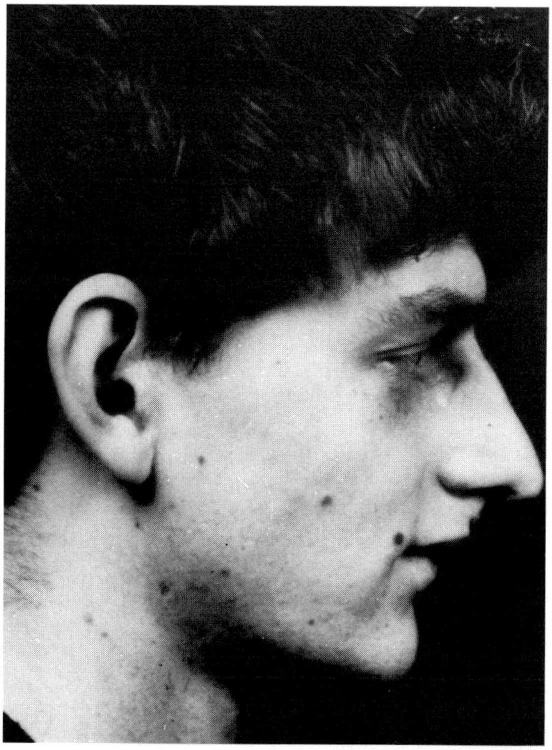
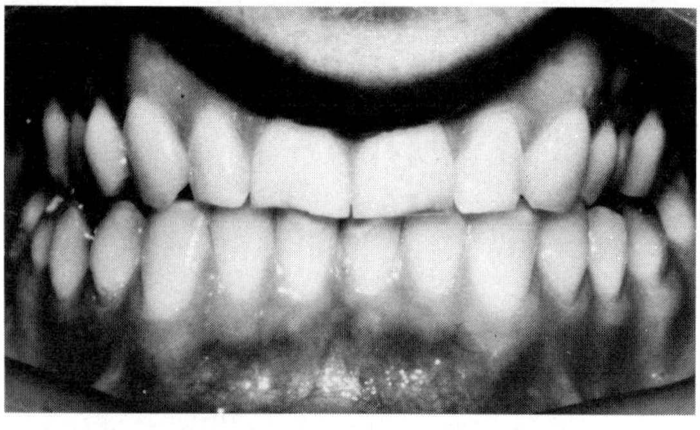
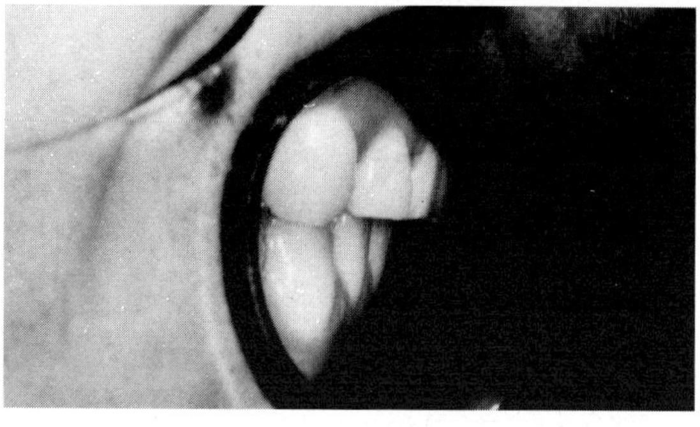
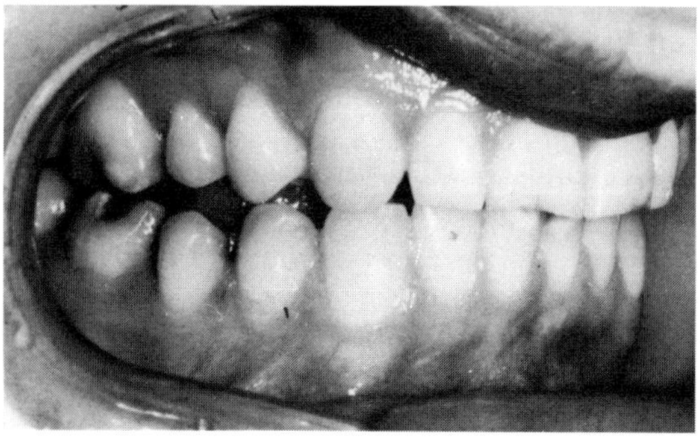
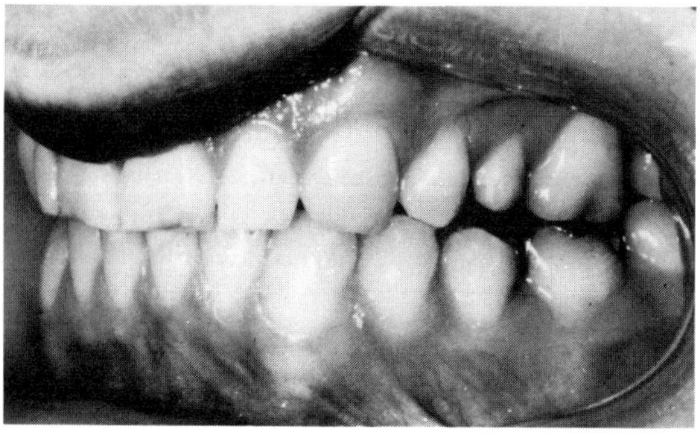

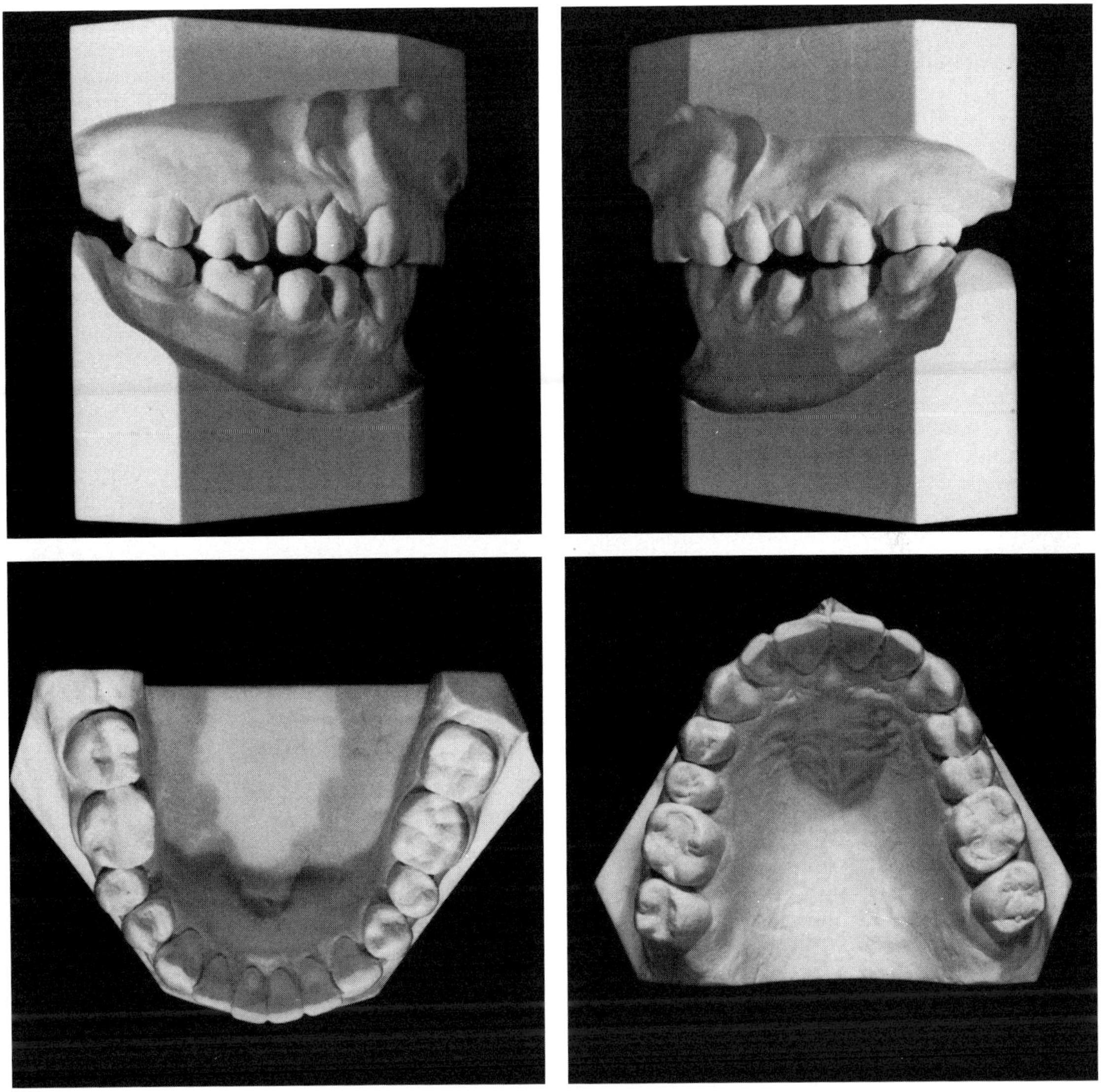

Figs 29-5 and 29-6 At the age of 21 y, 1 m.o, five years after completion of treatment, the profile has become straighter and the nose and chin have developed more to ventral. The mandibular arch has taken up a more mesial position in relationship to the maxillary arch than it had five years earlier, but still without matching of the occlusion. The increase in width obtained by the treatment has been partly lost due to the absence of an interlocking occlusion. The tongue still lies at this age between the teeth when at rest, swallowing, and speaking.

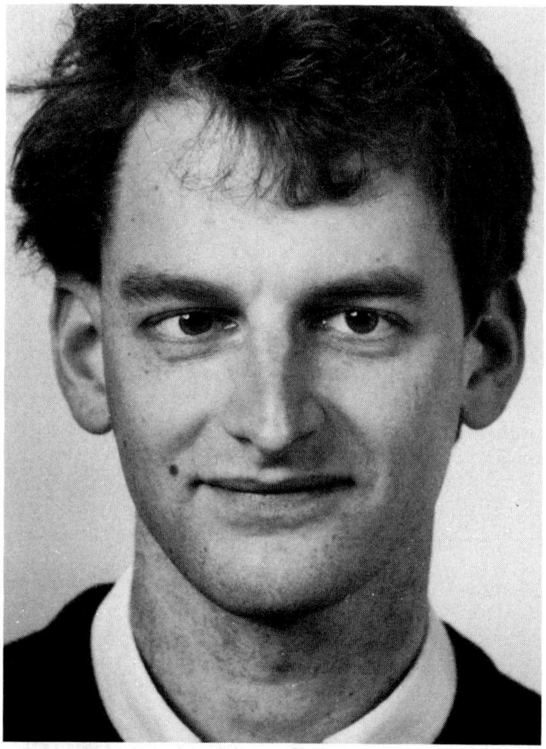

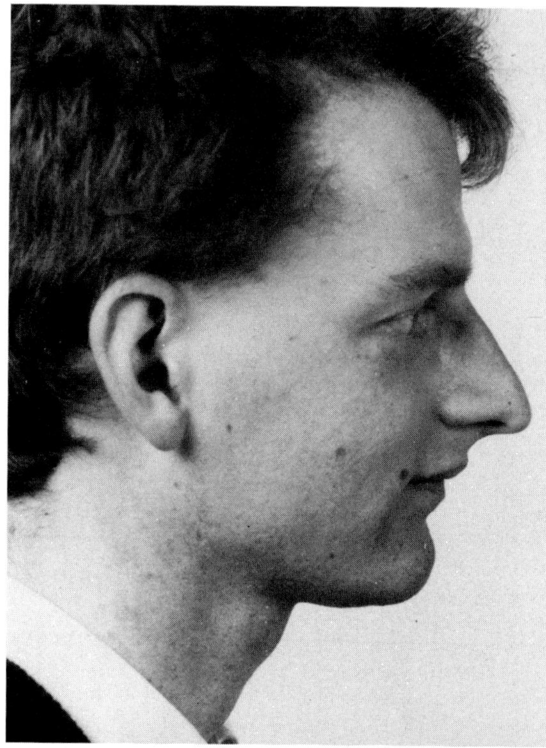

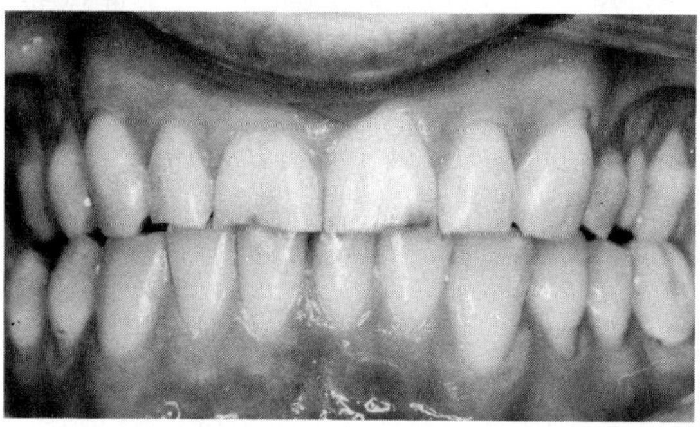

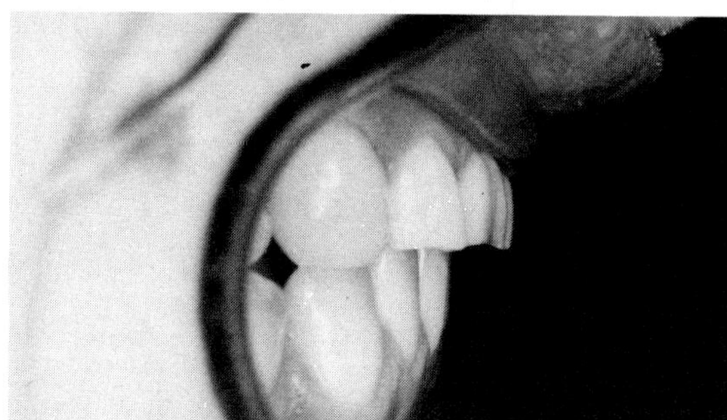

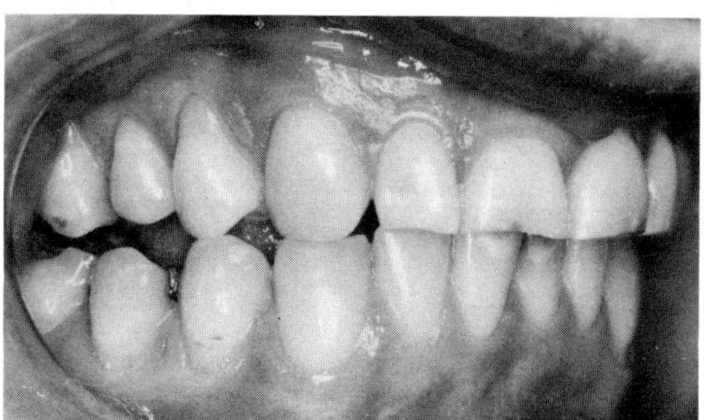

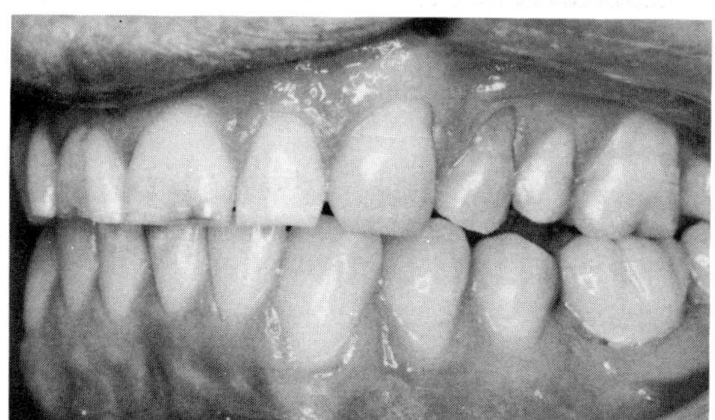

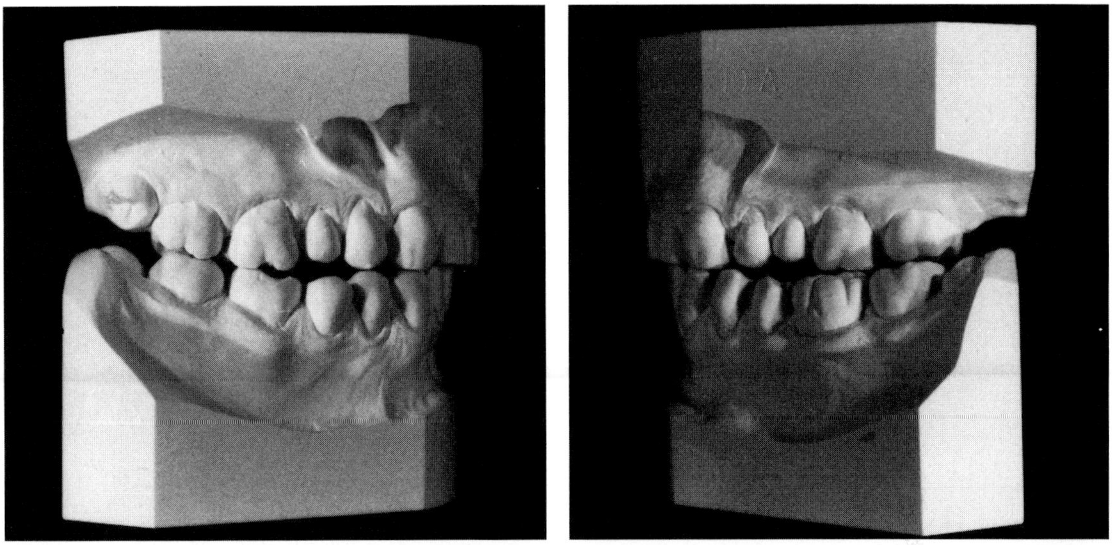

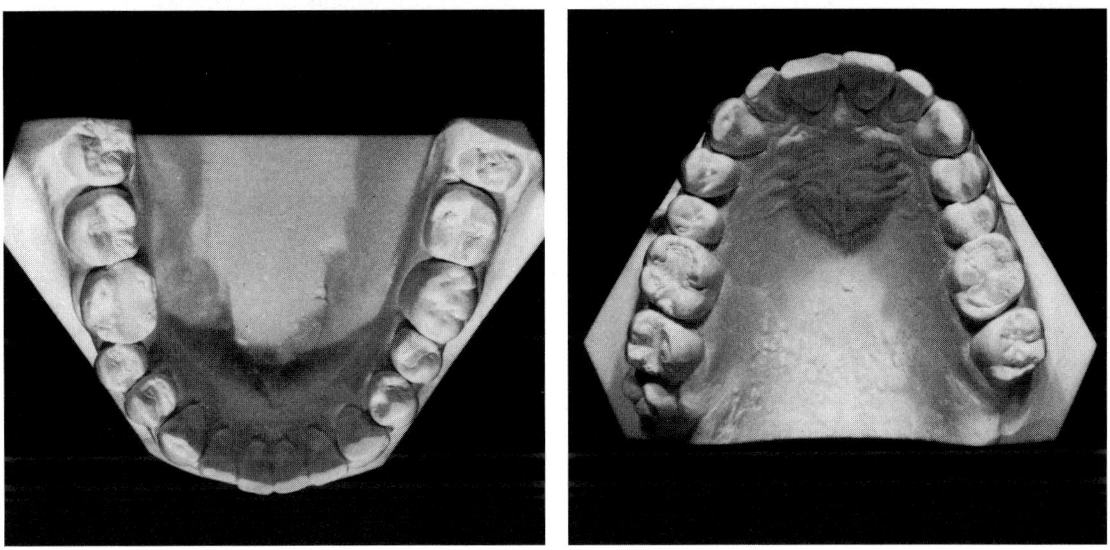

Figs 29-7 and 29-8 At the age of 26 y, 2 mo, ten years after treatment, the face has matured further. The ventral development of the mandible has led to a neutro-occlusion and an improved profile. The posterior teeth contact each other here and there. The diastema in the maxillary anteriors has vanished and the incisors are no longer in labioversion. The incisal edges of the mandibular and maxillary anteriors have been noticeably flattened by bruxism.

Figure 29-9a

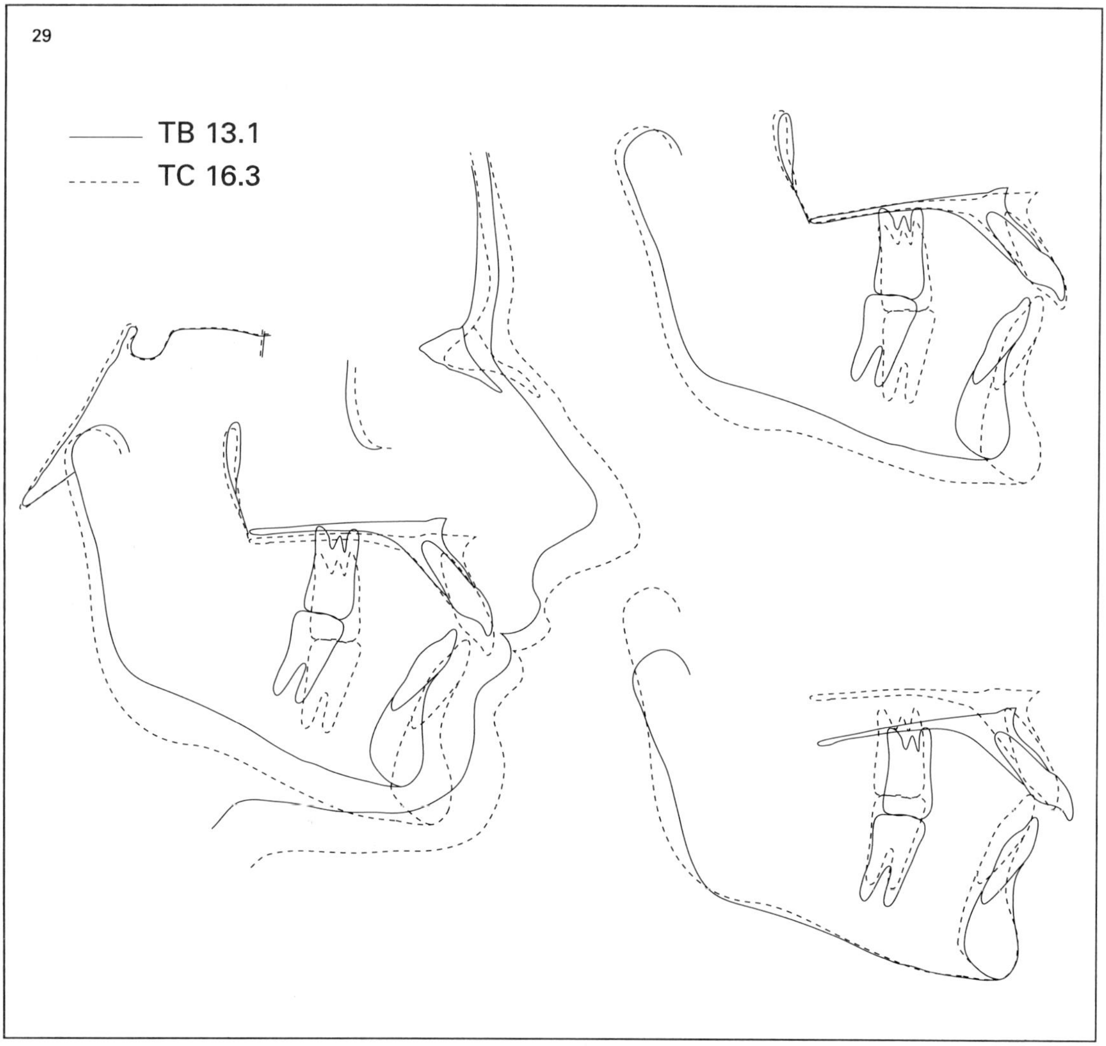

Fig 29-9 Superimposition of tracings from cephalometric radiographs shows that during treatment the ventral development of the maxilla had been inhibited and that the mandible came forward without the height of the face increasing excessively. The development of the lower face was also to ventral in the ten years following treatment, and the slope of the lower border of the mandible did not increase.

Figure 29-9b

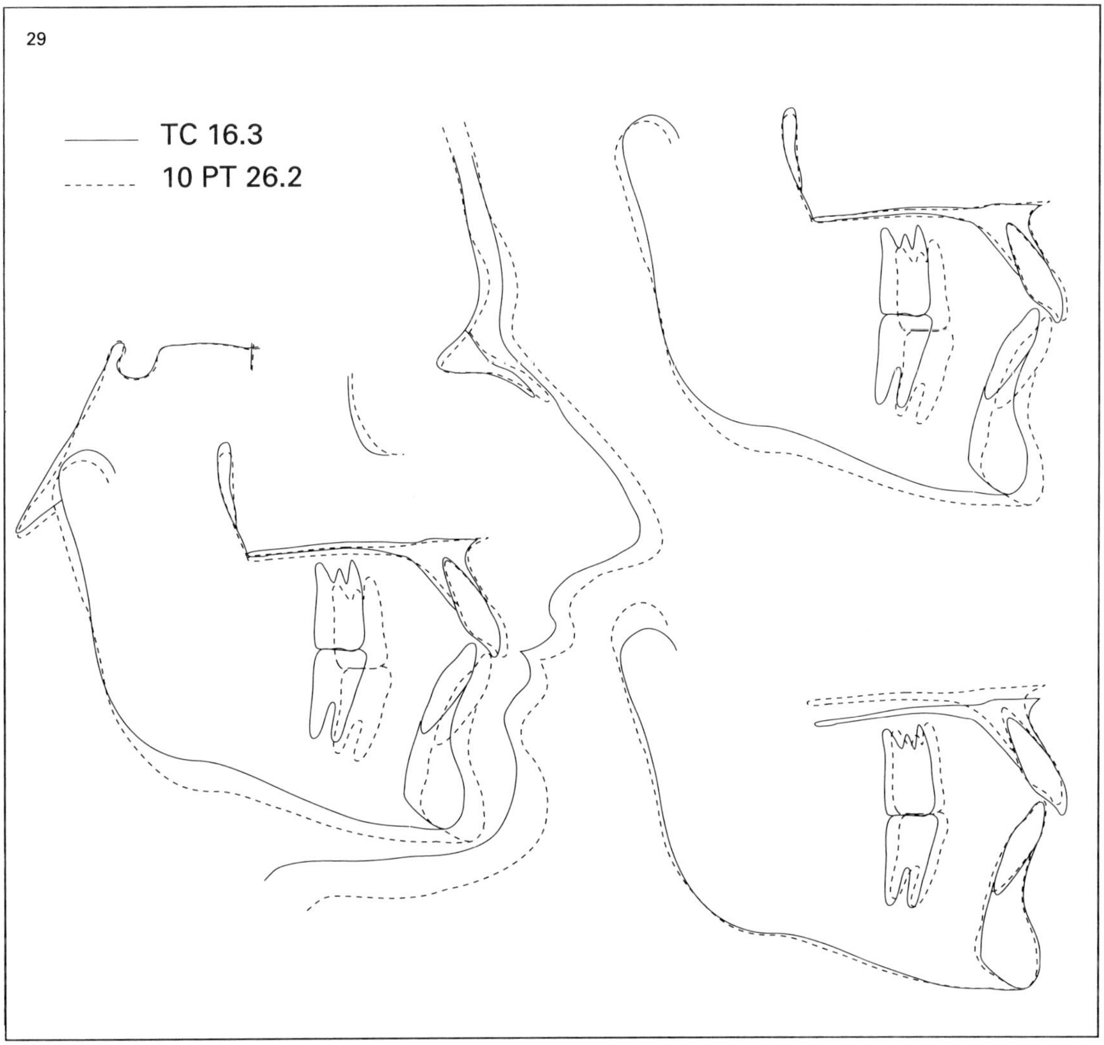

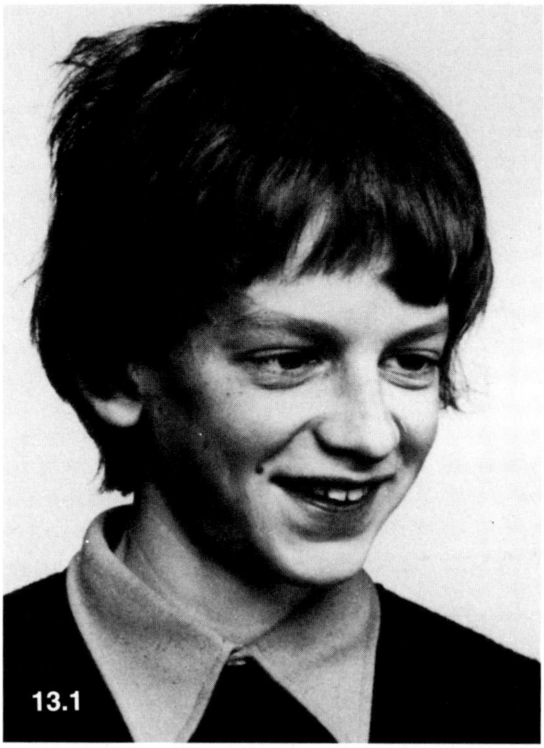

13.1

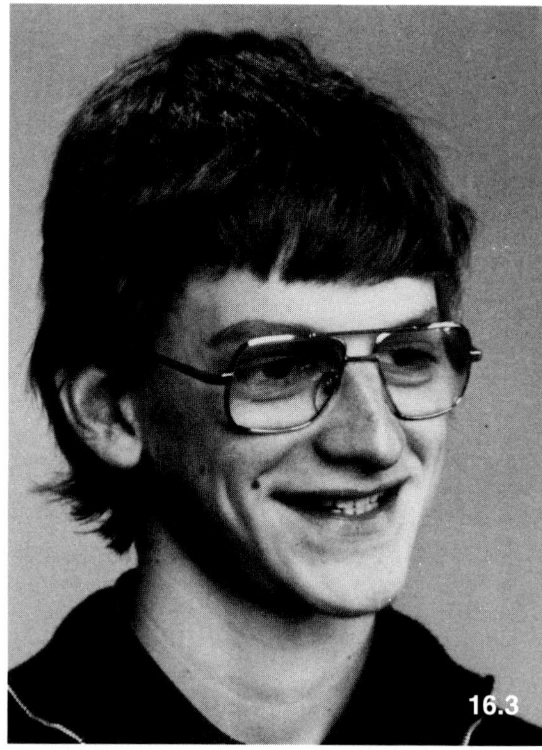

16.3

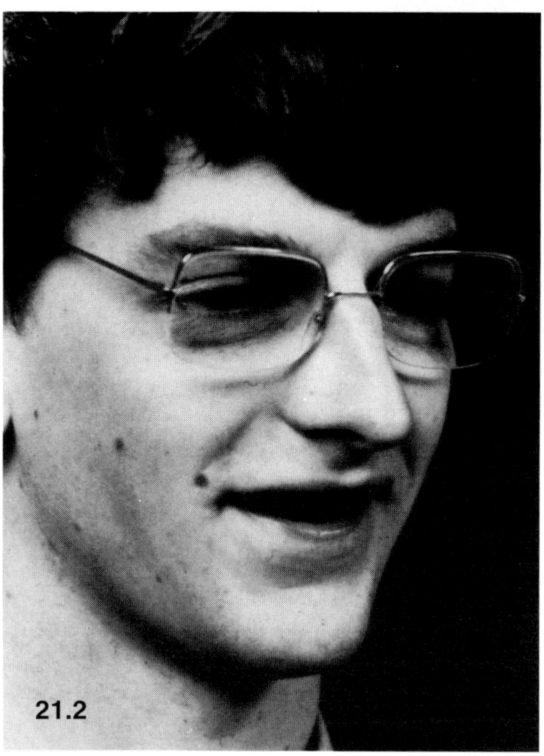

21.2

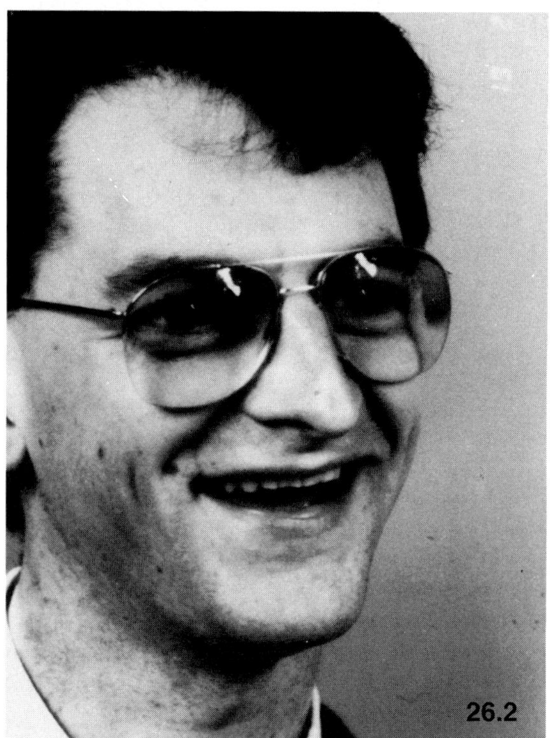

26.2

Fig 29-10 Nothing seen here indicates that there is a total open bite. Due to the treatment and the favorable growth, the outer appearance has improved over the years.

The internal volume of the oral cavity had been increased by the suture expansion, so that it should be possible for the tongue now to be accommodated within the dental arches; however, this did not occur, even after the ends of the tongue barriers that extended down to the lingual side of the mandibular alveolar process were made sharp. After six months the tongue barriers which appeared to have had no effect at all, were removed and the plate continued to be worn, with the headgear, only for retention purposes. At the same time, speech lessons were begun, resulting in a notable improvement in tongue behavior during speech.
At the age of 16 years, 2 months orthodontic treatment was terminated. The disto-relation had been partly eliminated, the maxillary dental arch corresponded with the mandibular one in width, but an adequate occlusion had not been attained (Figs. 29.3 and 29.4).
Because of the lack of interdigitation, the widening of the maxillary dental arch was partly lost during the years after treatment. There was also no rail mechanism working as the mandibular arch grew mesially. Five years after treatment the nose and chin had become dominant facial features and the overjet had diminished (Figs 29.5 and 29.6).
The tongue interposition, which was the origin of the total open bite and the lack of occlusal coordination between the opposing posterior teeth, showed no signs of lessening ten years after treatment at the age of 26 years, 2 months. The consequences of the situation were evident. The profile had improved as a result of facial development. The situation regarding intraoral function had not changed apart from the fact that a tooth grinding habit had caused attrition of the incisal edges of the anterior teeth (Figs. 29.7 and 29.8). The oblique facial photographs, but particularly the superimposed cephalometric tracings, show the predominance of ventral over vertical growth during treatment and the following ten years. This applied particularly to the mandible. The growth pattern before, during, or after treatment was by no means unfavorable (Figs 29.9 and 29.10).

Total open bites are associated with an entire lack of vertical contact between opposing teeth in the anterior and posterior regions of the dental arches during the act of swallowing. In addition, the tongue is found to lie between the dental arches at rest and during speech. The tongue interposition impedes eruption and the functioning of the cone-funnel mechanism is prevented. This can be confirmed by holding the corner of the mouth a little open with two instruments, and observing the tongue position at rest and during swallowing and speaking. Furthermore, either by watching or palpating it can be seen that a patient with a total open bite swallows without the temporal or masseter muscles contracting obviously. A contracting of these muscles only shows up when such a patient is asked to bite the teeth together.

A B C D E F G H

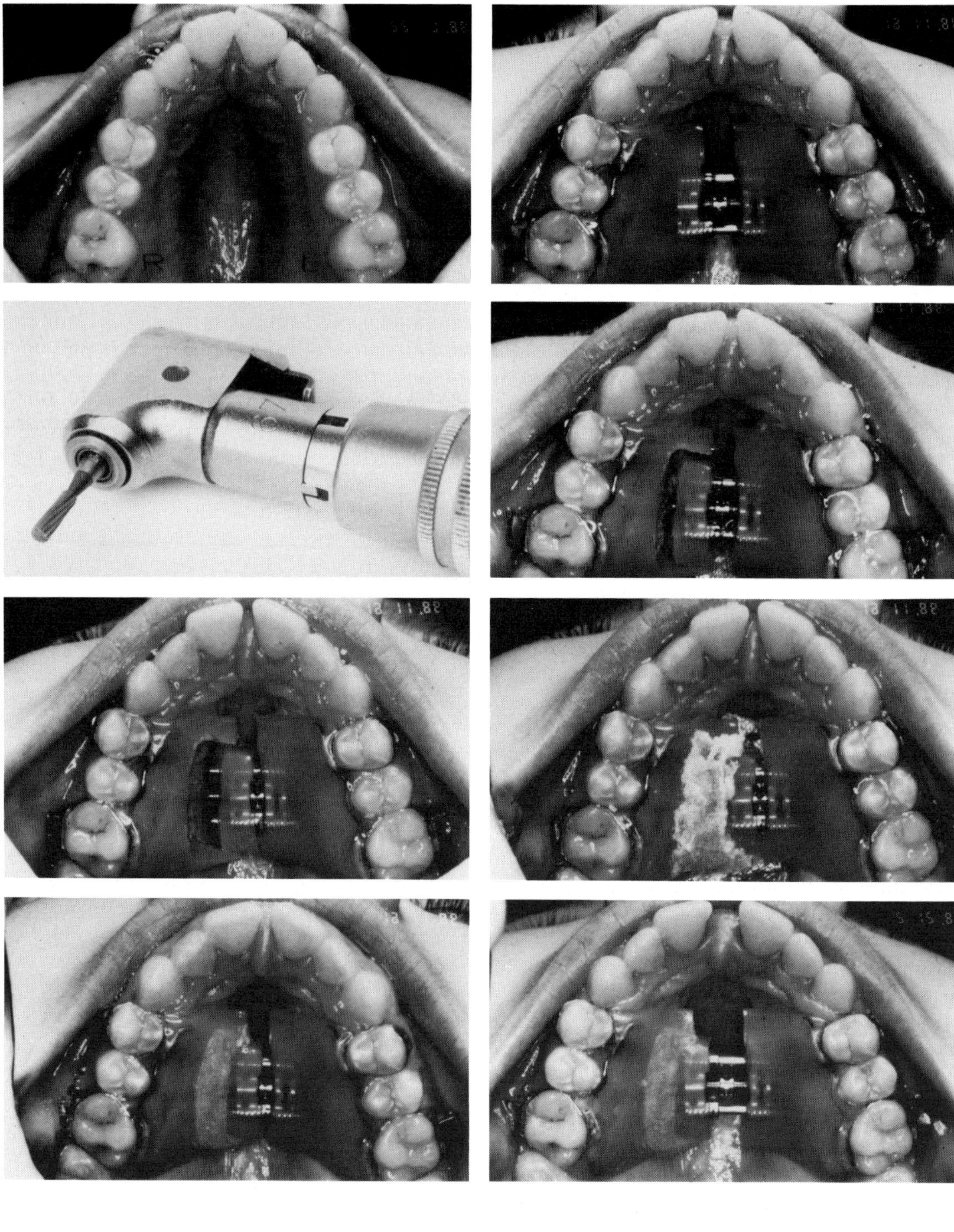

Fig 29-11 Technique for increasing the range of action of an acrylic appliance for rapid maxillary expansion without removing it from the mouth.
A First, premolars and first molars are provided with bands carrying palatal extensions for fixation in the acrylic parts.
B The appliance in the mouth after the screw has been turned over 90 degrees for 32 of the maximal 36 times.
C "Acrylic bur" for cutting free the screw from the acrylic on one side.
D The cut out part of the screw can be turned back.
E After the screw has been turned back a strip of soft wax is inserted between the palate and the prepared area.
F With self-polymerizing resin, the open area is filled in.
G The smoothed plate after removing the wax strip.
H The screw is now used maximally for the second time. If needed, the procedure can be repeated on the other side.
The plate could also haven been cut through in a straight line from front to rear. However, such a cut can easily involve the mucosa particularly in the anterior region. Cutting is safer in the way illustrated because the acrylic in the prepared area is at some distance from the palate. In addition, stronger new construction is provided in this manner.

Generally, what is seen is not a real total open bite, since the tongue is held only between the lingual cusps of the first molars or the premolars and the buccal cusps make contact.
If the maxillary dental arch is narrow in comparison with the mandibular arch, it is usually due to tongue interposition. A too narrow maxillary dental arch is often the first symptom noticed in a lateral or total open bite, followed by the lack of occlusal contact.
When patients with a total open bite (that nonetheless includes contact between the buccal cusps) are asked to close their teeth together, their mandible will glide off to one side. It would not be correct to diagnose that lateral gliding to be a forced bite, because a habitual occlusion would be lacking. Moreover, this lateral gliding does not occur in patients with a forced bite when closing the mandible from central toward habitual occlusion, but the mandible moves from the open position directly to habitual occlusion.[13]
Another characteristic of patients with a total open bite is the lack of a sharp, hard sound when they are asked to close their teeth together with a "clap". Such a noise is clearly heard when an individual has solid vertical contacts, also when it is associated with a forced bite.
In hindsight, it can be asked if rapid maxillary expansion was appropriate for this patient. The increase in width thus gained eventually was lost to a significant extent through lack of any solid interdigitation. In view of the broad mid-face it had been hoped that by securing extra space by means of the expansion the tongue would have been held between the dental arches, something which — as already stated — did not occur. It is not clear if tongue interposition changes as the result of an

increase in intraoral volume. If it is indeed the case, then the possibility should be admitted that it might also happen without arch expansion. On rare occasions, tongue interposition may disappear with time.
Surgical reduction of the tongue also offers no certain elimination of tongue interposition. The indication for such an intervention is limited to excessively large tongues (macroglossia) to which unacceptable malformations of the dental arches can be attributed.
Tongue barriers and sharp pieces of orthodontic wire fixed to teeth can cause the tongue to assume different positions temporarily. As soon as those obstacles are removed, the tongue will in almost all cases return to its former position. In this patient, the tongue barrier was used to no avail.
As previously mentioned, myofunctional therapy that aims to alter tongue position at rest and during swallowing does not appear to secure an improvement. This is in contrast to speech lessons, which can indeed procure a permanent change in tongue behavior during speaking.
Finally, the technique by which suture expansion can have its range of action increased in the mouth is worthy of mention. By cutting the acrylic part of one side of the appliance free, the screw can be turned back. Then the plate can be reconstructed in the mouth with self-polymerizing resin. This procedure can be repeated on the other side at a later date if required (Fig 29.11).

Chapter 30

Class II/1 subdivision, crossbite 26 and 27
Extraction 24, maxillary removable plate
Male: 14 years, 3 months to 25 years, 6 months

A boy aged 14 years 3 months exhibited a class II/1 subdivision anomaly with a neutro-occlusion on the right and a ¾ PW disto-occlusion on the left side. Moreover, the maxillary left first and second permanent molars were in crossbite. The mandibular dental arch and the maxillary arch on the right were more or less free of abnormality. In the second quadrant, crowding existed in the canine region and the permanent molars were positioned too far to palatal. The patient had good facial configuration, adequate lip closure, and overall he enjoyed normal function and no sign of temporomandibular joint problems. In accordance with the asymmetric occlusion, the midline of the maxillary arch was 2 mm to the right of the one in the mandible. The maxillary incisors were also too far to the right in relationship to the nose and upper lip. The midline deviation was clearly localized in the maxillary arch (Figs 30.1 and 30.2).

The decision was taken not to treat the mandible and to let the crossbite remain. The maxillary left first premolar was extracted, which provided room for better alignment of the lateral incisor and the mesially angulated canine. In addition, the teeth distal to the extraction space could drift mesially into a disto-occlusion of a full premolar width with a good mesiodistal interdigitation. To obtain the desired tooth movements, a maxillary plate with labial arches and a buccal spring onto the left canine were fitted at the age of 14 years, 6 months after the extraction had been performed two months earlier. The deep bite was reduced with a biteplane, after which the incisors were retracted with the labial arches. After 1½ years, the desired result had been obtained and treatment was terminated. The deviation of the midlines of the dental arches had been corrected and good interincisal contact was reached. The maxillary left second premolar interdigitated well with the mandibular premolars; the maxillary left permanent molars occluded with their antagonists in a disto-occlusion of 1 PW and in crossbite (Figs 30.3 and 30.4).

Five years later, little of the improvement had been lost and the result was still acceptable (Figs 30.5 and 30.6). The same applies to the situation at the age of 25 years, 7 months, approximately ten years after treatment (Figs 30.7 and 30.8). The photographs of his smiling face show little of the improvements in the dentition because the left side, on which the faults appeared, is not visible (Fig 30.9).

In class II/1 anomalies with an asymmetric occlusion and a midline deviation toward the side of the neutro-occlusion, extraction of a maxillary tooth on the side of the disto-occlusion should be considered. In situations with a disto-occlusion of ½ PW,

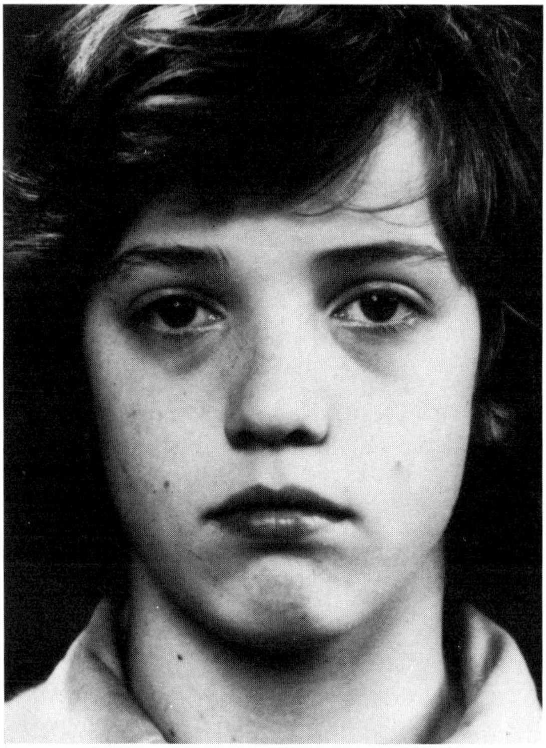

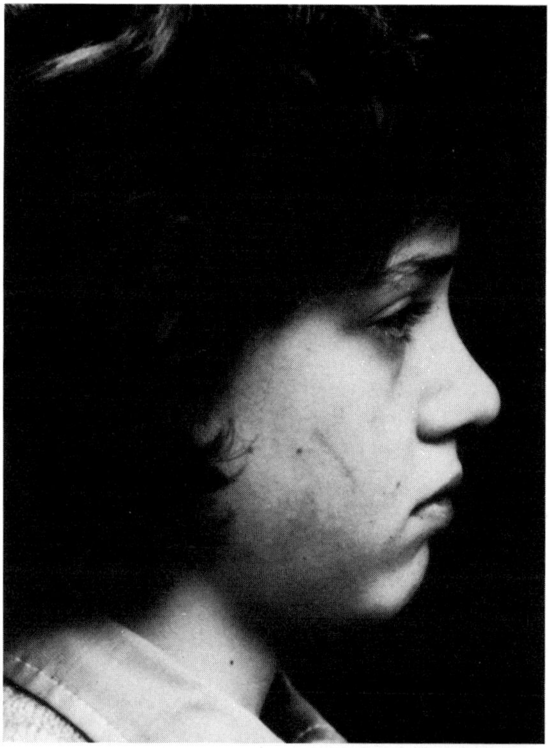

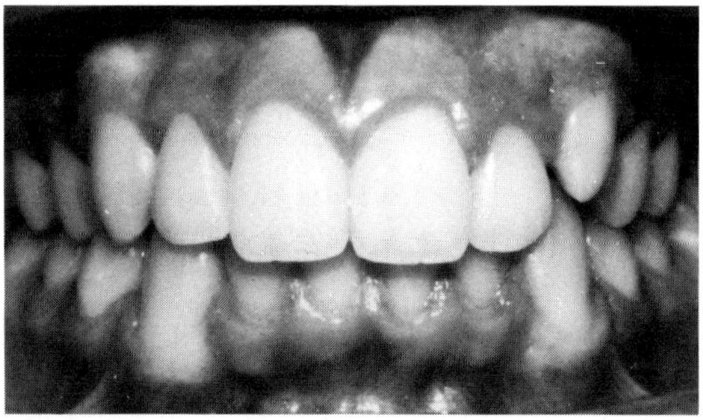

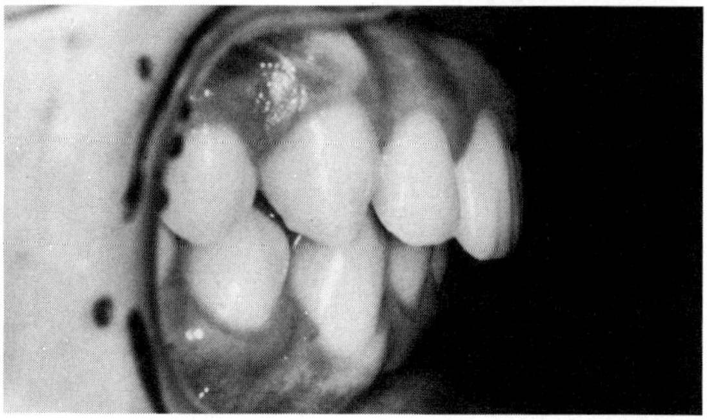

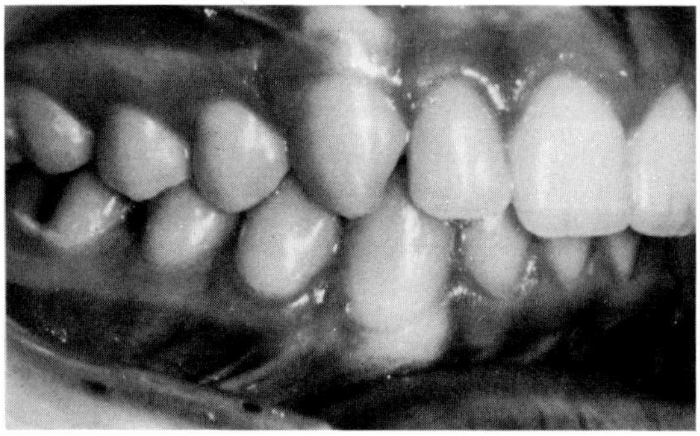

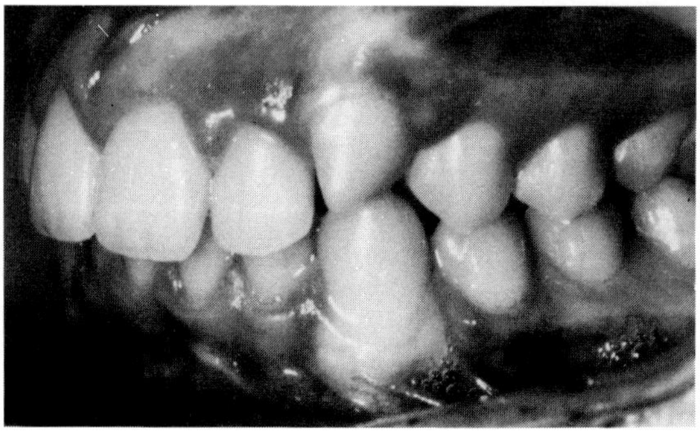

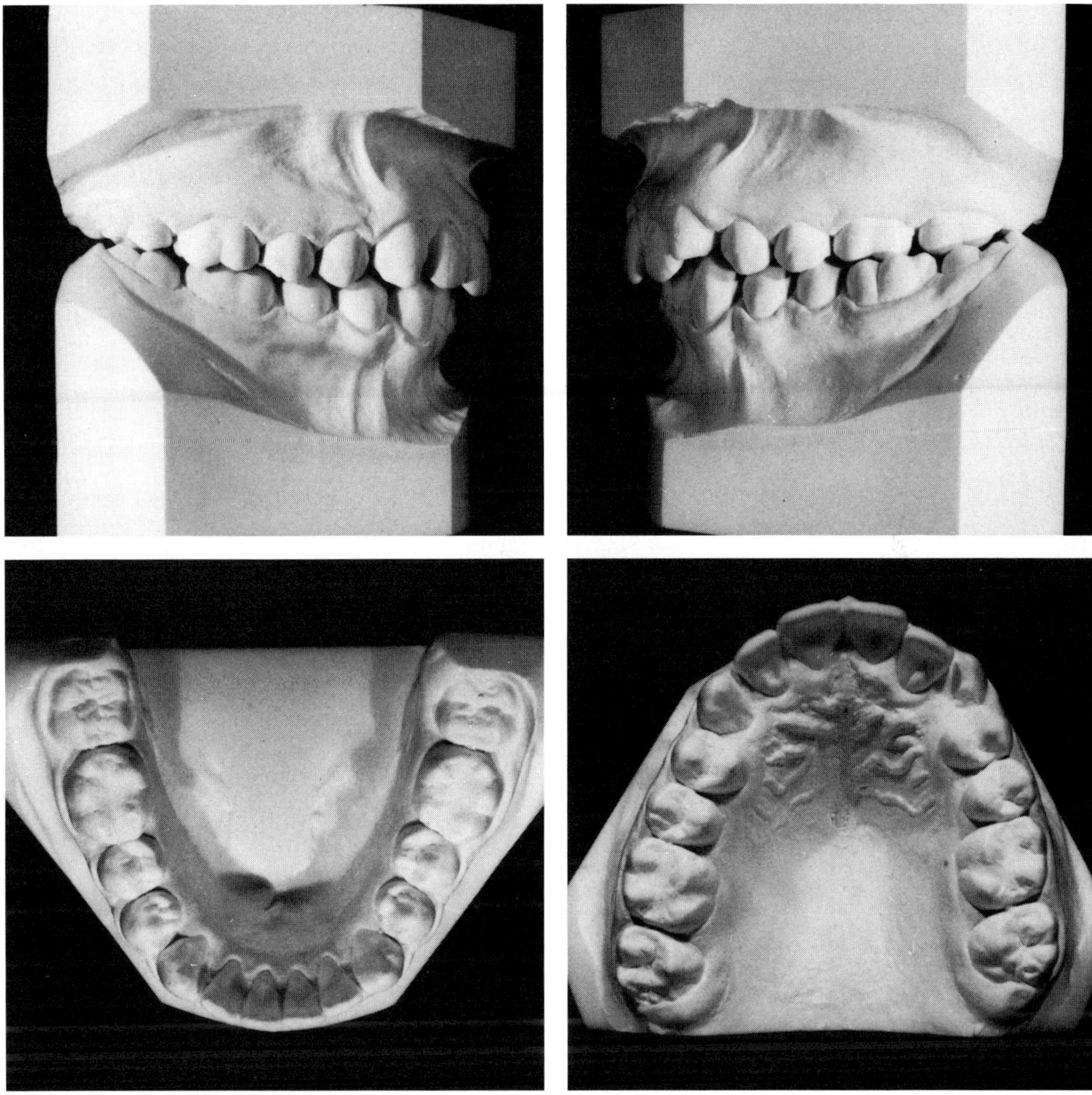

Figs 30-1 and 30-2 A boy aged 14 y, 3 mo with a good facial structure has a class II/1 subdivision anomaly (right neutro-occlusion, left ¾ PW disto-occlusion) and a crossbite of the maxillary left molars. The mandibular first molar is positioned a little to the buccal and is in buccoversion. There is solid interdigitation, including in the region of the crossbite, with crowding of the maxillary left lateral incisor and the adjacent canine. The midline of the maxillary dental arch is displaced 2 mm too far to the right in relationship to the overall structure of the face and the mandibular arch in particular. It is not possible to discern any facial asymmetry.

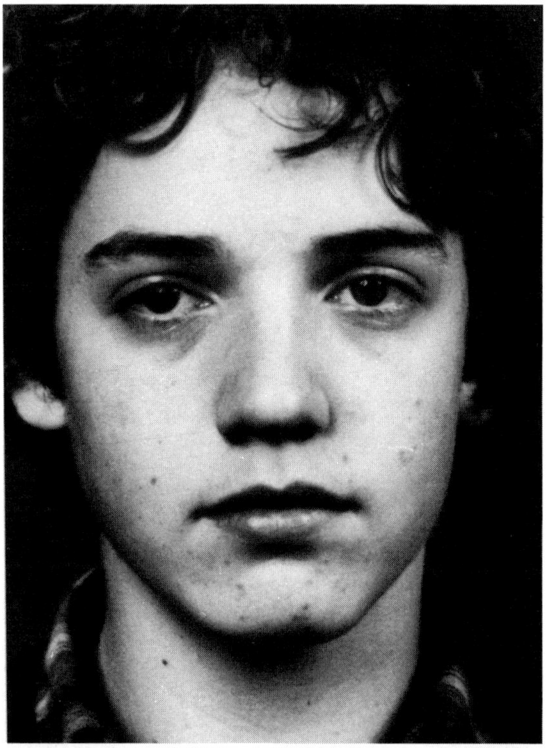

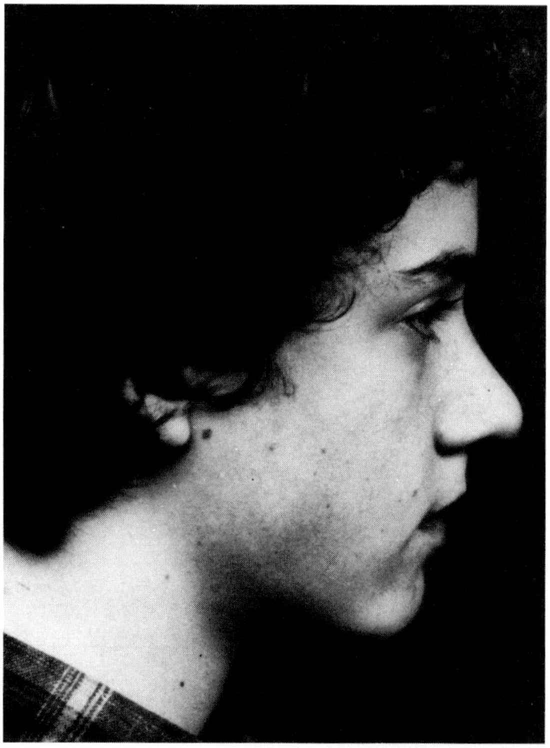

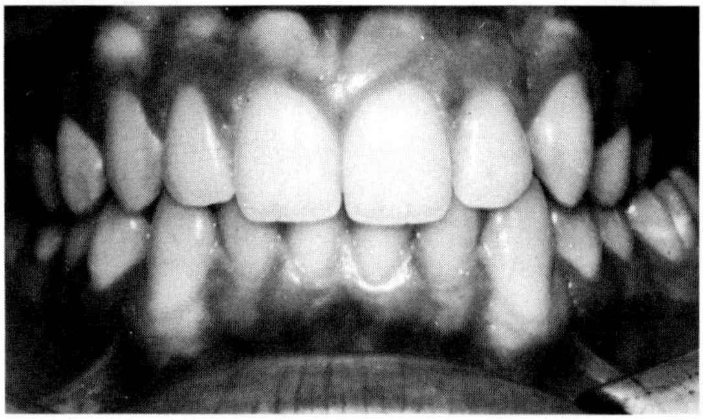

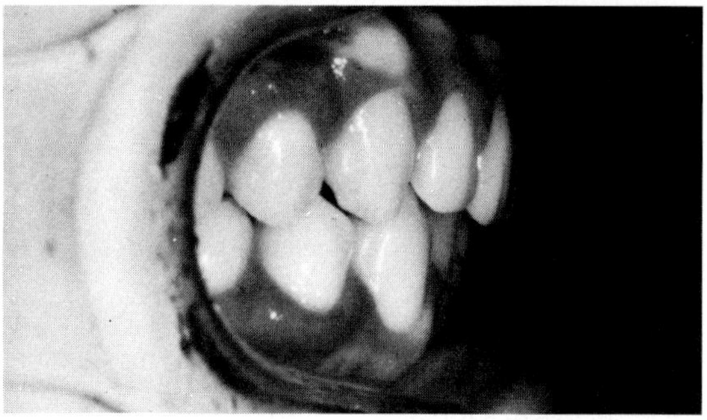

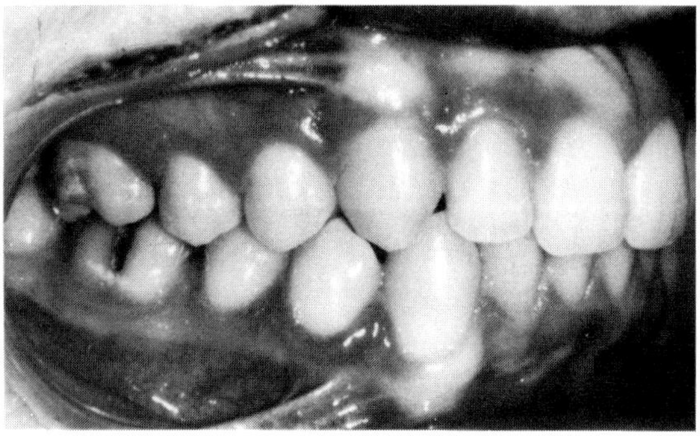

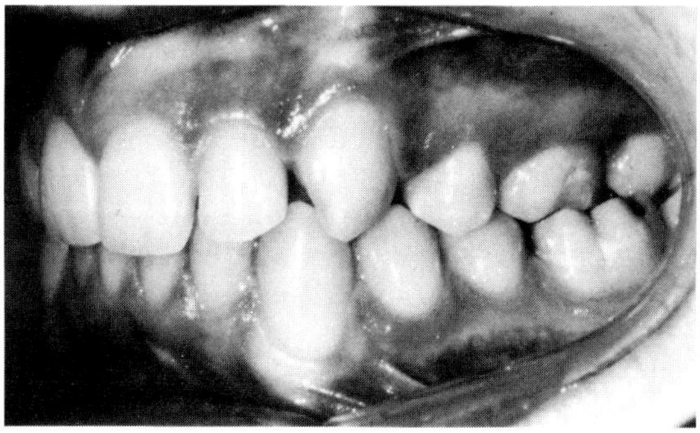

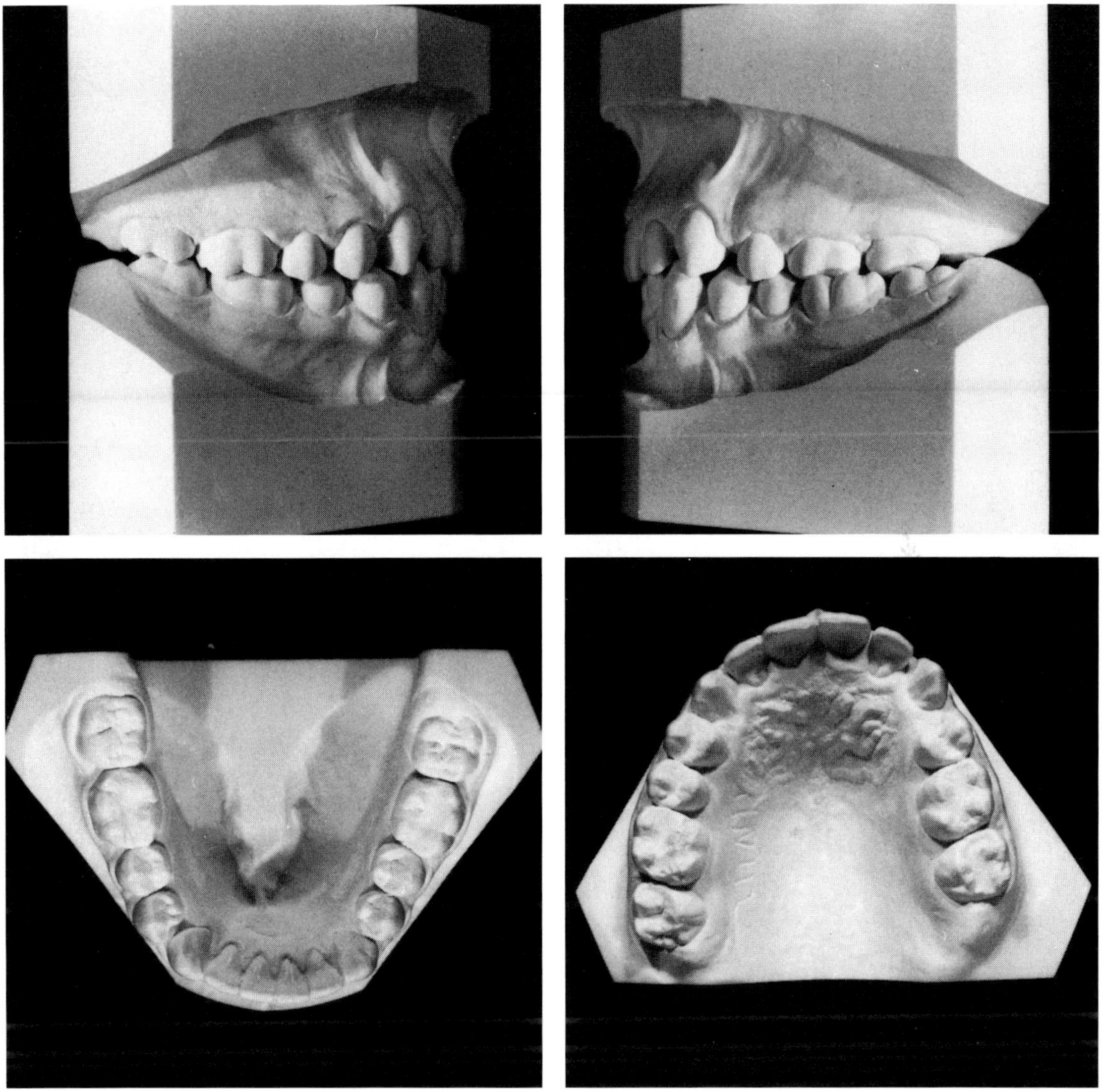

Figs 30-3 and 30-4 At the age of 16 y, 0 mo after 1½ years of treatment following extraction of the maxillary left first premolar, use of a maxillary plate has successfully corrected the midline deviation, secured proper contact between the anterior teeth, and moved the maxillary left canine into good alignment. On the left side, the crossbite has remained and the molars and second premolars interdigitate in a disto-occlusion of 1 PW. The extraction space where the first premolar was removed has not been totally eliminated.

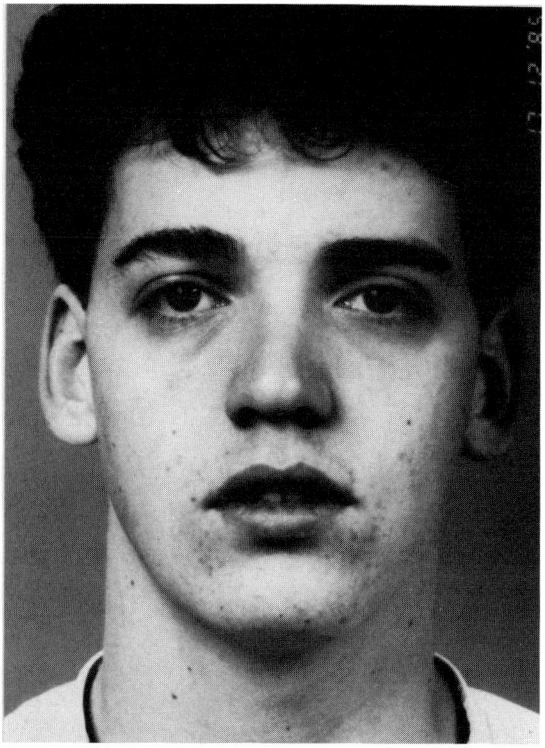

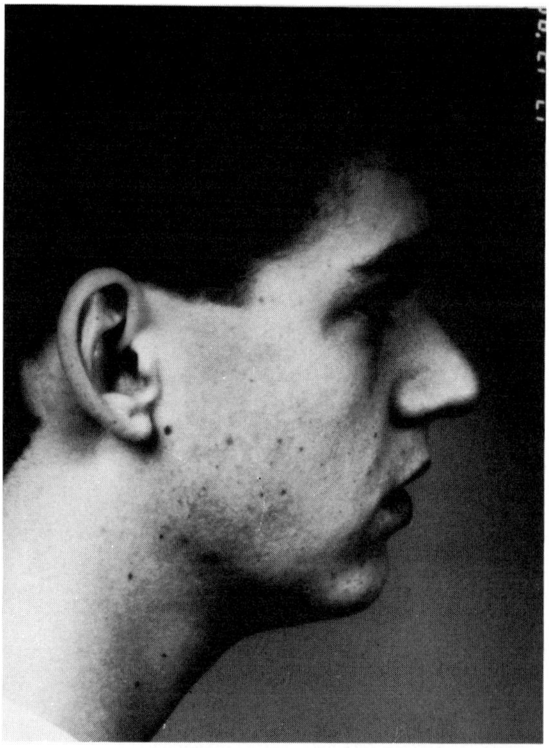

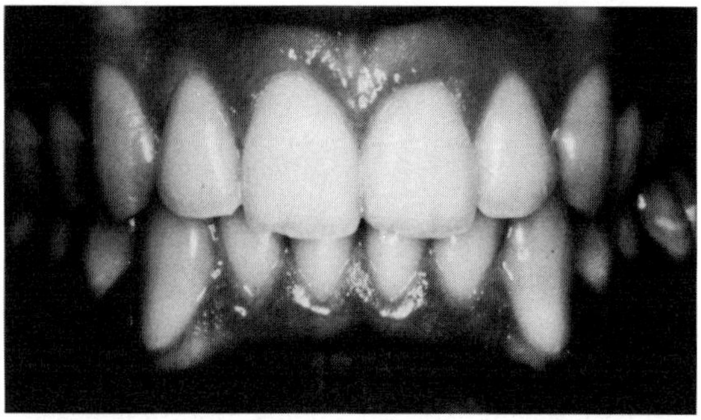

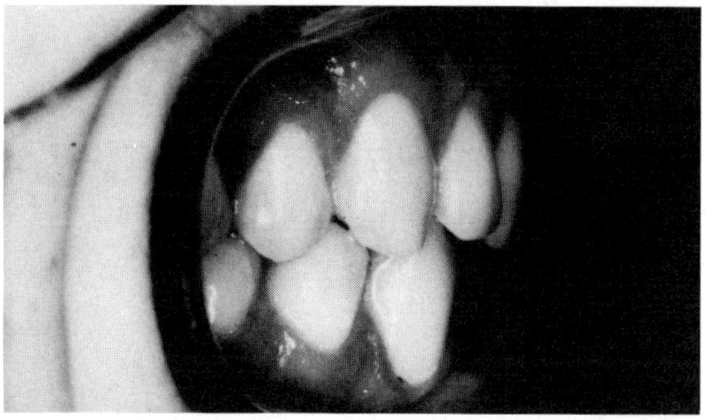

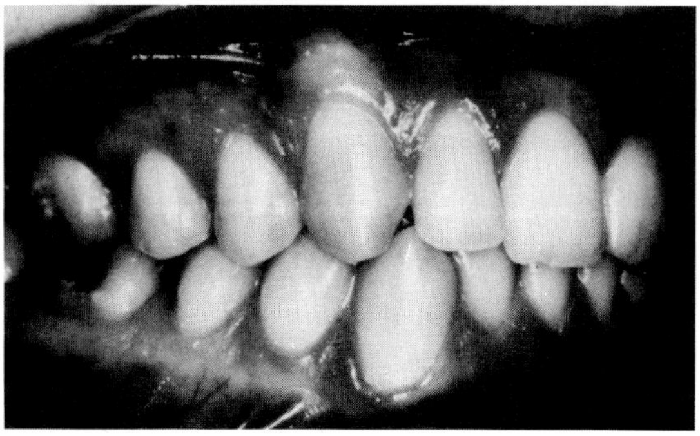

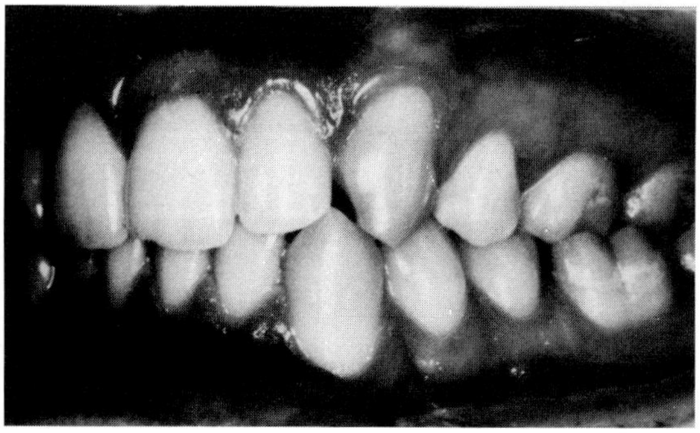

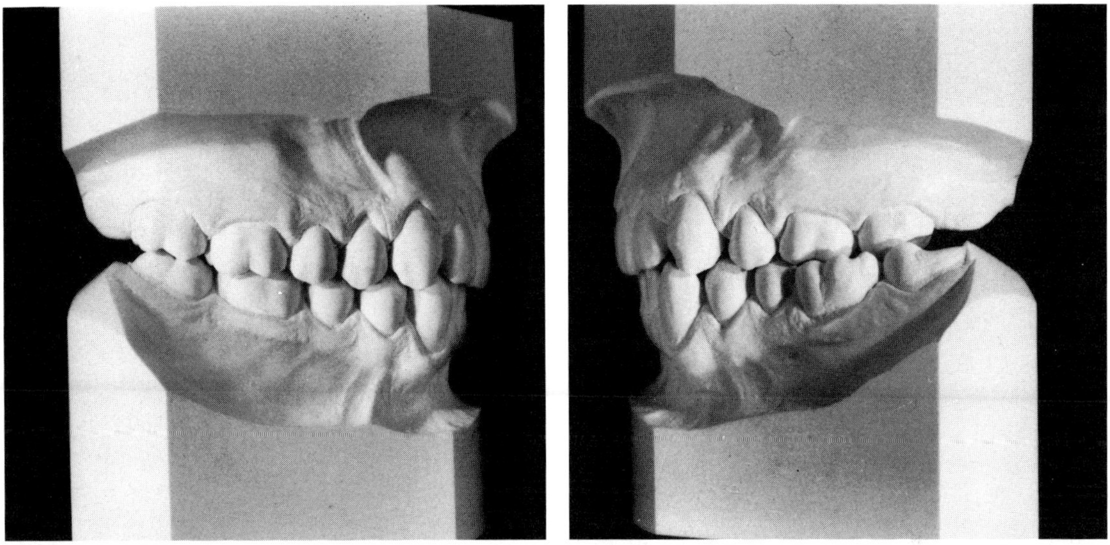

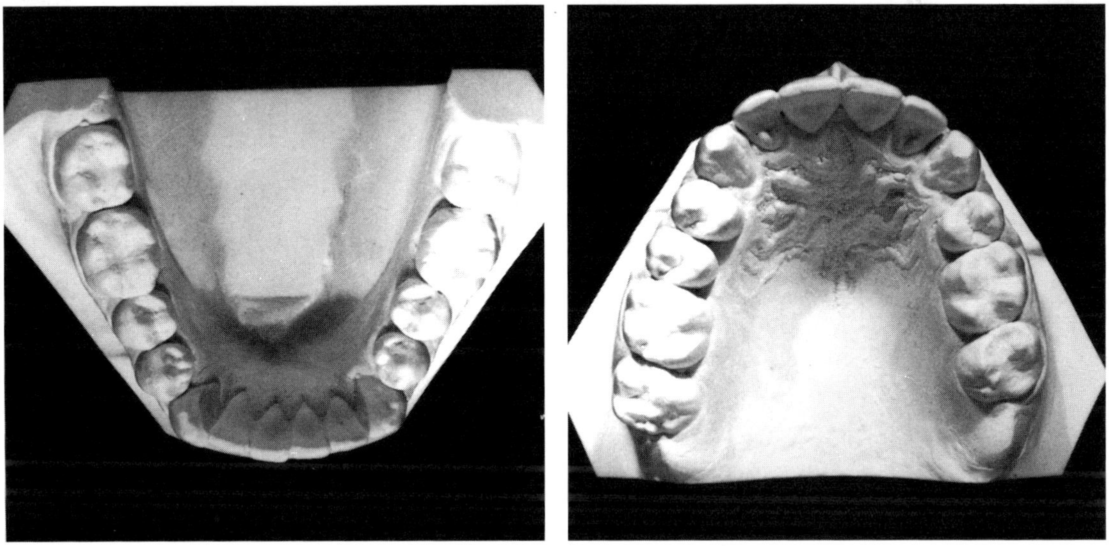

Figs 30-5 and 30-6 *At the age of 21 y, five years after treatment, the face is acceptable. The dentition also fulfils requirements in esthetics and function. There is solid interdigitation in the posterior segments. The residual extraction space has almost vanished. Minor tertiary crowding is evident in the mandibular anteriors.*

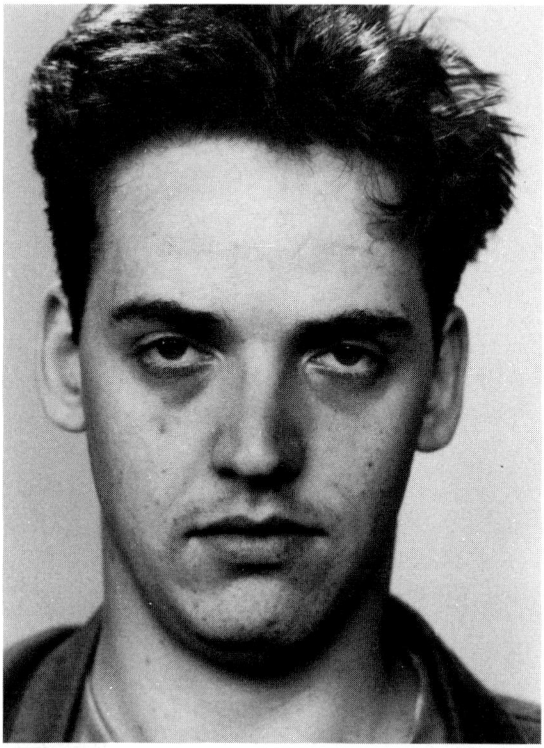

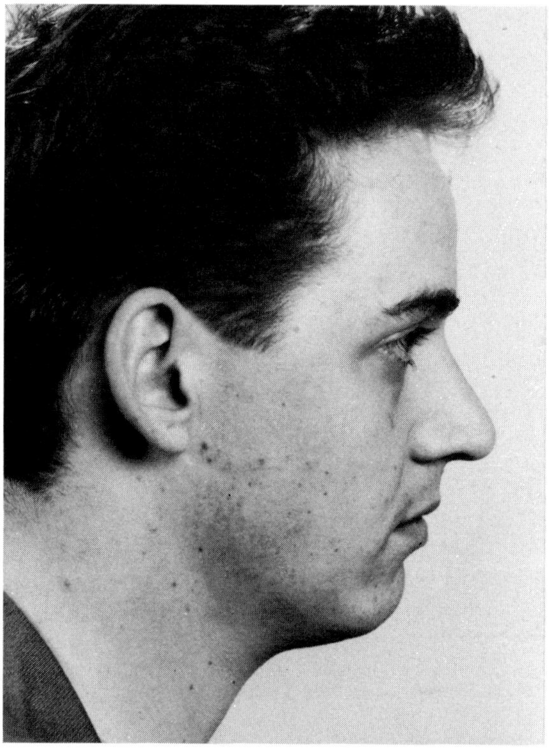

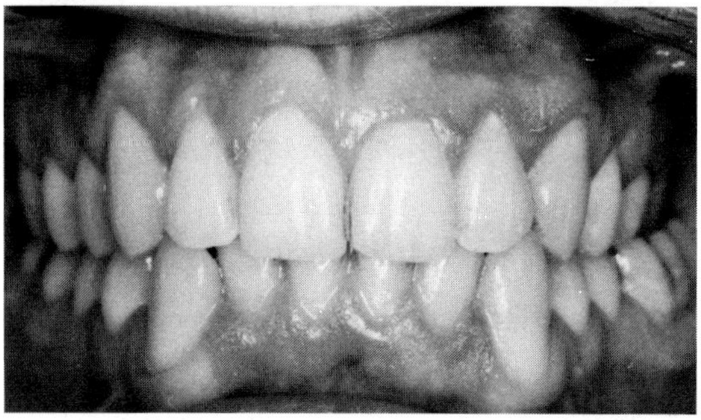

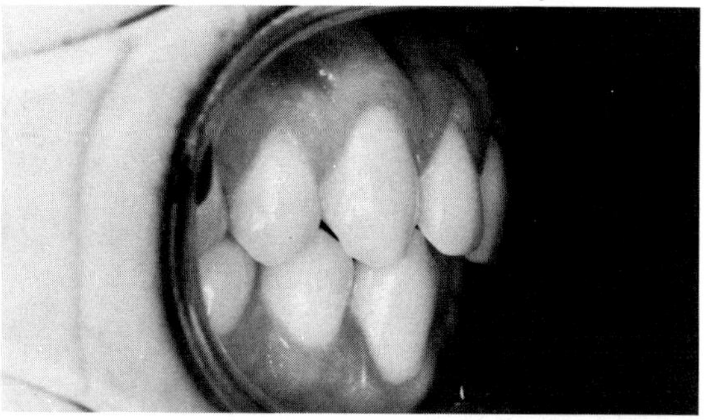

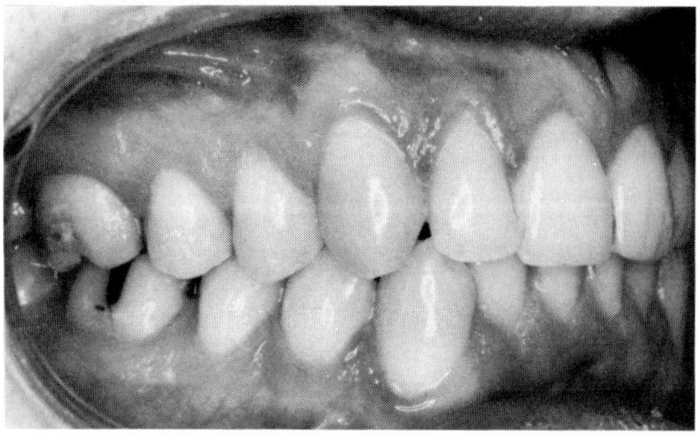

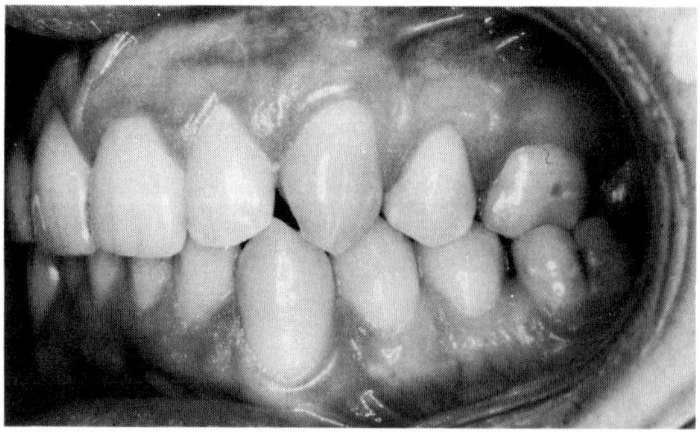

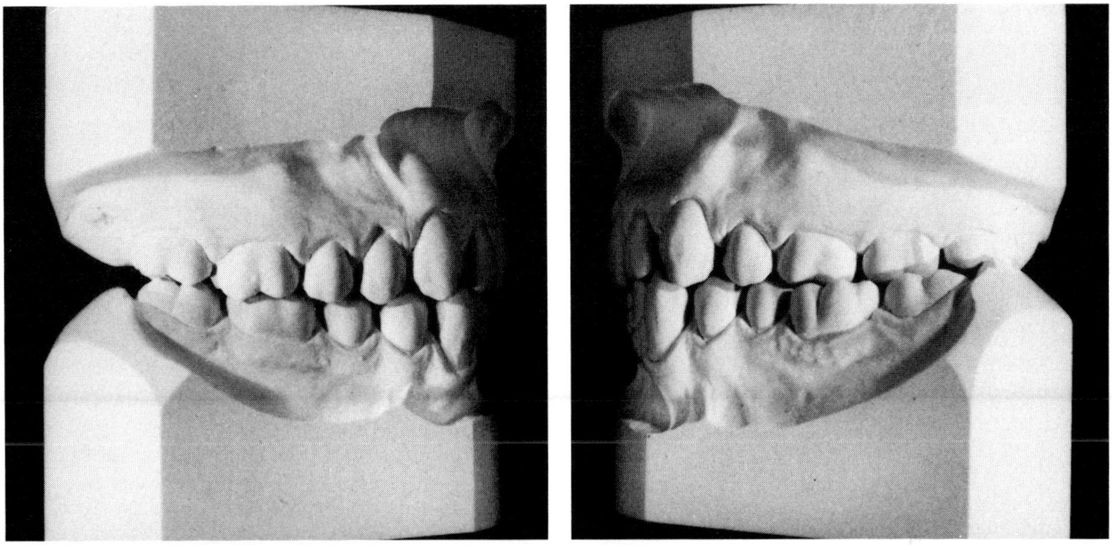

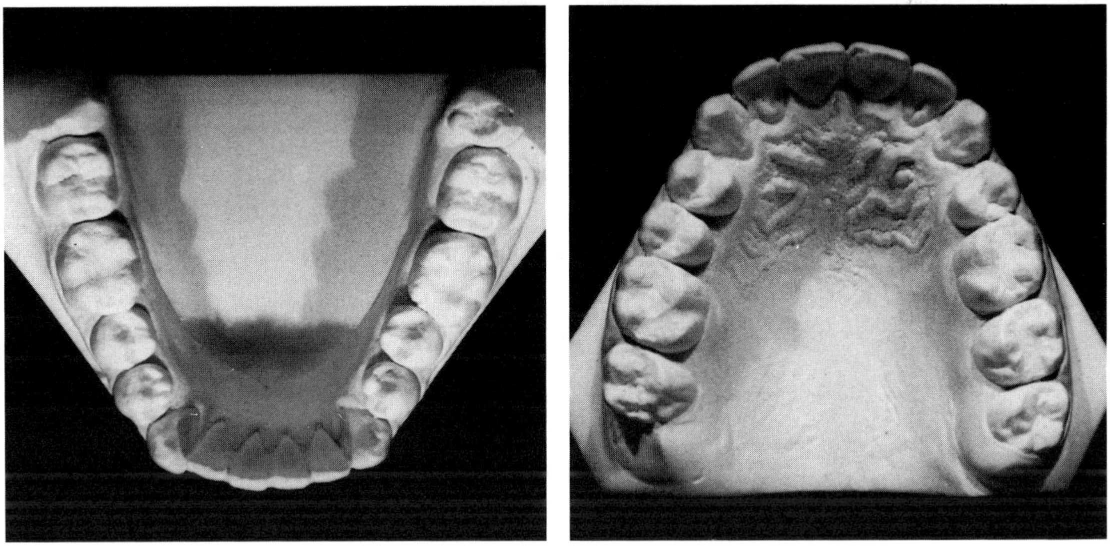

Figs 30-7 and 30-8 *At the age of 25 y, 5 mo, nearly ten years after the conclusion of treatment, there is a harmonious face with a dentition that is esthetically and functionally satisfactory. In the three quadrants with two premolars present insufficient space for the third molars is available and their removal is indicated. The fact that in lateral excursions the maxillary molars, which are in crossbite lose contact with their antagonists is of no concern to the patient (see Fig 30.10).*

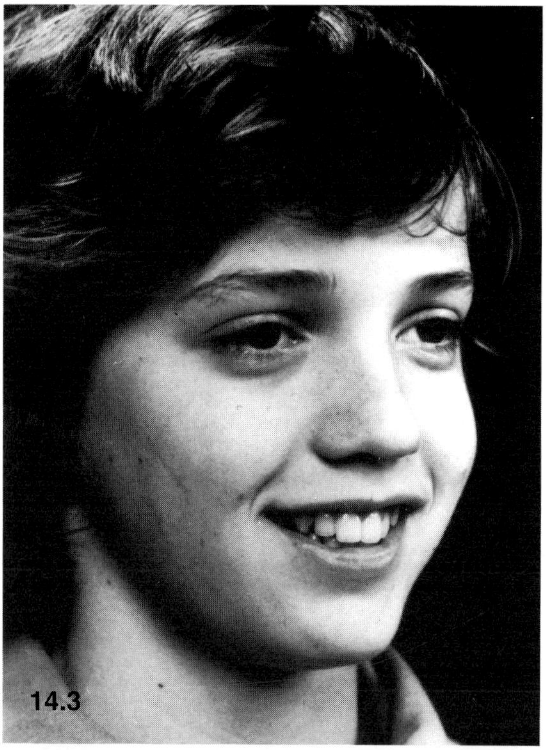

14.3

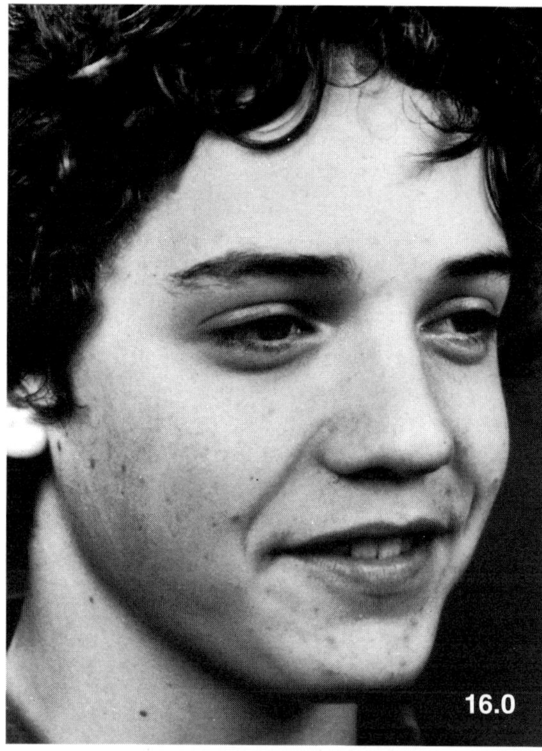

16.0

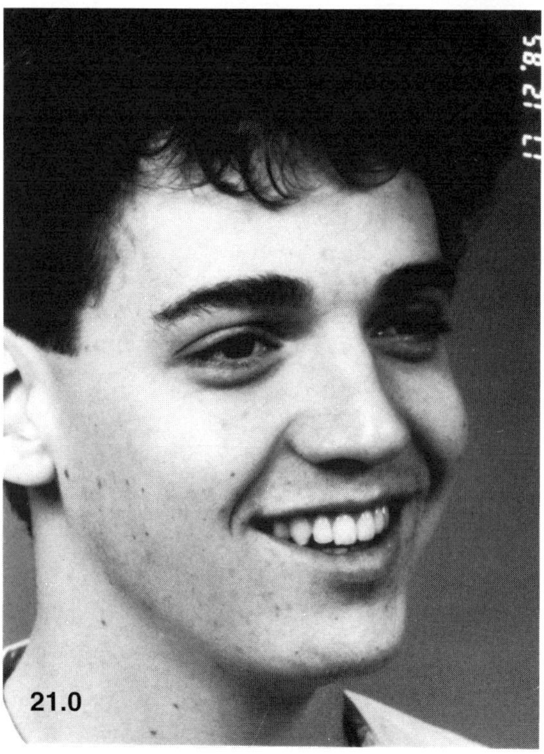

21.0

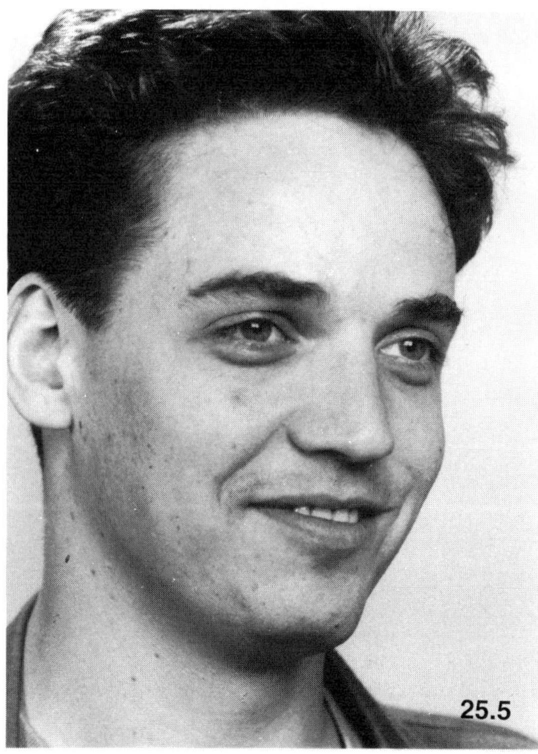

25.5

the second premolar would be the tooth of choice; then an excess of space can be filled more easily from the distal than if the first premolar had been extracted, since then both the second premolar and the molars would have to move mesially. Moreover, an unwanted residual space in the second premolar region would probably not be noticed.

Another possibility in such cases of asymmetry is the extraction of the maxillary first or second molar. Here the quality of the teeth and the presence or absence of the third molars and their positions would be taken into account. Closure of a first molar extraction space would require a fixed appliance. If the second molar were removed, the task would be simpler. The first molar can be moved distally with a plate or a lip bumper. The third molar, at least if it is well-located, will subsequently assume the place and function of the second molar. If the disto-occlusion is greater than ½ PW, and the more posterior teeth are able to migrate mesially only a little, then it would be better to extract the first premolar. That would be the case particularly where crowding is concentrated in that area or if the canine is severely angulated to the mesial.

A typical aspect of crossbites is that during lateral excursions, contact between antagonists is quickly lost (Fig 30.10). Other drawbacks are not involved, and evidence is lacking that crossbites might lead to temporomandibular joint problems. However, crossbites of first premolars, and to a lesser degree second premolars, can be esthetically objectionable. The oblique view of the dentition reveals a step inward behind either the canine or the first premolar, which can be ugly. This did not apply to this patient.

Fig 30-9 Little of the original problem and its improvement are noticed, since they are on the left side and the standard photographs are taken on the right.

A

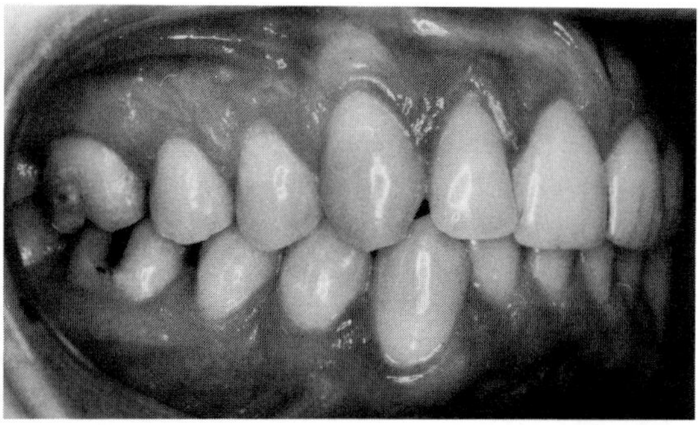

B

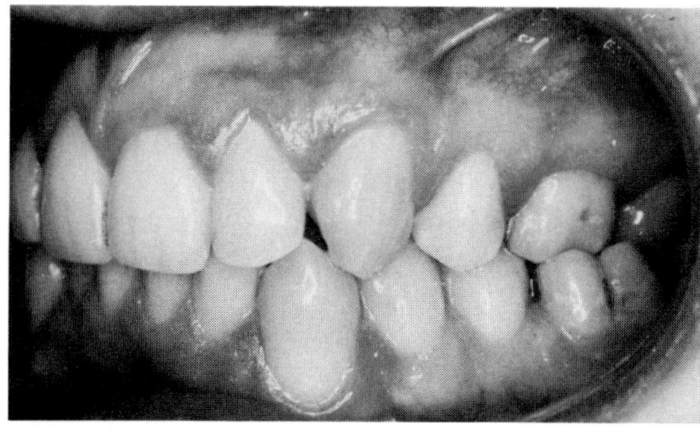

C

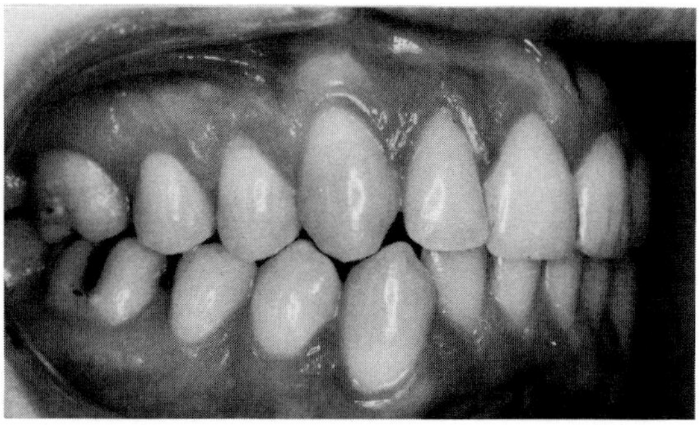

D

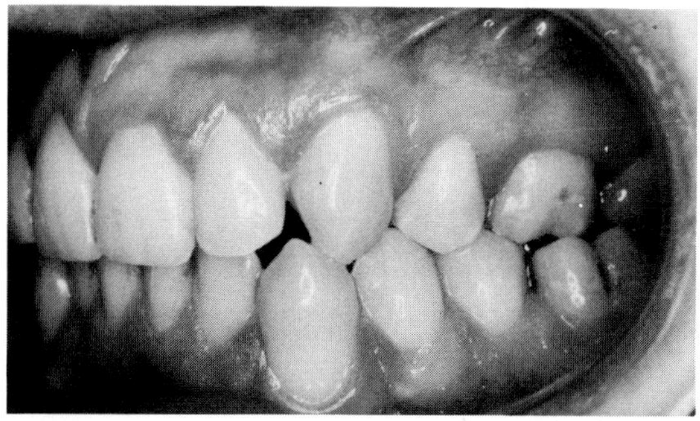

E

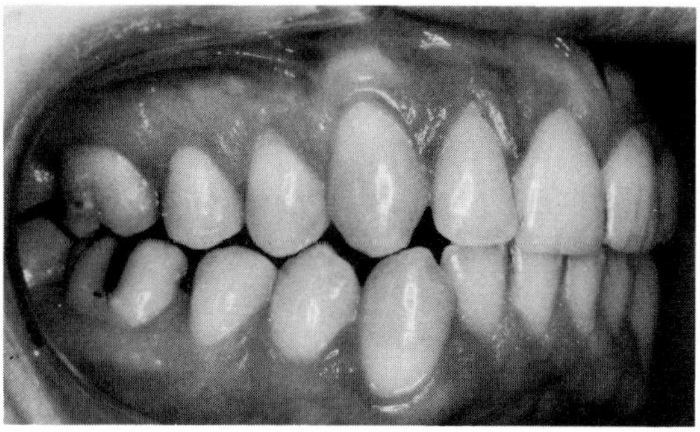

F

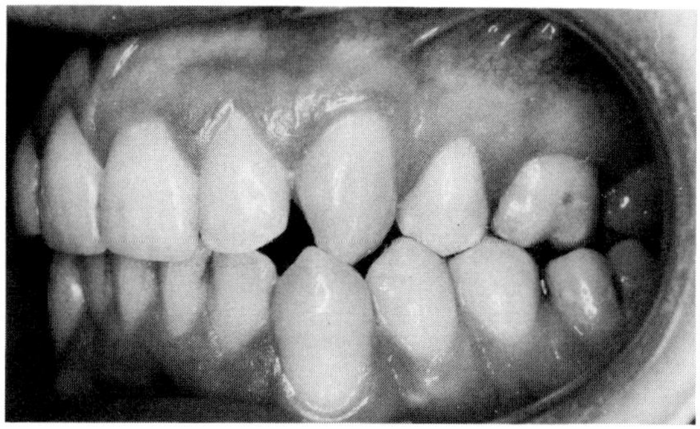

G

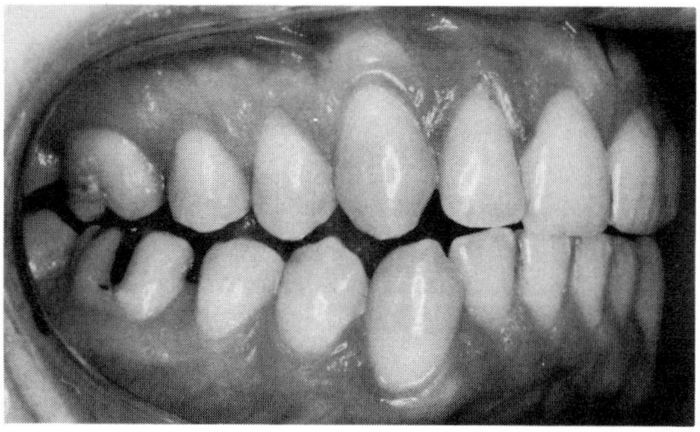

H

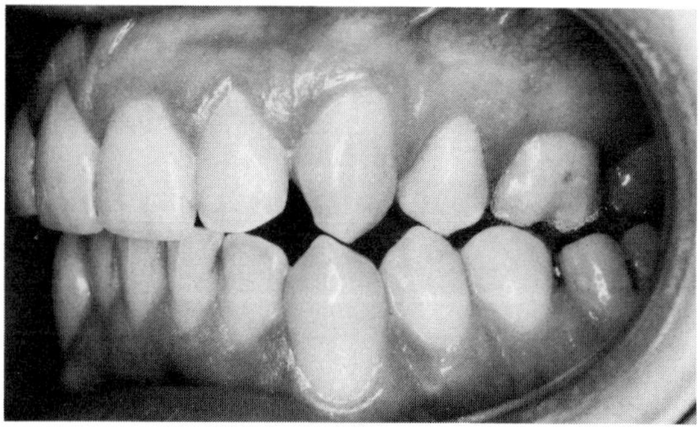

Fig 30-10 A series of lateral excursions.
A–D Excursion to the right shows occlusal guidance between canines, premolars, and molars.
E–H Excursion to the left shows the molars that are in crossbite lose contact ,while the remainder of the teeth in the region exhibit occlusal guidance.
This series of photographs demonstrates that molars in crossbite lose contact during lateral excursions. This also applies to premolar crossbites.

Chapter 31

Class II/1, agenesis 35
Extraction 75, cervical headgear, maxillary removable plate
Female: 8 years, 7 months to 34 years 0 months

A girl aged 8 years and 7 months exhibited a class II/1 anomaly with normal function; she occasionally sucked her thumb. She could breathe easily through her nose and usually kept her lips together. The mandibular left second premolar was congenitally absent and some of the deciduous molars were carious. In the maxilla, the right deciduous canine had exfoliated prematurely and the permanent incisors had drifted to the right. Consequently the middle of the maxillary dental arch was located 2mm too far to the right (Fig. 31.1). The prognosis for the mandibular left second deciduous molar was unfavorable: the crown was carious and the roots were resorbed to about the same extent as those of the contralateral tooth despite there being a successor erupting beneath the latter (Fig. 31.13). Since there was normal lip closure and a disto-occlusion of just half a premolar crown width, early intervention was not indicated. Therefore it was decided to postpone orthodontic treatment for a few years and in the meantime to proceed with the extraction of the mandibular left second deciduous molar. In the second transitional period, a cervical headgear would be used to correct the disto-occlusion and to increase the space available for the maxillary right canine. It was expected that the mandible would not need active treatment, but that a removable plate would be needed in the maxilla in addition to the headgear.

At the age of 9 years, 2 months, the mandibular left second deciduous molar was removed. Two years later, a cervical headgear was fitted. By that time, the first permanent molar in the third quadrant had drifted mesially and also tilted a little to lingual. Furthermore, the second permanent molar and the first premolar in that quadrant had emerged. The premolar had large diastemata mesially and distally. In the maxilla, the transition of the posterior teeth was complete on the left, with the first premolar emerging in a good transverse occlusion on the right. The space available for the right canine had increased somewhat (Fig 31.2).

After one year and three months, the disto-occlusion had been corrected and there was almost sufficient room for the maxillary permanent canine to take its place, although it had emerged rather too far mesially (Figs 31.3 and 31.4). After that time, the headgear was worn less, just at night. Finally a maxillary plate was worn at all times for four months to improve the alignment of the incisors.

At the age of 13 years, 9 months, all appliances were removed. The diastemata on each side of the mandibular left first premolar had diminished. On the right side, all

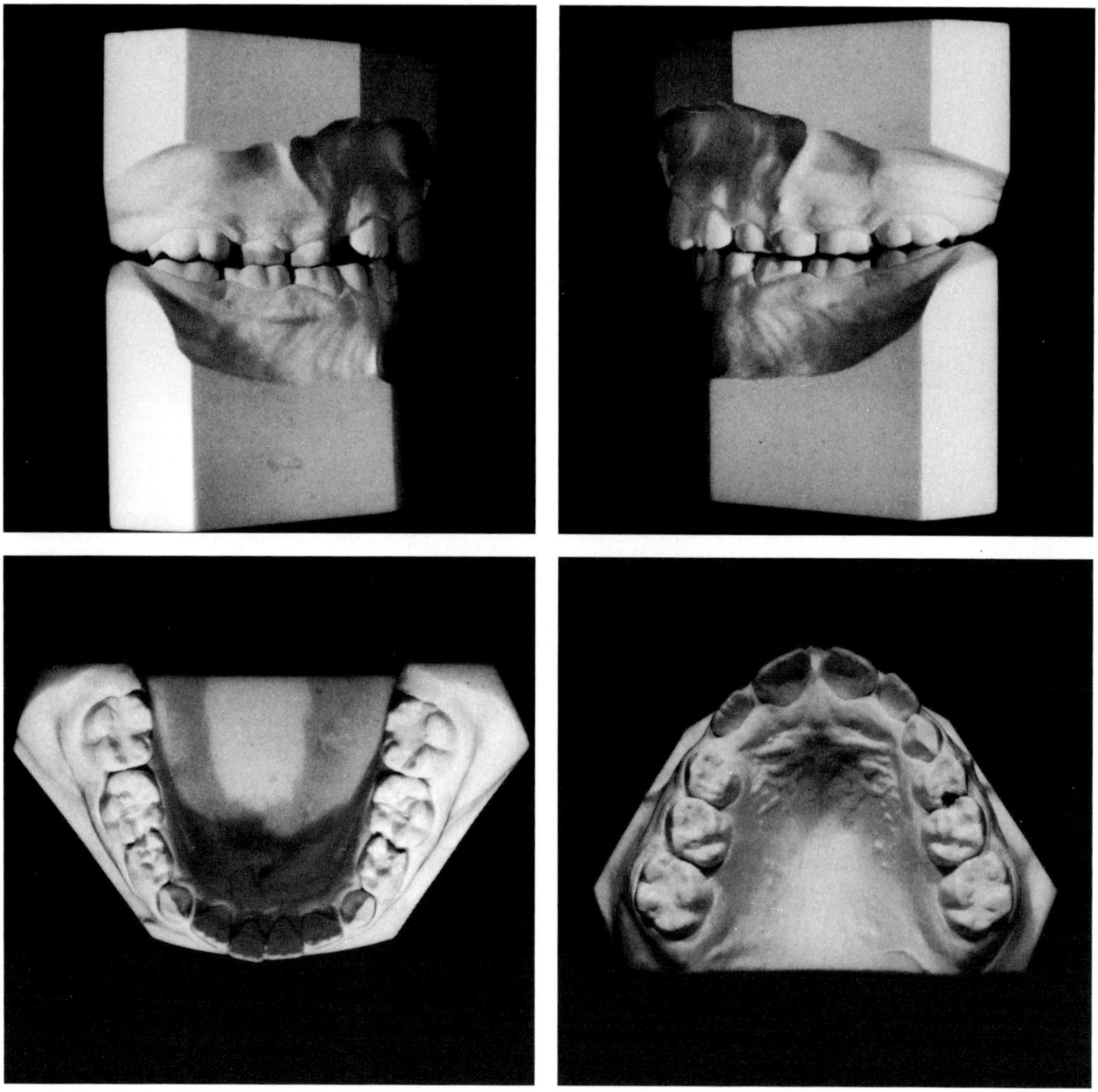

Fig 31-1 Dental casts of a girl aged 8 y, 7 mo with a class II/1 anomaly and disto-occlusion on the right of ¾ PW and on the left of ½ PW (the facial and intraoral photographs are missing). The mandibular dental arch shows no abnormality, except a reduction in the arch length due to caries of the deciduous molars. Anteriorly there is excess space, while the mandibular left second premolar is congenitally absent. The maxillary arch is narrow, the maxillary right deciduous molars occlude in crossbite, the maxillary right canine has exfoliated prematurely and partly due to the incisors having drifted to the right, the space for its successor is inadequate. The overjet is only slightly greater than normal because the disto-occlusion is combined with a deficiency in the maxillary arch length.

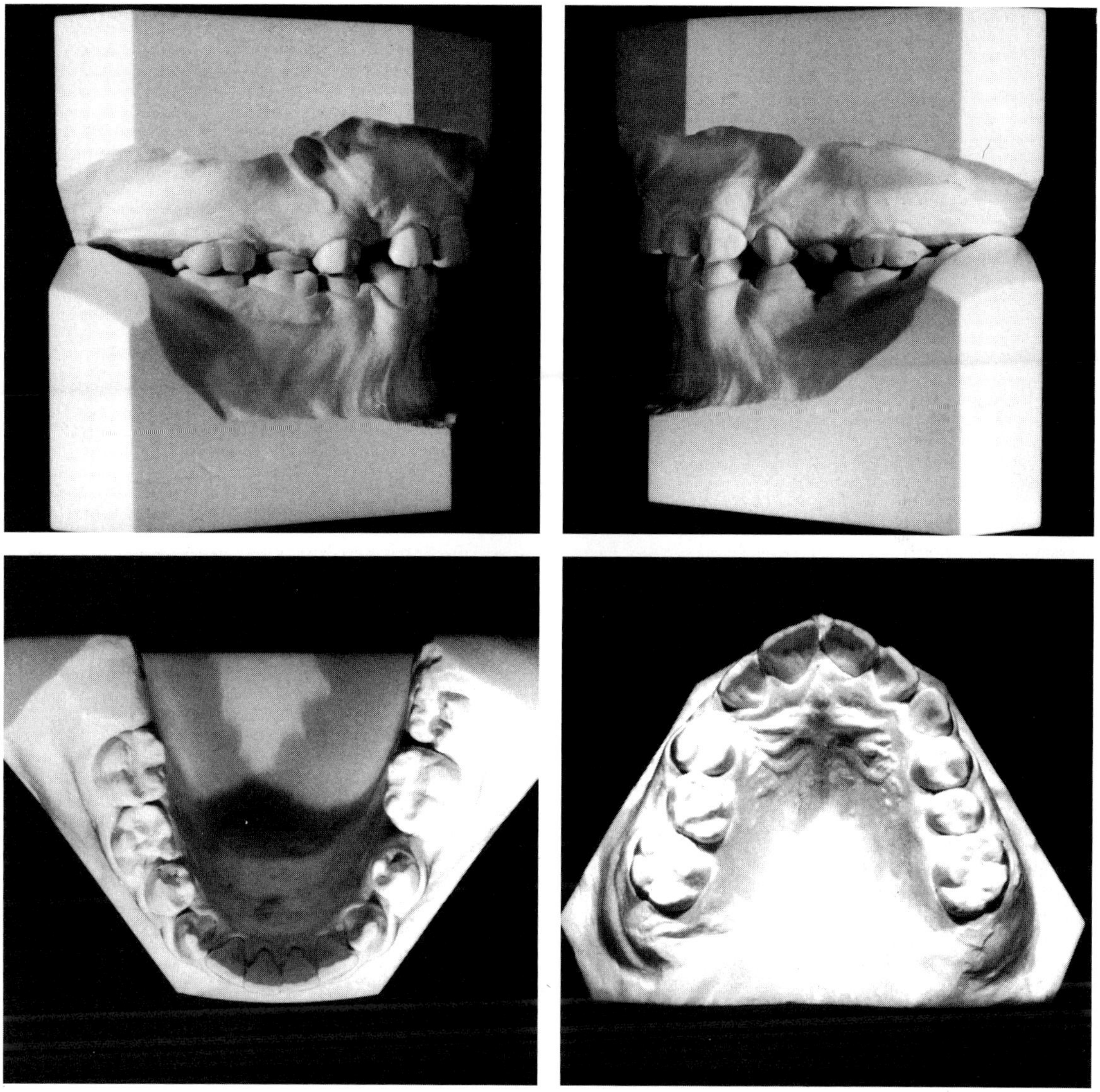

Fig 31-2 At the age of 11 y, 2 mo, two years after extraction of the mandibular left second deciduous molar, the first permanent molar on that side has drifted mesially and tipped a little lingually. Large diastemata can be seen on either side of the mandibular left first premolar. The mandibular left second permanent molar has emerged early. The mandibular right second deciduous molar has lost so much of its crown from caries that it now is the same width as its successor. (In the 1960s, carious deciduous teeth were seldom restored and often not extracted either.) In the maxilla, the premolars and canines have emerged without problems on the left. On the right, the second deciduous molar is still present and the first premolar has come into good transverse occlusion. The right permanent canine has only 3 mm space available for it in the arch, while the spaces in the anterior part of the arch have gone.

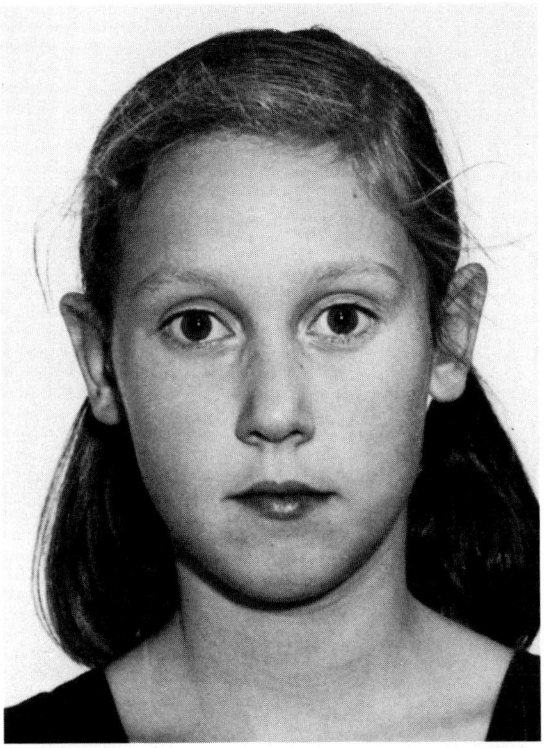

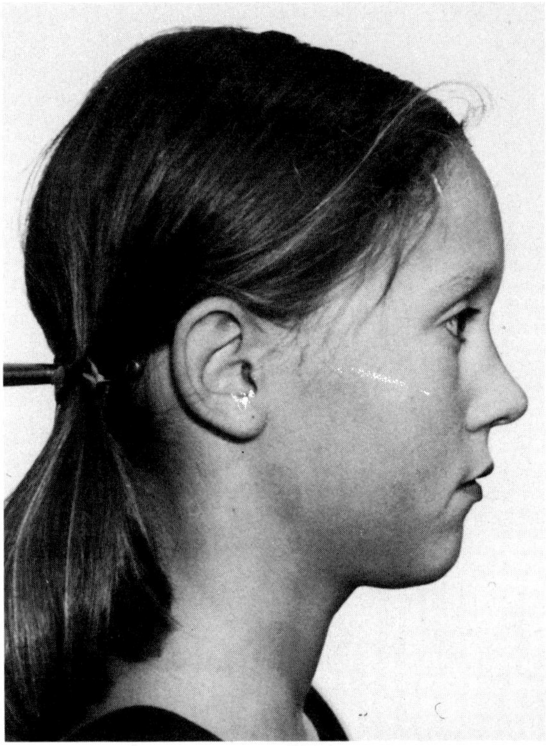

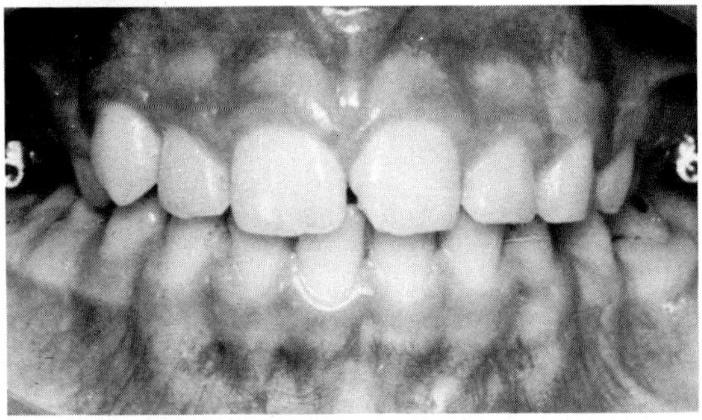

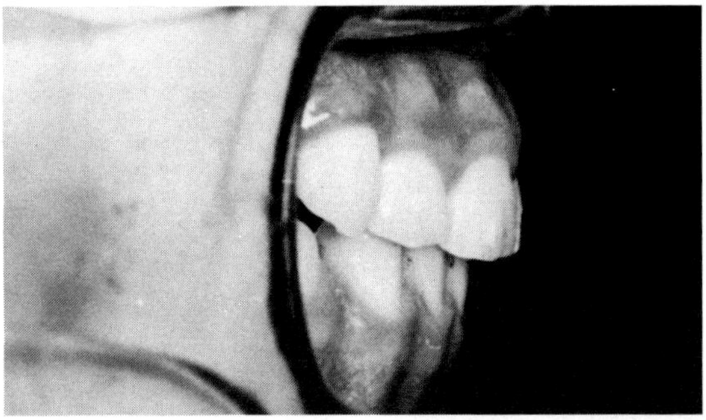

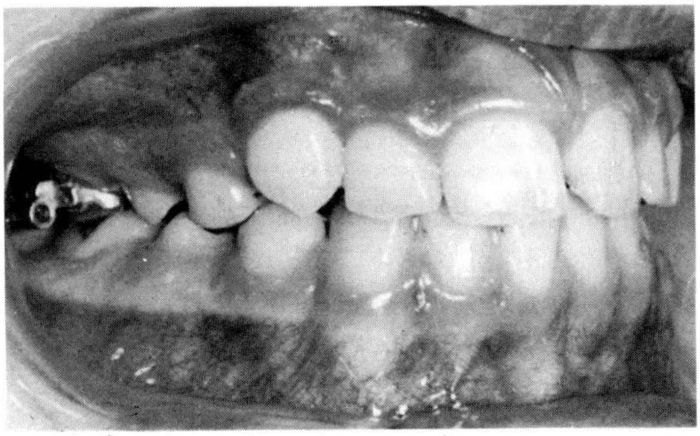

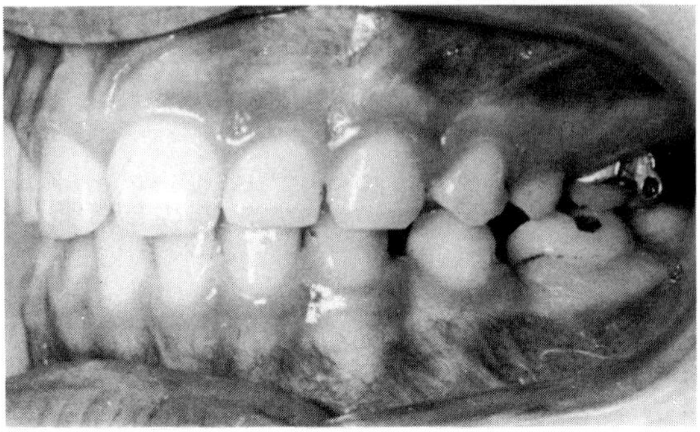

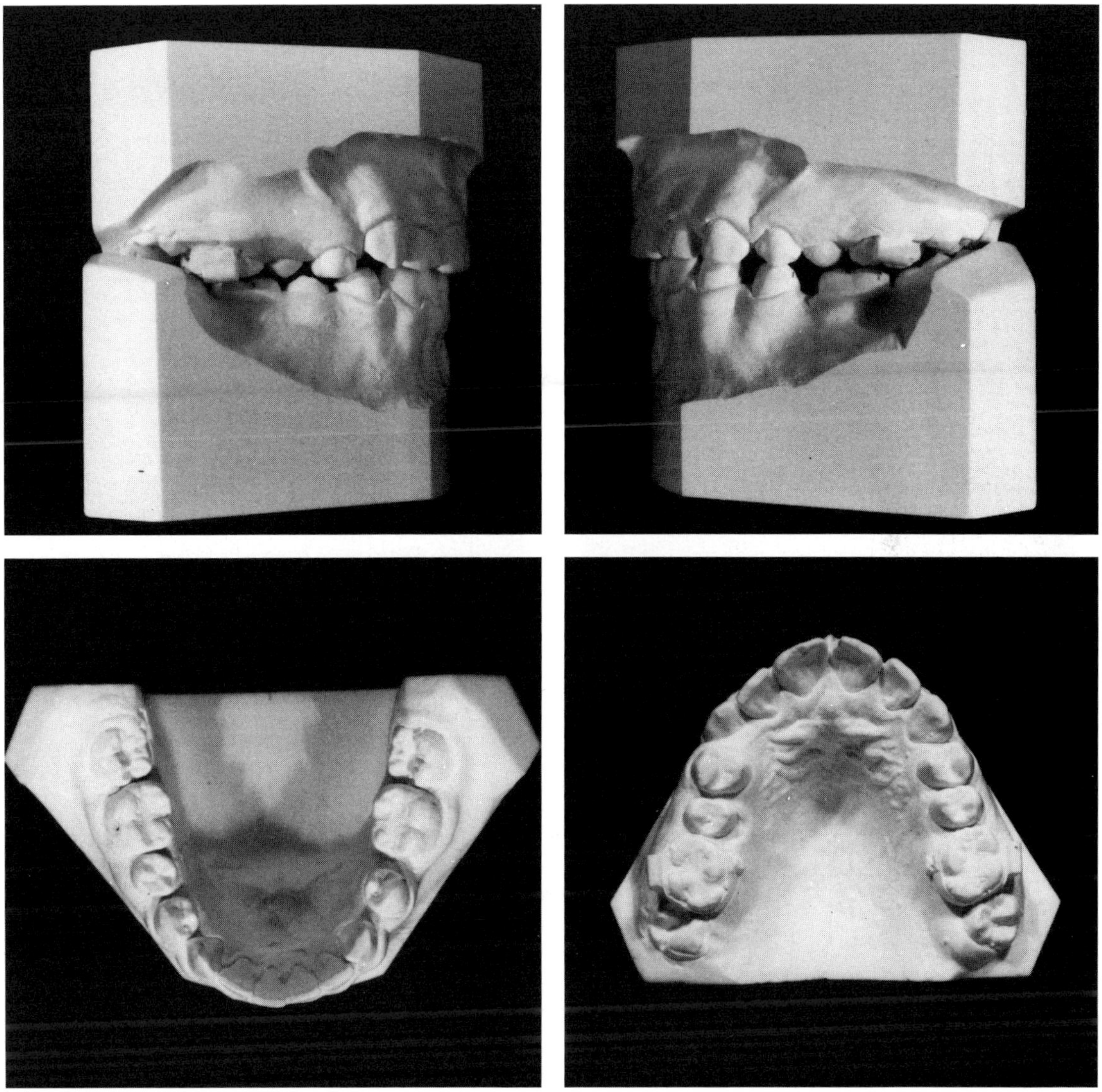

Figs 31-3 and 31-4 *At the age of 12 y, 5 mo after treatment for one year and three months with a cervical headgear that was worn 14 hours per day, the disto-occlusion has been eliminated. More space has been provided for the maxillary right permanent canine. This increase in space is related to the narrowness of the second premolar, which despite the crossbite of its predecessor has emerged in correct transverse occlusion. The diastemata in the third quadrant have become smaller. The mandibular incisors have been displaced to the left, resulting in a midline deviation of the dental arches. Most of the deviation was due to the maxillary incisors having drifted too far to the right; it has now undergone spontaneous correction.*

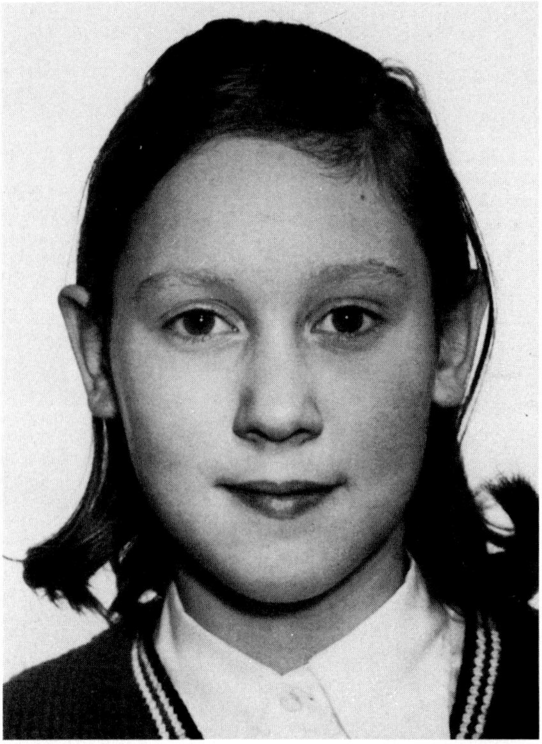
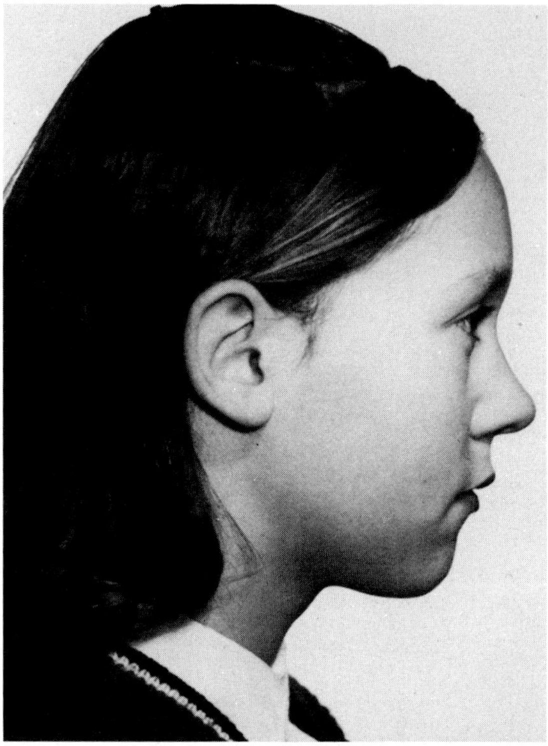
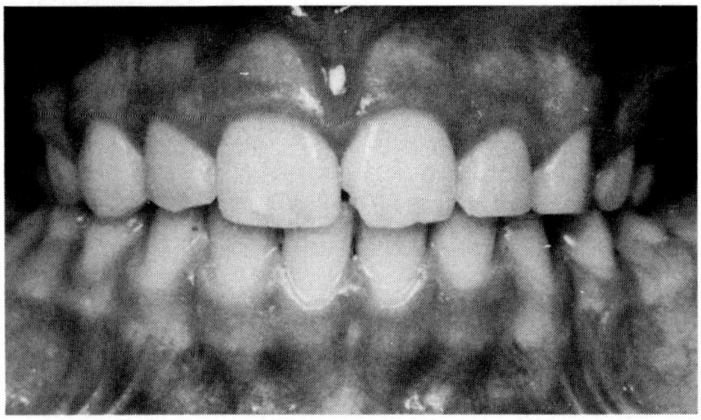
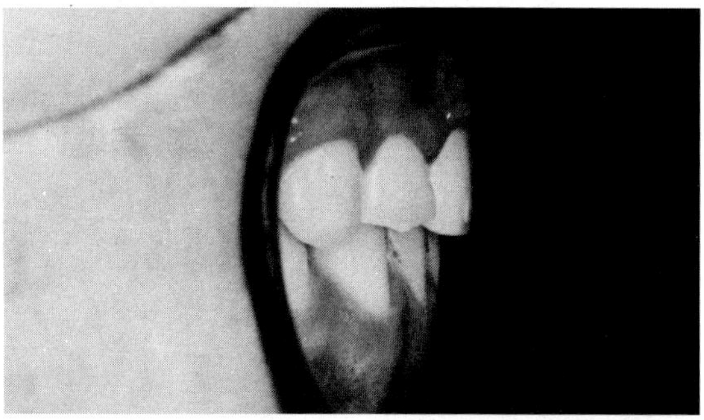
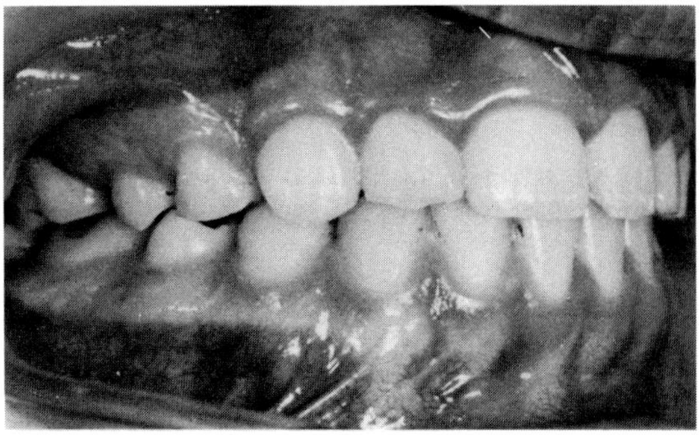
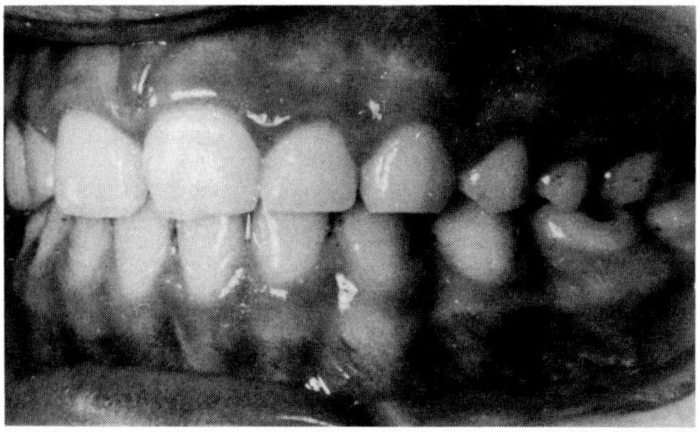

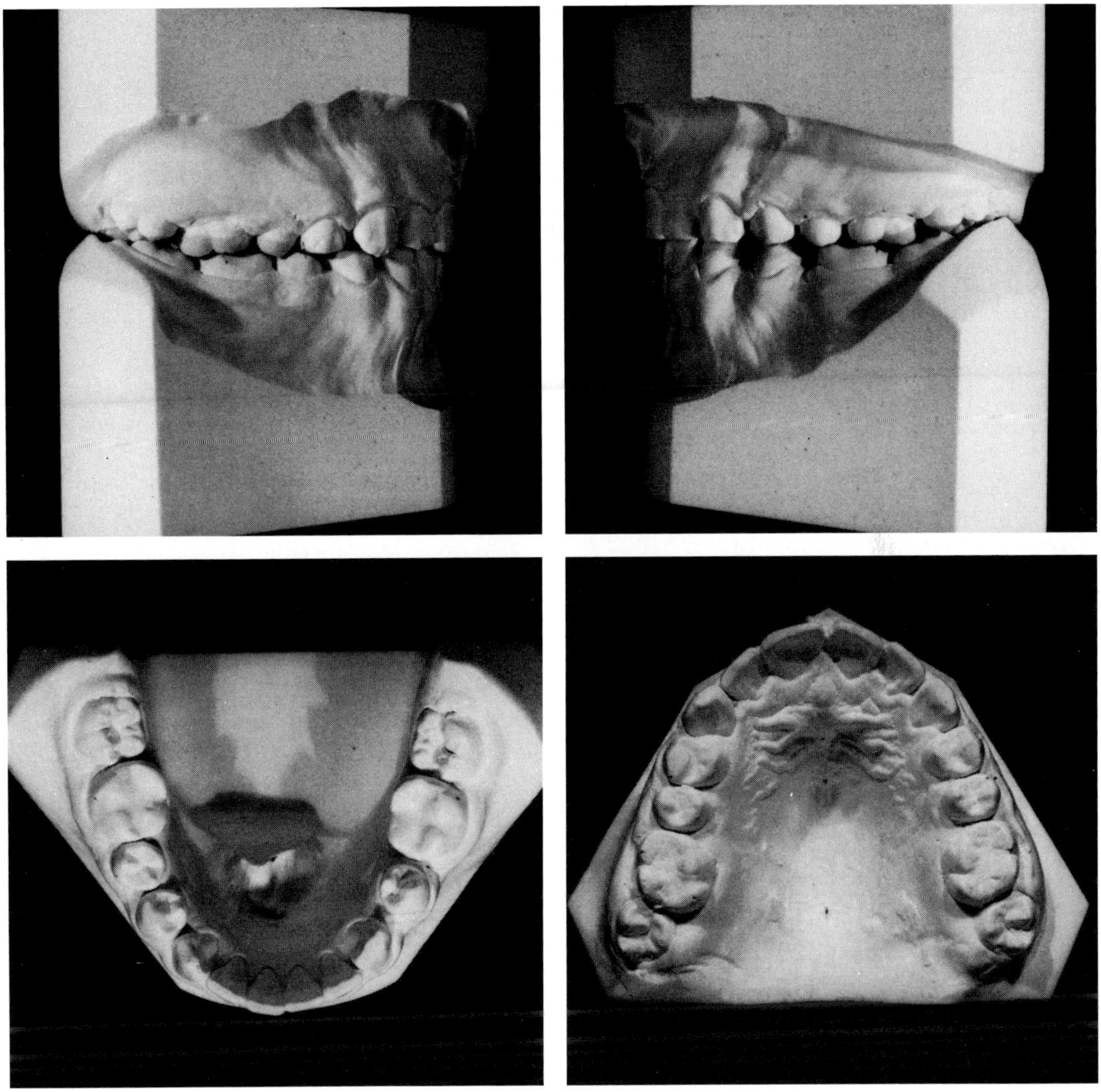

Figs 31-5 and 31-6 *At the age of 13 y, 9 mo, the treatment was concluded with an acceptable result. The occlusion on the left is not ideal. The canines and first premolars are placed more or less directly opposite each other and the molars are just in mesio-occlusion. Nonetheless, there is no disturbance in the articulation since the teeth on the left, particularly the canines, are well ground in.*

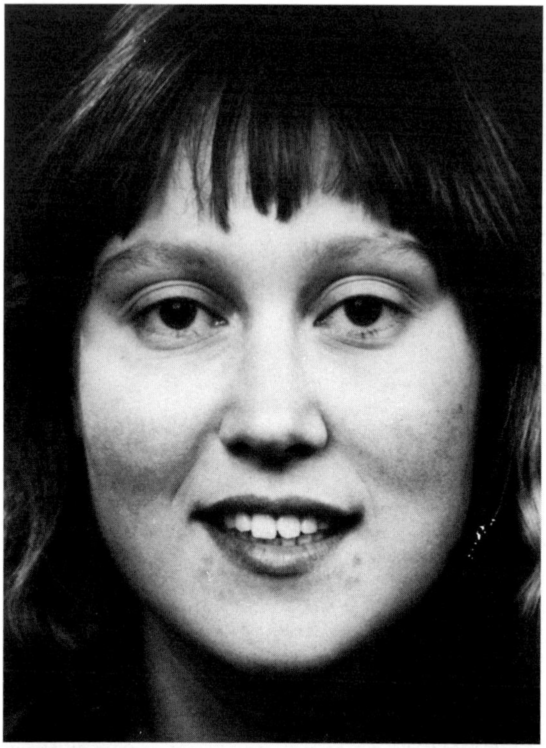
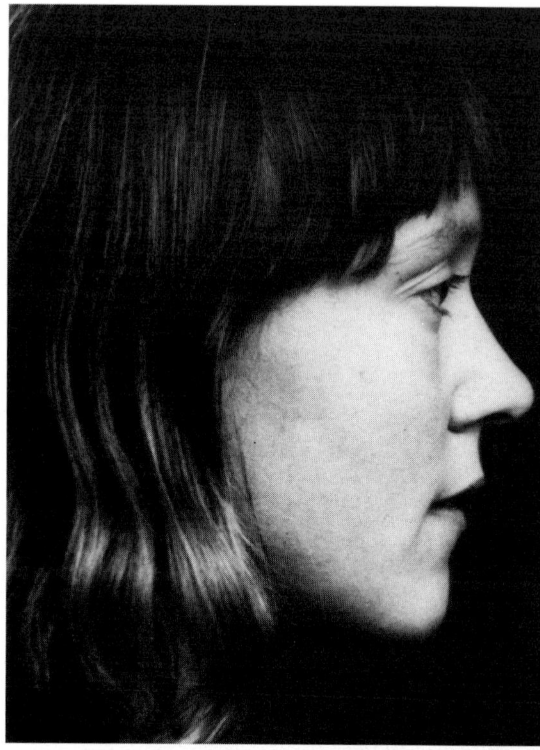
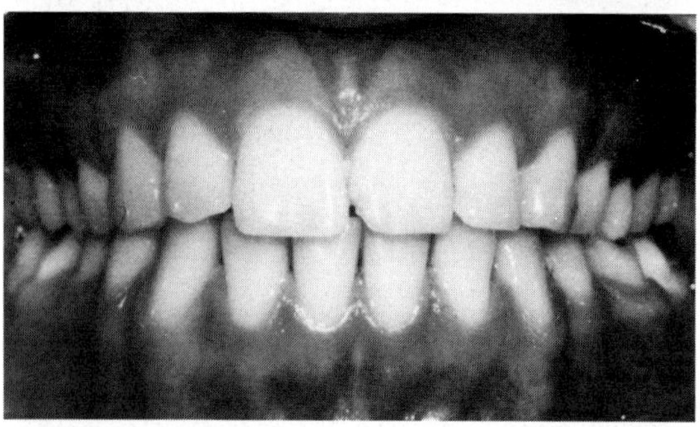
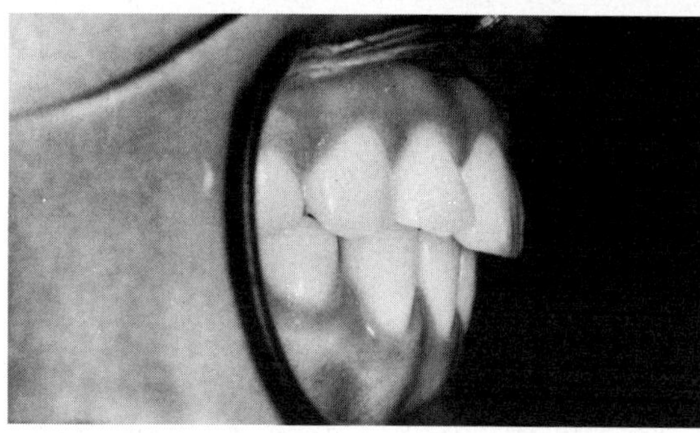
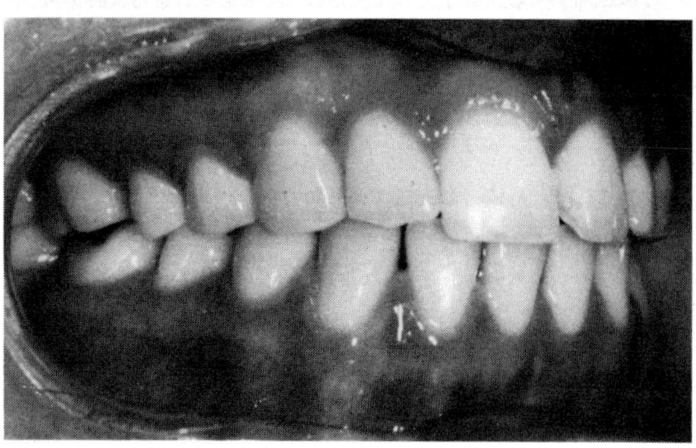
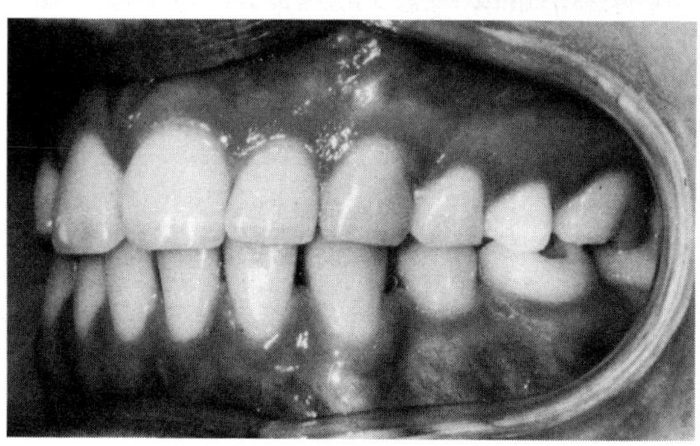

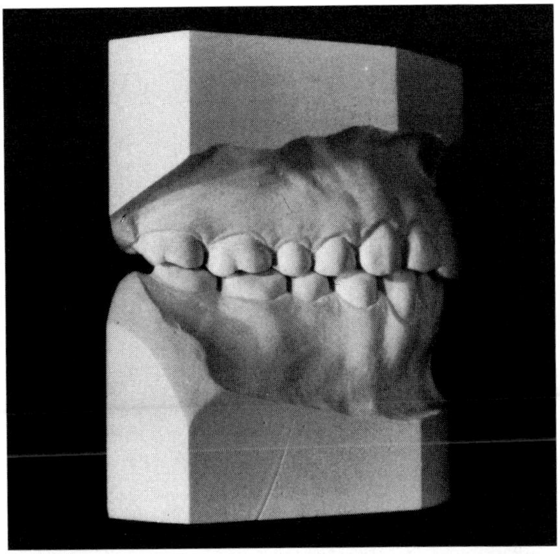
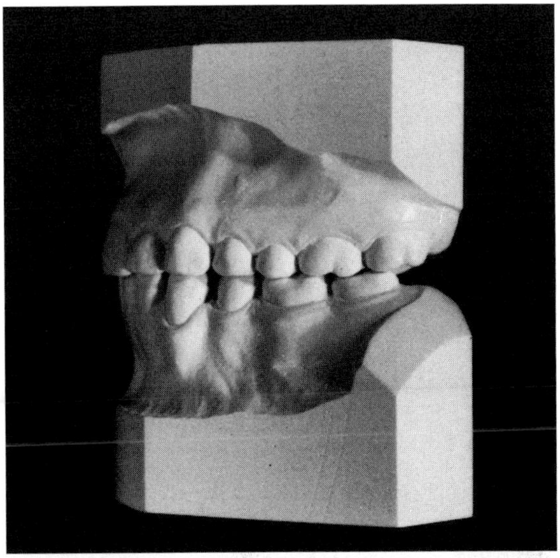
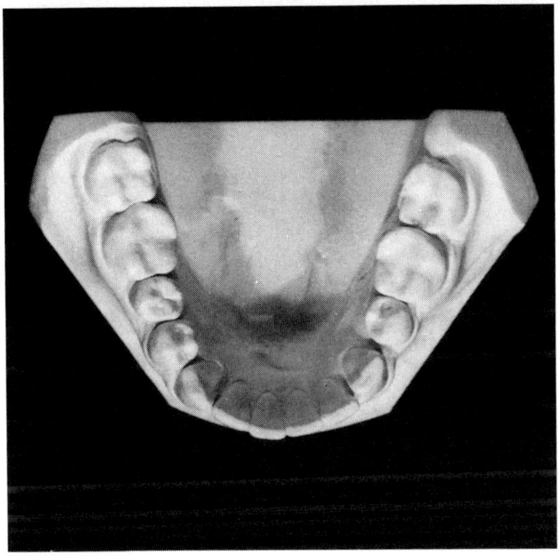
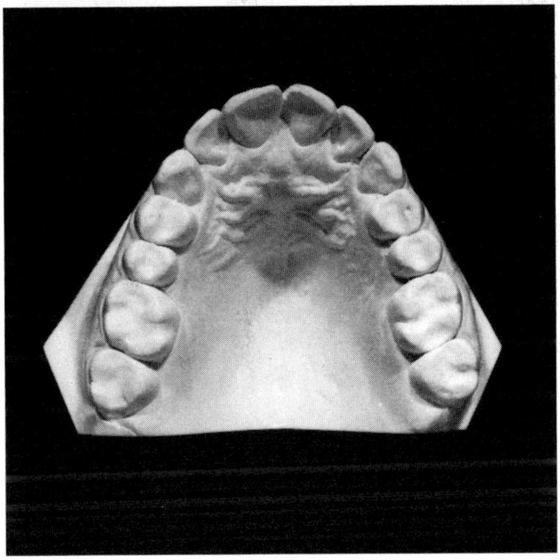

Figs 31-7 and 31-8 *At the age of 24 y, 7 mo, ten years after the end of treatment, the face has developed more, and the chin point is now more ventral with respect to the rest of the face. Little change has occurred in the dentition. On the left in the mandible the first premolar and the first molar are in contact, while there is a small diastema on each side of the canine. That now is also the case with the mandibular right canine. On the left side, the mandibular dental arch has moved mesially with respect to the maxillary dental arch, which led to an improvement in the occlusion.*

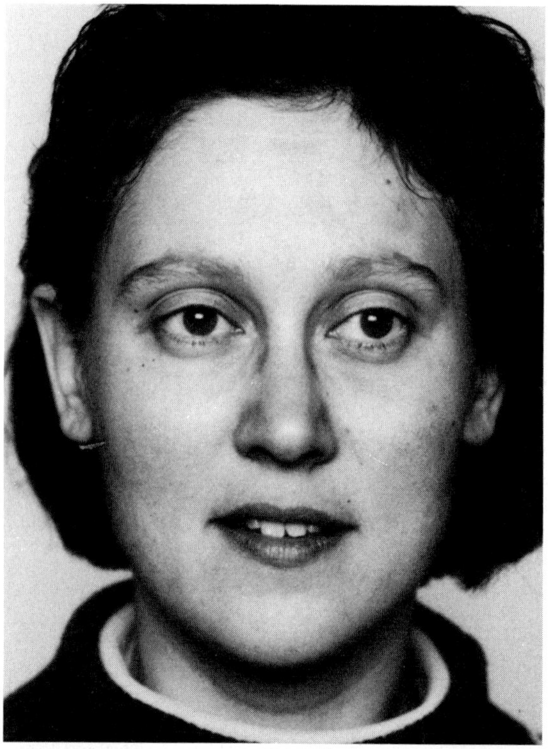

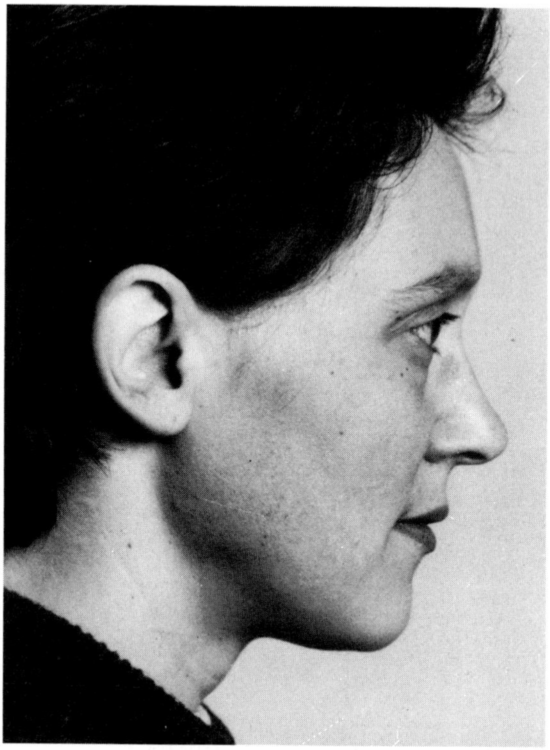

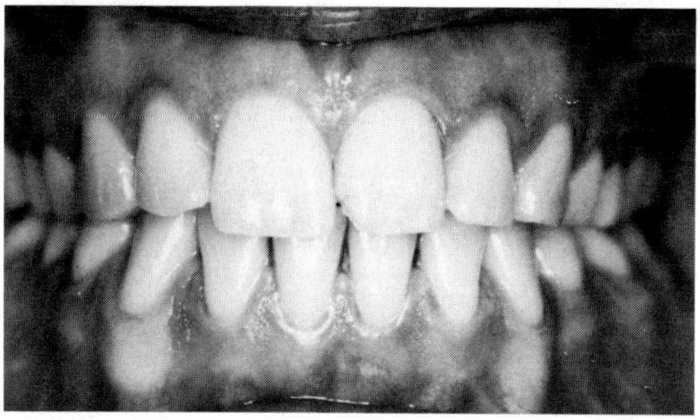

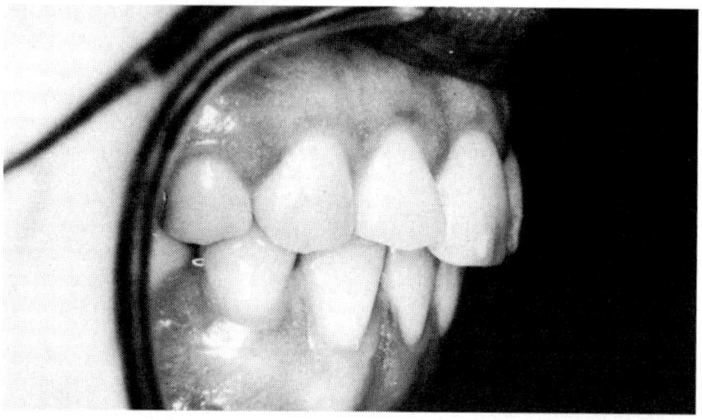

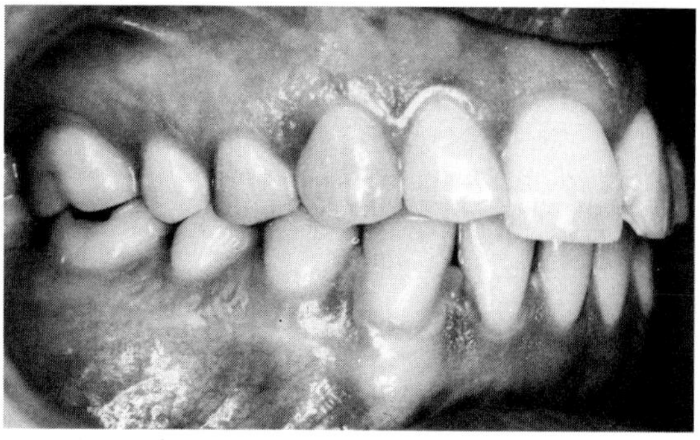

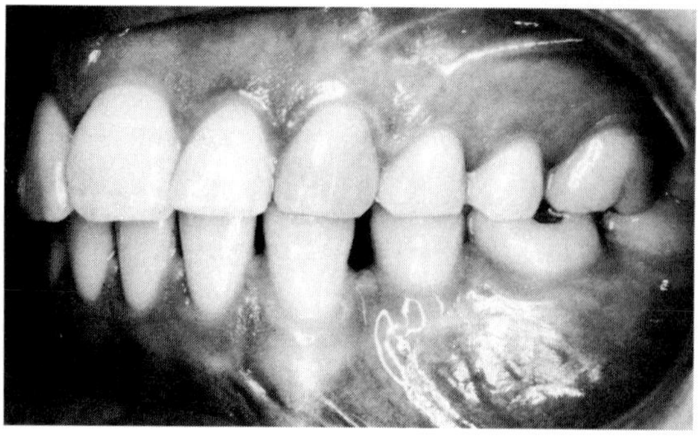

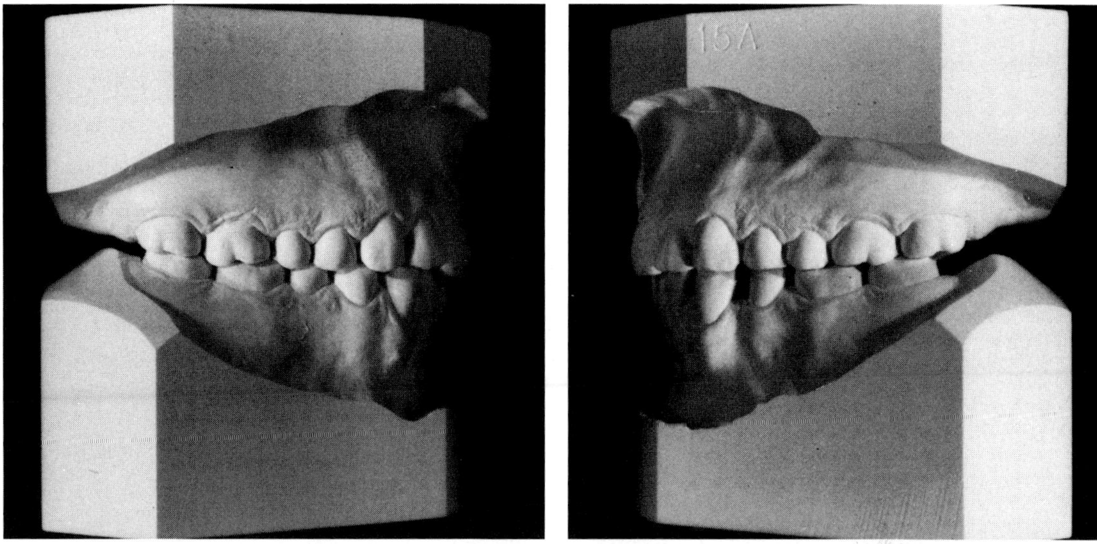

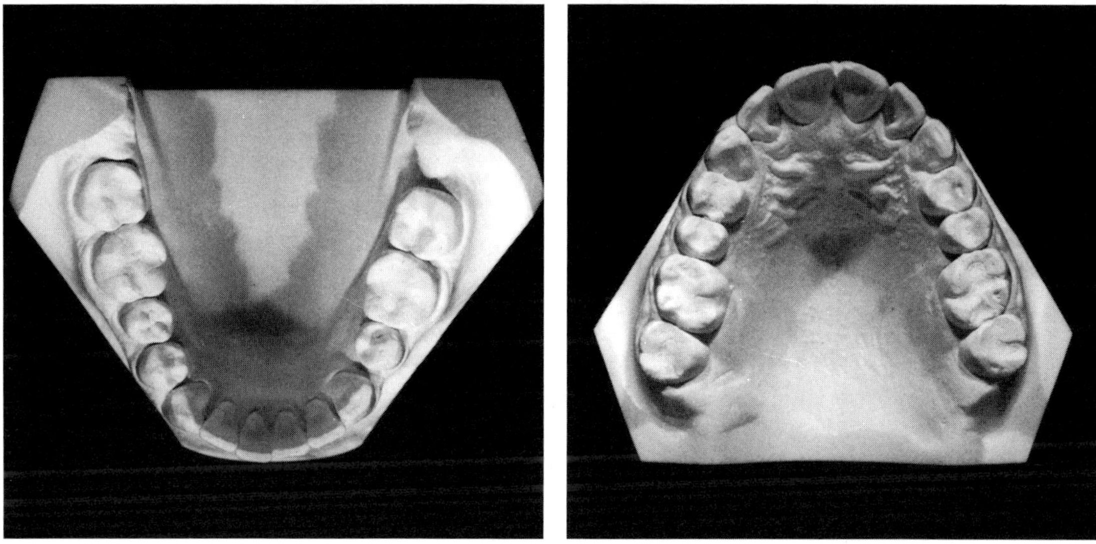

Figs 31-9 and 31-10 *At the age of 34 y, 0 mo, twenty years after treatment, the dentition functions well and has an excellent appearance in a harmonious face. Although the occlusion on the left deviates from the ideal, that is in no way disturbing. The opposing teeth have been well ground in through use, and movements during articulation cause no problems. Temporomandibular joint problems have never been experienced.*

Figure 31-11a

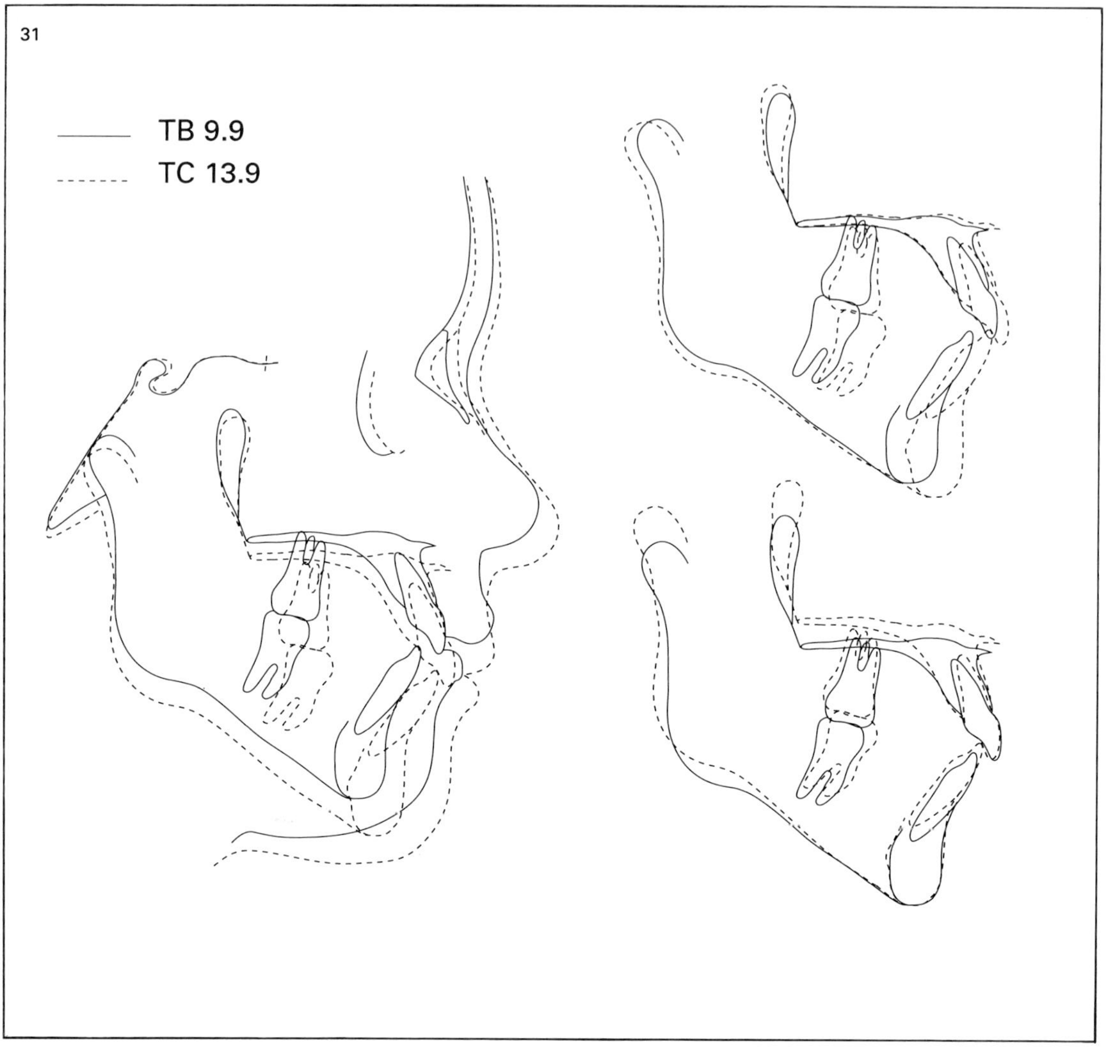

Fig 31-11 Superimposition of tracings of different cephalometric lateral radiographs gives an impression of the changes that took place during treatment and subsequently.

Figure 31-11b

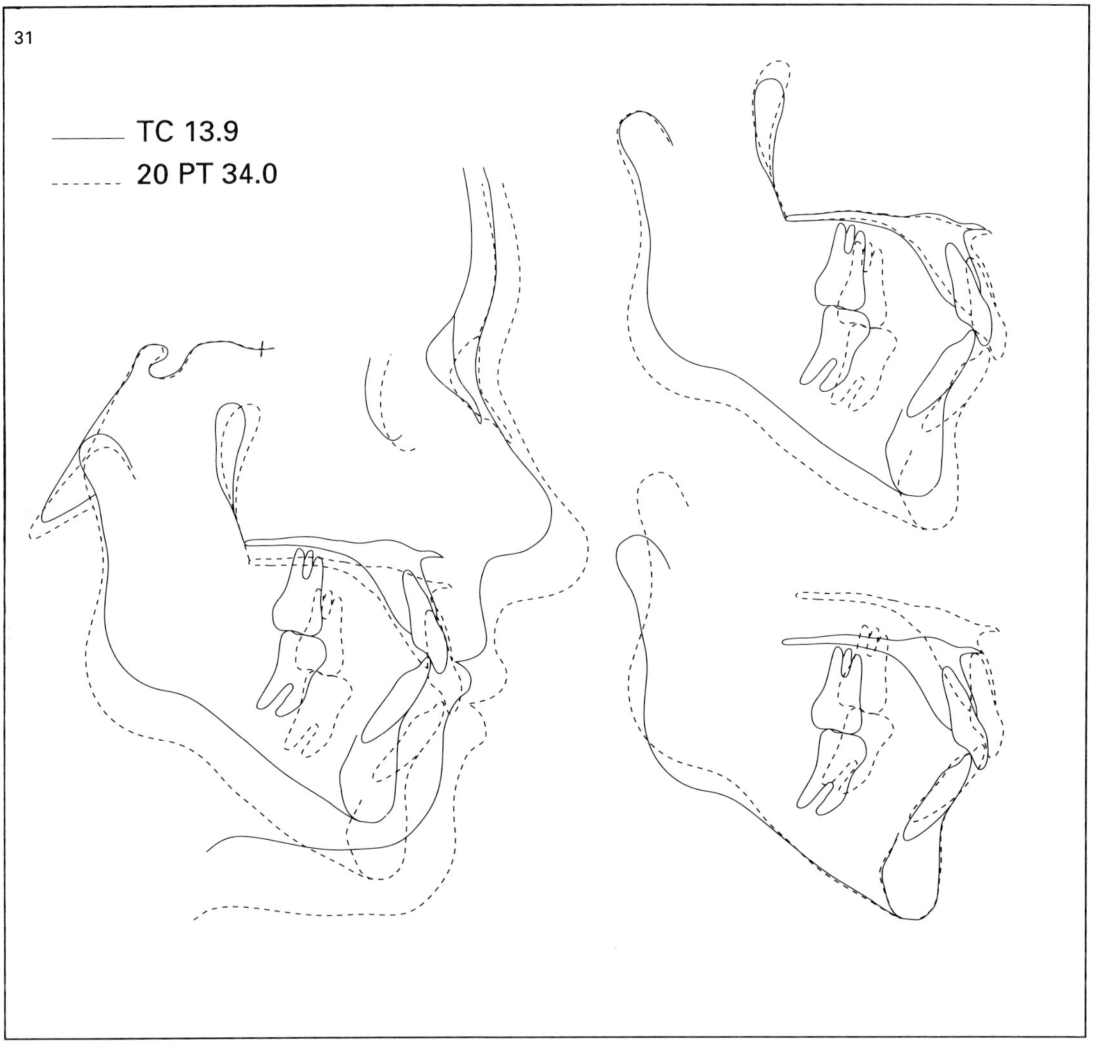

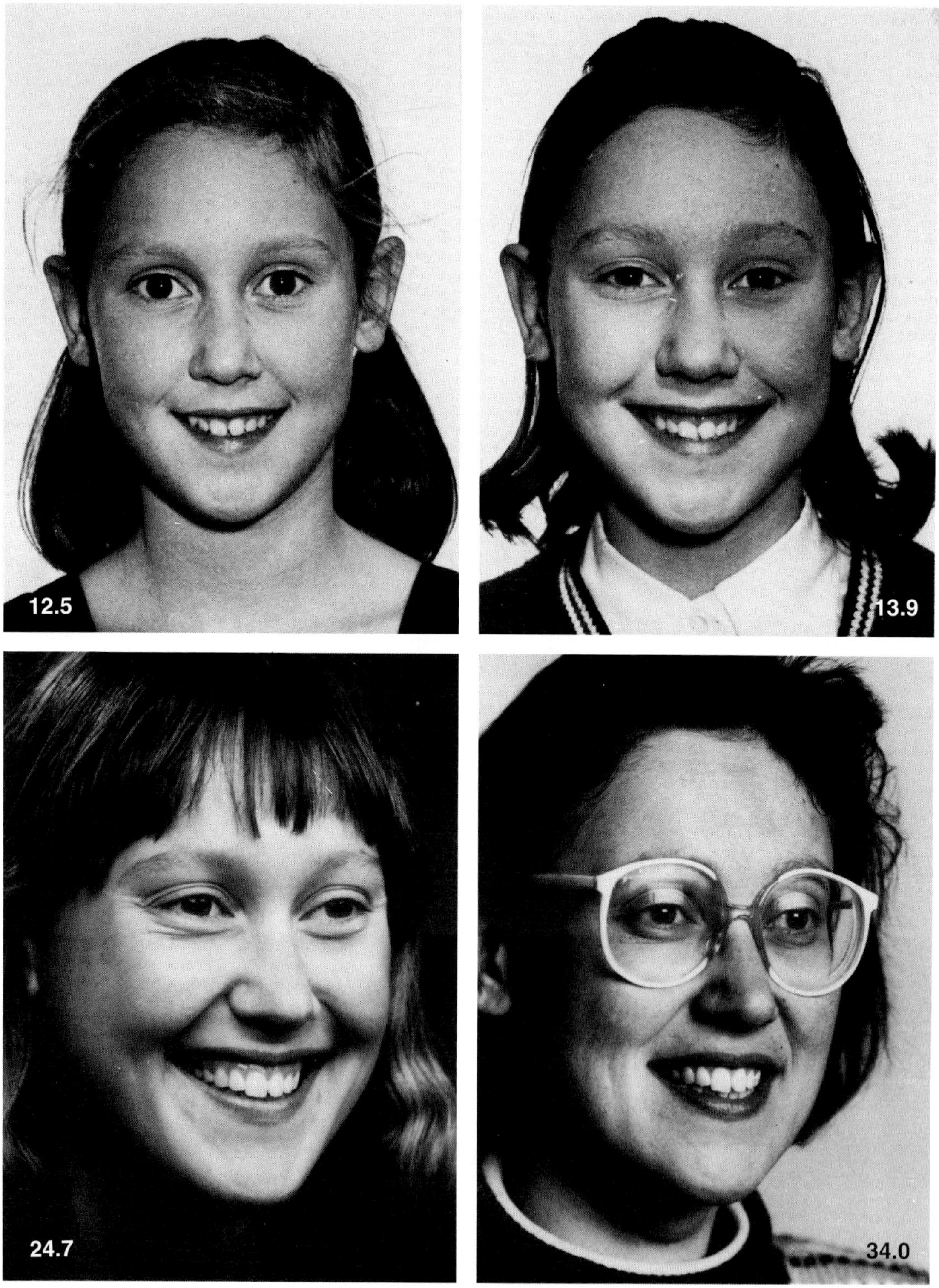
12.5
13.9
24.7
34.0

Fig 31-12 Note the changes that have occurred in the dentition.

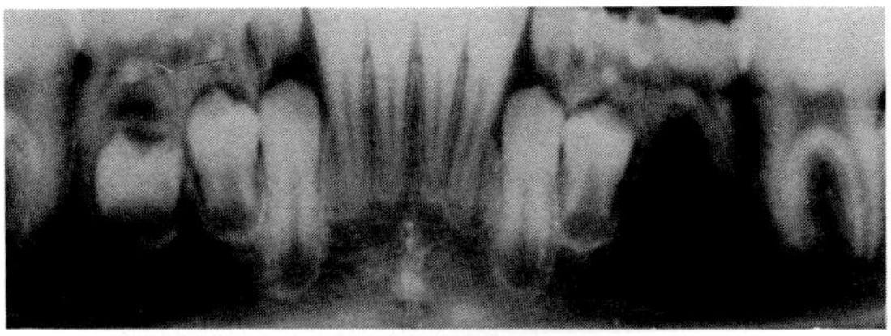

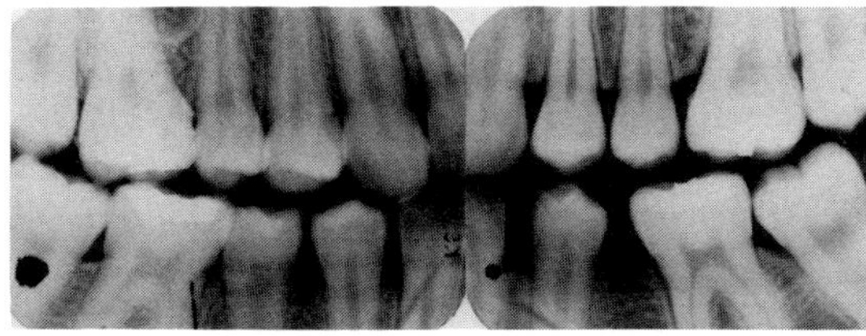

TB 8.7 TC 13.9

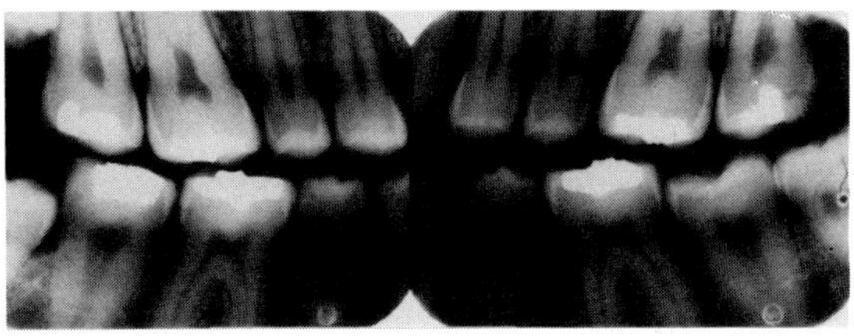

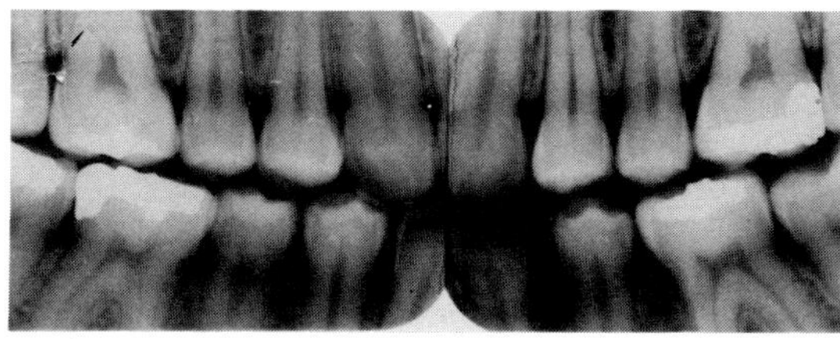

5 PT 19.7 10 PT 24.7

Fig 31-13 Intraoral radiographs at different ages show that at the age of 8 years, 7 months, the roots of the mandibular left second deciduous molar were almost as much resorbed as those of the contralateral tooth. Moreover, caries in the mandibular left second deciduous molar is evident. Five years later, after extraction of that tooth at the age of 9 y, 2 mo, the mandibular teeth on the left have taken up acceptable positions and used up the reduced amount of space quite evenly. In subsequent years the situation has improved further. The bone structure is healthy.

the teeth occluded well; on the left the occlusion was only fair due to the absence of the mandibular left second premolar. Associated with that, the midline deviation had not improved. However, there was no disturbance of the articulation of the teeth (Figs 31.5 and 31.6).

Ten years after treatment, the alignment of the maxillary and mandibular anteriors had barely changed. The mandibular left first premolar was in contact with the first molar, with only the diastema distal to the canine remaining (Figs 31.7 and 31.8).

At the age of 34 years, twenty years after treatment, the picture is almost the same. The dentition is completely satisfactory in esthetic and functional aspects (Figs 31.9 and 31.10).

The superimposition of the cephalometric tracings and the photographs of the smiling patient display the changes that have taken place over the years (Figs 31.11

and 31.12), while the individual radiographs show the conditions in the third quadrant at different ages (Fig. 31.13).

In chapters 22 and 23, two patients were described in whom second deciduous molars that had no successors were retained. The criteria that have to be considered in the decision-making process for such cases were discussed in those cases. In the case described here, the roots of the pertinent deciduous molar were as much resorbed as those of the contralateral deciduous molar beneath which a successor was indeed present, and in addition the crown of the deciduous molar was carious. Its long-term survival could not be expected.

If a deciduous molar without a permanent successor is removed from a dental arch with adequate room, then it should be done promptly so that an opportunity is afforded during subsequent dental development for spontaneous correction of the untoward results of the extraction. Moreover, eventual crowding in the anterior part of the dental arch can be reduced. If the extraction is done before the second permanent molar has emerged, then the first molar will drift more to the mesial.

If for other reasons, treatment of the mandibular arch is not indicated, then it is necessary to maintain regular observation of the spontaneous corrections that may follow the extraction to judge how acceptable the final conditions might be. It is especially desirable in the case of an extraction of a mandibular deciduous molar to watch for overeruption of the opposing maxillary tooth occurring to such a degree that it impedes the mesial movement of the mandibular first permanent molar. In favorable circumstances such as in this case, active intervention can be avoided.

The provision of appliances to correct the disto-relation and to increase the available space in the maxillary arch was deliberately delayed for some time. As has been reiterated several times, the cervical headgear is particularly effective for reaching those treatment objectives. Beginning earlier would have been pointless. The treatment would then have been needlessly prolonged, since it could only have been concluded after the premolars and canines had fully emerged.

Finally, it must be mentioned that a natural dentition can provide satisfactory life long function even if there is not an ideal occlusion. Excursions of the teeth during function can enjoy interference-free articulation even when the antagonists are positioned cusp to cusp, provided that they have been subjected to natural attrition or deliberate occlusal grinding that will provide the cusp-height and form required for undisturbed movements.

Chapter 32

Class II/1, impacted 45, scissorbite 14 and 24
Cervical headgear, maxillary removable plate, brackets 12, 11, 21, and 22, mandibular lip bumper, extraction 45, lingual arch, maxillary removable retainer
Female: 11 years, 8 months to 26 years, 3 months

A girl aged 11 years, 8 months exhibited a class II/1 anomaly with a large lower face height. She could breathe easily through her nose but usually kept her mouth open. Her oral hygiene was only fair. The mandibular right deciduous molars had been lost prematurely and there was no longer sufficient room for the second premolar which was wedged between the first premolar and the first permanent molar. Some degree of crowding existed in the remainder of the mandibular dental arch, with an ALD of –9 mm. The maxillary lateral incisors had emerged too far to palatal and the maxillary first permanent molars were rotated mesio-palatally. Nonetheless, the ALD was only –2mm due to the presence of diastemata. The maxillary first premolars were in scissorbite. The first permanent molars on the right were in normal occlusion. If allowance were made for three-quarters of the loss of space being due to mesial drifting of the molars, the occlusion of the molars could be estimated to have been ¾ PW disto on the right and ½ PW on the left. All the third molars were forming (Figs 32.1 and 32.2).

The decision was taken to correct the disto-occlusion by means of a cervical headgear and at the same time to use it to rotate back the first permanent molars. At a later stage, a removable plate would be used for other corrections in the maxilla and if necessary it would be followed by a partial fixed appliance. An attempt would be made to regain the space lost for the mandibular right second premolar, with a lip bumper, and in conjunction a lingual arch would be used to improve the positions of several teeth in the mandibular arch.

A cervical headgear was fitted at the age of 11 years, 11 months. Seven months later, a maxillary plate was provided and three months later a mandibular lip bumper was fitted. Although the lip bumper was worn well, the increase in available space in the mandibular arch after six months seemed to be negligible. The mandibular right second premolar had erupted a little further and could be palpated lingually. At the age of 13 years, 4 months, radiographs were taken and impressions obtained for dental casts. From the study of the additional records it was clear that indeed hardly any space had been gained in the mandibular arch, and that on the right the mandibular third molar was mesially inclined and lay against the second molar. It was decided to make no further attempt to gain space for the mandibular right

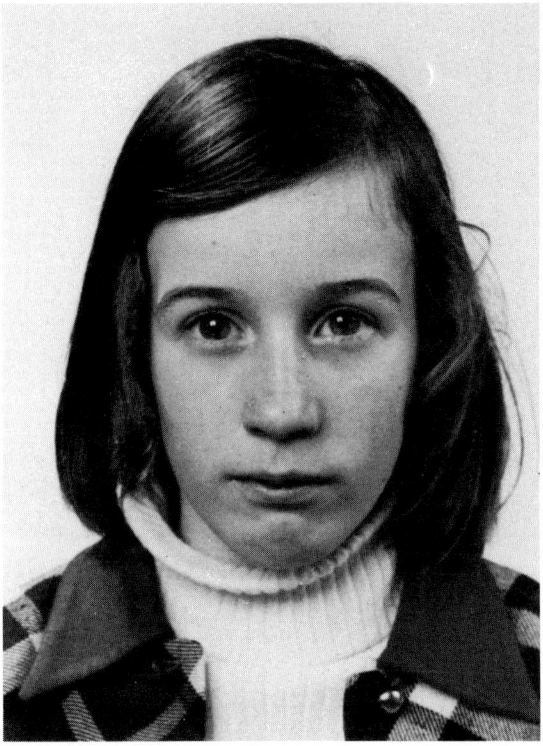
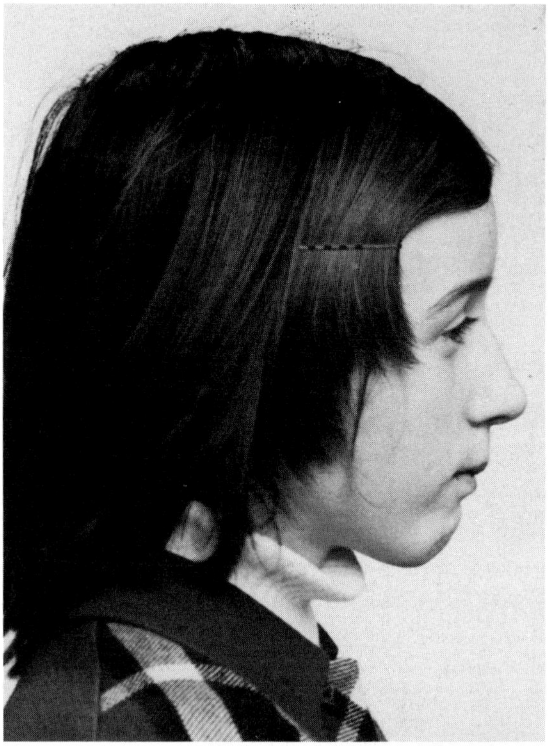
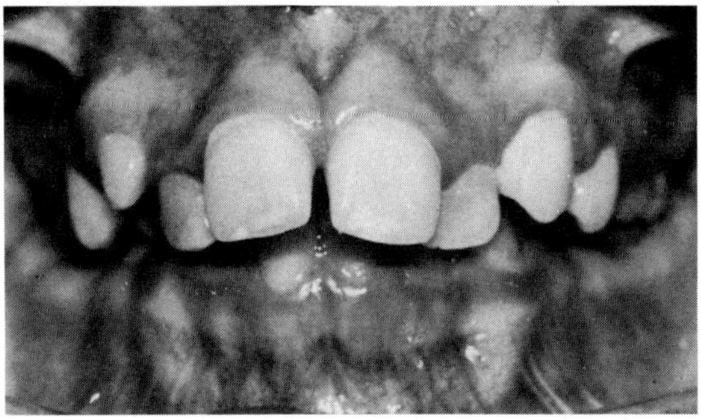
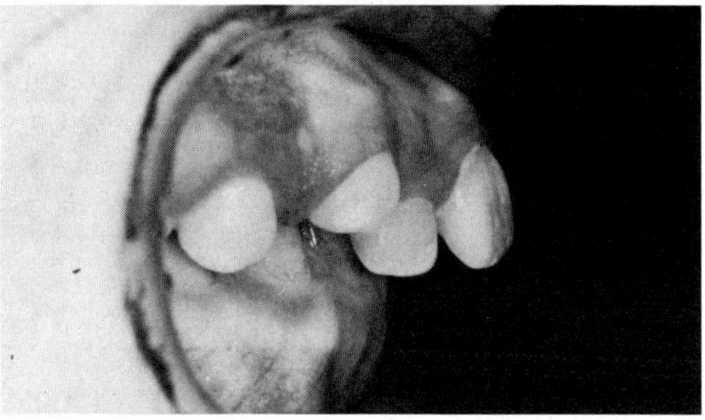
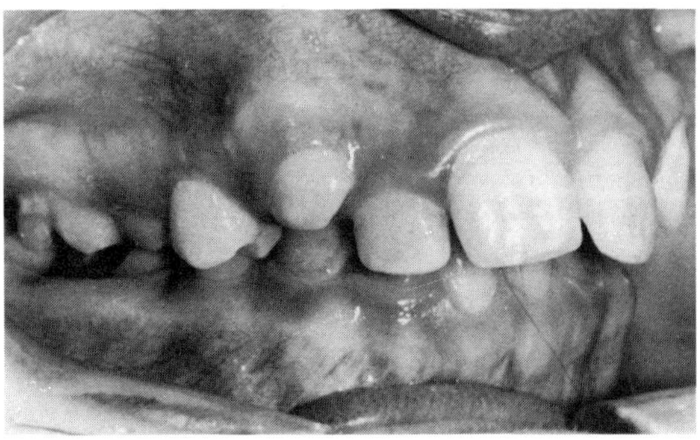
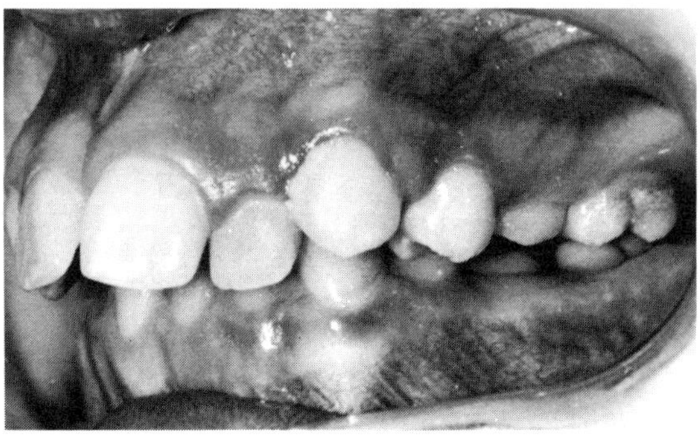

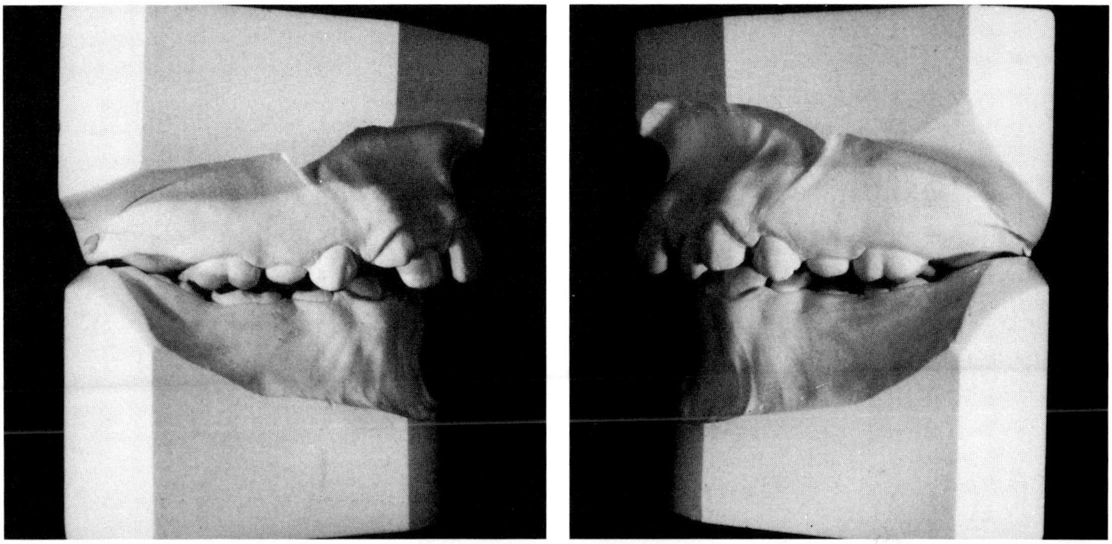

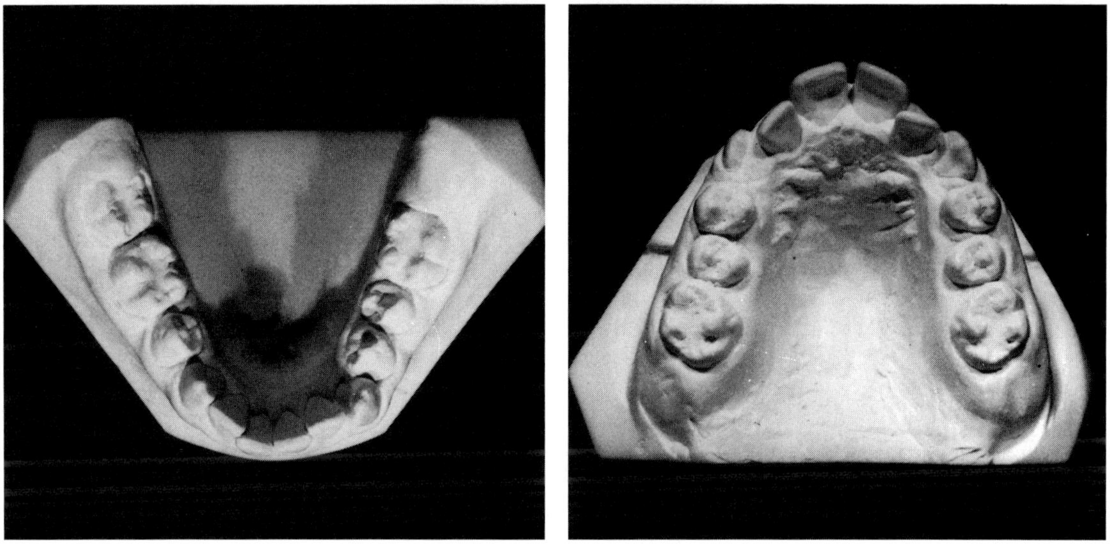

Figs 32-1 and 32-2 *A girl aged 11 y, 8 mo with a class II/1 anomaly, in which the space for the mandibular right second premolar has vanished due to the early loss of the deciduous molars. Her oral hygiene is unsatisfactory and the gingiva is congested and slightly inflamed. The mandibular dental arch is narrow. The mandibular right first premolar is almost contacting the first permanent molar, and the second premolar is unerupted, impacted between those two teeth. There is still some crowding in the remainder of the mandibular arch; the ALD measures –9 mm. In the maxillary arch, the first permanent molars are rotated mesio-palatally, the lateral incisors are positioned too far to palatal, and the first premolars are buccally displaced and in scissorbite. After mentally repositioning the teeth that migrated as a consequence of the premature loss of the deciduous molars, there would be a disto-occlusion of ¾ PW on the right and ½ PW on the left.*

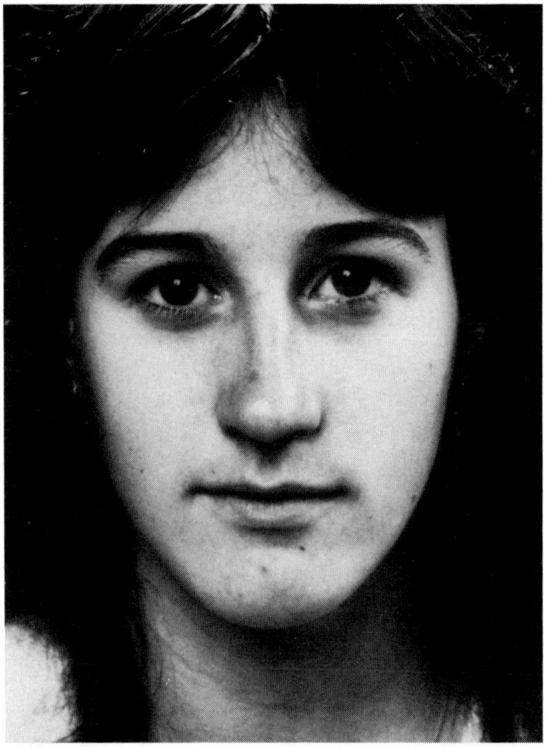
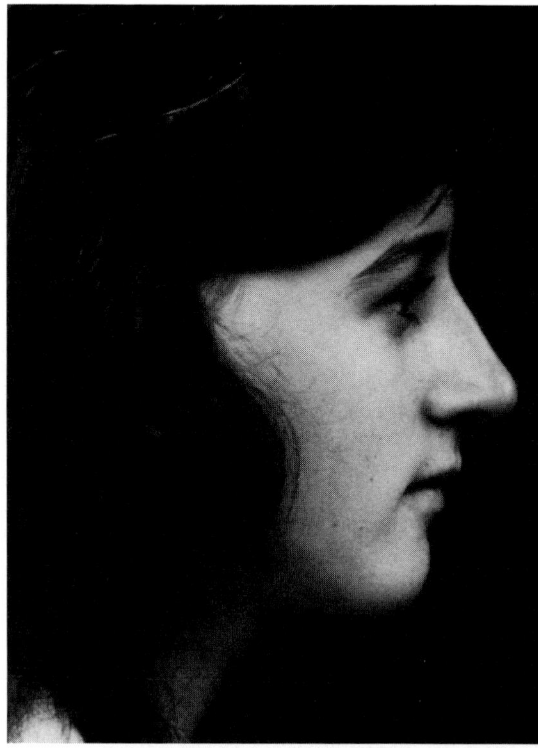
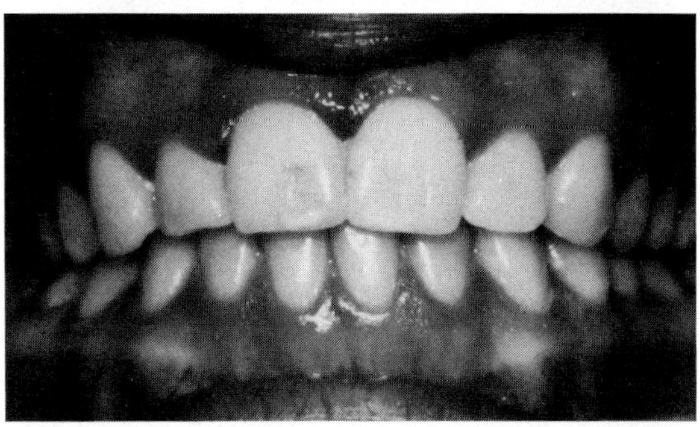
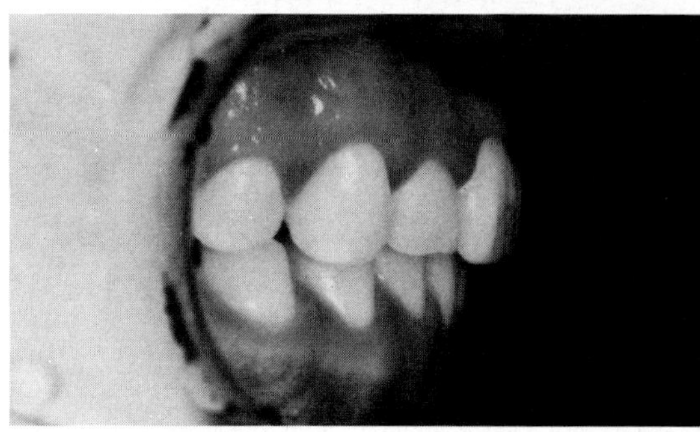
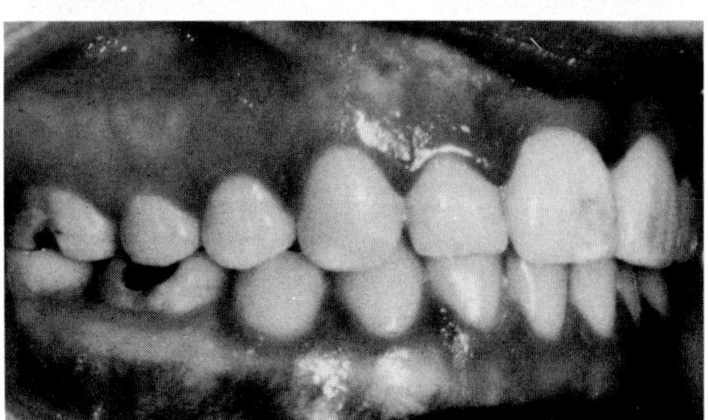
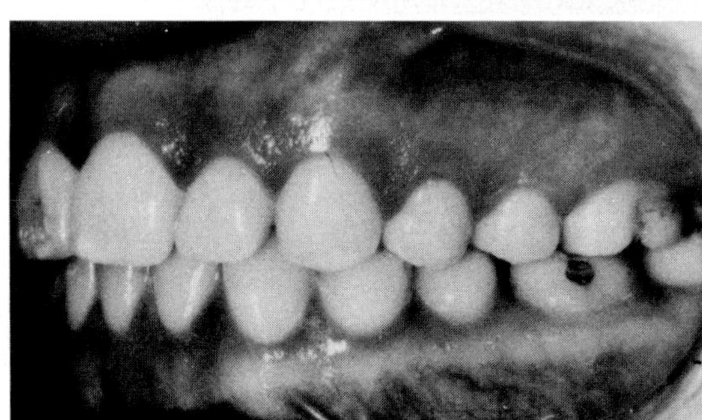

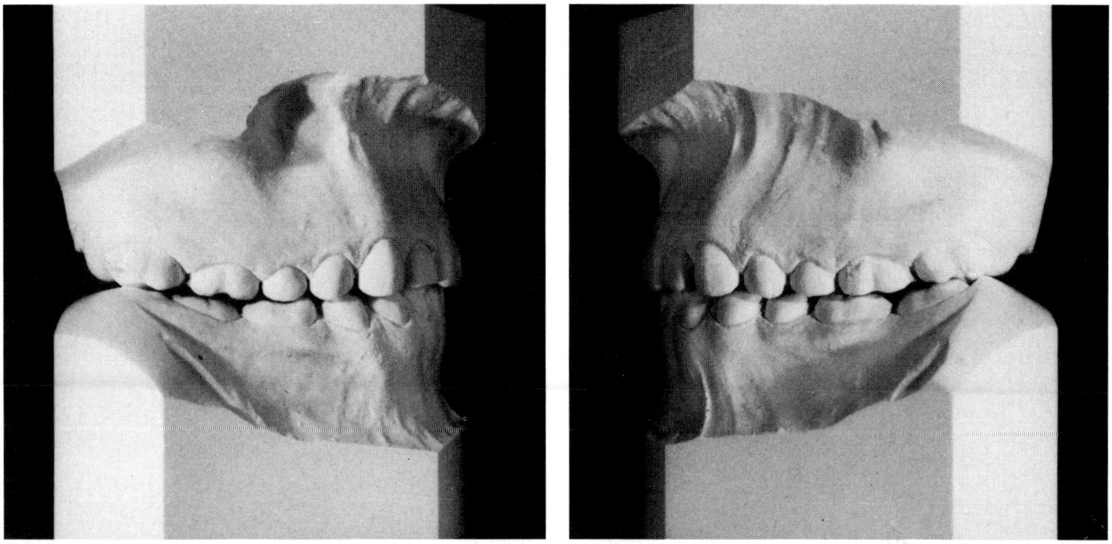

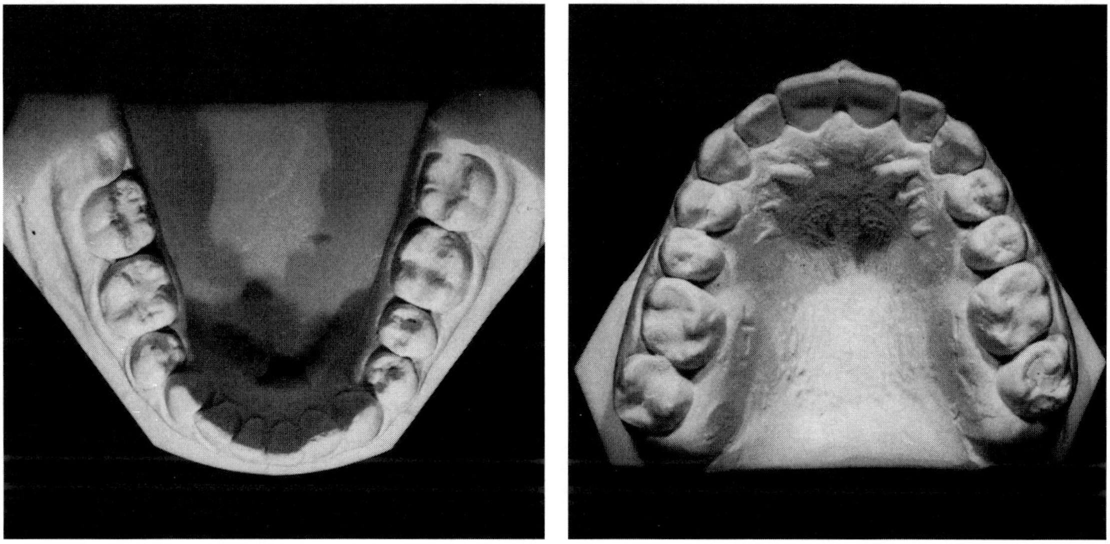

Figs 32-3 and 32-4 *At the age of 16 y, 1 mo, after treatment for 3½ years and a retention period of eight months, the result obtained is good. The face is harmonious and the dentition is esthetically and functionally satisfactory. However, the mandibular right second premolar is missing and the premolar occlusion on the right is not normal; namely, the maxillary second premolar occludes with the central fossa of the mandibular first permanent molar. Because of the shallow cusp heights, the excursions of the mandible are free of interference. There is bilateral group guidance in lateral excursions. Except for the slight mesiopalatal rotation of the maxillary left canine, the maxillary dental arch is excellent. The minor abnormalities of the mandibular arch, specifically the linguo position of the right canine, are connected with the unusual occlusion on the right side.*

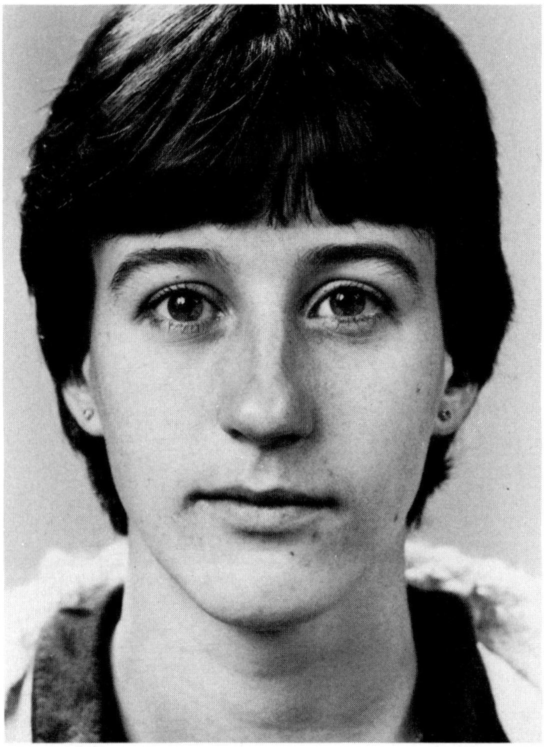

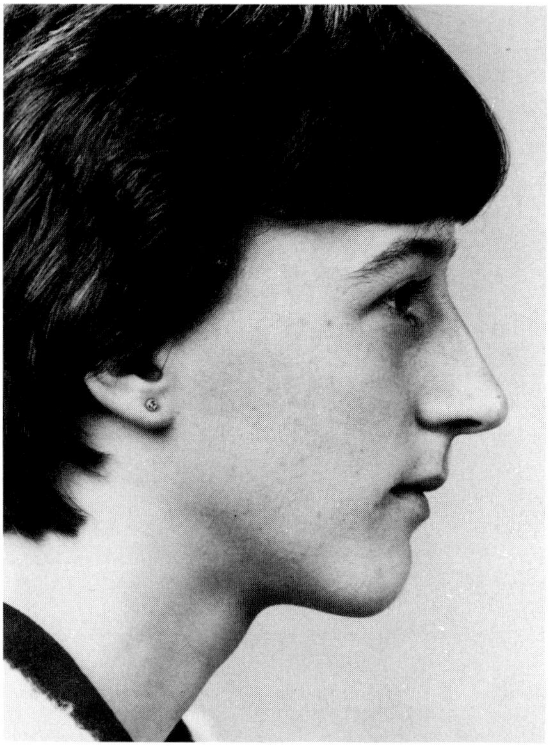

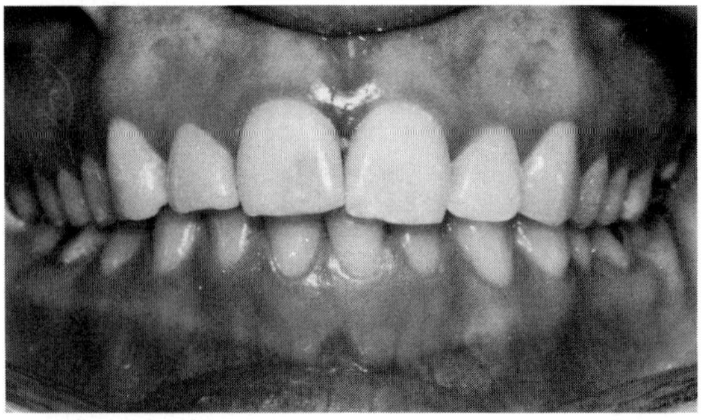

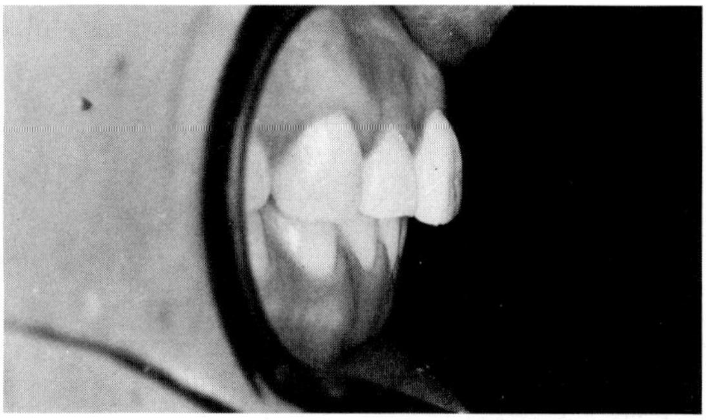

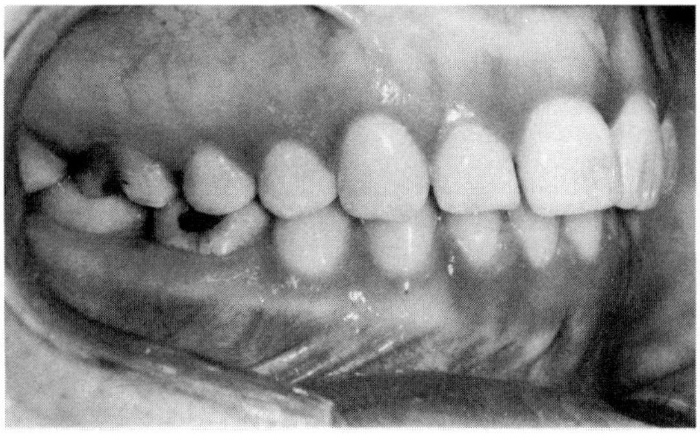

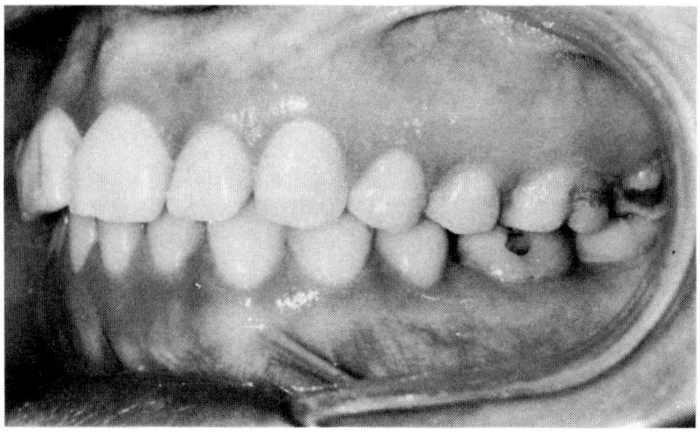

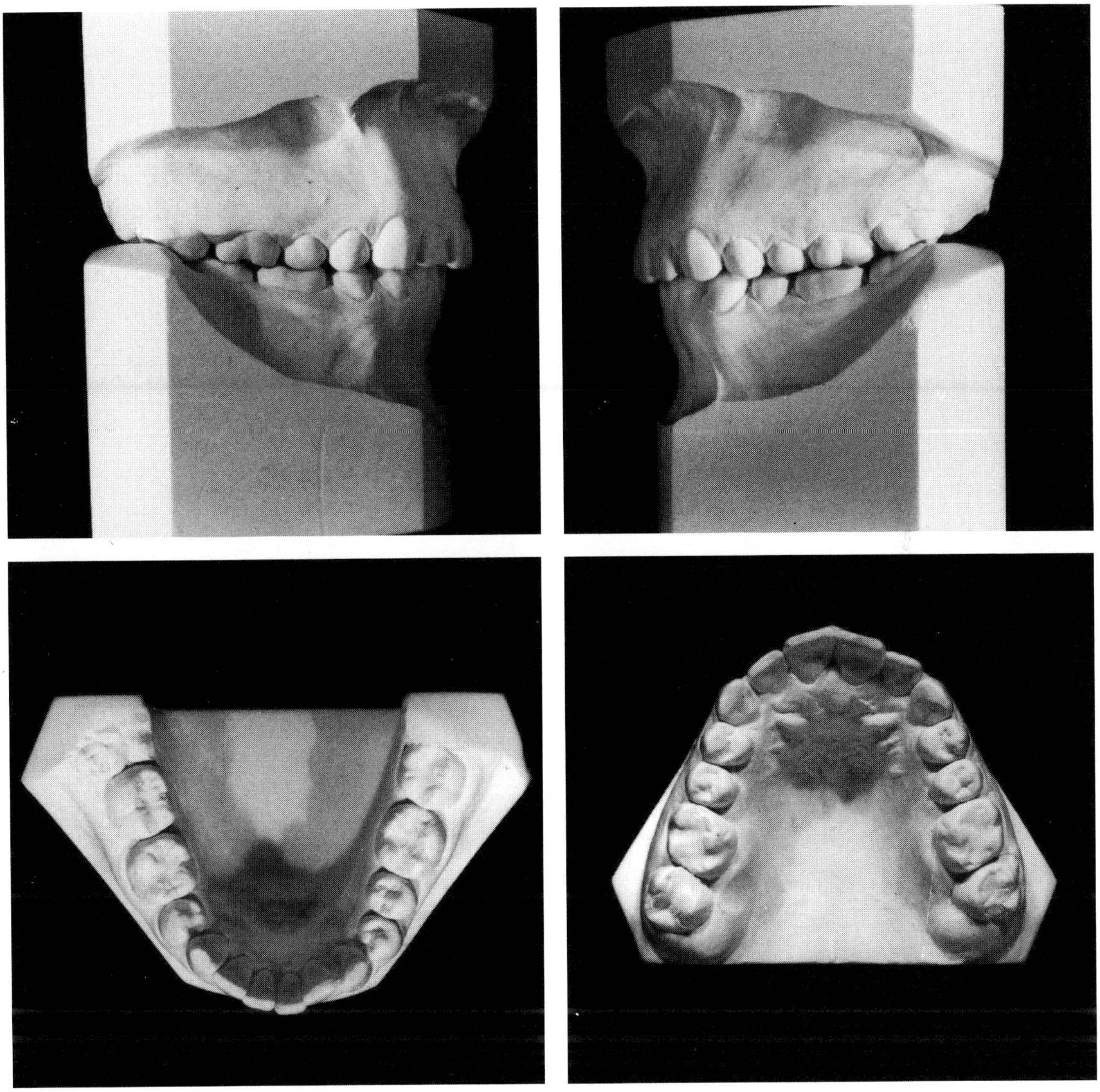

Figs 32-5 and 32-6 *At the age of 21 yr, 1 mo, five years after discontinuing retention, there has been little change. The facial growth had already finished and had no influence on the situation of the dentition. There is insufficient space in both jaws for the third molars, and it was advised that the mandibular third molars of which the right one had partially emerged, be removed. The face has clearly matured and this may have contributed to the appearance of some tertiary crowding in the mandibular incisors. As mentioned earlier, a mesio-palatally rotated maxillary canine seldom is esthetically objectionable. This was the case on the left side of this patient.*

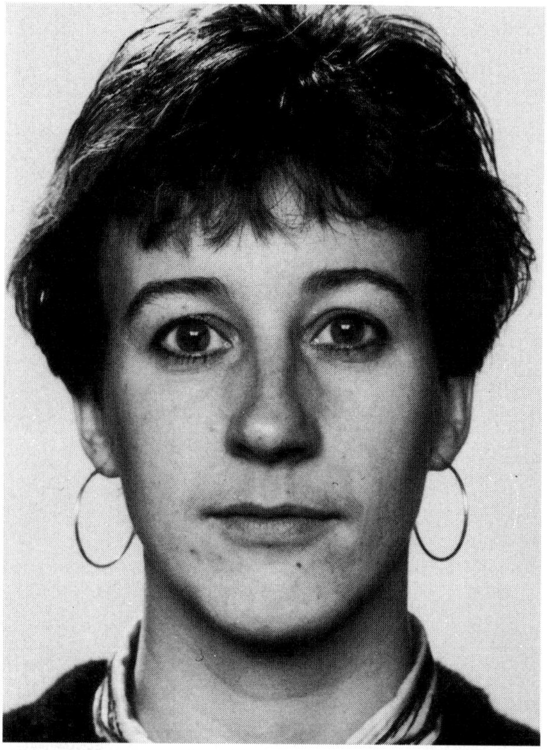

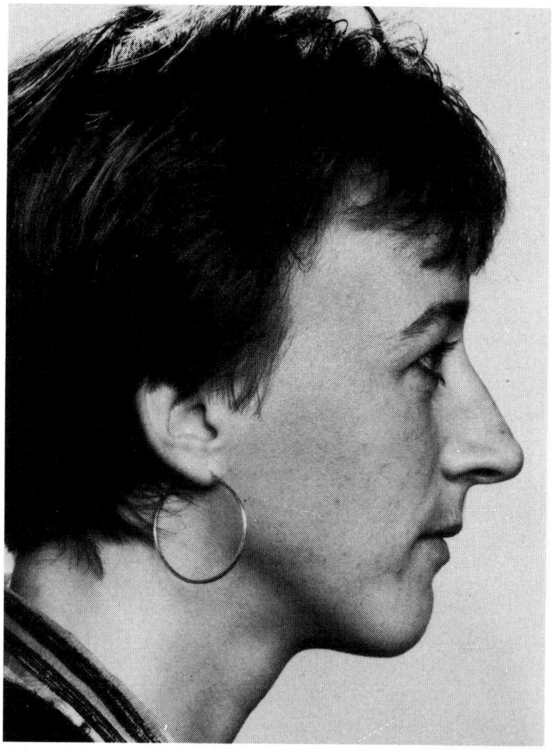

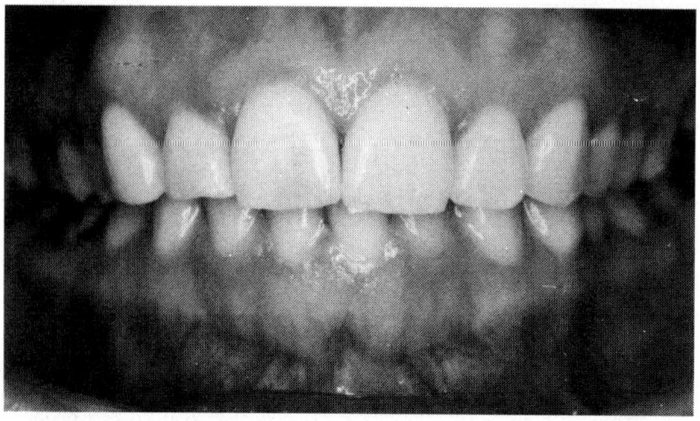

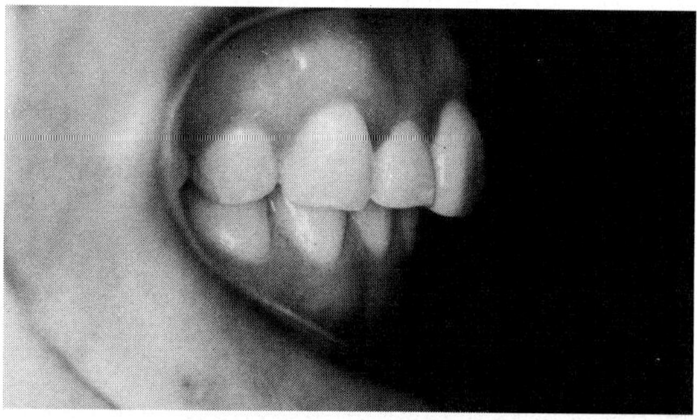

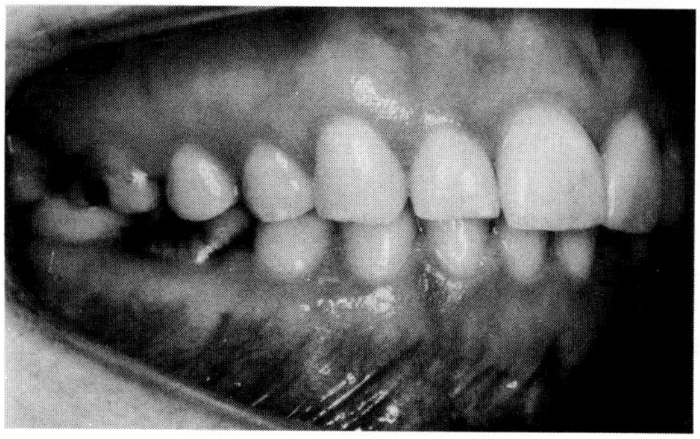

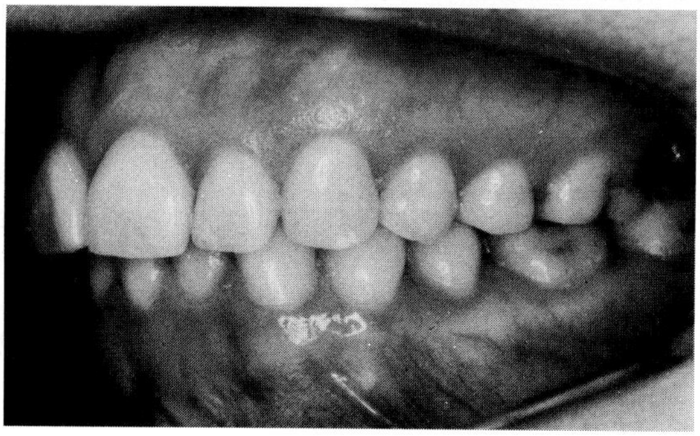

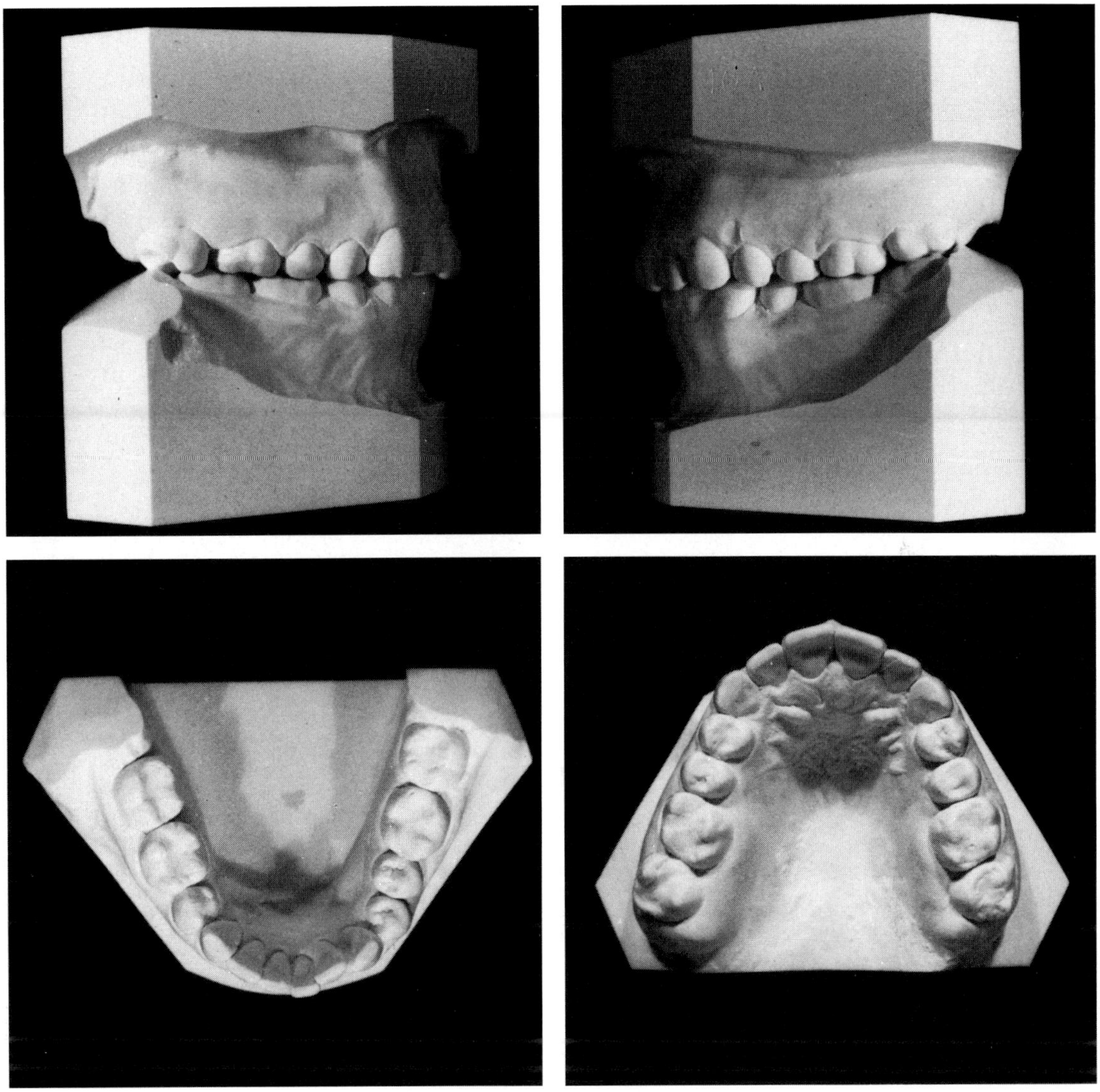

Figs 32-7 and 32-8 *Aged 26 y, 3 mo, ten years after retention, the teeth have been worn down with normal use, particularly the canines on the right side. The crowding in the mandibular anteriors has increased slightly but is not considered objectionable. The maxillary incisors are in good alignment and have contact with the mandibular incisors. It was a pity that the mandibular right third molar had to be removed; the maxillary right second molar has as a result less than half of its occlusal surface in contact with an antagonist. The movements in articulation suffer no interference (see Fig 32.11). Temporomandibular joint problems have not developed.*

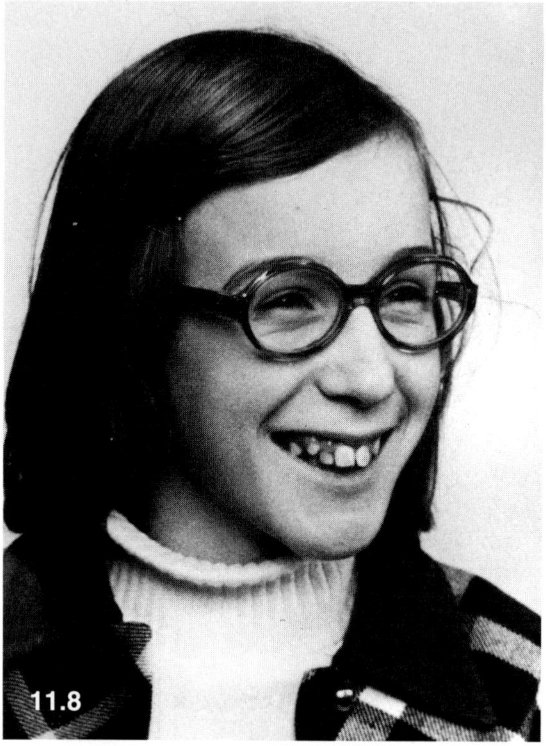
11.8

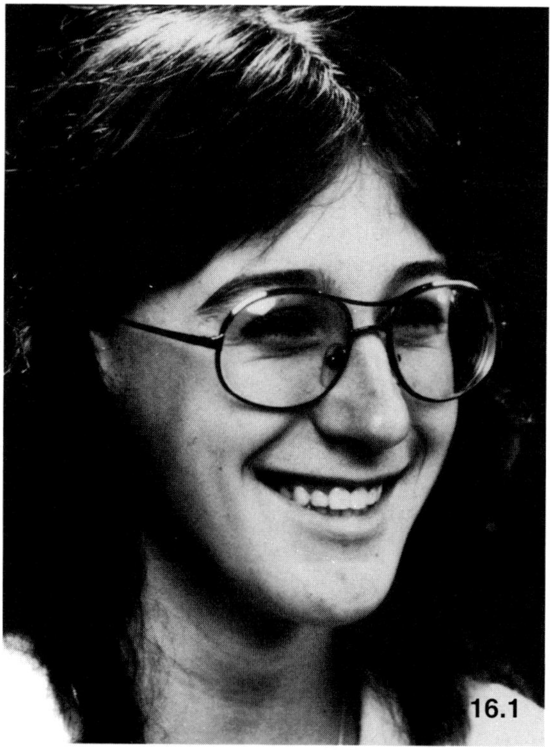
16.1

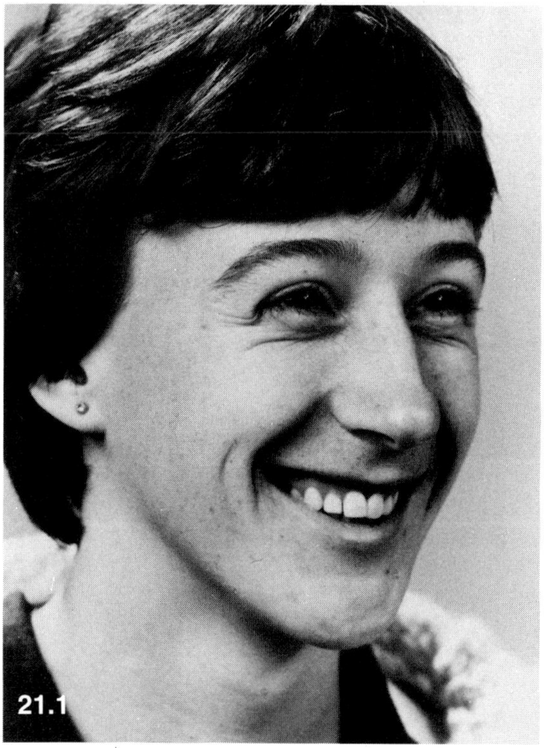
21.1

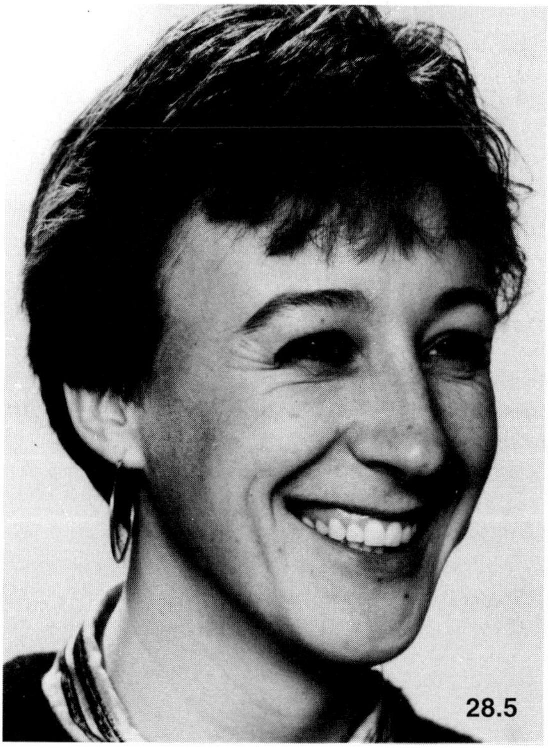
28.5

Fig 32-9 Note the improvements in the dention at different ages.

second premolar and to remove that tooth instead. A month later, a lingual arch was placed incorporating springs to move both the mandibular left premolars and the right first premolar to buccal. Three months later, a new maxillary plate was made, using buccal springs to move the maxillary first premolars to palatal.

When the patient was 14 years, 2 months old, the lingual arch broke. Since the tooth movements for which the lingual arch had been intended had been obtained some time previously, the lingual arch was not replaced. The mandibular molar bands were removed. To improve the alignment of the maxillary anteriors and to torque them, brackets were placed on the maxillary incisors at the age of 14 years, 5 months. First a twistflex arch of 0.0175" was placed in the brackets and subsequently a solid 0.017" × 0.0215" arch was fitted. A year later, the appliances were removed and a maxillary plate provided for retention. This plate was worn continuously for three months and then just at night with diminishing frequency for another five months. The records taken at the age of 16 years, 1 month show a result that was satisfying in all respects (Figs 32.3 and 32.4). Despite the fact that the occlusion on the right certainly was not normal, excursions in the articulation were free of interference (Fig 32.10).

Five years after treatment ,hardly any change was to be seen except for minor crowding developing in the mandibular anteriors (Figs 32.5 and 32.6). At the age of 28 years 5 months, twelve years after treatment, little more had been lost of the good treatment result. There had been a slight increase in the mandibular incisor crowding (Figs 32.7 and 32.8). The oblique photographs of the patient's smiling face show the improvements that became evident during and after treatment (Fig. 32.9).

In retrospect, the question can be posed as to whether the extraction of the mandibular right first permanent molar instead of the second premolar might not have been better. This arises because there is a large restoration in the first molar and the position of the third molar is unfavorable, leading to its eventual removal. The third molar would have been able to emerge properly since the second molar would have drifted mesially, which would have resulted in a better occlusion for the maxillary second molar. However, there would have been some risk involved in this reasoning: not all mesially tipped third molars move vertically and emerge well if the first molar in that quadrant is extracted early.

Likewise, the question can be asked if all four first premolars could have been extracted and full fixed appliances used. Taking into consideration the only fair oral hygiene and especially the possibility that a fallen-in mouth might have resulted, this treatment plan was dismissed.

A further question that can be asked is whether or not it was realistic to plan on regaining the space for the mandibular right second premolar with a lip bumper, particularly as the third molars all were forming. It often occurs that a mandibular second premolar does in the course of eruption regain its place in the dental arch without the use of any appliances. For that reason, ten months were allowed to pass

Figure 32-10a

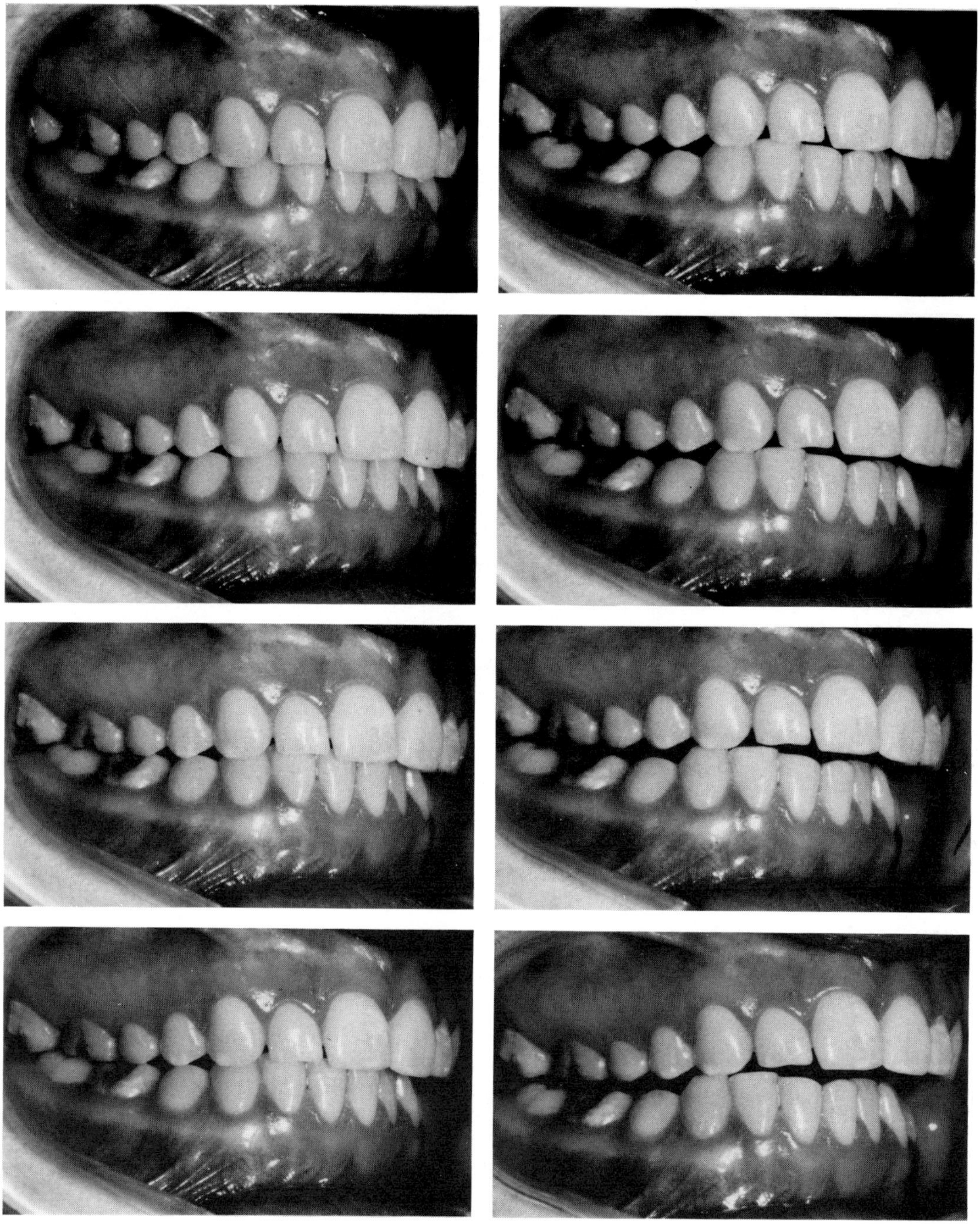

Fig 32-10 At the age of 16 y, 1 mo following cessation of retention, photographs were taken of the articulation of the dentition in various excursions. Group guidance exists in lateral excursions. In protrusive movements, no interferences are encountered.

Figure 32-10b

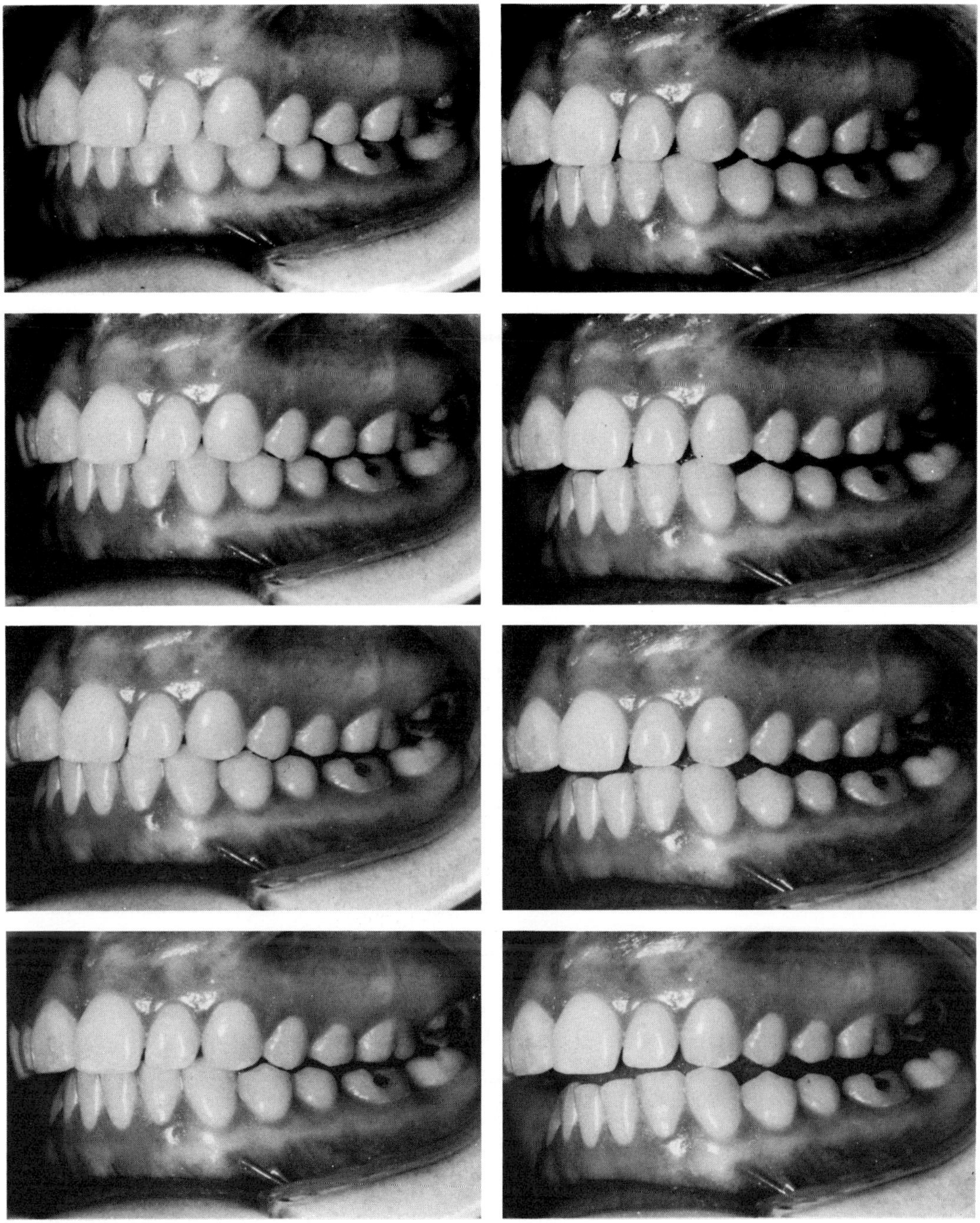

Figure 32-11a

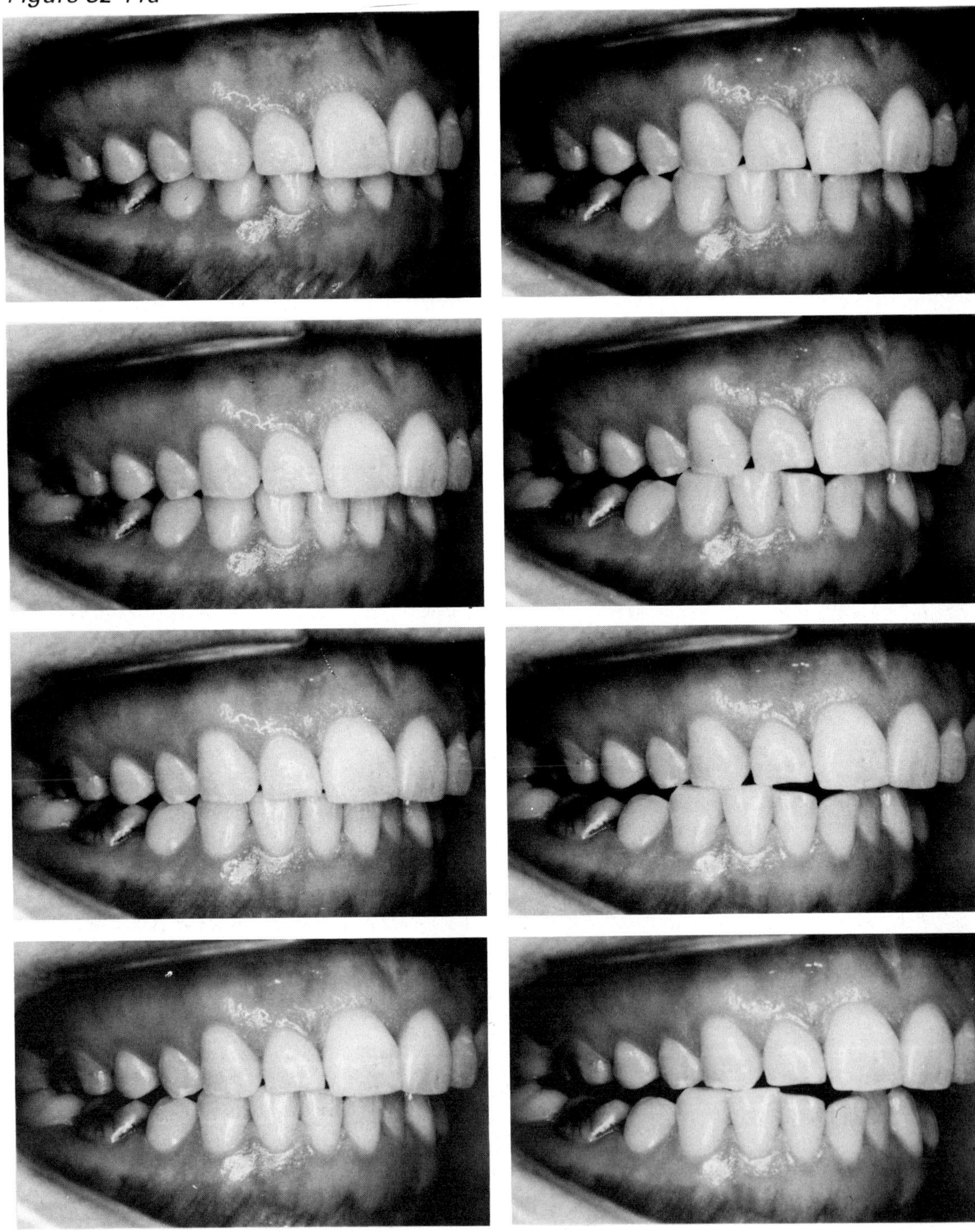

Fig 32-11 At a check-up at the age of 28 y, 5 mo, photographs of the articulation were taken for a second time. The situation has not noticeably changed in the preceding twelve years.

Figure 32-11b

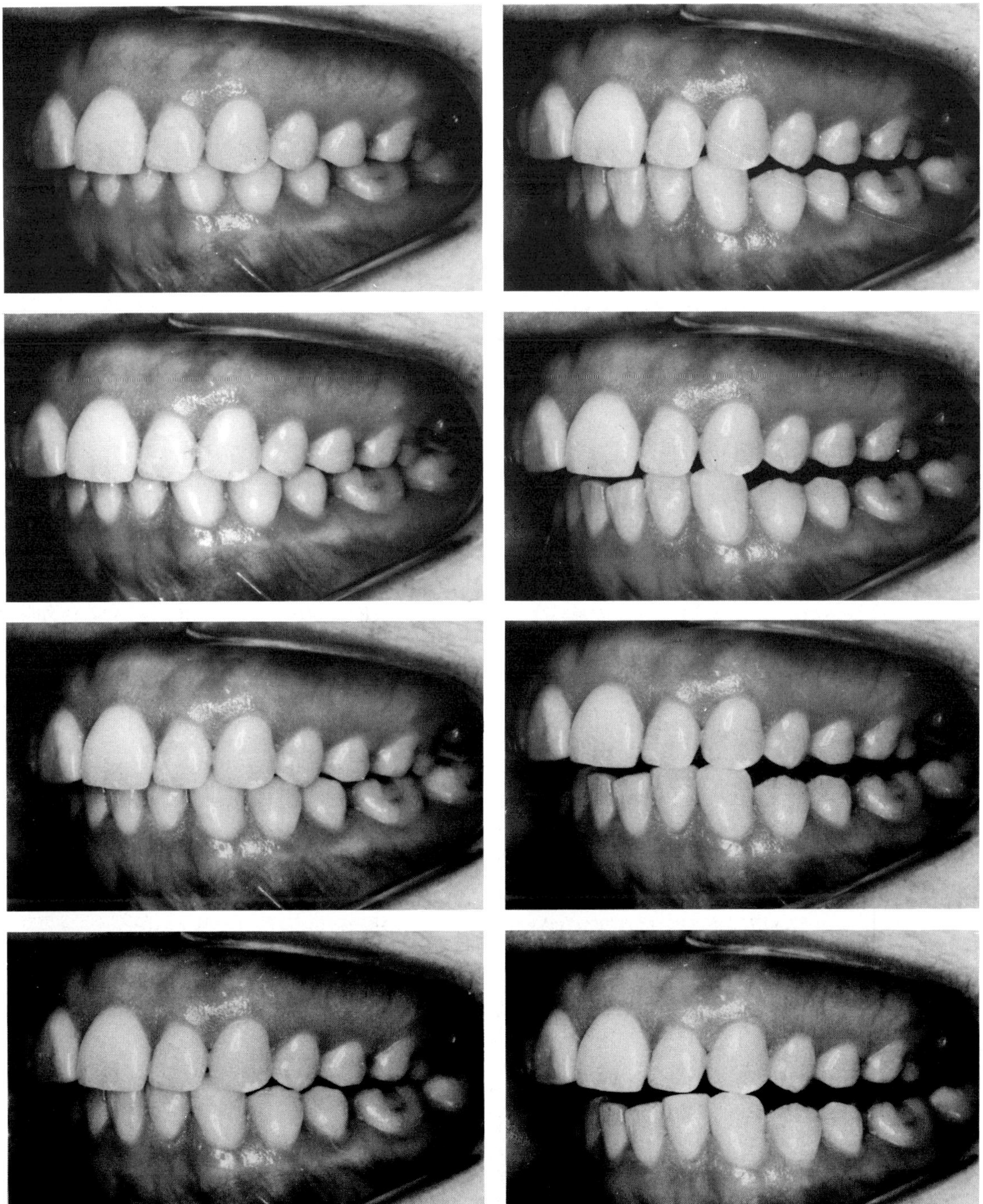

before fitting the lip bumper. Because no additional space was noticed over that period, it should have been an indication that not much success was to be expected from the lip bumper.

In the previous chapter, a patient was described who had agenesis of a mandibular second premolar, for whom the end result corresponds closely with this result. For both patients, there is a midline deviation of the maxillary and mandibular dental arches after treatment, with a mesio-occlusion of the molars on one side yet no occlusal disturbance in lateral excursions. Both patients also have a good overjet and overbite, implying that the maxillary teeth must be slightly too narrow (TSD), or that the mandibular anteriors must be somewhat crowded. Otherwise, where there is a neutro-occlusion on only one side, the middle of the mandibular arch has to deviate more to the other side with respect to the maxillary arch as was the case in both patients.

It has to be emphasized yet again that even where the occlusion is imperfect, the movements during articulation can be quite satisfactory so that it is not always necessary to adapt the slopes of the cusps by grinding. Furthermore, it has never been shown that disto-occlusions that come into being when a premolar is removed from each side of the maxillary arch in a class II/1 anomaly function less well than neutro-occlusions. That applies also to unilateral mesio-occlusions of first molars as described here and in the previous Chapter. Generally some adaptation in the size and shape of the maxillary second premolar and the mandibular first molar are called for. In the realm of disturbances in articulation, the importance of correcting the scissorbite of the maxillary premolar should be mentioned again. These teeth displayed a supra-occlusion already at the beginning of treatment. Without treating the incorrect bite, this supra-occlusion would probably have increased and as a result interfered with excursions of the articulating surfaces. Of course, trauma to the gingiva by teeth in supra-occlusion is a substantial additional risk.

Chapter 33

Class II/1, impacted 35 and 45

Extraction 34 and 44, cervical headgear, maxillary removable plate, elastics through the bite to the lingual of 45 and 46

Male: 13 years, 2 months to 36 years, 9 months

A boy aged 13 years, 2 months appeared with a mild class II/1 anomaly, which was complicated by the fact that in the mandible the deciduous molars had been lost prematurely and the second premolars on both sides were impacted. Most of the time he kept his mouth open; the lower lip was not held behind the maxillary incisors. In the mandible, the incisors were tipped forward and the first premolars almost lay against the first permanent molars. Diastemata were present distal to the mandibular canines. The ALD for the mandible was –10 mm. In the maxilla the left lateral incisor was palatally displaced and the ALD was –3 mm. The overjet was somewhat too large, being 4mm. The dentition had many restorations, cavities, and decalcifications (Figs 33.1, 33.2, and 33.11).

The mandibular incisors were everted and the space for the second permanent molars was limited. Moreover, the third molars were forming and were located close to the second molars. It was therefore decided to obtain space in the mandible for the second premolars by extraction. It was decided to extract the first premolars rather than just to eliminate the second premolars, since the latter procedure would require a considerable amount of bone to be removed. In addition, second premolars usually occlude better than first premolars. Extraction was rejected in the maxilla, since only a little extra room was needed and this could be gained mainly by rotating back the first permanent molars. Furthermore, it was feared that extraction of premolars would lead to a falling-in of the mouth, certainly if the nose and chin developed significantly, as is seen more in boys than girls. Extraction of maxillary premolars would have the additional consequence that the use of full fixed appliances would be required to attain a good result. This would have been unwise in the presence of the high caries activity in this patient.

The rotations of the first permanent molars would be corrected with a cervical headgear, simultaneously obtaining more space in the maxillary dental arch and eliminating the disto-relation. At a later stage, a maxillary plate would be utilized to provide any further corrections that might be needed. It was assumed that the development of the mandibular arch would proceed favorably after the extraction of the first premolars, so that no further appliances would be needed there.

Both mandibular first premolars were extracted at the age of 13 years, 5 months. Five months later the mandibular second premolars had emerged and a cervical headgear was fitted. Six months after that, it was noticed that the mandibular right first molar

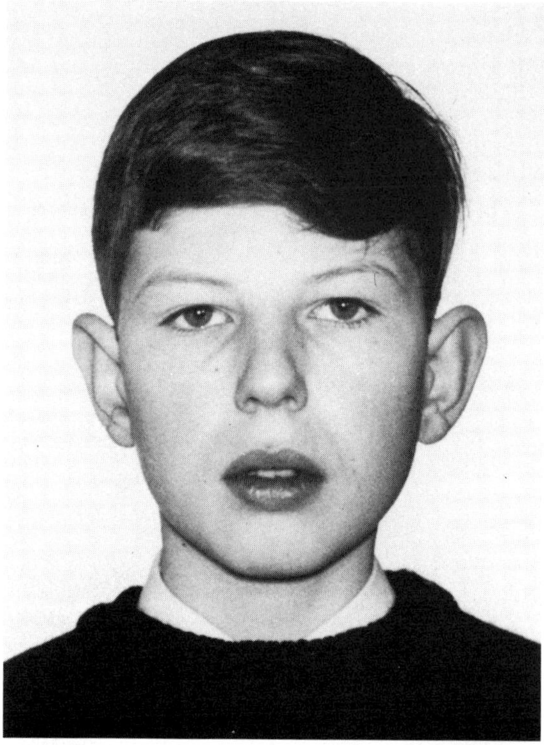
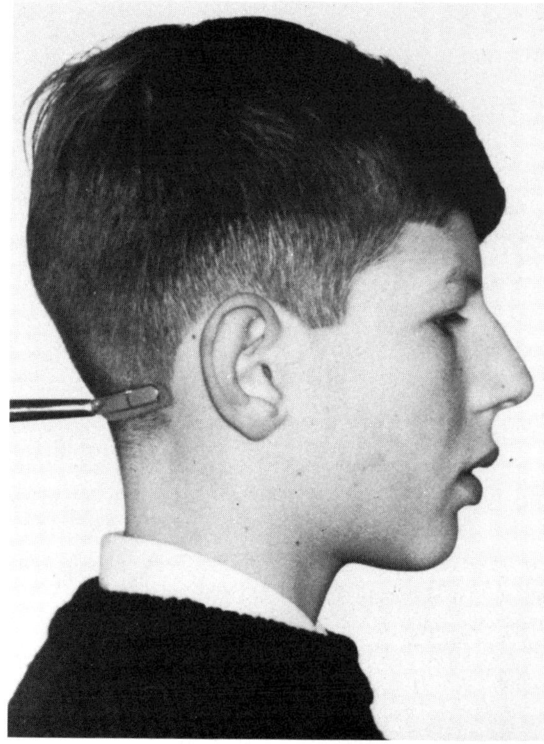
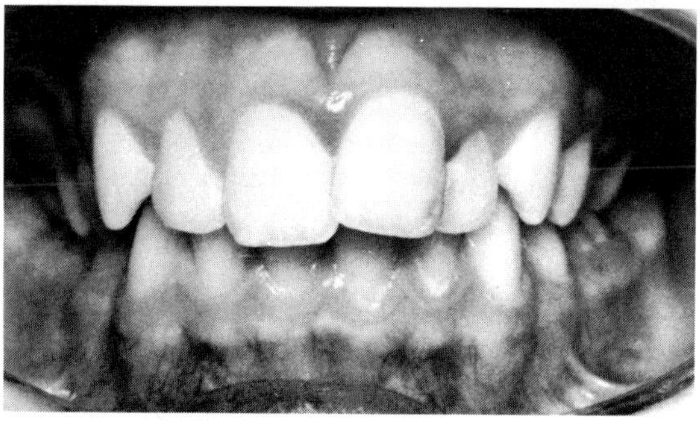
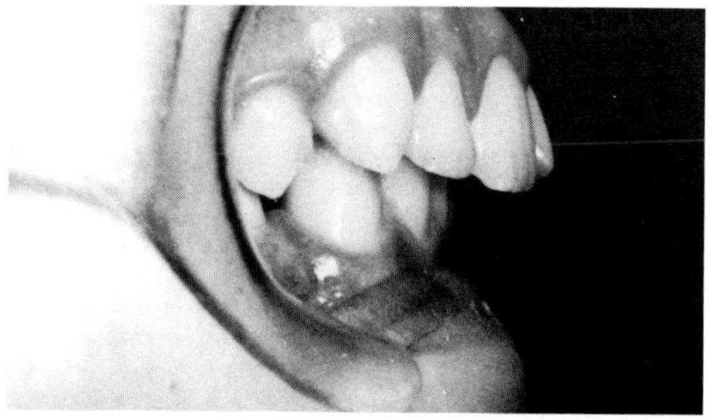
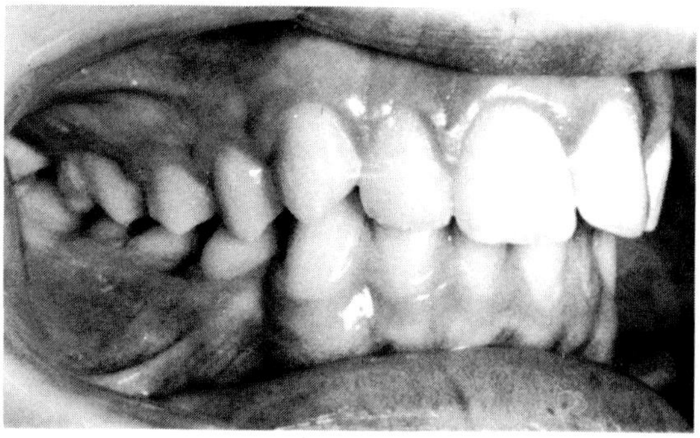
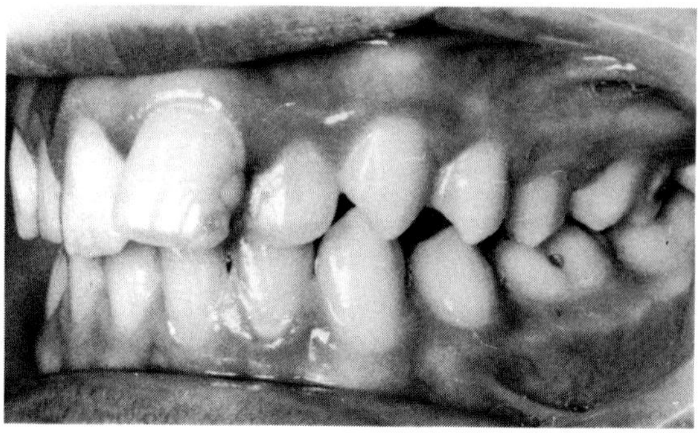

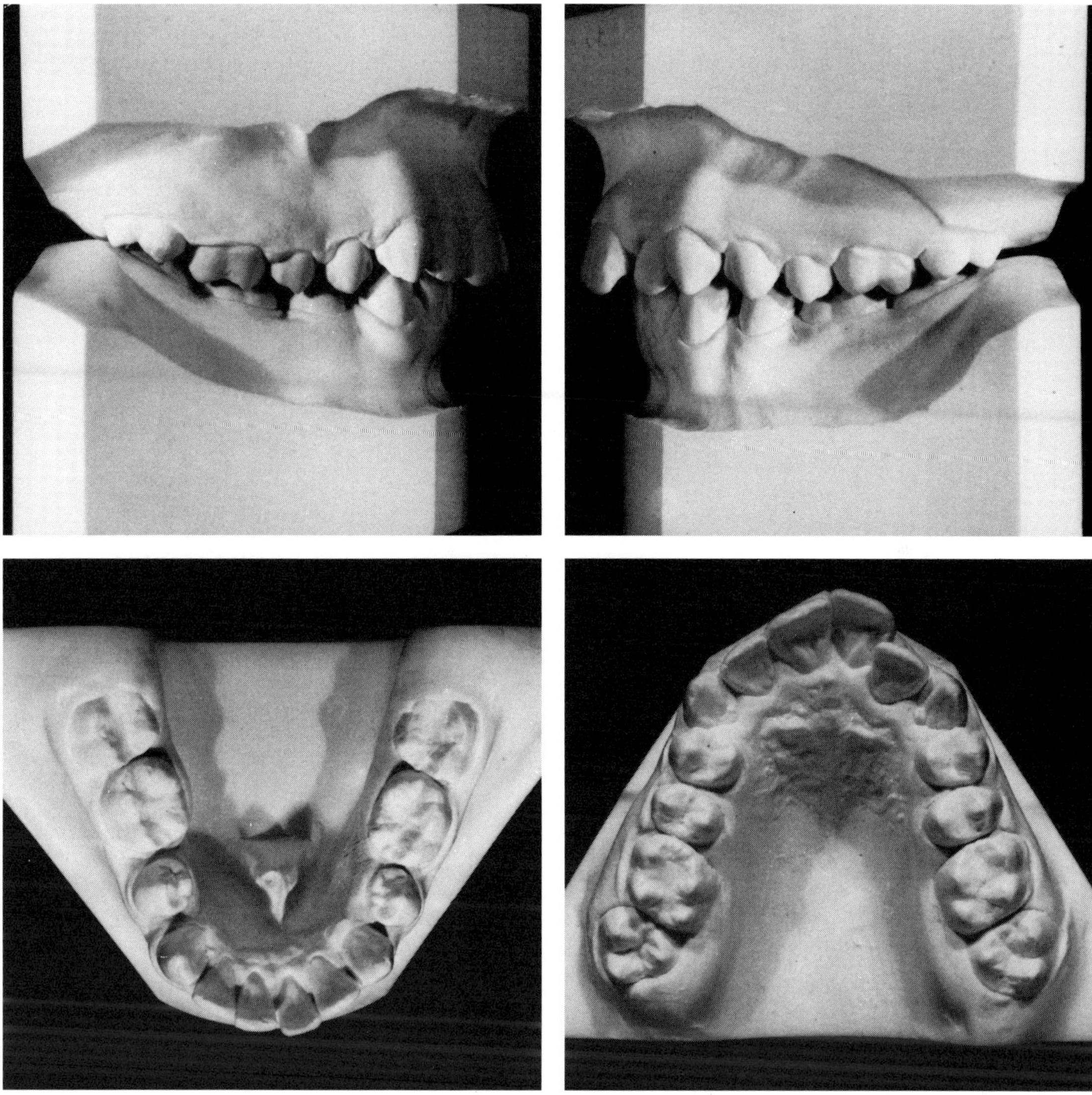

Figs 33-1 and 33-2 *A boy of 13 y, 2 mo with a mild class II/1 anomaly, a slight disto-relation, and an overjet of 4 mm. The quality of his dentition leaves something to be desired. Besides many restorations, there are several cavities and decalcifications. Both mandibular first molars have three amalgam fillings, but also three cavities. The deciduous molars in the mandible were lost prematurely and the second premolars are impacted. The mandibular incisors are everted and the mandibular first permanent molars have tipped lingually and are rotated mesio-lingually. Both jaws barely have space for the second permanent molars, which have already emerged. The occlusion in the canine/premolar region is ¾ PW disto-occlusion, while the molars are in slight mesio-occlusion because they drifted mesially after the loss of the deciduous molars.*

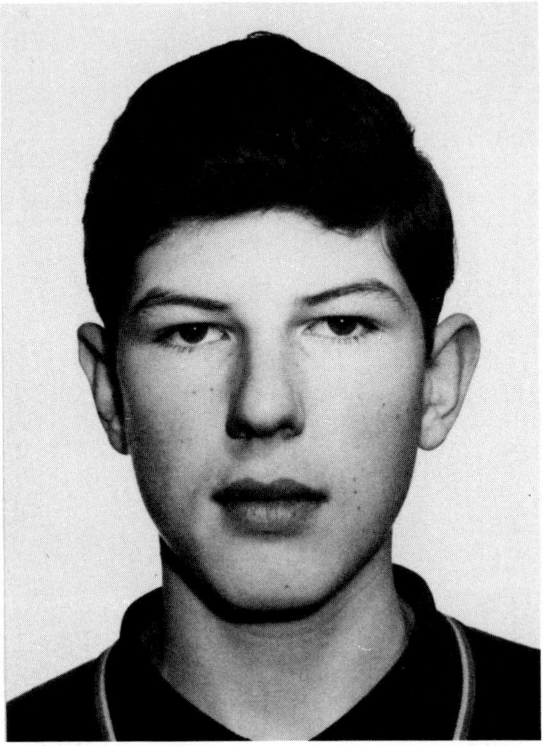

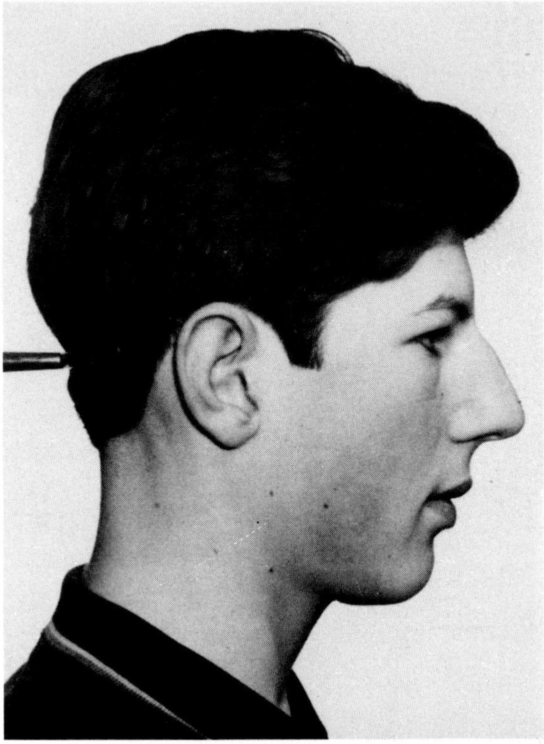

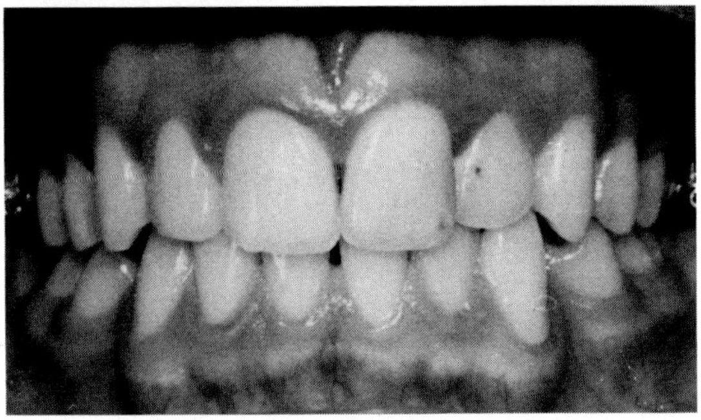

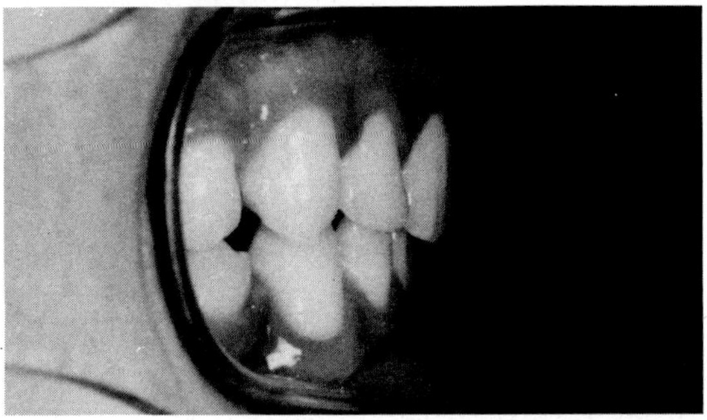

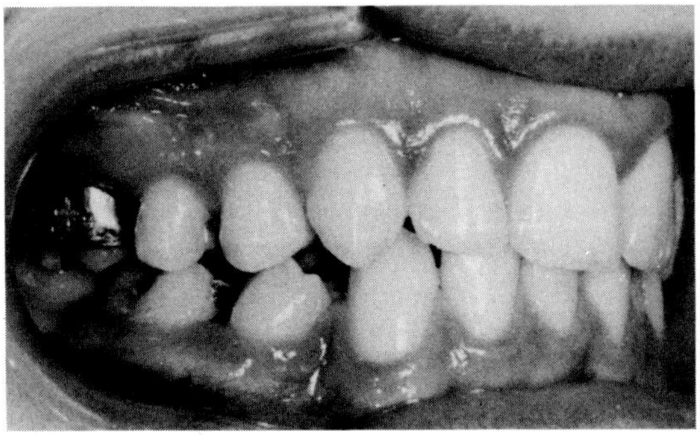

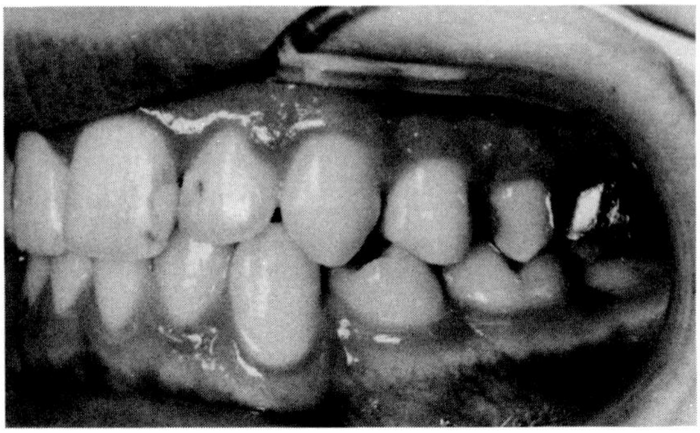

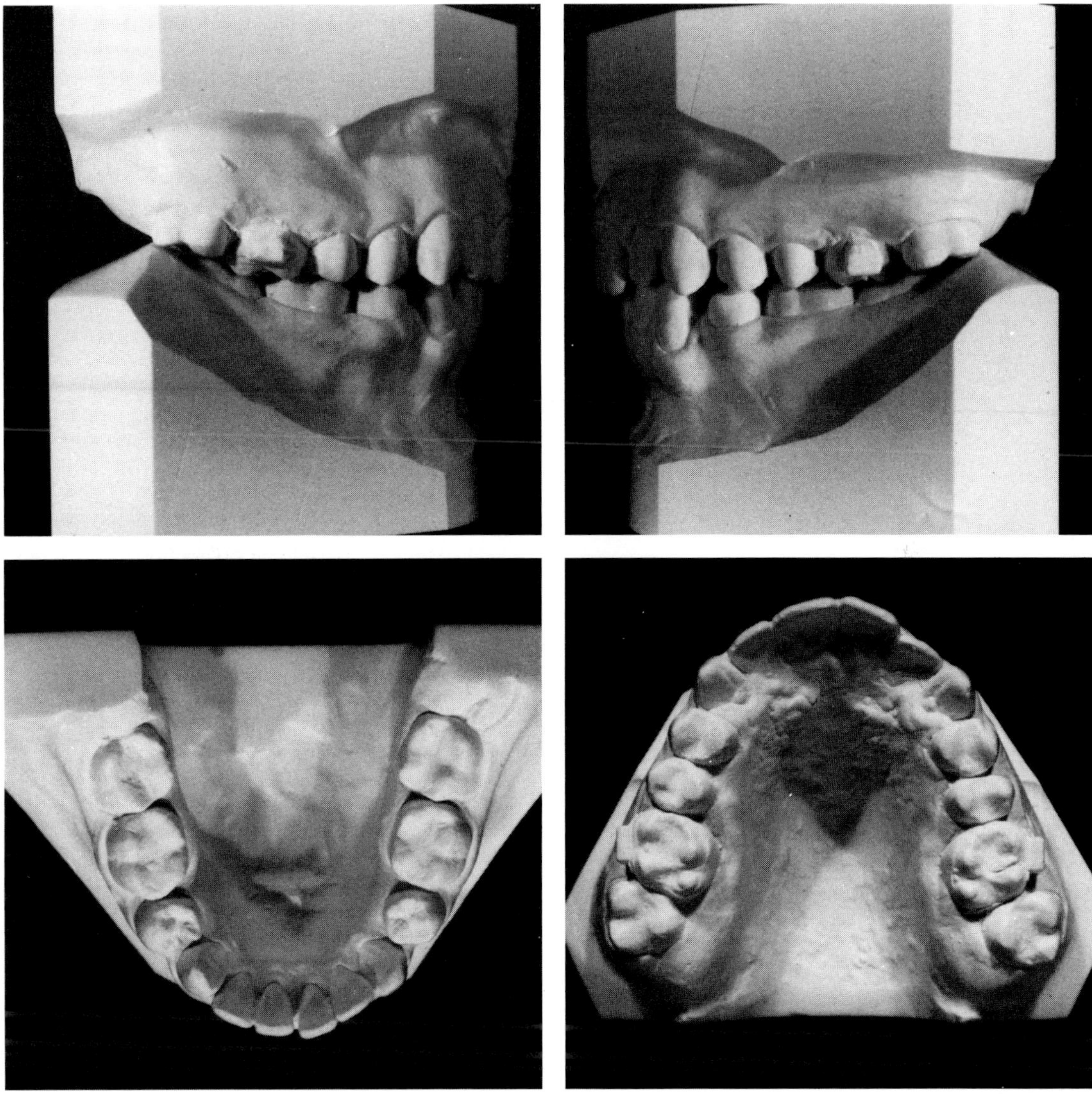

Figs 33-3 and 33-4 *Aged 16 y, 1 mo active treatment has finished. The plate is being worn for retention for another six months. The face has grown appreciably; the nose is much larger and the mandible has developed to ventral. Since a premolar is missing on both sides of the mandible but not in the maxilla, the maxillary second premolars occlude only with the mandibular first molars. This does not have to cause problems as has been pointed out in the past two chapters. Despite the removal of the first premolars, there is still insufficient room in the mandible for the third molars to emerge in good positions. This can be seen on the left. In the maxilla, the posterior section of the apical area is too small as is reflected in the bucco-position of the second molars.*

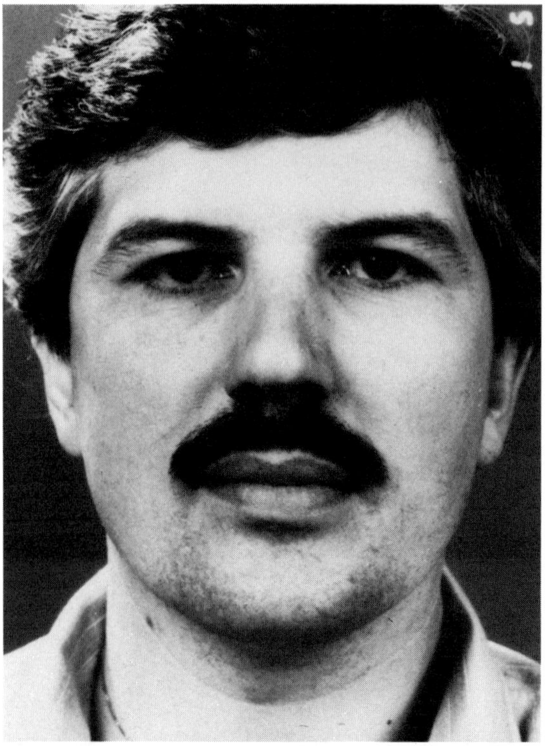

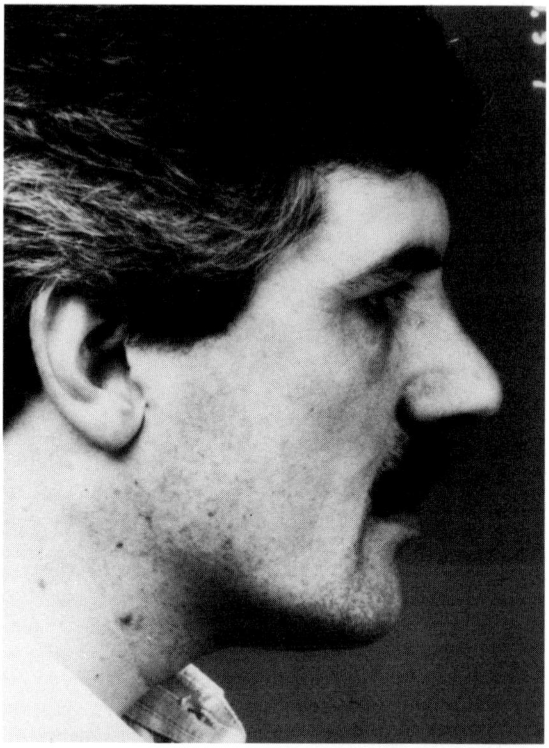

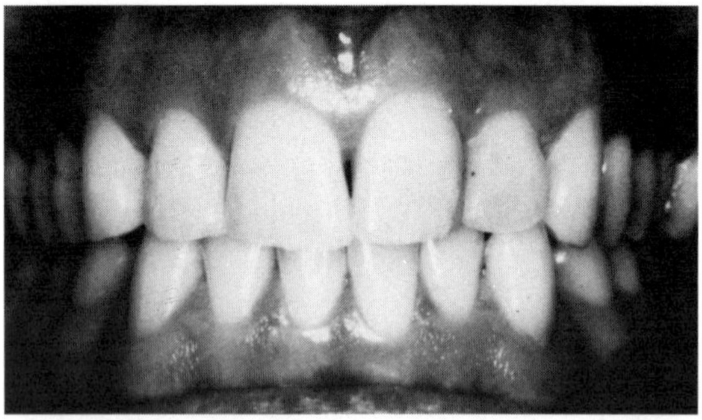

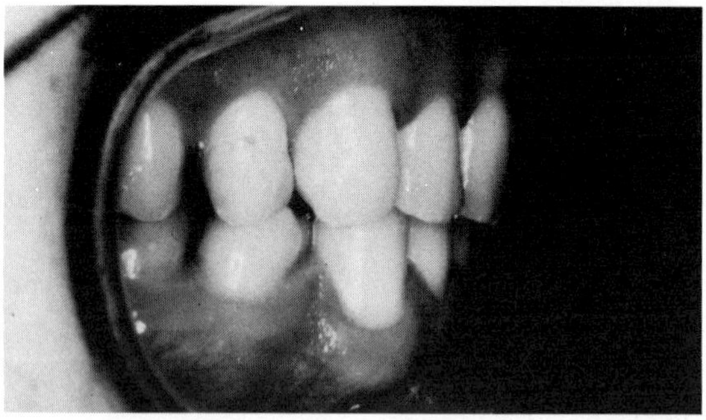

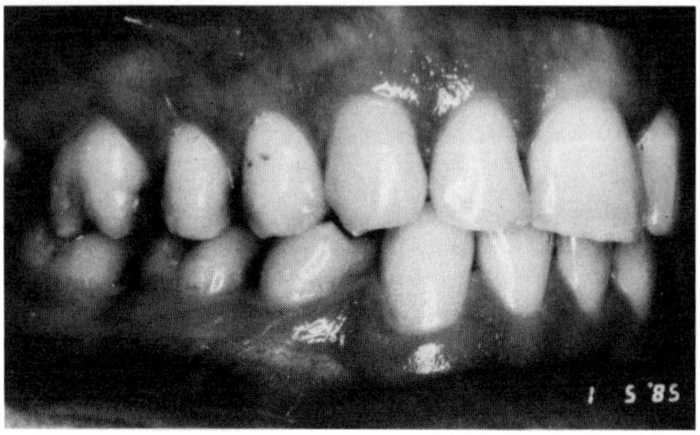
1 5 '85

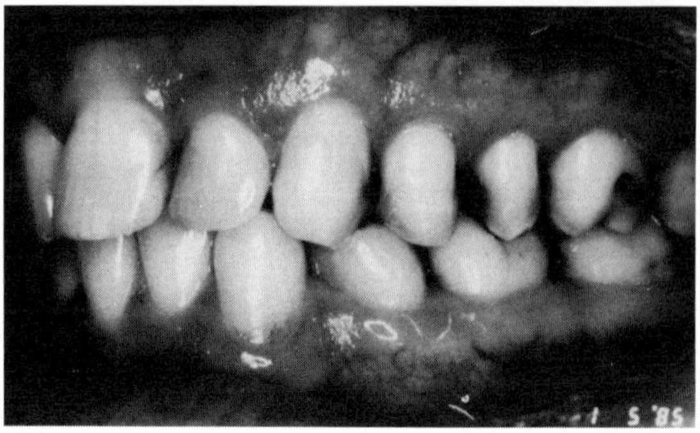
1 5 '85

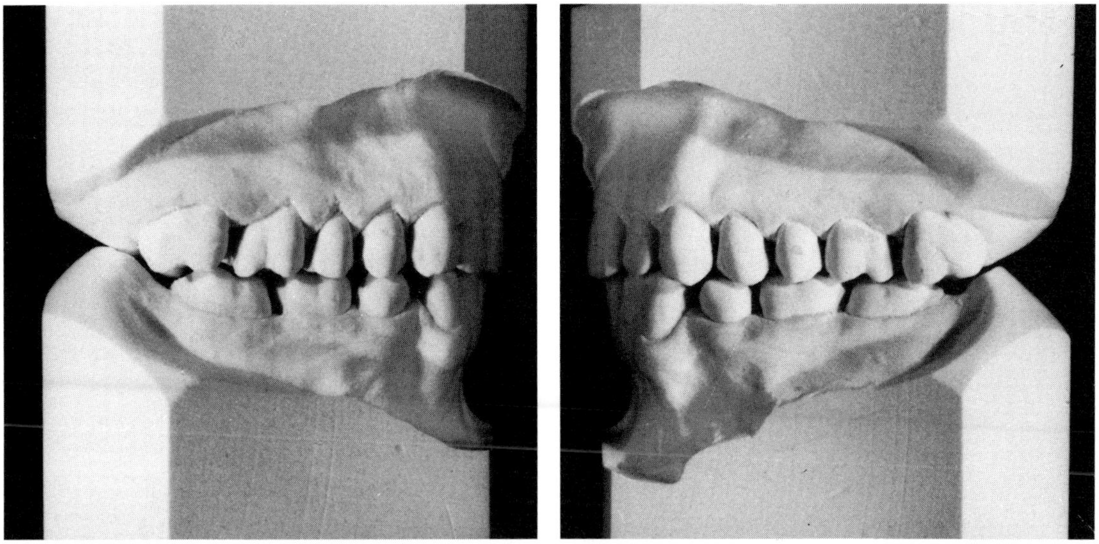

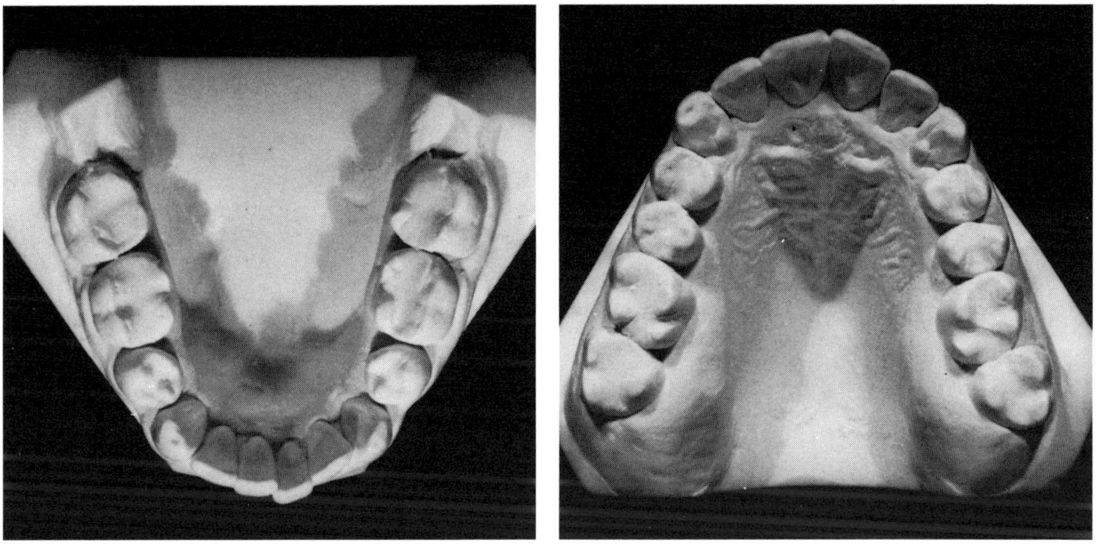

Figs 33-5 and 33-6 *At the age of 32 y, 4 mo there is a harmonious facial appearance with an esthetically and functionally satisfactory dentition. The mandible has developed to ventral with respect to the maxilla, the chin has become more prominent, and the teeth occlude more mesially. In the mandibular anteriors some crowding has occurred, although it is not found objectionable. After removal of the mandibular third molars, the second molars have moved vertically and their mesial sides have moved buccally so that they now are better aligned. In the maxilla, on the right side, the positions of the lateral incisor and the canine have improved. That does not apply to the second molars, which probably is related to the continued presence of the third molars which lie high in the alveolar process (see Fig.33-11).*

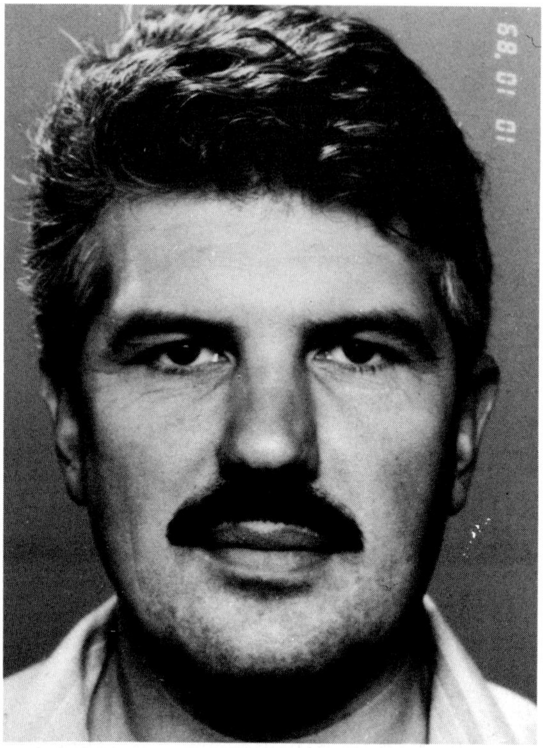

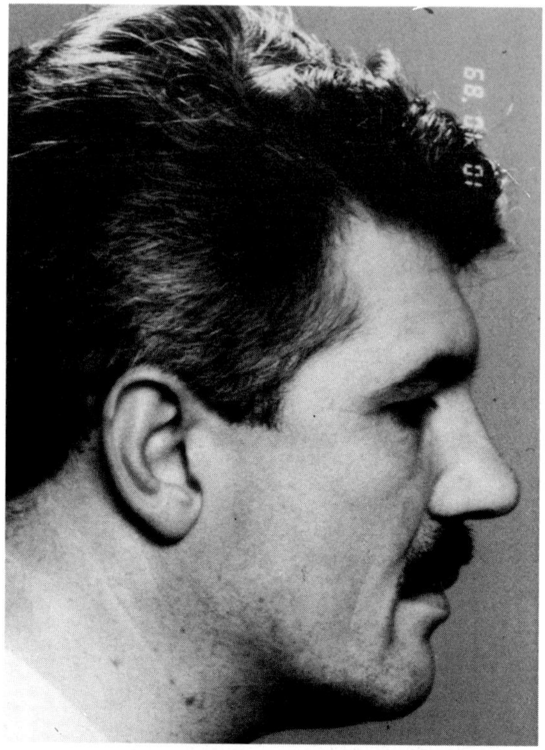

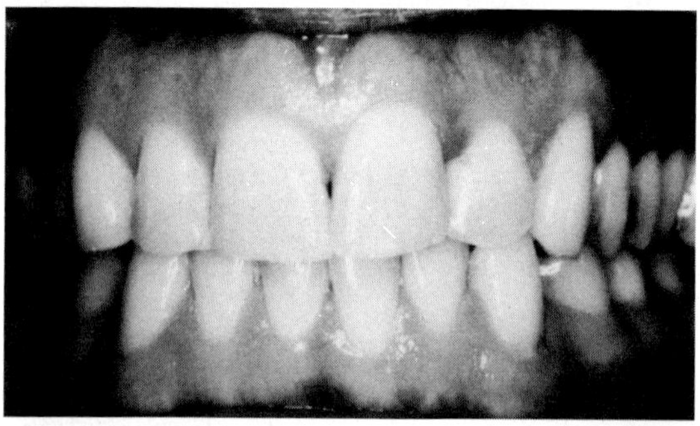

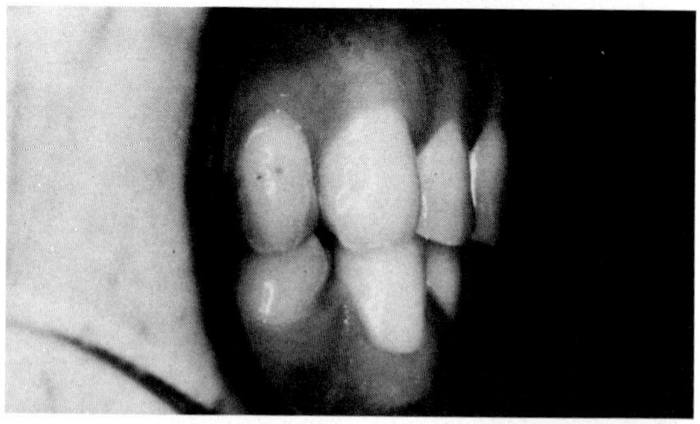

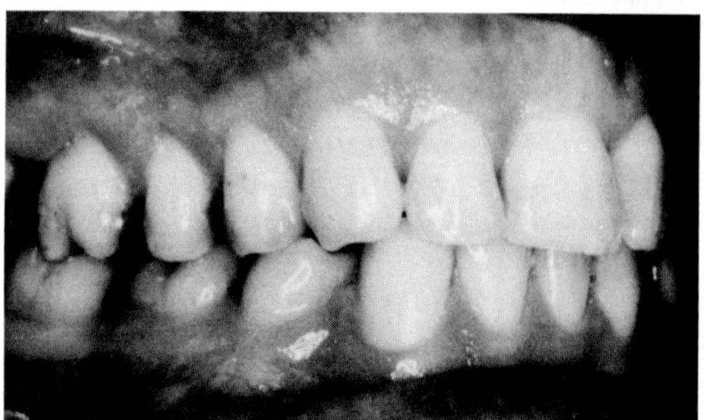

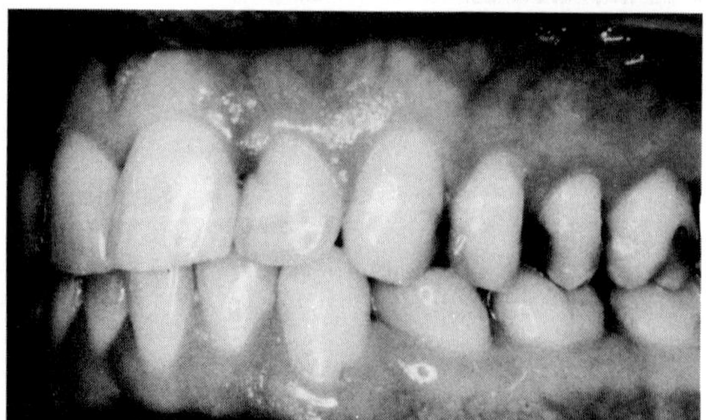

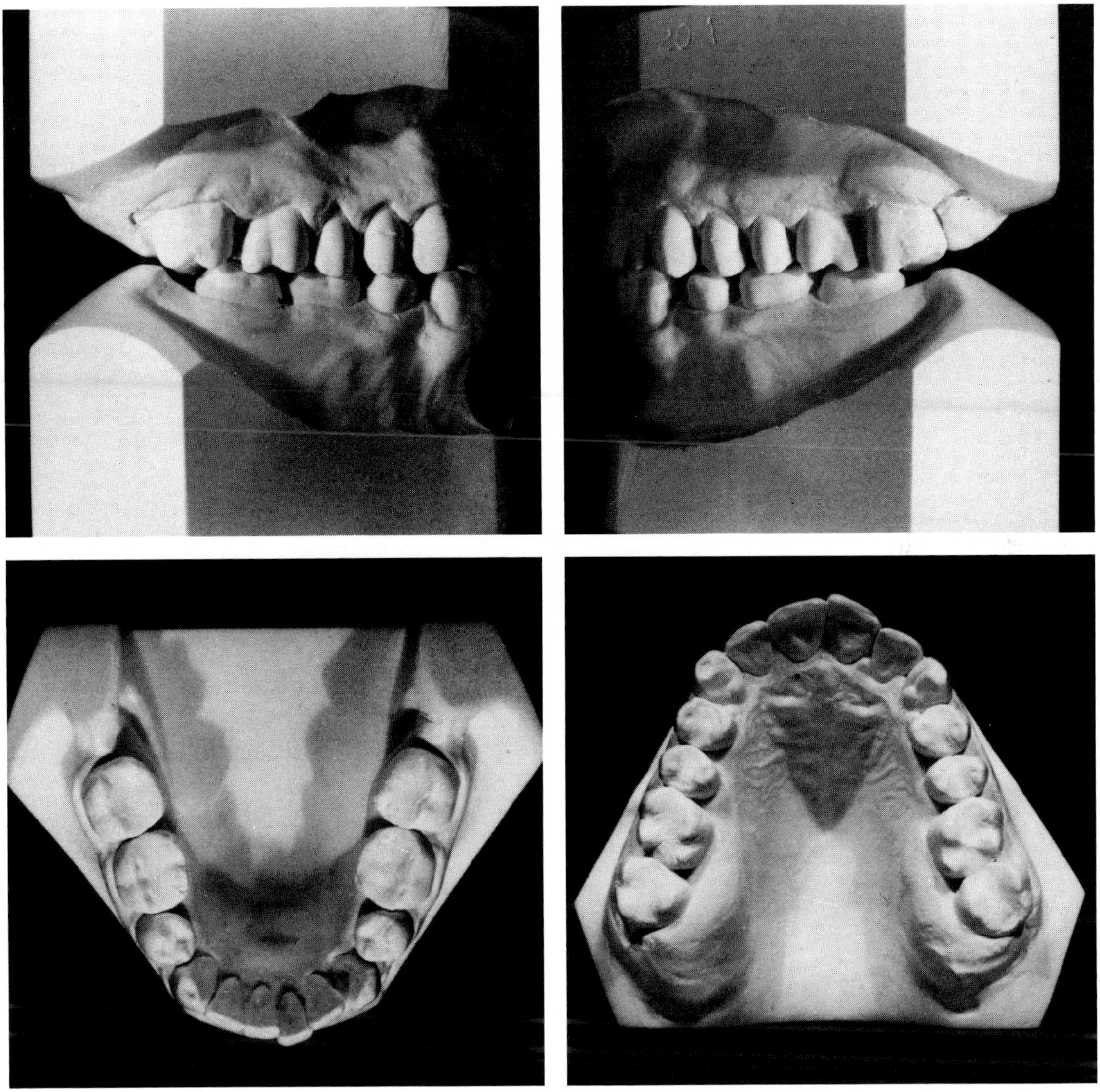

Figs 33-7 and 33-8 *At the age of 36 y, 9 mo, the face, with all the hallmarks of a harmonious structure, begins to exhibit the specific signs of age. Light creases and wrinkles are evident. There are also signs of age in the dentition. The incisal edges and cusps are more worn down and the contact during mandibular excursions has increased. Gingival recession is to be seen in the premolar/molar regions. The dentition gives the impression of being in good health. There are no temporo mandibular joint complaints despite the occlusion clearly being far from ideal.*

Figure 33-9a

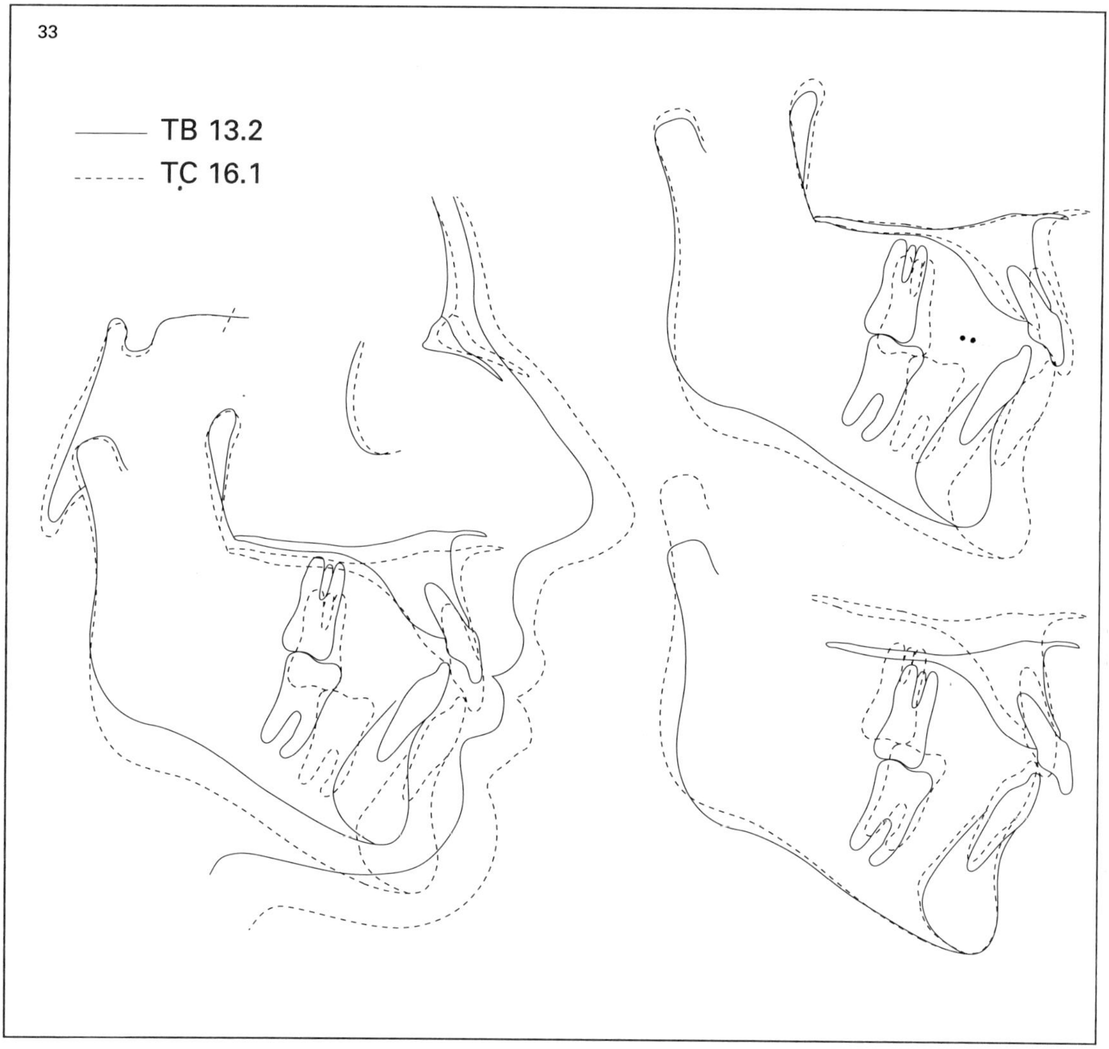

Fig 33-9 Superimposition of tracings from different cephalometric radiographs gives an indication of the changes that have taken place during and after treatment.

Figure 33-9b

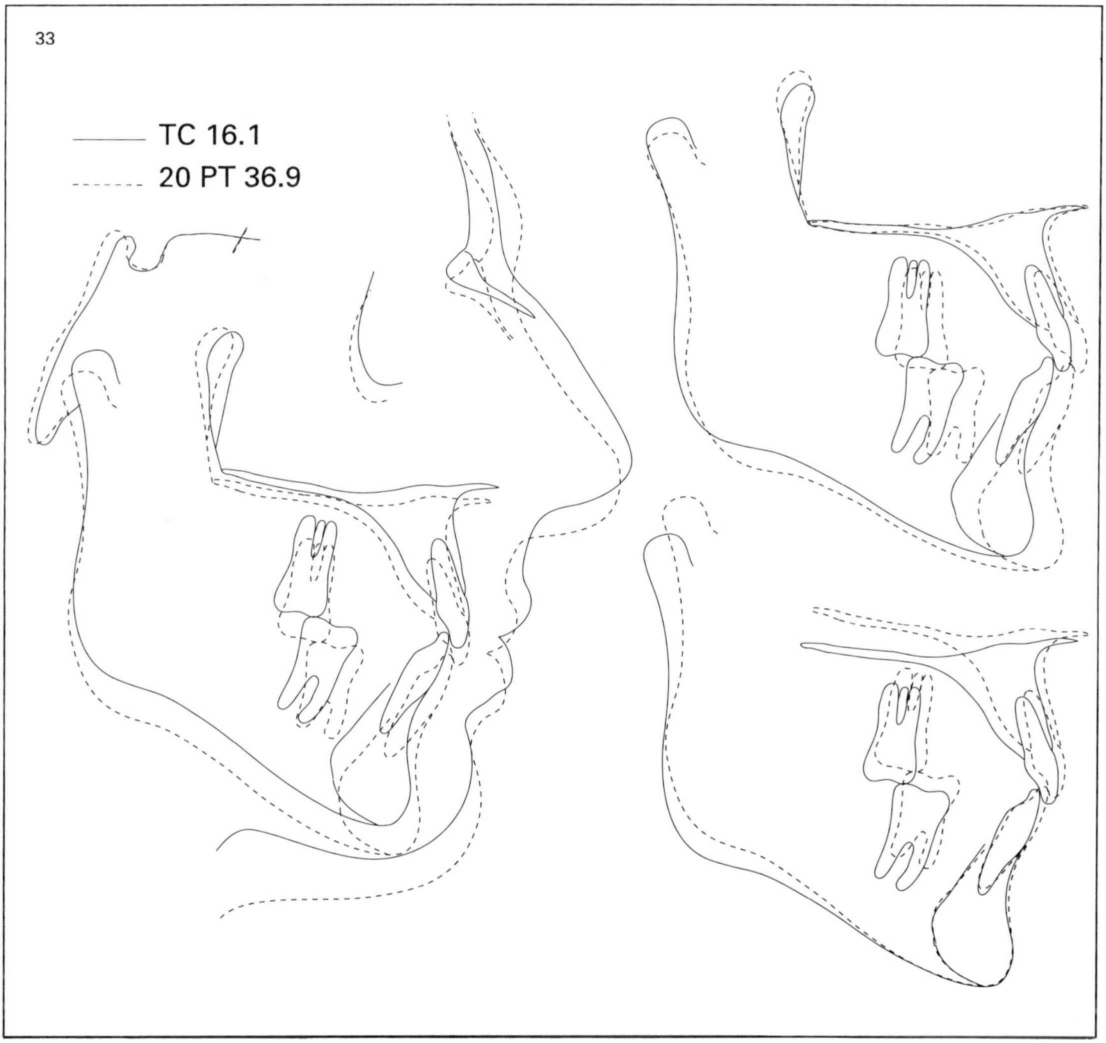

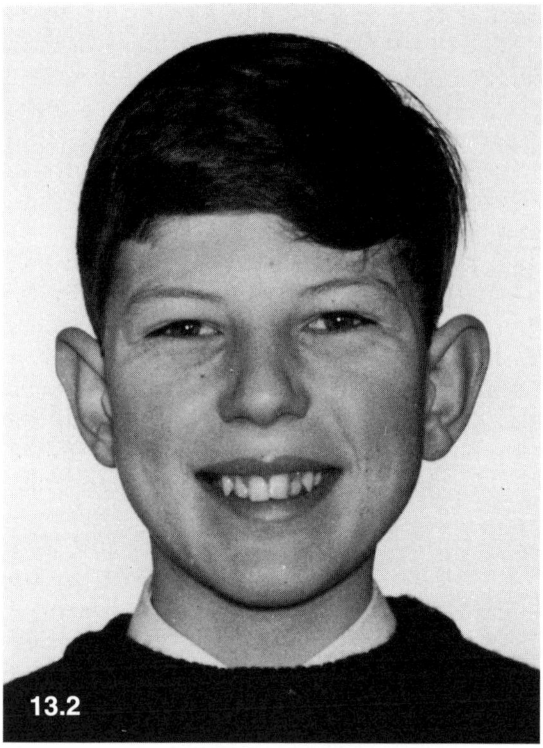

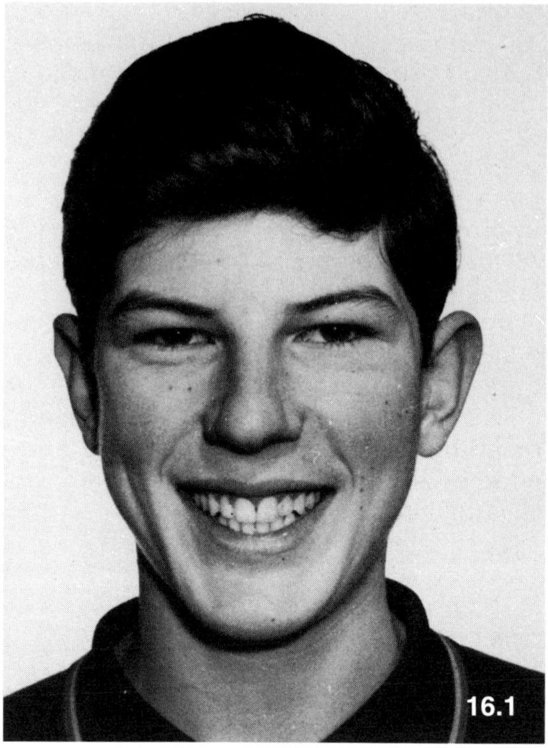

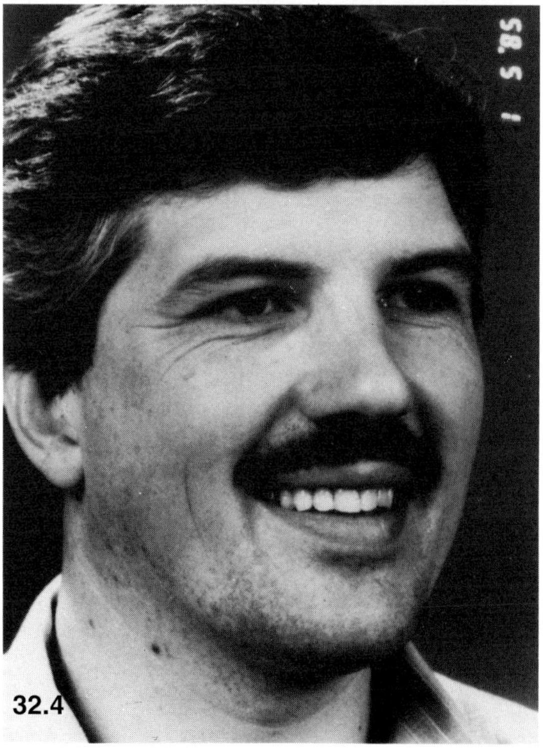

Fig 33-10 Note the appearance of the dentition.

and the second premolar had not spontaneously moved vertically as had the teeth on the left; therefore, lingual hooks were attached to those teeth. Elastics were then hooked from them to the buccal of the maxillary right first molar. For that purpose a short piece of rectangular wire was placed in the edgewise tube on the molar and the ends of the wire turned cervically to form hooks. To prevent these molars from tipping to palatal and also to make some corrections in the maxillary anteriors, a plate was fitted. Three months later, the position of the mandibular teeth had improved and the hooks for the elastics were dispensed with.

After active treatment for two years and three months, an acceptable occlusion and facial appearance had come about by the age of 16 years, 1 months. The mandibular arch had developed well and exhibited little irregularity. This applied also to the maxillary arch. Moreover, there was a good overjet and overbite. The posterior occlusion was decidedly out of the ordinary since a mandibular premolar was missing from each side. The second premolars in the maxilla occluded only with the mandibular first molars (Figs 33.3 and 33.4). The plate was worn for retention a another six months, the last three months of which were nighttime wear only, gradually reducing in frequency.

Fifteen years later, the breadth of the face has increased and the mandible has moved further ventrally in relationship to the other facial structures. This shows up among other things in the fact that the mandibular dental arch has taken up a more mesial relationship to the maxillary arch. The diastemata in the mandibular arch had vanished and the mandibular anteriors exhibited slight crowding despite the fact that the third molars had been removed (Figs 33.5 and 33.6).

The records obtained 4½ years later give an indication of the changes that may become evident in a patient's 30s. The clinical crowns of incisors, canines, and first premolars have become somewhat shorter due to natural attrition. The clinical crowns of the second premolars and molars have become longer due to some recession of the gingiva. There has been little change in the alignment of the various teeth; however, the mandibular arch does appear to occlude more mesially against the maxillary arch (Figs 33.7 and 33.8).

The superimpositions of the cephalometric tracings reveal the changes that have occurred over many years. That also applies to the facial photographs that not only show what effect orthodontic treatment but also aging can have on facial appearance (Figs 33.9 and 33.10). The various points mentioned previously are clarified by reference to the lateral skull radiographs (Fig 33.11).

In retrospect, the decision not to extract any premolars in the maxilla can be seen to have been correct. Had extractions been done, then the lips would have fallen back and the maxillary arch would have been narrower across the canine/premolar regions with a resultant accentuation of the nasolabial fold and increase in the nasolabial angle. In a face in which there was an increase in the size of the nose, the prominence of the chin, and the breadth of the mid-face, this would certainly have led to a reduction in facial animation.

A better result might possibly have been obtained if the maxillary second molars had been extracted. It would then have been easier to rotate the first molars and gain space in the maxillary arch. Furthermore, the third molars would then probably have emerged and taken up a better position in the arch than the two heavily restored

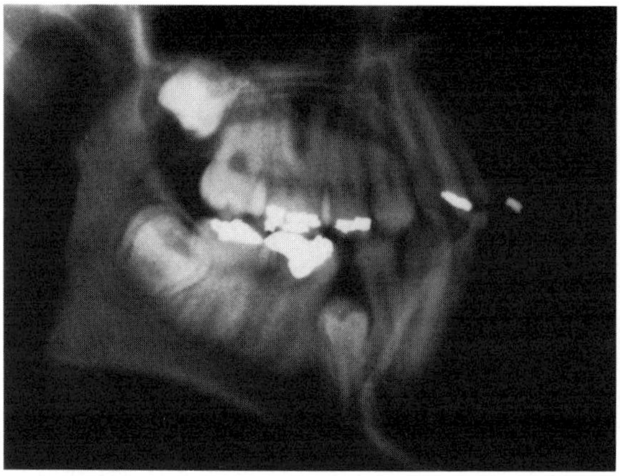

TB 13.2

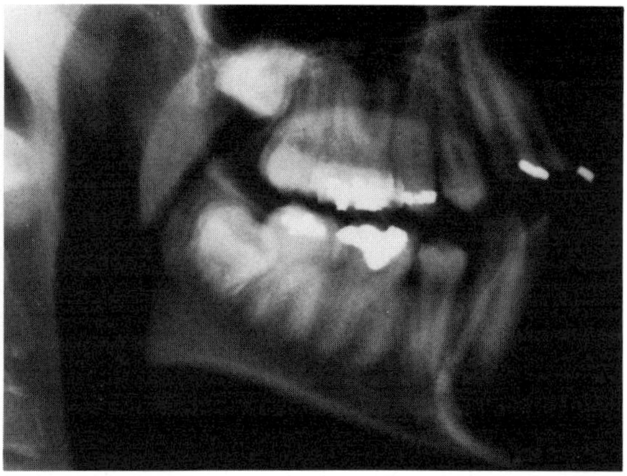

DT 14.1

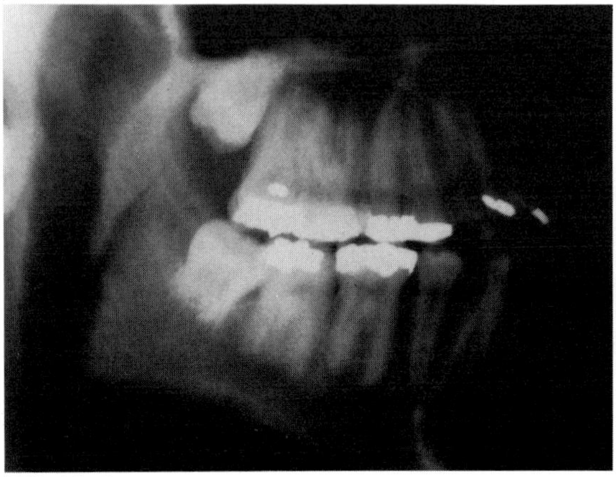

BR 16.1

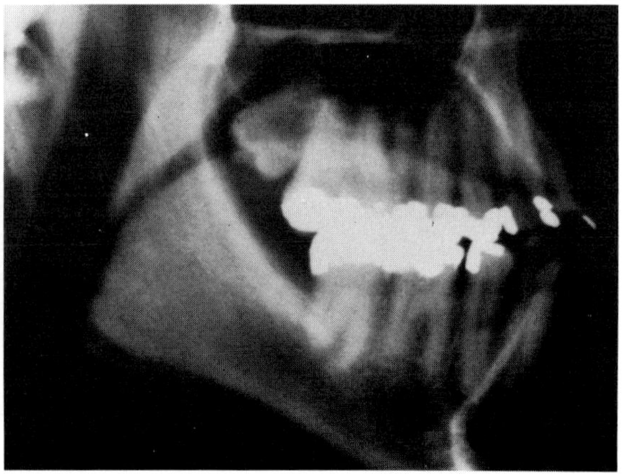

10 PT 26.11

Fig 33-11 Illustrations taken from the dental structures portrayed in lateral cephalometric radiographs at various ages.
At the beginning of treatment (TB 13.2), the second premolars in the mandible are impacted. Maxillary and mandibular incisors are everted; many restorations can be seen.
During treatment (DT 14.1) the jaw relationship improved and eight months after removal of the mandibular first premolars, the second premolars have emerged and nearly reached the level of the occlusal plane.
At the beginning of retention (BR 16.1), there is inadequate room (also seen clinically) for the mandibular third molars. Later they could not emerge properly and had to be removed.
Ten years after treatment (10 PT 26.11), the maxillary third molars are still located high in the tuberosities and obstruct a change in the positions of the second molars. Ten years later, this picture was unchanged. The impacted third molars however were symptomless.

molars now present. There is also the risk that the impacted molars may yet cause problems. The radiographs that were taken at the beginning and the end of treatment do not indeed give the impression that the posterior sections of the apical area in the maxilla are small. On the basis of that it might justifiably have been expected that the third molars would have emerged (see Fig. 33.10).

One can also wonder if another approach might have been warranted with respect to the mandible. Both the clinical and radiographic evidence gave the impression that insufficient room would be available for the third molars there, even if a premolar had been removed on each side. In hindsight, it seems that removing the first permanent molars with their defective crowns would have been better than removing the premolars with their sound crowns. The proper emergence of the second premolar could then have been expected and in the meantime the second molar would have drifted mesially, making room for the eventual emergence of the third molars. Against that is the risk that the second molar would have tipped more mesially and demanded the use of fixed appliances for remedy.

When the treatment plan had been devised 25 years ago, the knowledge of the development of the human dentition, third molar eruption patterns, and the relationships between such factors and treatment were still limited. For example, it was not recognizsed that the extraction of premolars in the mandible had only minimal effect on increasing the chance of third molars erupting well. At the same time, it has become clear since then that in class II/1 anomalies being treated with facial orthopedic measures, initiation of treatment should in general be earlier, specifically prior to the exfoliation of the second deciduous molars.

Chapter 34

Class II/1, crowding, defective 16, 26, 36, and 46 Extraction 16, 26, 36 and 46, cervical headgear Female: 10 years, 9 months to 25 years, 7 months

A girl aged 10 years, 0 months displayed a class II/1 anomaly, otherwise having normal function. Significant crowding had developed after premature loss of deciduous molars. The incisors, particularly the maxillary ones, were steeply inclined. There was hardly any room for the maxillary canines. In the mandible, the crowding was concentrated mostly in region of the impacted second premolars. In habitual occlusion the incisors were in contact, but with an overjet of 3 mm and an overbite of 6 mm. After taking into account the drifting of the posterior teeth, a disto-occlusion of ½ PW between the molars was estimated. The problem was complicated by a high caries activity with the consequences of decalcifications, cavities in the first permanent molars, and probably the early loss of the deciduous teeth (Figs 34.1 and 34.2).

It was decided to extract all four first permanent molars because due to their poor quality they were most unlikely to be able to be conserved for long. After the second permanent molars had come into occlusion, a cervical headgear would be fitted to the maxillary molars to improve the intermaxillary relationship and to secure more space for the maxillary canines. Depending on the oral hygiene and cooperation of the patient, other appliances might be used in due course.

At the age of 10 years, 10 months, the first permanent molars on the right side were removed, and four weeks later, those on the left also were extracted. It is possible to see on the models provided six months later when aged 11 years 5 months, that the mandibular second premolars had emerged with all the second permanent molars (Fig. 34.3). Six months later, the second molars were in occlusion and the space between the second premolars and the second molars in both jaws had diminished, although those teeth were tipped and rotated. The space in the maxilla for the canines had scarcely increased as a result of the extractions and the canines had emerged ectostomatically (Fig 34.4). At this stage, the maxillary second molars were banded and a cervical headgear was fitted. It was the intention to improve the molar occlusion by this means, and meanwhile to correct the rotations of the maxillary second molars and increase the space available for the canines.

After 2½ years, during which the wearing of the headgear was not satisfactory, treatment was concluded. The patient was satisfied with the result and had previously indicated, despite the oral hygiene having greatly improved, that she did not desire full fixed appliance therapy. The corrections aimed for had not been fully

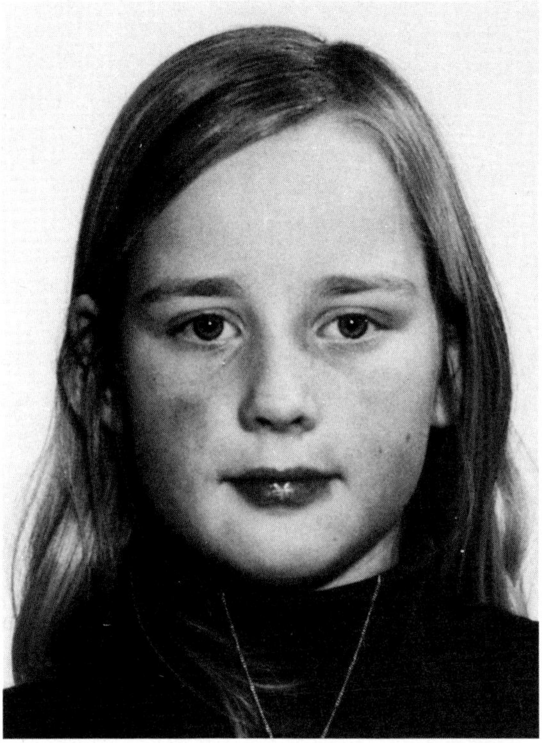

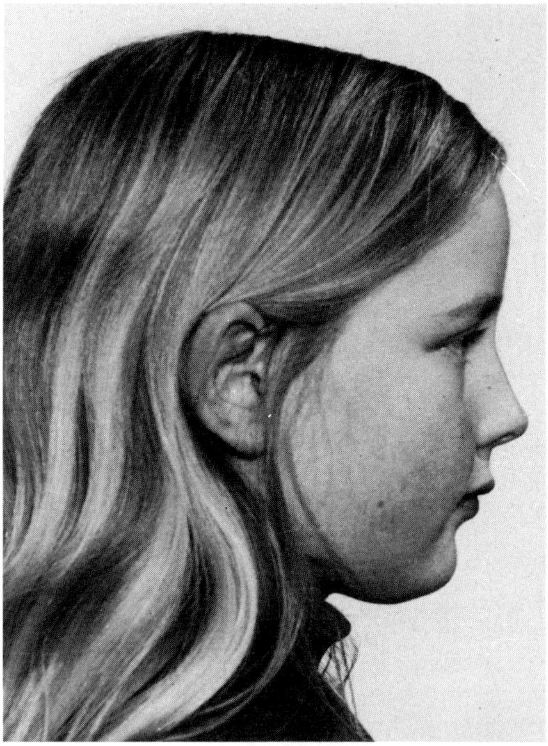

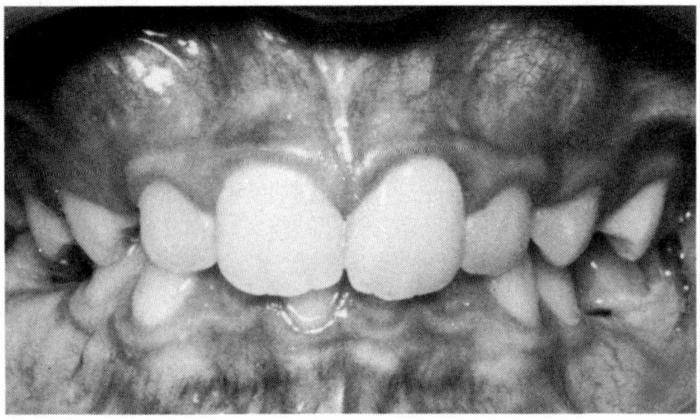

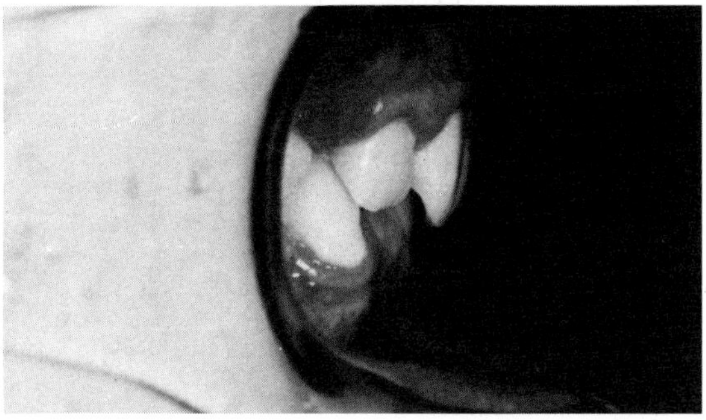

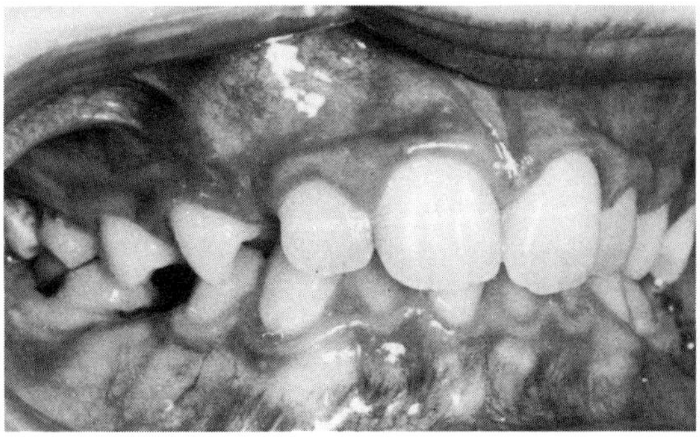

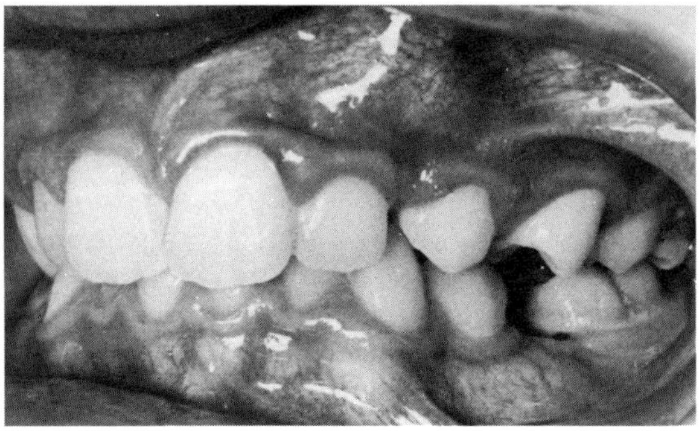

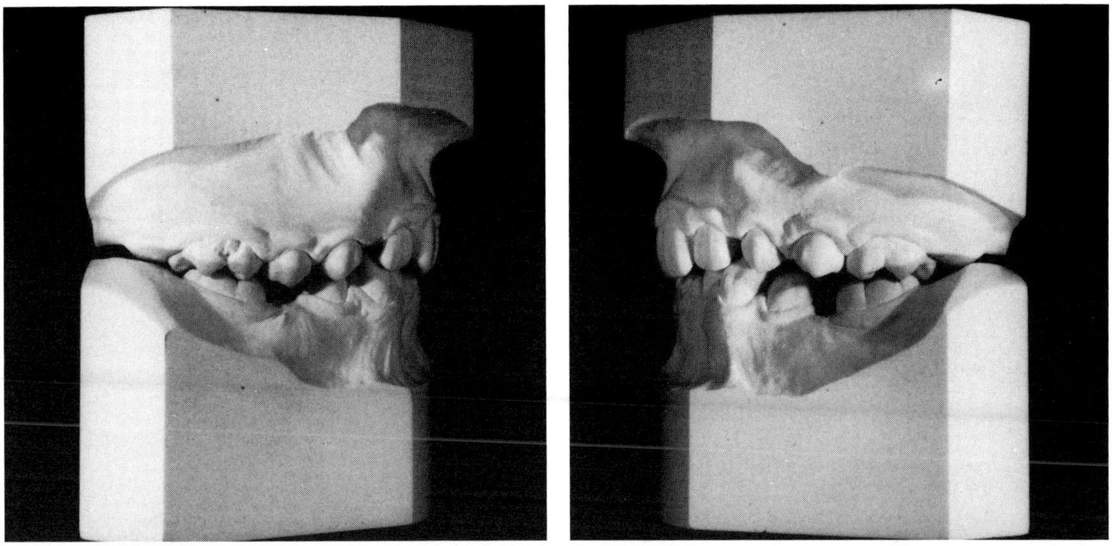

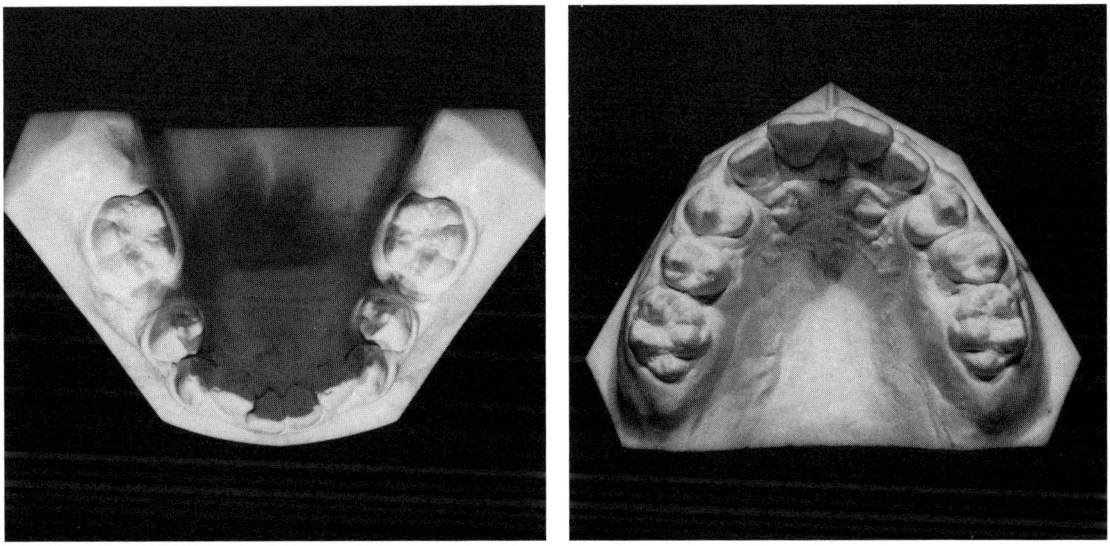

Figs 34-1 and 34-2 *A girl aged 10 y, 9 mo with a class II/1 anomaly and marked crowding in both dental arches, which is attributable mainly to the early loss of the deciduous molars. The mandibular incisors and the maxillary ones to a greater degree are tipped back. There is an ALD of –9 mm in the mandible and the crowding is localized primarily in the second premolar region. In the maxilla, the ALD is –10 mm; the first permanent molars have migrated mesially and rotated and there is almost no space for the canines which are located buccally high in the vestibule. The dentition is poorly cared for. Plaque is found in many situations and the gingiva are congested. The first permanent molars have deep caries and decalcification buccally and lingually. Even the maxillary incisors have been attacked, although to a lesser extent.*

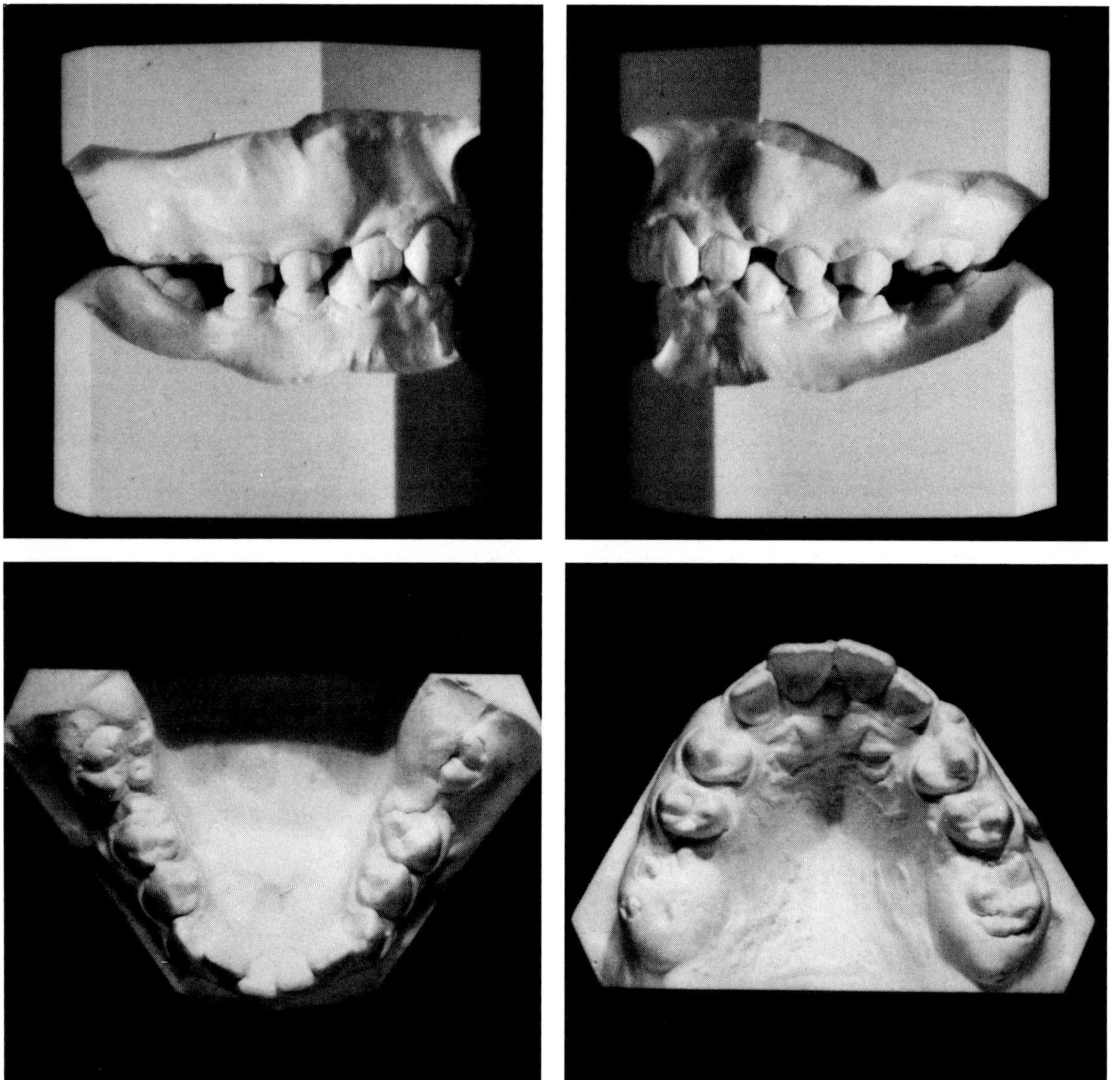

Fig 34-3 *Six months after extraction of the first permanent molars, the second premolars in the mandible and all the second permanent molars have either fully or partly emerged. The first premolars and the canines in the mandible have drifted a little distally, enabling the lateral incisors to move to labial. In the maxilla, the extraction of the first permanent molars has not contributed much to increasing the room available for the canines. The lateral photographs were not taken perpendicular to the median plane but are perpendicular to the molar/premolar arch segments.*

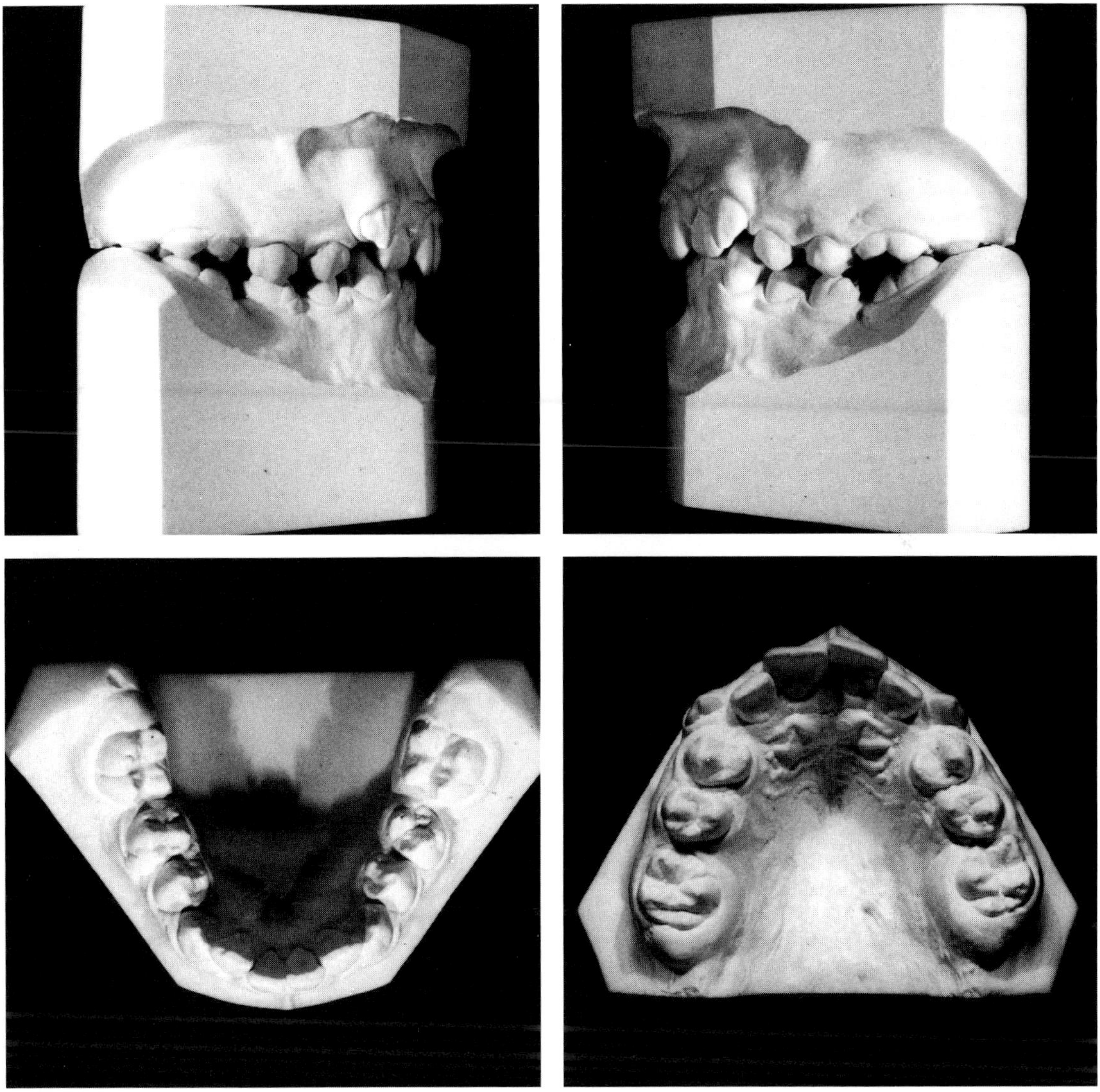

Fig 34-4 A year after the extraction of the first permanent molars, both the mandibular left second molar and that on the right in the maxilla have fully emerged. The space available for the maxillary canines has increased only slightly; the canines have emerged ectostomatically. The mesio-palatally rotated second molars are located close to the second premolars.

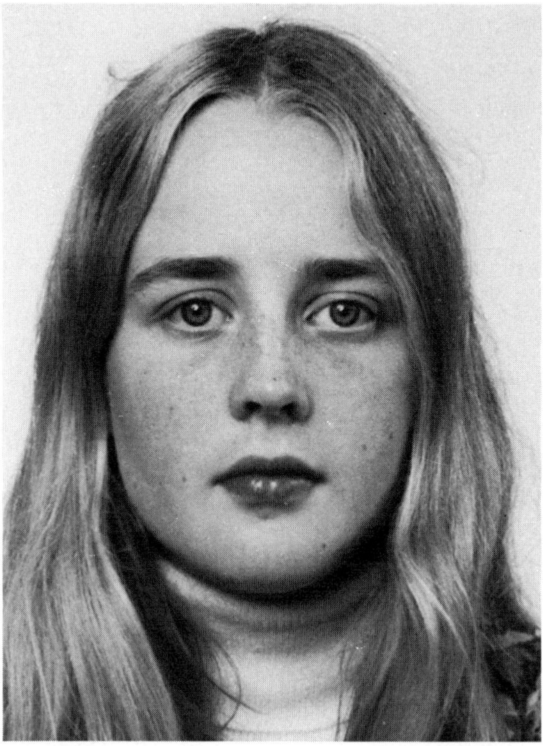

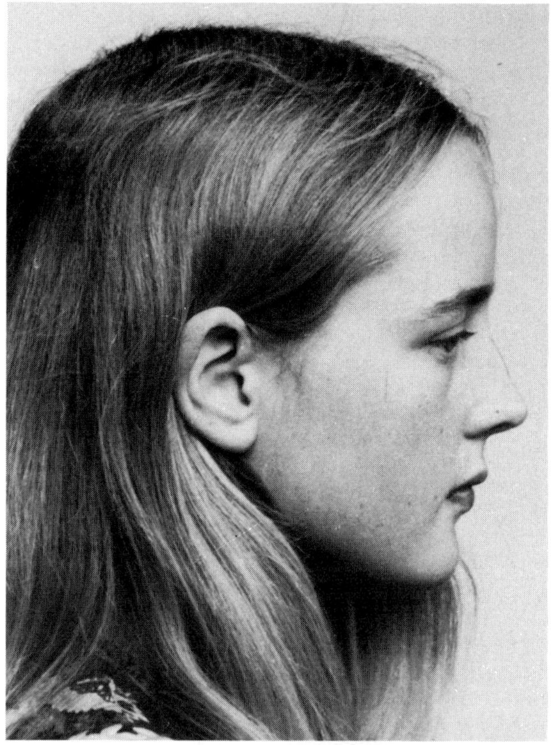

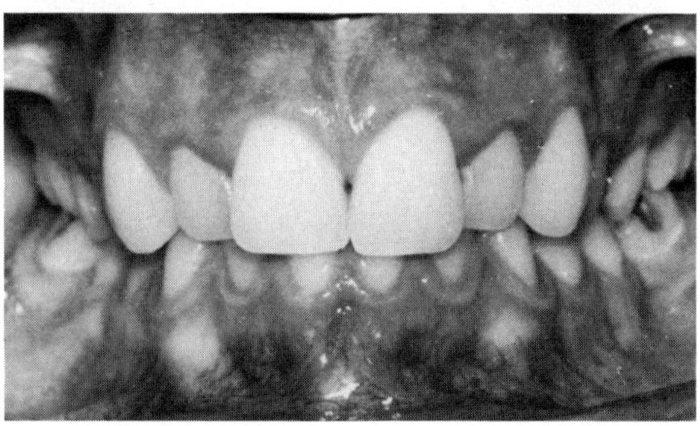

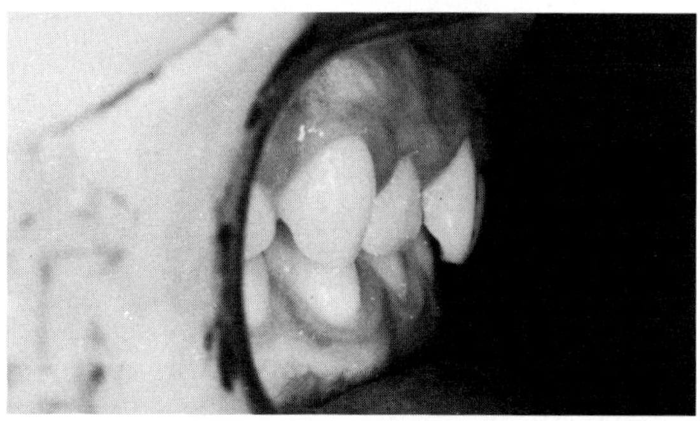

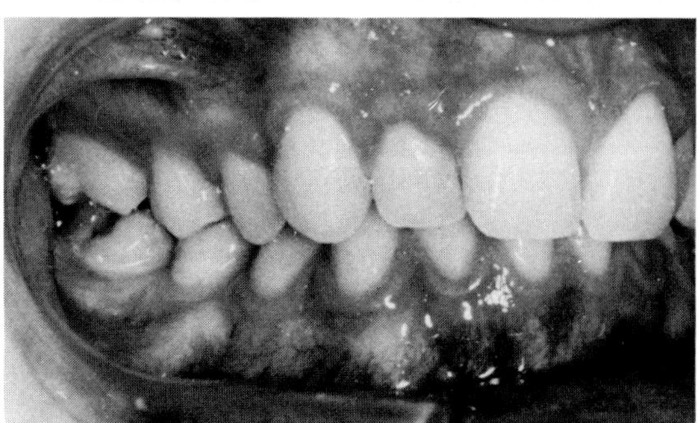

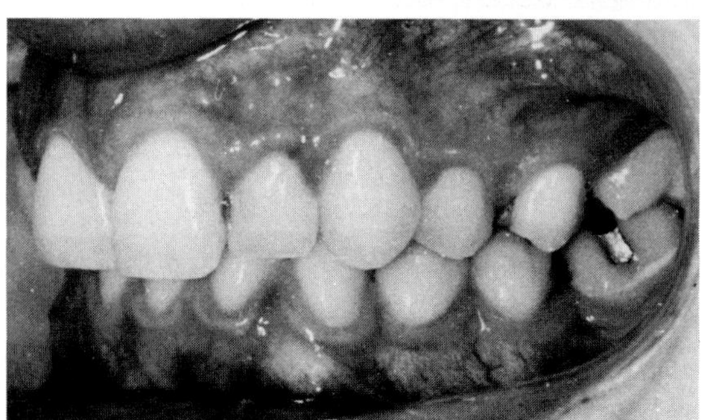

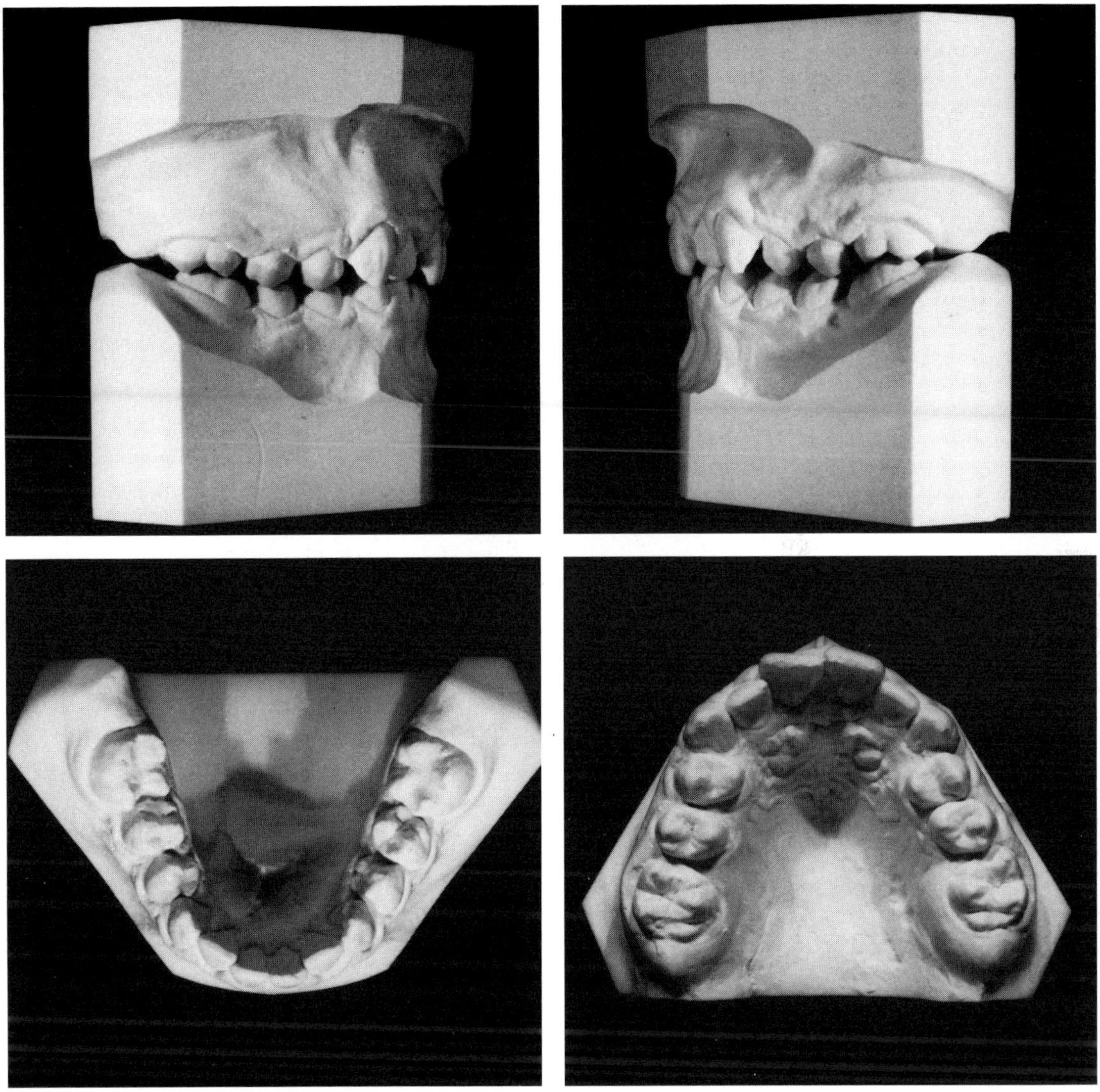

Figs 34-5 and 34-6 At the age of 14 y, 4 mo the treatment involving a cervical headgear was terminated at the request of the patient. The space required in the maxillary arch has not been attained. The canines are located too far to buccal and the incisors are crowded. In the mandible, the second molars have uprighted under the influence of the occlusion and function satisfactorily. The disto-occlusion has not been fully corrected; the steep inclination of the maxillary incisors and the deep bite show little improvement.

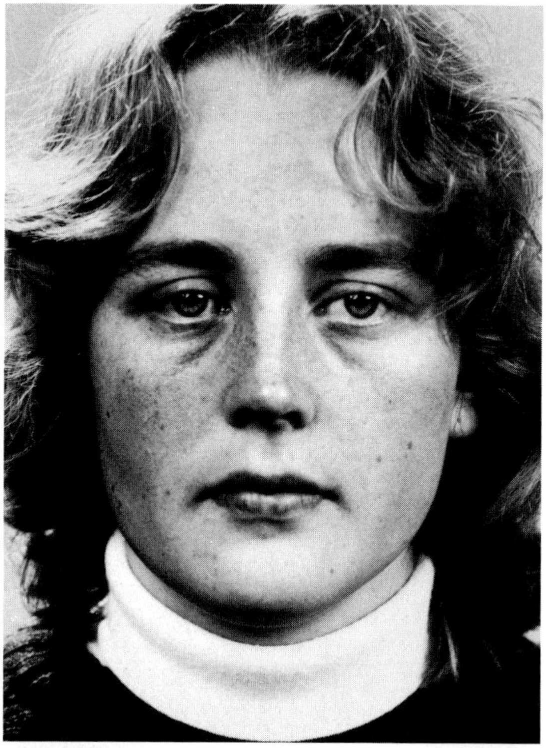

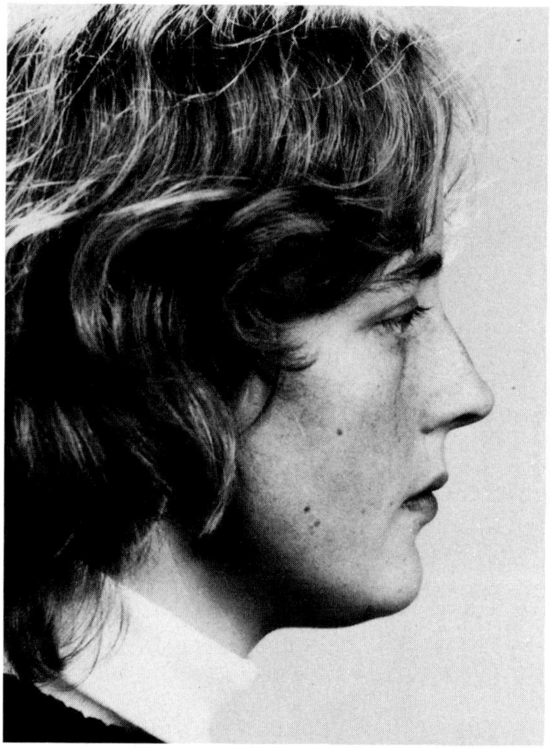

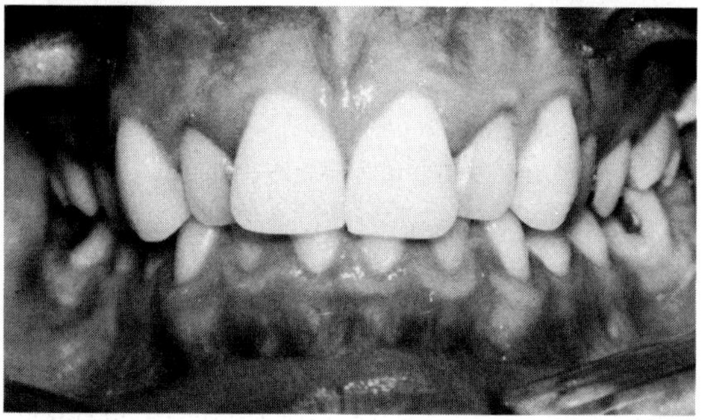

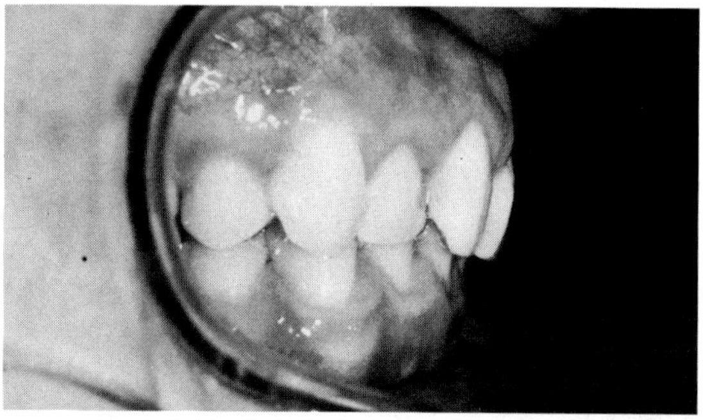

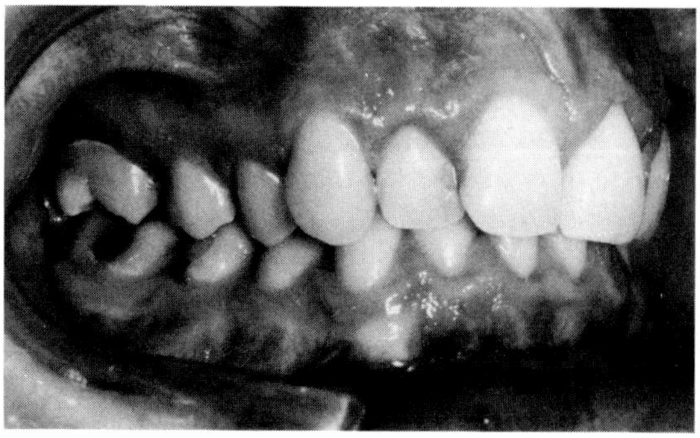

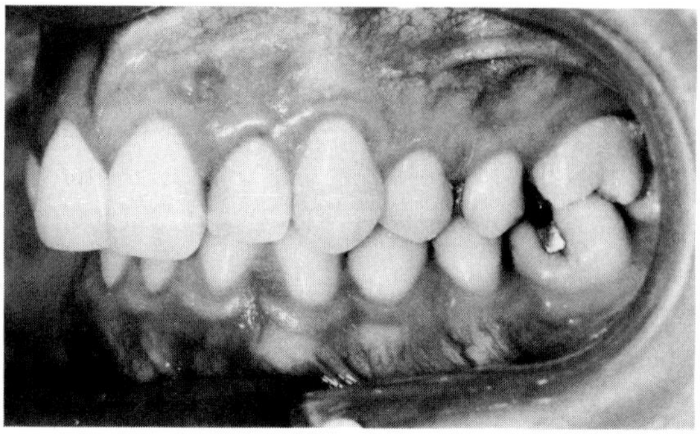

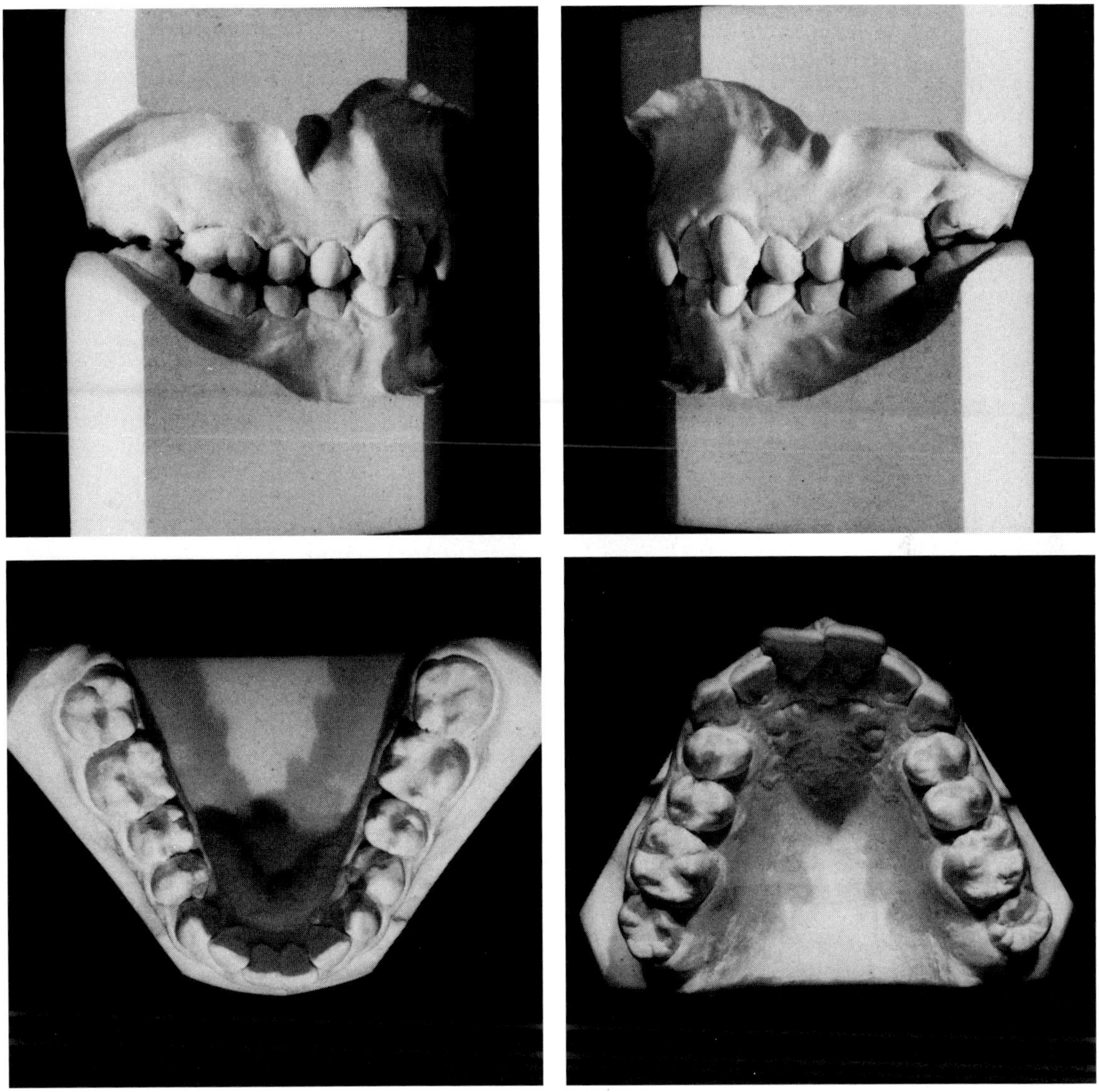

Figs 34-7 and 34-8 *At the age of 25 y, 7 mo, eleven years after the end of treatment, the patient is still satisfied with the result. The adult face is harmonious in form with a good profile and an acceptable appearance of the teeth. The steep inclination of the anteriors and the depth of the bite have not increased. All third molars have emerged; little else has changed.*

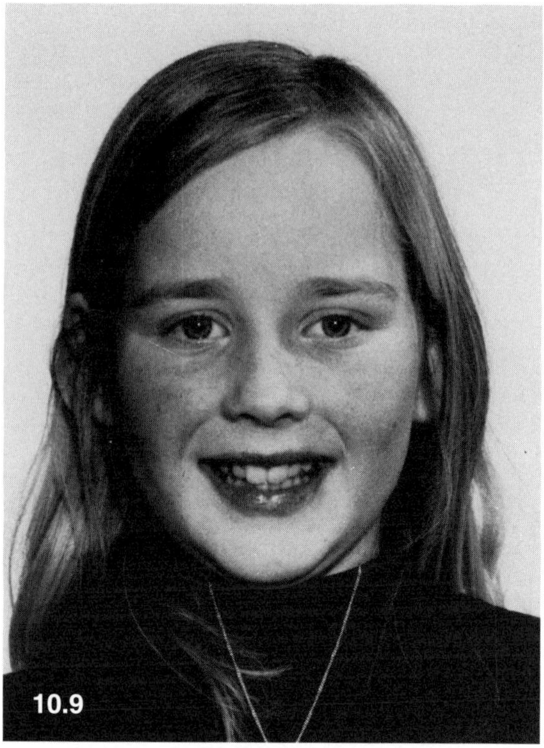

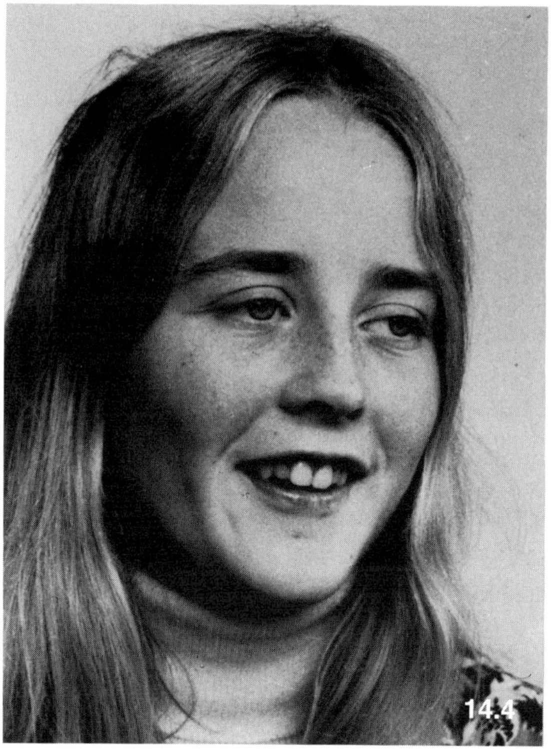

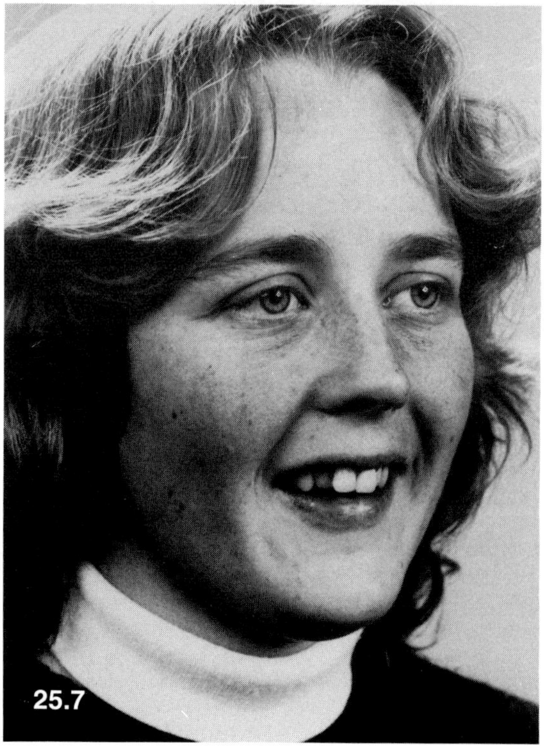

Fig 34-9 Note the limited change in the dentition.

realized. The room for the canines remained inadequate and a disto-occlusion of ¼ PW remained. In particular, the overbite had been little reduced and the steep inclination of the maxillary incisors remained. The angulation of the mandibular second premolars had improved and particularly that of the second permanent molars. The profile had become straighter (Figs 34.5 and 34.6).
At the age of 25 years, 7 months, ten years after treatment had ended, the face was harmonious and showed good facial animation. The mouth had not fallen in and no exagerated nasolabial fold is seen. The patient is satisfied with the alignment of her teeth and the dentition functions well (Figs 34.7 and 34.8).
The photographs of her smiling face at various ages illustrate the changes that took place during the fifteen years (Fig 34.9).

In *Problems and Procedures in Orthodontics*[33] a separate chapter is devoted to the problem of whether or not to extract first permanent molars of poor quality at an early age. Further information on this topic should be sought there. Some remarks will be made that are pertinent to this case.
Where the first permanent molars are of outstandingly poor quality and there is normal occlusion, the early extraction of those molars should be seriously considered. In patients with marked crowding in both arches, such extractions are definitely to be favored. Nonetheless, crowding seldom occurs in the molar regions and usually occurs more mesially. Extraction of the first molars instead of premolars certainly significantly complicates any orthodontic treatment, especially because it almost always involves the use of full fixed appliances over a long period.
It is worth noting that particularly in the maxilla the extraction of the first permanent molars does little to reduce crowding in the canine areas. For instance, if the second permanent molars can move freely to mesial after emergence then, as has been described in this case, any extra space made available by the extractions can quickly be lost from the distal. Moreover, even if the mesial drifting of the second molars is prevented, the premolars have to be moved actively to distal with appliances to increase the space for the canines.
Regarding the treatment described here two aspects can be mentioned that would have provided a better result but which were at that time not known.
First, the effects of an intervention such as the extraction of first permanent molars are to a large extent dependent on the time the extractions are done and the order in which they take place. The molars in the mandible need to be extracted first, and then a considerable time later those in the maxilla can be removed.[14, 15] The rules governing this matter are outlined in Figure 34.10. In cases with crowding, it is essential to be alert to the possible loss of the space that is needed just for the relief of the crowding. Where the occlusion is abnormal the rules sometimes need to be modified since vertical contact may occur in different areas. In this case, it would have been better if the first permanent molars had been extracted in the mandible and those in the maxilla had been left until after the maxillary second molars had been in occlusion with their antagonists, the mandibular second molars, for some time.
Second, the use of a maxillary plate could have procured a significantly better result if it had been used to hold the second molars back, move the premolars to distal and

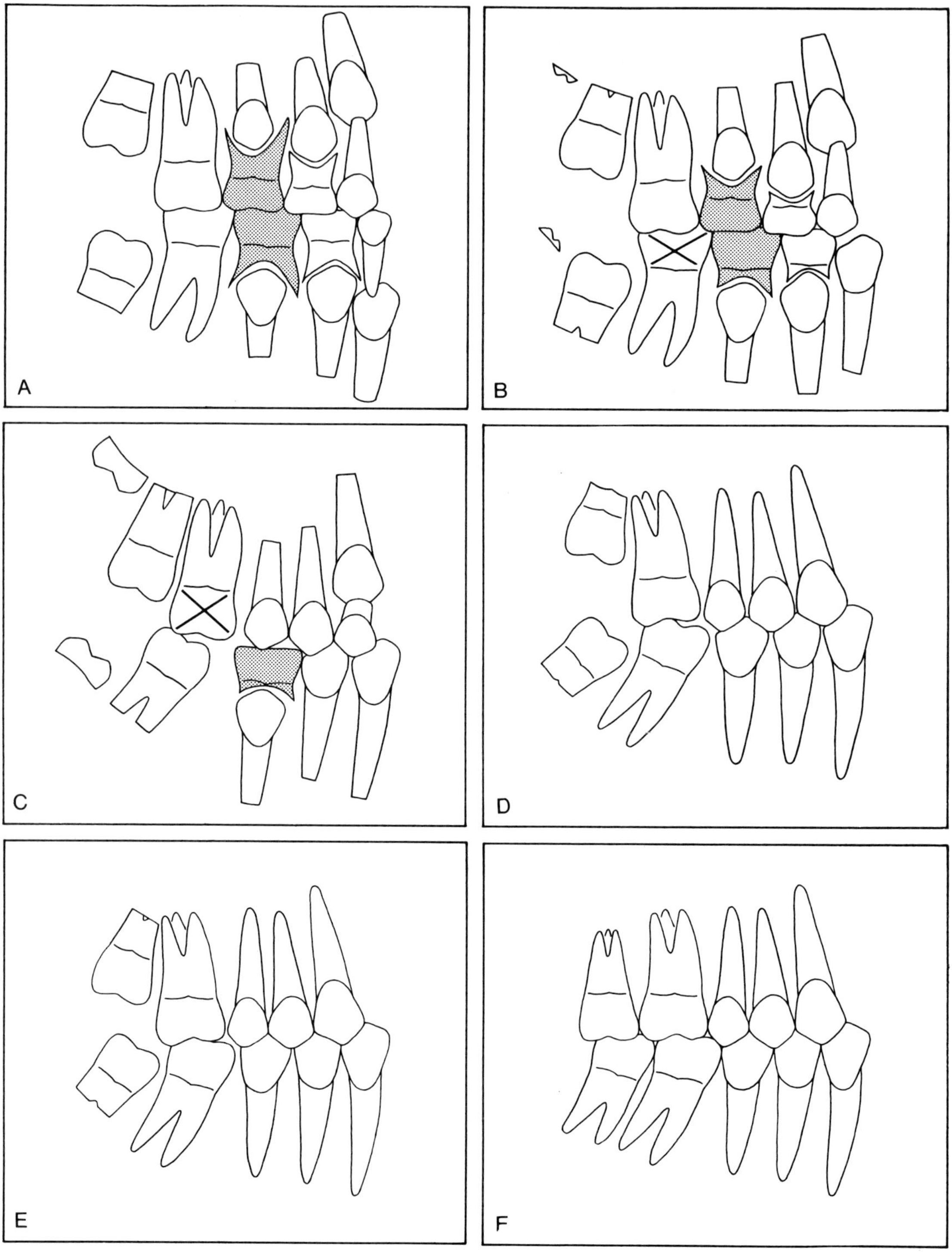
A
B
C
D
E
F

Fig 34-10 Schematic representation of the decision-making process in a class I situation involving early extraction of first permanent molars in maxilla and mandible. At the same time, the situations that normally are seen five (E) and ten (F) years afterward are portrayed.

A At about the age of 8 years the second premolars are found at a considerable distance from the occlusal plane. Extraction of the first permanent molars at this stage could lead to an abnormal path of eruption of the second premolars. In particular, the mandibular second premolar often has a tendency to tip distally. Moreover there is still uncertainty at this time regarding the state of formation of the third molars. The furcation of the second permanent molars is not yet calcified.

B Before extraction of the mandibular first permanent molar, the situation depicted here should be awaited. The second premolars are now closer to the occlusal plane, the furcations of the second molars are now visible and the third molars appear to be forming. The mandibular first permanent molar should be extracted when the second molar is about one crown height distant from the occlusal plane. To wait longer before extraction is not desirable. At this time, the second molar can move not only horizontally but vertically, permitting a better mesio-distal angulation to develop later.

C After emergence of the mandibular second permanent molar, it will develop contact between its disto-buccal cusp and the maxillary first permanent molar. As a result its mesial migration will be associated with some uprighting. The timing of the extraction of the maxillary first permanent molar is less critical; it can wait about one year or longer after the removal of the mandibular molar. The maxillary second molar drifts much more rapidly mesially than does the mandibular second molar. Furthermore, less undesirable tipping will occur, this being due to the more favorable original axial direction of the maxillary molar. Shortly after emergence, the maxillary second molar will make contact with the mandibular second molar.

D After full emergence of the maxillary second molar, occlusal contact is established between the distal cusps of second molars. The uprighting effect on the mandibular molar is continued. The maxillary second molar is also subjected to a favorably directed force. In both jaws, diastemata are present between the premolars and molars, those in the mandible being greater. The third molars have largely followed the movements of the second molars.

E The diastemata in maxillary and mandibular arches have been reduced in size. The mandibular second molar has uprighted itself and moved more mesially. A better sagittal occlusion has been established between it and the maxillary molar. The third molars have come further to mesial and approached closer to the occlusal plane than when the first permanent molars had not been extracted early. They will also emerge about eighteen months earlier.

F The third molars are well positioned. Full occlusal contact exists between them. The angulation of the maxillary second permanent molar is more or less normal. The mandibular second molar is still mesially tipped. This position will not improve measurably later. The space between the mandibular second premolar and second molar remains unfavorable from a periodontal viewpoint. The occlusion of the second molars is also not optimal. This applies also, however to a lesser extent, to the premolars, the rotations of which will not correct themselves naturally. The diastemata in both dental arches have closed. In the maxilla, this happens almost always as a rule. In the mandible they quite often will remain open.[33]

improve the positions of the incisors and canines. In addition, the deep bite and the steep inclination of the maxillary incisors, by tipping them labially, could have been corrected. The high caries activity had been accepted then as a definite contraindication for the use of appliances, either fixed or removable. Since then it has been recognized that good oral hygiene, sensible eating habits, and daily rinsing with fluoride solutions can largely prevent decalcifications and caries accompanying the use of orthodontic appliances. However, that not all patients can be motivated to cooperate.

Chapter 35

Class II/1, lower lip behind maxillary incisors, over-erupted maxillary and mandibular incisors

Cervical headgear, maxillary removable plate, mandibular lip bumper, activator

Male: 10 years, 4 months to 18 years, 10 months

A boy aged 10 years and 4 months showed a pronounced class II/1 anomaly. He had sucked his thumb until the age of five years, was able to breathe through his nose, and kept his lower lip behind his maxillary incisors. The lower border of his mandible was horizontally oriented and the bony chin was strongly developed. The sagittal discrepancy between the jaws was fairly small and the overjet of 14 mm was largely the result of the linguo-version of the mandibular incisors and the marked eversion of the maxillary incisors. The crowding in the mandibular incisors (ALD -3 mm) and the excessive space in the maxillary incisor region (ALD +3 mm) are associated with the interposition of the lower lip. The overbite measured 8 mm, with the mandibular incisors contacting the palate. On the right, the disto-occlusion was ¾ PW; on the left it was 1 PW. Oral hygiene was bad. The permanent molars and the mandibular incisors were heavily restored. The patient was frightened of the dentist and seemed very much opposed to orthodontic treatment (Figs 35.1 and 35.2).

Taking into consideration the attitude of the patient and the quality of his dentition, the choice of treatment would be the least taxing. With the use of a cervical headgear and a maxillary removable plate with a biteplane, the disto-occlusion could be corrected and the overjet and overbite reduced. Meanwhile, a mandibular lip bumper would be fitted to prevent the lip being interposed between the mandibular and maxillary incisors and to provide the opportunity for the mandibular incisors to move ventrally.

At the age of 10 years, 6 months, the maxillary first permanent molars were banded and a cervical headgear was fitted. A week later, a maxillary plate was provided, while two months after that a lip bumper was fitted to the mandibular arch. During the first four months of treatment loose bands had to be recemented six times, the headgear had to be replaced due to breakage, and a labial arch on the plate had to be replaced twice. The oral hygiene remained inadequate and the gingiva behind the maxillary incisors became hypertrophic. In addition, the palatal surfaces of the maxillary incisors were decalcifying.

It was decided to replace the lip bumper and maxillary plate with a less potentially damaging and vulnerable appliance — an activator — but to continue to use the headgear. By this means, two facial-orthopedic approaches would be combined and the chance that caries or decalcifications would develop would be reduced. Regular oral hygiene instruction was given throughout the treatment.

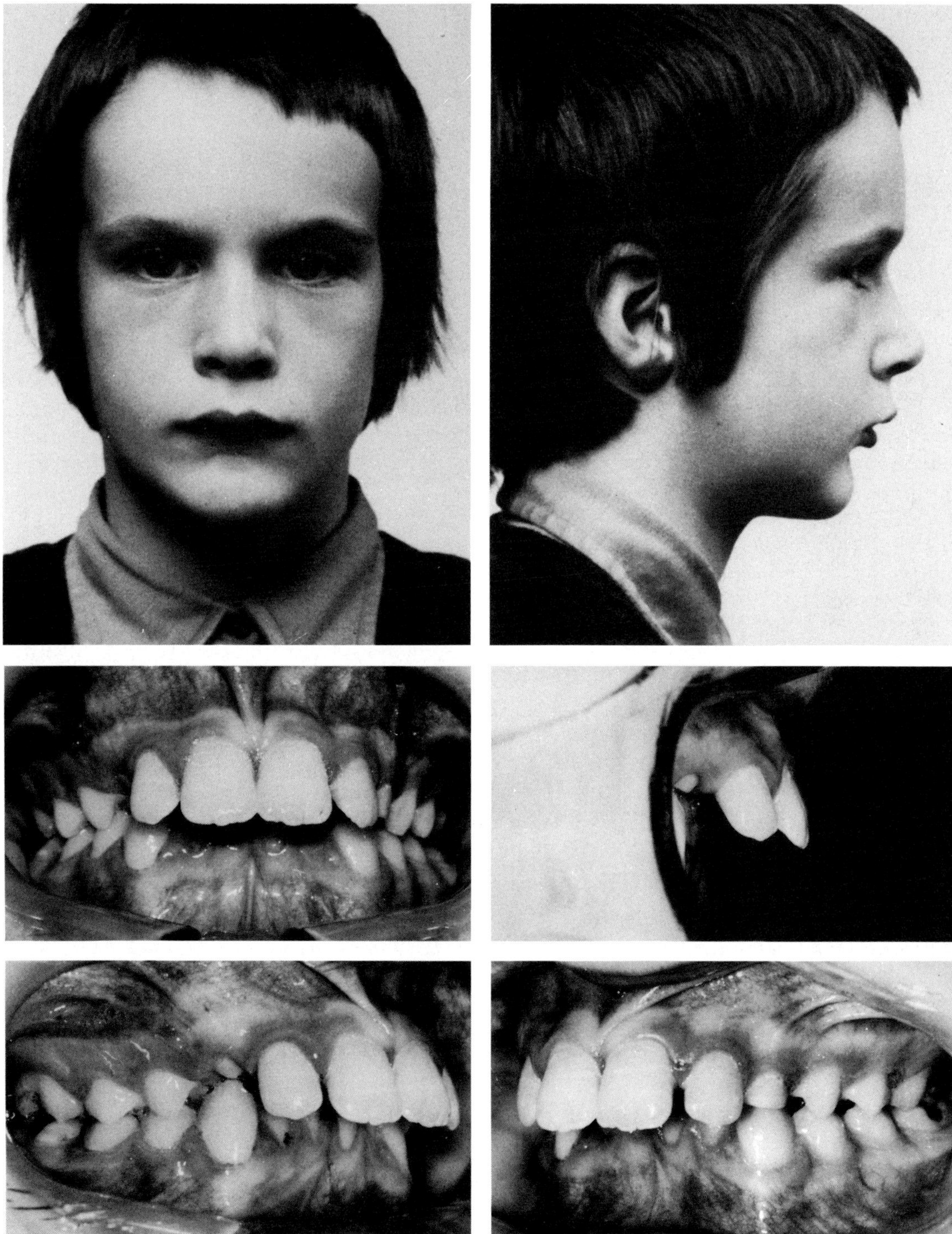

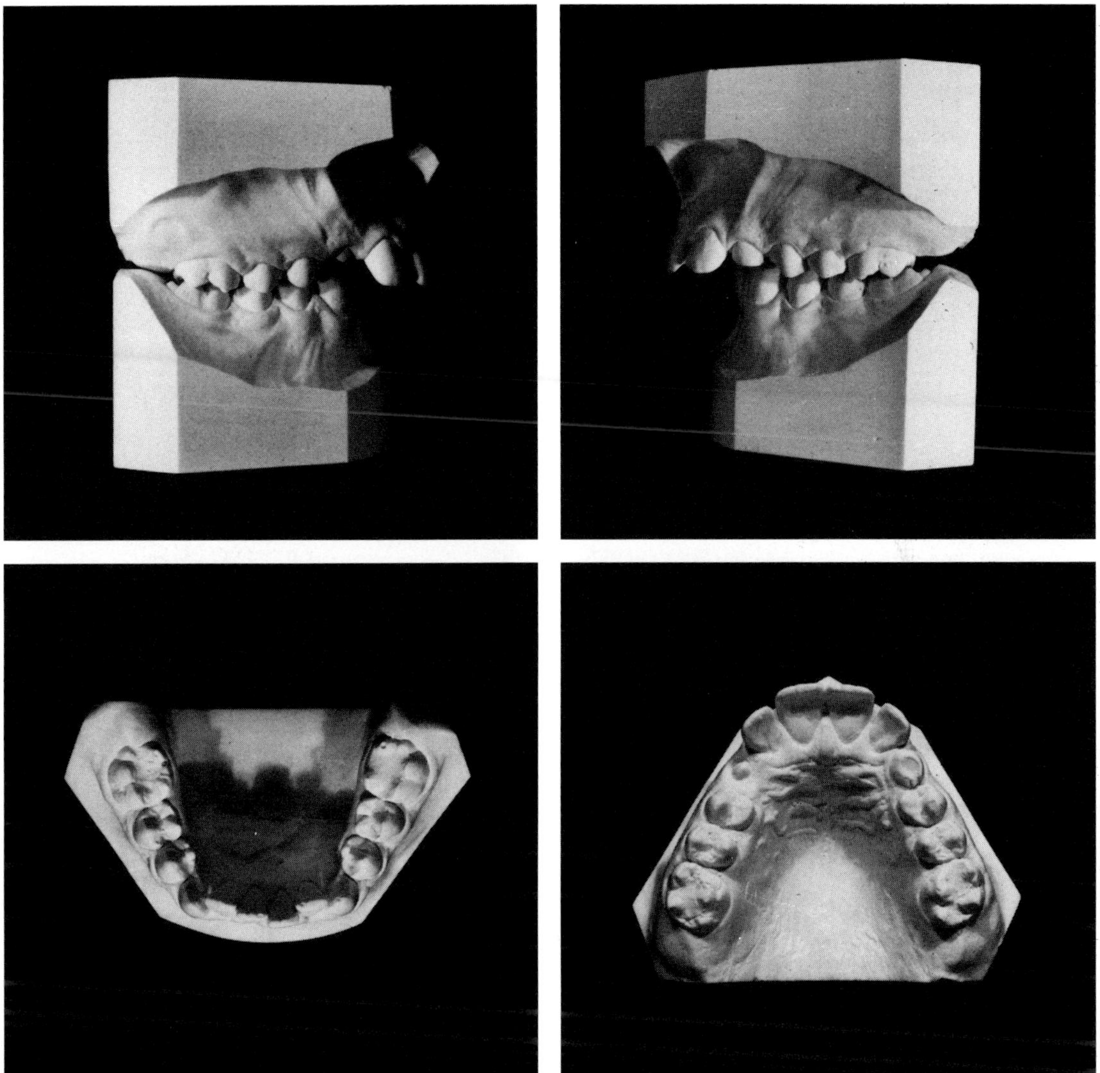

Figs 35-1 and 35-2 A boy aged 10 y, 4 mo with a pronounced class II/1 anomaly that is based not so much on the disto-relation of the jaws but on abnormal positions of the teeth. The lower lip is held behind the everted maxillary incisors and the mandibular incisors are tipped lingually. The ALD of the mandibular arch is –3 mm, and of the maxillary arch is +3 mm. The middle of the mandibular arch is 2mm to the left, compared with that of the maxillary arch. This asymmetry corresponds with the difference in the disto-occlusion, which is ¾ PW on the right but 1 PW on the left. The mandibular incisors contact the palate. The overjet is 14 mm, the overbite 8 mm. The attachment of the labial frenum is low but there is no central diastema.

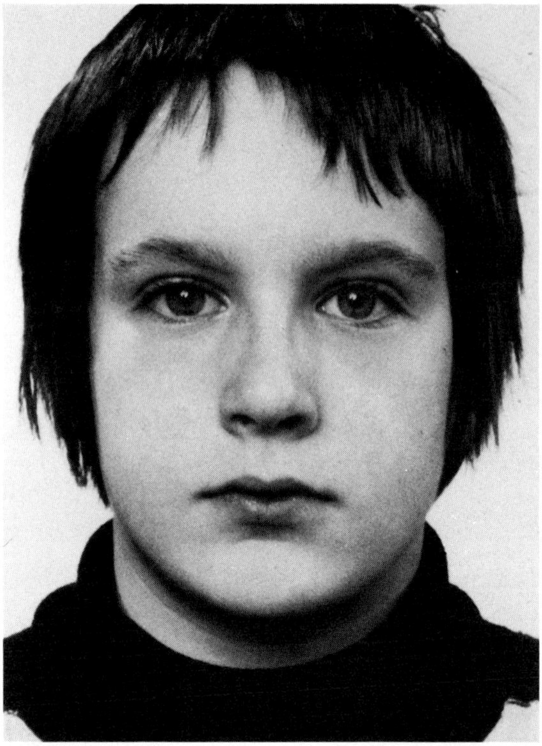
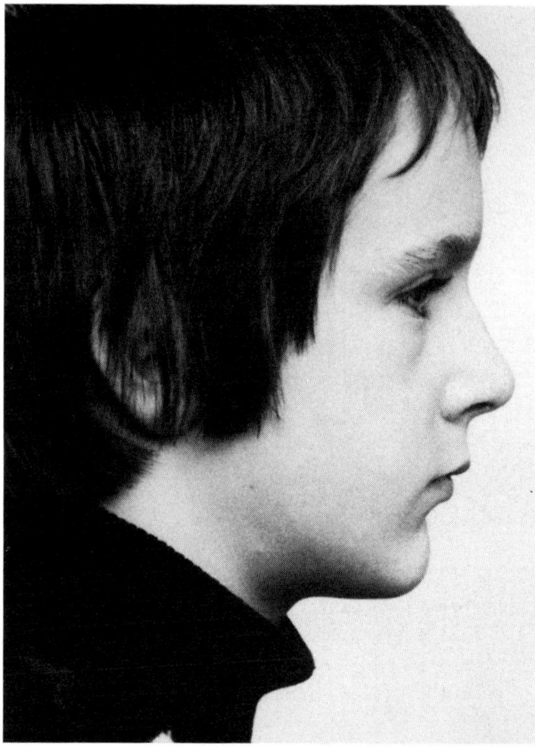
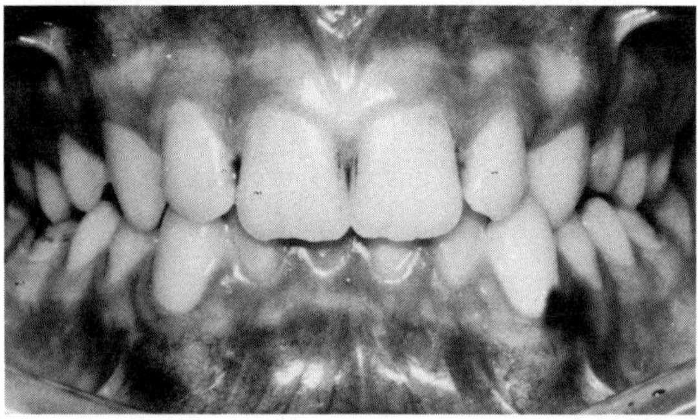
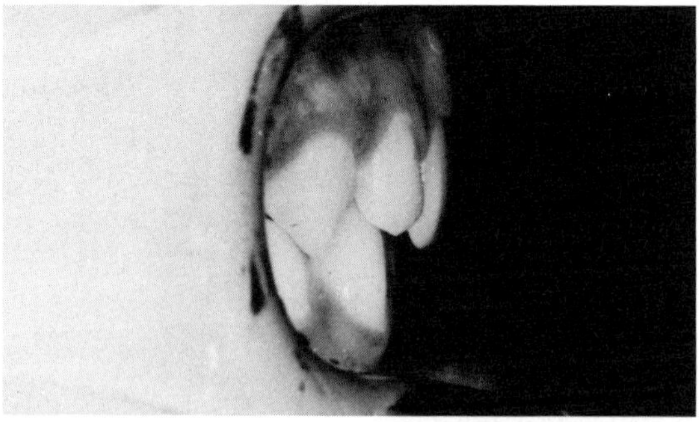
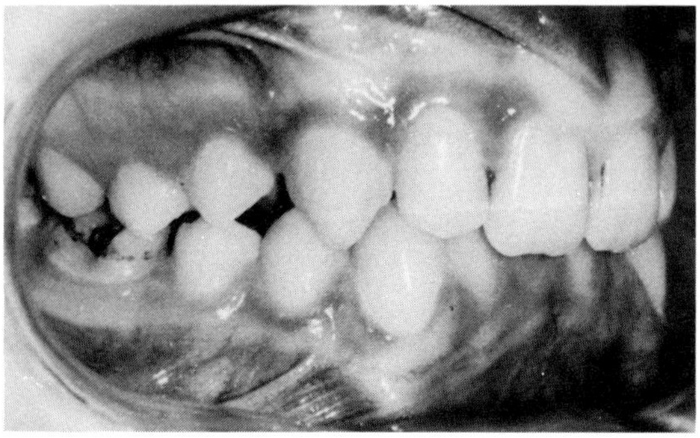
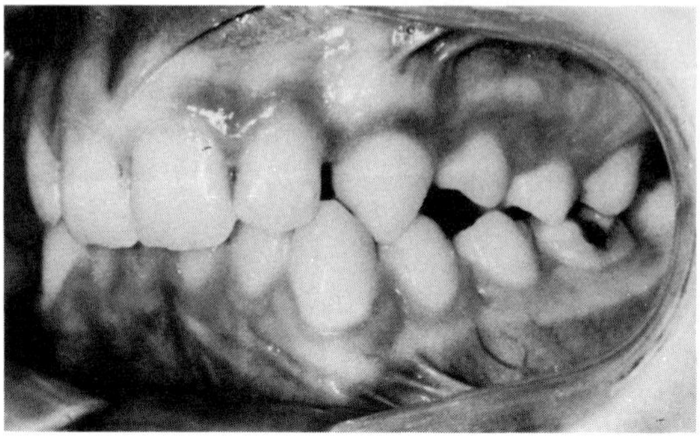

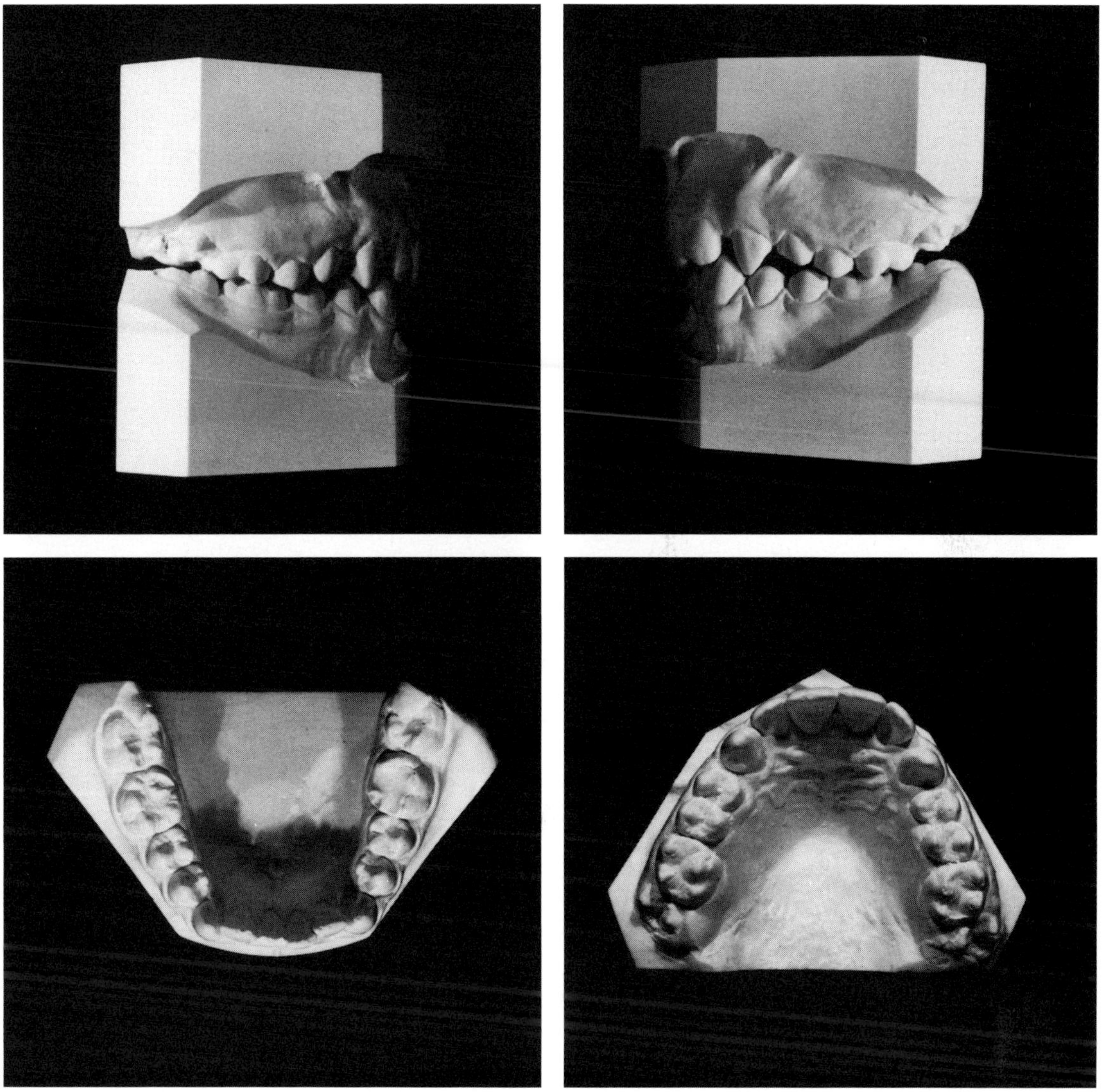

Figs 35-3 and 35-4 *At the age of 12 y, 6 mo, after two years of treatment with primarily a cervical headgear and an activator, a significant improvement has been achieved. The first molars and second premolars occlude well, the mandibular anteriors have moved to ventral, and the mouth is kept closed. The mandibular anteriors exhibit mild crowding still, the maxillary incisors are steeply inclined, and the bite is deep. It can be expected that the maxillary first premolars will erupt further and come into good occlusion.*

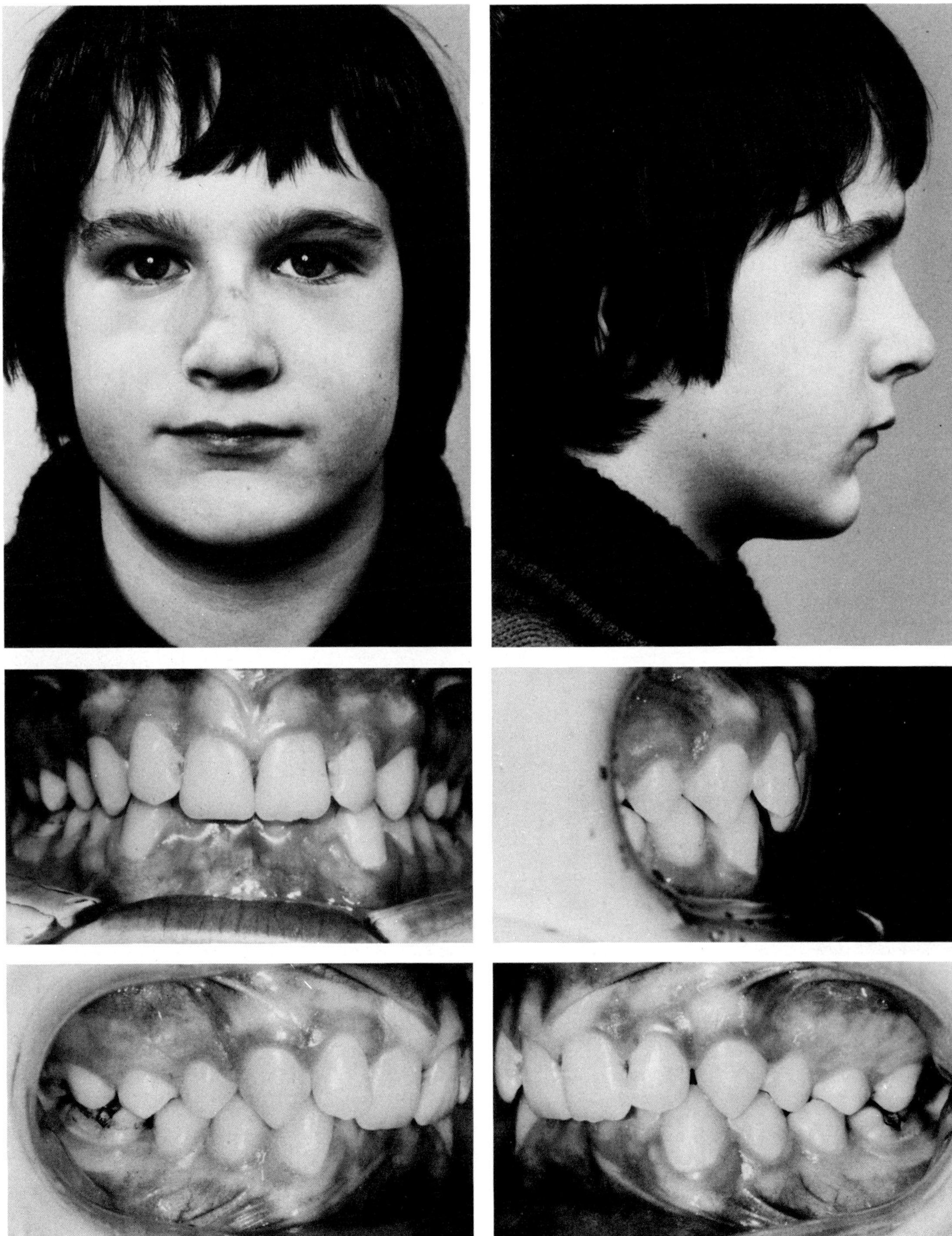

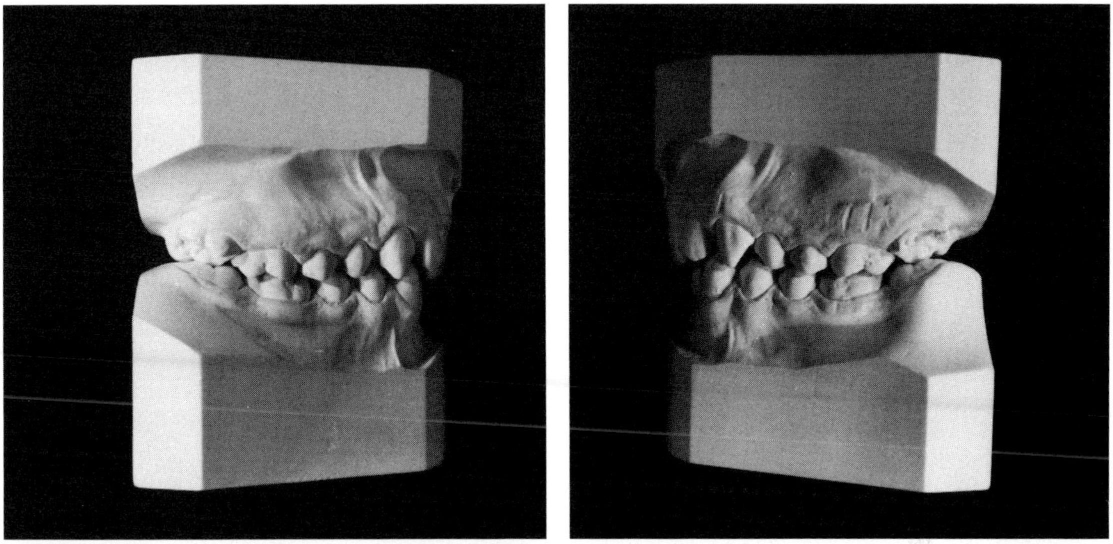

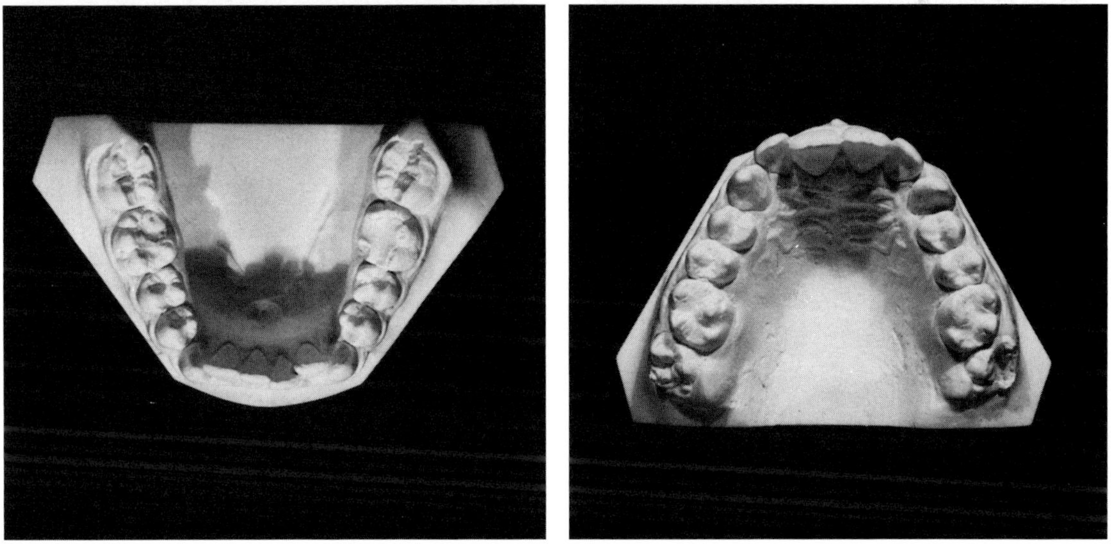

Figs 35-5 and 35-6 *At the age of 13 y, 6 mo, 1 year after finishing treatment, the maxillary central incisors are tipped palatally and the maxillary left lateral incisor, but more so the right one, have moved labially. The mandibular anteriors are more crowded and the incisors have tipped lingually between the canines. The overbite has increased. In contradistinction to the changes anteriorly those in the posterior regions have been improvements. The occlusion on the right has become better consolidated, although that on the left has regressed slightly toward disto-occlusion.*

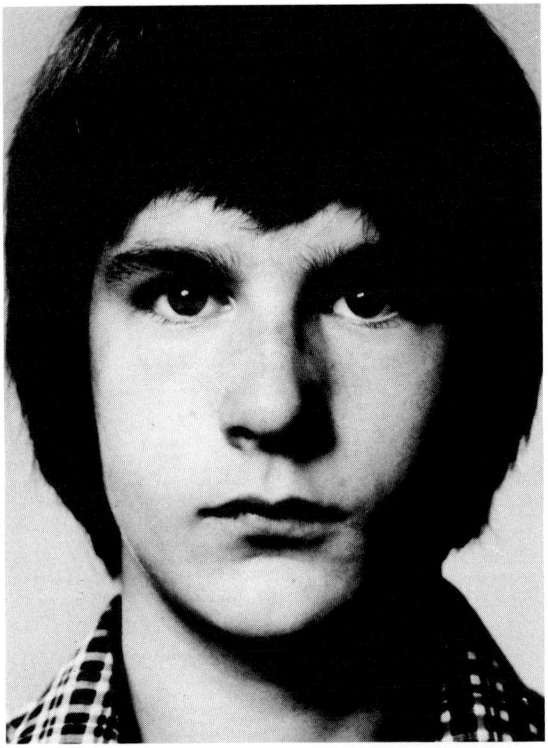

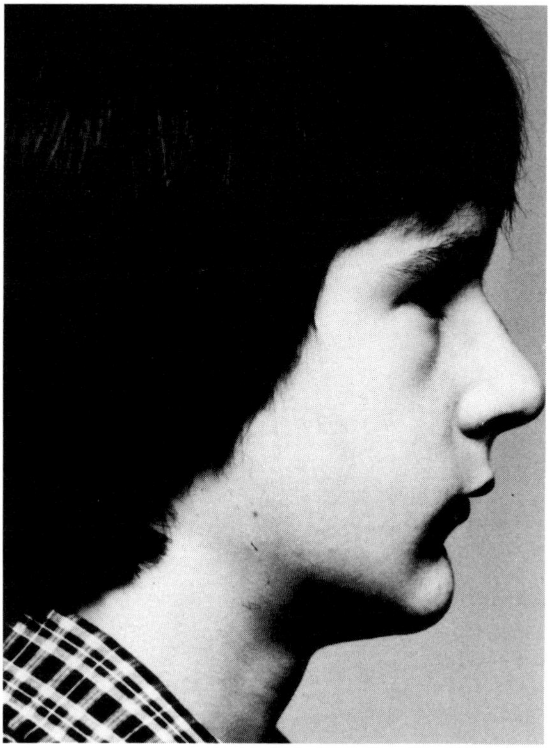

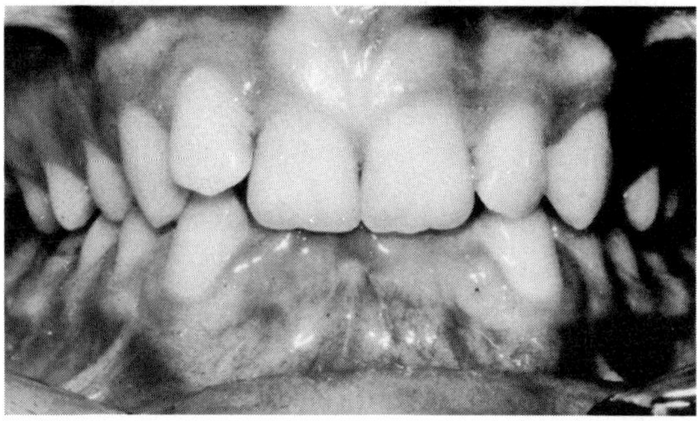

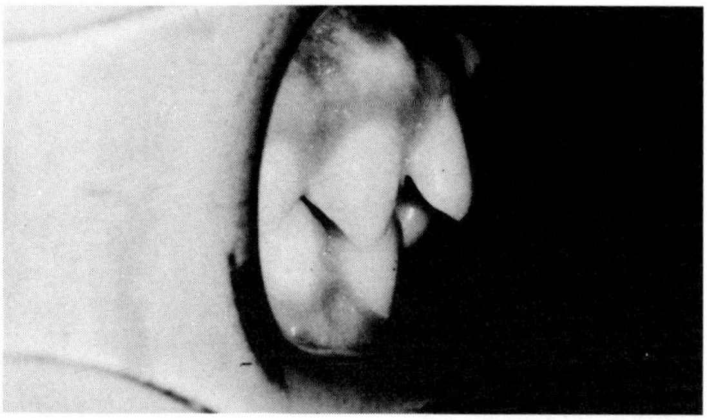

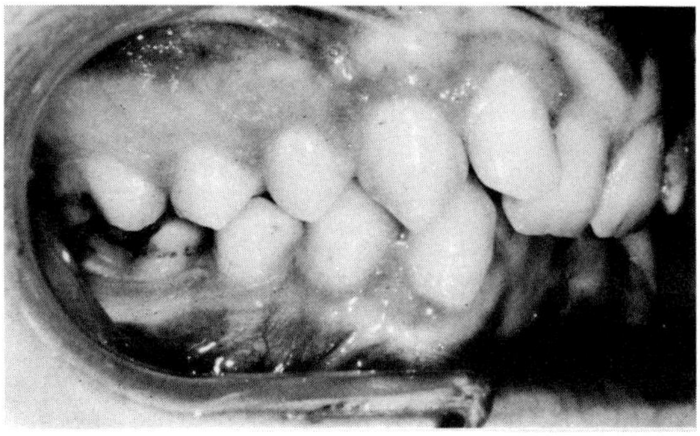

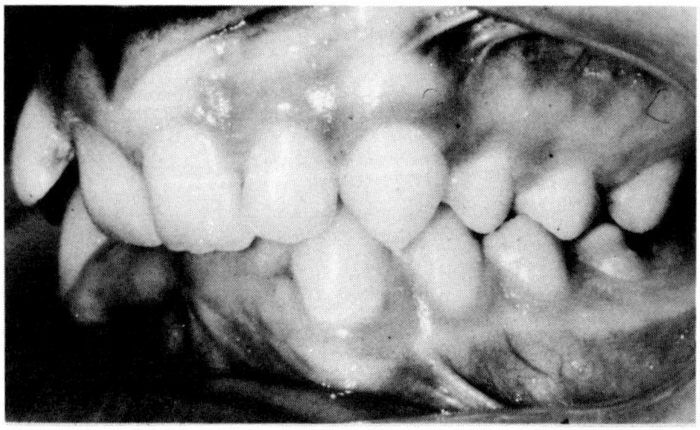

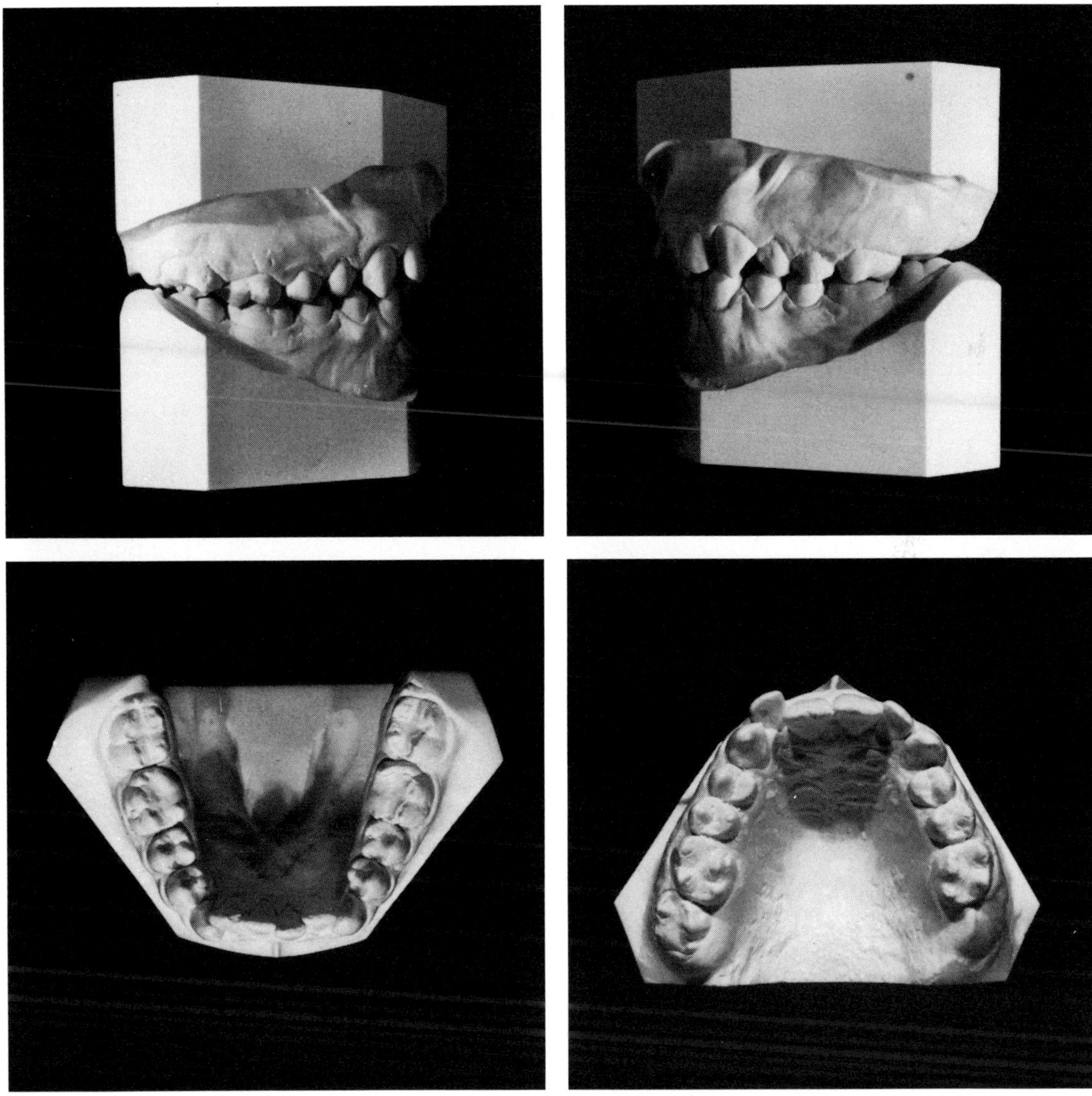

Figs 35-7 and 35-8 *At the age of 14 y, 6 mo, the tipping backward of the maxillary central incisors has increased so much that their palatal surfaces lie in contact with the labial surfaces of the mandibular incisors and fully cover them. The mandibular right lateral incisor overlaps the lingual surface of the adjacent canine more than halfway. The mandibular teeth on both sides occlude now more distally than the year before; this might be ascribed to the dorsally directed force that is exerted on the mandibular incisors by the backward-tipped maxillary incisors. The maxillary right second molar has moved palatally and aided by the cone-funnel mechanism can come better into occlusion. The maxillary left second molar was so far buccally displaced the previous year that it would have gone entirely outside occluding with*

(continued on page 593)

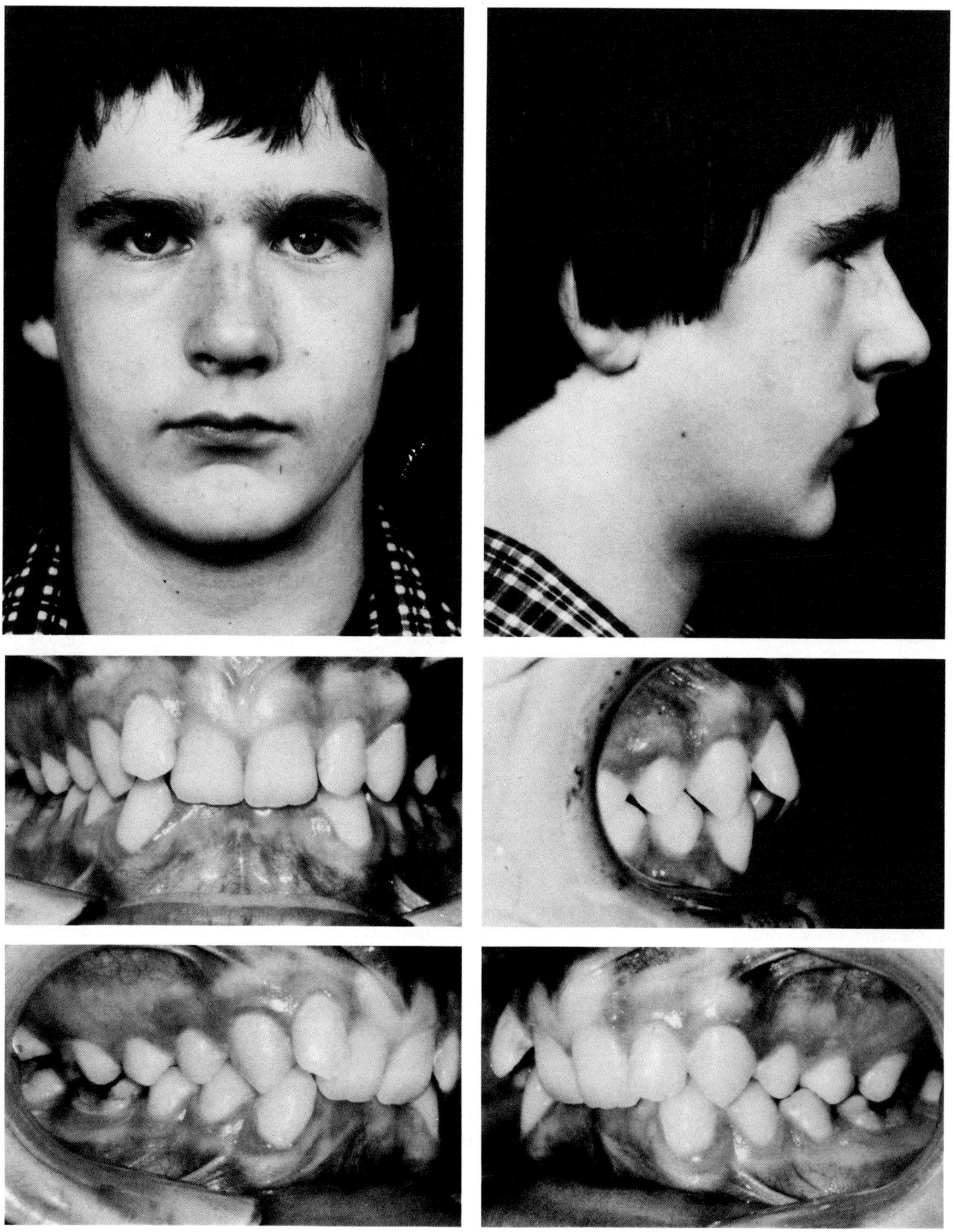

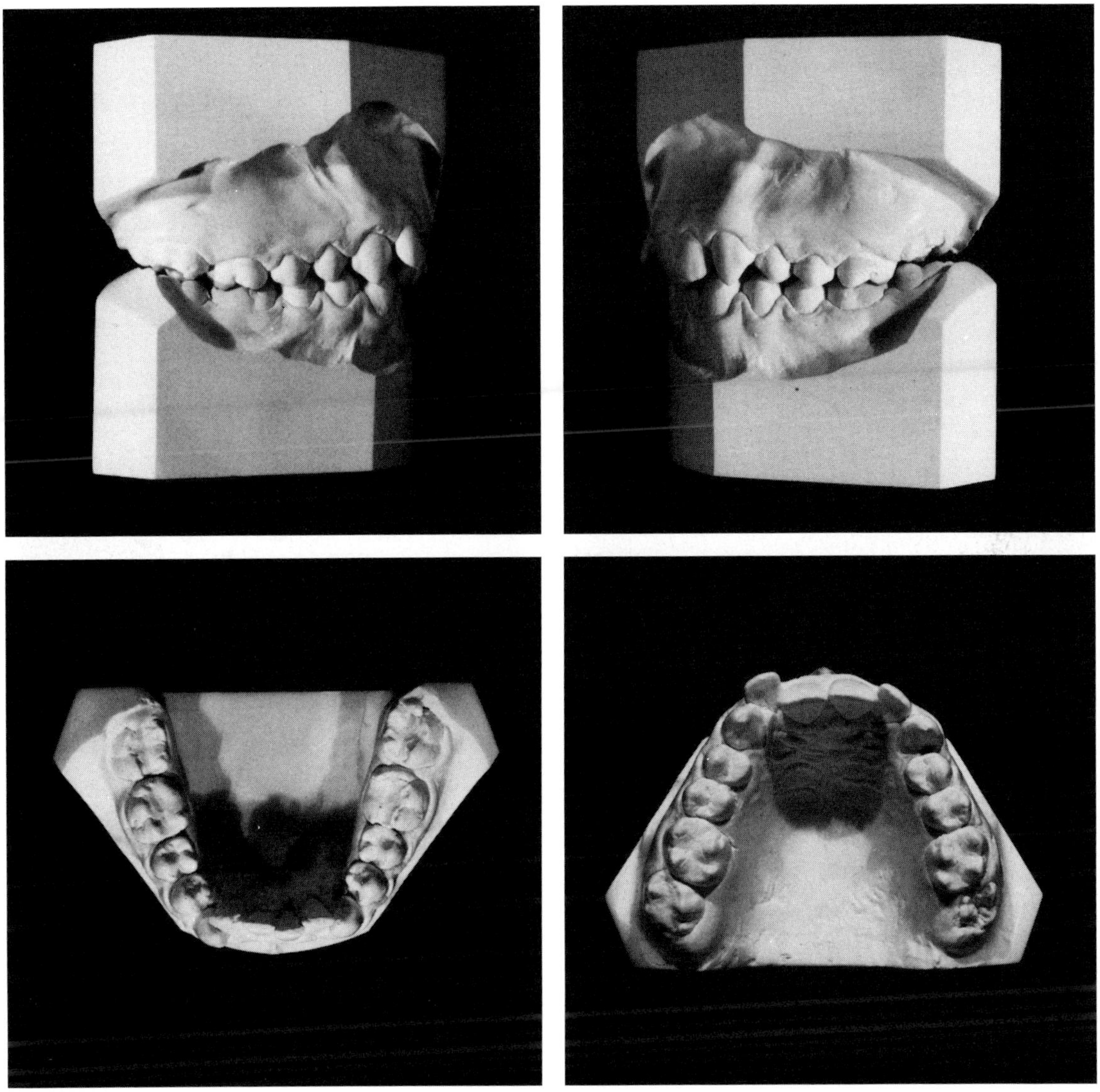

Figs 35-9 and 35-10 At the age of 15 y, 10 mo, the changes that were producing the coverbite had continued but less dramatically. The maxillary central incisors have tipped further backward and the mandibular incisors have moved more to lingual. Both maxillary lateral incisors protrude further labially than they did a year previously. In the place of the extracted second molar in the maxilla on the left the third molar has emerged, although there is barely room for it. The growth of both the mandible and the maxilla has been insufficient to accommodate three adjacent molars. The dentition has possibly been moved dorsally en bloc, this leading to increased crowding in the molar regions.

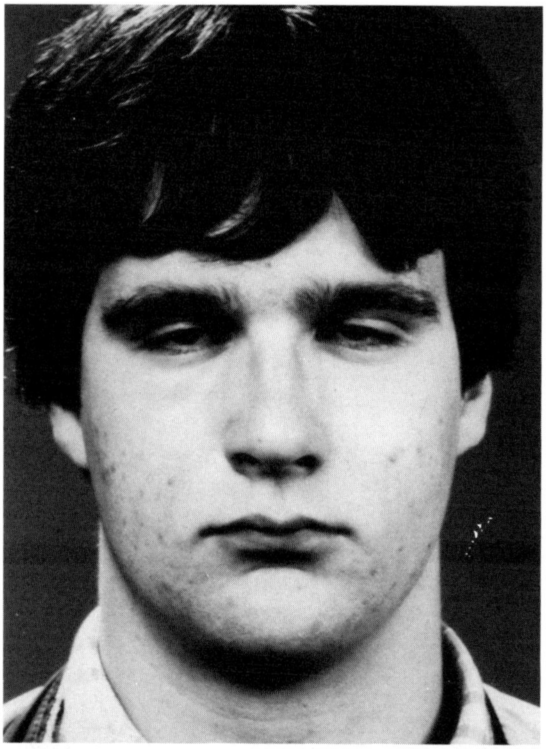
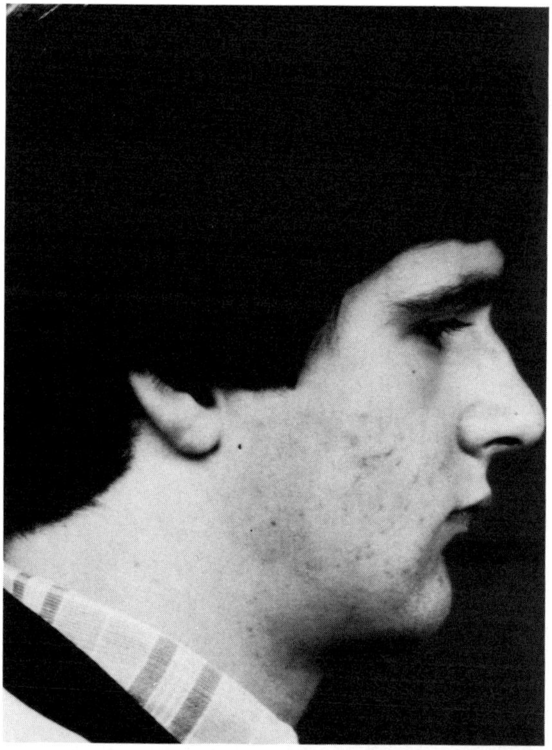
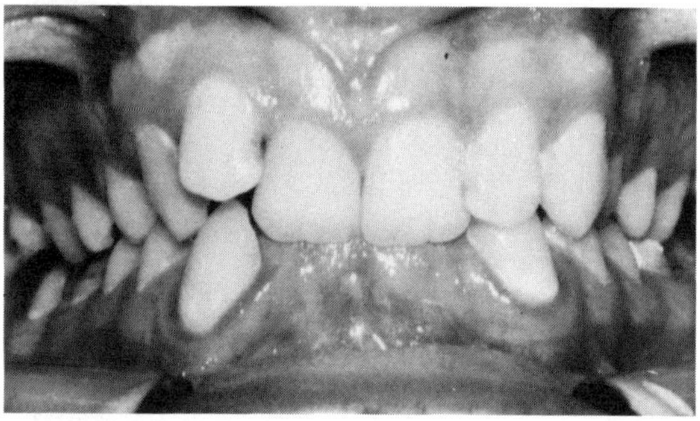
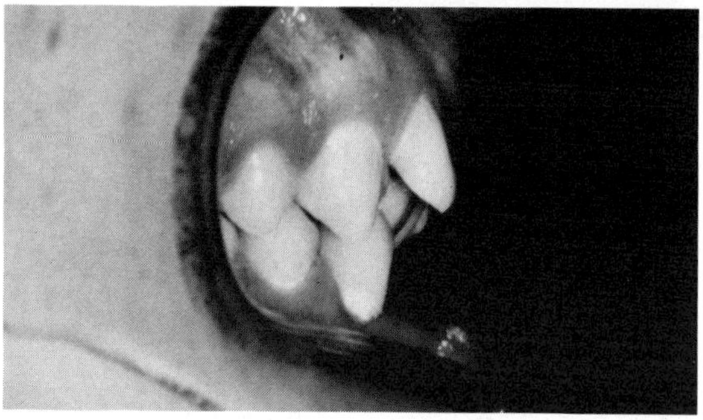
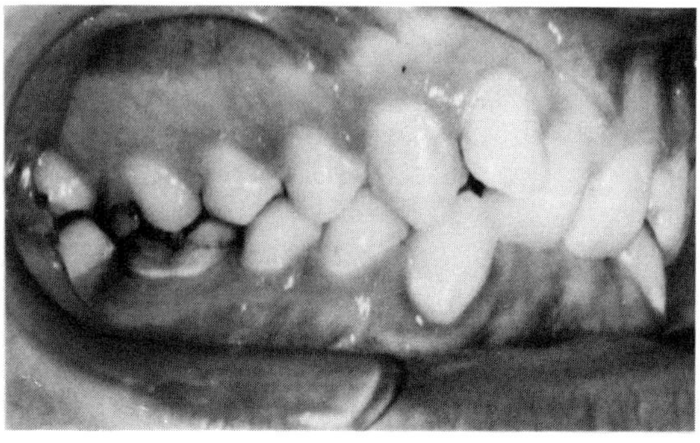
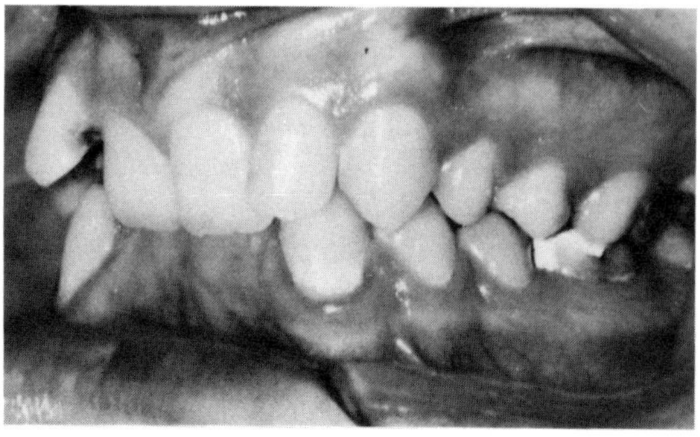

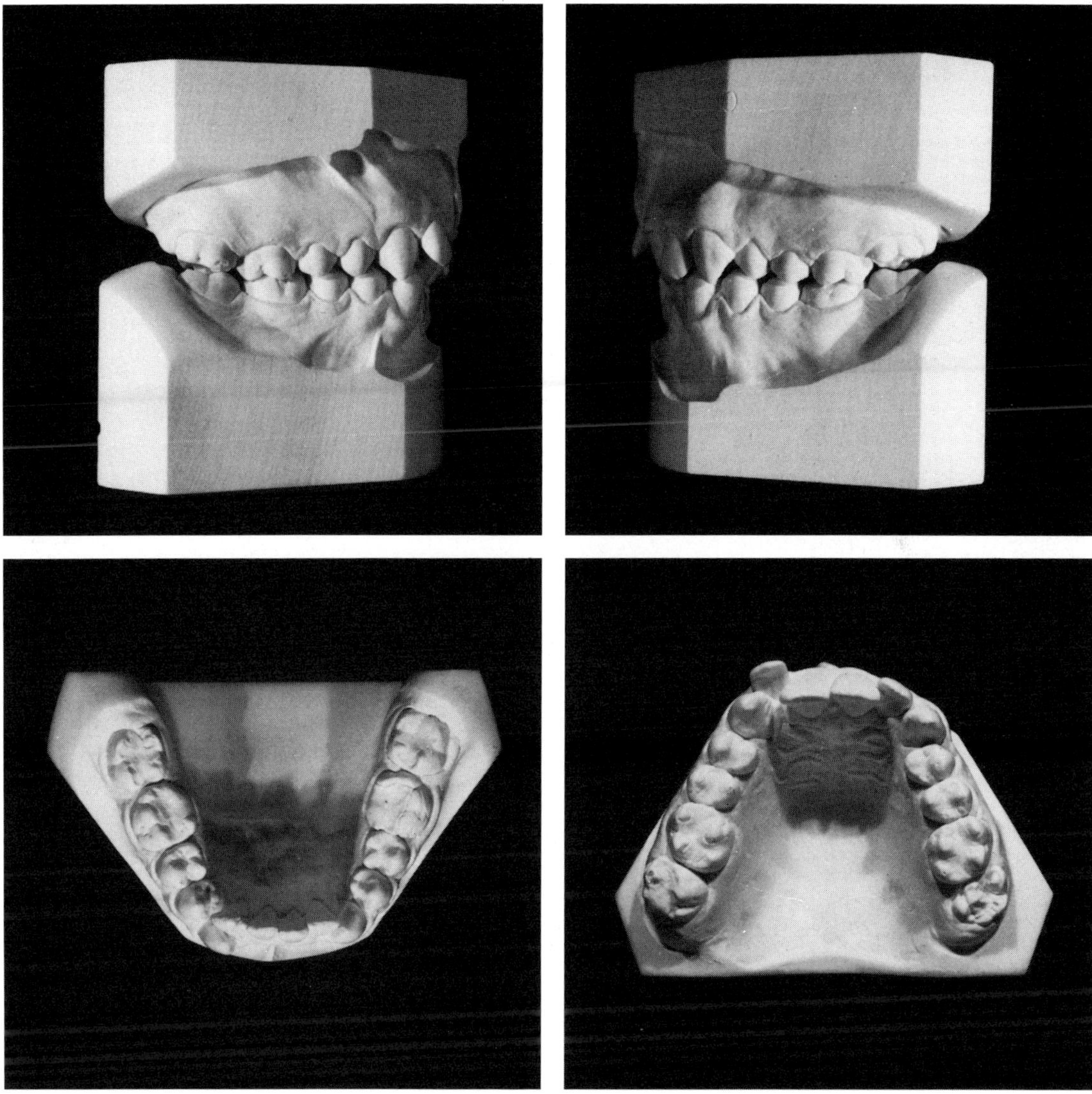

Figs 35-11 and 35-12 *At the age of 18 y, 10 mo it appears that a stable situation has developed and the deterioration of the coverbite has ceased. The maxillary central incisors have tipped further back and contact the gingiva labial to the mandibular incisors, which also have moved further lingually. Those mandibular incisors now bite into the palatal tissues. In the maxilla on the right side, the lateral incisor on the right has tipped further labially and the distance between the central incisor and the canine has diminished. In the mandible on the right side the lateral incisor is in contact with the first premolar and the canine is totally excluded from the arch. The maxillary left third molar will come into occlusion after further eruption. The other three wisdom teeth are impacted.*

Figure 35-13a

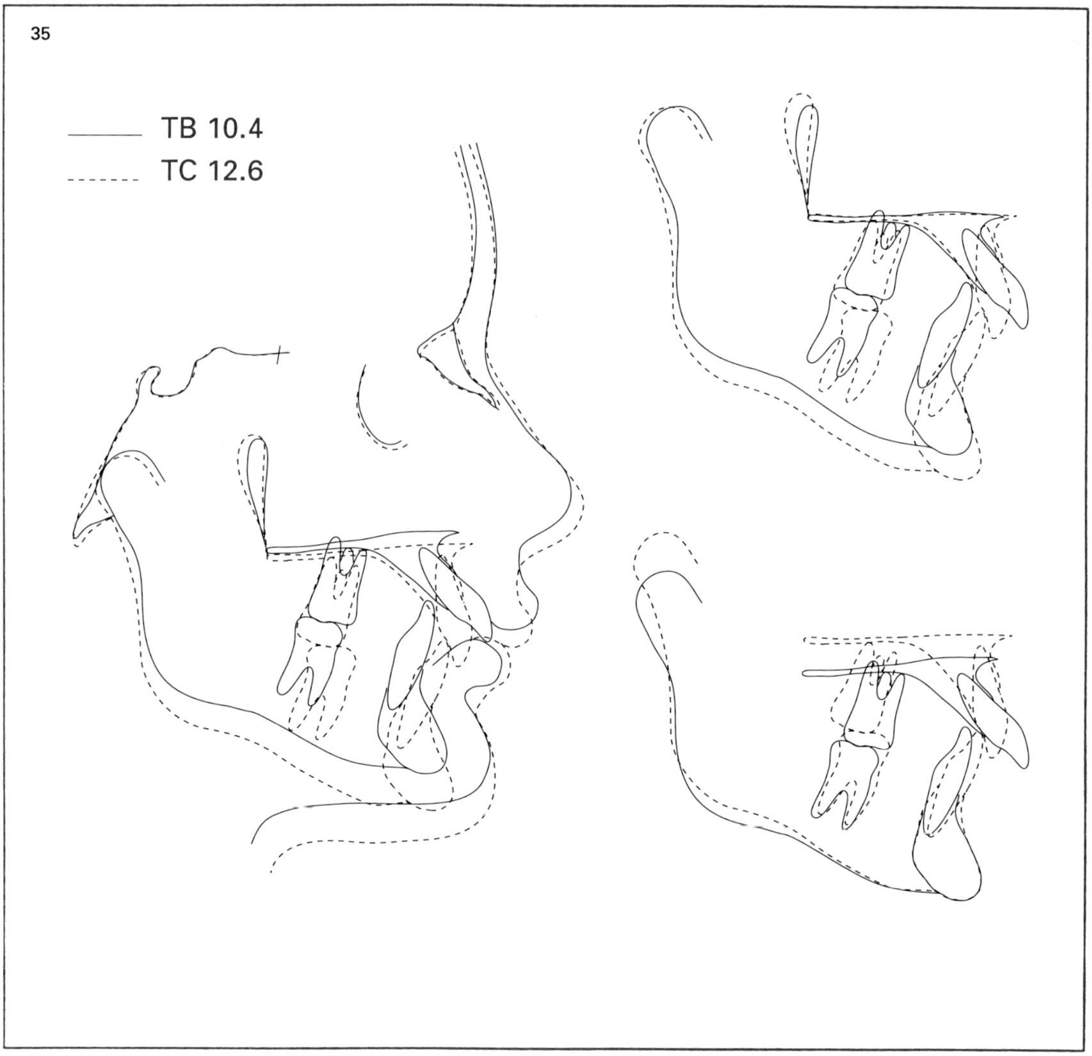

Fig 35-13 Superimposition of tracings from different cephalometric radiographs provide an overview of the changes that took place during treatment and of those associated with the subsequent development resulting in a coverbite.

Figure 35-13b

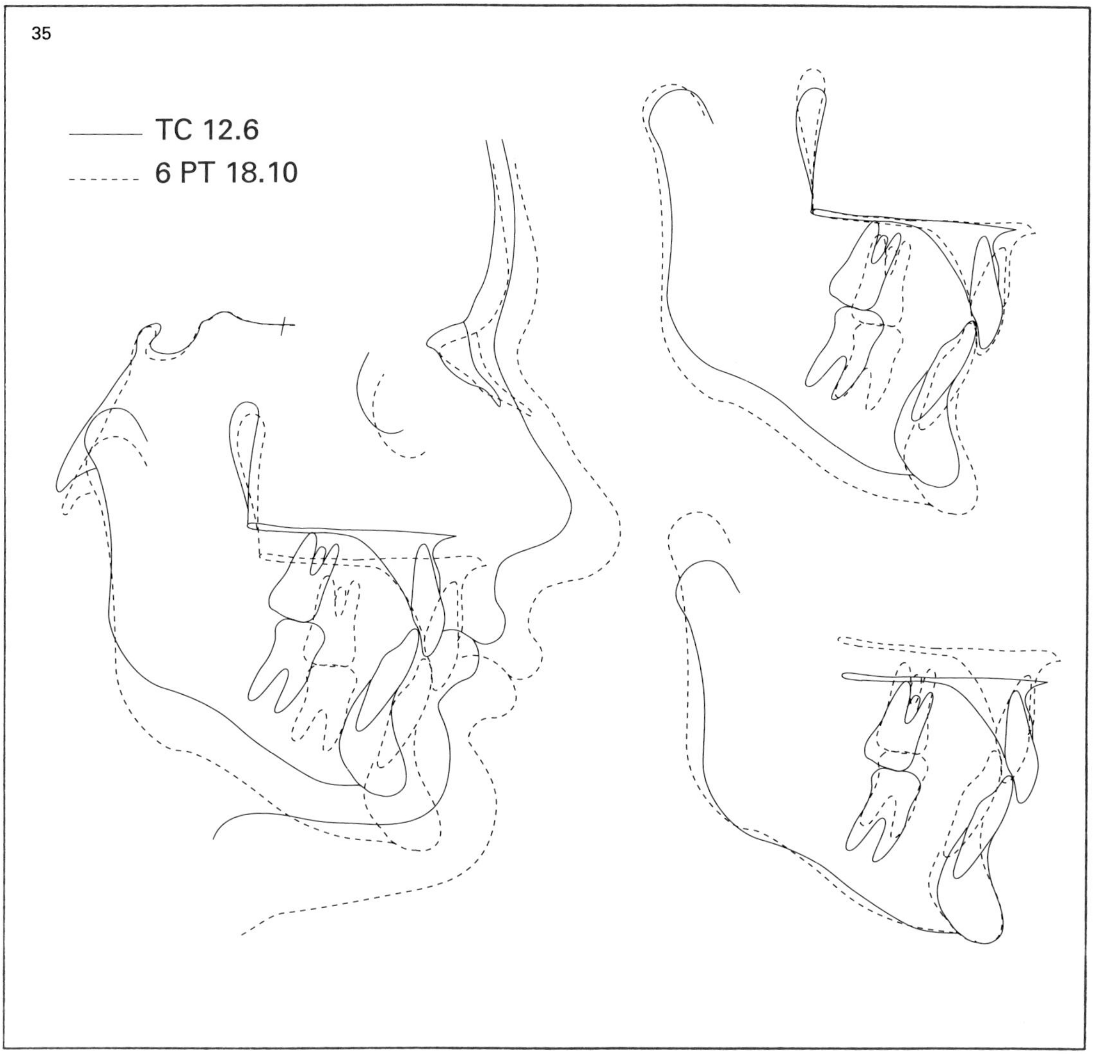

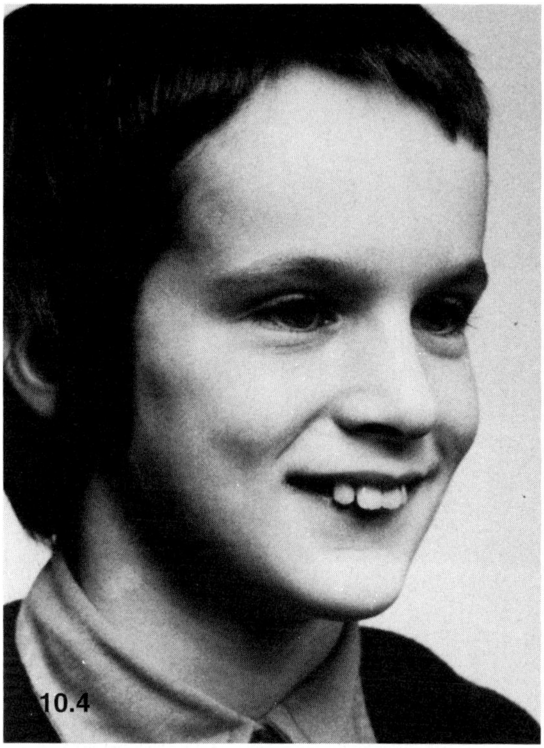

10.4

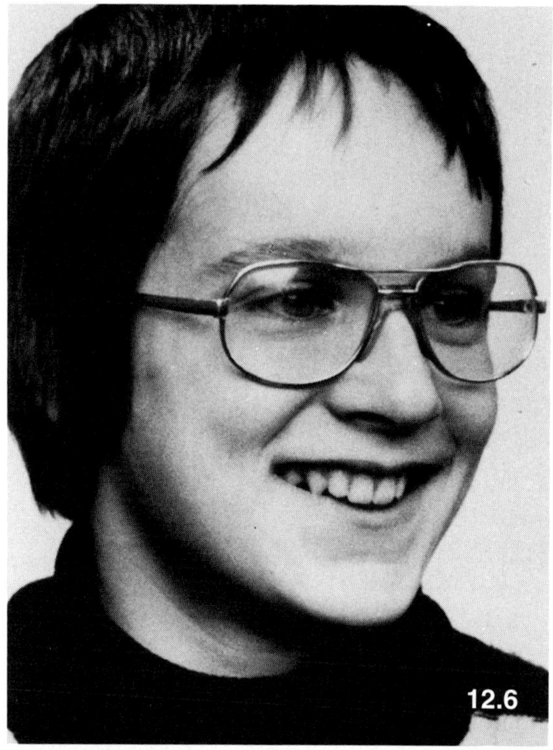

12.6

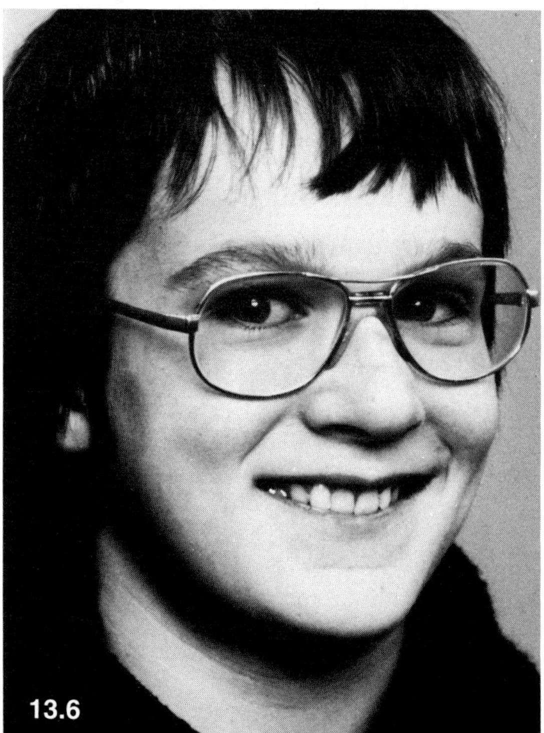

13.6

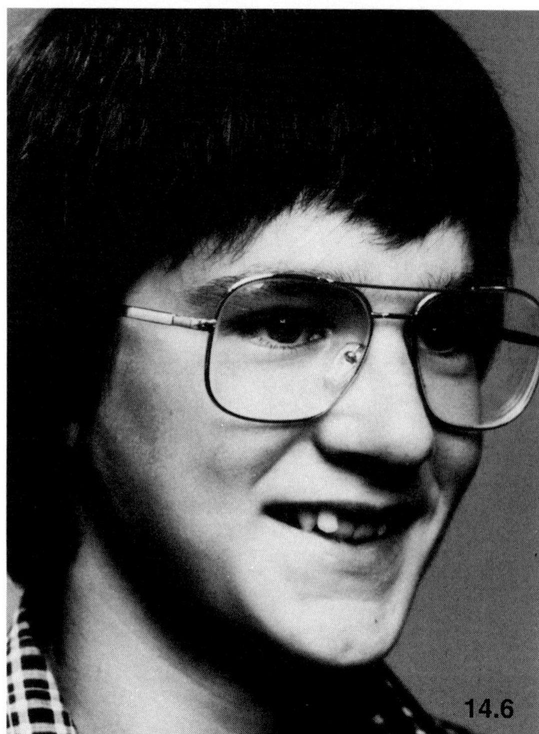

14.6

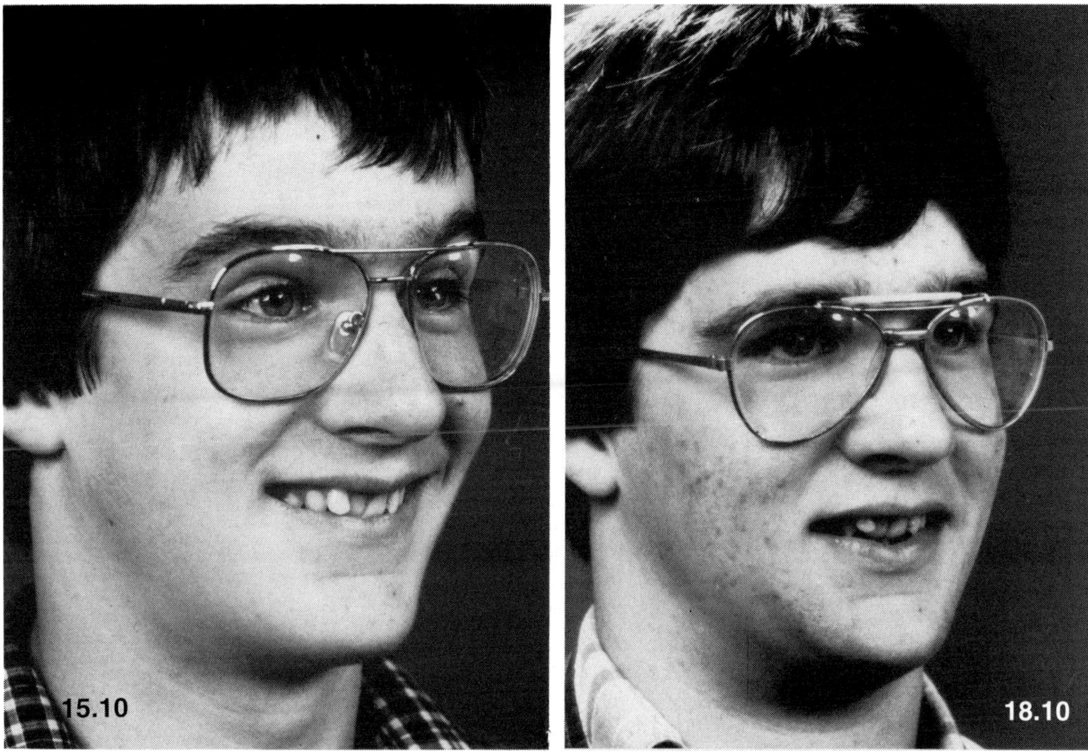

Fig 35-14 Note the improvement that occurred during treatment, and in subsequent years, a pronounced coverbite that gradually developed, which would be characterized as a class I with class II/2 symptoms.

Figs 35-7 and 35-8 (continued, see page 585)
the mandibular arch unless corrected with an elastic through the bite. Prior to doing that, it was necessary to restore a large cavity in that molar, but the patient refused to have it done. When he was seen a year later the tooth had been removed due to pain.

The activator was fitted by grinding in the usual manner; in addition, the acrylic was removed from the labial aspects of the mandibular incisors to permit them to move ventrally.[4]

After the activator and headgear had been worn approximately 12 hours each day for ten months, neutro-occlusion had been achieved on both sides. The molar bands were removed and the treatment was continued with the activator alone for another eight months. At the age of 12 years, 6 months, an acceptable result had been attained. The profile was improved, the mouth was kept closed and the molars and second premolars occluded in neutro-occlusion. The mandibular anteriors had moved ventrally, but the maxillary incisors were steeply inclined and the overbite was too great (Figs 35.3 and 35.4).

Four months later, the first premolars also were occluding well. Another eight months later, a year after terminating treatment, the depth of bite had increased and the central incisors in the mandible, but even more the maxillary central incisors, had tipped lingually (Figs 35.5 and 35.6). This tendency increased while at the same time the maxillary right lateral incisor tipped to labial (Figs 35.7 and 35.8). After the cessation of treatment, a "coverbite" had gradually developed (class I with symptoms of class II/2). This development can be ascribed to the high lip line that is associated with that anomaly. The lower lip fully overlapped the clinical crowns of the maxillary central incisors (Fig 35.17). A year later the symptoms were more pronounced (Figs 35.9 and 35.10).

By the age of 18 years, 10 months, it appeared that a stable situation had evolved (Figs 35.11 and 35.12). In the mandible, the lingual tipping of the incisors had led to such an ectostomatic position of the right canine that the lateral incisor and the first premolar contacted each other. In the maxilla, the right lateral incisor had come right out of the dental arch. The maxillary central incisors impinged on the gingiva labial to the mandibular incisors and the mandibular incisors bit into the palatal mucosa. However there were no signs of lesions in the soft tissues.

It can be seen from the superimpositions of tracings of cephalometric radiographs that during treatment the mandible had grown ventrally and caudally. The incisal edges of the mandibular incisors had moved about 3 mm to labial. The incisal edges of the maxillary incisors had moved 7 mm to palatal in a tipping movement with the center of rotation in the root about 8 mm from the apex. Because of this tipping movement, the incisal edges had moved 3 mm occlusally. By the end of treatment, three-quarters of the clinical crown length of the maxillary central incisors was overlapped by the lower lip. The consequences of this will be described more fully. In the six years after treatment, the face grew noticeably both caudally and ventrally, while the mandibular anteriors went further to dorsal and the maxillary incisors tipped steeply back and overerupted (Fig 35.13). The photographs of the smiling face show the changes that took place during treatment and also the development of the coverbite that came into existence subsequently (Fig 35.14).

This patient has been presented because fundamental errors of judgement in both diagnosis and treatment were made. It was not recognized after treatment had finished that an entirely different and serious anomaly could now develop.

With class II/1 anomalies in which the lower lip takes up a position behind the maxillary incisors, there is no vertical support for the maxillary incisors so that they are able to over-erupt. If the lip gives support to those teeth in the direction of their root axes, then the over-eruption can be resisted (Fig 35.15).

When over-erupted maxillary incisors are tipped back they come to stand more steeply and their incisal edges are situated more caudally. If the lip then comes to lie in front of those incisors then the overlapping becomes excessive and as a result an abnormally large palatally directed force is applied to the maxillary incisors. A coverbite can subsequently develop as it did in this case (Fig 35.16).

In a growing individual, the height of the lower face can increase during treatment, the lip line can descend, and the overlapping of the maxillary incisors by the lower lip can decrease. That is especially evident in the course of facial-orthopedic treatment associated with a marked vertical development of the lower face. However,

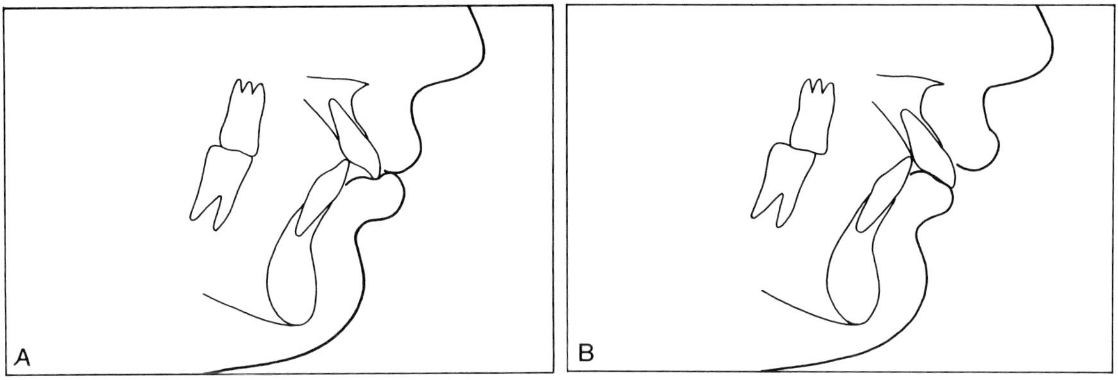

Fig 35-15 In cases of increased overjet, the vertical position of the maxillary incisors depends partly on the posture of the lower lip.
A If the lower lip rests against the incisal edges of the maxillary incisors, then eruption will be stopped by it; this is usually the case in mild class II/1 anomalies (½ PW disto-occlusion).
B In more serious cases (1 PW disto-occlusion) the lower lip can be placed behind the maxillary incisors, which deprives them of support along their root axes and permits further eruption.

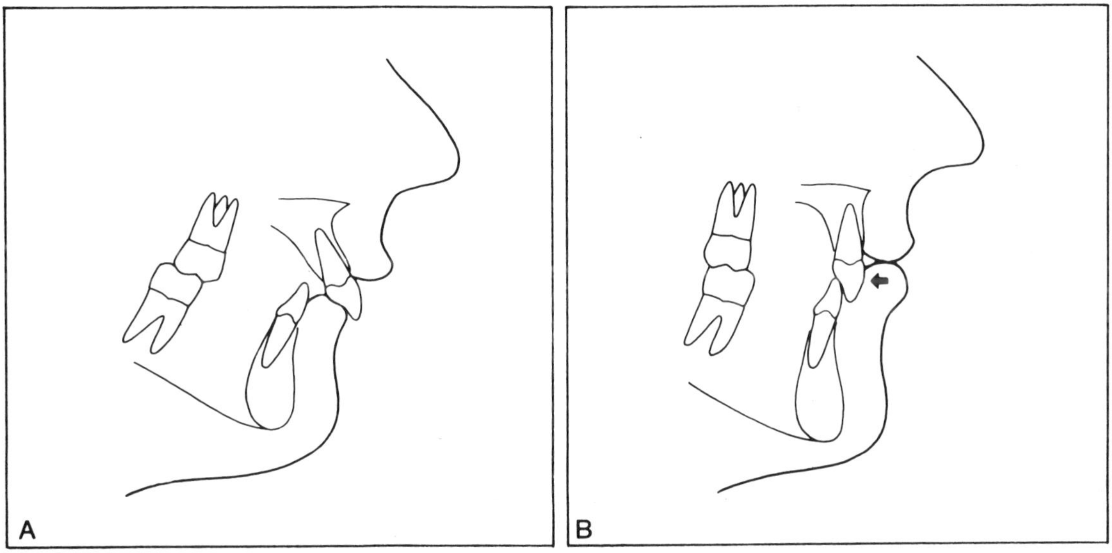

Fig 35-16 Aspects of palatally tipping of over-erupted maxillary incisors in the treatment of class II/1 anomalies.
A If the maxillary incisors are tipped backward, their incisal edges will move relatively further to caudal.
B After such movement, the maxillary incisors will be excessively overlapped by the lower lip and an abnormally large palatally directed force will be imposed on them through which a coverbite may develop.

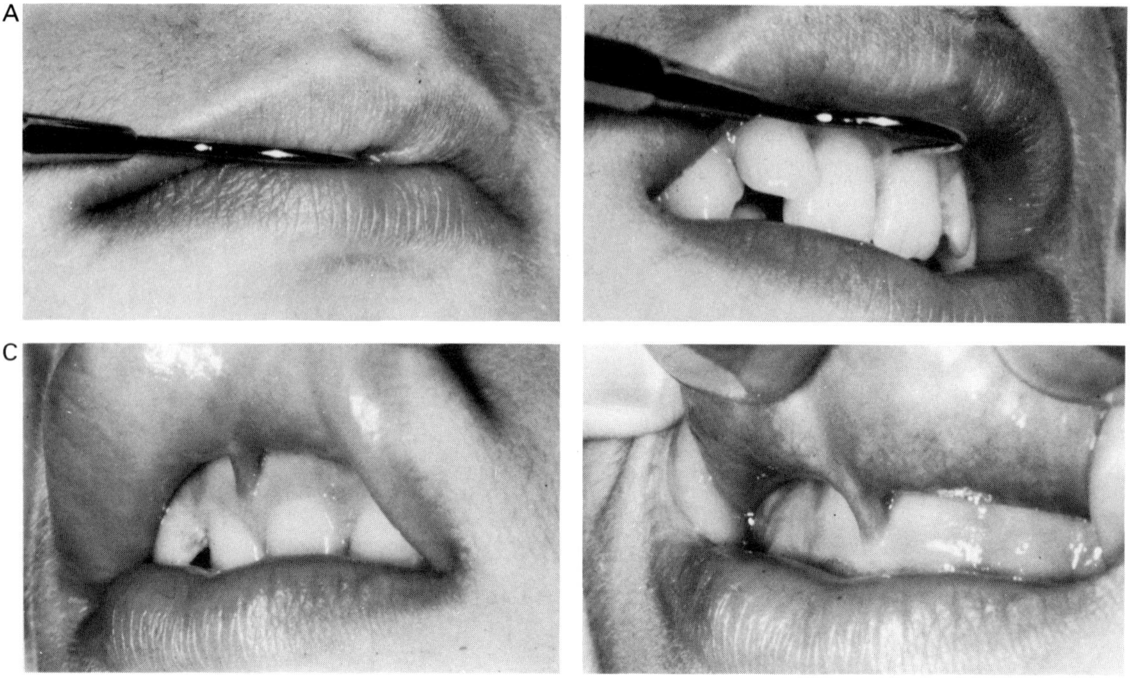

Fig 35-17 Judging the lower lip's vertical position in relationship to the maxillary central incisors.

A While the patient holds his posterior teeth together a thin instrument such as a sickle-shaped probe or periodontal probe is carefully placed between the lips in the median plane parallel to the occlusal plane, until it contacts the teeth.

B After pulling up the upper lip it is clear what level the lower lip had reached.

C It is also possible to lift the upper lip when the mandible assumes its rest position.

D The degree of lip cover in the same patient when the teeth are in habitual occlusion.

this vertical development is seldom sufficient, and generally the maxillary incisors will need to be intruded to further reduce the extent to which the lower lip overlaps them. In the treatment of adults, coverage by the lower lip can only be reduced by intruding the maxillary incisors unless a combined orthodontic/surgical technique is used.

At the time this treatment was begun, the previous information was not available and the unfavorable development after treatment was not foreseen. Besides, the bad oral hygiene, the attitude of the patient, and his carelessness with the appliances would have made the use of fixed appliances most unwise. Therefore any alternative treatment really was not open to consideration. Furthermore, the excessive overlapping of the maxillary incisors by the lower lip would not have been so pronounced if the lower face had grown more caudally during treatment.

The most important conclusion to be drawn from the course of events described here is that it is essential to determine the height of the lip line both before and during treatment. The manner of doing this was described previously but is presented again in Figure 35.17.
An additional remark might be made that it is not always possible to foresee an unfavorable development such as that described in this patient. However, if such a situation is likely, a more complex treatment including full fixed appliances should be used.

Chapter 36

Class III, ventral forced bite
Chin cap with vertical posts, maxillary removable plate
Female: 7 years, 3 months to 23 years, 5 months

A girl aged 7 years 3 months exhibited a class III anomaly. Her eyes were deeply recessed in her face, which was correlated with the lack of development of the midface to ventral. The mandible was not exceptionally large but the chin was the predominant feature in her face. There was no abnormal function except for a prognathic forced bite. When the mandibular dental arch in its most dorsal position was brought into contact with the maxillary arch, the mandibular incisors touched the maxillary incisors slightly labial to the incisal edges. As the teeth were closed further together the mandible slid ventrally before the posterior teeth made full occlusal contact. Both dental arches showed no signs of abnormality. There was a clear mesio-occlusion when in habitual occlusion (Figs 36.1 and 36.2).

It was decided to stimulate the development of the maxilla, through which incidentally the abnormal occlusion and the ventral forced bite both could be corrected. For this purpose the first permanent molars had bands with buccal tubes cemented in place at the age of 7 years 4 months while the first deciduous molars were provided with bands bearing buccal hooks. Following this a plate was made for the maxilla which fitted the palatal surfaces of all the teeth accurately and bore 3/4 clasps that buccally engaged the first permanent molars and the first deciduous molars. Apically extending hooks of rectangular wire (.0125" × .027" were fixed into the molar tubes, reaching buccally about 5 mm above the cervical margins. These hooks could hold the elastics that would provide the force to ventral on the molars preferrably at the level of the centre of resistance of the molar roots. The elastics were stretched from the hooks on the molars and also first deciduous molars to hooks mounted on the vertical posts from a chin cap (Fig 36.17B). The patient was asked to wear the plate and the chin cap during sleeping hours only. The elastics were chosen so that each had a force of about 100 grams so that the total force exerted ventrally on the maxilla was approximately 400 grams.

After six months the midface had clearly moved forward and the class III anomaly with its ventral forced bite had been eliminated. There was good sagittal interdigitation of the posterior teeth. Retention was judged not to be necessary although the interdigitation of the well worn deciduous molars was not totally satisfactory (Figs 36.3 and 36.4).

Two years later the jaw relation was more or less the same as when treatment concluded (Figs 36.5 and 36.6). The permanent canines, premolars and molars came into neutro-occlusion after emergence (Figs 36.7 and 36.8).

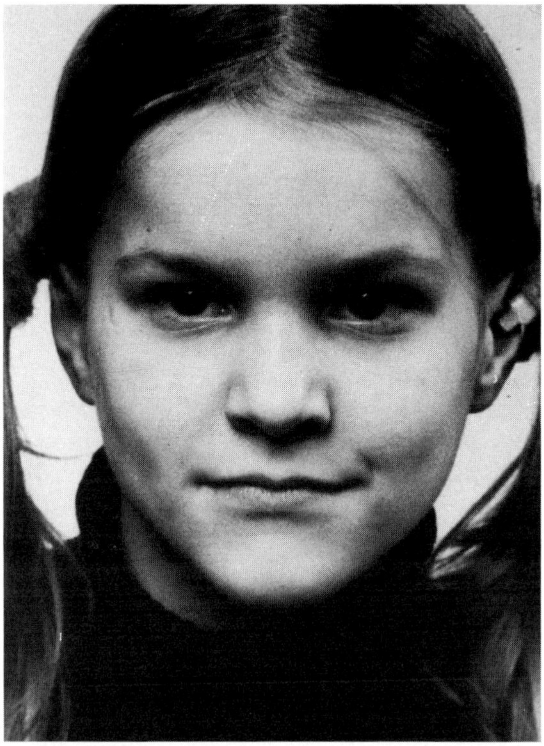
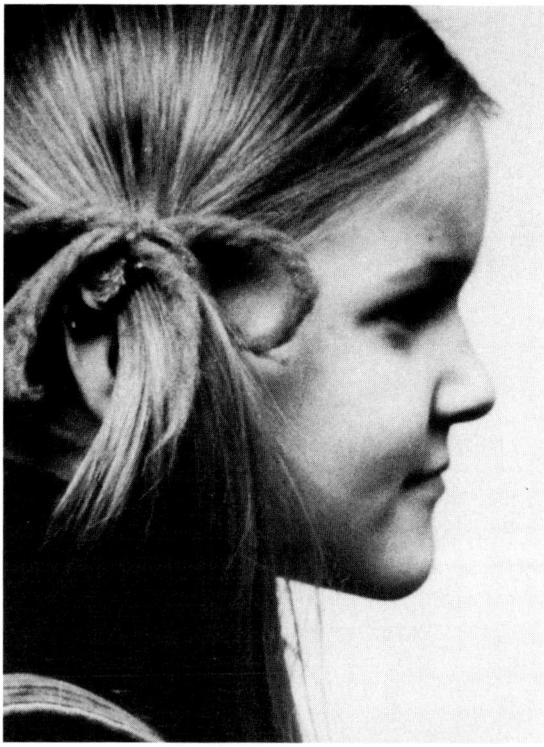
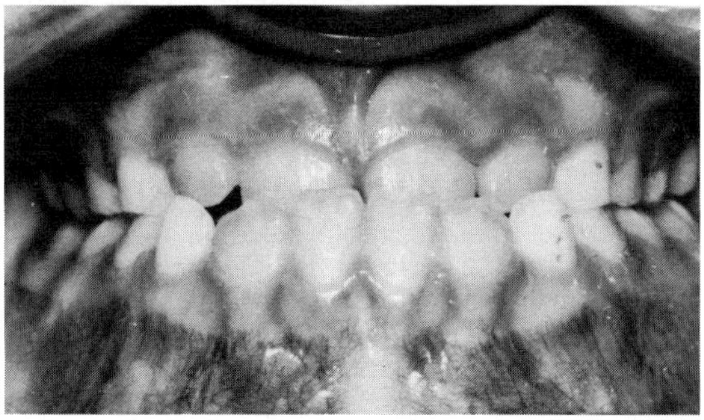
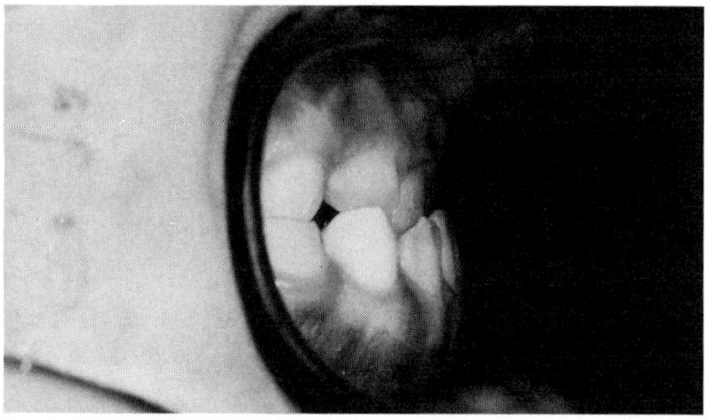
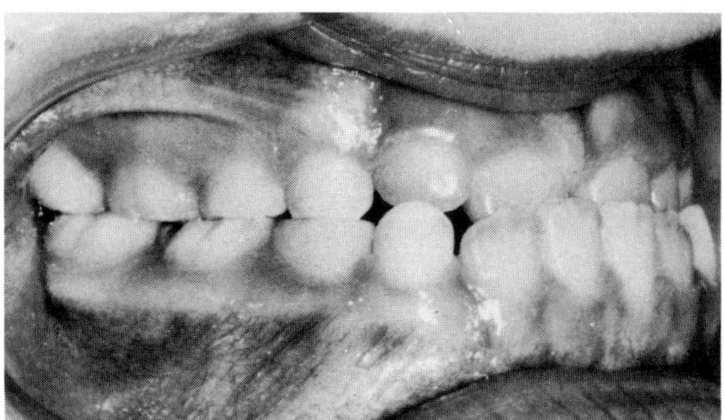
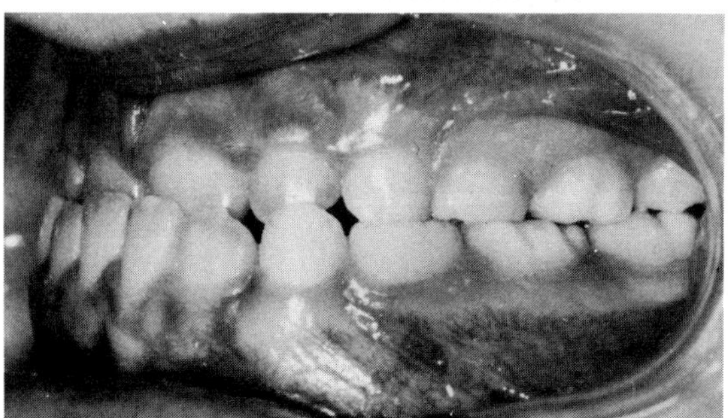

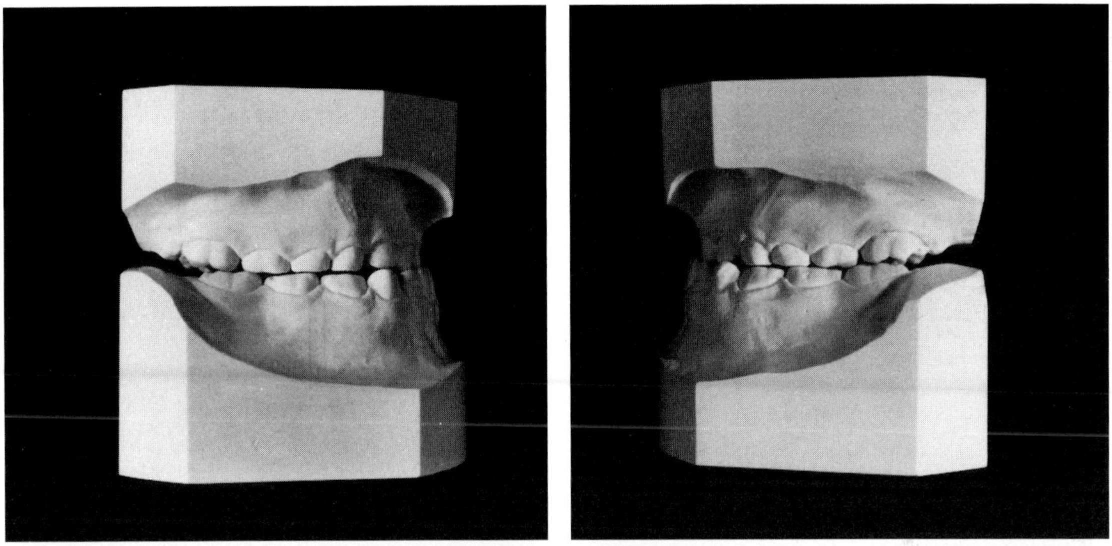

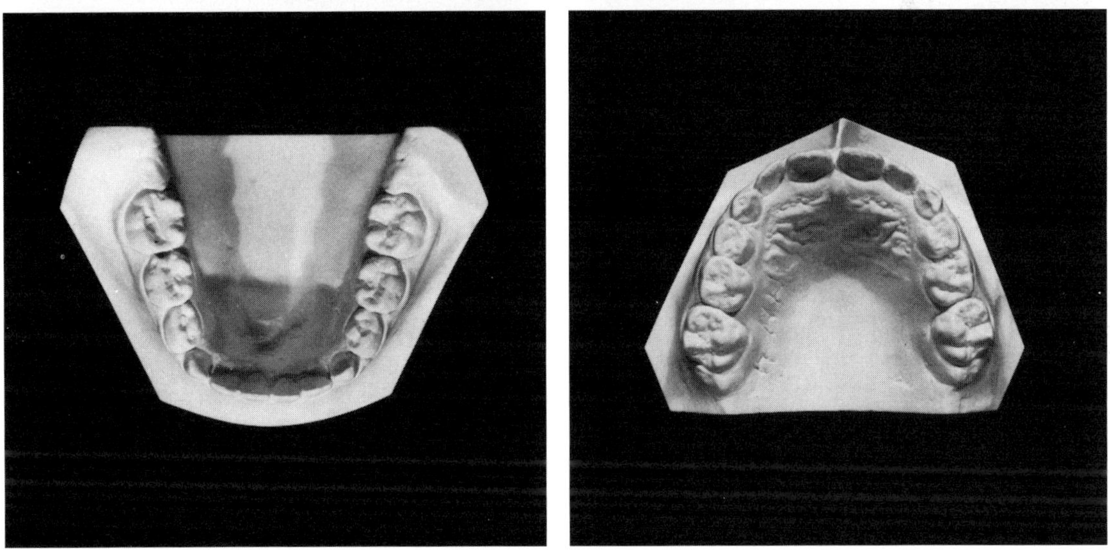

Figs 36-1 and 36-2 *A girl aged 7 y, 3 mo whose midface lacked ventral development and whose mandible was not unusually large exhibited a mild class III anomaly combined with a ventral forced bite. When closing in the maximum retruded position, the mandibular incisors met the maxillary incisors a little labial to the incisal edges of the latter. The lower lip protruded slightly in front of the upper lip but the profile gave no real indication of there being a reversed overbite. The dental arches were free of abnormalities. In habitual occlusion, the mandibular arch was located slightly mesial in relationship to the maxillary arch, more on the right than the left. This corresponded with a deviation to the left of the midline of the mandibular arch.*

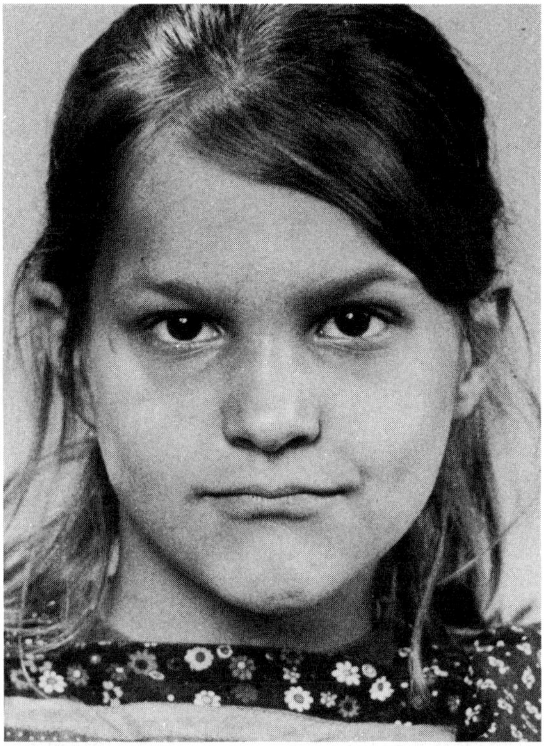

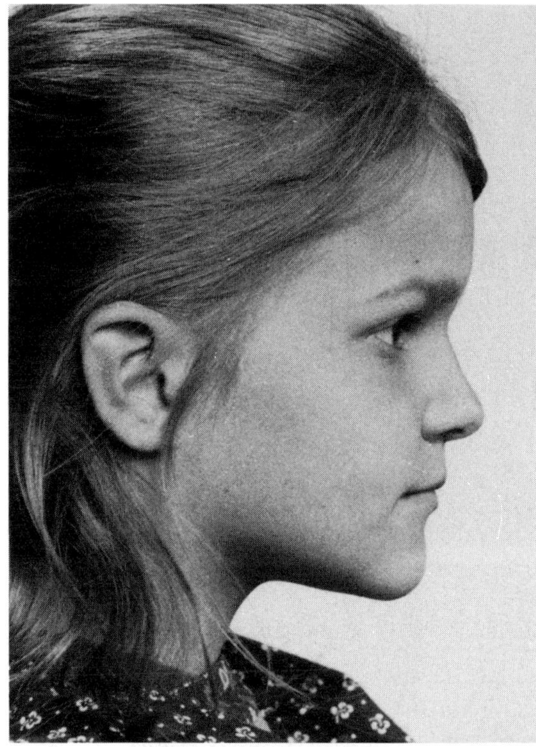

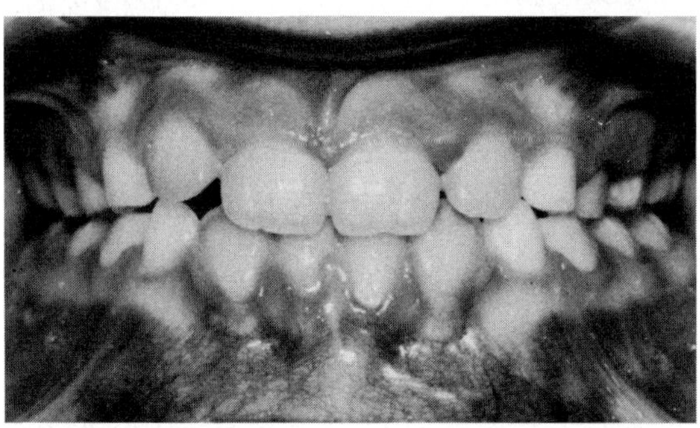

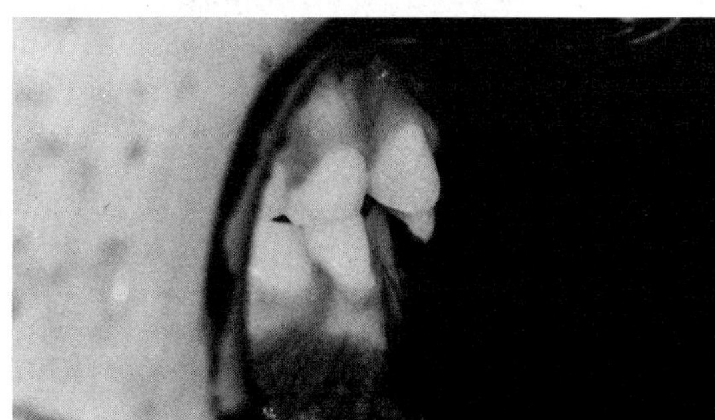

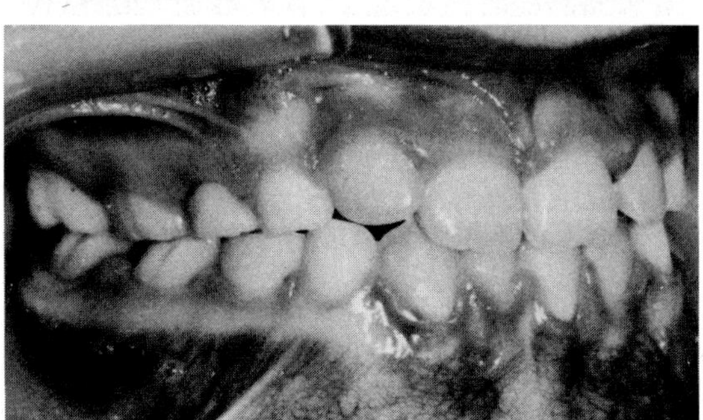

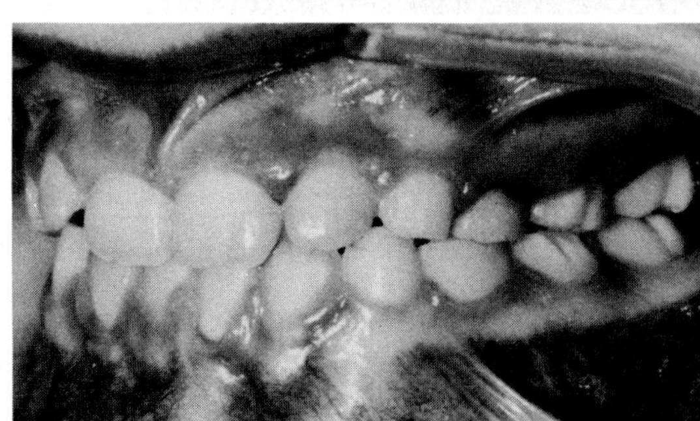

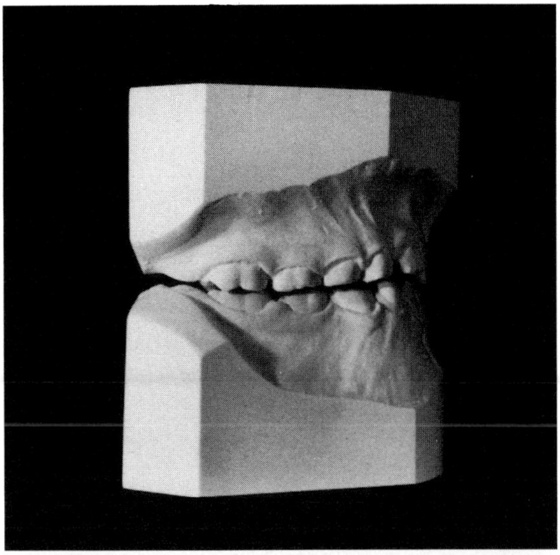

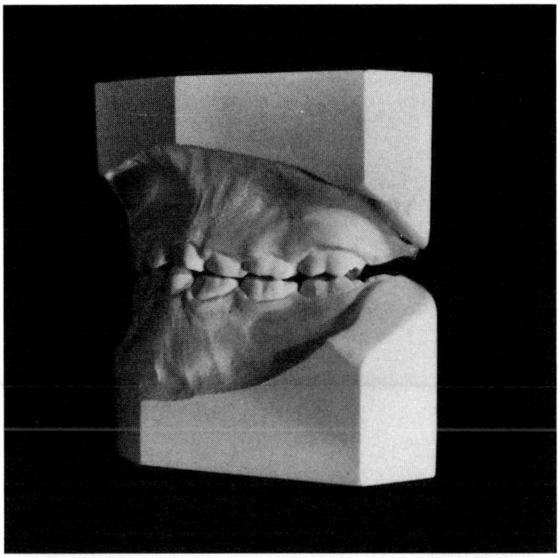

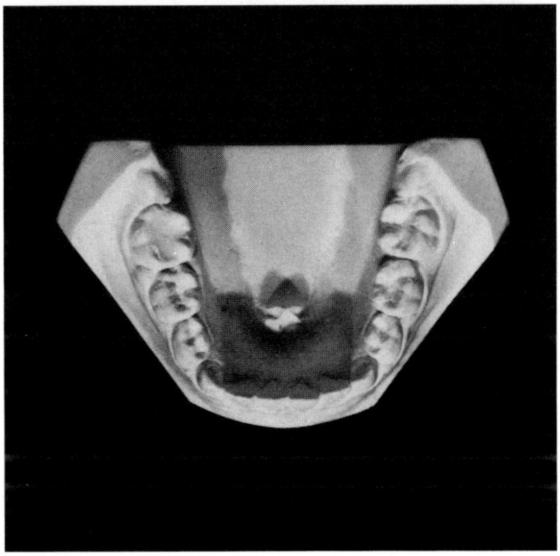

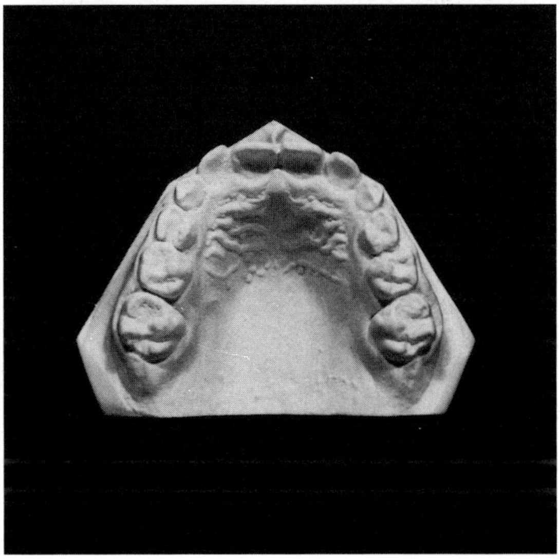

Figs 36-3 and 36-4 *At the age of 7 y, 10 mo, the midface has clearly moved ventrally after treatment for six months. This change had been accomplished by wearing a chincap with vertical posts during sleep, with elastics from those posts to the maxillary first permanent molars and first deciduous molars applying forward traction. The teeth were held as well as possible in a solid unit with a maxillary removable plate. The class III anomaly and reversed anterior overbite have gone. The deciduous canines are in neutro-occlusion, although the first permanent molars are in edge-to-edge occlusion. This is accounted for by the fact that the deciduous molars, which have a greater mesio-distal width in the mandibular arch than in the maxillary arch, are still all present. During treatment ,the maxillary lateral incisors tipped a little to labial, while the inclination of the central incisors hardly changed.*

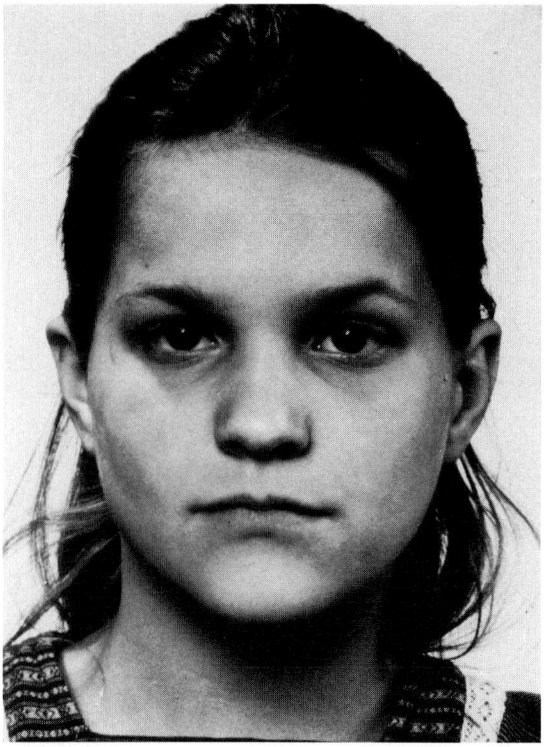

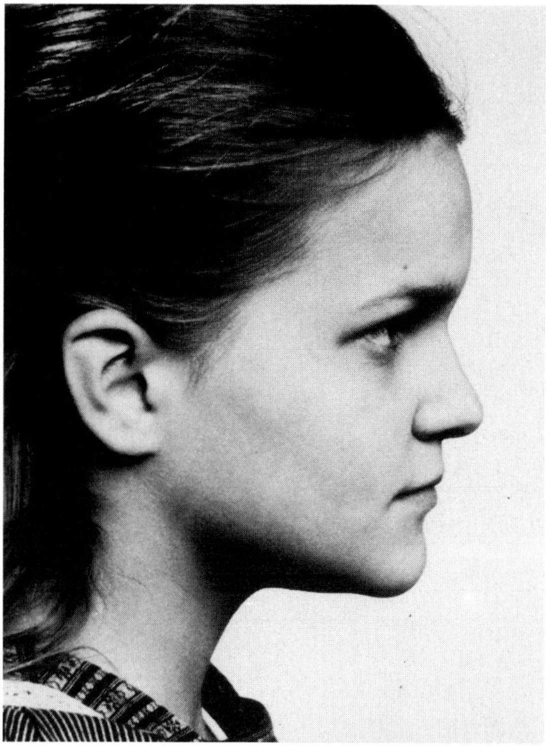

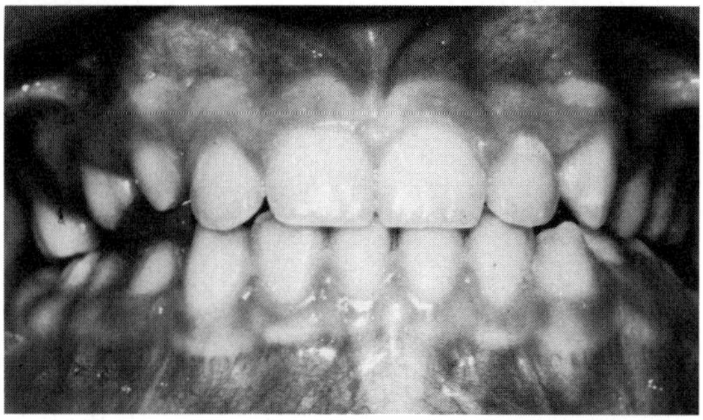

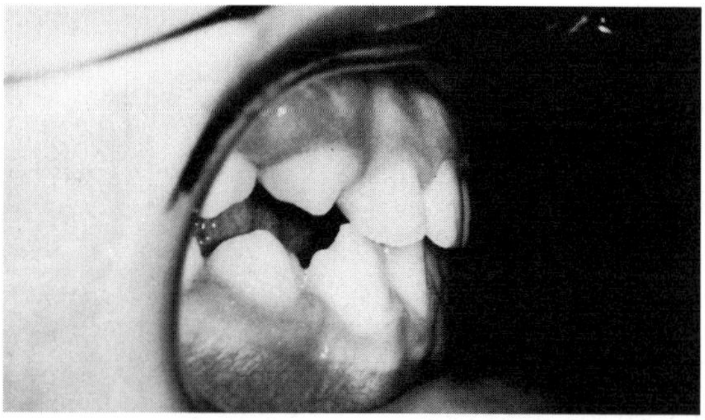

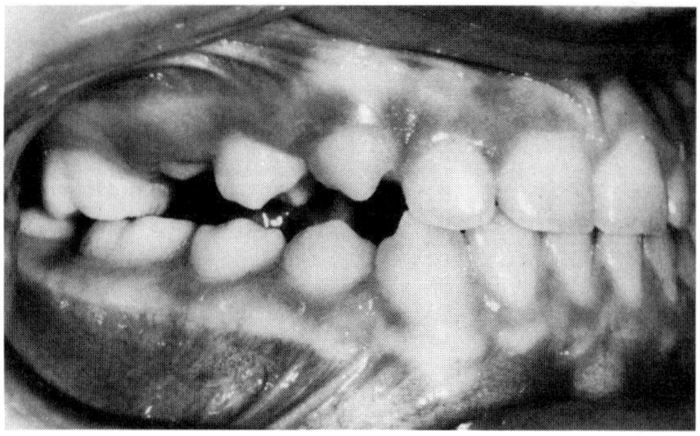

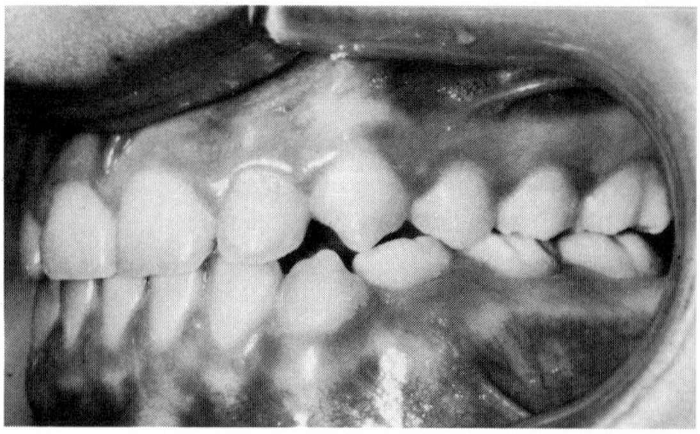

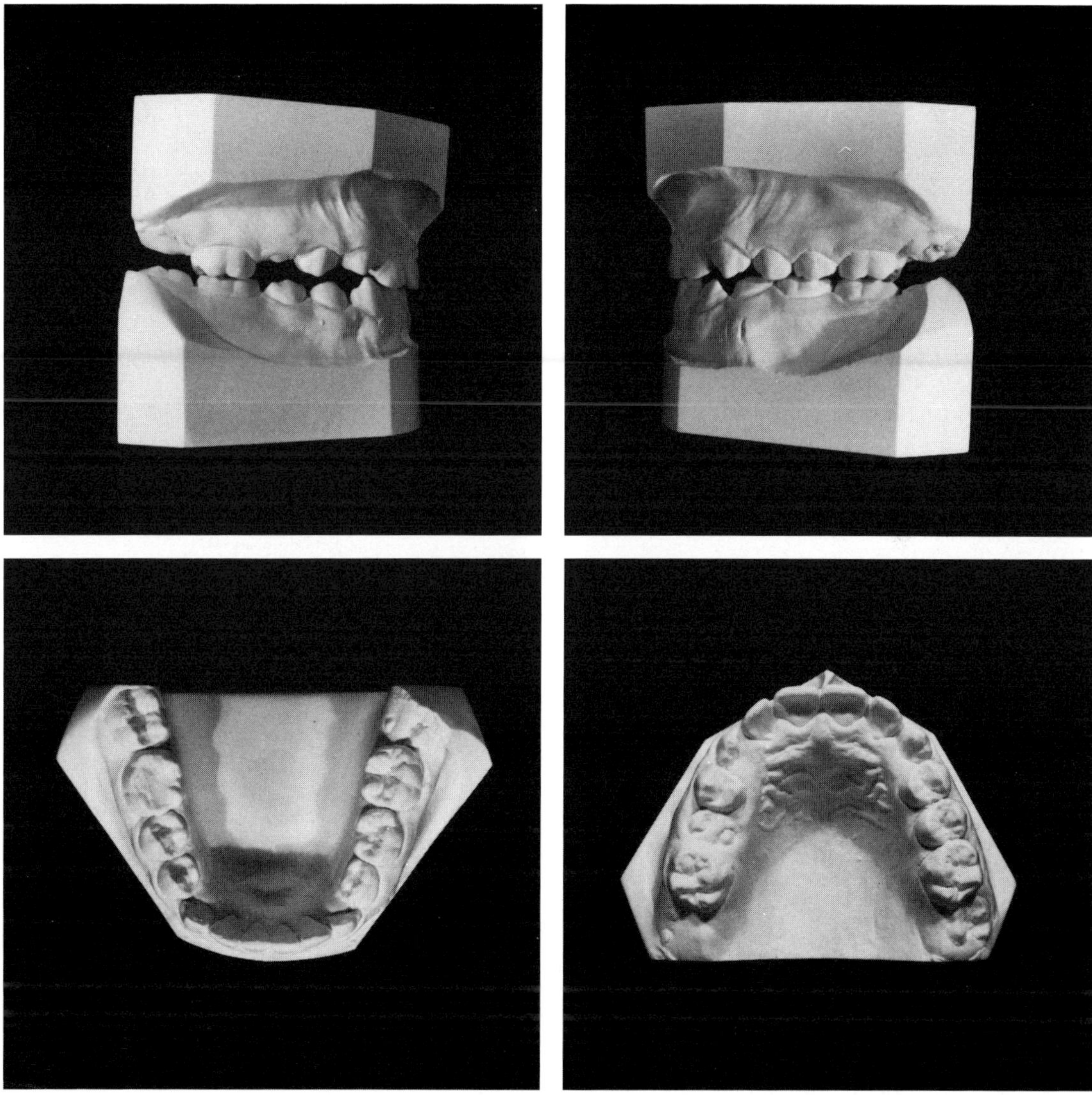

Figs 36-5 and 36-6 *At the age of 9 y, 10 mo, there has been little change in the face and the anterior occlusion. The permanent canines have emerged as have the premolars, except for the mandibular left ones. During the intertransitional period, some crowding developed. The permanent canines in the mandible emerged rotated. The midline of the mandibular dental arch deviated to the left in relationship to the maxillary arch. This midline discrepancy was present prior to treatment and will not grow less in the course of further development of the dentition.*

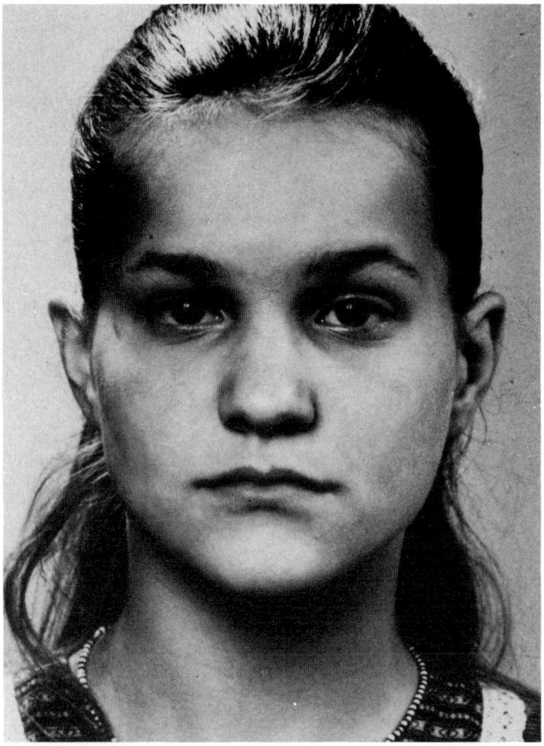
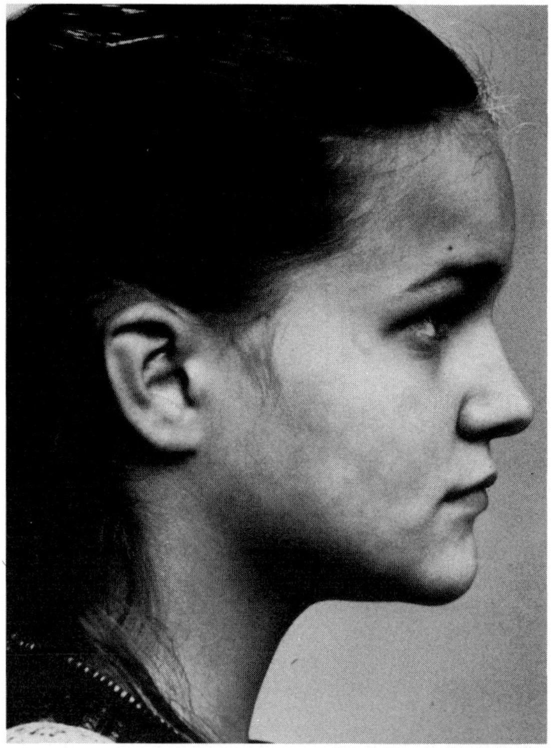
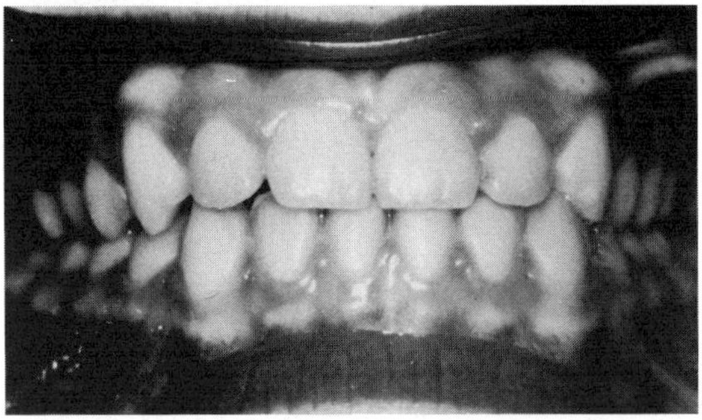
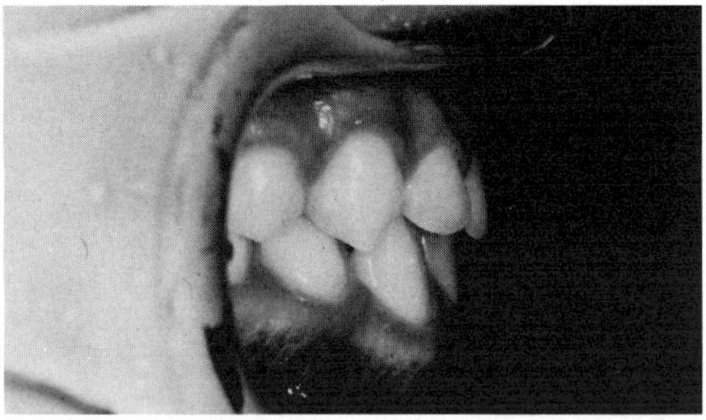
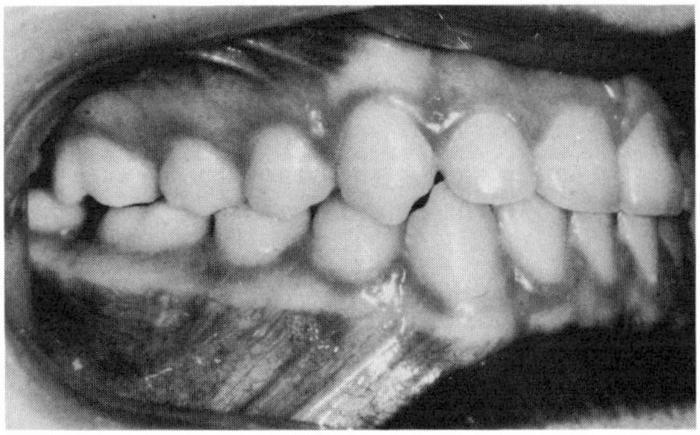
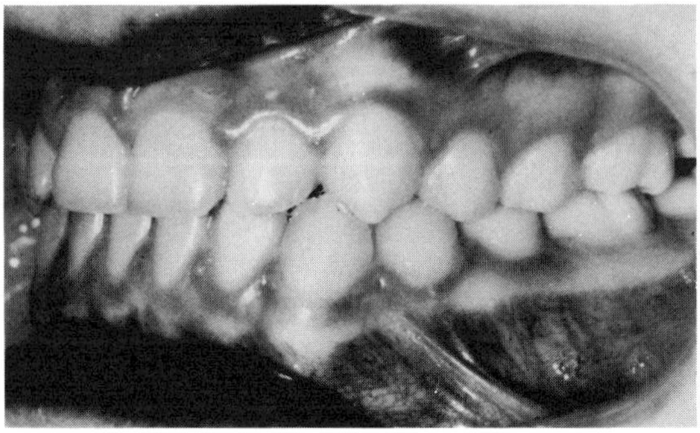

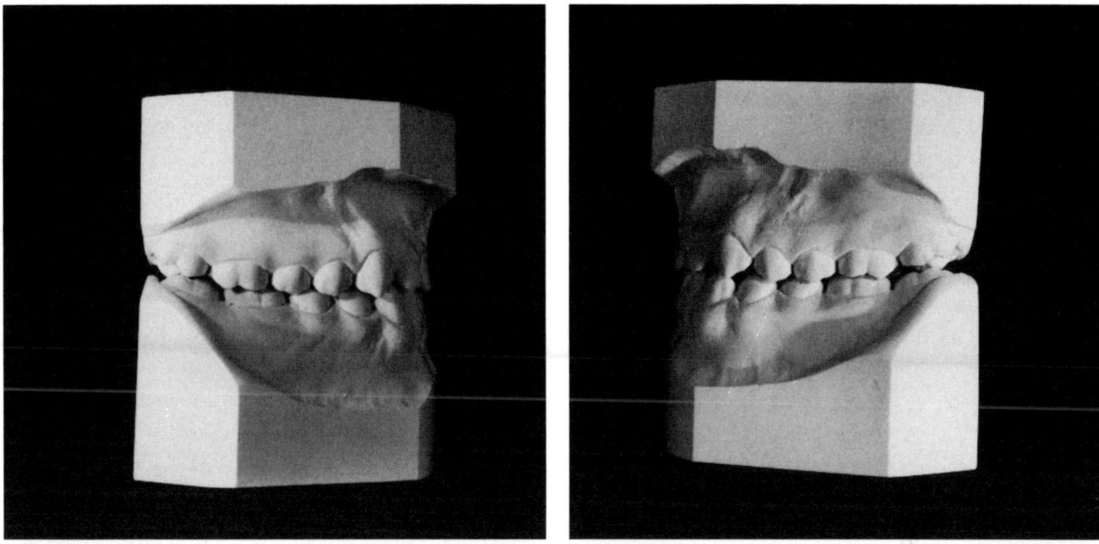

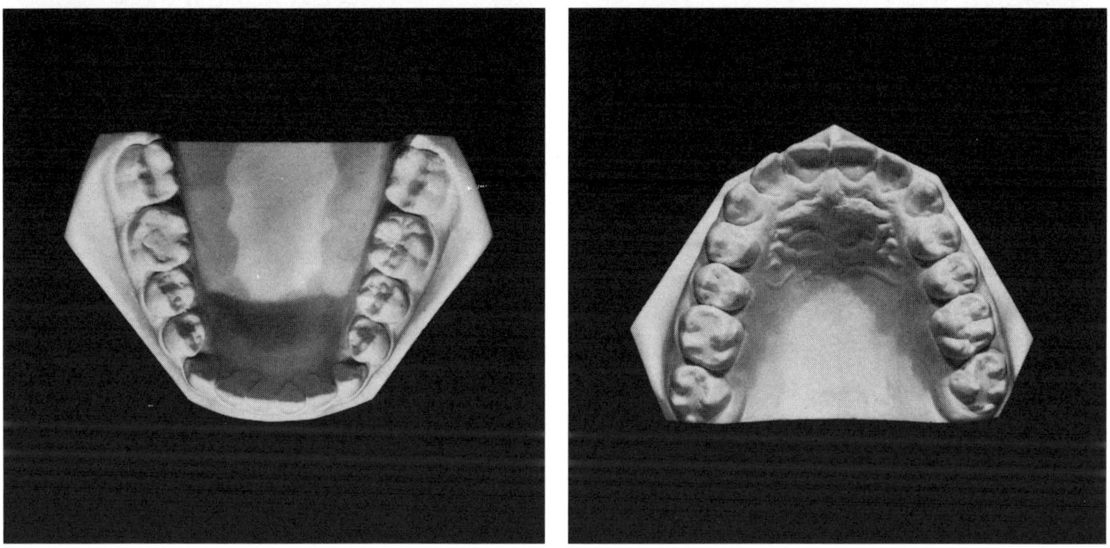

Figs 36-7 and 36-8 *At the age of 10 y, 10 mo the second transitional period is complete and the second permanent molars have emerged well and are nearly in occlusion. In the maxillary arch, the teeth are correctly aligned and have normal contacts. In the mandible, there is mild crowding in the region of the canines which, with the premolars, are slightly rotated. Neutro-occlusion is seen on the right, a mild disto-occlusion on the left.*

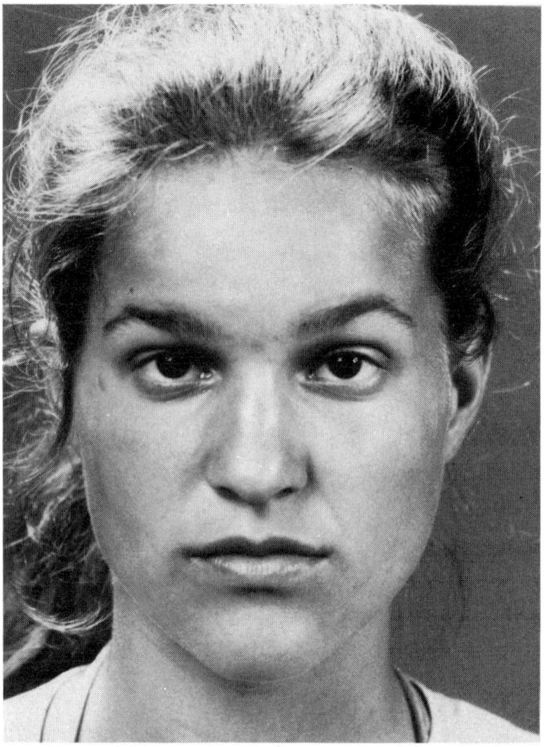
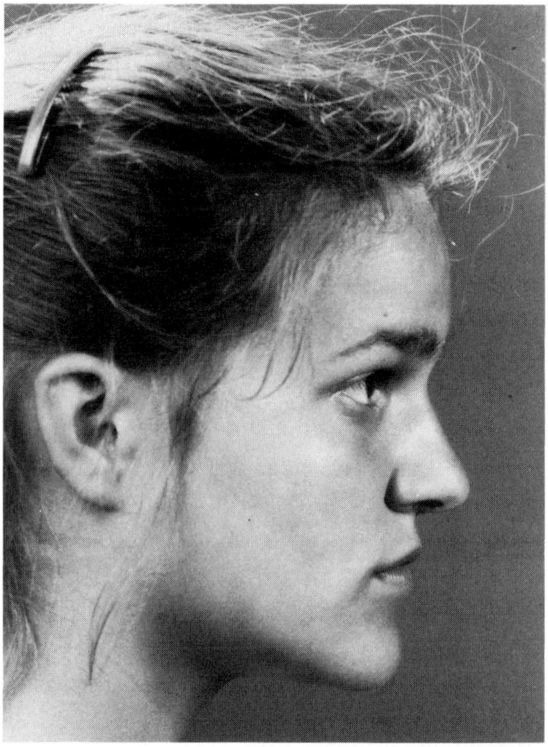
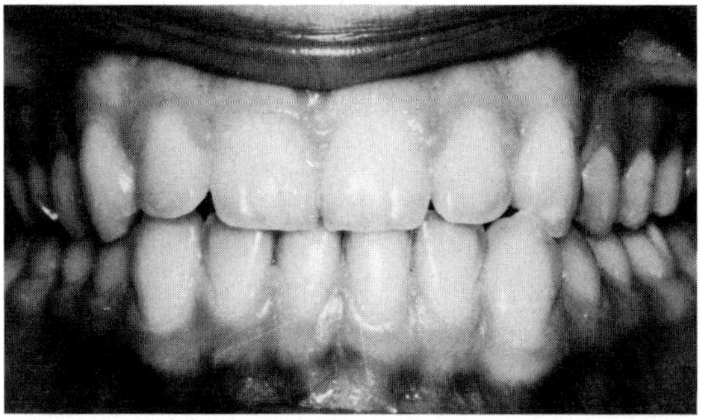
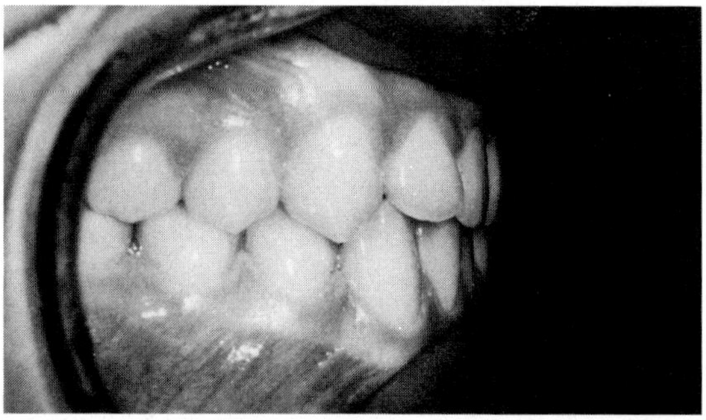
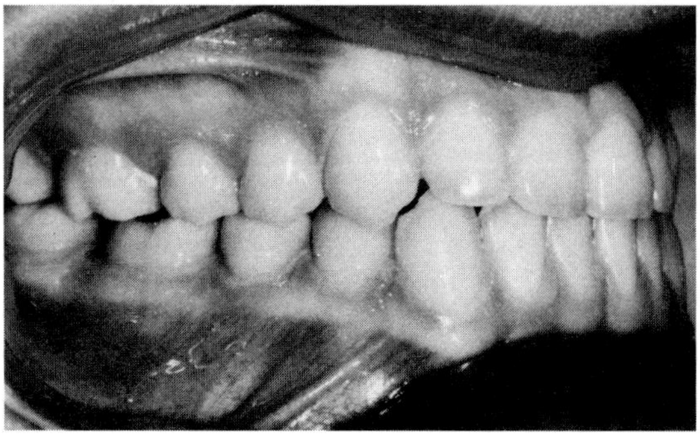
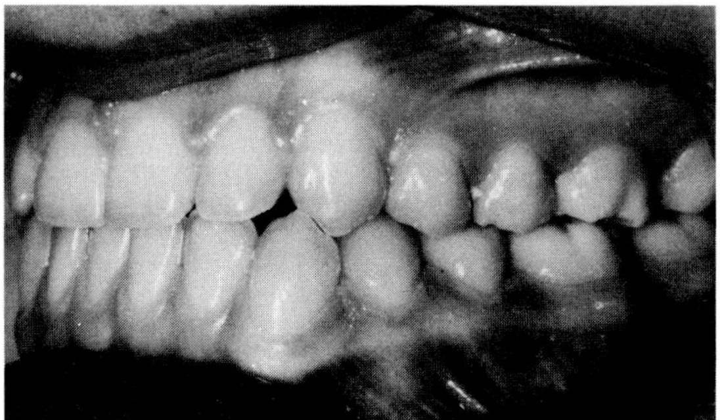

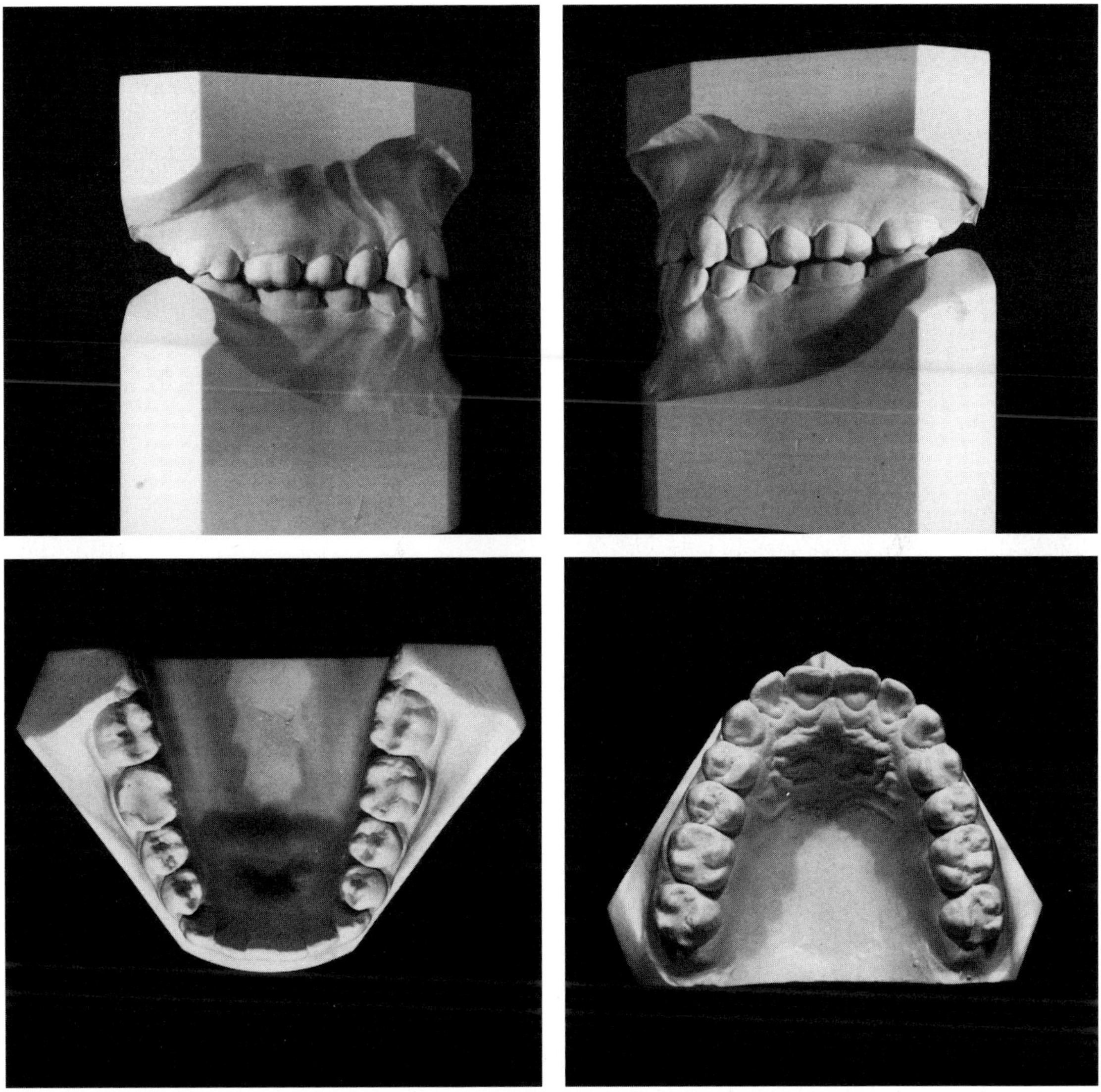

Figs 36-9 and 36-10 *At the age of 14 y, 11 mo, the growth of the face is now more or less complete. In the years following treatment, the mandible had still grown significantly while the ventral development of the maxilla had been meager (Fig. 36.13). In correspondence with those changes, the mandibular arch now occludes more mesially, the overjet and overbite have diminished, and the labioversion of the maxillary anteriors has increased.*

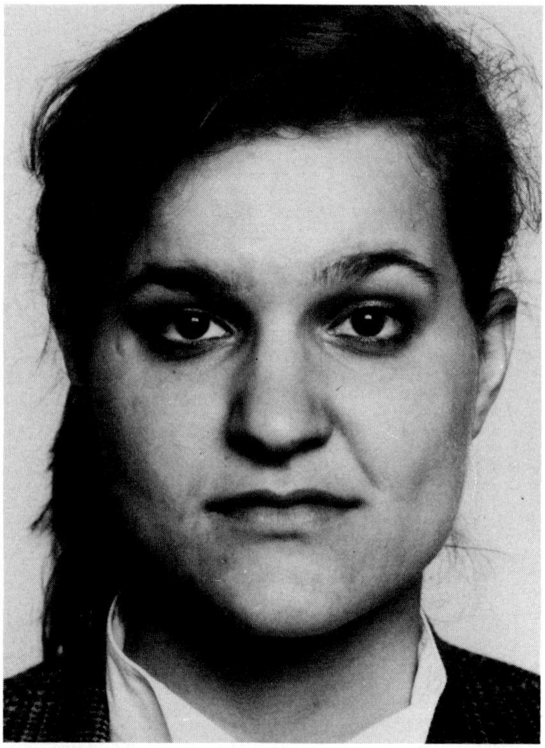
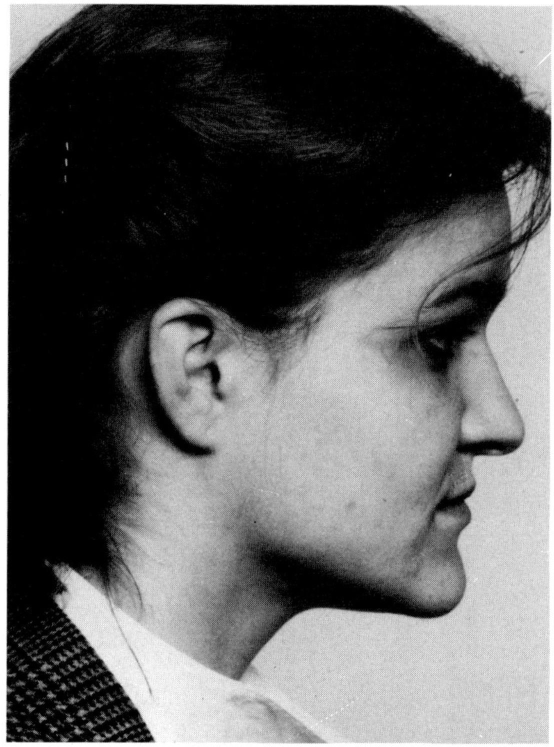
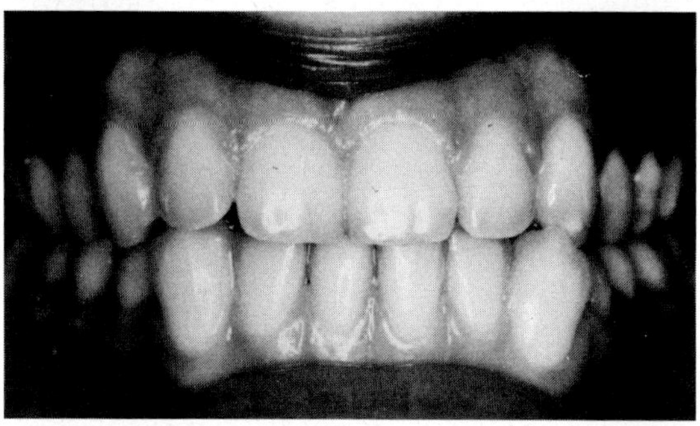
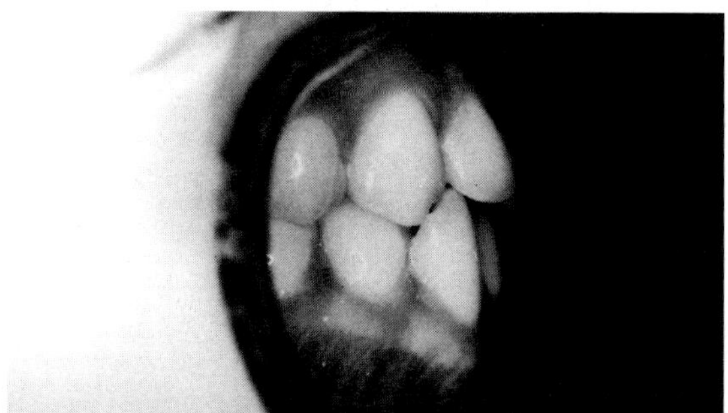
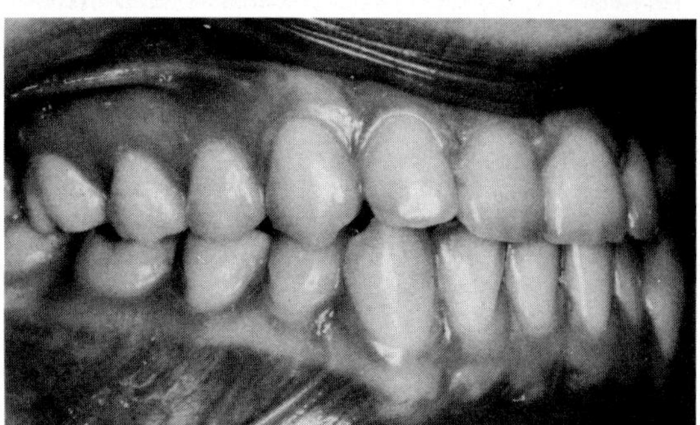
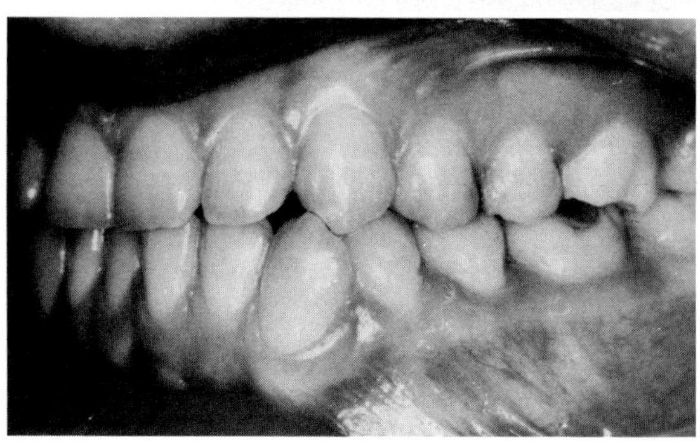

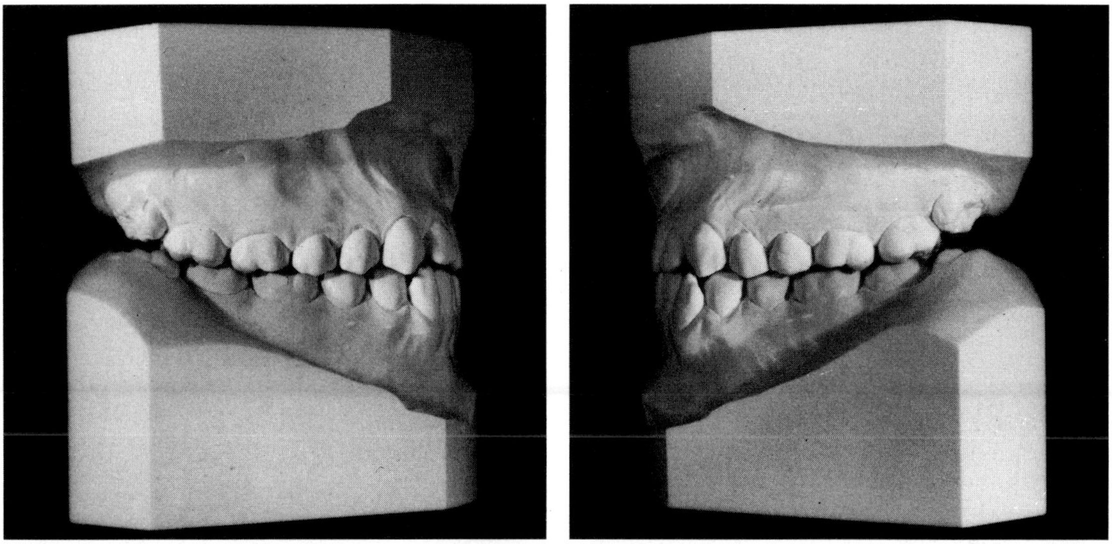

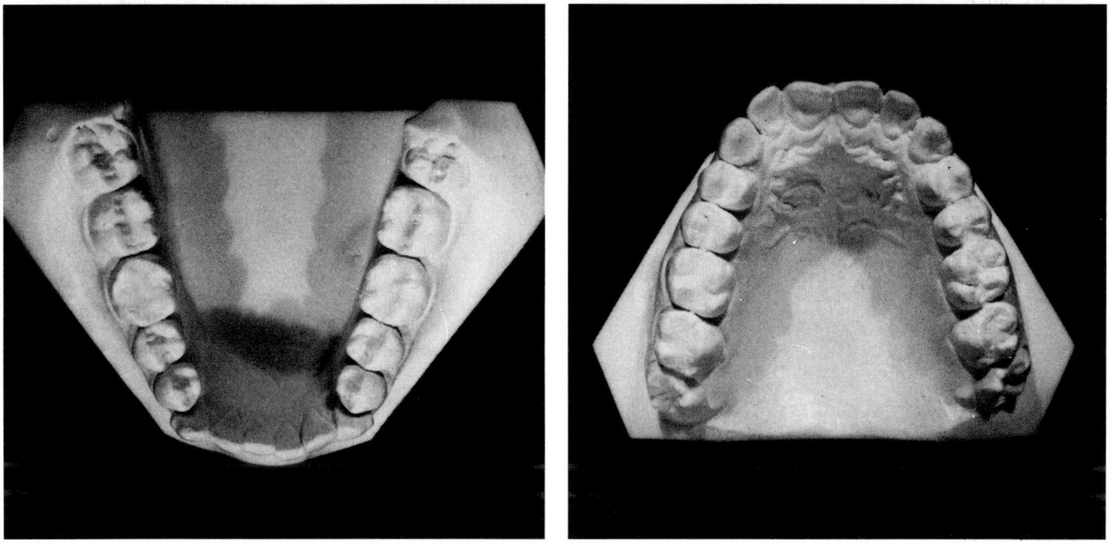

Figs 36-11 and 36-12 *At the age of 20 y, 9 mo, thirteen years after the facial orthopedic treatment had finished, there is a stable occlusion with the mandibular dental arch occluding a little more mesially than six years previously. The maxillary central incisors have been tipped somewhat more labially now, the mandibular ones going to lingual. The crowding has increased in the mandible in the canine areas and there is also some crowding now in the mandibular incisors. In the meantime, the third molars have emerged; there is too little room available for them in the jaws to permit them to come into good occlusion.*

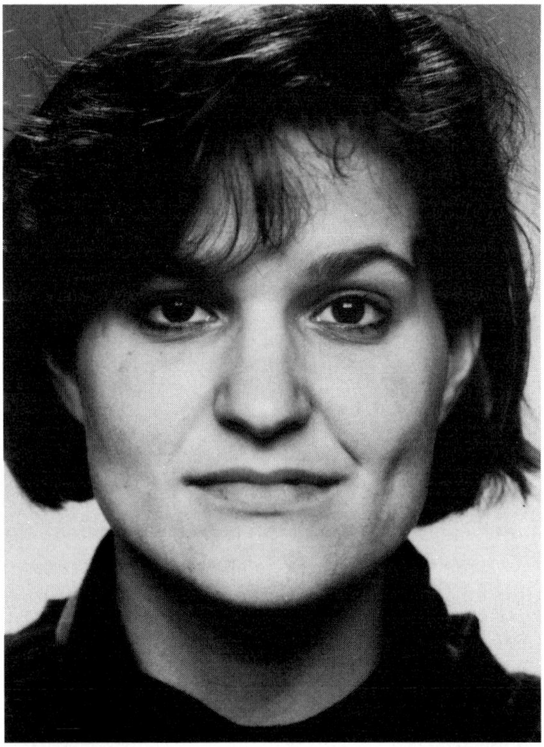

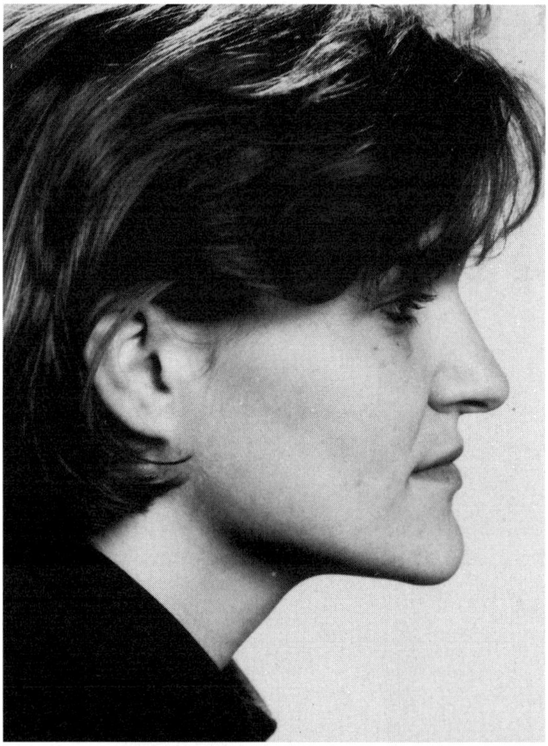

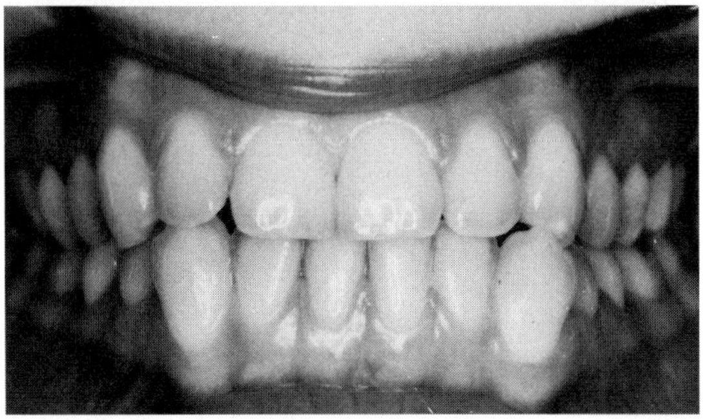

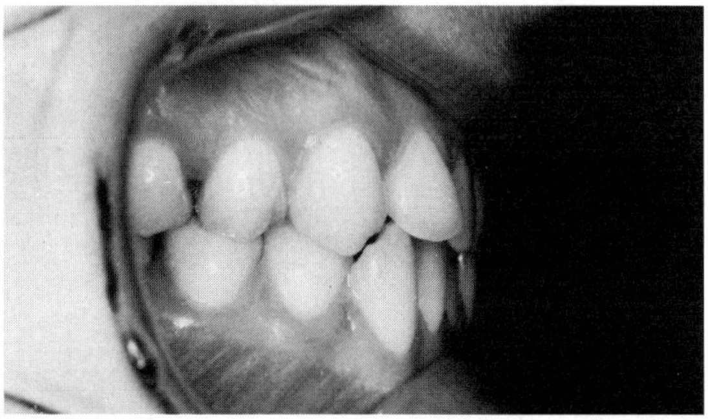

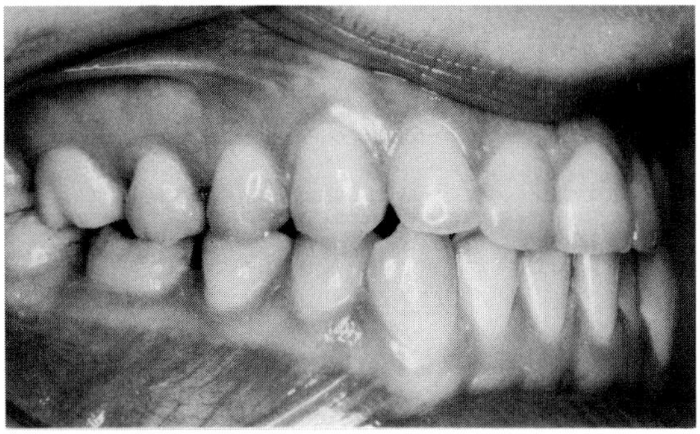

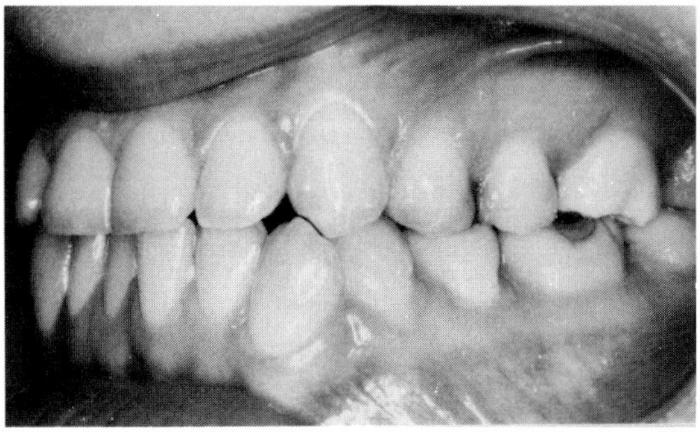

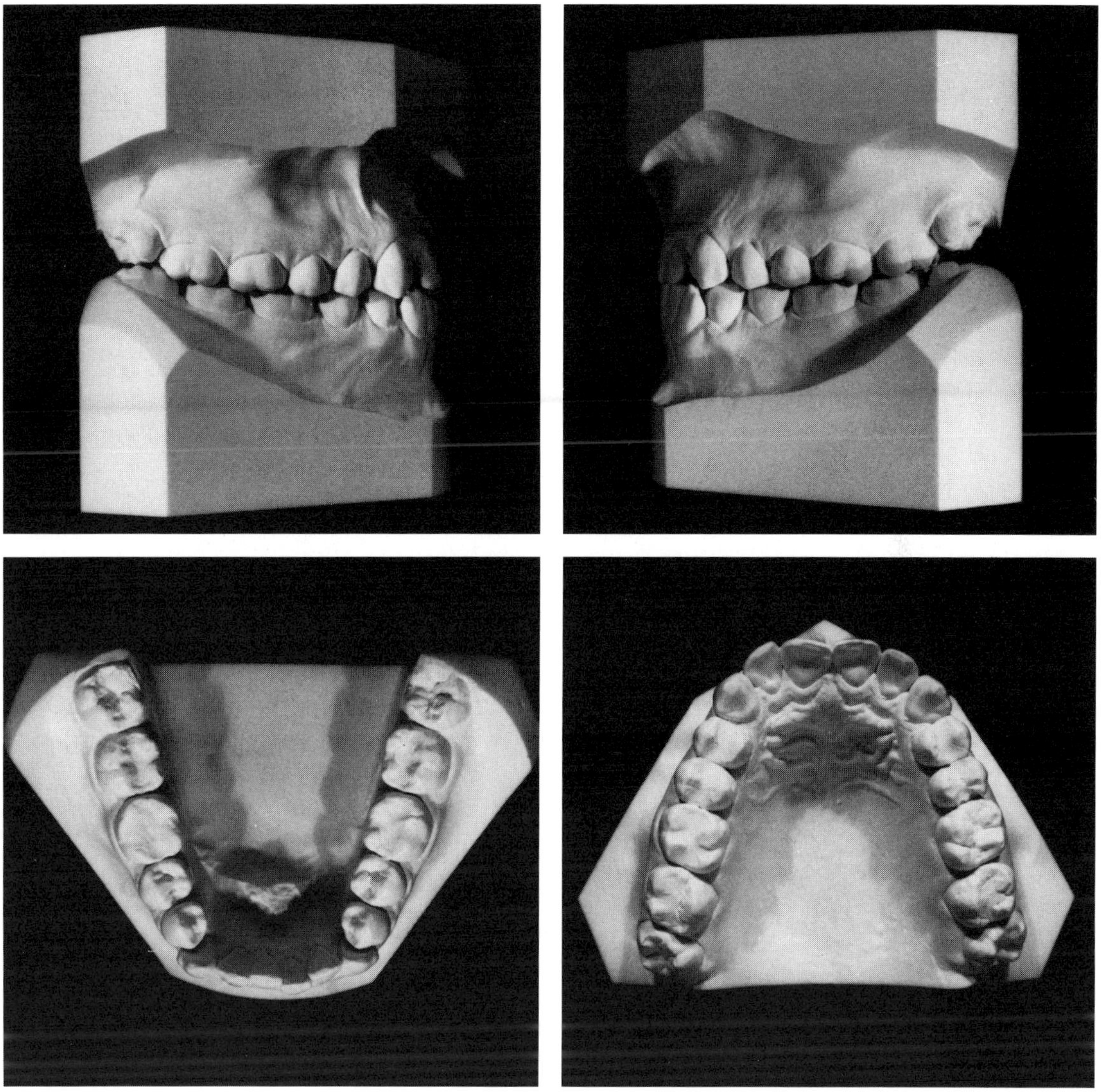

Figs 36-13 and 36-14 At the age of 23 y, 5 mo, the chin prominence appears to have increased and the mandibular arch has moved slightly more mesially into occlusion. The mandibular incisor crowding has increased a little and the maxillary right lateral incisor has moved more labially.

Figure 36-15a

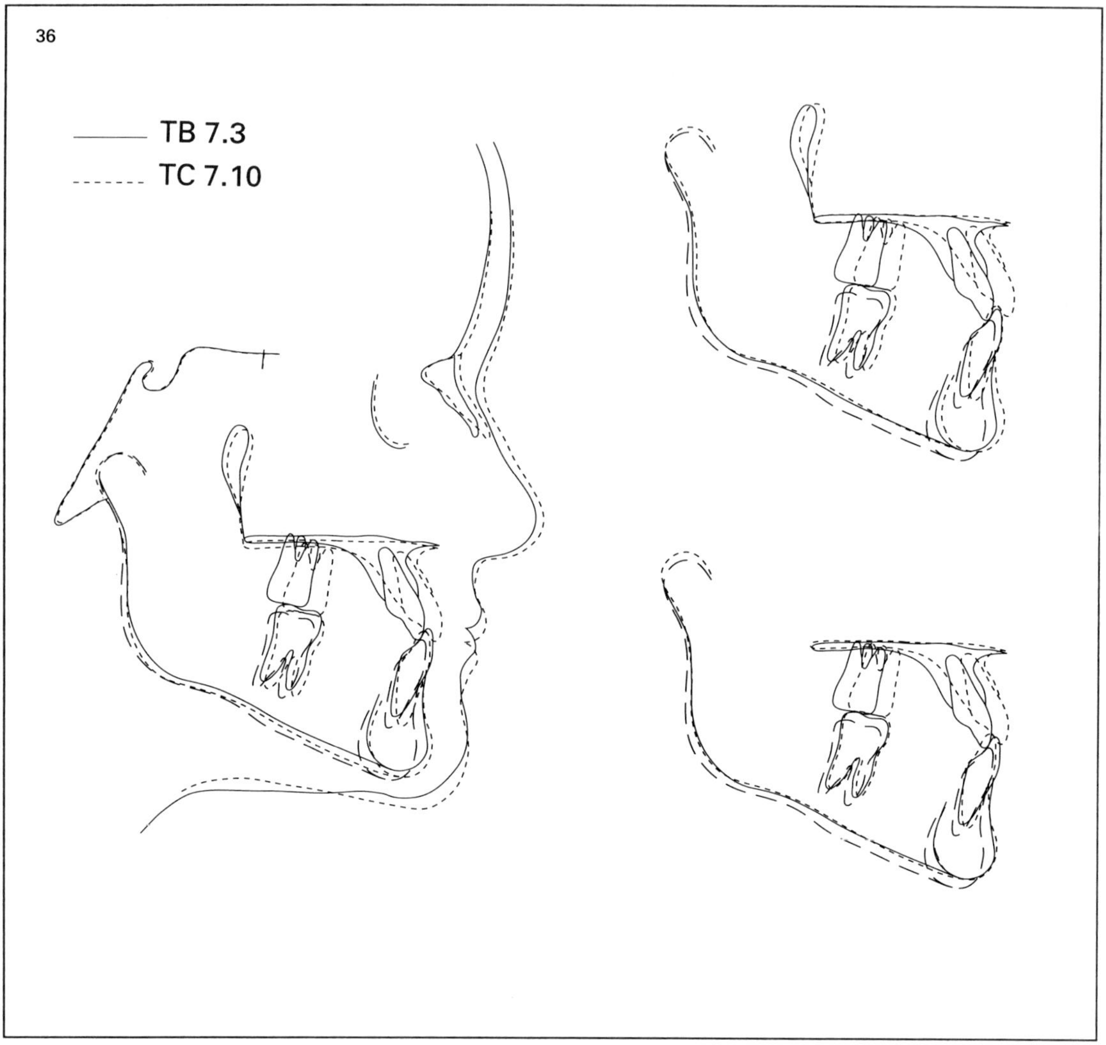

Fig 36-15 Superimposition of the tracings of cephalometric radiographs demonstrates well the marked ventral development of the maxilla during treatment. In addition, the original difference between central relationship (broken lines) and habitual occlusion is shown. The posterior section of the apical area of the maxilla, where the permanent molars are located, has become noticeably larger. In the five years subsequent to treatment the mandible continued to grow considerably, while the maxilla developed only slightly to ventral. The inclination of the anterior teeth has altered in response to the dento-alveolar compensatory mechanism. This tendency continued to be seen subsequently, although to a lesser degree.

Figure 36-15b

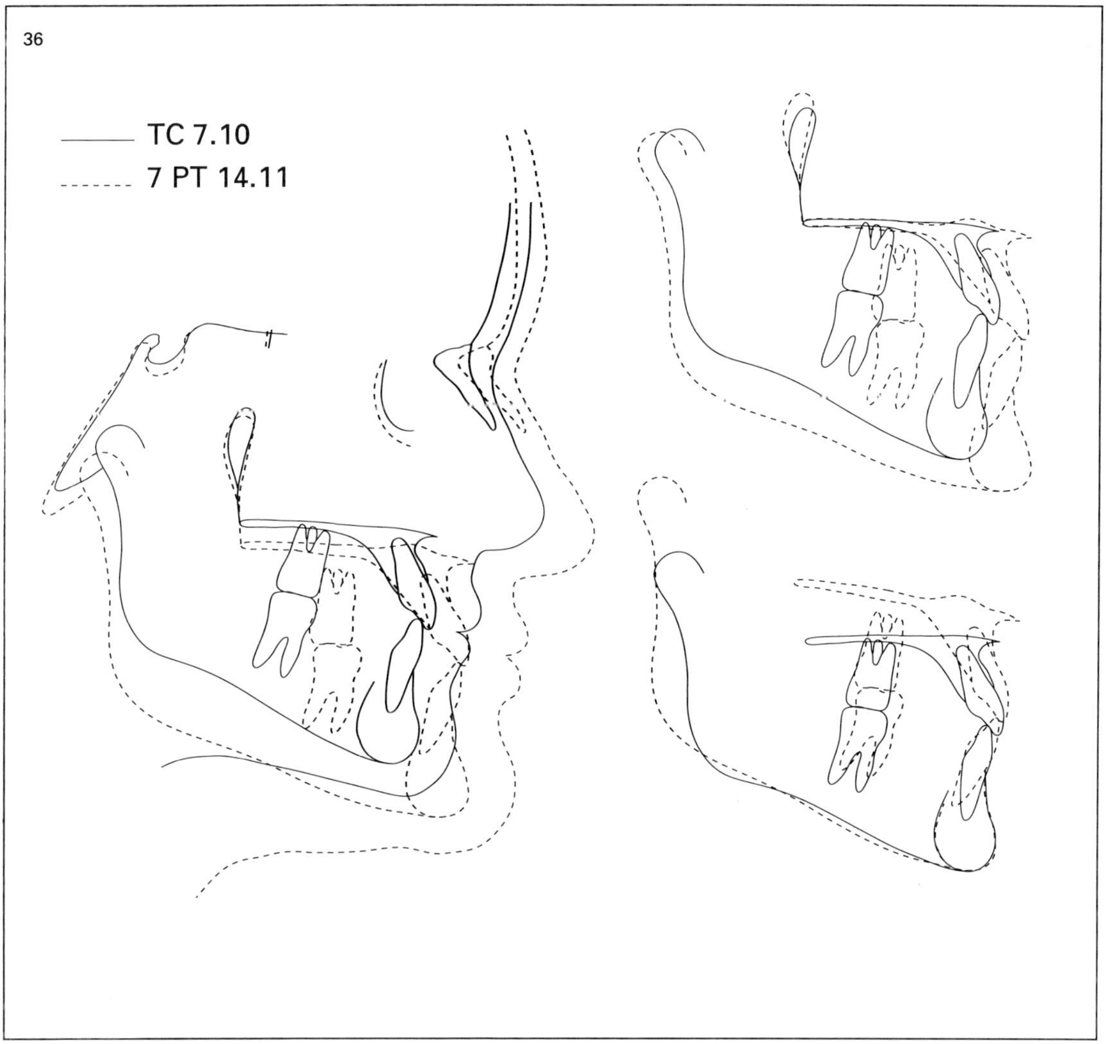

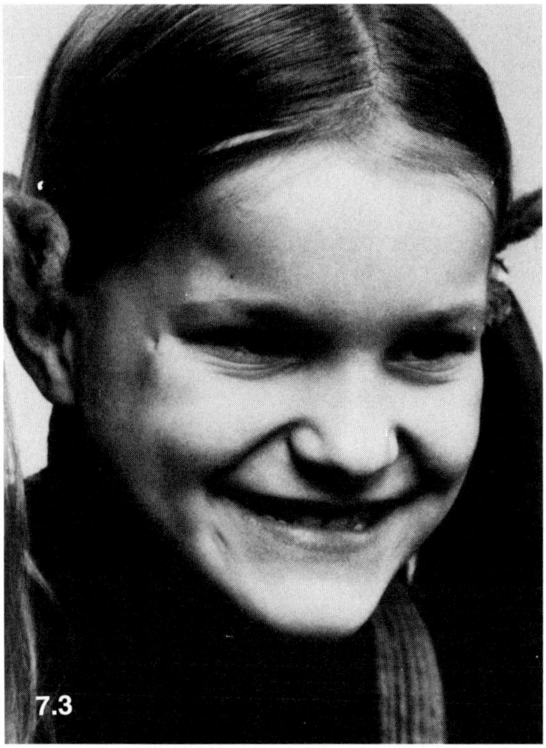
7.3

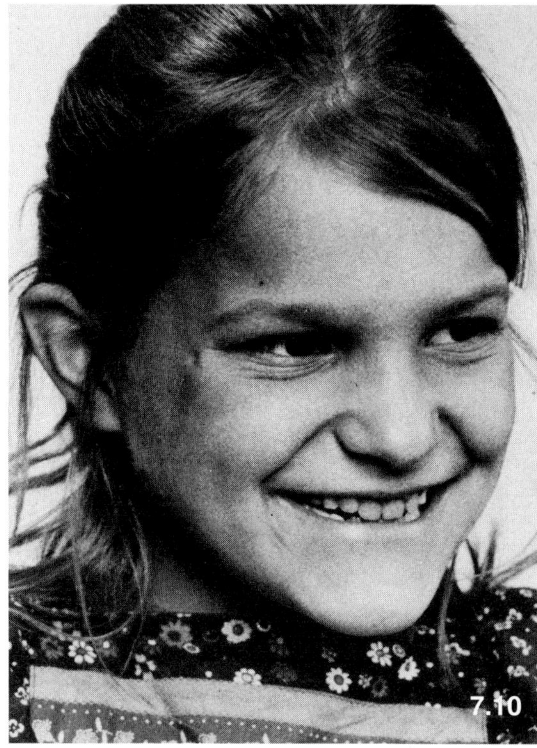
7.10

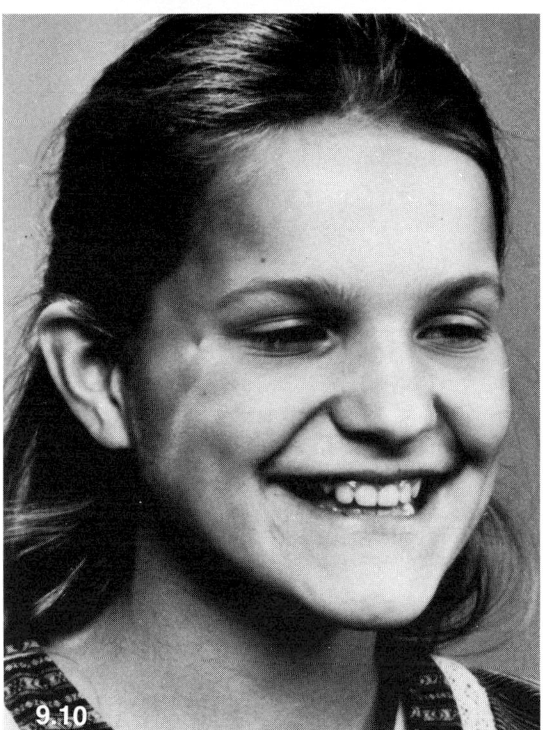
9.10

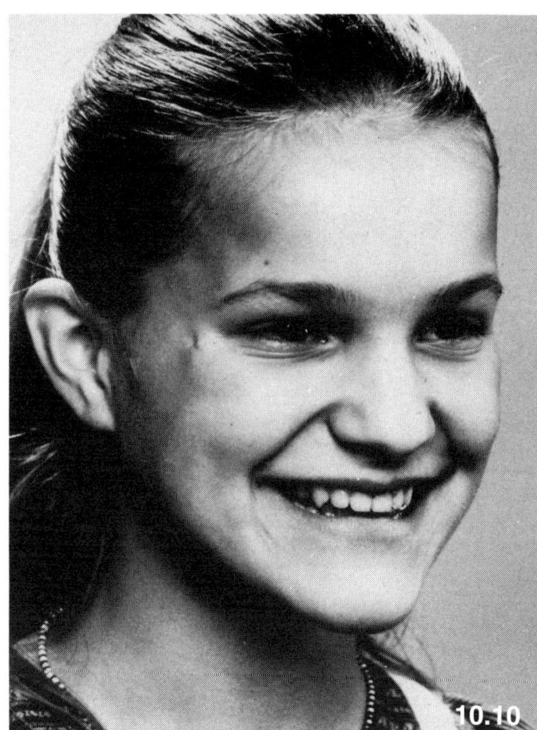
10.10

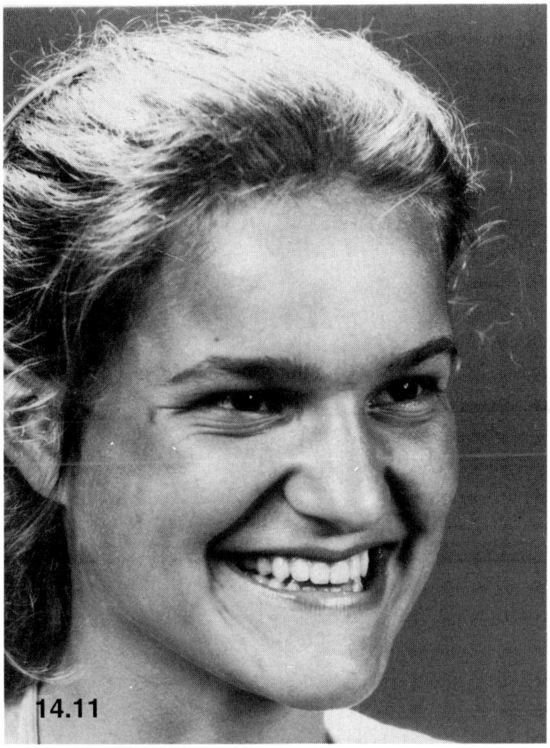

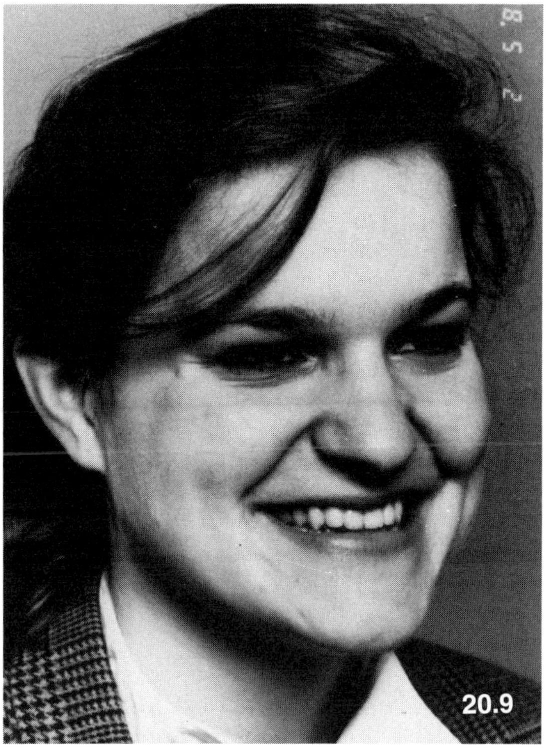

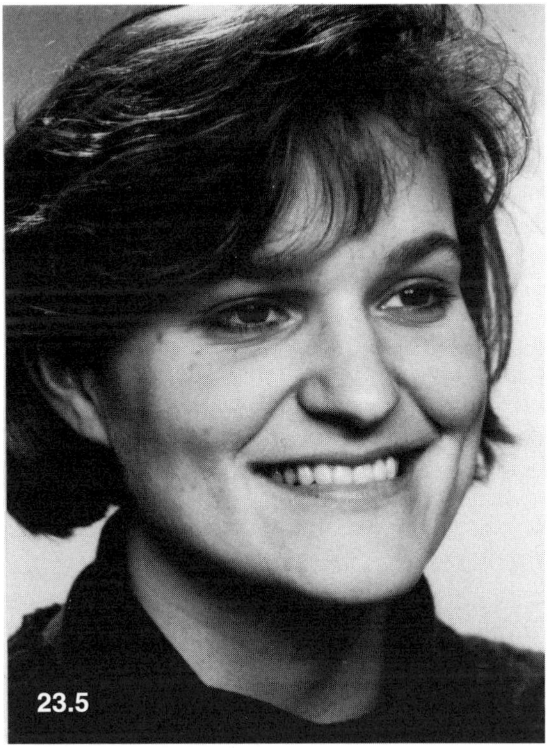

Fig 36.16 *The oblique facial photographs reveal the changes that can be attributed to growth and treatment. The midface originally was obviously under developed but was moved ventrally by the facial orthopedic therapy. In subsequent years, the mandible grew considerably while the maxilla grew ventrally very little, and this is clear from the conformation of the adult face of this patient.*

In the subsequent five years the facial growth was still significant, particularly with reference to the mandible, while the maxilla grew ventrally only slightly. The dento-alveolar compensatory mechanism led to a change in the inclination of the incisors and tipped the mandibular incisors a little backwards, this leading to a degree of crowding while the vertical overbite became less (Figs. 36.9 and 36.10).
Thirteen years after treatment it appeared that the mesial movement of the mandibular arch and the mandibular dental arch crowding had still increased a little. An adequate overjet and overbite was still evident and more than a minimal further change was not to be expected (Figs. 36.11 and 36.12). Yet subsequently the picture did change slightly, which was brought to attention when some two and a half years later the patient returned remarking that the right maxillary lateral incisor had become more prominent. To a limited extent this indeed proved to be the case. Moreover, the crowding in the mandibular anteriors had increased slightly and the mandibular arch was now occluding a little more mesially (Figs 36.13 and 36.14).
The tracings of the cephalometric radiographs illustrate the difference between central relation and habitual occlusion at the beginning of treatment, and in addition the marked ventral movement of the maxilla seen during the facial orthopedic therapy. Accompanying this was a considerable increase in size of the posterior section of the apical area as a consequence of accelerated bone formation as the maxilla moved ventrally. On the basis of these tracings it is possible to assess the growth of the face and changes in inclination and occlusion that were associated with these phenomena. The tracings also show how, after treatment, the mandible developed substantially to ventral while the maxilla moved forward less (Fig 36.15).
The photographs of the patient smiling show the originally underdeveloped midface, the increase in its prominence that occurred during therapy, and the domination of the growth of the mandible over the ventral development of the maxilla in the following years. The midface gradually has come to lie relatively retruded in relationship to the rest of the face. The solid interdigitation of the teeth has brought about an adaptation of the dentition, which has preserved the overjet and overbite (Fig 36.16).

Class III anomalies, and ventral forced bites, merit early treatment when possible. Rendering functional and jaw relationships normal leads to a more favorable situation within which development can proceed. That is not to say that where normal conditions have been achieved by the time treatment is finished it necessarily will be the case that no untoward events will occur. The ventral movement of the maxilla may prove to have been insufficient, but also the mandibular growth may become excessive and lead to a relapse of the reversed overbite and the manifestation of a class III profile. Even where no excessive mandibular growth takes place, the maxillary growth often will be relatively retarded with respect to that of the mandible and may produce the same relapses. Even when there is solid interdigitation, there will be a stronger tendency for mesial movement of the mandibular arch than would occur normally. This mesial displacement becomes evident most during adolescence.[27,28] Maxillary incisors tip more to labial and mandibular incisors more to lingual than normally.
If a class III anomaly is of genetic origin, there will be a good chance that an improvement obtained by early treatment subsequently will be at least partly lost.

Nonetheless, it is sensible to intervene at an early age and attempt to bring about a normal set of circumstances. This has not only psychological advantages, but also provides a better starting point for any future treatment even if it involves combined surgical and orthodontic therapy. If it is clear that surgical intervention cannot be avoided, then to reduce the incidence of "treatment fatigue," it is wise to provide as large a rest period as possible between the two phases of treatment. Furthermore, it is disappointing if after a rather long treatment episode the patient has to be told that surgical treatment is still required.

Lack of ventral development in the maxilla needs to be recognized early, although that is not a simple matter. The differentiation between the various types of class III anomalies and the recognition of whether or not progressive development is to be expected demands much insight and experience and must therefore, just as this also applies to the execution of the treatment, be left in the sphere of the orthodontic specialist.

For the correction of a class III anomaly with facial orthopedic therapy, the preference is for extraoral appliances, which are available in various forms (Fig 36.17). Their use varies according to age and circumstances. A summary of different indications and applications will be presented. At the same time, some practical suggestions will be given, some of which have appeared previously.

Class III anomalies in which the ventral development of the midface has lagged behind (not so much those that are the result of excessive mandibular growth) can be corrected in children at an early age by applying elastic traction ventrally from the maxillary arch to hooks either on vertical posts from a chin cap (Fig 36.17B) or on a facial mask following the design of Delaire (ventral headgear) (Fig 36.17C).

The sutures between the bony components of the maxillary complex have tension applied by the elastic traction in the direction of growth. In a relatively short time the maxilla can be brought forward a considerable distance at an early age with the appliance being worn only during sleep.

Ventral traction on the maxillary complex results in an increase in size of the posterior sections of the apical area in the maxilla through additional formation of bone at the tuberosities and from the mesial movement of the maxillary first molars. The latter movement will be associated with a corresponding reduction in the size of the middle section of the maxillary apical area.

Delaire's facial mask is supported by the forehead and the chin (Figs 36.17C and D). In this manner, a force is applied to the mandible that is comparable to that obtained from a chincap supported by the back of the head (Fig 36.17A). It is possible that the direction of growth in the condyles is influenced. This would be more applicable to the chincap with vertical arms, since all the force applied for ventral traction of the maxilla would be absorbed by the chin alone. The superior margin of such a chin cap has a tendency to rotate inward, which not only can cause skin irritation but can also tip the mandibular incisors lingually, something that is not always desirable.

For treatment in the deciduous dentition, a chincap providing traction from the back of the head is the method of choice. If there is a possibility that the midface is deficient in development, the use of a Delaire face mask can also be considered.

During the first transitional period, the sole objective can be to prevent or to correct a ventral forced bite. If there is also a mesio-relation, then a chincap or facial mask can be used for correction of that.

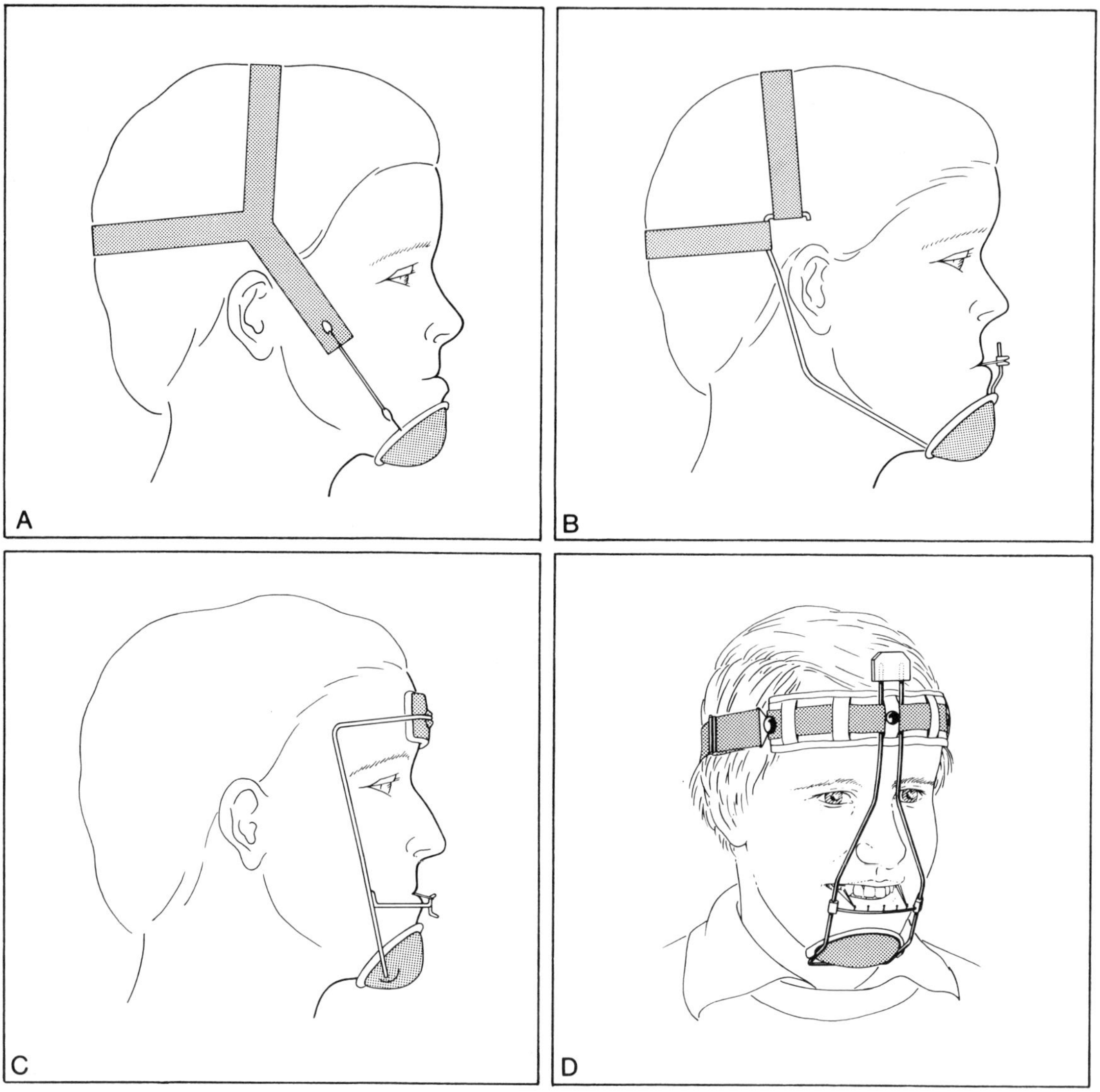

Fig 36-17 Appliances for treatment of class III anomalies.

A A chincap with dorsocranial traction on the mandible.

B A chincap with vertical posts from which ventral traction can be applied to the maxilla with elastics (Hickham's model). The straps across the head are not elastic, exerting no active dorsocranial force.

C A facial mask according to Delaire, with ventral traction to the maxilla using the forehead and chin for anchorage.

D The Tübingen model of Delaire's facial mask.[36]

During the intertransitional period, a facial mask or a chin cap with vertical posts is preferred. In this procedure, the ventral force needs to be applied as much as possible to the maxilla as a whole. This can be attempted with a well-fitting plate that has clasps and a labial arch that embrace all the teeth from all aspects. The traction can, depending on the direction wished for, be applied to the first permanent molars or deciduous molars to which hooks have been attached. Traction can also be applied successfully to ankylosed deciduous teeth.

In class III anomalies with an increased lower-face height and/or an anterior open bite, the application of ventral traction to maxillary molars (which will then tend to rotate) requires much care to avoid introducing a vertical component since extrusion of the molars is undesirable. When the force is derived from other teeth it is still necessary to watch for any possible undesired vertical changes.

During the second transitional period a facial mask or a chincap with vertical posts would be preferred even more. Use of these appliances for a longer time than just during sleep would be required.

If the permanent dentition is fully emerged (except for the third molars), then there is little likelihood of improvement with facial orthopedic therapy, certainly not when facial growth has reached a late stage and the anomaly is pronounced.

Where the maxilla requires significant broadening of the dental arch, combining ventral traction with rapid expansion of the midpalatal suture can be advantageous.

Finally it might be noted that the effect of ventral traction is much greater than that of dorsal traction. A marked improvement can be achieved in six months with ventral traction although the appliance is only worn while sleeping. The correction of a disto-relation with a headgear lasts much longer, while the appliance must be worn more hours each day.

Chapter 37

Class III
Chincap with vertical posts, maxillary removable plate
Male: 7 years, 9 months to 23 years, 9 months

A boy aged 7 years, 9 months displayed a class III anomaly with a slightly large lower face and an underdeveloped midface. His general growth was retarded, as was the development of his dentition; the latter was illustrated by the fact that his first deciduous tooth did not emerge until after his first birthday. The transition of his dentition also appeared to be slow. For example, the first permanent molars had not yet emerged. However, the mandibular permanent central incisors were indeed present in the mandible. They were tipped lingually and crowded. Diastemata were present in the maxillary anteriors. There was a mesio-occlusion of 1 PW on both sides. The deciduous molars and canines in the maxilla were in endo-occlusion and the incisors had a reversed overbite without incisal contact. The overbite was +1 mm, the overjet –3 mm, while the mandible could not be moved distally more than ½ mm past the position of habitual occlusion. The oral hygiene was poor, and there were various decalcifications and cavities; most of the deciduous molars had restorations already (Figs 37.1 and 37.2).

It was decided that for the moment no treatment would be given but that both the development of the dentition and facial growth should be kept under observation, particularly since at present, the boy had no trouble with the anomaly. After emergence of the permanent incisors, sagittal contact was established between them. At the age of 10 years, he could get the incisal edges of the opposing incisors to meet.

At the age of 11 years, there was still a full crossbite except where the maxillary left lateral incisor closed labial to the mandibular deciduous canine on that side. The facial appearance showed only mildly the characteristics of a class III anomaly because the reversed relationship of the upper and lower lips was limited in degree and the chin was not excessively dominant (Figs 37.3 and 37.4).

Shortly after his eleventh birthday, bands were placed on the first permanent molars and the deciduous canines, with molar tubes and elastic hooks, respectively, to attach elastics with which to provide ventral traction from vertical posts on a chincap. At the same time, the projections on the bands provided undercuts that would improve the retention of the plate to be fitted for the purpose of fixing the maxillary teeth into one unit. The patient was asked to wear the plate and the chin cap with elastics while sleeping.

At the age of 11 years, 7 months, the reversed overbite and the crossbite in the

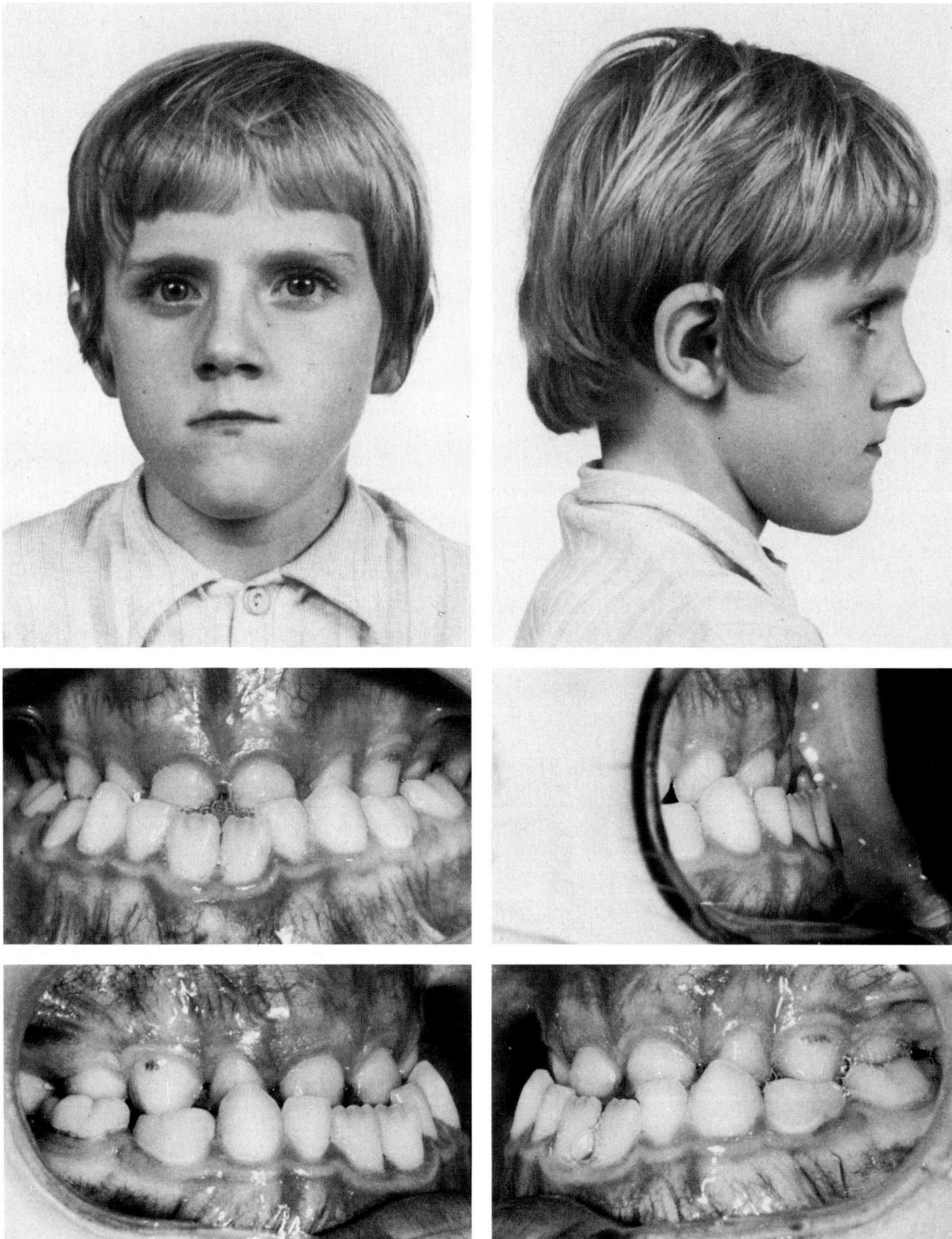

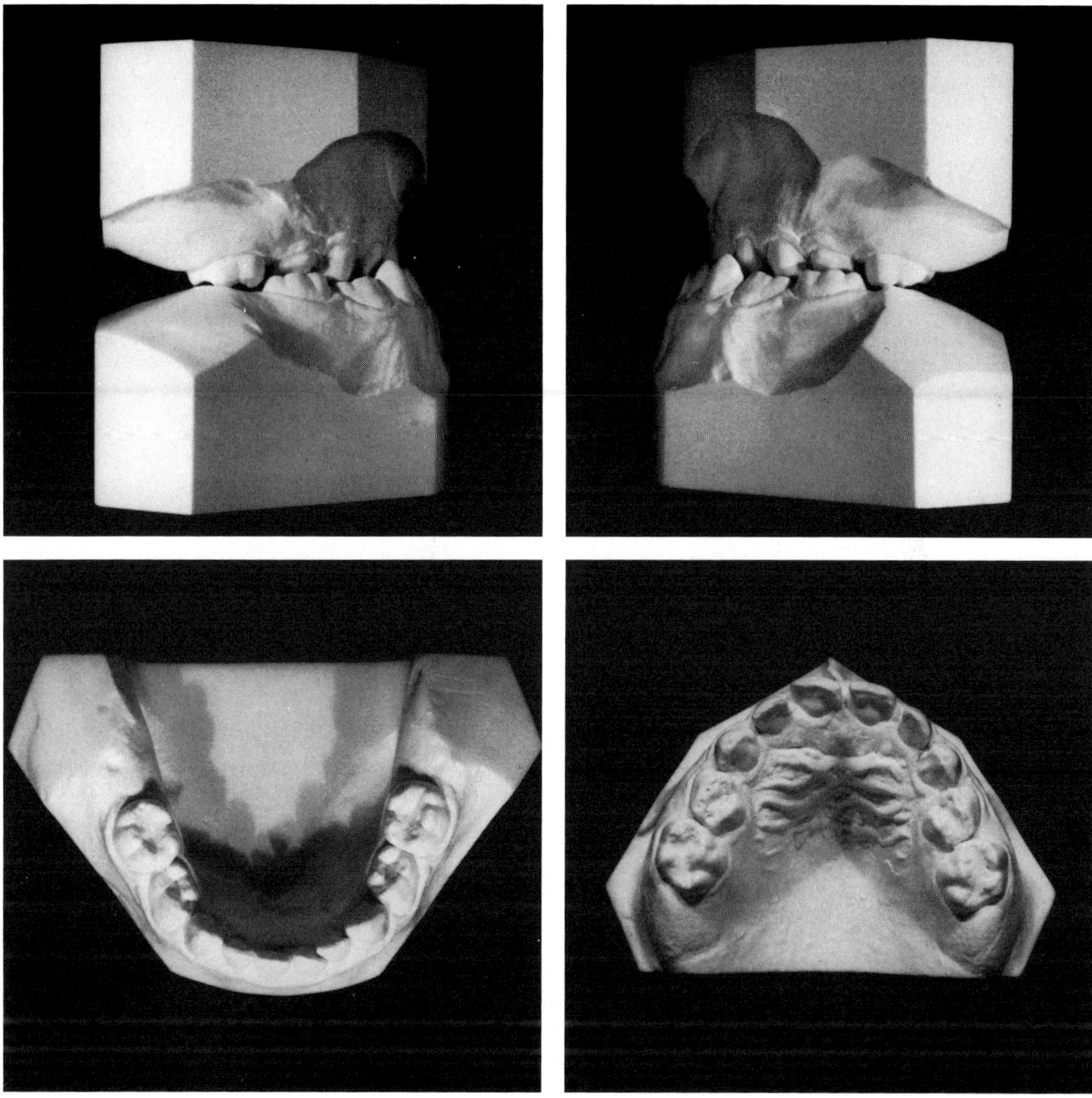

Figs 37-1 and 37-2 A boy aged 7 y, 9 mo with a class III anomaly, a slightly large lower face, an underdeveloped midface and a large mandible. All the maxillary teeth occlude inside the mandibular arch. The mandibular anteriors do not contact the maxillary ones. There is a mesio-occlusion of 1 PW on each side. Except for the mandibular central incisors, which have already exfoliated, the deciduous dentition is still totally present, while the permanent molars have not yet emerged. The mandibular anteriors are lingually tipped and crowded; the maxillary anteriors show spacing.

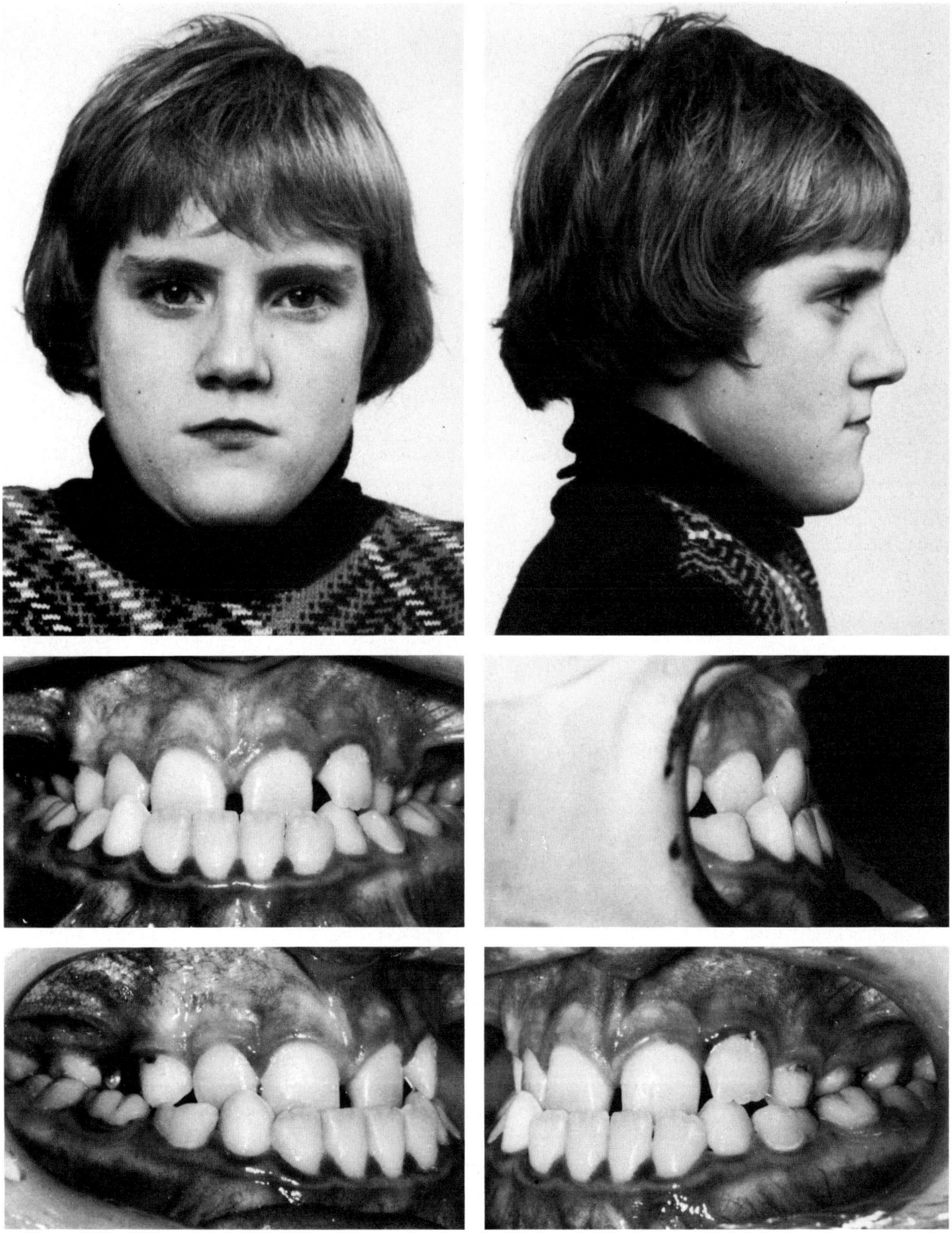

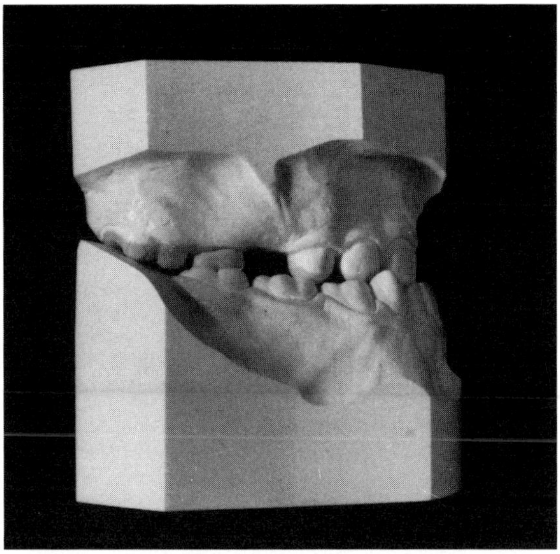
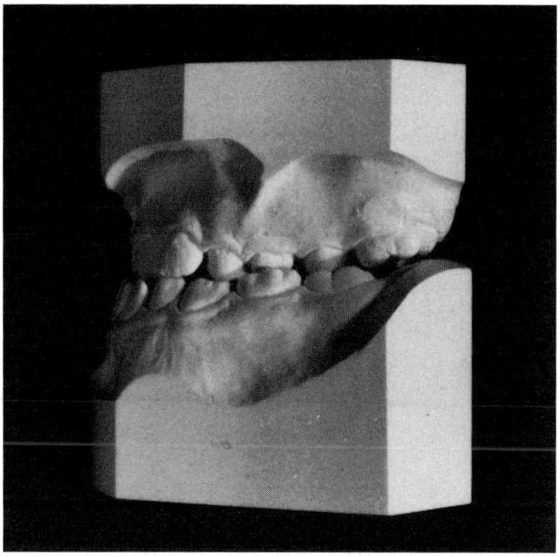
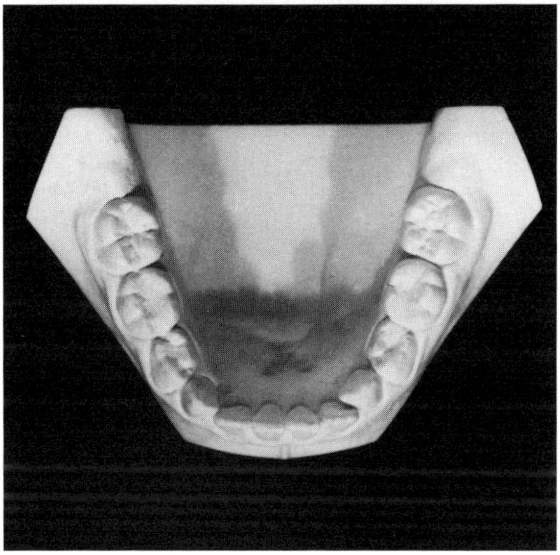
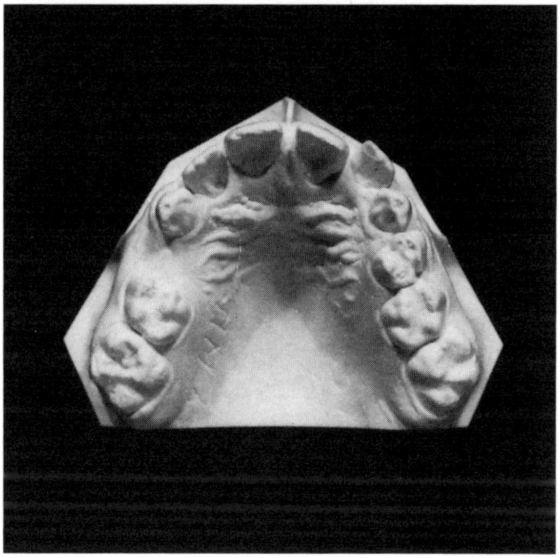

Figs 37-3 and 37-4 *At the age of 11 y, 0 mo there is a class III profile evident to a limited extent. The lower lip protrudes a little in front of the upper lip and the chin is a fairly dominant facial feature. The midface certainly is relatively underdeveloped, although it is less so than three years previously (Fig 37.15). The incisors have erupted fully and are in contact, although the maxillary left lateral incisor is the only tooth in the maxillary arch that does not fall inside the mandibular dental arch. There is just sufficient room in the mandibular arch to accommodate the teeth, while in the maxillary arch there are anterior diastemata. On both sides the first permanent molars are in mesio-occlusion to the extent of 1 PW.*

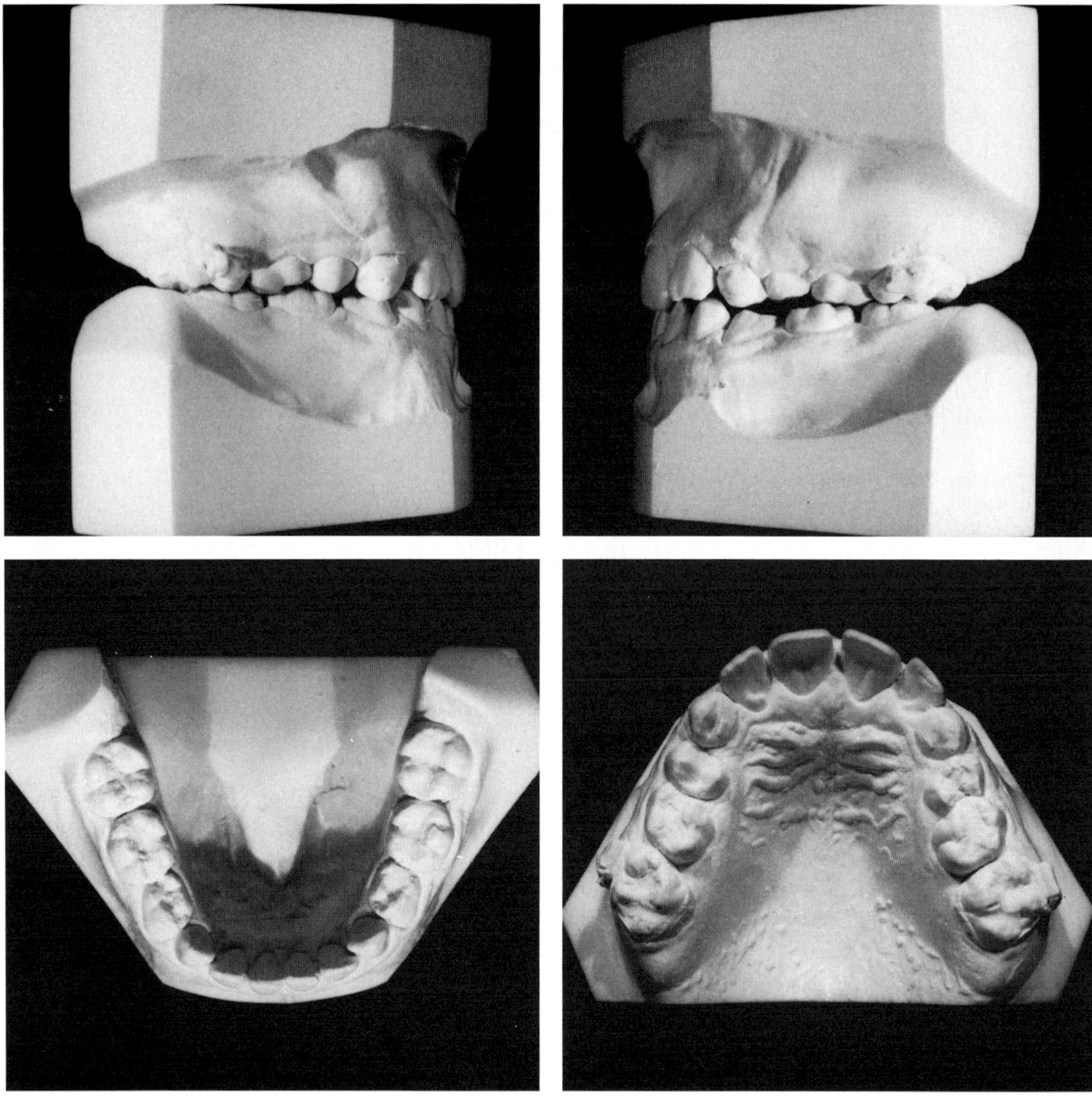

Fig 37-5 At the age of 11 y, 7 mo the maxilla had been brought obviously forward (Fig.37.15). The posterior teeth are in neutro-occlusion. A normal transverse occlusion has occurred on the right side but on the left side an open bite and an edge-to-edge transverse relationship between the deciduous molars exists. The overjet and overbite are normal.

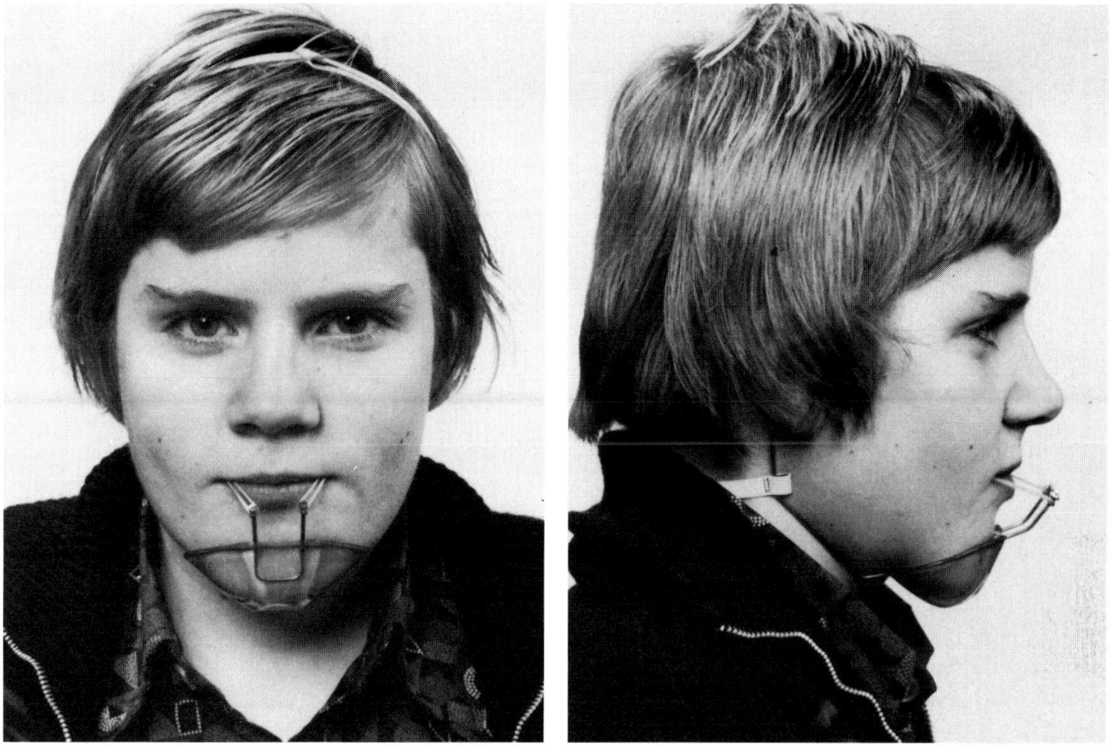

Fig 37-6 The patient wearing the chincap with vertical posts on the day treatment was terminated for the first time. The chin cap is held in place with leather thongs, with one behind the head or neck and the other across the crown of the head. The height at which the elastics are attached to the vertical posts can be adjusted by sliding the hooks up or down the posts. The projecting ends of the posts can then be removed. The direction in which the traction is applied to the maxilla depends also on the location of the intraoral attachment of the elastics. The elastics should run as horizontally as possible, and at the level of the center of resistance of the roots if that can be done. If they are attached only to the molars, the maxilla will have a tendency to rotate and an anterior open bite can develop. This will not happen to any extent if the elastics are hooked only to the canine region.

An effect that is seen with the use of a chincap with vertical posts and elastics is that the mandibular incisors are often tipped lingually. The elastic traction pulls the upper margin of the chincap backward and it exerts pressure on those teeth lingual to it. If such tipping of the mandibular incisors is not desired, then it would be better to use a facial mask such as that of Delaire.

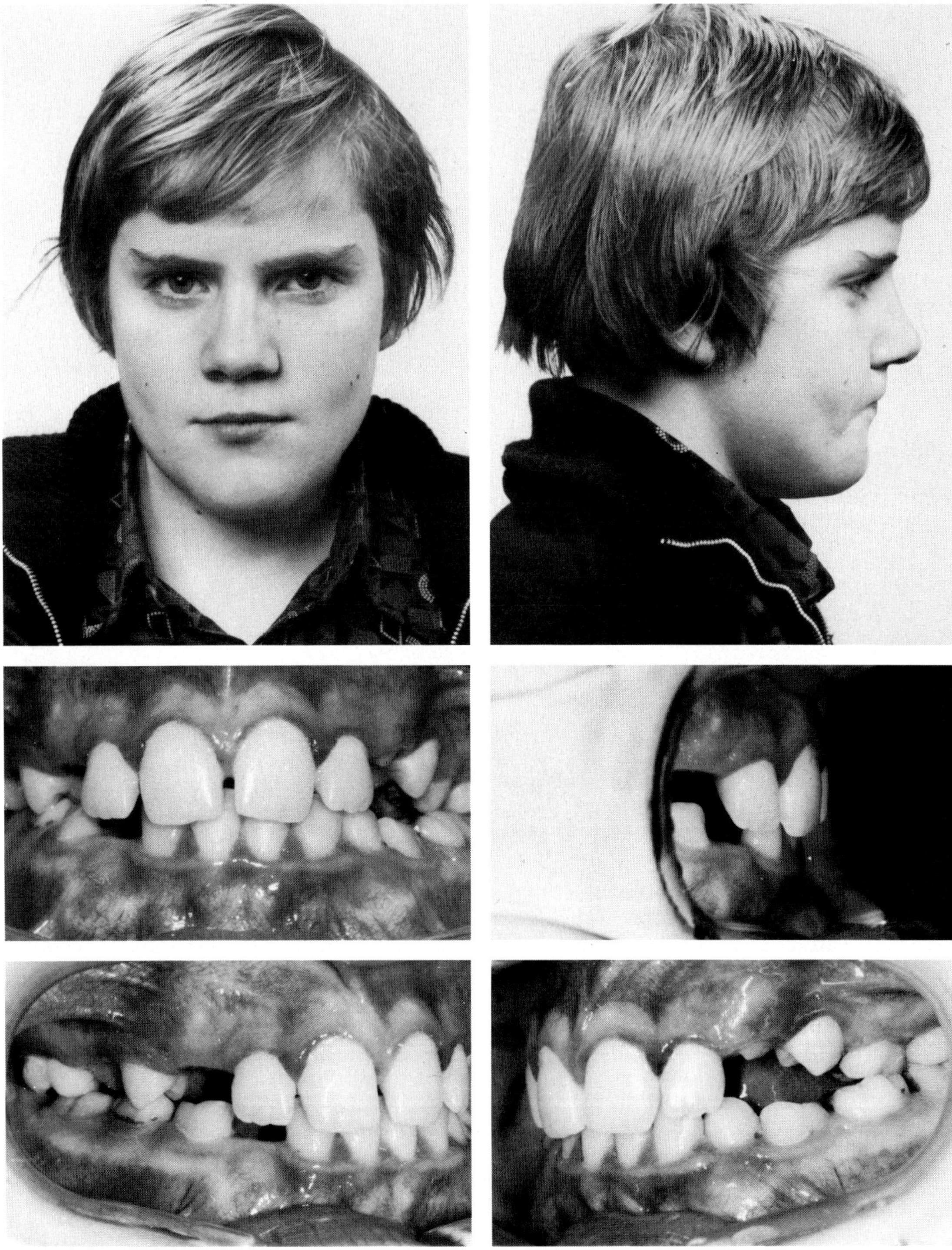

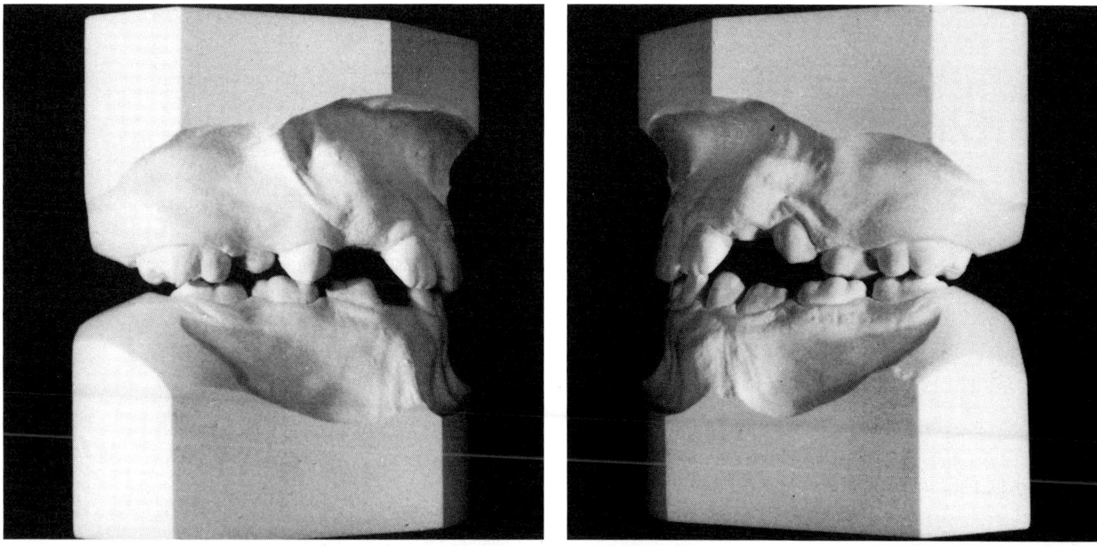

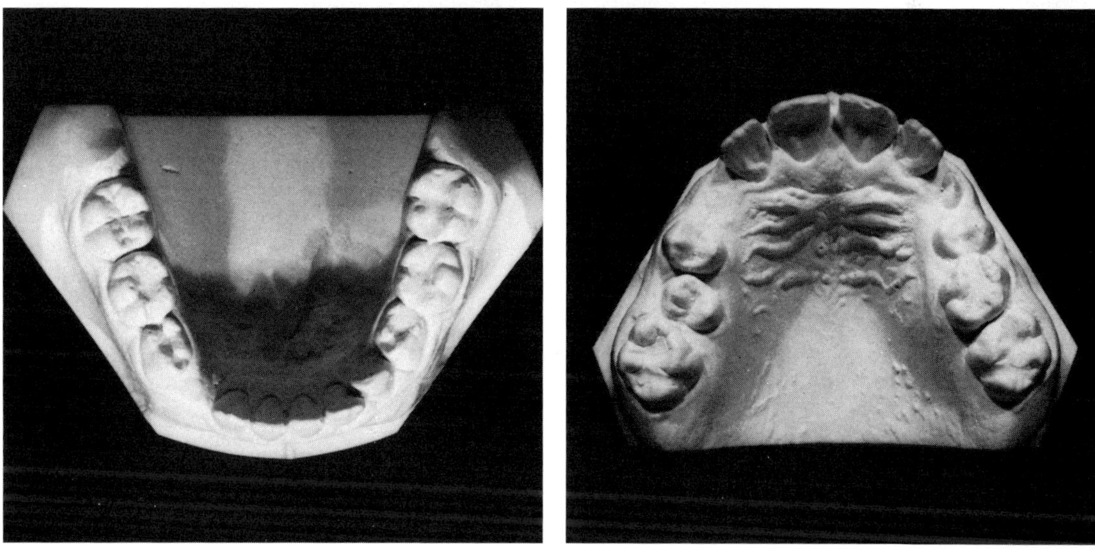

Figs 37-7 and 37-8 At the age of 13 y, 1 mo, treatment is terminated for the second time. The midface is sufficiently far to ventral and there is a good overjet and overbite. (The profile is not easily judged from the photograph because the lips are not relaxed; the photograph in Figure 37.6 taken on the same day gives a relaxed picture.) The middle of the mandibular dental arch is situated to the left in relationship to the maxillary arch, something that seems to have been the case from the beginning. No attempt was made to correct this deviation. The first molars on the right occlude in neutro-occlusion and on the left in a mild disto-occlusion, which corresponds with the midline situation.

All the deciduous molars are still present in the mandible. In the maxilla three premolars have emerged, of which two are tending to develop in crossbite. There is still a lot to be desired with regard to oral hygiene.

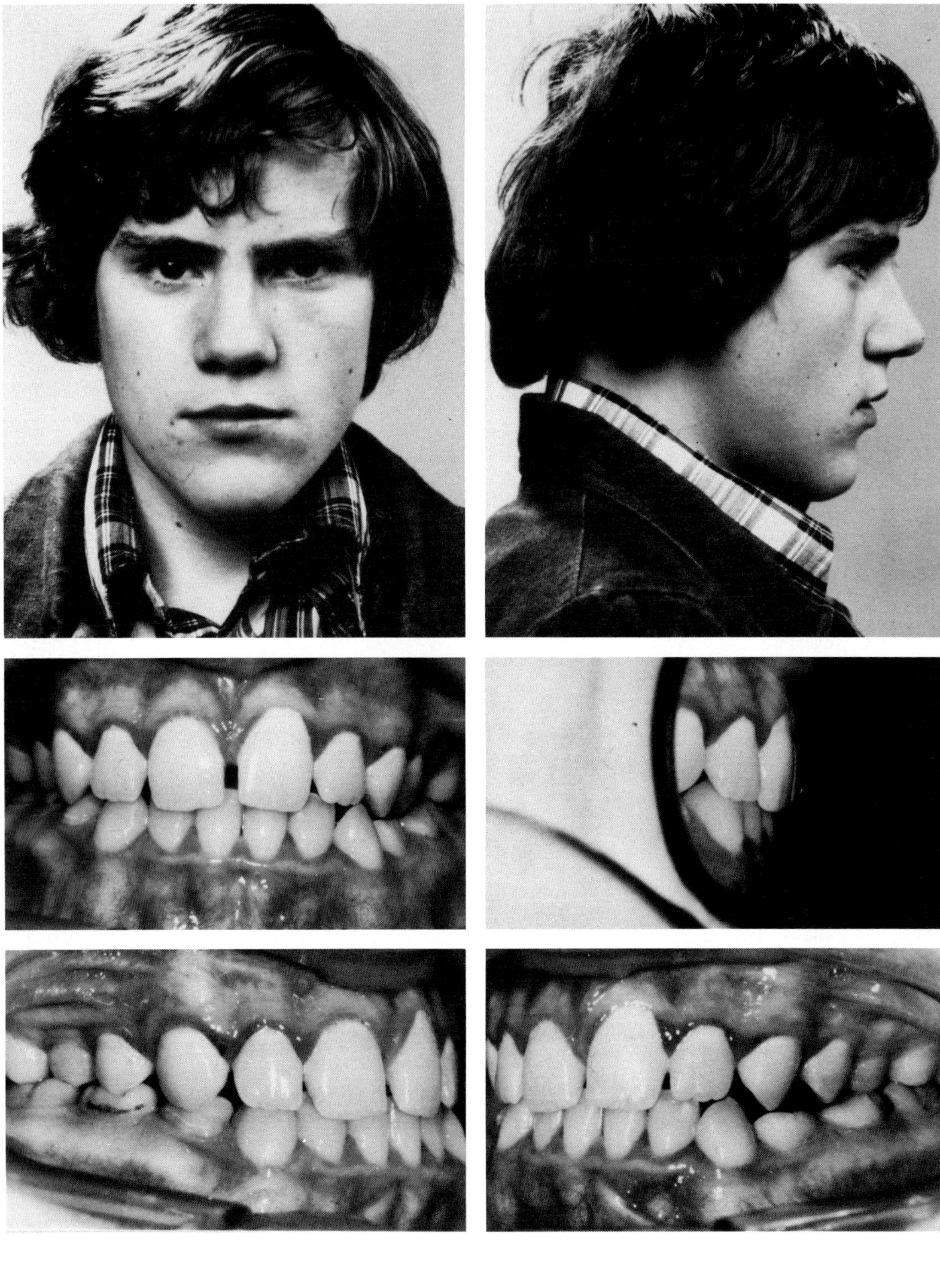

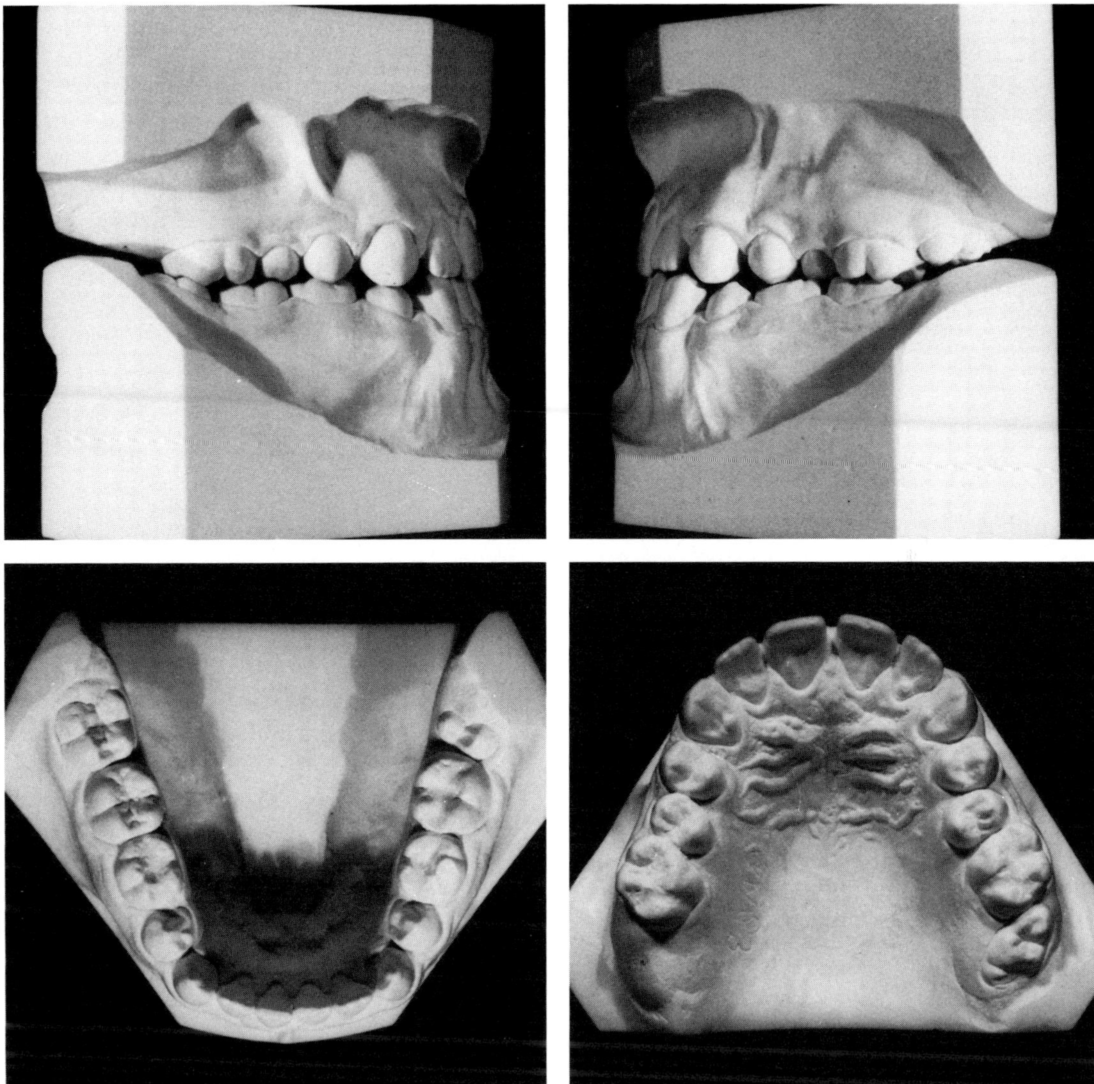

Figs 37-9 and 37-10 *At the age of 15 y, 7 mo, 2½ y after the end of treatment, little has been lost of the improvements gained with facial orthopedic therapy. As the result of growth that occurred after treatment, the anterior aspect of the maxilla has moved ventrally together with that of the mandible (Fig 37.15). The overjet and overbite have become only slightly smaller. The maxillary premolars did not move into crossbite, despite the fact that on the left still no occlusal contact exists. The maxillary left second premolar emerged rotated by 180 degrees, which causes no problem. (The dental casts depicted were made six months after the intraoral photographs; the first premolars in the mandible had then emerged.)*

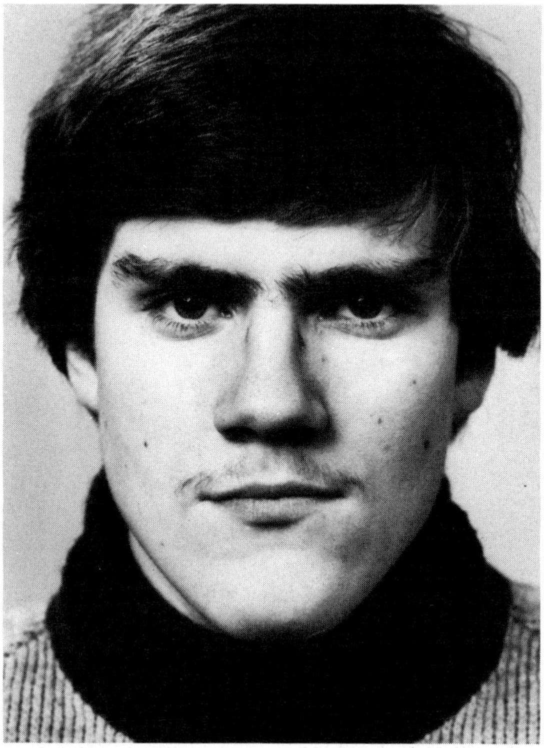

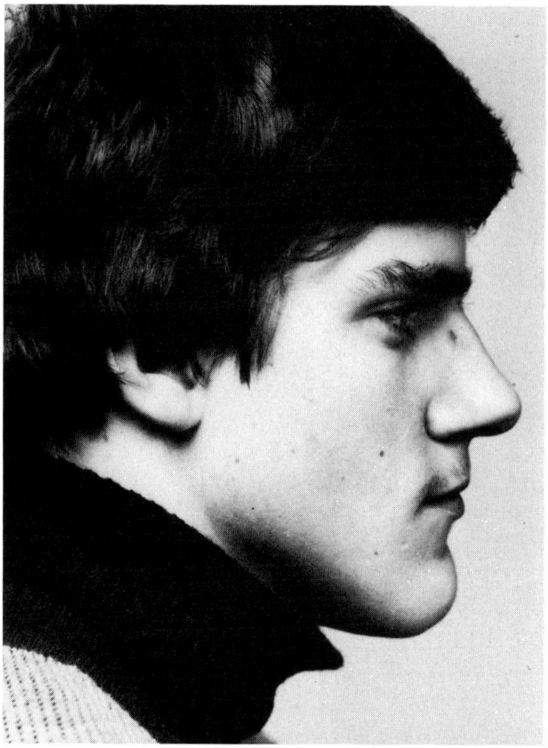

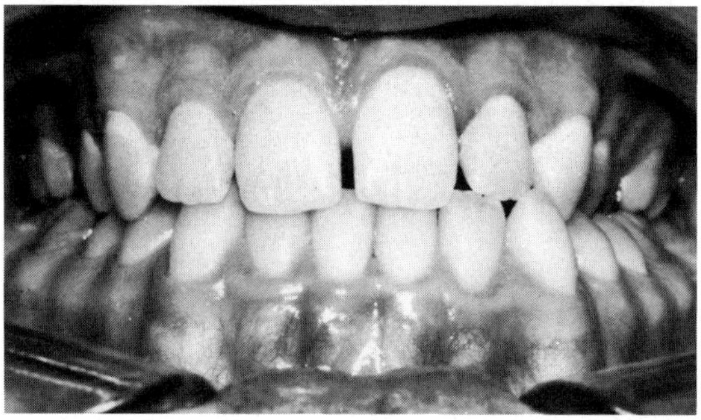

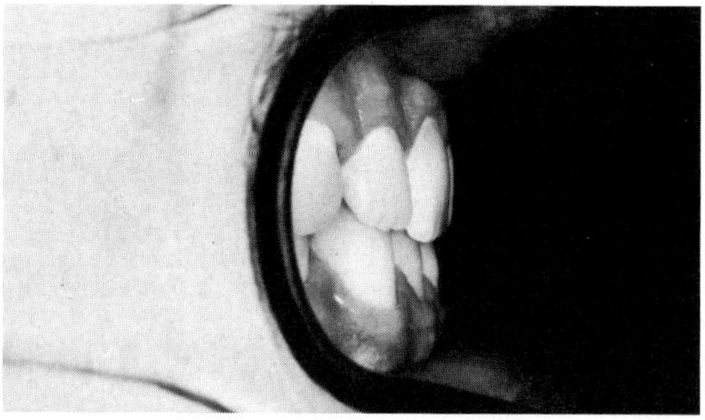

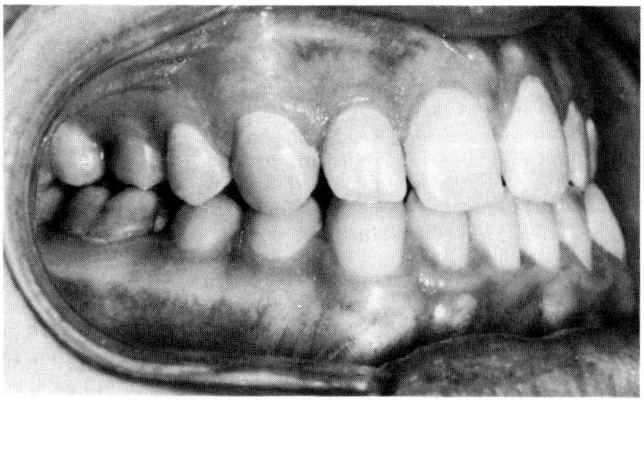

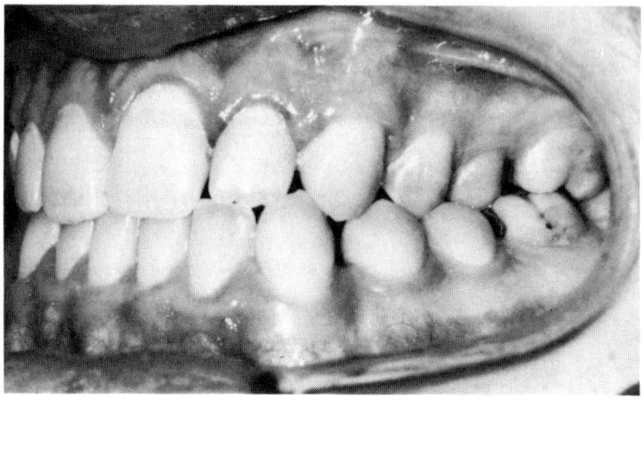

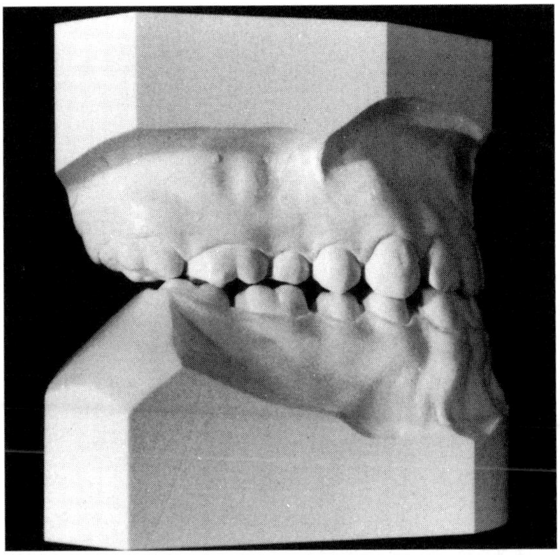
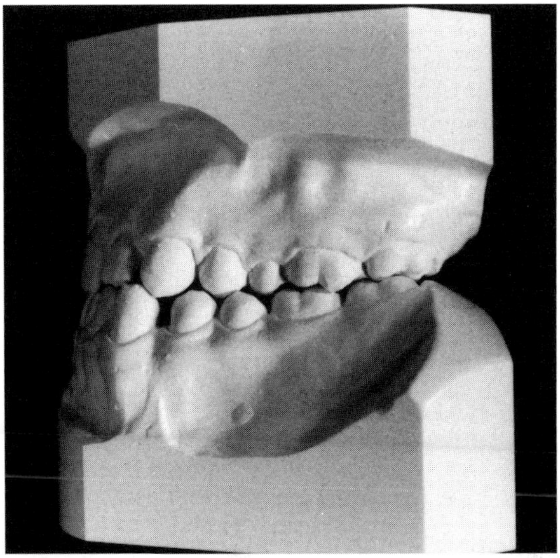
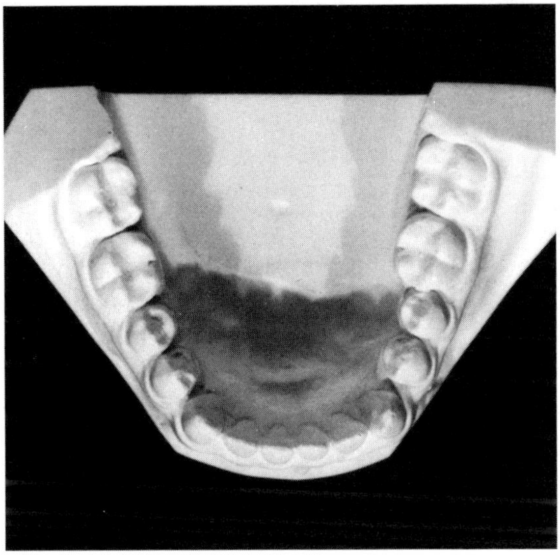
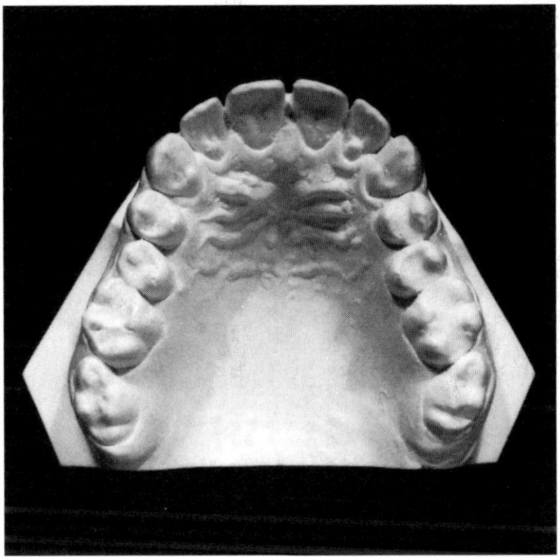

Figs 37-11 and 37-12 At the age of 18 y, 2 mo, there is still an acceptable profile, though the mandible has moved further ventrally than the maxilla. The overjet and overbite have diminished and the maxillary incisors are now showing more labioversion than 2½ years previously. The posterior teeth occlude more mesially and the maxillary premolars are palatally displaced. Meanwhile the permanent second molars have fully emerged and come into occlusion; those on the right do not occlude fully because there is a mesio-occlusion of ½ PB.

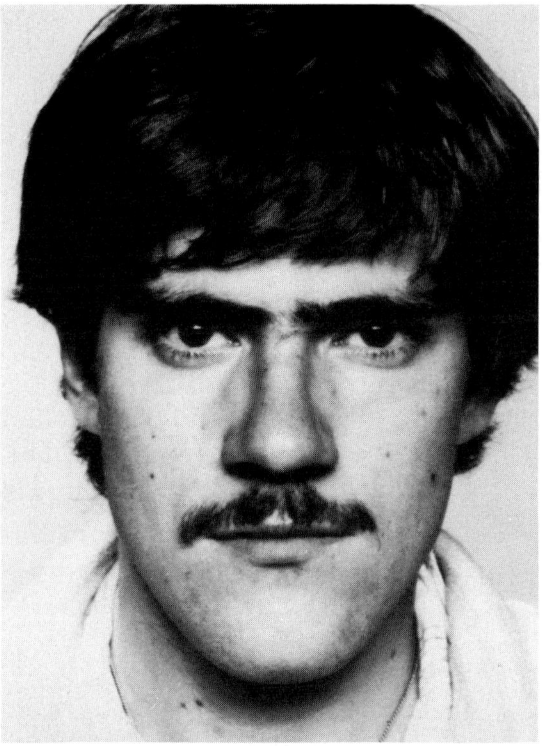

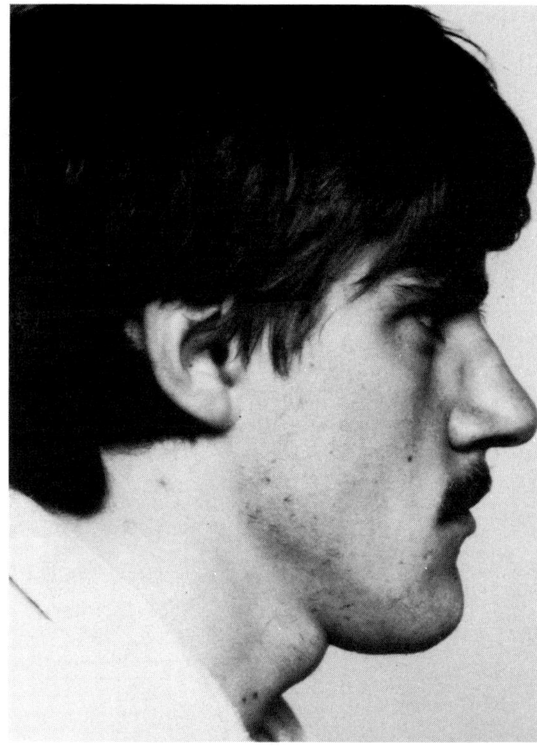

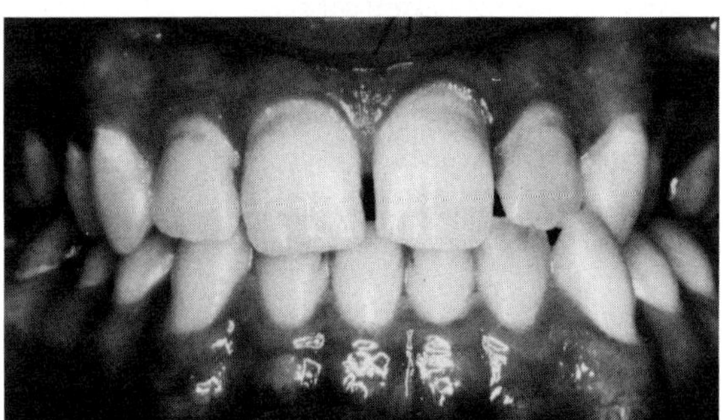

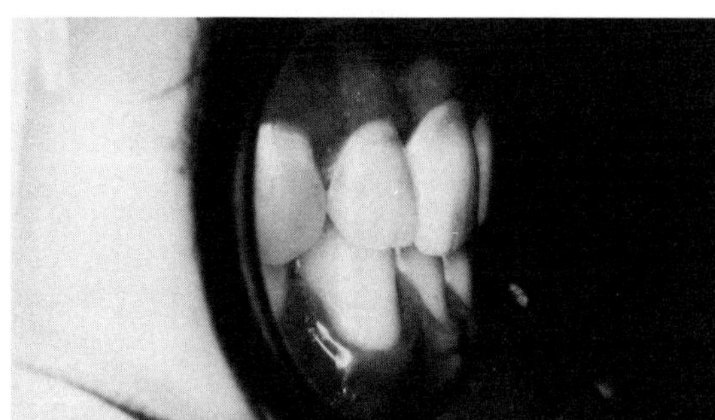

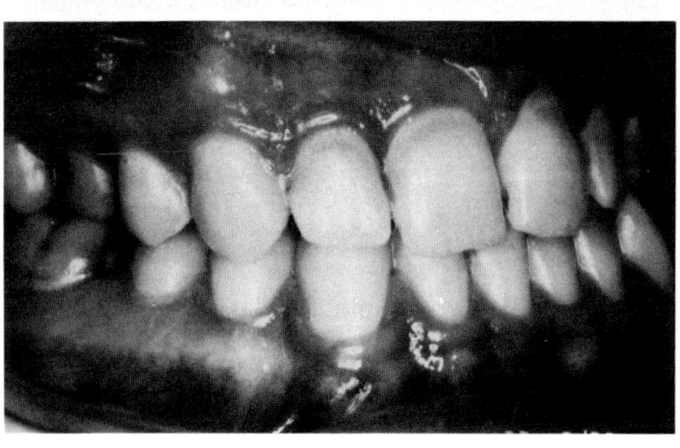

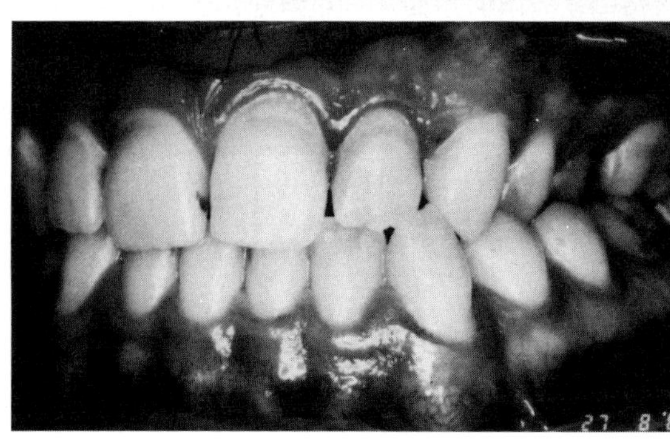

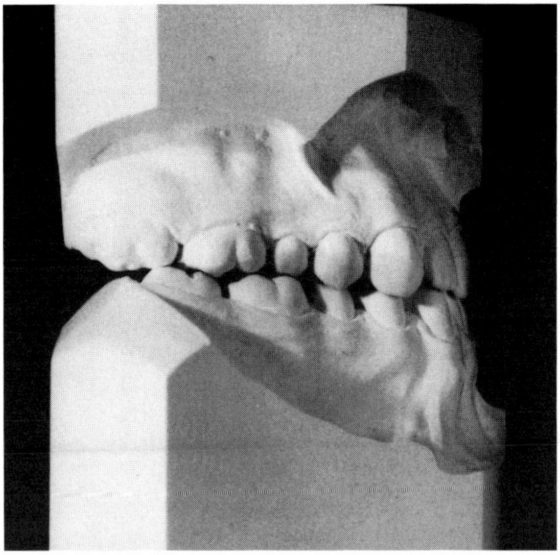
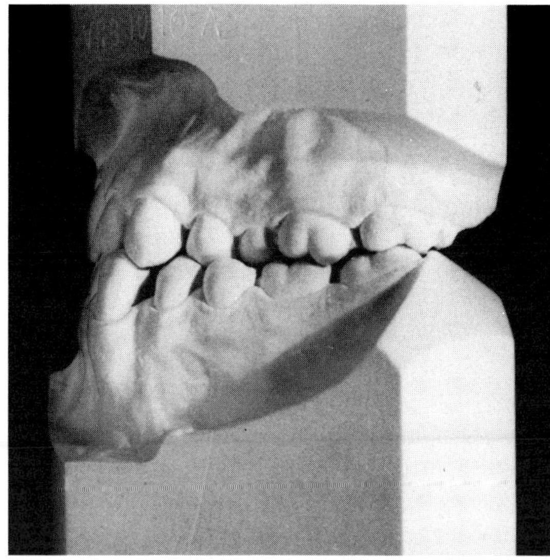
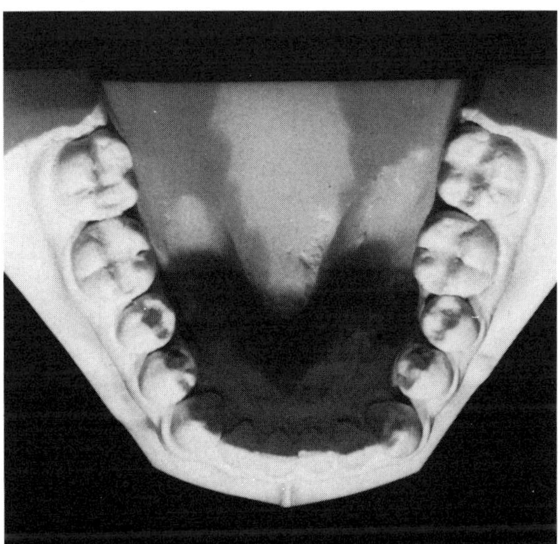
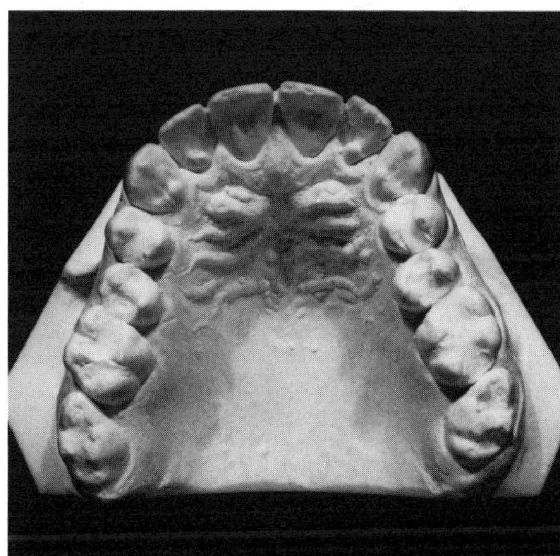

Figs 37-13 and 37-14 *At the age of 23 y, 9 mo, ten years after the end of treatment, the result is acceptable in all respects, certainly considering the simplicity of the appliances used and the short duration of the therapy. In comparison with the conditions five years before, only minor changes have taken place; not an unfavorable situation.*

Men have an advantage if their midface is recessive, which really was not the case for this patient, that they can camouflage it by growing a moustache.

posterior teeth had been eliminated. The maxilla had developed significantly to ventral and it was considered acceptable to end the facial orthopedic therapy (Figs 37.5 and 37.15). Six months later, a slight mesio-relation of the jaws was found and some of the improvement in the occlusion that had been gained was now lost. It was decided to replace the molar bands, make a new maxillary plate, and wear the chincap with vertical arms and elastics again. Four months later, a neutro-occlusion existed again and the patient was asked to wear the appliances every other night. Four months later, the frequency of wearing was reduced to every third night.

At the age of 13 years, 1 month, treatment was ended for the second time, hoping that the mesio-occlusion would not return and that the further development of the dentition in the posterior regions would proceed favorably. With respect to this, it was important that the premolars would come into occlusion in a good transverse relationship (Figs 37.6 to 37.8).

Two and a half years later, the mandibular second deciduous molars were still present and there was still no occlusal contact in the premolar region on the left. Not only was the transition of the dentition late, but eruption was slow also. The overjet and overbite were reduced only slightly, this being linked with favorable facial growth (Figs 37.9, 37.10, and 37.15).

At the age of 18 years, 2 months, five years after ceasing treatment, the mandible had moved further ventrally. The overjet and overbite had reduced still further and the maxillary anteriors had tipped a little to labial. On the right, there is a mesio-occlusion of ½ PW, and of the four maxillary premolars, three tend to occlude in a crossbite. From the points of view of function and esthetics, there are no complaints (Figs 37.11 and 37.12).

Ten years after treatment at the age of 23 years 9 months, the picture has not deteriorated in comparison with that of five years earlier; on the contrary,the bite has deepened somewhat (Figs 37.13 and 37.14).

The superimpositions of the tracings have been reproduced in more detail than in other chapters, because the favorable growth that preceded the therapy and the notable ventral movement of the maxilla due to the facial orthopedic treatment are in that way made more apparent (Fig. 37.15).

The photographs of the smiling face also reveal the effects of growth and the influences on that growth (Fig 37.16).

The question now can be asked as to whether or not it would have been better to start with facial orthopedic therapy at once. A chincap could have been used, although the effect of such an appliance is usually limited and the anomaly was located primarily in the maxillary complex, where at that time no permanent teeth had emerged. A period of observation had the advantage that an idea could be obtained of the growth pattern of the face. The initiation of treatment at an early age has however — especially for children whose growth and development of the dentition is delayed — the disadvantage that the treatment often may last much longer.

The treatment described in this chapter shows that it is sometimes necessary to guide the growth of the maxilla over a lengthy period. Attainment of a normal jaw relationship in a short time gives no guarantee that the result will be stable. In general, corrections that are obtained rapidly have a greater tendency to relapse than

Figure 37-15a

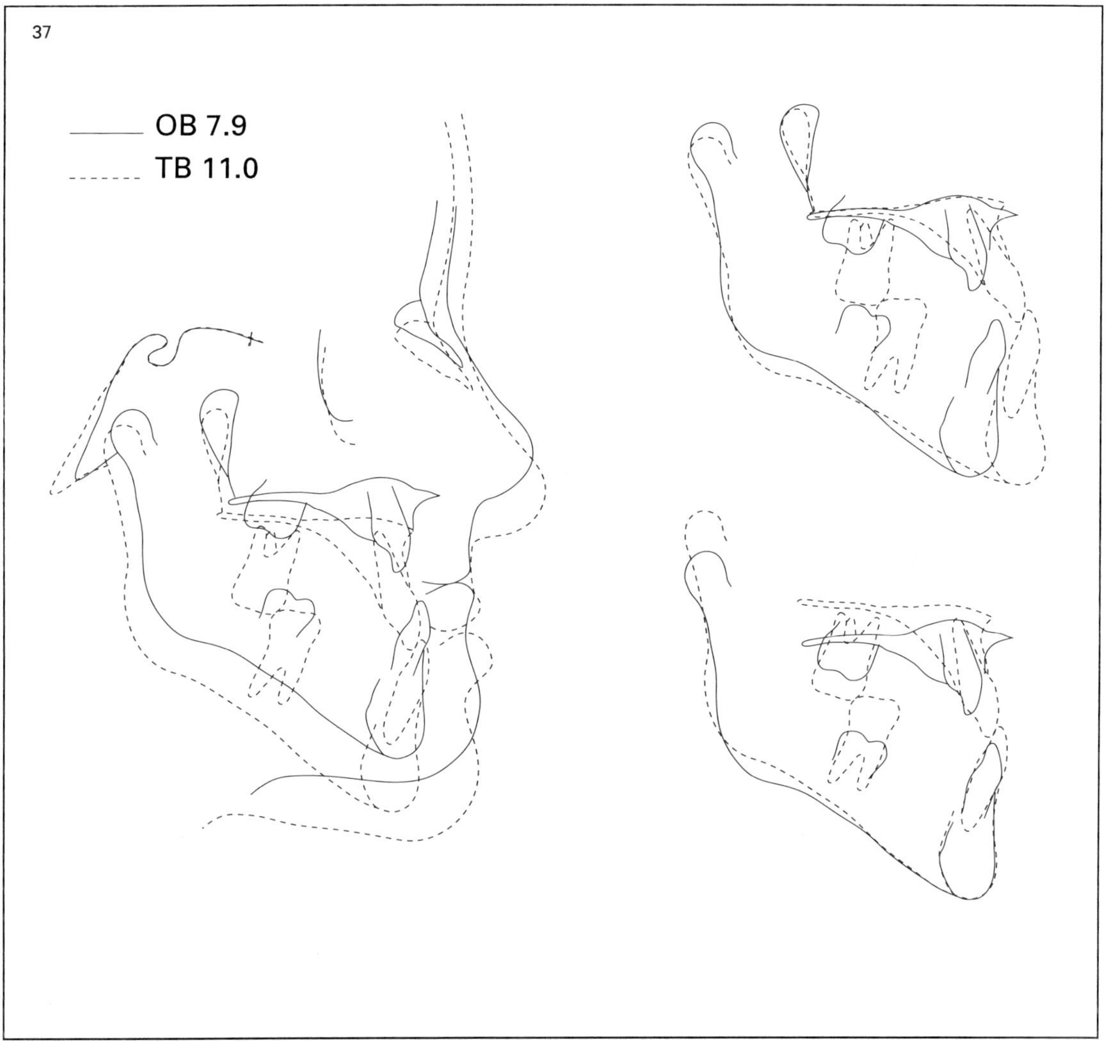

Fig 37-15 The superimpositions from different phases in treatment and growth show that the growth was not unfavouable in the observation period before treatment (a: 7.9–11.0). Much was achieved in a short time with facial orthopedic therapy (b: 11.0–11.7; 12.1–13.1), and after treatment the results obtained were hardly lost at all (c: 13.1–23.9).

Figure 37-15b

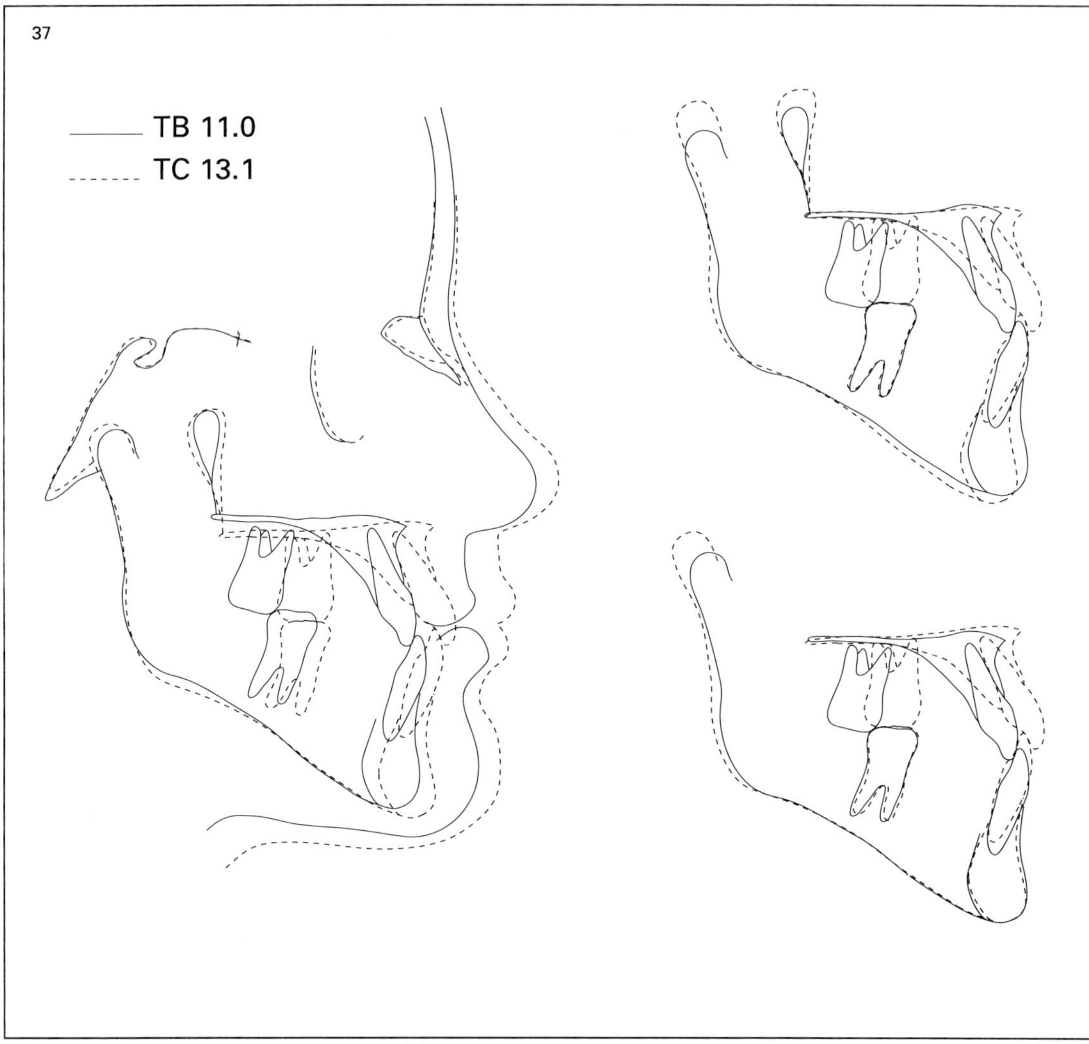

Figure 37-15c

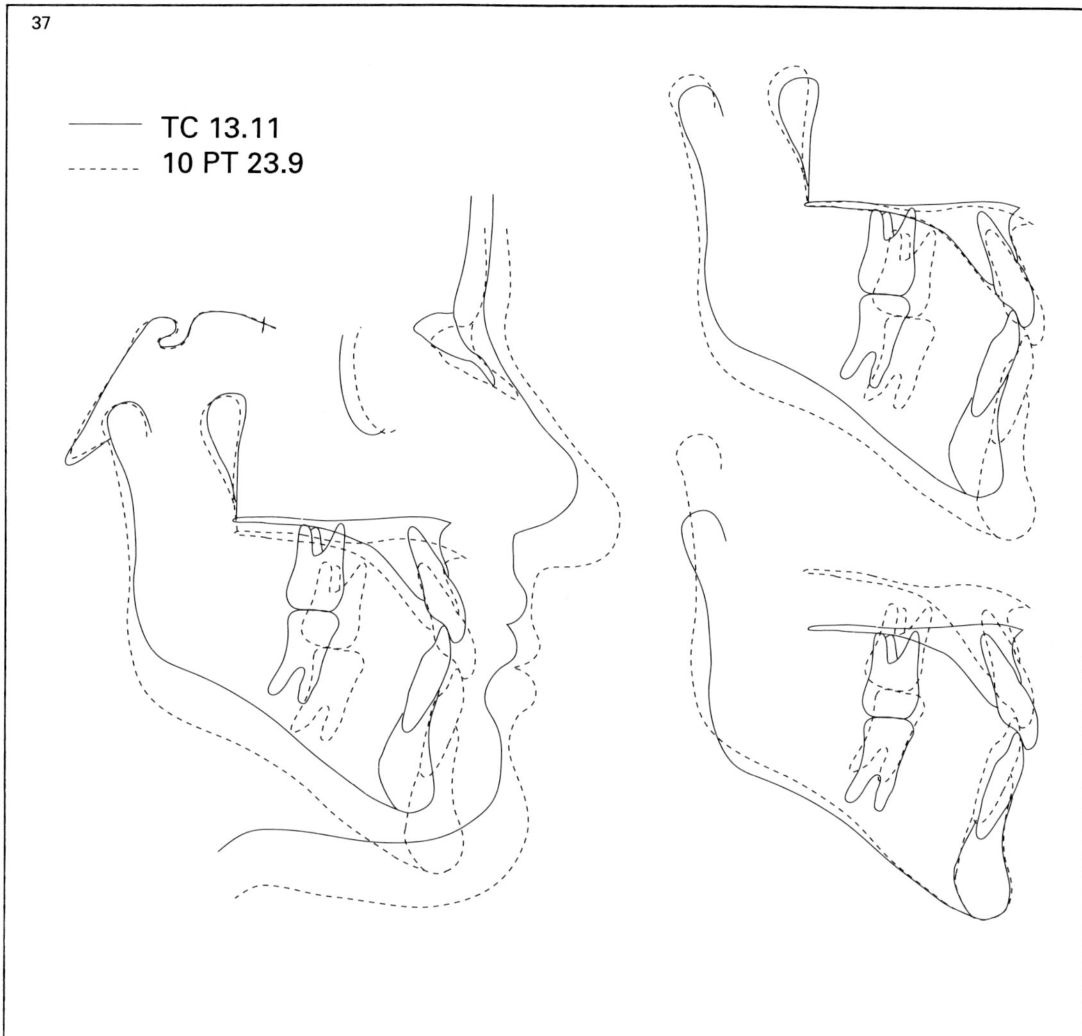

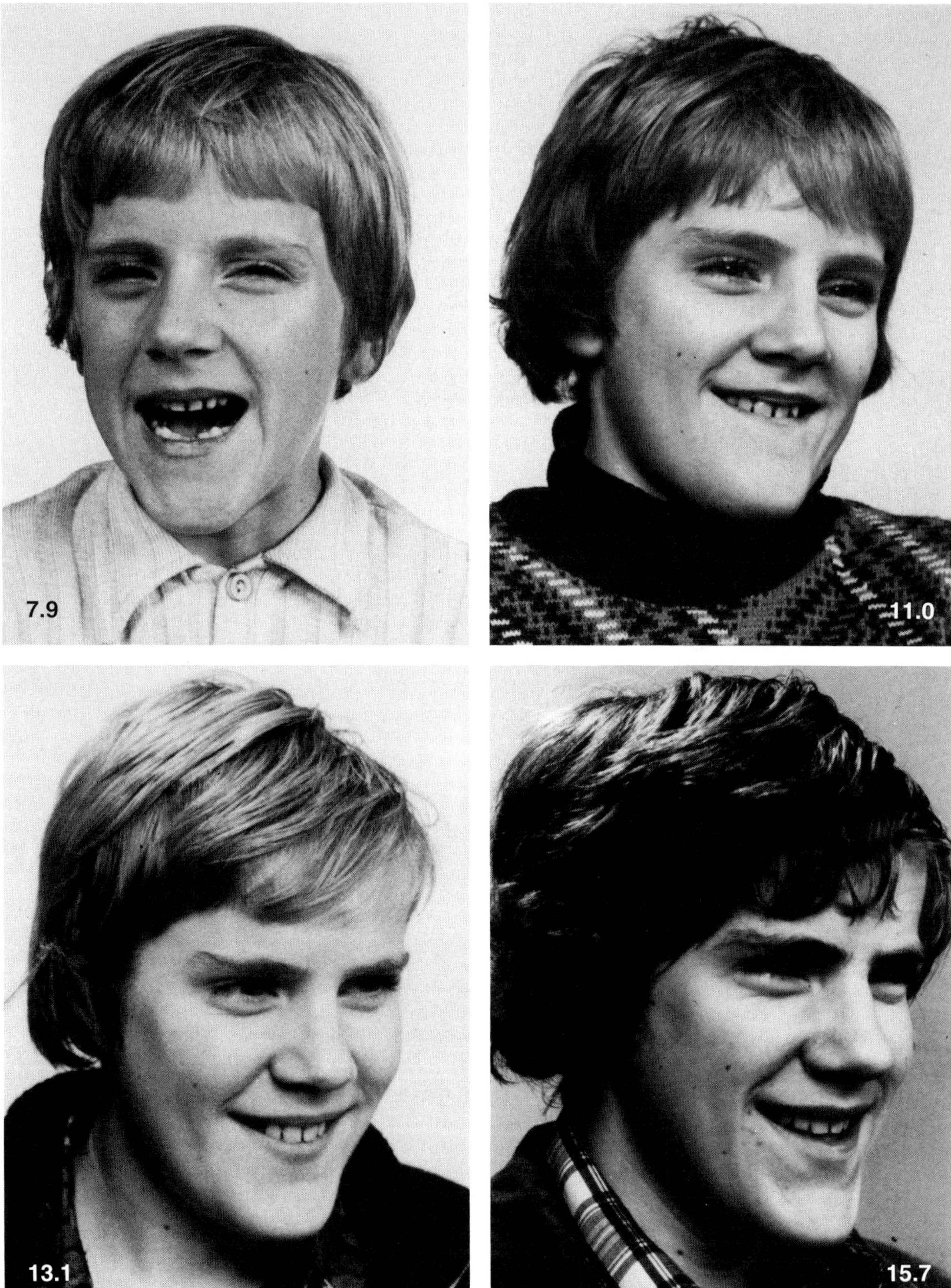
7.9
11.0
13.1
15.7

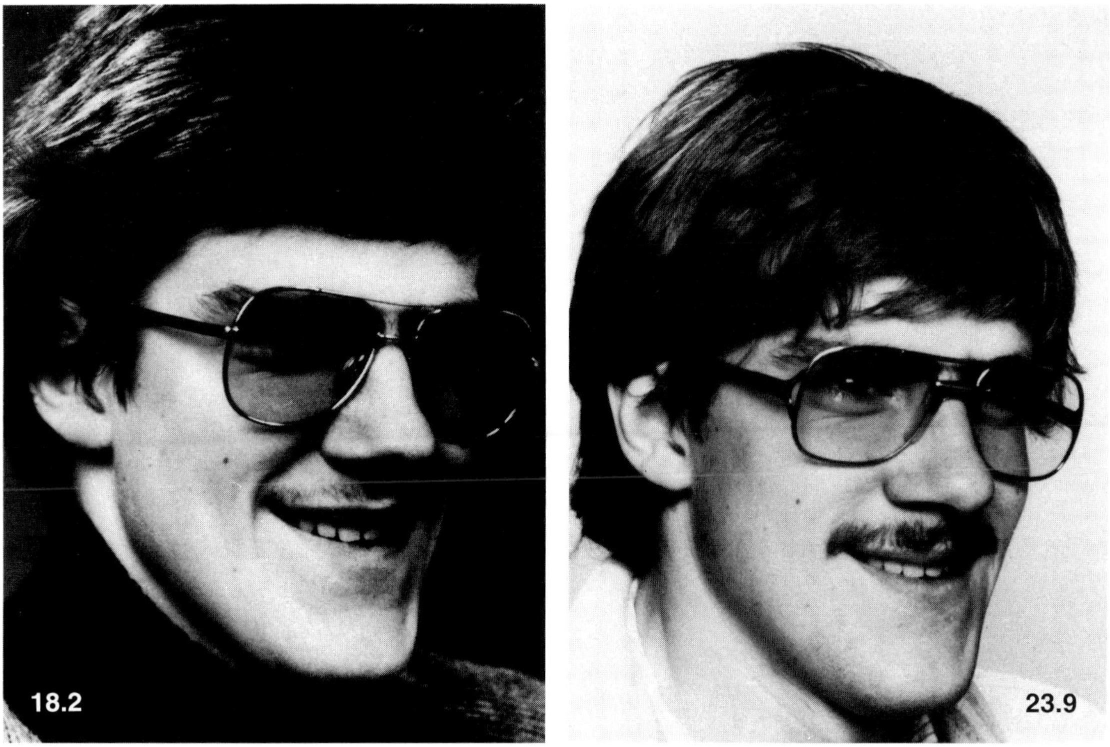

Fig 37-16 Note the effects of treatment and facial maturity.

those obtained over a longer time. In addition to that, an underdeveloped midface always remains to some extent less prominent than the rest of the face, even when the jaw relationship has become normal. Certainly, when there is an insufficiently solid interdigitation in the canine and premolar regions, some relapse must be allowed for. By continuing with the traction on the maxilla, eventually on alternate nights, the ventral growth of the maxillary complex can be stimulated just enough to keep pace with the mandibular growth.

If there is indeed a solid interdigitation between the premolar and canine teeth complete with a good sagittal contact, the dento-alveolar compensatory mechanism will cause changes in the axial directions of the teeth if facial growth is still proceeding. The facial development of the patient described in the previous chapter is a good example of this development. By continuing the ventral traction on the maxilla, the tooth movements that otherwise would have taken place as the result of the dento-alveolar compensatory mechanism could be wholly or partly prevented.

Finally, it is noted that the maxilla was not only set back in the face, but it also was narrow. Suture expansion was perhaps indicated here because it would have favorably influenced the transverse development of the occlusion. Indeed it is quite likely that it would have led to a less deep bite, with the risk that a reversed overbite could have developed again. Whenever one intends to use suture expansion, then consideration should be given to first expanding, then applying ventral traction directly afterward to the maxilla, before the disrupted sutures consolidate.

Chapter 38

Class III, mandibular laterognathia
Facial mask, maxillary removable plate, later mandibular surgery without orthodontic treatment
Female: 10 years, 4 months to 25 years, 8 months

A girl aged 10 years 4 months exhibited a class III anomaly with an underdeveloped maxilla, a slightly large lower face, the lower lip in advance of the upper, and a dominant chin. The mandibular lower border was very steeply angulated and was almost in line with the posterior border of the ascending ramus. The left side of the mandible was longer and higher than that on the right, which caused the lower part of the face to be asymmetric. The chin point and the middle of the mandible deviated to the right. During opening and closing movements of the mandible the asymmetry remained constant. Habitual occlusion and central relation coincided and there was no ventral forced bite. The anteriors were in an edge-to-edge occlusion on the left side and in a reversed overbite on the right side. Two millimetres of gum was exposed in the maxillary anterior region when smiling. The anomaly had already been treated with a chincap for 18 months without any noticeable improvement (Figs 38-1 and 38-2).

It was decided to attempt to stimulate the ventral development of the maxillary complex twith use of a facial mask according to Delaire, with the complementary force in a dorsal direction on the mandible. The chance of success was limited, considering the form of the mandible and the fact that the earlier treatment with the chincap had not been a success. Orthodontic and surgical intervention at a later age was taken into consideration bearing in mind that the asymmetry of the mandible could not be corrected with facial-orthopedic means.

At the age of 10 years, 9 months, the first permanent molars and first premolars in the maxilla were banded with appropriate tubes, hooks were attached, and a maxillary plate was provided. Elastics were used between the first molars and premolars and a facial mask. After six months, a neutro-occlusion had been achieved with an adequate overjet and overbite. The traction on the maxilla was not reduced since there was not yet a solid interdigitation in the premolar areas. At the age of 12 years, 2 months, the patient was asked to wear the appliances every alternate night only, but after two months the occlusion had deteriorated, so the appliance was worn every night. Three months later, an acceptable situation had been regained (Figs 38.3 and 38.4). Once more wearing was changed to alternate nights but yet again nightly wearing had to be resumed because the ventral development of the maxilla remained behind that of the mandible and the posterior teeth were tending to move into crossbite. Once neutro-occlusion was established again, the apparatus

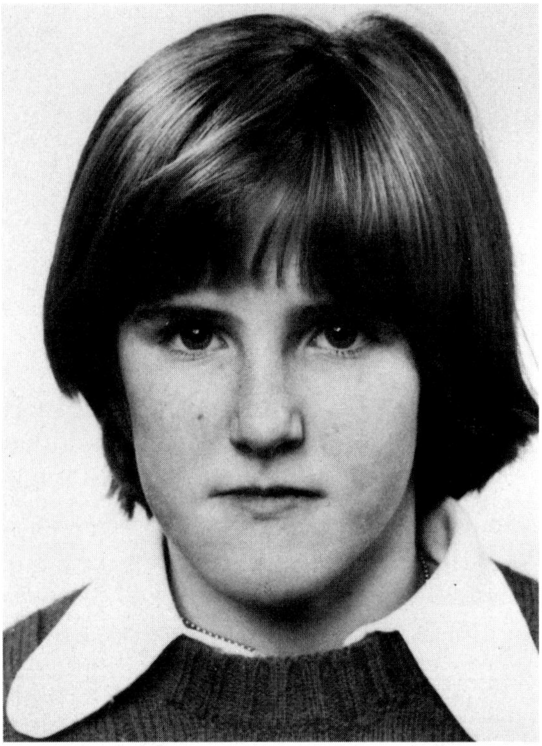

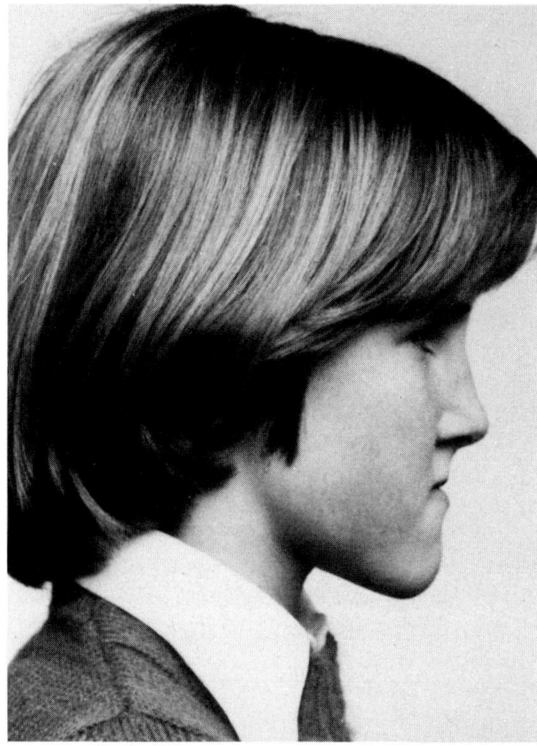

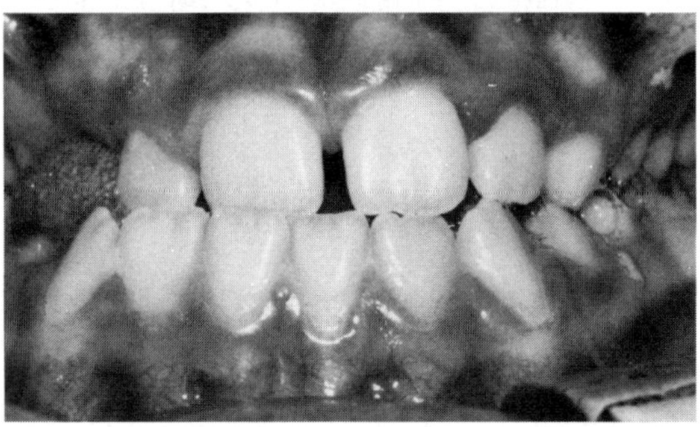

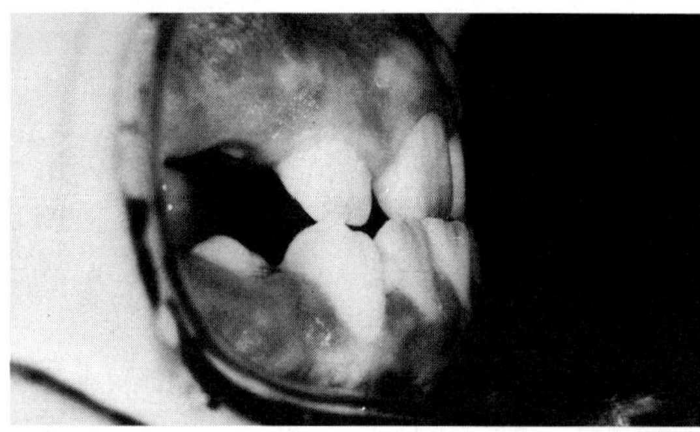

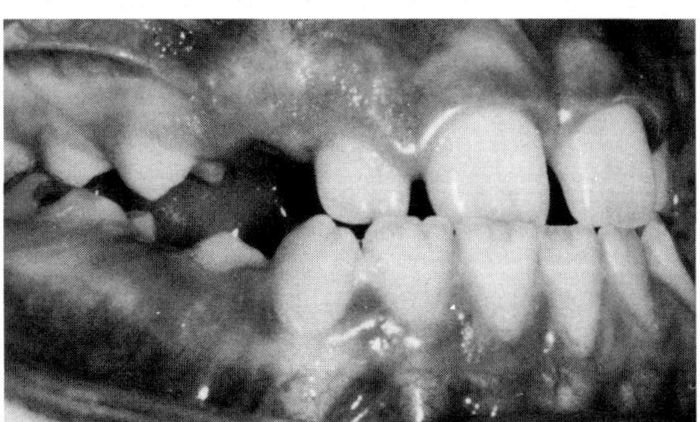

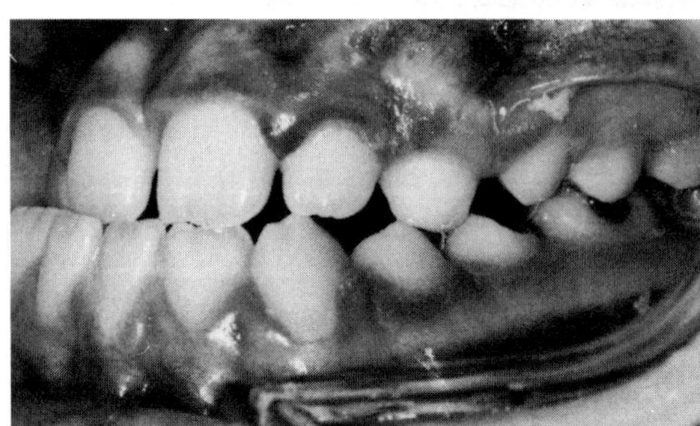

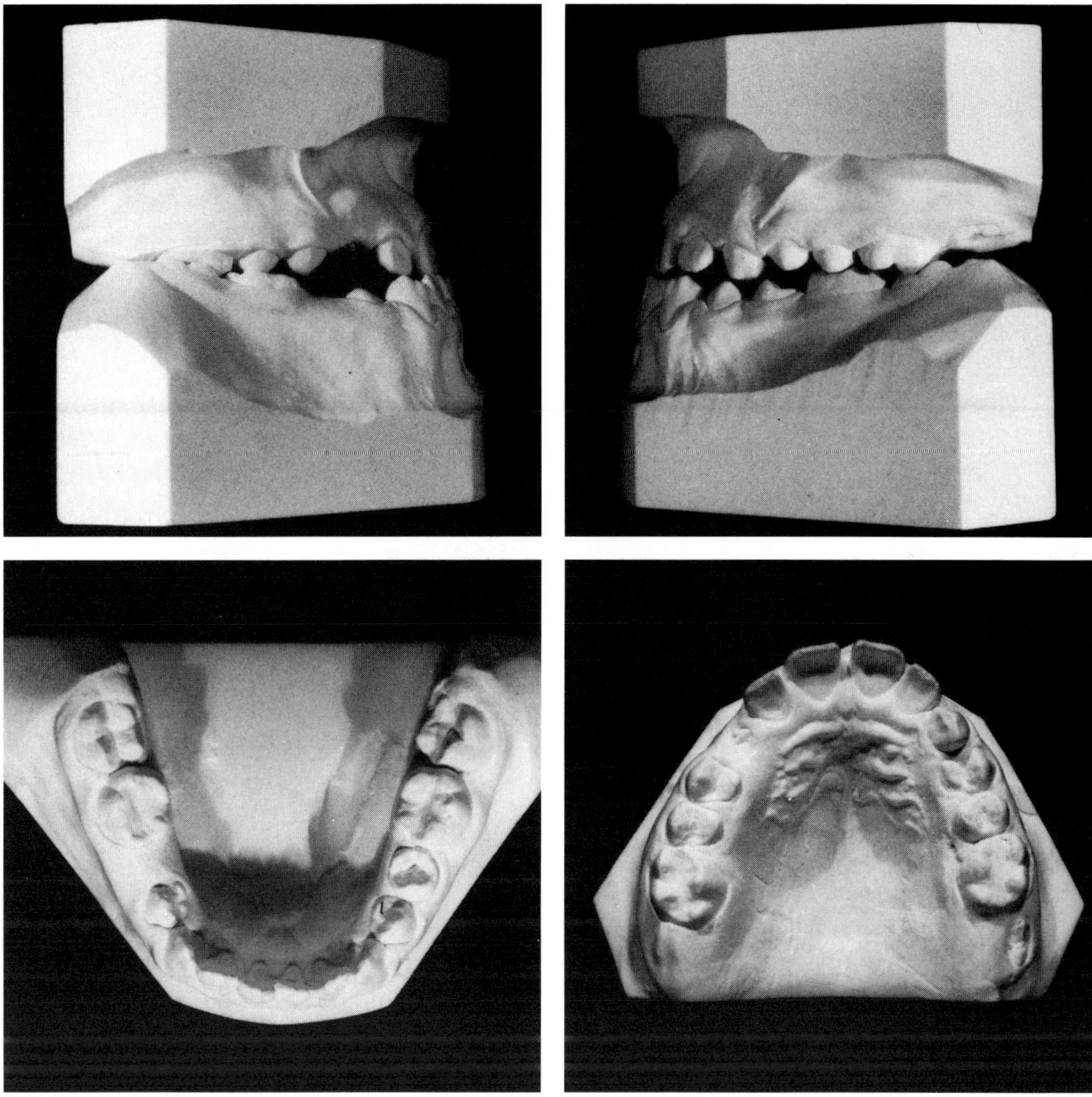

Figs 38-1 and 38-2 *A girl aged 10 y, 4 mo with a class III anomaly, a prominent lower lip, a dominant chin, and facial asymmetry. The mandible is long and the angle between the lower border of the body and the posterior border of the ramus is about 150 degrees. The left half of the mandible is longer and higher than the right. The chin and the middle of the mandibular dental arch deviate to the right. The dental arches are well formed and have sufficient space for all the teeth. The mesio-relation of the jaws is associated with a mesio-occlusion of ½ PW on the left and 1 PW on the right. The right side of the maxillary arch is contained within the mandibular arch and on the left the maxillary incisors and canine are positioned directly above their antagonists.*

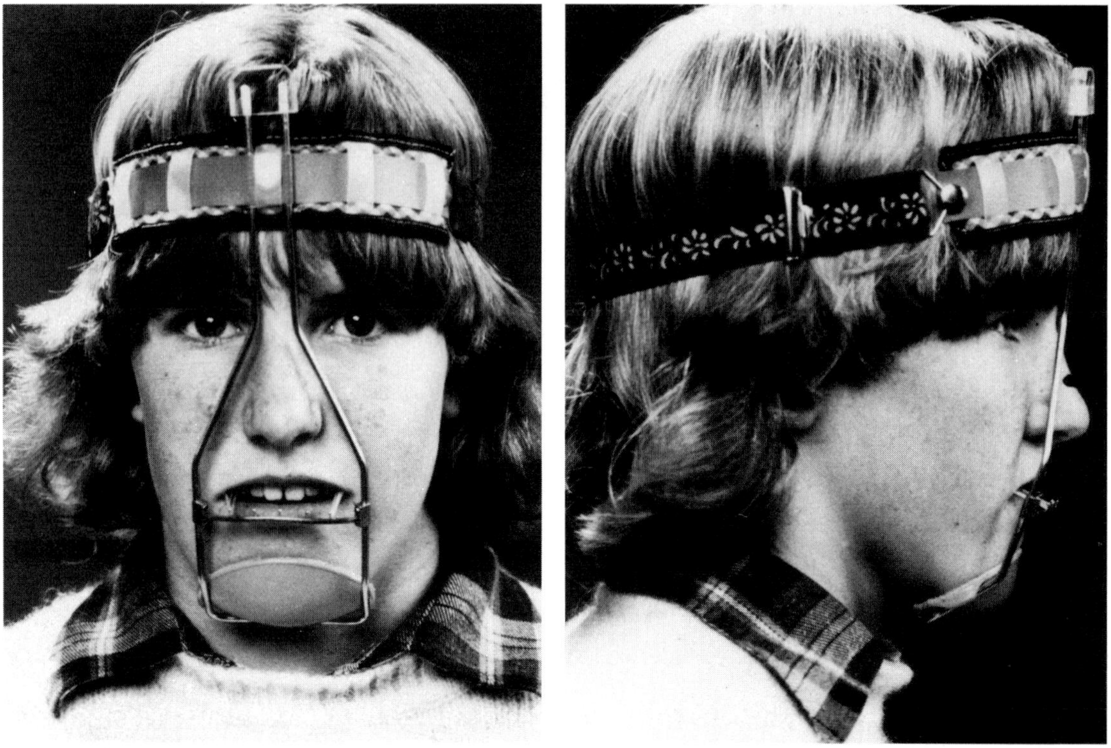

Fig 38-3 Facial mask, Tübingen model.
The appliance is supported by the chin and forehead. The parts of the vertical bars that run parallel above the bridge of the nose need to be contoured to the curvature of the forehead. Then they can be shortened so as not to project above the forehead. The horizontal component in front of the mouth can be moved up or down to the desired position and then secured with the screws. It carries five short projections with ball-ends, which are used to attach elastics. The posts used depend on the width of the mouth and the way the elastics run along the maxilla.
Besides the model illustrated here, there is another facial mask available that runs lateral to the eyes, and this one is more acceptable if the appliance needs to be worn when the patient is not in bed (see Fig 36-17C, page 620).

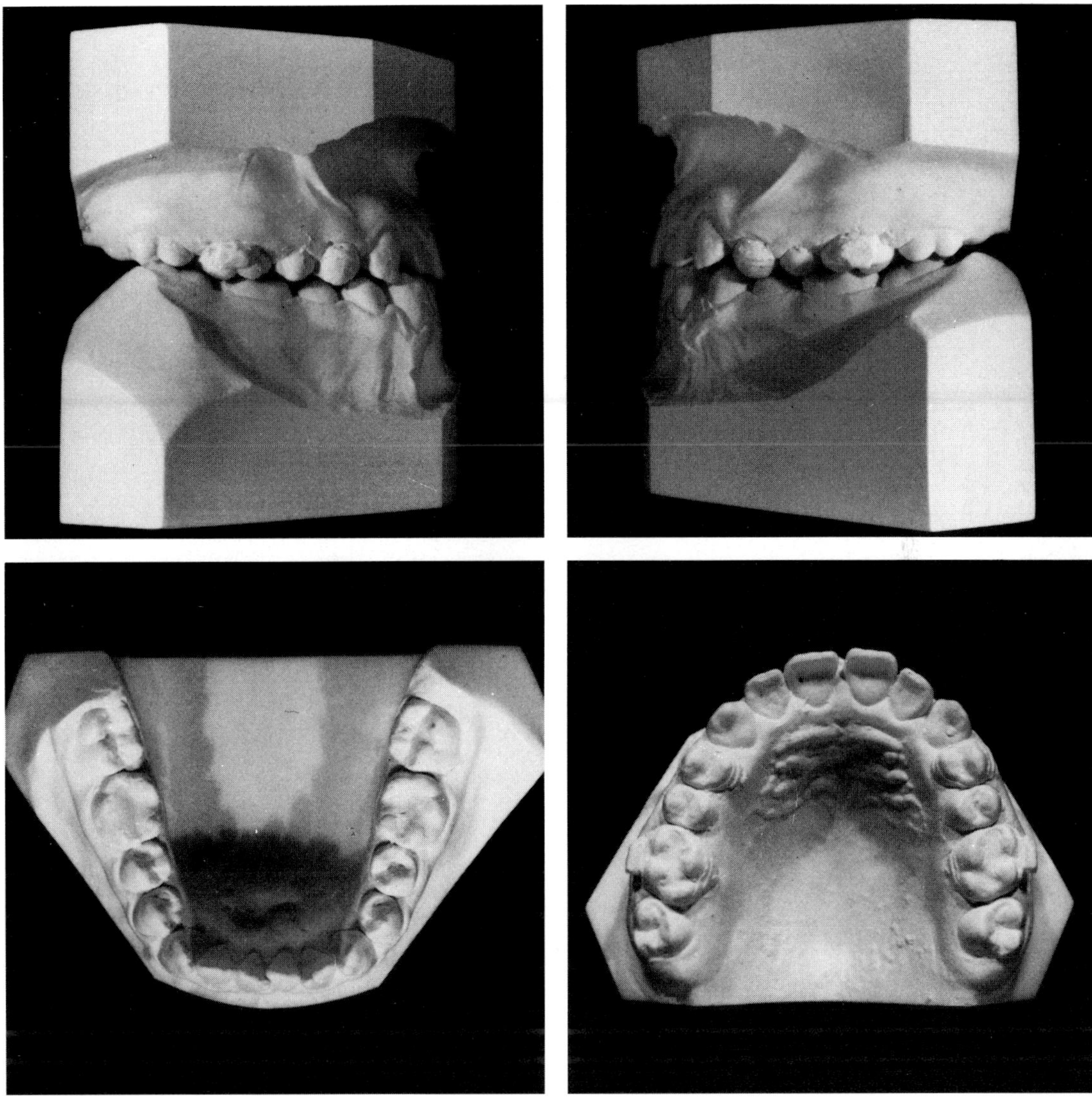

Fig 38-4 At the age of 12 y, 7 mo, a reasonable result has been obtained. The first permanent molars and premolars interdigitate properly sagittally and transversely, and the incisors are in normal contact. The crowding in the mandibular anteriors has increased.

This result proved not to be stable, as became apparent when the appliance was worn less. The ventral development of the maxilla lagged behind that of the mandible and a mesio-occlusion returned, while the teeth in the posterior regions showed a tendency to go into crossbite.

This development corresponded with the occurrence seen when after another seven months a neutro-occlusion was reached and it was assumed that the appliance could be worn less. On that occasion too, it was necessary to return to wearing the facial mask every night.

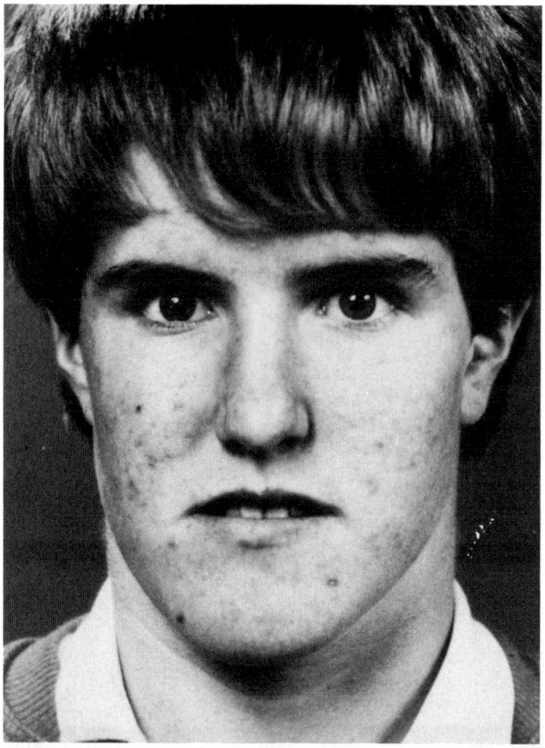
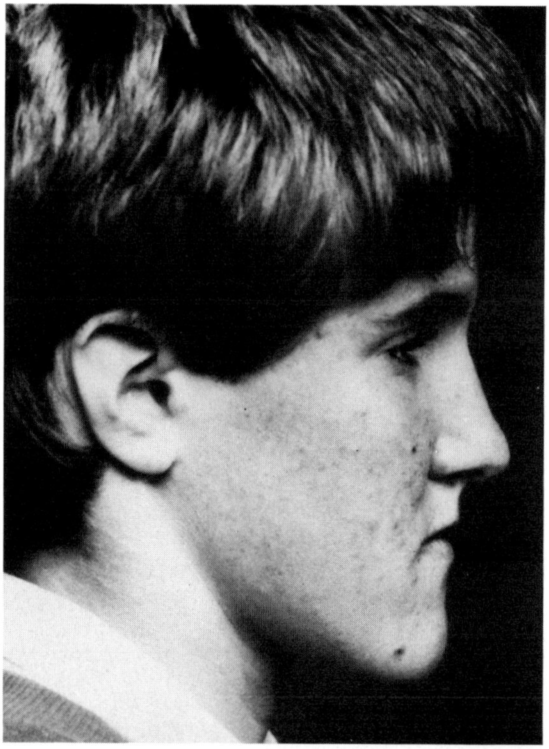
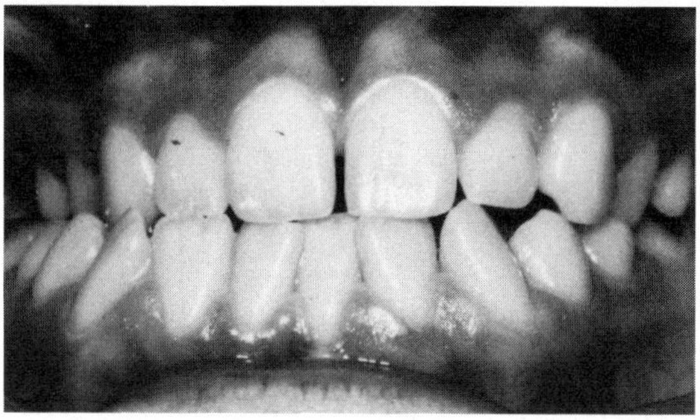
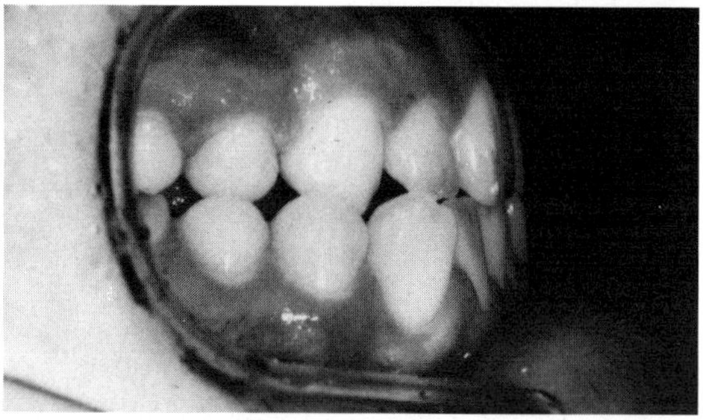
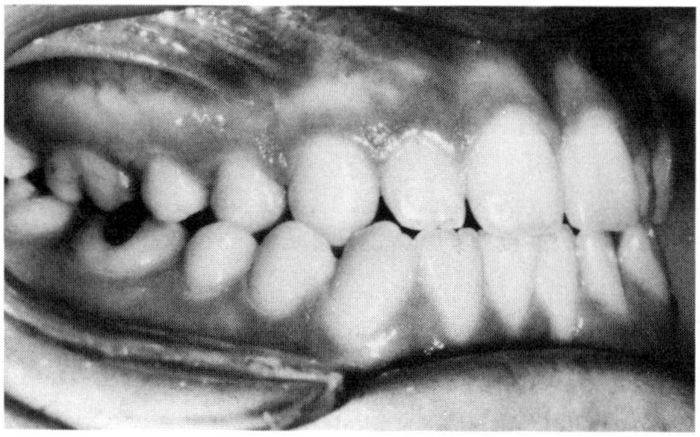
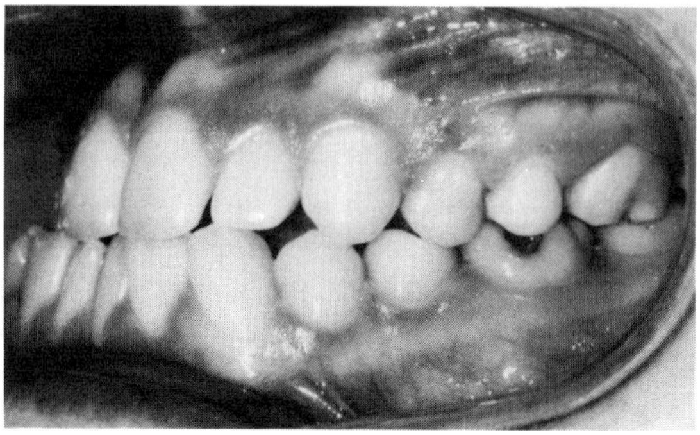

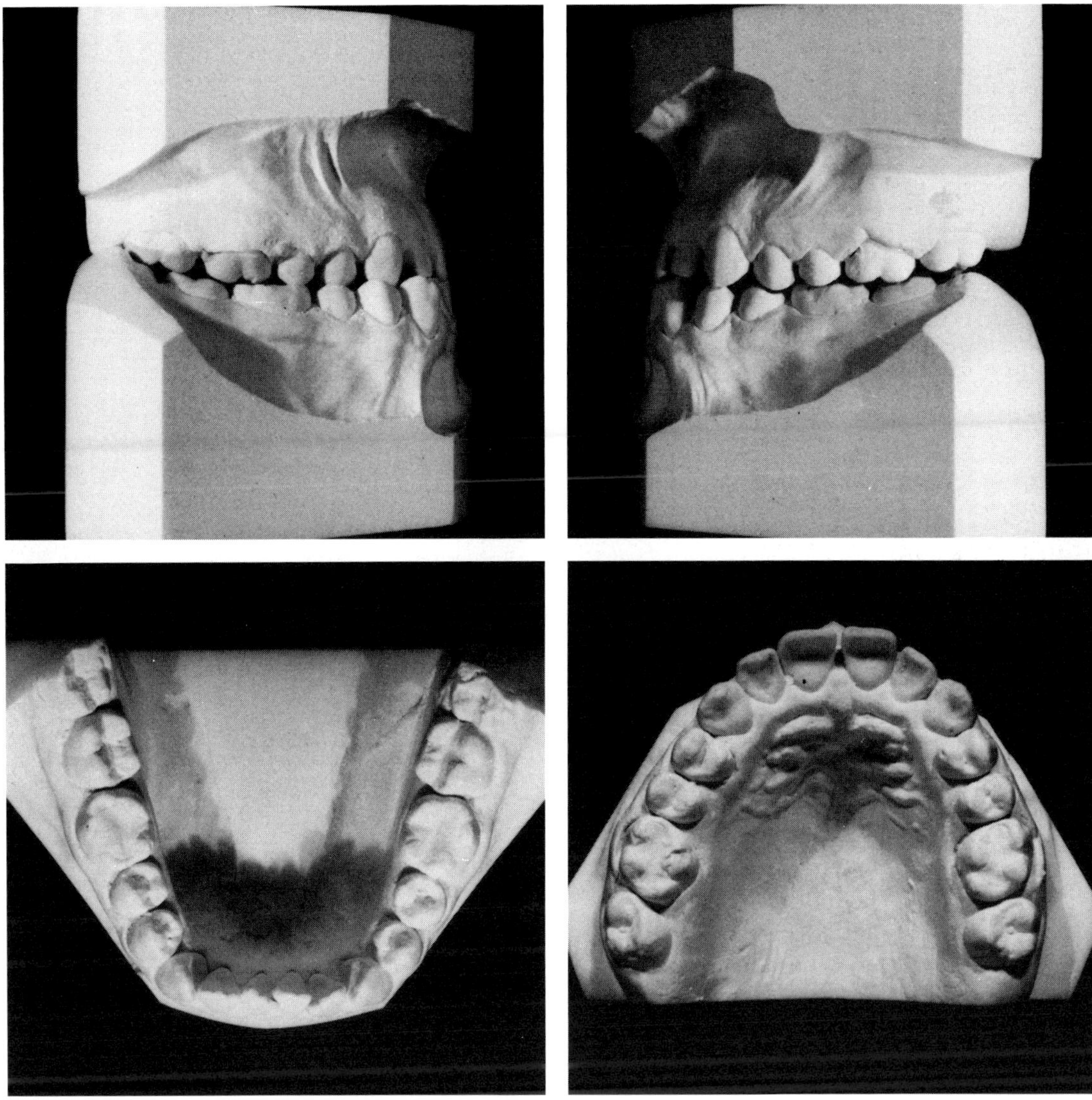

Fig 38-5 and 38-6 *At the age of 17 y, the facial orthopedic treatment was terminated without having achieved a satisfactory result. Although at different times during the previous years there had been a good occlusion, it was clear that the maxilla could not be brought forward enough to keep pace with the mandibular growth produced during the adolescent growth spurt. Moreover the face is still asymmetric; neither the growth nor the therapy had brought about an improvement.*
Because of the fact that the maxillary dental arch is positioned too far to dorsal with respect to the mandibular arch (on both sides there is a mesio-occlusion of ½ to ¾ PW and anteriorly the incisal edges are in contact), a number of the teeth in the posterior regions, particularly on the right, are now in endo-occlusion.

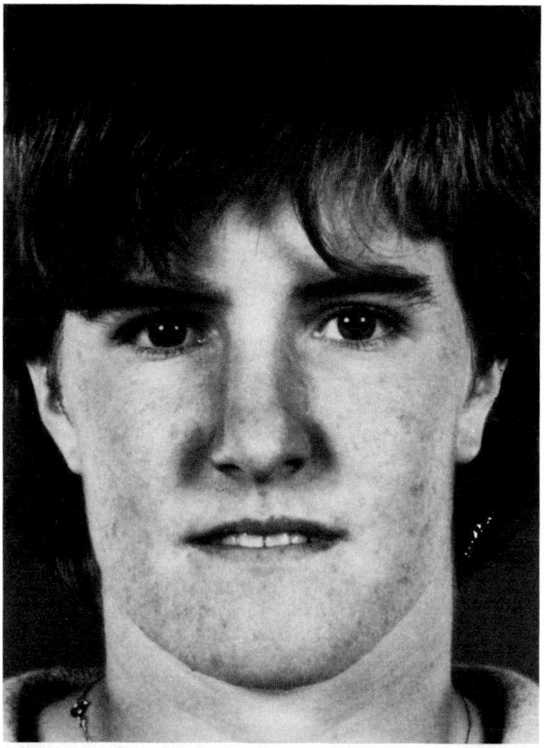

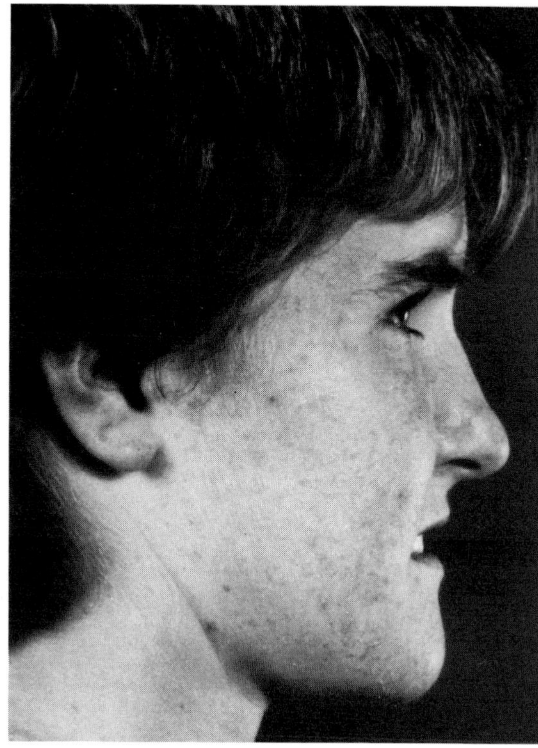

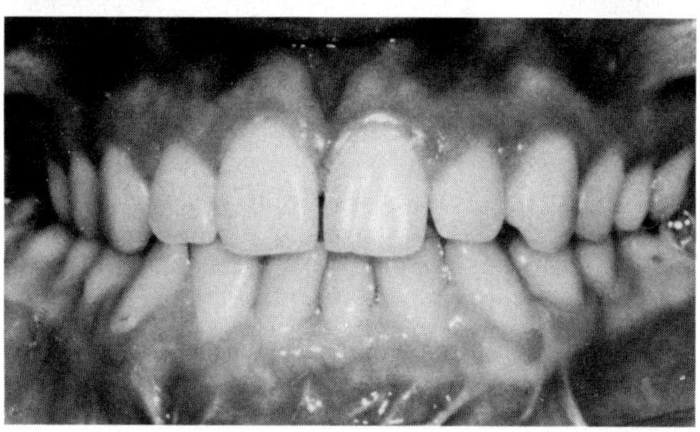

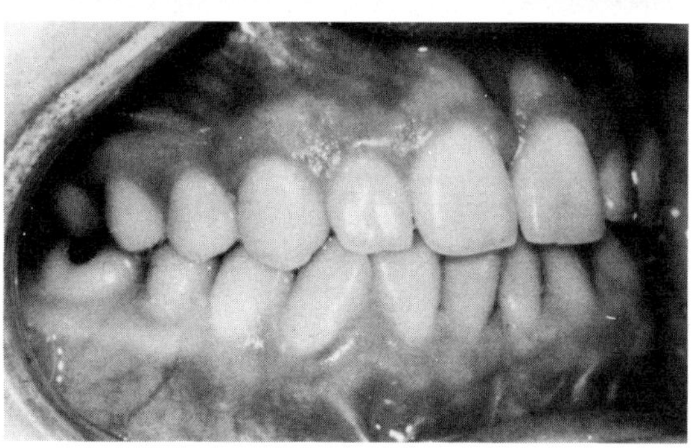

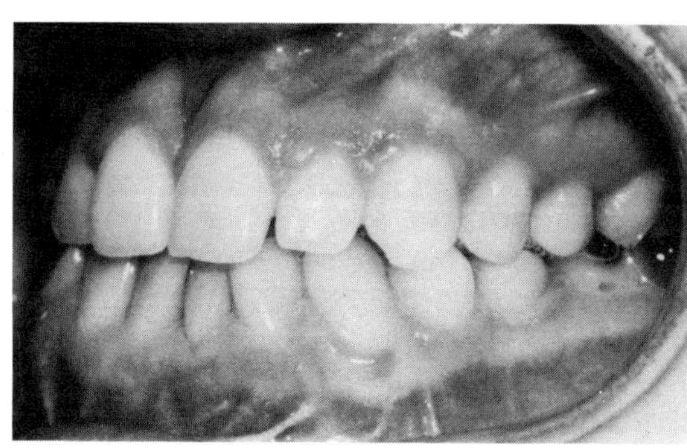

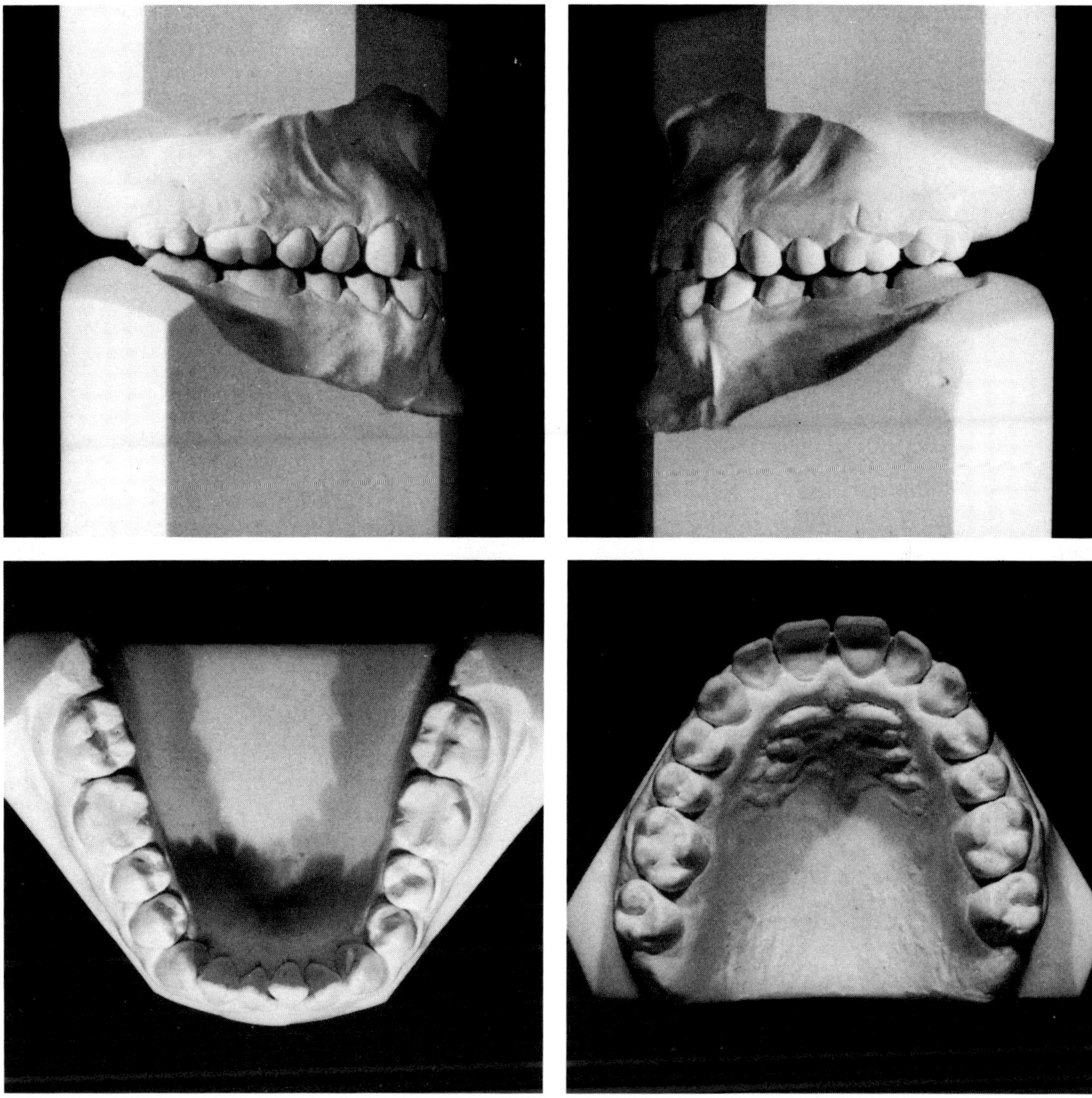

Figs 38-7 and 38-8 At the age of 19 y, a good result has been achieved with surgical correction of the mandible three months previously, in which the horizontal part of the mandible was brought back, the asymmetry done away with, and the bony chin reduced in height. Both dental arches proved to match each other so well after treatment that neither before nor after the operation was any tooth movement required.

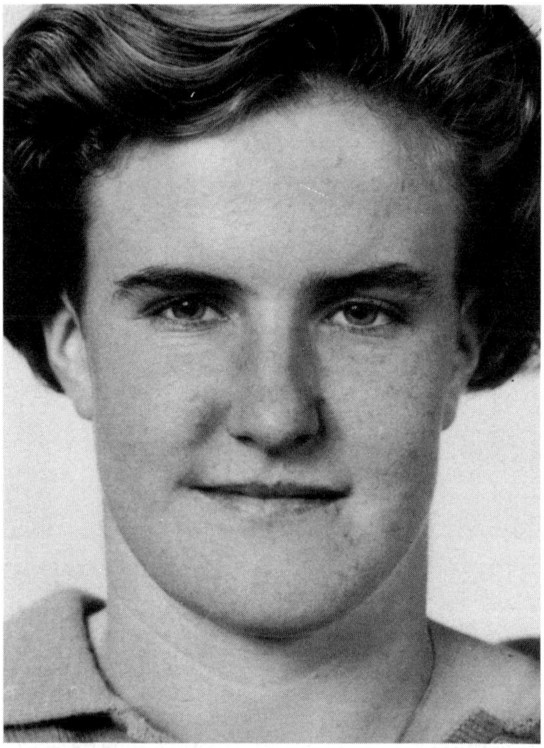
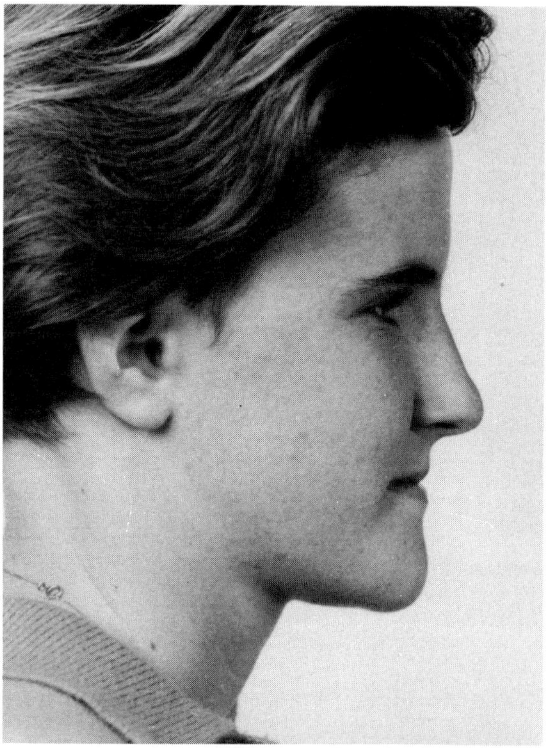
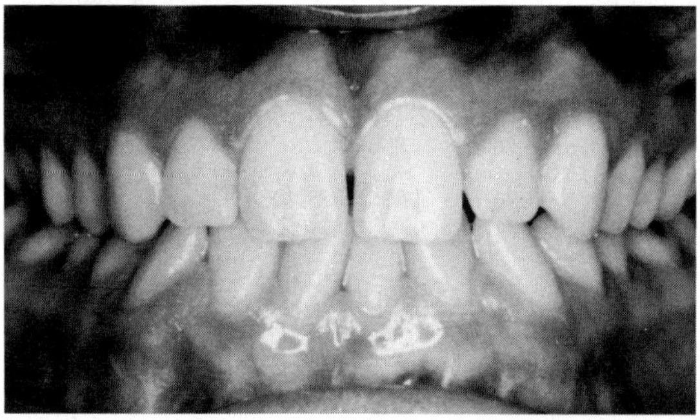
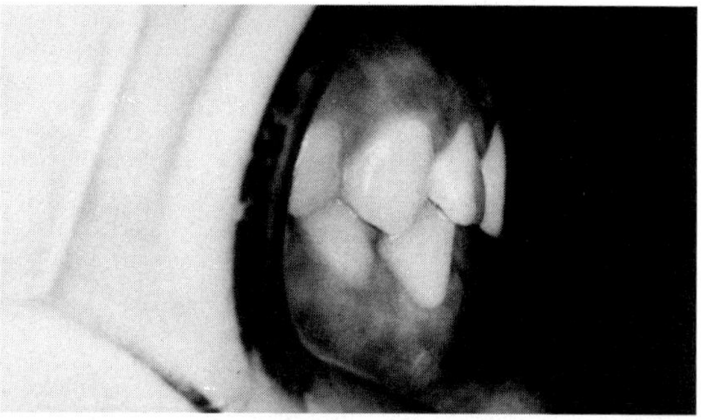
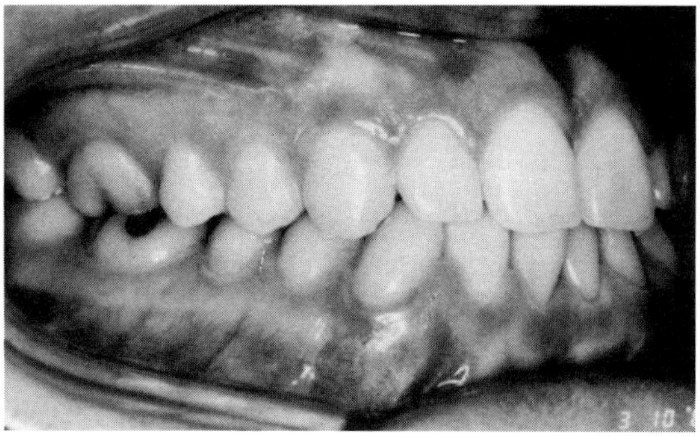
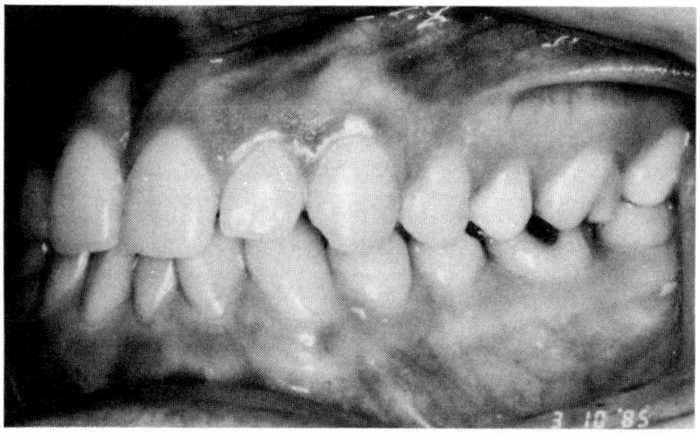

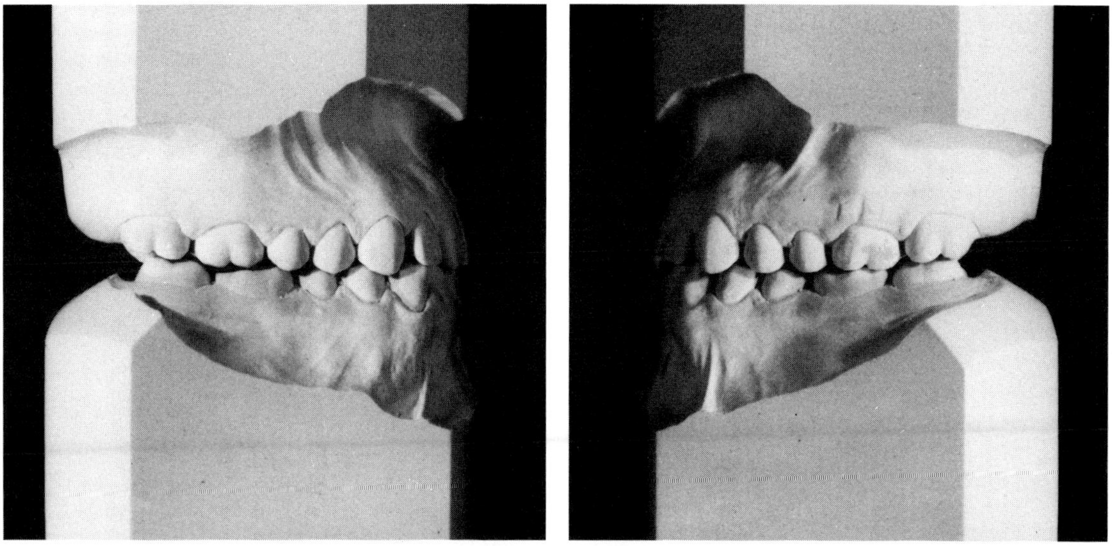

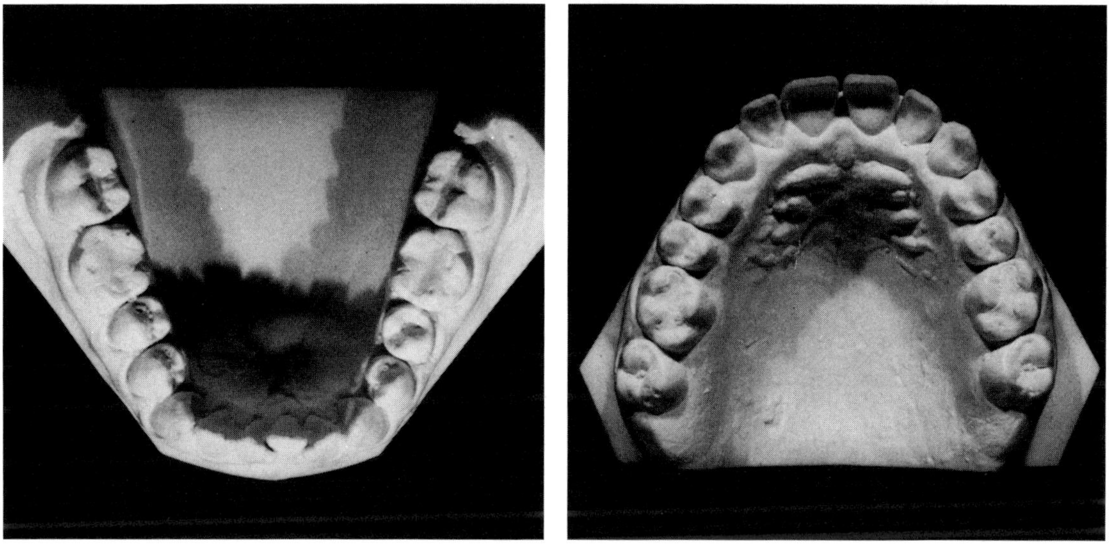

Figs 38-9 and 38-10 *At the age of 21 y, two years and three months postoperatively, it could be seen that none of the improvements gained by the operation had been lost, neither in the face nor in the dentition. The sagittal and vertical overbites have not diminished, the midlines of both dental arches still match, and there is neutro-occlusion in the posterior regions where all premolars and molars are solidly interdigitating. The crowding in the mandibular anteriors has not increased; the central diastema in the maxilla has not become larger.*

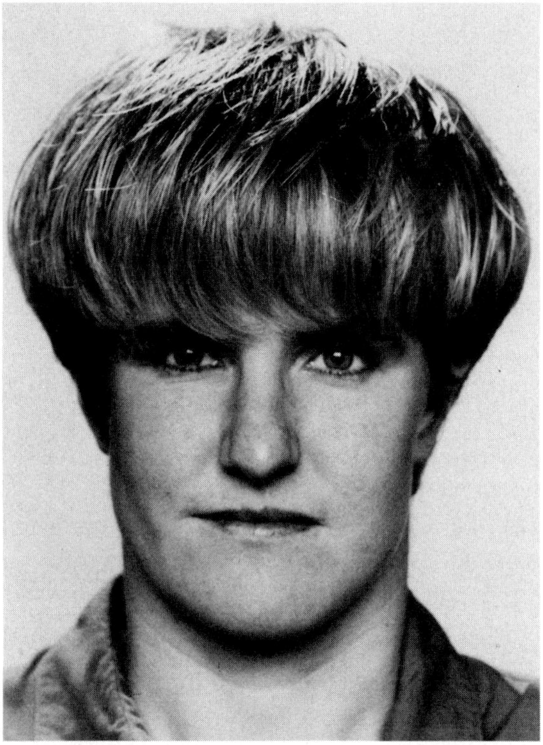

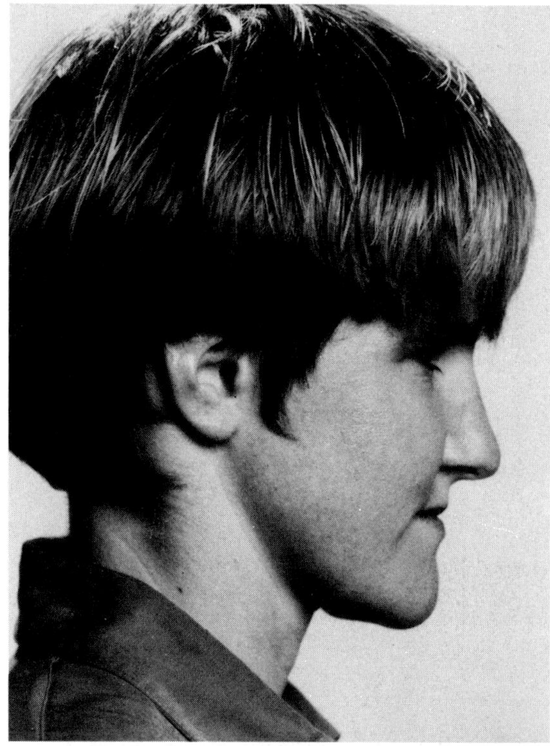

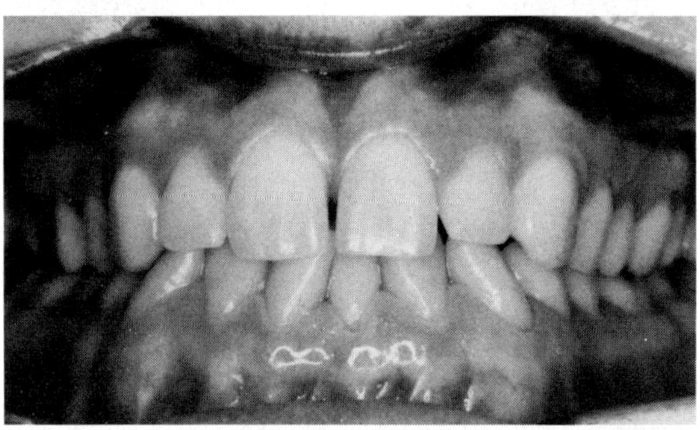

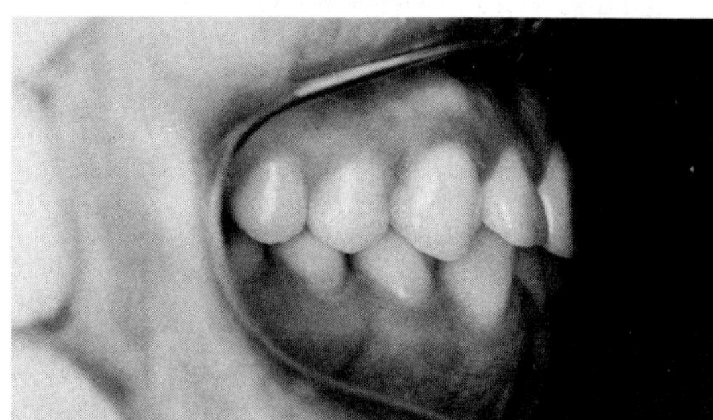

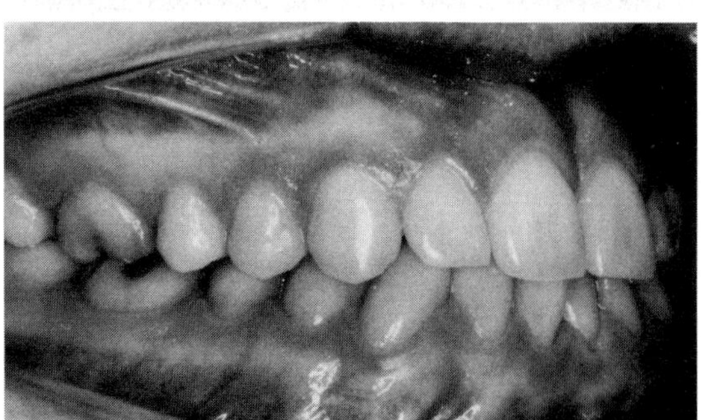

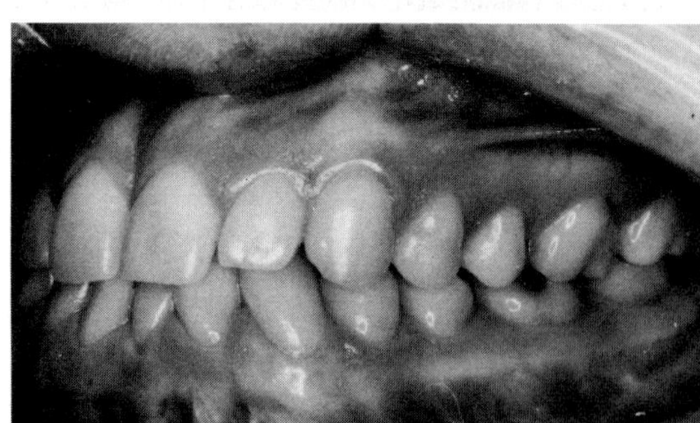

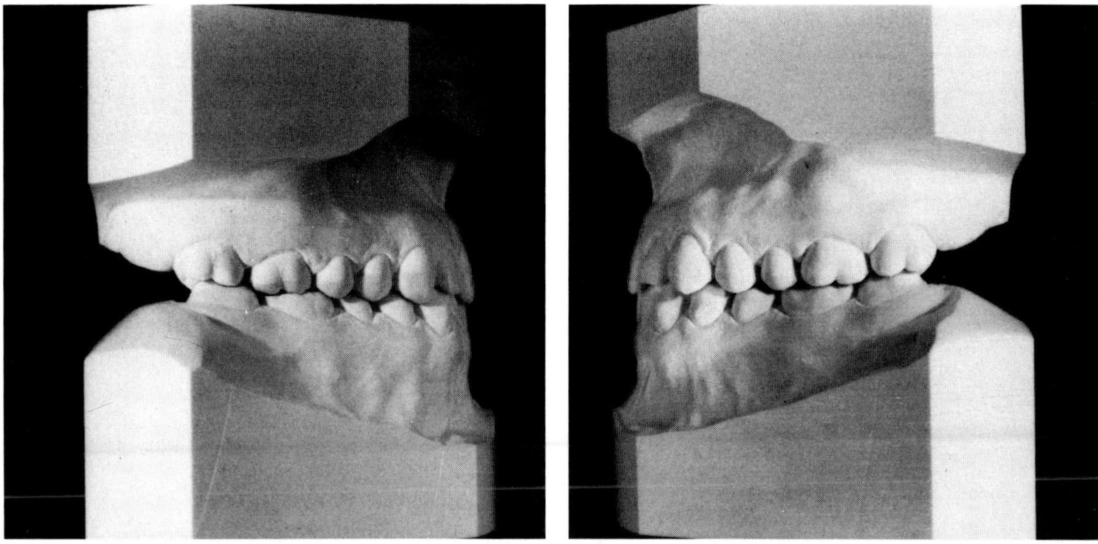

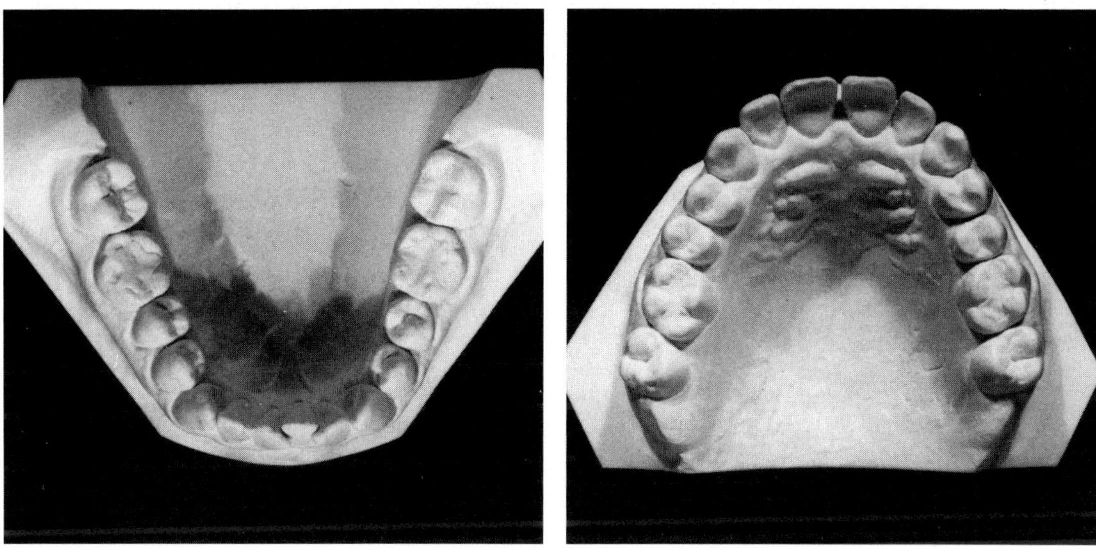

Figs 38-11 and 38-12 *At the age of 25 y, 9 mo, seven years after the operation, the picture is not noticeably different from what it was three years previously. The dentition functions well in all respects and the patient is pleased with her teeth and her appearance.*

Figure 38-13a

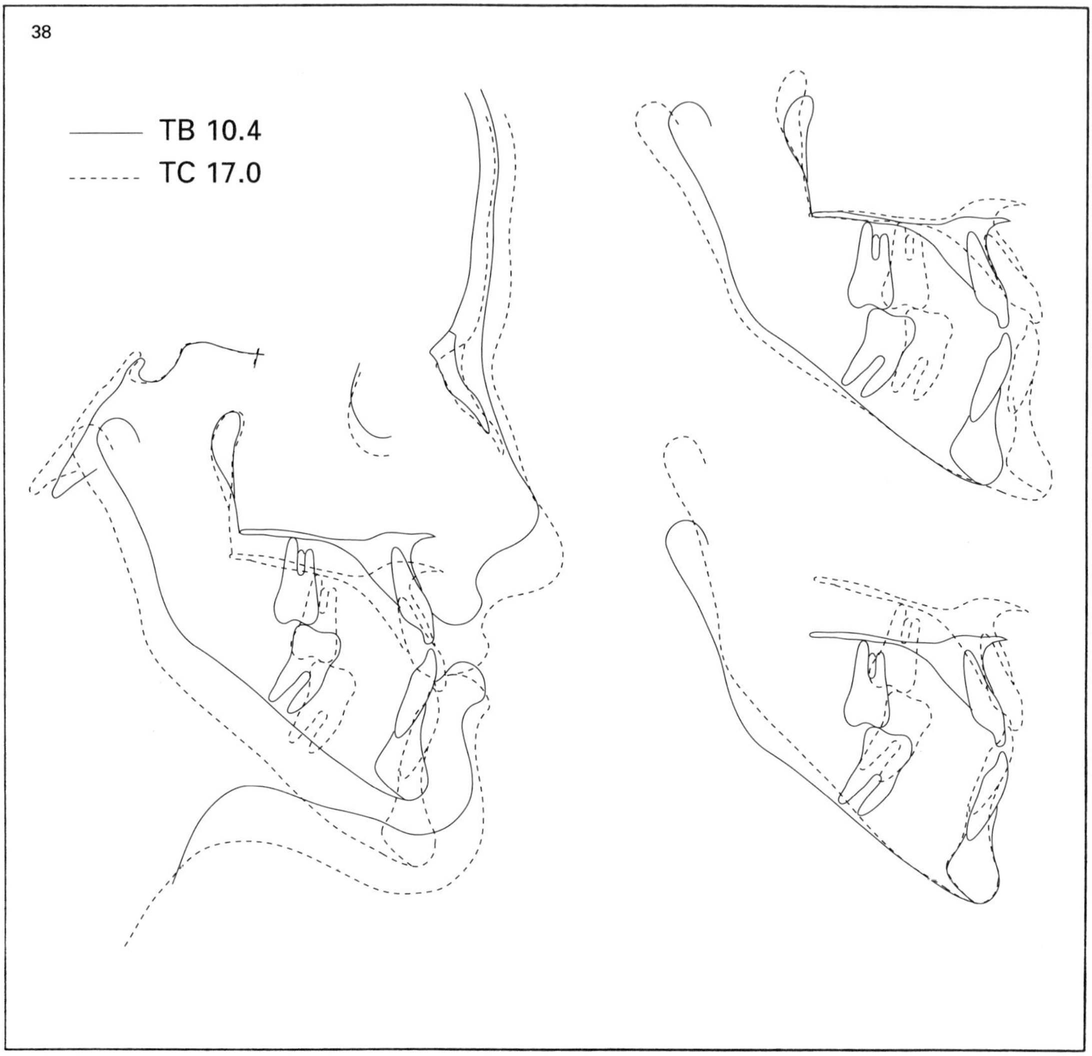

Fig 38-13 The superimpositions of the tracings from cephalometric radiographs show the abnormal morphology of the mandible. The originally dorsally situated midface and the effects from the facial orthopedic therapy that had little success and the surgical treatment that did achieve success can all be compared.

Figure 38-13b

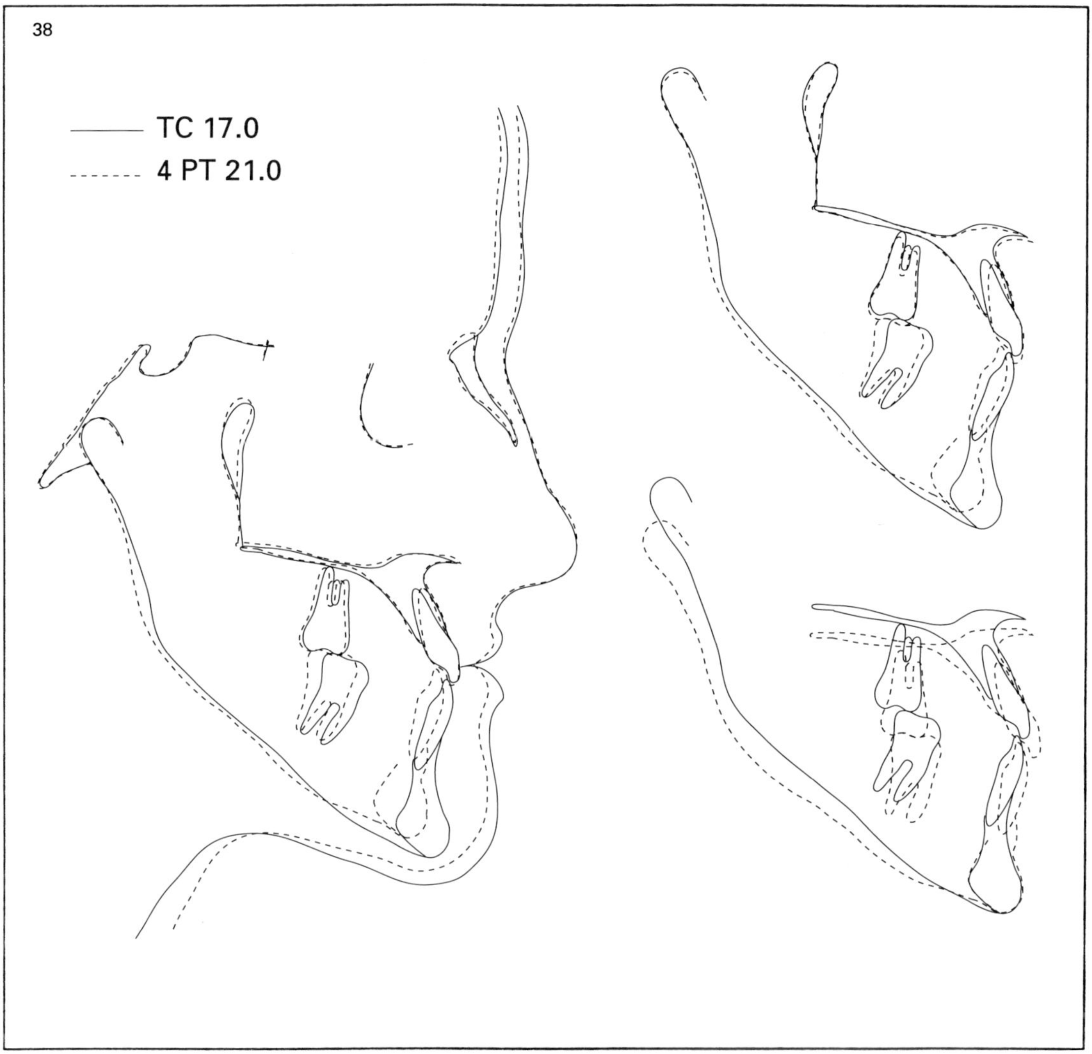

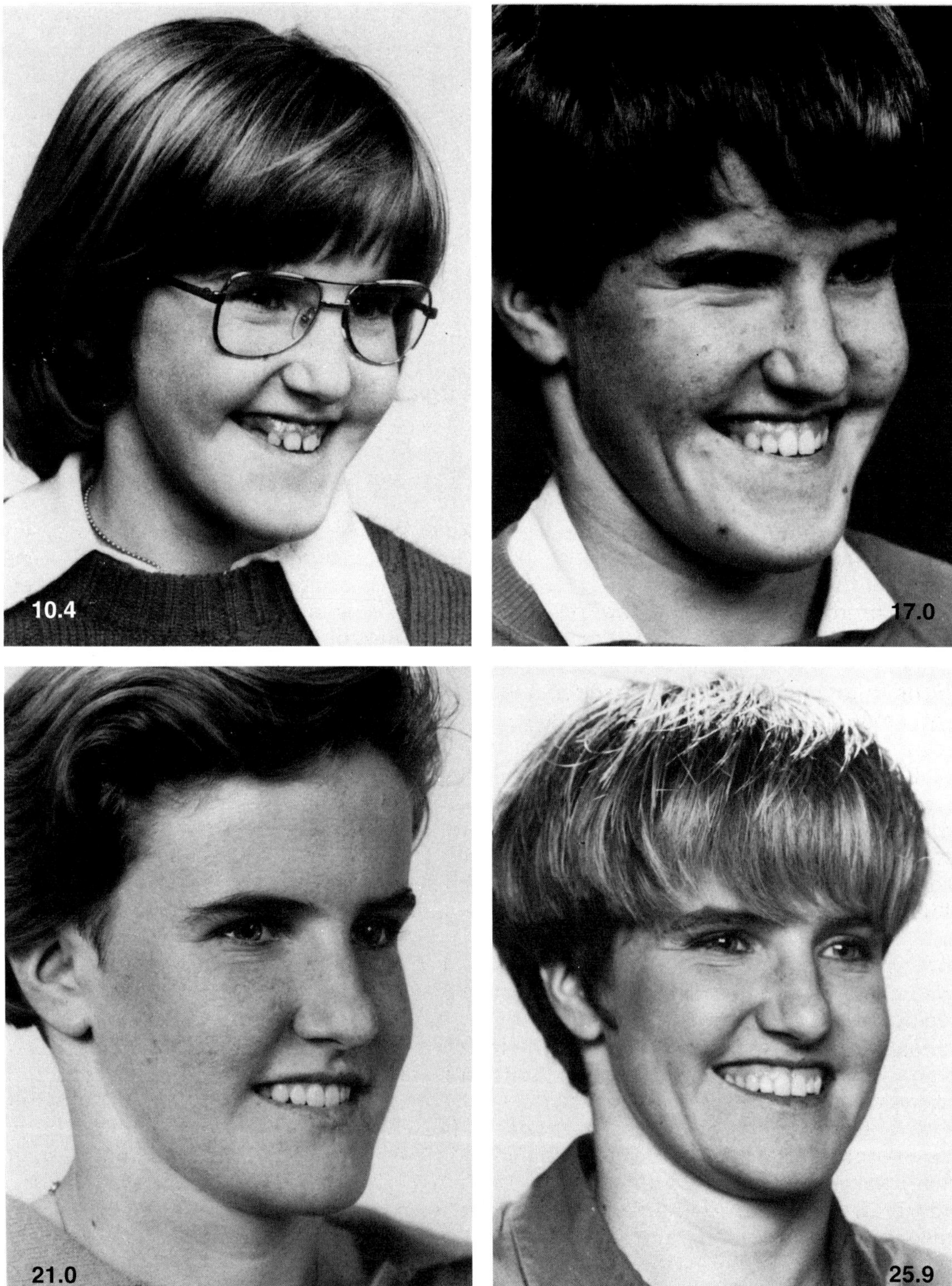

10.4 17.0 21.0 25.9

Fig 38-14 Note the changes before treatment, after facial orthopedic therapy, and after surgery.

was still worn every night. This could not prevent the development ventrally of the maxilla lagging behind that of the mandible. The chin became more dominant and it was clear that an acceptable result could not be reached without surgery.

At the age of 17 years, the treatment with the facial mask was concluded. There was no sagittal or vertical overbite and the incisal edges of the mandibular and maxillary incisors met. The maxillary premolars and canine on the right were in palatal crossbite. A mesio-occlusion of ½ to ¾ PW was present on both sides. The facial asymmetry was still obvious and the middle of the mandibular arch still deviated to the right in relationship to that of the maxillary arch (Figs 38.5 and 38.6).

A year later when the face had fully grown and the occlusion had not changed further, the possibilities for improvement surgically were brought up again. After a month in which to consider this, it was decided to consult a surgeon who might perform a suitable operation in due course. This could be done without further orthodontic treatment, since both dental arches would match each other well once the mandible was brought back and rotated.

At the age of 18 years, 9 months, a mandibular osteotomy (Obwegeser-Dal Pont, Fig 38.15) was performed during which more bone was removed on the left than the right. At the same time, the height of the bony chin was reduced. The records taken three months later show the result. The profile is significantly improved, the asymmetry has gone, and the occlusion — ignoring the mandibular anterior crowding — is nearly ideal (Figs 38.7 and 38.8).

In the following years, little changed and at 21 years of age the picture is functionally and esthetically satisfactory (Figs 38.9 and 38.10). The same applies to the situation seven years after the operation, at the age of 25 years, 9 months (Figs 38.11 and 38.12).

The superimpositions of the tracings from the cephalometric radiographs clearly show the unfavorable mandibular form, the lack of success with facial orthopedic therapy, and the improvements secured with surgery (Fig 38.13).

The changes brought about by growth, facial orthopedic therapy, and surgery are illustrated in the photographs of the smiling patient (Fig 38.14).

In contradistinction from the patients with class III anomalies described in the two previous chapters, a satisfactory result could not have been obtained by means of facial orthopedic treatment alone.

It has already been pointed out that the lack of success with chincap therapy is a bad sign. However, ventral traction on the maxilla influences the sutures, not the condyles. So, at the time, it was sensible still to attempt to attain an acceptable result with ventral traction, despite the abnormal shape of the mandible and the large lower-face height associated with it. This was the more so because it was assumed that a surgical solution with the risks it entailed might have been avoided. At present , however, it is more obvious that the facial form and skeletal conformation in this case present too many unfavorable indications. Moreover, laterognathias usually become worse with growth.

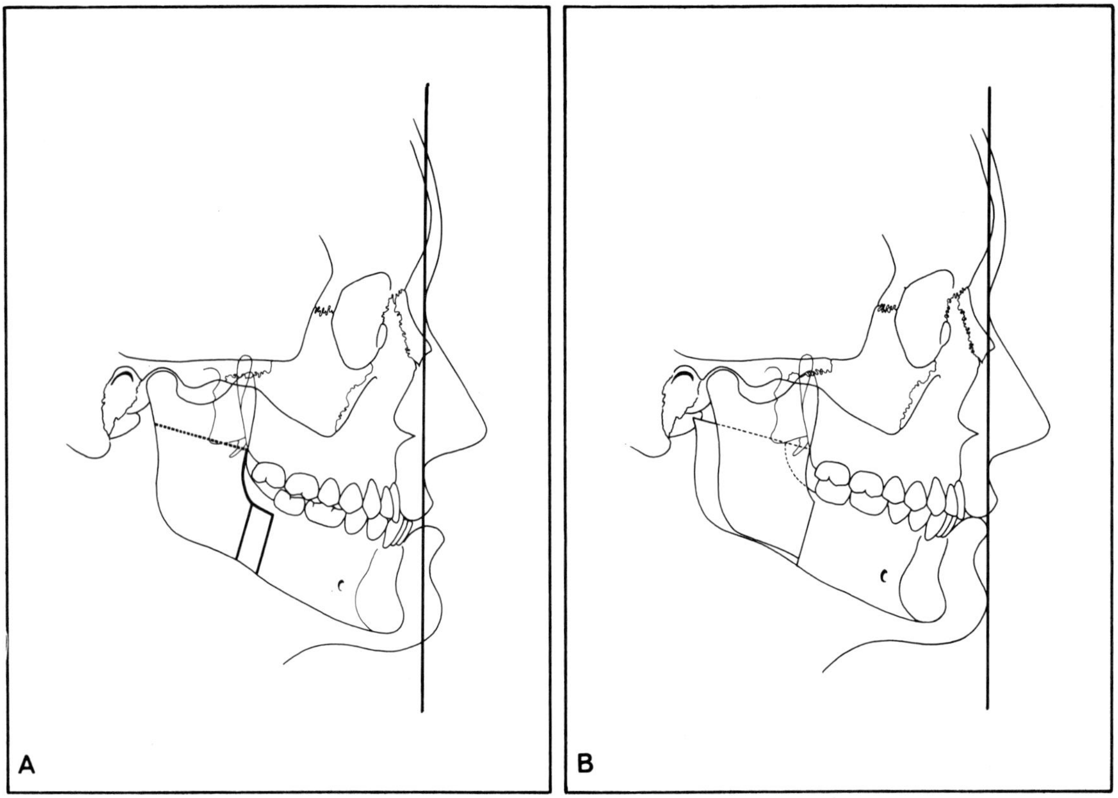

Fig. 38-15 Osteotomy of the mandible according to Obwegeser-Dal Pont for a Class III anomaly with mandibular prognathism.

A The ramus needs to be reduced in width ventrally by removing a strip of bone buccally. This is followd by a sagittal split.

B After dispacement and fixation, the lingual plate of the ascending ramus projects dorsally. This will resorb naturally.[37]

It is difficult to forecast whether or not prolonged facial orthopedic treatment in class III anomalies will lead to a satisfactory result. With severely deviant facial configurations, high lower-faces, and abnormal mandibular forms, it is necessary to take account of the subsequent possible need for surgical procedures. It then requires consideration of whether or not to go through with facial orthopedic treatment, since a difficulty can be that prolonged ventral traction can pull the dentition forward in relationship to the maxillary base. Such a situation prejudices the success of the surgical intervention. The jaws can then be translated less far and any orthodontic corrections that need to be done may be greater in magnitude.

As far as orthodontico-surgical reasoning is concerned, there have been changes in the interim. A mandibular and a chin operation would no longer be considered satisfactory. Also, the position of the midface would be changed with use of a Le Fort I operation to enable the maxilla to be displaced ventrally.

It seldom occurs that a good occlusion can be obtained just with surgery. In that respect, the case just described is exceptional. Usually prior to surgery both dental arches require extensive orthodontic treatment so that immediately postoperatively they match properly. Often it is still necessary to correct details after surgery.

An attempt has been made in the description of this patient and the two previous patients to bring out some aspects of the treatment of class III anomalies and the difficulties that can arise. Two comments need to be added.

Not all patients who give the impression at an early age that they will develop a class III anomaly proceed to do so, as was shown in Chapter 2: the boy who was left untreated.

With class II anomalies that have been corrected with facial orthopedic therapy, and a solid interdigitation of the premolars and permanent canines has been achieved, it can be assumed that there will be no relapse of the disto-occlusion. As jaw growth proceeds, the mandible does not lag behind the maxilla despite the mandible in class II/1 anomalies being relatively shorter initially and remaining so after treatment when compared with class I situations.[16] That also applies to the marked development associated with adolescent growth, which can be quite marked particularly in boys. With class III anomalies, however, where a solid interdigitation of premolars and permanent canines has been obtained, the effect of growth following treatment can involve the loss of the neutro-occlusion. The development of the maxilla to ventral is stimulated during treatment, but can be inadequate subsequently, certainly when there is still significant growth of the mandible. Sometimes, and more so in boys than in girls, it is necessary to carry on wearing a facial mask for some years two or three nights per week to prevent the mesio-occlusion from returning too much and an anterior reversed overbite to reoccur.

Chapter 39

Class I, ventral forced bite, everted maxillary incisors
Maxillary removable plate
Female: 43 years, 3 months to 53 years, 8 months

A woman aged 43 years, 3 months had enjoyed a fairly normal dentition until five years previously, when the maxillary incisors had become everted and on both sides of the right central incisor large diastemata had developed. The central diastema was not particularly pleasing to the patient. In habitual occlusion, the anterior teeth made contact. The anomaly gradually developed after a dentist had constructed a bridge in the maxillary arch on the right and the articulation was deflected to ventral. In addition, the gingiva had retracted in many places. Periodontal pockets of 5 to 6 mm were to be found interproximally and 3- to 4mm palatally around the maxillary incisors. Mesial to the maxillary right first premolar, which functioned as an abutment for the bridge, was a 7mm pocket. The mandibular premolars had pockets 5 to 6mm deep and the maxillary left second molar had paradontitis that had progressed so far that it was doubtful if the tooth could be kept. The gingiva overall was swollen and bled easily if touched (Figs 39.1 and 39.2).

Prior to embarking on any orthodontic treatment the periodontium needed to be brought into as healthy a state as possible. The initial treatment comprised supragingival and subgingival plaque and calculus removal, root planing, and polishing. In some places, the pockets were surgically eliminated. After four months, the paradontal tissues were healthy and optimal oral hygiene was being maintained.

It was decided to provide a maxillary removable plate; the premature contact on the bridge was ground away. Because the mandibular incisors struck the plate, the bite in the posterior regions was slightly opened; this permitted the patient to close more easily in central occlusion. Moreover, it eliminated the contact between the maxillary and mandibular incisors, allowing the maxillary incisors to be retracted. This was done by means of divided labial arches. During the orthodontic therapy, the patient underwent professional scaling and polishing every two months. Despite this, it proved impossible to preserve the maxillary left second molar.

After orthodontic treatment for a year, the objective had been reached. The maxillary incisors had been retracted, the diastemata closed and habitual occlusion and central relation now coincided (Fig 39.4). After a period of six months' retention, bridges were provided in the posterior regions, which improved the occlusion considerably. In addition, the maxillary incisors and canines were bonded together with composite. From the records collected six months later, it seems that a satisfying result has been obtained. The dentition fulfils both functional and esthetic demands (Fig 39.3).

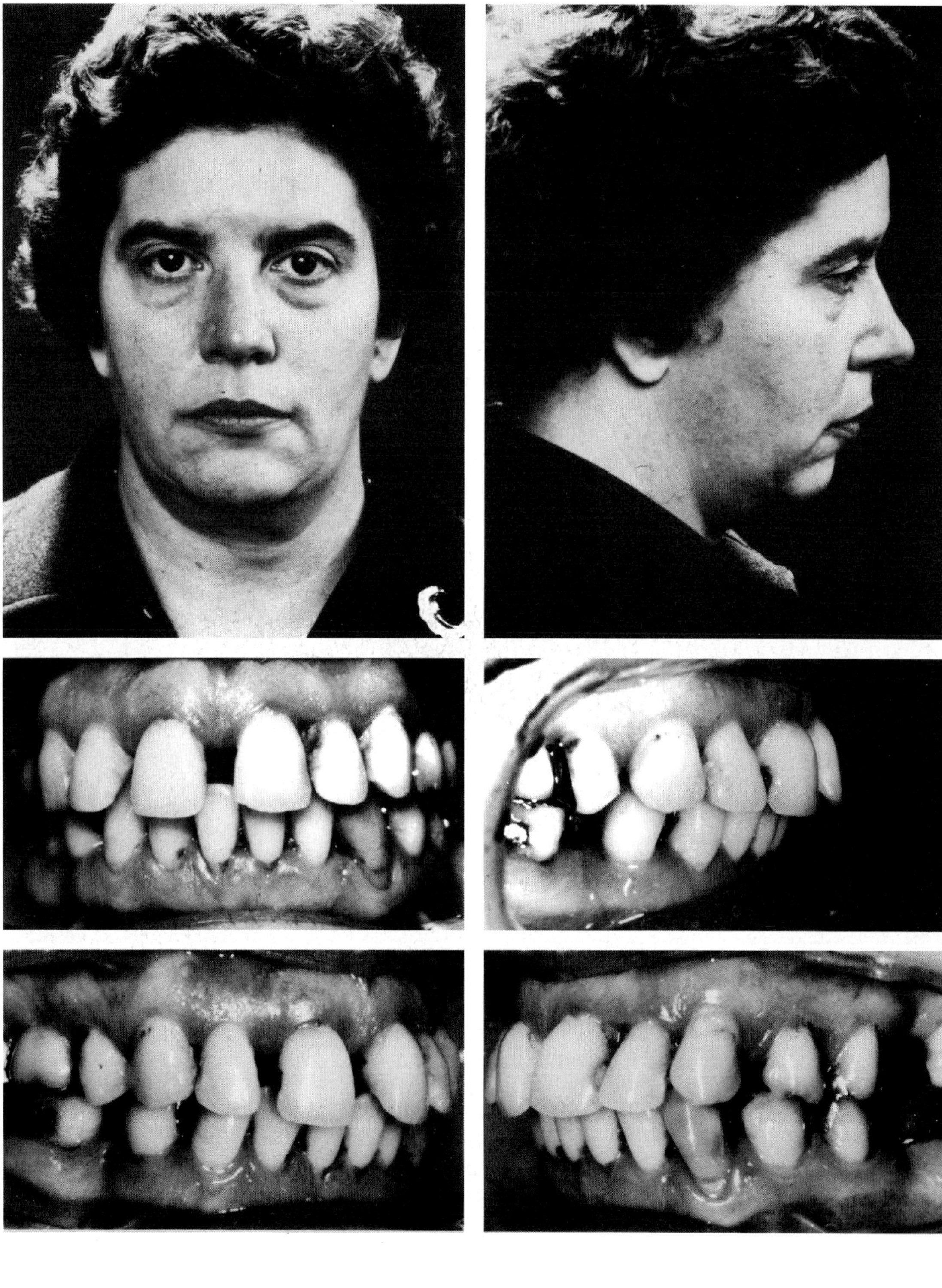

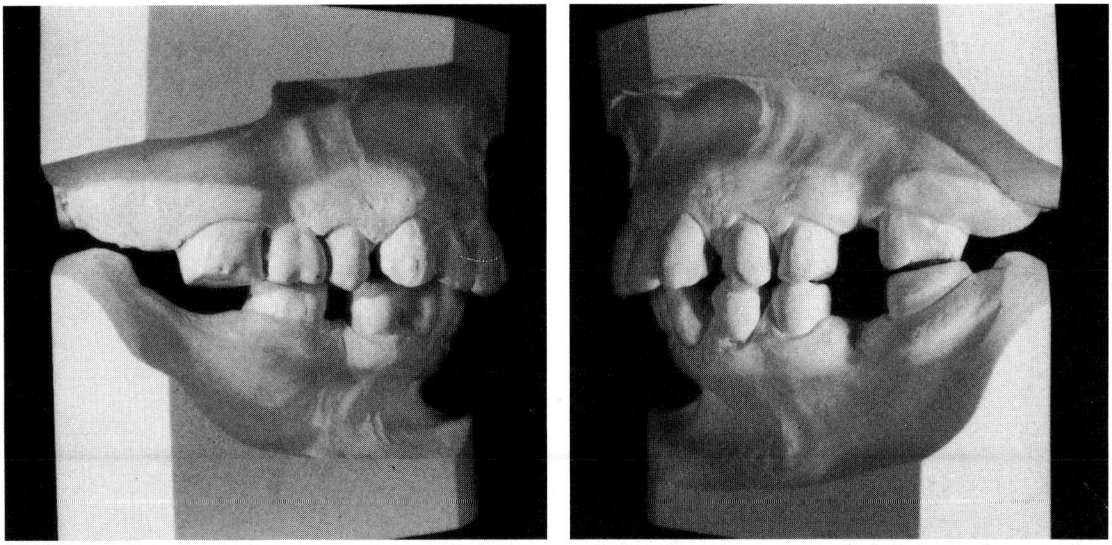

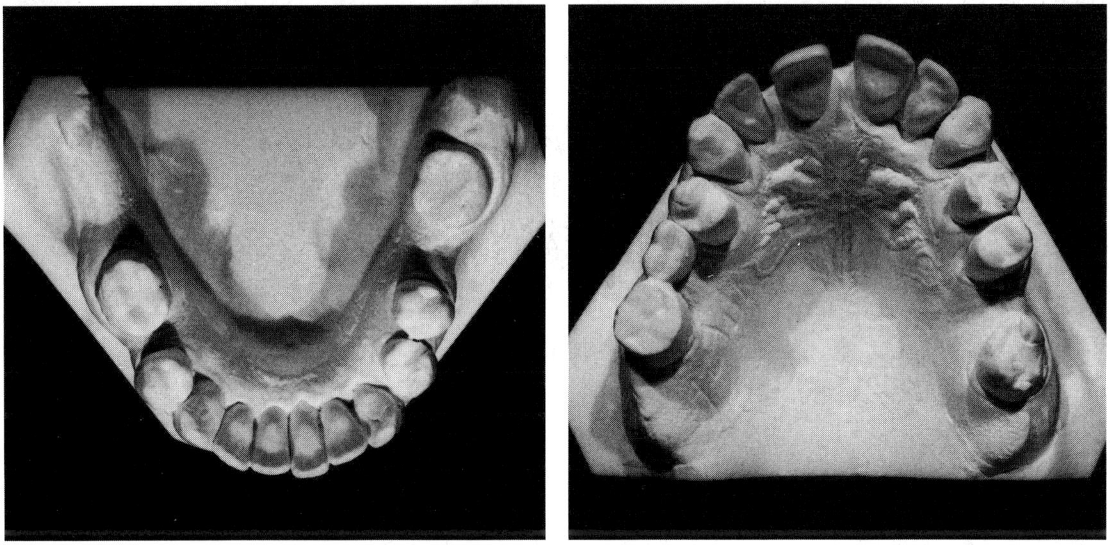

Figs 39-1 and 39-2 A woman aged 43 y, 3 mo presented with a poorly maintained dentition that showed no abnormalities until five years previously. The maxillary central incisors are everted, with large diastemata on both sides of the right central incisor. The gingiva are swollen and inflamed. At different places there are pockets of 5 to 6mm depth. There are several posterior teeth missing and a bridge has been placed in the maxillary arch on the right. Its presence provides a step in the occlusal surfaces in that region. When the teeth are closed from rest, the mandibular right first molar glides 2 mm to ventral over that step. Although this forced bite has been present for five years there are no symptoms of functional problems. However, the maxillary incisors, especially the central incisors, have been displaced to labial and large spaces have appeared between the incisors.

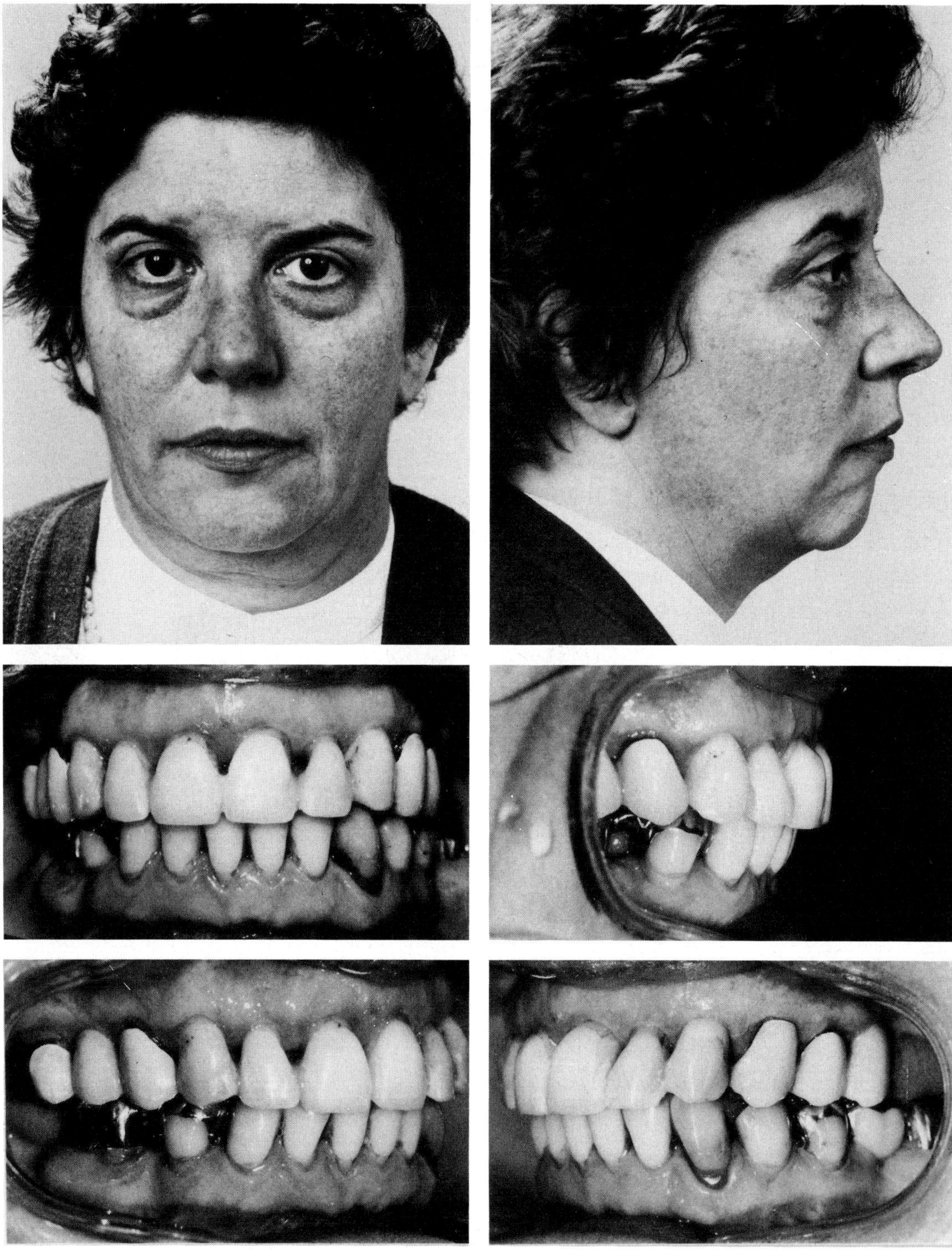

Fig 39-3 At the age of 47 y, 1 mo, orthodontic treatment had been finished 18 months previously and the posterior bridges subsequently made have been in service for one year. The six maxillary incisors have been bonded together at their contact points with composite resin as a form of permanent retention.

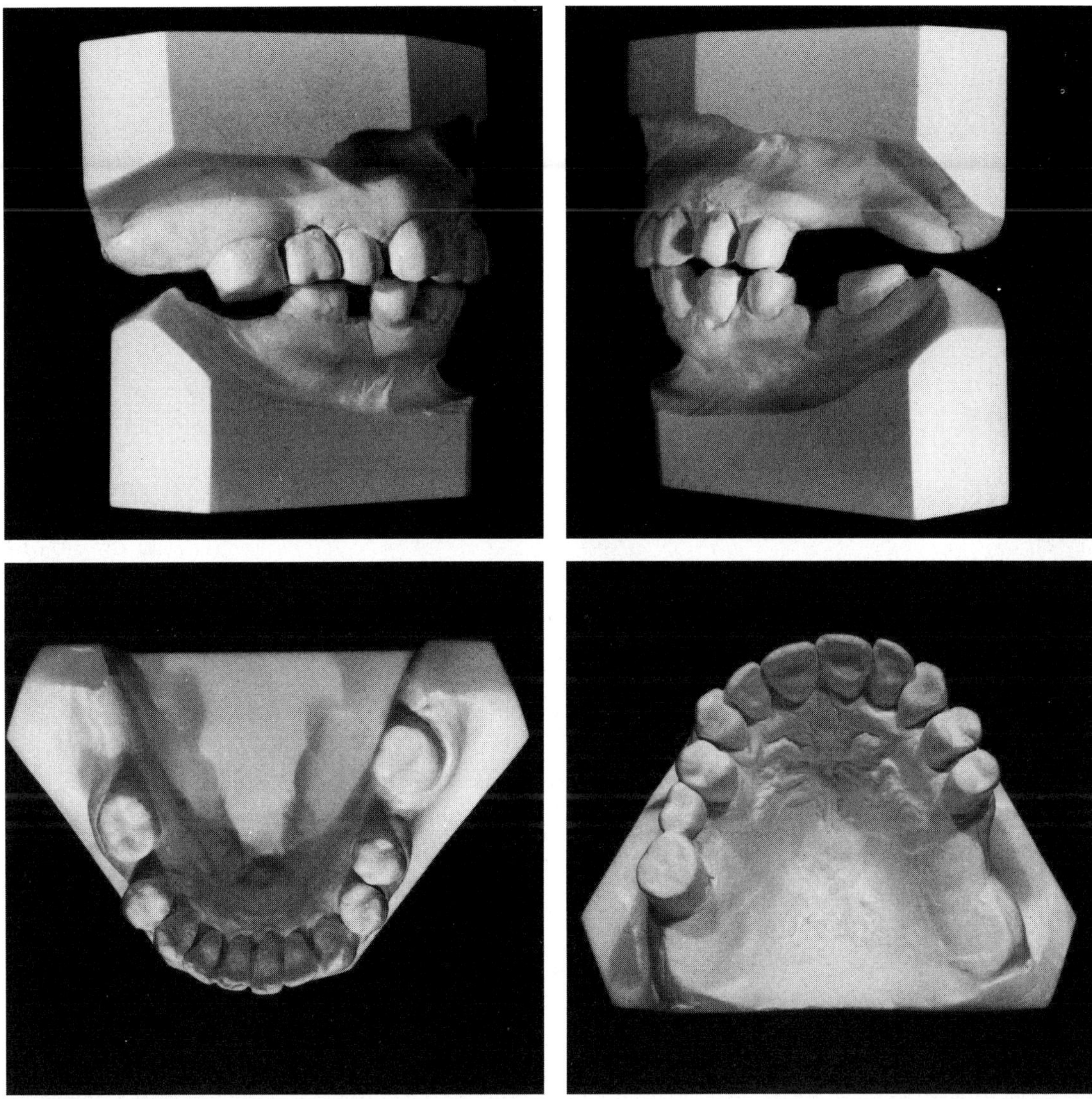

Fig 39-4 Dental casts obtained at the termination of orthodontic treatment and before the provision of bridges (age, 45 y, 7 mo).

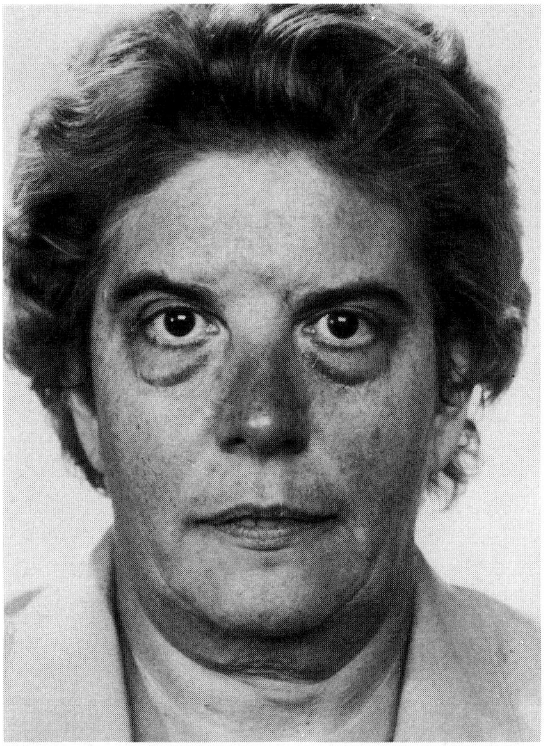
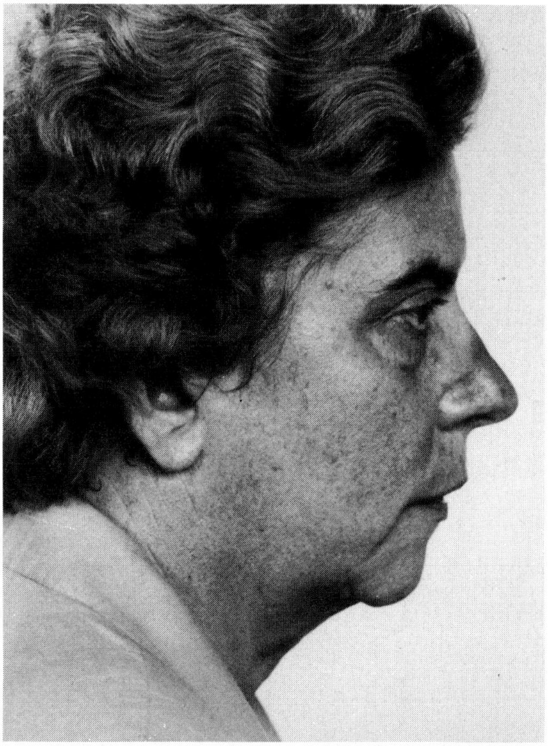
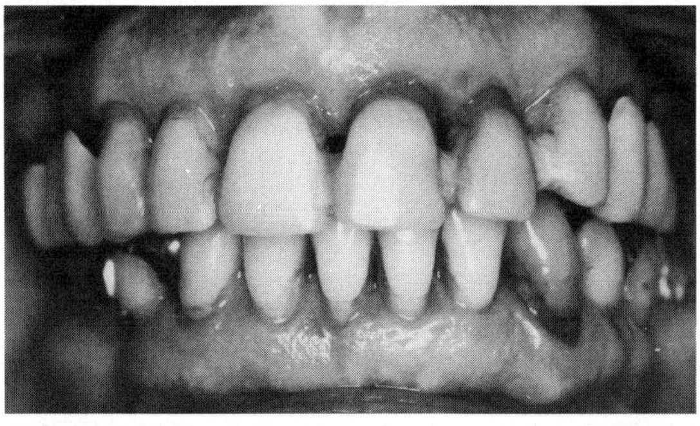
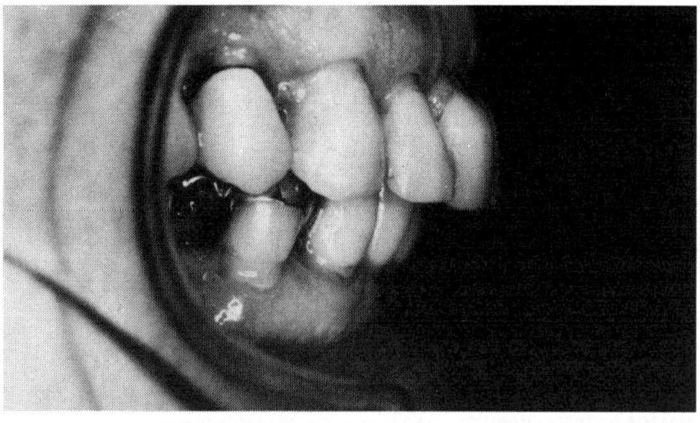
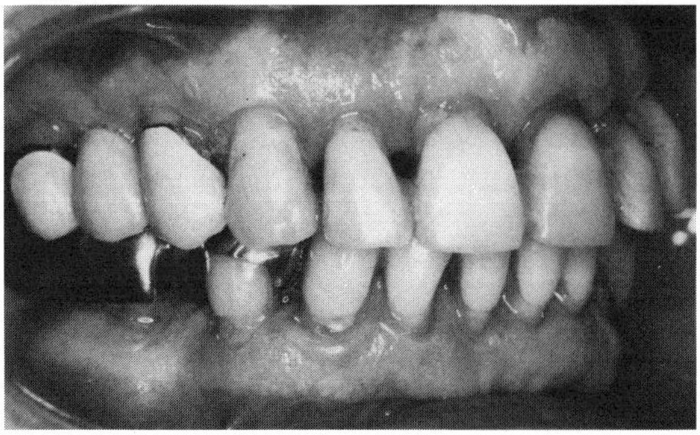
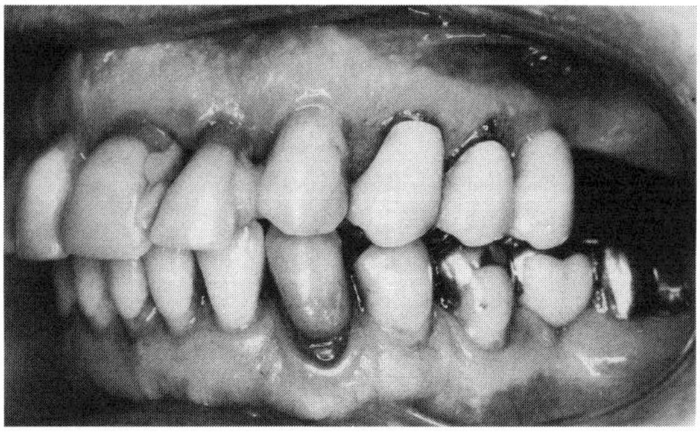

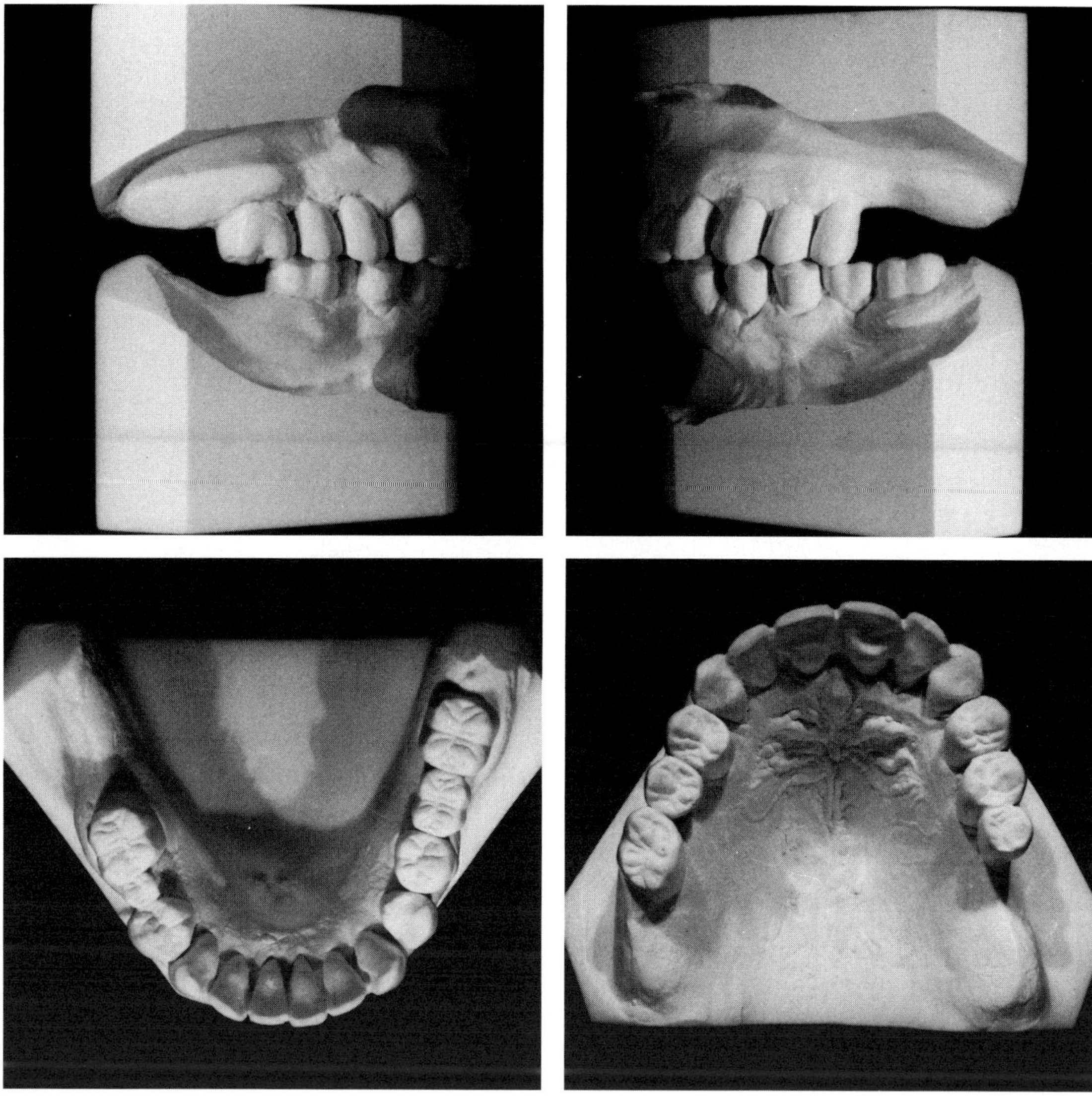

Figs 39-5 and 39-6 *At the age of 53 y, 8 mo the alignment of the teeth and their occlusion show little or no change. The composite bond first on the mesial and then later on the distal of the maxillary left lateral incisor broke down. Unfortunately, this was not noticed by the patient until after a diastema had opened up there. When the bond was renewed, this space was closed with more composite. In addition to the above, the gingival tissues and interdental papillae have receded further in various places and some exposure of cervical dentine has occurred.*

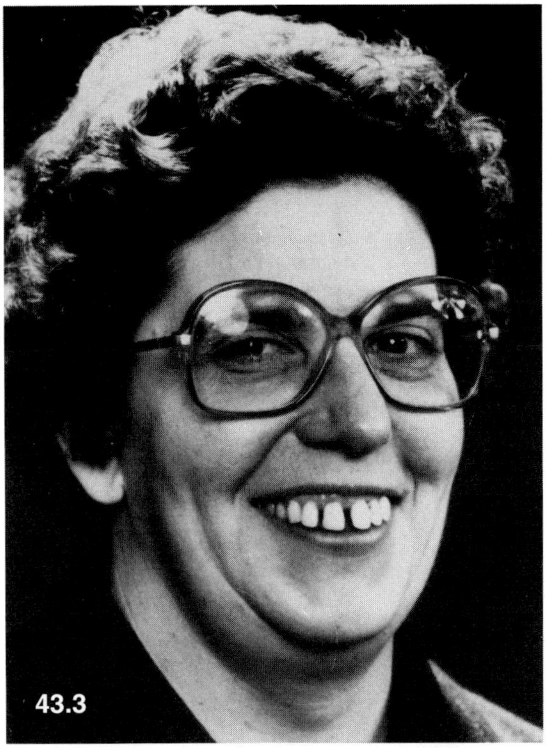
43.3

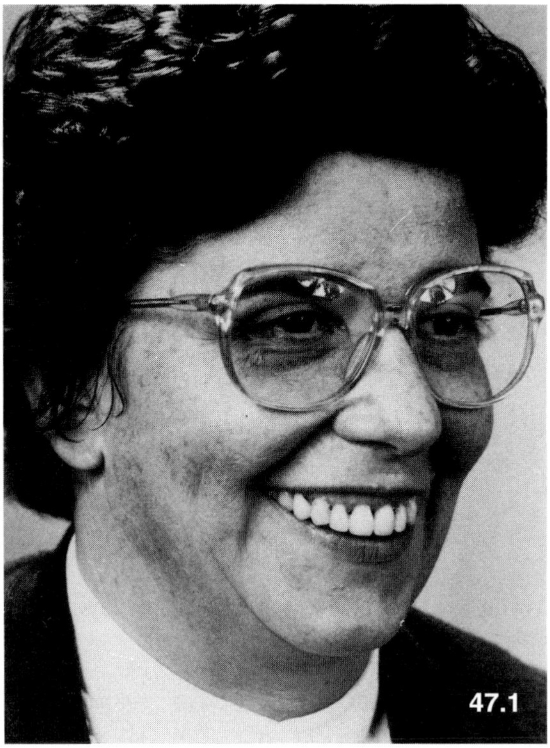
47.1

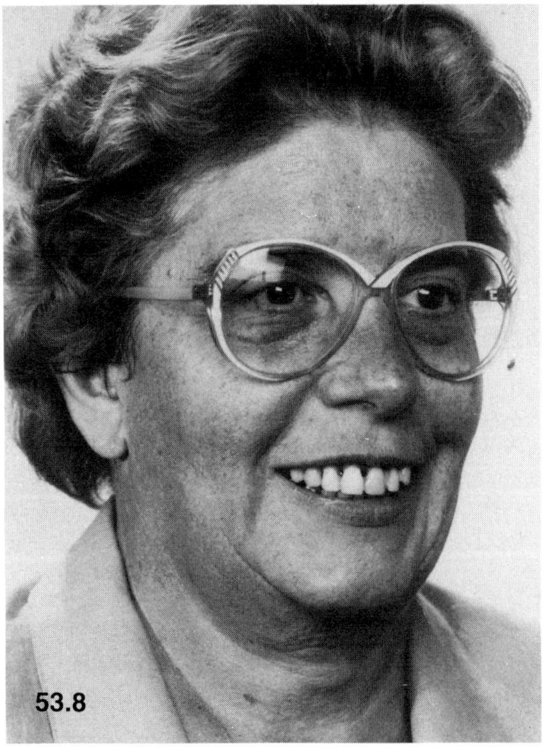
53.8

Fig 39-7 Notice the improvements the treatment has attained.

Composite bonding of the incisors however is fragile and can be broken. Therefore a plate was provided that the patient could insert immediately if one of the bonds broke down and could not be repaired on the spot (Fig 39.9). Unfortunately, it happened twice that a bond fractured without the patient noticing it until tooth movement had already taken place. The consequence of this was that the diastemata that returned on each side of the maxillary left lateral incisor had to be filled in with composite additions. The records at the age of 53 years, 8 months, 6½ years after treatment, show that this tooth movement reduced the standard of the original treatment result. This was somewhat accentuated by the discoloration of the composite at the junction of the enamel, and the further retraction of the gingiva and interdental papillae (Figs 39.5 and 39.6).
The photographs of the patient smiling display the effect of the treatment and the subsequent changes (Fig 39.7).

It is frequently found that adults who experience drifting of their anterior teeth after reduction of the periodontal attachment come with the request that the original alignment of their teeth be retrieved. Orthodontic treatment should never be undertaken until paradontal conditions have been rendered as good as possible and optimal oral hygiene is ensured.
For this patient, the possibility was first examined of merely eliminating the forced bite by occlusal grinding of the bridge and then waiting to see if when a more dorsal habitual occlusion was permitted the maxillary incisors would spontaneously move palatally. This plan was dismissed because the mandibular incisors would have been able to over-erupt and impede any palatal movement of the maxillary incisors. Above all, the patient was particularly anxious to have the distressing appearance of her teeth corrected as quickly as possible.
Had there been no forced bite — something which usually is the case —- then as the maxillary incisors splayed out the bite would have deepened correspondingly. Retraction of maxillary incisors and closure of diastemata would not be possible without first reducing the overbite. The necessary intrusion of the maxillary and/or mandibular incisors is difficult in adults, requiring fixed appliances and easily leading to periodontal damage and root resorption. In most cases, the approach would be to reduce the height of the mandibular canines and incisors by grinding. Moreover, this has the advantage that the proportion of the attached root to the rest of the tooth increases and becomes mechanically more favorable. By fitting a plate to the maxilla and building on it a biteplane into which the mandibular anteriors bite accurately (using self-curing acrylic to make that bite plane with the posterior teeth in occlusion), further eruption of the mandibular incisors will be prevented. Gradual retraction of the maxillary incisors can be accomplished while preserving the biteplane and the position of the mandibular incisors. As the maxillary incisors are retracted, the acrylic of the plate is ground away a small amount at a time parallel to the palatal surfaces of the incisors and to the palatal soft tissues covering the alveolar process.
Many adults are particularly anxious that the visibility of any orthodontic appliance be minimal. To satisfy this requirement, thin tooth-colored elastics can be used in place of a labial archwire to retract maxillary incisors. To ensure that the elastics are kept in their proper place vertically, small slots made of composite can be bonded to

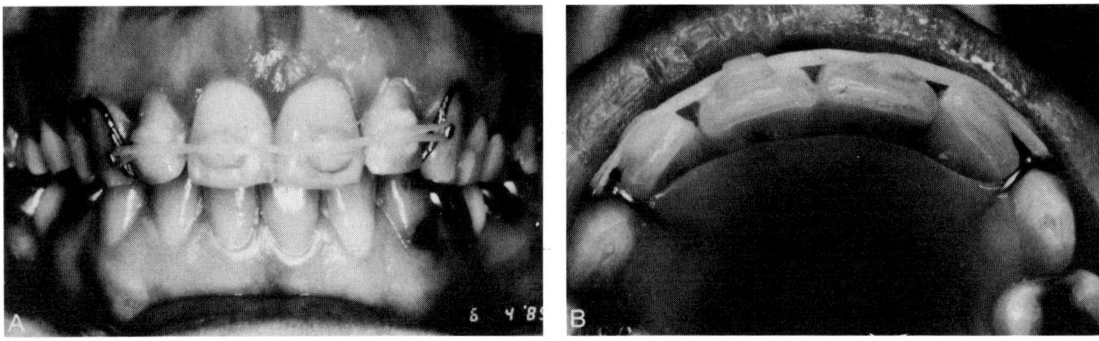

Fig 39-8 *Retraction and rotation of maxillary incisors can be achieved quite unobtrusively with elastics in combination with a removable plate. The plate incorporates three-quarter clasps for the canines with elastic hooks welded to the wire as shown. The elastics must be long and thin since otherwise too large a force is applied to the teeth. Composite can be used to build up a groove on the labial surfaces into which the elastic fits to prevent it from slipping cervically. By varying the height of the groove in relationship to the incisal edge, a vertical component can be introduced into the forces involved. It is also possible to vary the retracting force on individual teeth by increasing or decreasing the distance that the floor of the groove stands away from the labial surface of the tooth. By applying these principles to vary the force on the mesial or distal of the labial surfaces, rotating forces can be applied. Selective careful grinding of the palatal aspect of the plate behind each tooth encourages the desired tooth movements to occur.*

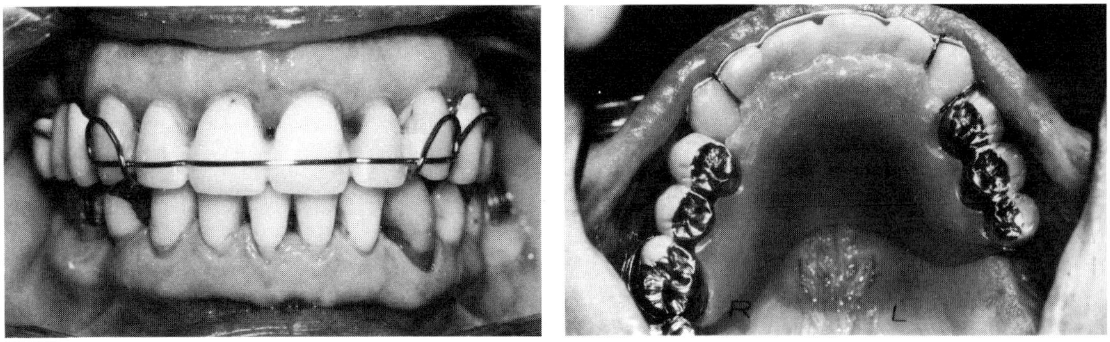

Fig 39-9 *A plate that can be used to retain the treatment changes. It might be worn at all times for a short period after treatment and subsequently reduced to wearing at night only.*
A similar device was used for this patient as a reserve to prevent movement of the maxillary incisors if one of the interproximal bonds unexpectedly should break. If the patient observed such an occurrence, the plate immediately should be worn every night until the bond is repaired. The labial arch is closely fitted to the labial surfaces of the incisors and embraces the canines with loops, thus improving the plate's retention.

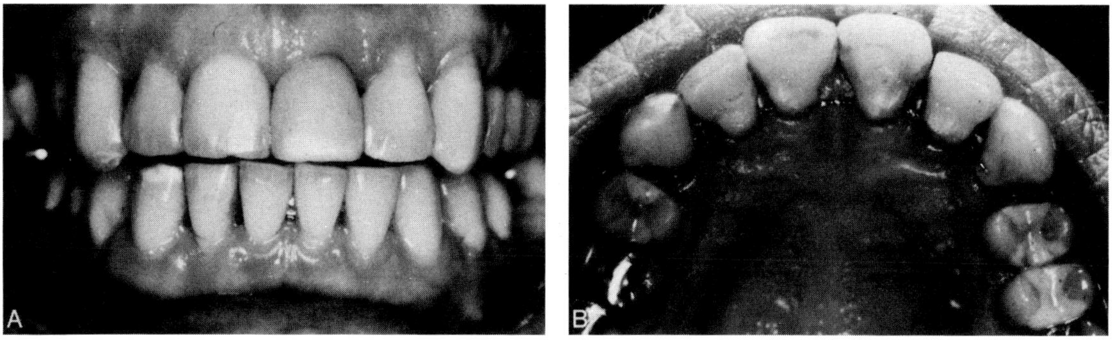

Fig 39-10 *After correcting the alignment of the incisors as shown in Figure 39-8, a 0.015" twistflex wire was bonded to the palatal surfaces of those teeth. To prevent it being bitten on, the wire was placed far to the cervical. Moreover, the incisors were individually built up interproximally to fill in the interproximal spaces. In this way the retaining wire was kept from being visible and it was possible to improve the shape of the crowns of the teeth.*

the labial surface of the incisors. The elastics can be attached to hooks welded to the three-quarter clasps embracing the canines. By varying the positions of the "grooves" and their thickness on the labial enamel, teeth can be subjected to differing forces. In combination with selective grinding of the acrylic of the plate the required retrusion and rotation can be obtained (Fig 39.8).

The reactive forces from the elastics can lead to undesired tooth movements and mobility of anchor teeth. For that reason, elastics should not be hooked onto buttons or hooks bonded to canines or premolars unless those teeth have been rigidly held in place. One might be inclined to use such buttons if there is an anterior open bite and no plate is required to control the vertical overbite. Nevertheless as many teeth as possible need to be involved in supporting the elastic forces to avoid undesirable movements. This can be achieved with a plate on the maxillary arch that embraces the canines and posterior teeth accurately and with good retention. Those teeth can also be splinted with orthodontic wire and composite resin, although it makes good oral hygiene much more difficult to attain.

Corrections that have been made to anomalies in maxillary incisors in a dentition that has periodontal lesions require lifelong retention. This can be provided with a plate that is worn only at night (see Fig 39.9), or by splinting relevant teeth. This latter can be done by etching and bonding the contact points, or by fixing thin twistflex wire (.015") to the palatal surfaces of the incisors and canines with composite. An advantage of this last method is that it permits a limited amount of movement by individual teeth so that the composite fixation is less readily lost. Therefore, the wire must be thin and flexible enough with sufficient free wire available between the attachment points. When the mandibular incisors make contact with the maxillary incisors, they must not strike the wire or composite. This can only be avoided if the wire is placed sufficiently far cervically or by insetting the wire into the enamel. If the interdental papillae do not completely fill the interdental space or if there is considerable recession, the twistflex wire may be visible. By filling up those spaces in such cases by separately adding composite cervical to the contact points, not only can the visible wire be hidden but also the often unsightly spaces can be reduced in obtrusiveness (Fig 39.10). A disadvantage of this procedure is that the area concerned becomes more difficult to clean and interdental brushes are less effective. Unless the oral hygiene is extremely good it can be best — as in this case — to splint the teeth by bonding the contact points which will also fill up the interdental spaces to some extent.

In retrospect, it might have been better to have this patient continue to wear the reserve retainer plate a few nights per week even though the incisors were splinted. Then an accidental unnoticed fracture of an interdental bond would not have been followed by drifting of the teeth. Once movement has occurred, either the treatment has to be repeated or a less satisfactory result has to be accepted. In either case, the splinting has to be renewed.

Chapter 40

Class I, everted 11 and 21, too narrow 12 and 22

Brackets 12, 11, 21 and 22, bands 16 and 26, maxillary removable retainer

Female: 49 years, 8 months to 57 years, 8 months

A woman aged 49 years, 8 months asked if it might be possible to do something about the alignment of her incisors. She had a harmonious face but the eversion of the maxillary central incisors and the large spaces distal to the centrals incisors offended her. The labiopalatal diameter of the maxillary central incisors was excessive and their eversion was largely the result of this. The existence of the spacing was due mainly to a TSD, which indicated a lack of tooth material in the maxillary incisors. The maxillary lateral incisors were narrow; they were even narrower than the corresponding mandibular incisors. The periodontal tissues were in good condition. There were no pockets in the incisor regions. In the posterior segments a few pockets not exceeding 4 mm in depth were found (Figs 40.1 and 40.2).

It was decided to correct the maxillary incisors and to use a partial fixed edgewise appliance rather than a removable plate. The most important reason for this was that the maxillary incisors would need to be intruded. At the age of 49 years, 10 months, the first permanent molars were banded, the central incisors provided with brackets and a twistflex .0175″ archwire inserted. Two months later these incisors were ground down palatally and retracted. Four months later, the palatal surfaces of the central incisors were reduced further and brackets were placed on the lateral incisors with the aim to move them mesially along a .019″ x .026″ archwire.

At 50 years, 9 months and after a treatment period of nine months, all appliances were removed and a removable plate supplied to retain the situation that had been established. The excess space in the maxillary anteriors now was divided in such a way that similar diastemata existed on either side of the lateral incisors. This was done to provide suitable conditions under which to build up the crowns of the lateral incisors with composite directly after the end of orthodontic treatment (Figs 40.3. and 40.4).

The photographs and dental casts at the age of 51 years, 11 months demonstrate the improvements that were obtained by building up the lateral incisors (Figs 40.5 and 40.6). The retainer was worn day and night for the first four months, but only at night after that. Nevertheless the central incisors moved a little to labial and small spaces opened up. At the age of 57 years, 8 months an esthetically and functionally satisfactory result still remained, partly because the discolored composite had been replaced and added to fully eliminate the spacing (Figs 40.7 and 40.8).

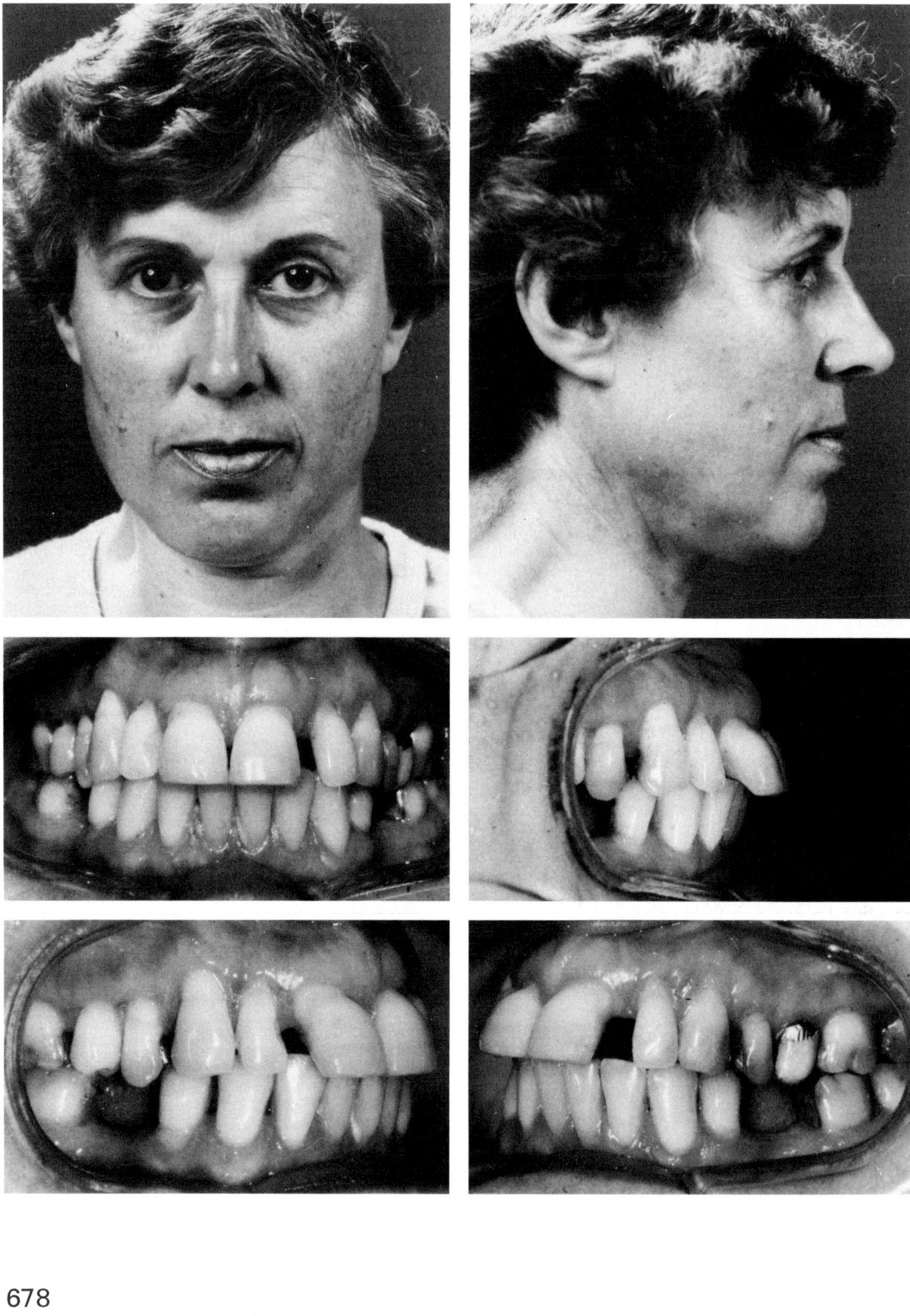

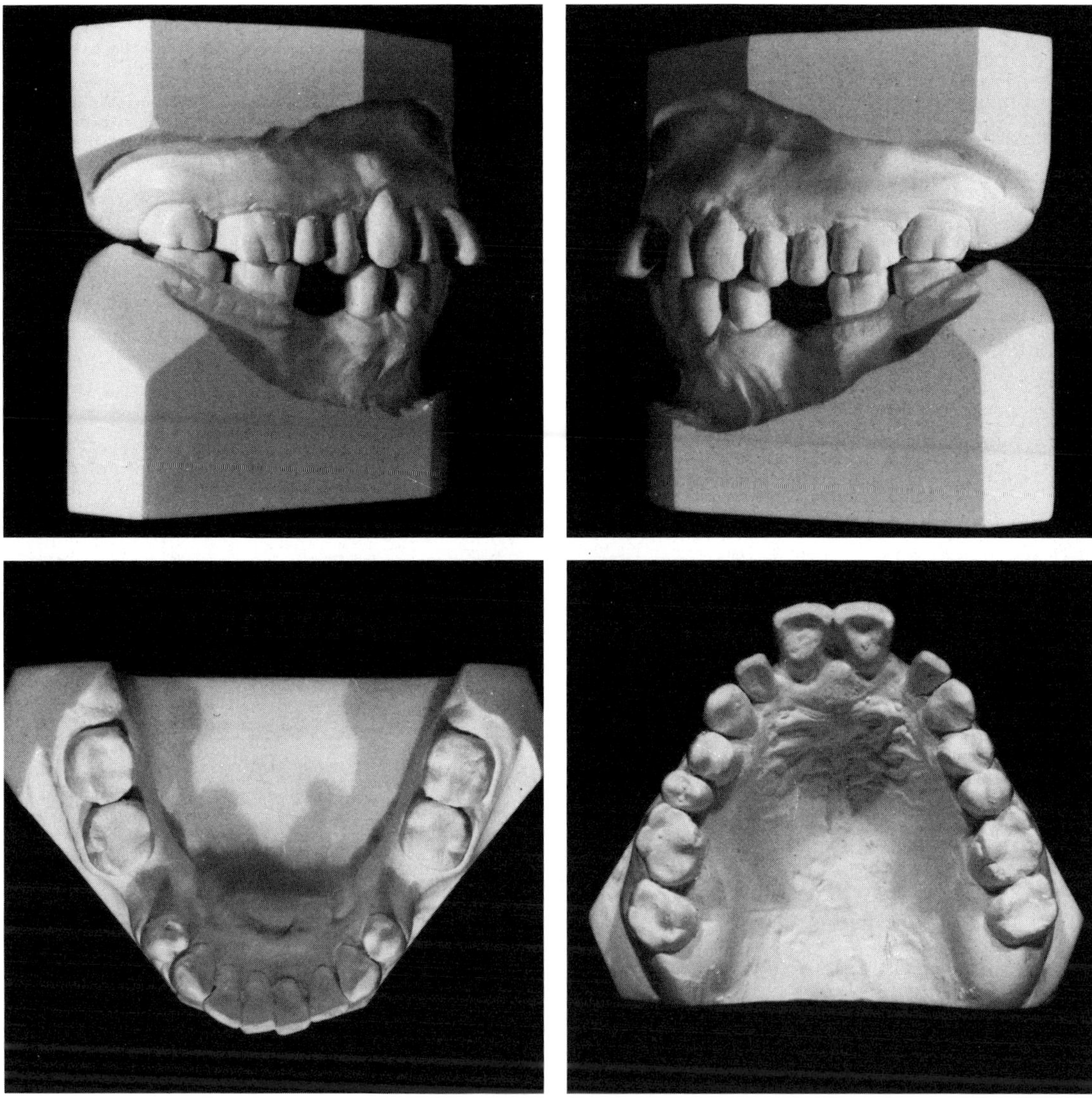

Figs 40-1 and 40-2 A woman aged 49 y, 8 mo presented with a pleasant face but with objectionably positioned maxillary incisors. The maxillary central incisors have abnormally thick crowns. The lateral incisors are narrow, which this is mainly responsible for the large diastemata between the central and tlateral incisors. The canines and molars are in neutro-occlusion and due to the lack of opposing mandibular posterior teeth the maxillary second premolar has overerupted somewhat.

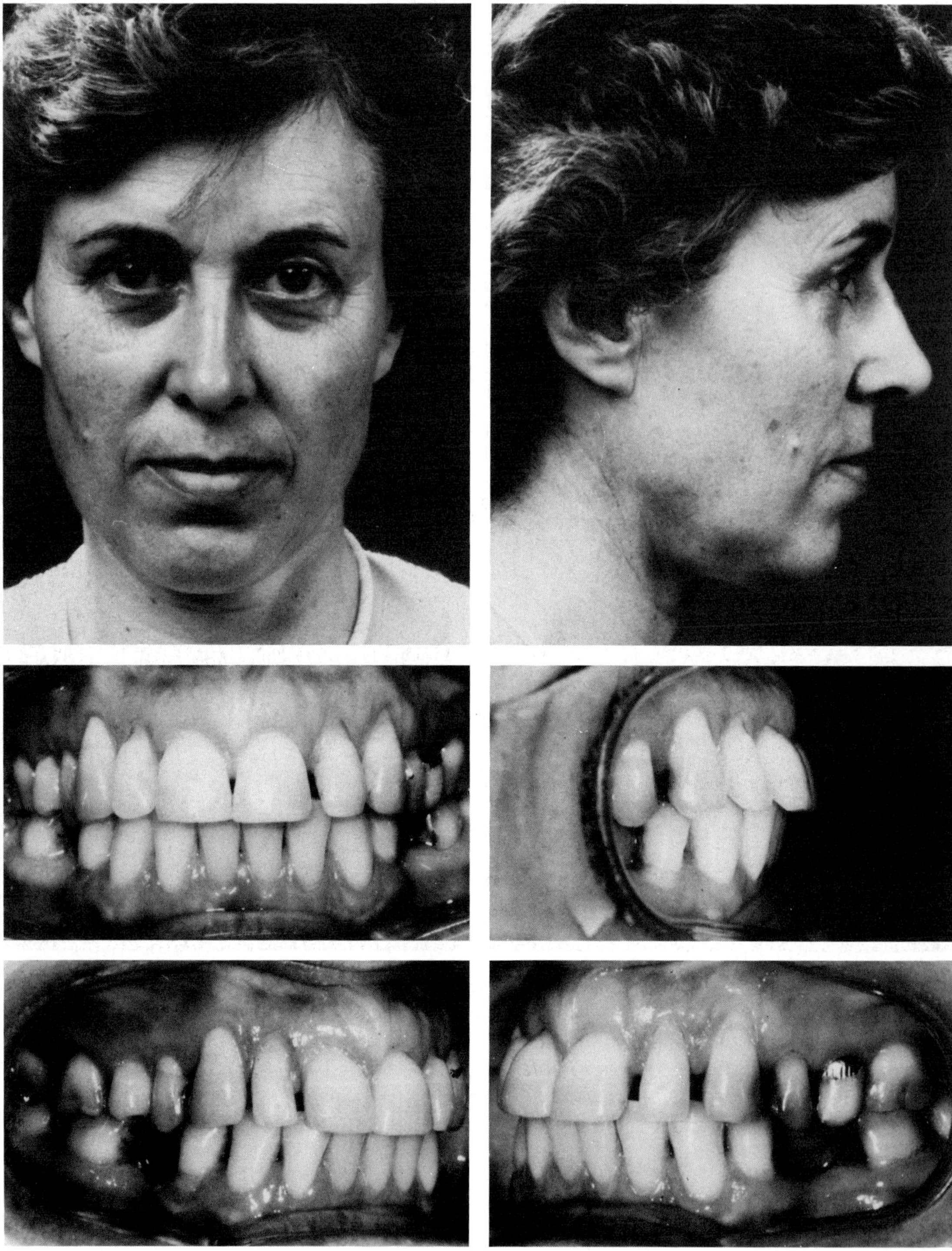

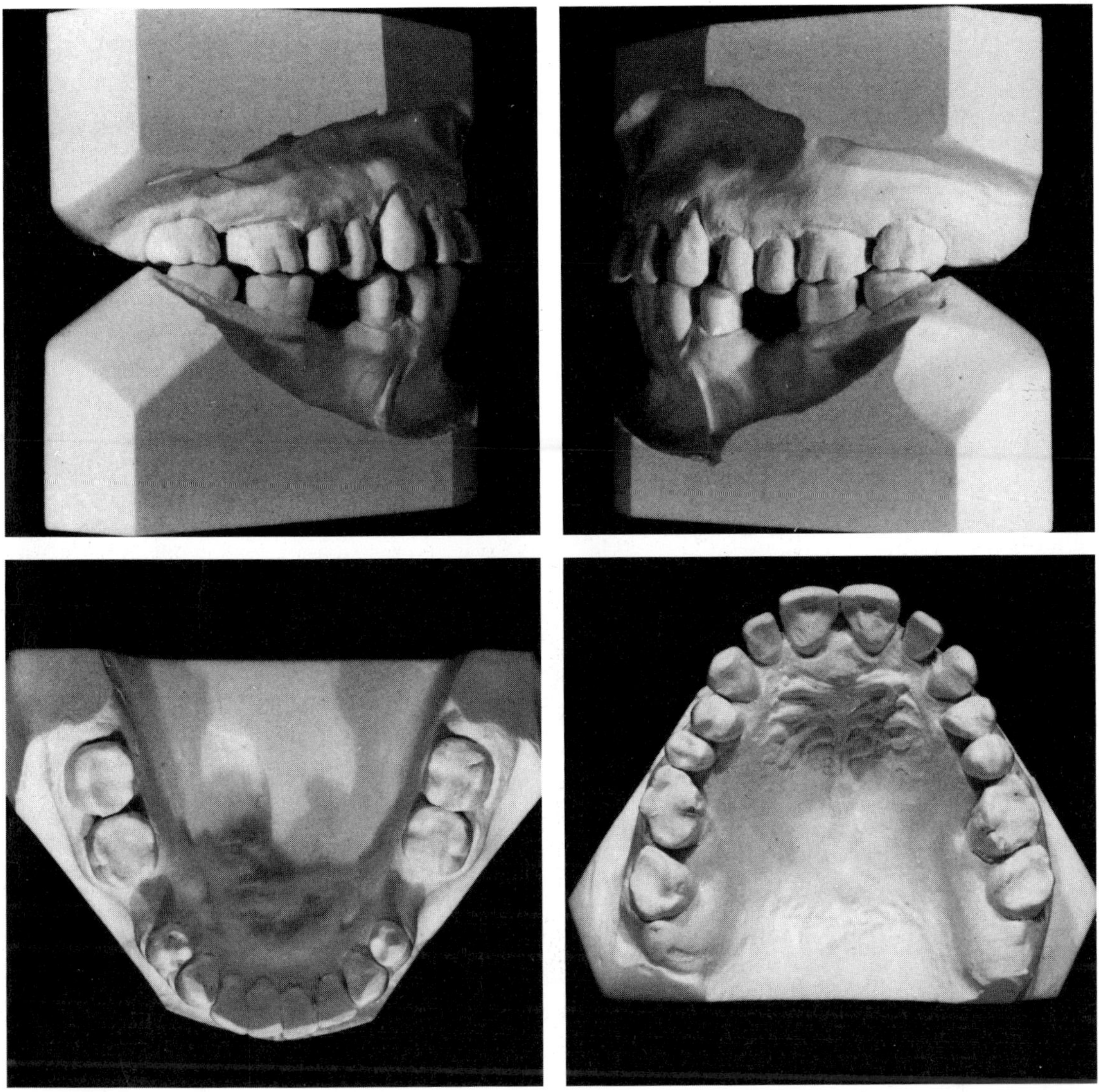

Figs 40-3 and 40-4 At the age of 50 y, 8 mo, the orthodontic treatment has been completed. The maxillary central incisors have been intruded and retracted and the diastemata that were attributable to a TSD are now located on either side of the lateral incisors. This makes a satisfactory elimination of the spacing possible by building up the lateral incisors with composite.

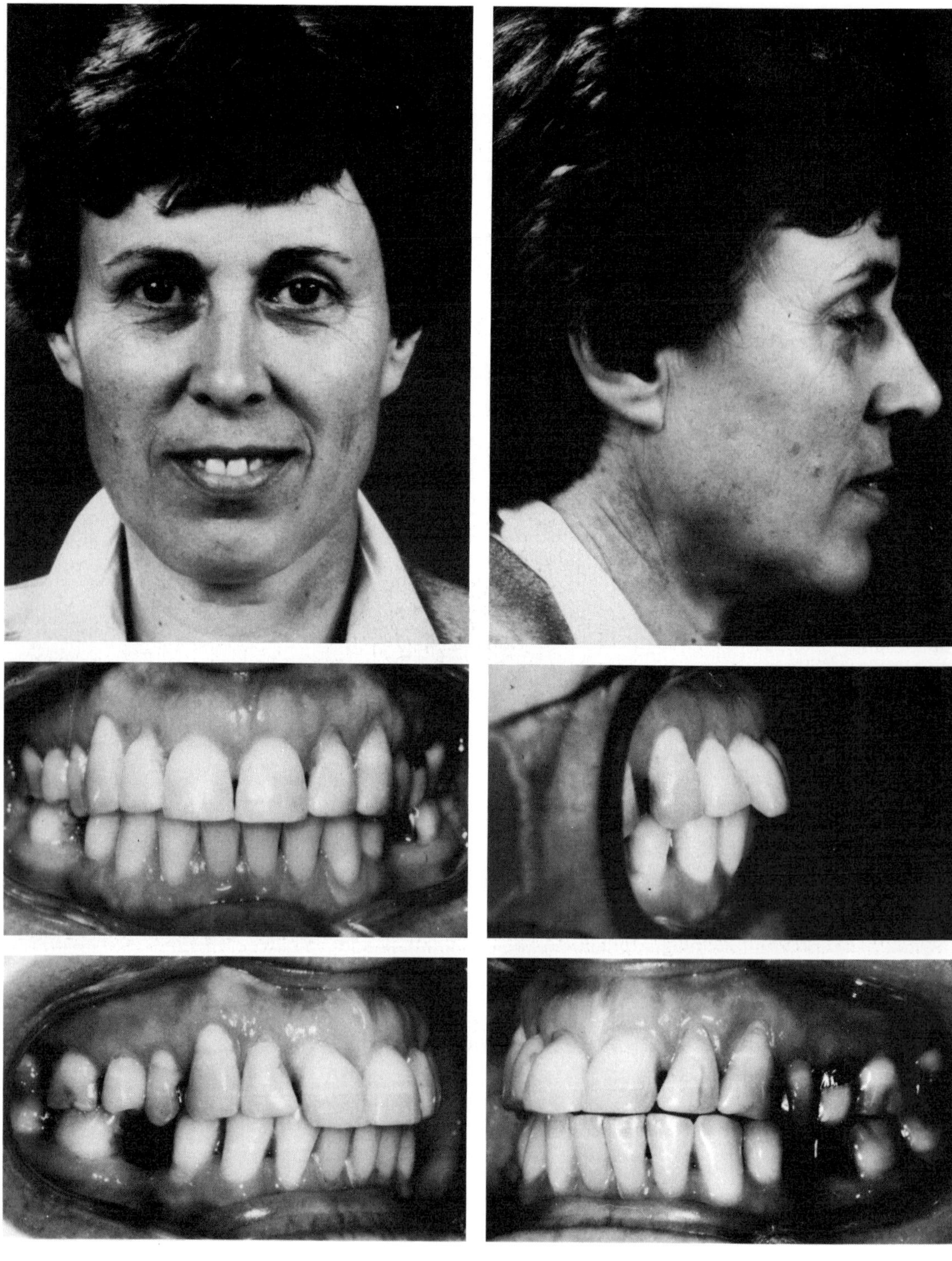

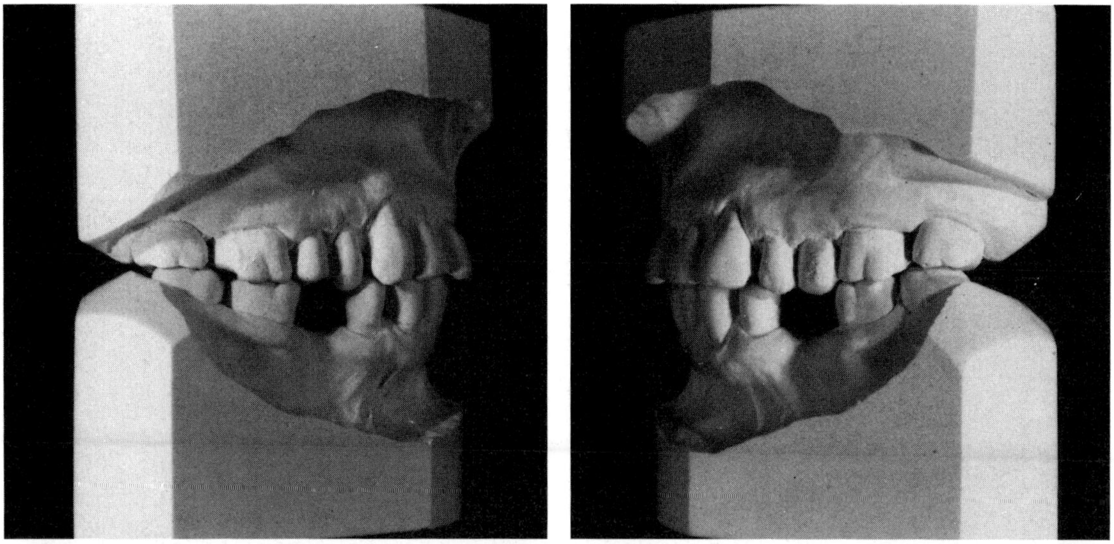

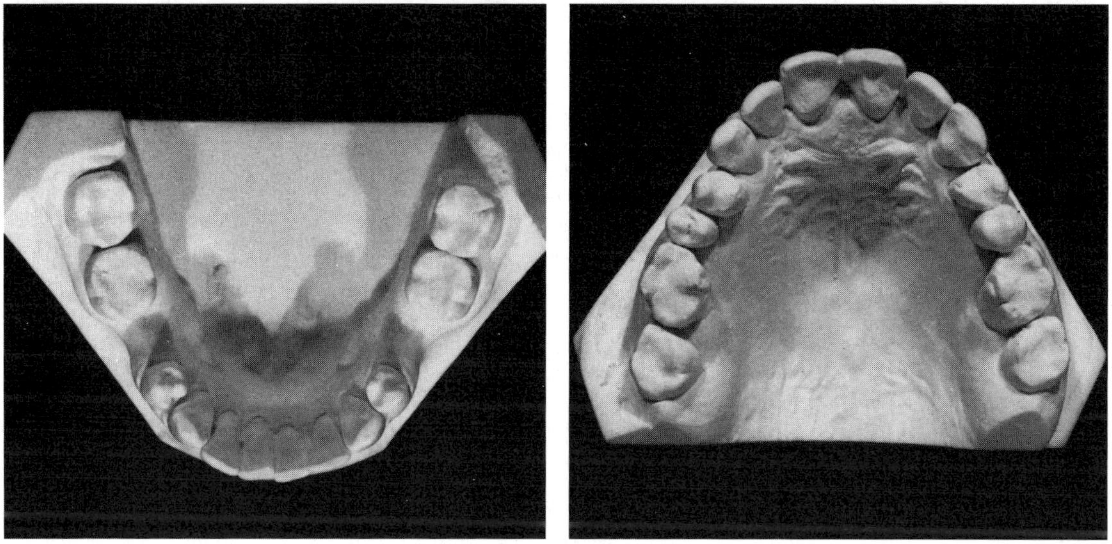

Figs 40-5 and 40-6 *At the age of 51 y, 11 mo, one year and three months after completion of orthodontic treatment the composite has discolored slightly. Otherwise the situation is quite satisfactory.*

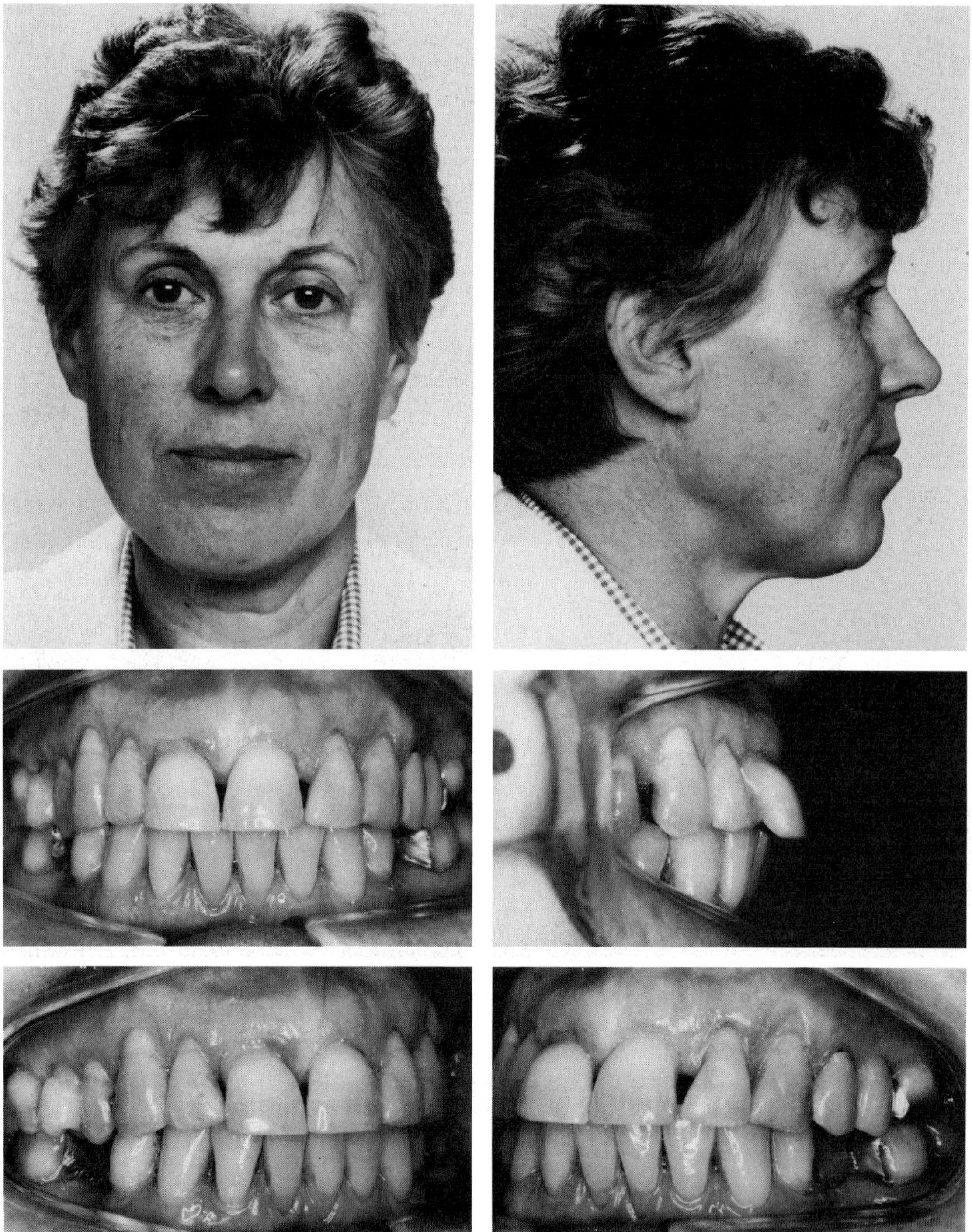

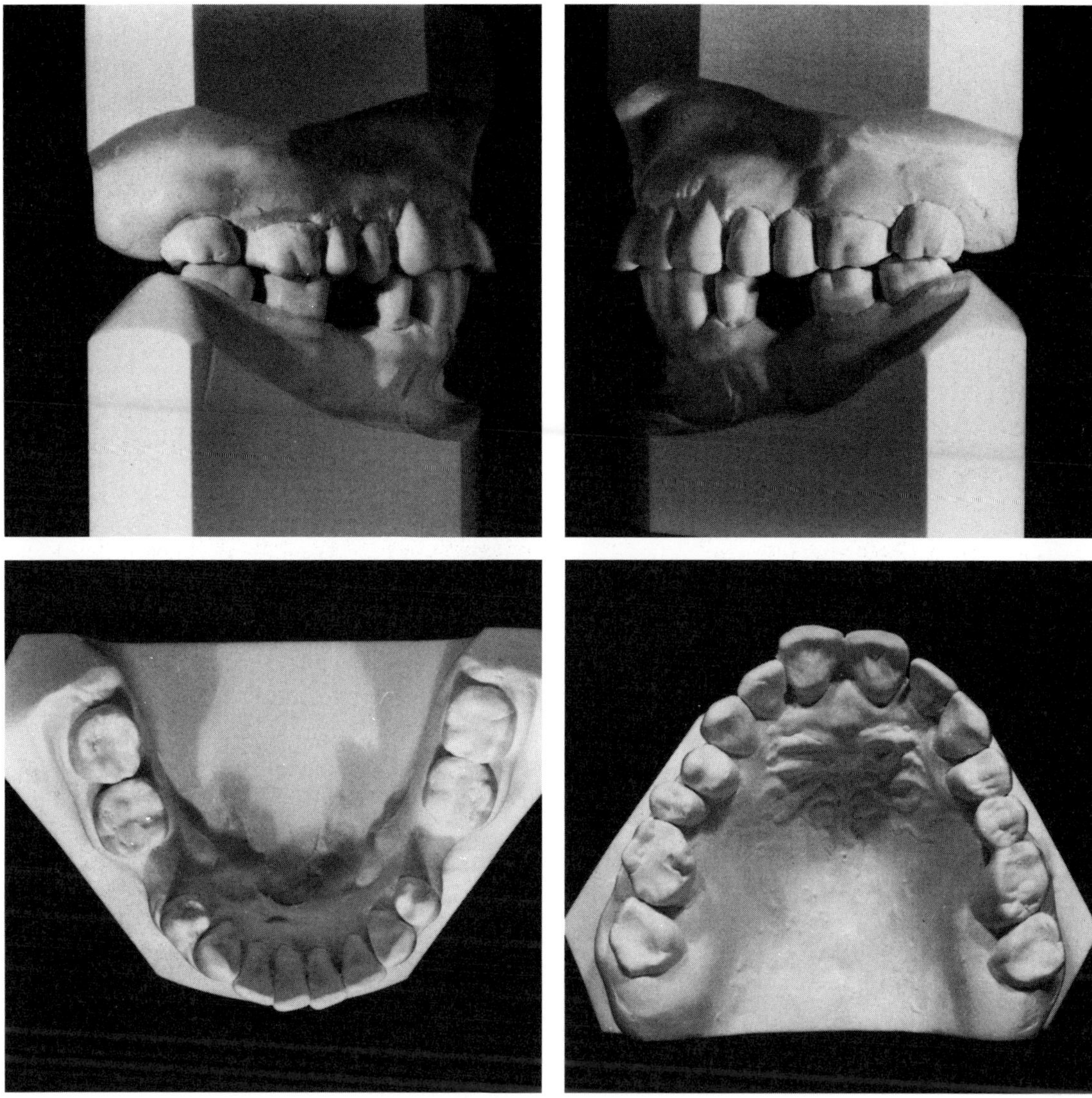

Figs 40-7 and 40-8 *At the age of 57 y, 8 mo, seven years after treatment ended, the maxillary central incisors have moved a little labially, despite wearing a retainer every night (Fig 40.10). On the left, a small space has opened up. The composite additions to the lateral incisors have been replaced in the meantime. In addition, the maxillary left second premolar was extracted and replaced with a bridge.*

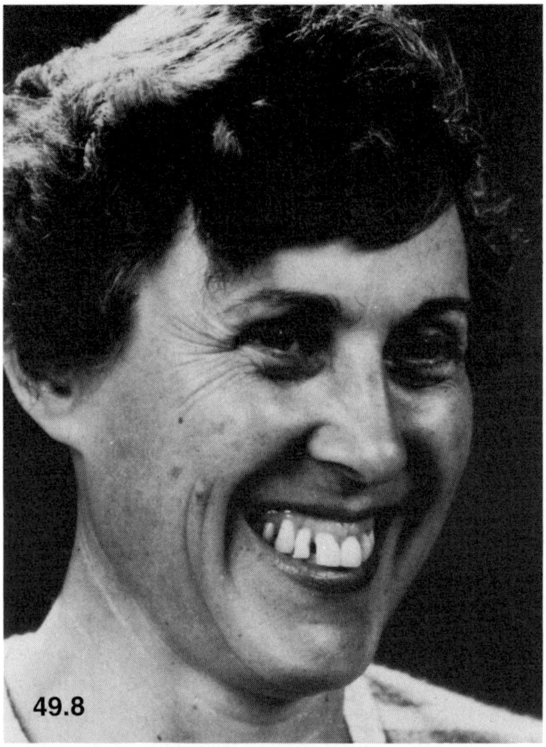

49.8

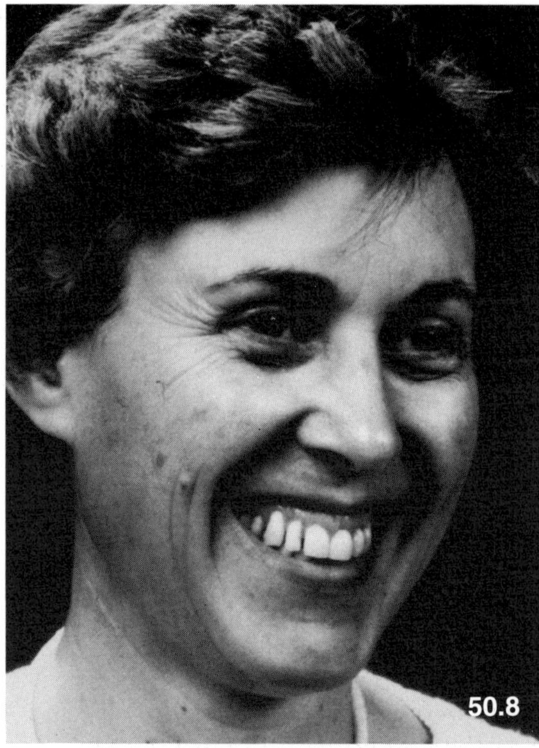

50.8

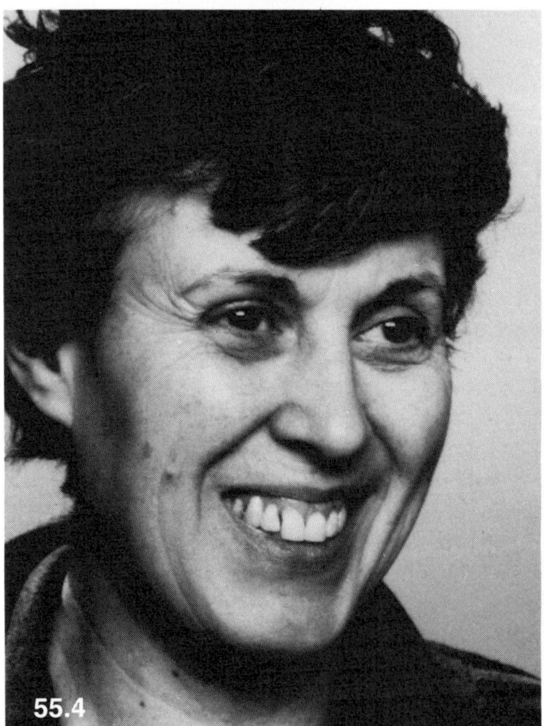

55.4

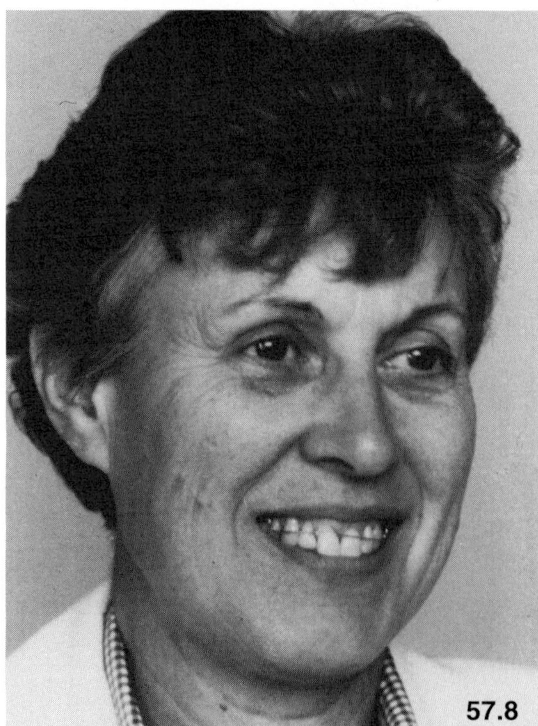

57.8

Fig 40-9 Note the changes, including a lowering of the lip line with age. When the last photograph was taken, the fact that the patient was wearing the retainer was overlooked.

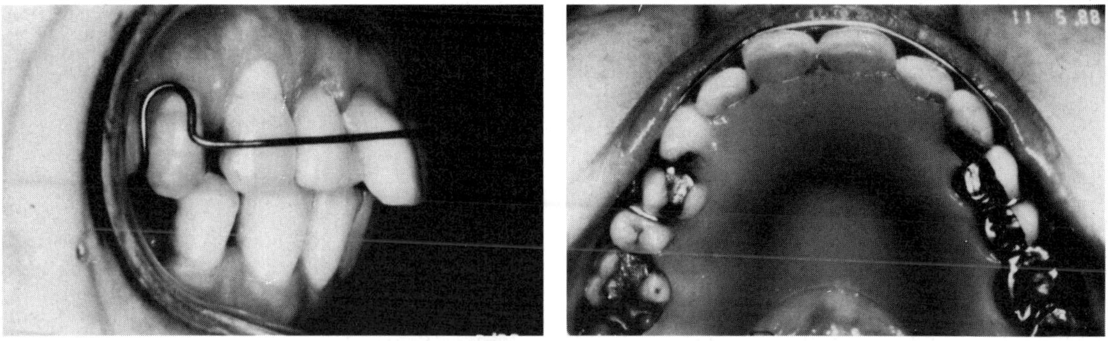

Fig 40-10 The retainer (plate) that the patient wore every night. It was checked every year along with the dentition overall. Because there was no space to run the wire of the labial arch across the incisal between the lateral incisors and the canines, the type of archwire illustrated in Figure 39-9 could not be used. That would hold the maxillary anteriors more firmly than a continuous labial arch with U-loops, as is seen here, which is less rigid and also provides no control over the canines.

The retainer will have to be worn every night in the future because it has been found that when it is not worn the central incisors do move labially despite their good periodontal condition (Fig 40.10). The photographs of the smiling face provide evidence of the changes that have occurred in the course of the years (Fig 40.9).

The abnormality in this patient did not arise when already advanced in years, as it did for the patient discussed in the previous chapter. Anomalies seen in adults can be divided into those present from the time the development of the dentition had been completed, and those whose presence became obvious at a later age as the result of degeneration of periodontal tissues or other causes. Corrections of all cases that have resulted from loss of periodontal attachment require permanent or semi-permanent (retainer worn nights only) retention.
When anomalies have existed from an early age, their correction may well be stable and not require permanent (or semi-permanent) retention. However, it is wise when tapering off the wearing of retainers to err on the side of caution. It sometimes comes to light that semi-permanent retention cannot be avoided, as was the case for this patient.

Anatomic crowns that are too thick or too narrow can influence the overall picture significantly. Unusual forms or sizes can be adjusted by well-directed grinding or building up with composite to obtain improvements relatively simply, just as was done for the patient described here. The application of this approach provided a noticeable improvement to the result obtained purely with orthodontic treatment.
It is also possible, without moving teeth at all, to mask an orthodontic anomaly with these procedures so that it becomes acceptable.[25] Such a relatively inexpensive treatment when compared with customary orthodontic treatment has considerable advantages, particularly for adults, since such treatment has a short duration and there is no fear of a relapse. Finally it might be noted that especially for patients with a high gum line, the esthetics of the maxillary incisors and the contour of the gingiva are of great importance. However, with increasing age, the lip line falls gradually and the maxillary incisors are displayed less.

Index

References

1. Baumrind, S., Korn, E.L., Molthen, R., West, E.W.: Changes in facial dimensions associated with the use of forces to retract the maxilla. *Am. J. Orthod.* 80: 17-30, 1981.
2. Behrents, R.G.: *Growth in the aging craniofacial skeleton.* Monograph No. 17. Craniofacial Growth Series. Center for Human Growth and Development. The University of Michigan, Ann Arbor, 1985.
3. Björk, A.: The principle of the Andresen method of orthodontic treatment, a discussion based on cephalometric X-ray analysis of treated cases. *Am. J. Orthod.* 37: 437-458, 1951.
4. Boersma, H.: *Eenvoudige orthodontisch therapie.* 4de druk. Samsom Stafleu, Alphen aan den Rijn, 1989.
5. Boese, L.R.: Increased stability of orthodontically rotated teeth following gingivectomy in Macaca nemestrina. *Am. J. Orthod.* 56: 273-290, 1969.
6. Brain, W.E.: The effect of surgical transsection of free gingival fibers on the regression of orthodontically rotated teeth in the dog. *Am. J. Orthod.* 55: 50-70, 1969.
7. Chipman, M.R.: Second and third molars: their role in orthodontic therapy. *Am. J. Orthod.* 47: 498-520, 1961.
8. De Kanter, R.J.A.M.: *Prevalence and etiology of craniomandibular dysfunction.* Doctoral thesis, University of Nijmegen, 1990.
9. Edwards, J.G.: A surgical procedure to eliminate rotational relapse. *Am. J. Orthod.* 57: 35-46, 1970.
10. Ericson, S., Kurol, J.: Early treatment of palatally erupting maxillary canines by extraction of the primary canines. *Eur. J. Orthod.* 10: 283-295, 1988.
11. Formby, W.A., Nanda, R.S., Currier, G.F.: Longitudinal changes in the adult facial profile. *Am. J. Orthod. Dentofac. Orthop.* 105: 464-476, 1994.
12. Frankenmolen, F.W.A.: *Orale gezondheid en zelfzorg van Nederlandse adolescenten.* Doctoral thesis, University of Nijmegen, 1990.
13. Hamerling, K., Naeije, C., Myrberg, N.: Mandibular function in children with a lateral forced bite. *Eur. J. Orthod.* 13: 35-42, 1991.
14. Holm, U.: Problems of compensative extraction in cases with loss of first permanent molars. *Trans. Eur. Orthod. Soc.* 46: 409-427, 1970.
15. Holm, U.: 25 Jahre Erfahrungen mit der Sechsjahrmolaren-extraktion in der Kieferorthopädie. In: *Studieweek 1980.* Pg. 99-112. Ned. Ver. Orthod. Studie, 1980.
16. Hooymaayer, J., Van der Linden, F.P.G.M., Boersma, H.: Post treatment facial development in corrected class II division 1-anomalies. *J. Dent. Res.* 68: 632, 1989.

17. Kuitert, R.B., Van Ginkel F.C., Prahl-Andersen B.: Long term stability of orthodontically corrected rotated teeth. *Eur. J. Orthod.* 14: 386, 1992.
18. Larsson, E., Schmidt, G.: The effect of the supra-alveolar soft tissue on the relapse of orthodontic treatment. *Br. J. Orthod.* 10: 50-52, 1983.
19. Mason, R.M., Proffit, W.R.: The tongue thrust controversy: Background and recommendations. *J. Speech Hearing Dis.* 39: 115-132, 1974.
20. McNamara, Jr, J.A., Seligman, D.A., Okeson, J.P.: Occlusion, orthodontic treatment, and temporomandibular disorders: A review. *J. Orofacial Pain* 9: 73-89, 1995.
21. Peck, S., Peck, L., Kataja, M.: The gingival smile line. *Angle Orthod.* 62: 91-100, 1992.
22. Proffit, W.R.: The proper role of myofunctional therapy. *J. Clin. Orthod.* 11: 101-115, 1977.
23. Proffit, W.R.: *Contemporary orthodontics.* 2nd edition. Mosby Year Book, St. Louis, 1993.
24. Rinaldi, S.A.: Changes in free gingival level and sulcus depth of the human periodontium following circumferential supracrestal fiberotomy. *Am. J. Orthod.* 75: 46-53, 1979.
25. Roeters, J.M., De Kloet, H.J.: *Kosmetische Zahnheilkunde mit Hilfe von Komposit.* Quintessenz Verlags-GmbH, Berlin, 1991.
26. Ruiken, H.M.H.M., Kuijpers-Jagtman, A.M.: De headgear, mechanische principes en klinische toepassing. *Ned. Tijdschr. Tandheelkd.* 98: 297-300; 1991.
27. Schols, J.G.J.H., Van der Linden, F.P.G.M.: Okklusale Anpassungen der Dentition in der Adoleszenz. *Inf. Orthod. Kieferorthop.* 20: 57-70, 1988.
28. Schols, J.G.J.H., Van der Linden, F.P.G.M., Prahl-Andersen, B.: Gesichtswachstum in der Adoleszenz. *Inf. Orthod. Kieferorthop.* 20: 71-94, 1988.
29. Subtelny, J.D., Subtelny, J.D.: Abnormal deglutition and myofunctional therapy: Facts and fallacies. In: *Pediatric dentistry.* Pg. 373-398. Eds. R.E. Stewart, T.K. Barber, K.C. Troutman, e.a. The C.V. Mosby Comp., St. Louis, 1982.
30. Van der Linden, F.P.G.M.: *Development of the dentition.* Quintessence Publ. Co. Inc., Chicago, 1983.
31. Van der Linden, F.P.G.M.: *Facial growth and facial orthopaedics.* Quintessence Publ. Co. Inc., Chicago, 1986.
32. Van der Linden, F.P.G.M.: Restrictions in clinical orthodontics for patients with deviating functional conditions. In: *Orthodontics: Evaluation and Future.* Pg. 319-332. Eds. C.F.A. Moorrees and F.P.G.M. van der Linden, Samsom Stafleu, Alphen aan den Rijn, 1988.
33. Van der Linden, F.P.G.M.: *Problems and procedures in dentofacial orthopaedics.* Quintessence Publ. Co. Inc., Chicago, 1990.
34. Van der Linden, F.P.G.M.: The role of the occlusion in the development of the dentition and facial growth, in orthodontic diagnosis and treatment, and in retention. In: *Essays in honour of Robert E. Moyers.* Monograph no. 24. Pg. 97-117. Eds. W.S. Hunter, D.S. Carlson. Craniofacial Growth Series. Center for Human Growth and Development. The University of Michigan, Ann Arbor, 1991.
35. Van der Linden, F.P.G.M.: Consequences of functional aspects and growth changes for retention and relapse. In: *Retention and long-term stability.* Pg. 19-27. Eds. Hösl,

E., Baldauf, A., Hüthig Buch Verlag, Heidelberg, 1993.

36. Van der Linden, F.P.G.M., Boersma, H.: *Diagnosis and treatment planning in dentofacial orthopaedics.* Quintessence Publ. Co. Inc., Chicago, 1987.

37. Van der Zwan, J., Boering, G.: *Operatieve kaakorthopedie.* Stafleu & Tholen, Alphen aan den Rijn, 1981.